Orofacial Pain & Headache
Second Edition

Orofacial Pain and Headache

Second Edition

Edited by

Yair Sharav, DMD, MS

Professor
Department of Oral Medicine
School of Dental Medicine
Hadassah Medical Center
The Hebrew University of Jerusalem
Jerusalem, Israel

Rafael Benoliel, BDS

Associate Dean for Research
Professor, Department of Diagnostic Sciences
Director, Center for Orofacial Pain and Temporomandibular Disorders
Rutgers School of Dental Medicine
Rutgers, The State University of New Jersey
Newark, New Jersey

Quintessence Publishing Co, Inc

quintessence books

Chicago, Berlin, Tokyo, London, Paris, Milan, Barcelona, Istanbul,
Moscow, New Delhi, Prague, São Paulo, Seoul, and Warsaw

Library of Congress Cataloging-in-Publication Data

Orofacial pain and headache / edited by Yair Sharav and Rafael Benoliel.
-- Second edition.
    p. ; cm.
Includes bibliographical references and index.
ISBN 978-0-86715-680-5 (softcover)
I. Sharav, Yair, editor. II. Benoliel, Rafael, editor.
[DNLM: 1. Facial Pain. 2. Headache Disorders. WE 705]
RC936
616'.0472--dc23
                              2015003559

© 2015 Quintessence Publishing Co, Inc

Quintessence Publishing Co, Inc
4350 Chandler Drive
Hanover Park, IL 60133
www.quintpub.com

5 4 3 2 1

Editor: Leah Huffman
Design: Ted Pereda
Production: Kaye Clemens

Printed in the USA

Contents

Preface to the Second Edition

When we published the first edition of this book, we felt there was a true need to bridge the fields of orofacial pain and headache with a textbook that could integrate the knowledge from both fields. While at the time we questioned the necessity for an additional book in the area of craniofacial pain, this worry soon became unnecessary. The book was accepted with great enthusiasm, and in 2009, the British Medical Association highly commended the first edition as one of the best books published in the medical field. Reviews were complimentary: "This textbook is a joy to read," proclaimed a 2008 review in the *Journal of Orofacial Pain* (Quintessence Publishing). The reviewers praised our success in integrating the broad topics of orofacial pain and headache. Furthermore, we were glad to see that this most important journal in the orofacial field changed its name in 2014 from the *Journal of Orofacial Pain to the Journal of Oral & Facial Pain & Headache,* pointing to what was already obvious to us; these two fields must continue to be integrated.

Integration ensures that we are consistent and relate all regional craniofacial pains to each other, thereby presenting the wider picture of craniofacial pain syndromes and the overlap between primary headaches and primary orofacial pain entities. Truly, the years since the first edition was published have seen some integration of the two fields, particularly through close collaboration between dental and medical professionals for the preparation of the 2013 International Classification of Headache Disorders. In spite of this, the International Headache Society's classification system does not yet adequately cover all currently accepted orofacial pain entities. Therefore, we added the recently reviewed classification of the Diagnostic Criteria for Temporomandibular Disorders (DC-TMD) and drew from our wide experience in the field. Certainly, in the diagnosis of acute dental and otolaryngological pain, we have continued to stress the importance of accurate, evidence-based diagnosis. This may seem oversimplistic at first, but consider the reports of misdiagnosis of cluster headache, paroxysmal hemicrania, migraine, and trigeminal neuralgia as dental pains or sinus headaches. The results to our patients are often devastating and unnecessary. Clearly as a profession, we still have hurdles to overcome.

While we preserved the well-structured format of the last edition, we updated the chapters to reflect current knowledge and added a new chapter on orofacial pain and sleep, as data continues to point to their interconnection. We have also made this edition friendlier to clinicians. In many chapters, we first address the clinical picture and treatment strategies and follow with a discussion of the underlying mechanisms. In addition, the design has been updated, and we have found that the esthetic layout of the present edition, made possible by the excellent editors and production staff of the Quintessence Publishing house, makes the excursion through the pages of this book a most pleasant experience.

Finally, as the first edition was highly praised, we felt that we were not in a position to disappoint our faithful readers and had to keep to the high standards that are expected. We very much hope we have succeeded in this mission.

Preface to the First Edition

For many years, the area of orofacial pain was completely dominated by the concept that most facial pains were due to "disturbed function" of the temporomandibular joint (TMJ). This was an approach established by an otolaryngologist named James B. Costen who linked etiology to derangements of the dental occlusion; facial pain was thus handed over to dentistry. As a profession, we enthusiastically adopted the treatment of facial pain but have for many years concentrated our efforts on a mechanistic approach to treatment. These events essentially segregated facial pain from headache and, in effect, from mainstream medicine. As a result, ideal conditions were established in each of the two disciplines for the development of different approaches to the understanding of mechanisms and therapy of craniofacial pain. However, as our understanding of pain mechanisms, and in particular chronic pain, developed, it became clear that facial pain has underlying neurophysiologic mechanisms common to headaches and other body areas. Masticatory muscle pain was examined in light of other regional muscle pains, and management of the TMJ was related to, and brought in line with, basic orthopedic principles. Most importantly, features of some facial pain entities are very similar to those of some headaches. Examples include masticatory myofascial pain and tension-type headache and a facial equivalent of migraine.

The dental profession has been slow in adopting medically based classification and approaches to therapy. In a similar fashion, the medical profession has been very resistant to incorporating established facial pains into current classifications; temporomandibular disorders are a prime example and currently unrecognized by the International Headache Society.

One may correctly claim that toothache is unique, but is it really? On a mechanistic level, pulpitis is an inflammatory process within a confined space—not very different from the inflammatory process of migraine confined within the skull. Indeed, we believe that migraine-like mechanisms exist within the pulp chamber mimicking pulpitis, in the paranasal sinuses imitating sinusitis, and in other confined cranial structures causing atypical symptomatology. In each of these cases, anti-migraine medications are the correct treatment.

Clearly the task required is integration of knowledge in this anatomically dense region, traditionally divided between many medical disciplines. Based on our extensive clinical experience with patients suffering from orofacial pain and headache as well as our thorough understanding of pain mechanisms specific to the trigeminal system, we feel that we are well equipped to fulfill this task. This textbook therefore deals with oral and facial pain as well as with headaches and aims to integrate the knowledge across these disciplines. We hope we have succeeded.

We appreciate the contribution of our teachers, colleagues, and students. Throughout our professional lives, we have interacted with many professionals worldwide, and each has enriched our understanding of pain mechanisms and our clinical knowledge. Being in the "business" of teaching, both undergraduates and residents, we have been consistently challenged by curious students with difficult questions. These have kept us up to date and enabled us to re-examine and reassess the way orofacial pain is understood and taught.

Last but not least, our warm gratitude and appreciation to our families for bearing with us through the long process of preparing, writing, editing, and publishing this book.

Contributors

Rafael Benoliel, BDS
Associate Dean for Research
Professor, Department of Diagnostic Sciences
Director, Center for Orofacial Pain and Temporomandibular
   Disorders
Rutgers School of Dental Medicine
Rutgers, The State University of New Jersey
Newark, New Jersey

Donald S. Ciccone, PhD
Adjunct Associate Professor
Department of Psychiatry
New Jersey Medical School
Rutgers, The State University of New Jersey
Newark, New Jersey

Marshall Devor, PhD
Professor and Chairman
Department for Cell and Animal Biology
Institute of Life Sciences
The Hebrew University of Jerusalem
Jerusalem, Israel

M. Franklin Dolwick, DMD, PhD
Professor and Division Head
Department of Oral and Maxillofacial Surgery
University of Florida College of Dentistry
Gainesville, Florida

Sharon Elad, DMD, MSc
Professor
Department of Dentistry
Eastman Institute for Oral Health
University of Rochester Medical Center
Rochester, New York

Ron Eliashar, MD
Professor and Director
Department of Otolaryngology, Head and Neck Surgery
Hadassah Medical Center
The Hebrew University of Jerusalem
Jerusalem, Israel

Eli Eliav, DMD, MSc, PhD
Professor and Director
Department of Dentistry
Eastman Institute for Oral Health
University of Rochester Medical Center
Rochester, New York

Joel Epstein, DMD, MSD, FRCD(C), FDS RCS(Edin)
Consulting Staff
Division of Otolaryngology and Head and Neck Surgery
City of Hope National Medical Center
Duarte, California

Charlene E. Gamaldo, MD
Medical Director
Johns Hopkins Sleep Disorders Center
The Johns Hopkins Hospital
Baltimore, Maryland

Richard H. Gracely, MS, PhD
Professor
Division of Rheumatology
Department of Internal Medicine
University of Michigan
Ann Arbor, Michigan

Menachem Gross, MD
Department of Otolaryngology, Head and Neck Surgery
Hadassah Medical Center
The Hebrew University of Jerusalem
Jerusalem, Israel

Gary M. Heir, DMD
Clinical Professor
Department of Diagnostic Sciences
Rutgers School of Dental Medicine
Rutgers, The State University of New Jersey
Newark, New Jersey

Bonnie Kaas, MD
Assistant Resident
Department of Neurology
The Johns Hopkins Hospital
Baltimore, Maryland

Zaza Katsarava, MD, PhD, MSc
Chair
Department of Neurology
University of Essen
Essen, Germany

Gary D. Klasser, DMD
Associate Professor
Department of Diagnostic Sciences
School of Dentistry
Louisiana State University Health Sciences Center
New Orleans, Louisiana

Dorrit W. Nitzan, DMD
Professor and Senior Surgeon
Department of Oral and Maxillofacial Surgery
Hadassah Medical Center
The Hebrew University of Jerusalem
Jerusalem, Israel

B. Lee Peterlin, DO
Associate Professor of Neurology
Director, Headache Research
Johns Hopkins University School of Medicine
Baltimore, Maryland

Karen Raphael, PhD
Professor
Department of Oral and Maxillofacial Pathology, Radiology
    and Medicine
New York University College of Dentistry
New York, New York

Zvi Harry Rappaport, MD
Director, Department of Neurosurgery
Rabin Medical Center
Petah Tikva, Israel

Rachel E. Salas, MD
Assistant Professor
Department of Neurology
Johns Hopkins University School of Medicine
Baltimore, Maryland

Yair Sharav, DMD, MS
Professor
Department of Oral Medicine
School of Dental Medicine
Hadassah Medical Center
The Hebrew University of Jerusalem
Jerusalem, Israel

Michael T. Smith, PhD
Professor of Psychiatry, Neurology, and Nursing
Director, Center for Behavior and Health
Co-Director, Center for Sleep-Related Symptom Science
Johns Hopkins University School of Medicine
Baltimore, Maryland

Herve Sroussi, DMD, PhD
Associate Professor and Chief of Oral Medicine
Director of Graduate Studies
Department of Oral Medicine and Diagnostic Science
University of Illinois at Chicago College of Dentistry
Chicago, Illinois

Peter Svensson, DDS, PhD, Dr Odont
Professor
Division of Orofacial Pain and Jaw Function
Department of Dentistry
Aarhus University
Aarhus, Denmark

Michael Tal, DMD, MS
Professor
Department of Anatomy and Cell Biology
School of Medicine
The Hebrew University of Jerusalem
Jerusalem, Israel

Luis Villanueva, DDS, PhD
Director of Research
Department of Dentistry
Psychiatry and Neurosciences Center
French Institute of Health and Medical Research
Paris, France

The Diagnostic Process

Yair Sharav, DMD, MS
Rafael Benoliel, BDS

1

Diagnosis and treatment of orofacial pain is a complex process compounded by the density of anatomical structures and the prominent psychologic significance attributed to this region. Management of orofacial pain thus demands the services of clinicians from various specialties, such as dentistry, otolaryngology, ophthalmology, neurology, neurosurgery, psychiatry, and psychology. Complex referral patterns to adjacent structures are common in orofacial pain and, indeed, one person's headache is another person's facial pain. In clinical practice, the two types of pain are often intimately related. Consequently, a patient with orofacial pain may wander from one specialist to another to try to find adequate help.

The second edition of this textbook continues to integrate the issue of orofacial pain with headache through contributions from practitioners in different disciplines, all of whom have extensive clinical experience and a thorough understanding of pain mechanisms specific to the trigeminal system. Accordingly, the authors address all regional craniofacial pains together and aim to present a wider picture of orofacial pain syndromes, including the overlap between primary headaches and primary orofacial pain entities. Many patients with chronic orofacial pain suffer primary headache variants in the orofacial region, and a lack of familiarity with these syndromes is likely a factor in misdiagnosis by dental practitioners and medical specialists. Other patients may suffer from primary orofacial pain entities that remain unclassified by the International Headache Society (IHS) and are unknown to neurologists, otolaryngologists, other medical practitioners, and even dentists.[1–3] The integration of headache and orofacial pain classifications is of paramount importance. In the past, about half of the patients in tertiary-care craniofacial pain clinics were labeled as "idiopathic" or "undiagnosable" when the previous IHS classification was applied.[2–5] The hope is that the current classification, which has witnessed a novel collaboration between orofacial pain and headache specialists, will improve the situation.

Moreover, there is considerable overlap in the clinical presentation of headaches, such as tension type with regional myofascial pains of the face, and generalized pain syndromes, such as fibromyalgia (see chapter 8). The relationship between isolated facial neurovascular pain (see chapter 10) and migraines or trigeminal autonomic cephalalgias remains unclear and is not accounted for by the recent IHS classification.[6] Furthermore, a growing patient population has chronic craniofacial pain from trauma associated with traffic accidents or from invasive dental procedures, such as dental implants, which demands a multidisciplinary approach. This book bridges the gap between medically trained headache and dentally trained orofacial pain specialists. It will be useful to readers at different stages of their careers—undergraduate students, residents, practitioners, and dental and medical pain specialists.

Epidemiology: The Silent Crisis

Statistics from the United States indicate that 100 million adults suffer from chronic pain[7] at an estimated annual cost of around $600 billion—higher than the cost for heart disease, cancer, or diabetes. However, chronic pain is a worldwide epidemic that has been termed "the silent crisis."[8] Examining relevant prevalence estimates gives important insight into the scope of the problem. Orofacial pain, of which about 10% is chronic, affects around a quarter of the general population.[9–11] Painful temporomandibular disorders (TMDs) are quite prevalent; 4.6% of the population reports this type of pain (6.3% of women, 2.8% of men).[12] This finding is in agreement with the 2009 National Health Interview Survey, which found that 5% of adults reported pain in the face or jaw over a 3-month period. Persistent facial pain, which has a reported incidence of 38.7 per 100,000 person-years, is more common in women and increases with age.[13] Syndromes identified included trigeminal neuralgia and cluster headache, which are the most common forms. Paroxysmal hemicrania and glossopharyngeal neuralgia were among the rare syndromes. Clearly, orofacial pain is more prevalent than previously thought.

Therefore, diagnosis and management of orofacial pain and headache have become important subjects in medicine and dentistry.

Both acute and chronic presentations may be benign or may signify serious underlying disease. The emphasis of this book is on the four major clinical families of orofacial pain: acute orofacial, neurovascular, musculoskeletal, and neuropathic (see chapters 6 and 8 to 12). In these chapters, the current etiology, diagnosis, and treatment are reviewed. The book includes many case presentations that are largely virtual, that is, created by integrating data from a number of cases seen in the clinic; thus, any resemblance to specific cases is purely coincidental. They are real, however, in that they reliably duplicate the type of cases seen in orofacial pain clinics. Typical textbook cases are rare, and each relevant section includes information related to the changes in presentation that may cause diagnostic confusion. Atypical cases may be difficult to manage; many have superimposed trauma and consequent neuropathic pain. Some of these cases present patients with a history of misdiagnosed acute pains in the orofacial region who have undergone repeated and unsuccessful interventions that slowly escalated and resulted in dental extractions and surgeries. Accurate diagnosis of acute dental and orofacial conditions is therefore essential (see chapter 6). The importance of acute and chronic otolaryngologic syndromes in the differential diagnosis of facial pain, particularly migraines and cluster headache, is paramount (see chapter 7). The growing number of older, often medically compromised, patients with orofacial pain deserves special attention (see chapter 14): Is orofacial pain in these patients related to their medical condition? Although this is essentially a clinical book, anatomy and neurophysiology are covered in a manner specifically relevant to the topic of orofacial pain (see chapter 2).

One of the mainstays of pain management is indisputably pharmacotherapy. Because many drugs are commonly used to treat many syndromes, two separate chapters on pharmacotherapy are included: acute and chronic (see chapters 15 and 16). The management of pain relies on accurate diagnosis and reliable follow-up that demonstrates objective improvement. Chapter 3 covers the important area of pain measurement as well as the assessment of pain modulatory systems and peripheral nerve function. Unfortunately, we are a long way from optimal patient care, and some of the best drugs offer notable relief for only a fraction of our patients, with some having disturbing side effects. Many patients inquire about complementary and alternative medicine and often actively search out these practitioners independently (see chapter 17). Neurosurgical approaches, including neuromodulation, remain relevant options for selected syndromes (see chapters 11 to 13). No diagnosis and treatment of orofacial pain would be complete without understanding its emotional undercurrents and having a thorough knowledge of its psychologic aspects and treatment possibilities, which are covered in chapter 4. A novel and welcome addition to this second edition is a description of the interactions between sleep and orofacial pain and headaches.

Chronic Pain Is a Disease

Pain is a multifaceted experience with physical, cognitive, and emotional aspects (Table 1-1). Three mechanistically distinct types of pain are distinguishable: nociceptive, inflammatory, and neuropathic. Nociceptive pain is the baseline defensive mechanism that protects us from potential harm. Inflammatory and neuropathic pains are characterized by altered and often aberrant function of the nervous system as a result of persistent pathology or plastic changes in the nervous system.

Thus, although we tend to call any sensation that hurts "pain," many types of pain exist that subserve various biologic functions. For example, acute pain from extreme heat initiates a reflex withdrawal and ensures minimal tissue damage (nociceptive pain). This type of pain is a survival mechanism and may be termed "good" pain. Consequently, if tissue has been damaged, the local inflammatory response causes increased sensitivity in peripheral nociceptors (peripheral sensitization) and dorsal horn neurons (central sensitization) associated with pain transmission. As a result, the hand is sensitive to touch and more sensitive to pain (allodynia and hyperalgesia; see Table 1-1) so that the person protects and immobilizes the limb to aid rapid healing. Essentially, the system has been altered to behave differently. In most cases, tissue injury is followed by a healing period associated with ongoing pain that ultimately resolves with no residual problems.

In contrast, pain with no biologic advantage to the person is termed "bad" pain. For example, chronic pain that is not associated with ongoing tissue damage, but inflicts severe physical and emotional suffering on the person, offers no survival value. Chronic pain is often the result of primary or reactive changes in the nervous system that are associated with neuronal plasticity but are unable to modulate and thus actually serve to perpetuate the sensation of pain; in short, the system has malfunctioned, and maladaptive pain remains. Chronic pain is, therefore, a disease in its own right and often not a symptom. Additionally, chronic pain responds to therapy differently from acute pain and is associated with emotional and social behavioral changes (see chapter 4). Acute and chronic pains differ in many respects, and some of the major differences are presented in Table 1-2.

Patients, and sometimes physicians, find it hard to distinguish pain as a disease from pain as a symptom. The latter signifies an expression of a pathologic process that, if treated, will cause the pain to disappear. Unfortunately, the inability to perceive pain as a disease may result in repeated and unsuccessful interventions, all in an attempt to eradicate the cause of pain.

Table 1-1	Definition of pain terms	
Term	**Definition**	**Clinical implication**
Pain	An unpleasant sensory and emotional experience associated with actual or potential tissue damage, or described in terms of such damage.	Some patients may be unable to communicate verbally. Pain is an individually subjective experience.
Allodynia	Pain due to a stimulus that does not normally provoke pain (eg, touch, light pressure, or moderate cold or warmth).	Associated with neuropathy, inflammation, and certain headache states (see chapters 5, 9, and 11). A lowered threshold where the stimulus and response mode differ from the normal state.
Hyperalgesia	An increased response to a stimulus that is normally painful.	Associated with neuropathy or inflammation. Reflects increased pain on suprathreshold stimulation. The stimulus and response mode are basically the same.
Hyperesthesia	Increased sensitivity to stimulation, excluding the special senses. Includes both allodynia and hyperalgesia.	Associated with neuropathy or inflammation (see chapter 11).
Hypoalgesia	Diminished pain in response to a normally painful stimulus.	Typical of neural damage. Raised threshold: stimulus and response mode are the same (lowered response).
Analgesia	Absence of pain in response to stimulation that would normally be painful.	Commonly observed after complete axotomy or nerve block. Not unpleasant.
Hyperpathia	A painful syndrome characterized by an abnormally painful reaction to a stimulus, especially a repetitive stimulus, as well as an increased threshold. May occur with allodynia, hyperesthesia, hyperalgesia, or dysesthesia.	Typical of neuropathic pain syndromes (see chapter 11). Faulty identification and localization of the stimulus, delay, radiating sensation, and after-sensation may be present, and the pain is often explosive in character.
Paresthesia	An abnormal sensation, whether spontaneous or evoked.	Typical of neuropathic pain syndromes (see chapter 11).
Hypoesthesia	Decreased sensitivity to stimulation, excluding the special senses.	
Dysesthesia	An unpleasant abnormal sensation, whether spontaneous or evoked. Hyperalgesia and allodynia are forms of dysesthesia.	

Table 1-2	Major features of acute and chronic pain	
Features	**Acute pain**	**Chronic pain**
Time course	Short (hours to days)	Long (months to years)
Etiology	Peripheral (inflammatory)	Central (neuropathic)
Behavioral response	Anxiety, "guarding"	Depression, "illness behavior"
Response to treatment		
Local intervention	Good	Poor
Analgesic drugs	Good	Poor
Psychotropic drugs	Poor	Moderate to good

Approach to Diagnosis and Management

The need to base therapeutic approaches on evidence-based medicine is obvious, and the authors wholeheartedly agree with this approach. Thus, this book cites state-of-the-art research to support statements whenever possible. However, evidence-based medicine is a tasteless science unless peppered by clinical experience and judgment, careful appraisal of drug side effects and complications (especially in the medically compromised patient), the individual variability of patients, and a respectful approach to a patient's autonomy. Therefore, expert opinion also enriches this text.

As in most other textbooks of medicine, this book presents knowledge in a linear, disease-based manner. Pain syndromes are described and their signs, symptoms, and associated features outlined. This is very different from the circular process of clinical data collection; indeed, patients present with complaints rather than diseases. Knowledge of a disease does not automatically guarantee the ability to identify it from a given set of signs and symptoms. The process of accumulating clinical data in order to reach a diagnosis is as much a science as it is an art, and part of this chapter is devoted to understanding and applying this process.

Classification, Disease, and Diagnosis

In the clinical setting as much as in the research setting, classification systems are important. Diagnoses (based on classifications) usually dictate therapeutic options and indicate a prognosis. A number of relevant classifications are available for orofacial pain and headache, though they are not in complete accord.[14] The IHS,[6] the American Academy of Orofacial Pain (AAOP),[15] and the Research Diagnostic Criteria for Temporomandibular Disorders (RDC-TMD)[16] have all recently reviewed their classifications.

These classifications often have offshoots based on specific characteristics. Thus, chronic facial pain[17] or chronic daily headache[18] may be subclassified as temporal, and indomethacin-responsive headaches[19] may be subclassified as therapeutic. The former is probably most useful in epidemiologic and disease-burden studies, whereas the latter presents a treatment-dependent diagnostic challenge. However, both classification approaches offer little advantage in guiding clinical diagnosis and therapy.[17]

The concept that diseases are identifiable through their symptomatology is the basis of classifications.[20] Classifications aim to organize orofacial pains, some headaches, and TMDs into a logical and applicable system. The level of detail of the classification depends on its planned use or requirements. Over the years, research has enriched medical practice with specific diagnostic biomarkers, but these are largely unavailable in the field of orofacial pain and headache. In the absence of adequate biomarkers, the diagnosis of orofacial pain and headache is based on a clinician's ability to recognize a particular combination of signs and symptoms in a patient. Thus, diagnosis remains heavily reliant on the patient's story—the way it is related and how the clinician interprets it.

Of course, diagnosis should not be confused with disease, as in all areas of medicine diagnoses are often made for unknown underlying processes. Consider migraine, which was once thought to be a vascular headache. After further scientific investigations, we now appreciate the complexity of the underlying central nervous system events leading to a migraine and the vascular changes understood as epiphenomena.[21] As we elucidate exact processes underlying a disorder, diagnosis approaches etiology and, ultimately, the true disease.[22]

Clearly, in orofacial pain and headache the aim of diagnosing all entities is unattainable. Therefore, classifications commonly have one or more "other" diagnoses or categories. Indeed, we all have patients with chronic orofacial pain whose diagnosis remains elusive[3,23–25] and whose signs and symptoms cannot be neatly pigeonholed into established diagnoses. Many of these entities share temporal features, such as pain for most or all of the day that is long-standing or chronic (> 3 months). Past attempts at terminology have left us with diagnoses of such diseases as atypical odontalgia, atypical facial pain, and persistent idiopathic facial pain; these classifications are inadequate. More recently, Nixdorf et al[26] exercised the classification of such cases based on ontologic principles and suggested the term *persistent dentoalveolar pain disorder*. These general terms may be accurate in the symptomatic description but may also tend to lump together a number of underlying diagnostic entities that may present with similar, but subtly different, clinical phenotypes; thus, their contribution to management may be minimal.[27,28]

Existing classifications are not always accurate or adequate. Often syndromes overlap in their clinical phenotype, and these are dis-cussed in the clinical chapters. For example, a tension-type headache (TTH) may be extremely difficult to differentiate from a mild migraine without aura because of overlap in the appearance of ostensibly diagnostic features. Mild nausea and photo- and phonophobia may form part of the TTH phenotype,[6] TTH may be aggravated by exercise,[29] regional muscle tenderness is equally prevalent in both,[30–32] and even headache precipitants are identical between migraine and TTH.[33]

Problems occur even with specifically tailored classifications; recent reliability studies on the RDC-TMD conclude that the specified clinical tests identified as independent diagnostic criteria would be unacceptably susceptible to diagnostic misclassification. The more common diagnoses had good examiner reliability, but some lack of agreement was clearly present, even when well-trained examiners perform these procedures.[34]

Field-testing of classifications often reveal novel subtypes of the same diagnosis or new diagnoses hidden within previous ones. Thus, cluster headache was extracted from migraines, and paroxysmal hemicrania was subsequently subclassified from cluster headache. In the field of TMDs, the recognition and classification of separate joint and muscle disorders in the late 1980s and early 1990s[35,36] opened an opportunity to revise old and irrelevant terminology. Much of this work has been admirably completed in regard to joint disorders but is still lacking in regard to muscle pain, particularly chronic masticatory muscle pain, which is often termed *myofascial masticatory muscle pain*, a term based on an outdated premise that the muscle and surrounding fascia are the origins of pain.

Multi-axis systems recognize the biopsychosocial model of pain, which reflects the inherent complexity of the pain experience and the clear relationship between onset, treatment response, and psychosocial issues.[37–39] For example, the RDC-TMD includes a separate axis for the classification of psychosocial dysfunction/suffering. It would clearly be an advantage to have an integrated classification of orofacial pain and headache that takes into account psychosocial comorbidity. The assessment of psychologic distress may be performed with the RDC-TMD questionnaire or with established alternatives.[40,41]

ONTOlogic

As health care providers, we have become increasingly dependent on a wide array of laboratory and imaging studies to diagnose and subsequently manage patients' diseases.[42] We must, however, appreciate the limitation of diagnostic tests in any clinical setting but particularly in the diagnosis of orofacial pain and headache. Not only are diagnostic tests inherently limited as diagnostic tools, but there are also few biomarkers in current use for the diagnosis of primary orofacial pain[43–45] and headache[46–49] disorders. In the absence of biomarkers, classifications are self-defining and difficult to validate. However, as biotechnology improves, we may be able to incorporate specific biomarkers into classification criteria, whether as a separate axis or integrated. Biomarkers will aid in diagnosis and enable assessment of disease control or severity, much as levels of fasting glucose levels and glycated hemoglobin are used for diabetes. Ongoing research may change the situation, but currently the predictive value of available biomarkers in primary orofacial pain/headache diagnosis is very low.

All of these classification systems are integrated in this book according to their strengths in the following manner. The authors have no doubt that for headaches the IHS is the most comprehensive, so it is used throughout this book for all headache entities. For orofacial pain entities, the IHS classification is not detailed enough; thus, the AAOP's criteria is used, and specifically for TMDs, the Diagnostic Criteria for TMD (DC/TMD) is used. The strength of the International Association for the Study of Pain (IASP) lies in its regional and systems approach to pain classification (eg, musculoskeletal, neurovascular pain) and to the excellent approach to neuropathic pain entities. The integration of such internationally accepted systems into pain clinics and research studies is essential and ultimately an enriching endeavor.

Diagnosis of Orofacial Pain

Faced with a patient with a pain complaint, clinicians have to answer three major questions—where, what, and why—and if possible, ask them in this order. The first, *where*, is concerned with the location, such as the anatomical structure or system affected. The second, *what*, deals primarily with the pathologic process. The third, *why*, is about the etiology. The patient's decision to seek medical help is the first step in the diagnostic chain; surprisingly, not all patients with significant pain seek treatment. Based mostly on the pain *location*, patients will choose which specialist to consult. Naturally, if it is a toothache, the patient decides to consult the dentist, and most times the choice will be correct. However, suppose the patient's pain is referred to the oral cavity from a remote organ (such as the heart; see chapter 14) or is associated with migraine-like mechanisms (see chapter 10), and he or she consults a dentist. The patient has clearly, and understandably, missed or misinterpreted the "where" or the "what." The clinician's responsibility is to analyze the patient's complaints and reach the correct diagnosis. In other words, the clinician has to rigorously apply the diagnostic process to accurately define the location, identify the pathologic process, and ideally establish the etiology of the pain.

The natural starting point is a comprehensive gathering of information. Clinicians routinely start with history taking, the strongest tool when it comes to the diagnosis of pain. Pain symptoms should specify location, duration, pain characteristics, and other pertinent data (see the section titled "The Pain History"). In addition, a thorough personal history should include details on medical, drug, and psychosocial history; occupation; stress; family history relating to marital status and recent events (eg, bereavement); and any history of familial disorders (eg, migraine, diabetes). The physical examination is next, supplemented by other tests as needed. Once this process has been completed, a working hypothesis needs to be generated, namely, a diagnosis. Gathering information is a starting point but does not on its own make a diagnosis. In the sections that follow, the process of using the patient's clinical data to generate diagnostic hypotheses is described.

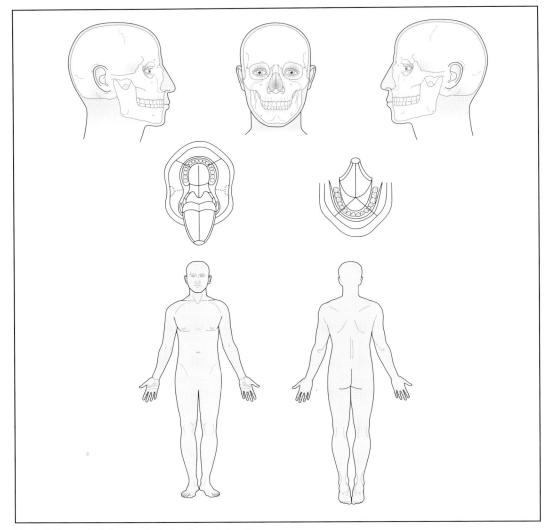

Fig 1-1 Suggested diagram for indicating pain location.

Getting to Know Your Patient and the Patient's Pain

Patients are normally willing to tell their story or pain history, but the clinician usually needs to supplement this information with specific questions concerning the location, temporal behavior, intensity, relation to function, and sensory modalities. A structured intake for the clinical interview and examination findings is useful (Fig 1-1 and Forms 1-1 and 1-2), particularly for teaching and training. The intake systematically records the basic information needed in a pain history (Box 1-1), and practitioners can design their own forms based on these principles. Additionally, the structured intake, or form, presents questions and examination procedures vital to the diagnosis of the more common clinical conditions (see chapters 8 to 12); for this, accepted classification systems such as those from the IHS, the AAOP, and the IASP are relied upon.

1. **Patient's details**
   Name _____ Age _____ Sex (M/F)
   Marital status _____ Occupation _____

2. **Medical status** Summary of relevant medical conditions, medications, etc *(patient must complete a detailed medical questionnaire, not shown here)* _____
   _____
   _____

3. **Pain complaint**
   • Pain location (also marked on pre-prepared drawing, see Fig 1-1) _____
   _____
   • Pain onset and duration _____
   • Age at onset of pain attacks _____
   • Pain attack frequency (mark continuous if no pain-free periods) _____
   _____
   • Pain attack duration _____
   • Pain severity (mark on scale below (10-cm line)

   No pain   Worst pain

   Factors that precipitate/aggravate pain _____
   Pain is eased by _____
   Pain quality (pressing/piercing/throbbing/burning/electric/sharp/other) _____
   _____

4. **Accompanying signs and symptoms**
   • Systemic: nausea/vomiting/photophobia/phonophobia/dizziness
   • Local: tearing/rhinorrhea/swelling/redness

5. **History of trauma** (Yes/No)
   If yes: date _____ Description _____

6. **Pain history summary** *(additional details including response to previous treatments)* _____
   _____
   _____

7. **Pain in other body regions** (also mark on Fig 1-1) _____
   _____

8. **How does your pain affect your quality of life?**

   No effect   Extremely

9. **How well do you sleep?**

   Very well   Extremely badly

10. **Does the pain wake you?** (Yes/No)   Frequency: times / night

Comments: _____
_____
_____

Form 1-1 Pain history.

1. **Extraoral examination**
   - Head and neck (mark any asymmetry, change in color, swellings, etc) _____
   _____
   - Lymph nodes _____

2. **TMJ and masticatory muscles examination** (mark tenderness to palpation on a scale from 0 to 3: 0 = no tenderness, 3 = very tender)

Muscles	Right	Left	TMJ	Right	Left	Opening	(mm)
Masseter			Lateral tenderness			Maximum open	
Temporalis			External auditory meatus tenderness			Deviation (right, left)	
Medial pterygoid			Right occlusal loading			Lateral movement (right)	
Lateral pterygoid			Left occlusal loading			Lateral movement (left)	
Suboccipital			Click*				
Sternocleidomastoid			Reciprocal click*				
Trapezius			Crepitation				

*Mark presence and the interincisal opening at which click occurs.

3. **Cranial nerves** (mark if examined and intact; findings to be summarized under "Remarks")
   - Corneal reflex ____
   - Pupillary reflex ____
   - III, IV, VI eye movements ____
   - Vth sensory ____
   - Vth motor ____
   - Facial (VII) ____
   - IX ____
   - XI ____
   - XII ____
   - Remarks: _____
   _____
   _____

4. **Intraoral examination** (summary) _____
   _____
   _____

5. **Ancillary tests, radiographs** (modality and summary of findings)_____
   _____
   _____

6. **Discussion of findings and suggested diagnosis** _____
   _____
   _____

7. **Treatment plan** (medications, other treatment modalities, follow-up planning) _____
   _____
   _____
   _____

Form 1-2 Physical examination. TMJ, temporomandibular joint.

Box 1-1 **Essentials of an orofacial pain history**

- Location
  - Local: head, neck, intraoral
  - Other body regions
- Attack onset
  - Time of day: morning, midday, evening
  - Month (menstrual)
  - Year (seasonal)
- Attack duration: seconds, minutes, hours, days
- Attack frequency
  - 24-hour distribution
  - Use of pain diaries
- Onset of present problem: age at onset, associated events, trauma
- Severity: verbal or visual analog scales
- Quality
  - Verbal descriptions: stabbing, burning
  - Structured questionnaires: McGill

- Associated features or signs: local, systemic
- Aggravating factors
  - Local: thermal, function
  - Systemic: dialysis, stress
- Alleviating factors
  - Endogenous: sleep
  - Exogenous: analgesics, massage
- Impact on daily function: lost work days, marital relations, wakes patient from sleep
- Personal and social history: occupation, stress, function; psychosocial evaluation
- Family history: headache, facial pain, bereavement
- Medical status: eg, hypertension
- Drug history: eg, analgesic drug abuse

The Pain History

Location

Precisely identifying location is a complex issue when specifically dealing with orofacial or craniofacial pain; the region is compact, and many important structures are close together (brain, eyes, nose, sinuses, and teeth), so pain spread is common. Notwithstanding, certain craniofacial pain syndromes have a propensity for particular areas and specific referral patterns. In order to record location, patients should point to the area where they feel the pain. Pain should also be marked on pre-prepared drawings of extraoral and intraoral regions (see Fig 1-1); these are helpful for communicating with the patient and serve as an important reference at a later stage. Pain can be *unilateral*, meaning on one side of the face, head, or mouth, or *bilateral,* that is, on both sides. Often pain is unilateral but may change sides from attack to attack (migraine), whereas in other conditions it may predominantly affect one side or even be *side-locked* (always on the same side). The patient should describe, and outline by finger pointing, whether the pain is *localized* or *diffuse*. Diffuse implies a large area with ill-defined borders and is usually outlined by patients with the whole hand rather than by finger pointing. Pain may *radiate*, which means the pain felt in a certain point spreads in a vectorlike fashion, or may *spread* in all directions. Pain radiation and pain spread are usually associated with severe pain (see chapter 6). When the source of pain is in one location but felt in another remote location, the pain is called *referred*. In many cases, the patient is usually aware only of the pain in the area of referral, and the primary source or location is identified by the clinician at a later stage (eg, myofascial trigger points; see chapter 8). The craniofacial symptoms may be associated with other body pains, and these are best recorded on a body drawing.

Temporal behavior

Another valuable descriptor is the behavior of pain in relation to time. The temporal behavior of the pain, once established, may be crucial in diagnosis. One of the essential features of many craniofacial pains is the *age of onset*; migraine typically begins early in life, whereas trigeminal neuralgia affects older subjects.

Pain may occur at specific times of the day, such as the morning or evening; thus, times of pain onset should be recorded. Moreover, pain onset may be associated with weekly (eg, weekends), monthly (eg, menstruation), or even yearly (eg, seasonal) events. Pain can be *intermittent* when it comes and goes, such as in pulpitis, or *continuous* when it lasts for long periods, such as in muscular pain. Episodic pain, also termed *periodic*, appears only during certain periods, and the patient is otherwise pain free. For example, pain appears for a day or two a couple of times in a month, as in migraine, or for a couple of weeks once a year, as in cluster headache (see chapters 10 and 11). Pain may become inactive for prolonged periods and be in remission, such as observed in cluster headache and trigeminal neuralgia. Of diagnostic significance is whether the pain wakes the patient from sleep, because this is related to pain intensity and often specifically to certain diagnoses.

Pain *duration* is often included in the classification of orofacial pain syndromes. Masticatory myofascial pain, for example, may last from a few hours to the best part of a day, with a mean of about 5 or 6 hours (see chapter 8). Very short pain attacks—from a few seconds to 2 minutes—are characteristic of trigeminal neuralgia. At the other end of the spectrum, TTHs may last a few days, though in the chronic form they are often continuous. Overlap in pain duration is common among related facial pain syndromes, such as the trigeminal autonomic cephalalgias (see chapter 11 and Fig 11-12a).

A further temporal aspect of pain behavior relates to the *frequency* of pain attacks. Frequency is the number of attacks over a defined period—per day, week, month, or months and in very frequent attacks in units of minutes to hours. As described later, pain may be evoked or initiated by external stimuli, in which case the frequency of pain is related to the frequency of the stimulus application. Although specific entities are associated with a characteristic *frequency* of attacks, there may be significant overlap (for example, see chapter 11 and Fig 11-12b). Frequency of attacks is easily obtained from conscientiously kept pain diaries (Form 1-3).

Modes of onset

When strong pain develops very rapidly and aggressively, such as in pulpitis or trigeminal neuralgia, it is termed *paroxysmal*. Pain is *evoked* when it occurs only after stimulation, for example, cold application to a tooth with a caries lesion; *spontaneous* when it occurs on its own with no external stimulus, such as pulpitis; or *triggered* when the pain response is out of proportion to the stimulus, such as is typical for trigeminal neuralgia. Pain is termed *progressive* when it becomes more severe, or stronger, over time.

Pain intensity

Pain intensity is valuable diagnostic information, and thus patients are asked to evaluate how strong their pain feels. A simple and quick way is to ask the patient to assess pain intensity on a scale of 0 to 10 (a verbal analog scale, where 0 means no pain at all, and 10 is the most excruciating pain imagined). The use of a visual analog scale, where the patient can mark the pain intensity, is also useful; a number of such scales are available. Chapter 3 gives detailed descriptions of the methods for evaluating and measuring pain intensity and unpleasantness. Note, however, that there is tremendous overlap between intensities reported for craniofacial pain syndromes (Fig 1-2).

Pain quality

Patients suffering from particular pain syndromes more often use certain descriptive terms. Trigeminal neuralgia presents with pain that is sharp or electric, and other neuropathies are characterized by burning pain (Fig 1-3). Neurovascular pain is usually throbbing in nature, although some forms of dental pathologies also possess this quality (Fig 1-4). Therefore, we as clinicians try to elucidate specific descriptions from patients with pain by conducting a verbal interview or using established questionnaires, such as the McGill Pain Questionnaire (see chapter 3).

Patient's name:_____

On a scale of 0 to 10, when 0 = no pain and 10 = worst pain imaginable, mark your pain for four periods in the day (morning, midday, afternoon, and night [only if it wakes you]).

Day and date	Pain intensity				Medication prescribed	Remarks	
	Morning	Midday	Afternoon	Night		Side effects, escape drugs (no., type)	Effect on quality of life
1							
2							
3							
4							
5							
6							
7							
8							
9							
10							
11							
12							
13							
14							
15							
16							
17							
18							
19							
20							
21							
22							
23							
24							
25							
26							
27							
28							

Form 1-3 Model of a pain diary used in a clinical setting.

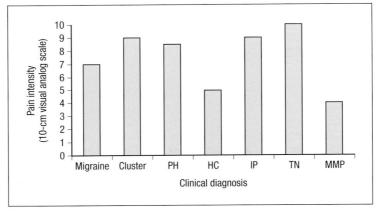

Fig 1-2 Mean pain severity in various craniofacial pain disorders. PH, paroxysmal hemicrania; HC, hemicrania continua; IP, irreversible pulpitis; TN, trigeminal neuralgia; MMP, masticatory myofascial pain.

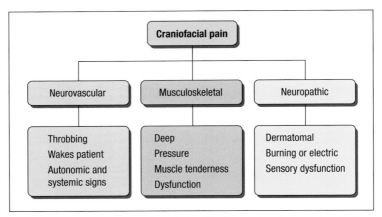

Fig 1-3 Symptomatic, system-based classification of chronic craniofacial pain.

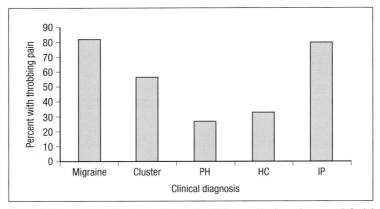

Fig 1-4 Percent of patients reporting a throbbing quality in various craniofacial pain disorders. PH, paroxysmal hemicrania; HC, hemicrania continua; IP, irreversible pulpitis.

Aggravating or alleviating factors

Another part of the pain history is an attempt to elucidate if the pain is aggravated by specific factors. These may be local factors, such as chewing; ingesting cold or hot drinks; or more generalized stimuli, such as exposure to cold air, bending down, physical activity, stress, or excitement. Certain syndromes are characterized by what alleviates or reduces the pain severity; for example, rest or sleep often alleviates pain for patients with migraine. The response to simple analgesics or specific medications may often aid in diagnosis (see chapters 11 and 12).

Impact on daily function and quality of life

Pain often interferes with basic orofacial functions, such as chewing, speaking, or tooth brushing. Secondary results may include detrimental dietary changes, social isolation, and dental neglect with ensuing pathology. Additionally, most chronic pain states produce an increasingly negative impact on the patient's general physical function and quality of life. This may reduce the patient's work capacity and affect the function of the surrounding family members.

Sleep disruption

Pain-related sleep disorders are very common and underlie many of the affective and cognitive problems in patients with chronic pain.[50] Prolonged periods of disturbed sleep induce daytime fatigue, sleepiness, difficulties with concentration, and reduced coping abilities.[51] Additionally, disturbed sleep per se may induce generalized muscle pain and reduced pain thresholds and endurance.[50] These are important factors to consider in the management of chronic orofacial pain.

Sleep disorders may occur directly because of pain or medical comorbidity.[52–55] Acute dental conditions, such as irreversible pulpitis or acute dentoalveolar abscess, may cause disturbed sleep. The association between such dental conditions and sleep is based on the intensity of pain and not a specific diagnosis.[56,57] Certain pain syndromes, such as the trigeminal autonomic cephalalgias (see chapter 11) and fibromyalgia (see chapter 8) may be pathophysiologically related to specific sleep disorders.[58,59] Pain diaries, where the patients record nighttime pain, are often the first sign that they suffer from disturbed sleep. However, patients often report getting a full night's sleep but awakening feeling not rested or unrefreshed. This pattern of unrefreshing sleep may aggravate the pain condition, and a vicious cycle is set up. Referral for a sleep study will determine the nature of the sleep disorder and help formulate a more comprehensive management approach. The orofacial pain specialist must be cognizant of the structure, control, and function of normal sleep and the effects of pain- or stress-related disruption. The relationship between pain and sleep is detailed in chapter 5.

Associated features

A number of local or general features consistently accompany pain attacks. These may be localized (as in swelling, redness, sweating, tearing, rhinorrhea, or ptosis) or generalized (such as nausea, photophobia, and dizziness). In addition, sensory changes *may* be associated with the pain complaint. Some patients may not be aware of a neurologic deficit, and thus the authors recommend a basic examination of the cranial nerves, outlined in Table 1-3. If there are findings, the specific modes of sensory changes are evaluated later, as discussed in detail in chapter 3.

Drug history as it pertains to the pain condition

Patients often forget the drugs and dosages they are taking, so they should bring documentation with them on their first visit. The most reliable method is to request a physician's summary, but a drug card, medical alert bracelets, and hospital release notes are also valuable sources of information. Recording what drugs the patient has tried in order to alleviate pain is imperative. These may be over-the-counter drugs or physician-prescribed drugs. Exact dosage, schedule, and duration for each drug will indicate whether the full therapeutic potential was exploited.

Table 1-3	Basic cranial nerve examination	
Test	**Result**	**Pathway/cranial nerve**
Group A (Cranial nerves I, II, III, IV, VI, and VIII)		
Shine a light into the patient's pupil (test both sides).	Tests the pupillary light reflex: Pupils should constrict bilaterally	Afferent is the optic nerve (I) and efferent the oculomotor (III)
Ask the patient to close his eyes, seal one nostril, and smell coffee, tobacco, or eugenol packed in unmarked containers.	Positive identification of smell	Tests olfactory nerve function (II); note that patients with colds or allergies may have a reduced ability
Ask the patient to seal one ear and whisper numbers contralaterally.	Accurate repetition	Tests the vestibulocochlear nerve (VIII)
Ask the patient to follow your finger with his eyes in the following directions:	Accurate and smooth tracking of finger movements by both eyes simultaneously	Tests the oculomotor (III), trochlear (IV), and abducens (VI) nerves
Group B (Cranial nerves V and VII)		
Ask the patient to look laterally and up with his eyes: gently stimulate the cornea with a wisp of cotton wool.	Tests the corneal reflex; causes immediate closure of the eyelids	Afferent is the trigeminal nerve and efferent the facial
With his eyes closed, ask the patient to identify sharp, blunt, and thermal stimuli in the upper, middle, and lower face.	Accurate identification of stimuli and area tested	Sensory branches of the trigeminal (V) nerve
Ask the patient to clench teeth.	Feel for symmetric contraction of masticatory (eg, masseter) muscles	Motor branch of the trigeminal (V) nerve
Ask patient to raise his eyebrows, close his eyes, smile, and whistle.	Symmetric movement; good muscle strength	Facial (VII) nerve function
Place sweet, salty, and sour stimuli on the patient's tongue.	Accurate identification	Chorda tympani branch of facial nerve
Group C (Cranial nerves IX, X, XI, and XII)		
Ask the patient to rotate his head to both sides, then raise his shoulders (all against mild manual resistance).	Symmetric movement; good muscle strength	Accessory (XI) nerve
Ask the patient to say "aah."	The uvula and soft palate should be raised symmetrically	Glossopharyngeal (IX) nerve
Ask the patient to perform tongue movements.		Hypoglossal (XII) nerve

Listening to the language of pain

Patients with similar pain conditions may describe their pain in very different terms. This may reflect differences in culture, education, or the actual physical experience of pain, no doubt influenced by genetic factors. Patients most often describe their pain in the physical dimension, for example, by severity and quality. Thus, a patient with trigeminal neuralgia may relate that the pain is severe and electric, or sharp. On the other hand, some patients may choose terms that describe an emotional dimension; the same patient with trigeminal neuralgia may add that the pain is unbearable to live with, frightening, or depressing. This multidimensionality of pain underlies its definition as an *experience* rather than as a *sensation*. The choice of words to describe pain is therefore important and offers an insight into the complete experience that a patient with pain endures (see chapters 3 and 4). Psychosocial assessment of patients with pain is therefore important (see chapter 4). The application of questionnaires typically used in such assessments is time-consuming but may be invaluable in preparing a treatment plan and assessing prognosis.

Physical Examination

The physical examination of a patient who complains of pain aims to identify the source and cause of pain, that is, the affected structure and the pathophysiologic process. Routine physical examination builds on the history to formulate a differential diagnosis and may require further special tests.

A routine physical examination of the head and neck should include observation, clinical examination (eg, palpation), and detection of functional and sensory deviations from the normal. Clinicians should look for facial asymmetry, change in color, and deviation or limitation of mouth opening. They should also palpate cervical and submaxillary lymph nodes, parotid and submandibular salivary glands, masticatory and neck muscles, and the temporomandibular joint to detect any abnormality in texture, mobility, or tenderness. A routine, basic examination of the cranial nerves (see Table 1-3) should also be performed. An intraoral examination seeks possible sources of pain (eg, caries lesions, mucosal erosions, or ulcerations) and includes examination modalities such as inspection, probing, palpation, and percussion. The authors summarize physical findings on a standardized form (see Form 1-2), though clinicians may want to devise their own form of examination according to personal preferences.

Confirmatory Tests

Several other tests, in addition to the routine physical examination, may be required to confirm or refute the suspected diagnosis. These may be as simple as the application of a cold stimulus to a tooth with suspected pulpitis or more elaborate sensory testing (see chapter 3). Radiographs and other means of imaging are still by far the most useful ancillary tests. These include the simple, relatively cheap, bitewing or periapical dental radiographs (see chapter 6) and more sophisticated, neuroimaging techniques such as computed tomography (CT) or magnetic resonance imaging (MRI).

The decision when to refer a patient with chronic orofacial pain for advanced neuroimaging is often complex, particularly under current financial constraints in health care systems. Most studies dealing with this issue relate specifically to headache or trigeminal neuralgia, but the guidelines may be easily adopted for orofacial pain in general.[60–62] Among patients with normal neurologic examinations and headaches diagnosed as migraine or tension type, the prevalence of significant intracranial abnormalities on neuroimaging is approximately 0.2% and 0%, respectively.[63] Undiagnosable headaches have a higher prevalence of intracranial abnormalities, but studies report varying, inconsistent figures ranging from 0% to 6.7%.[63] Positive neurologic findings are intuitively suggestive of an intracranial abnormality (see also chapter 12). However, the predictive value of an intracranial abnormality by a positive neurologic exam is surprisingly low, around 3%; this is due to the very low initial probability of intracranial abnormalities. Patient complaints of neurologic symptoms will significantly increase this risk.[63] The absence of findings on a neurologic examination notably decreases (but does not eliminate) the likelihood of finding a signif-

---

Box 1-2   **Indications for neuroimaging in headache**

Clear indication
- Unexplained abnormal neurologic finding (eg, numbness)

Possible indication
- Headache worsened by Valsalva maneuver
- Headache causing awakening from sleep
- New headache in the older population
- Progressively worsening headache or rapidly increasing headache frequency

---

icant lesion on neuroimaging.[63] When ordering neuroimaging, the orofacial pain practitioner should specifically ask that extracranial areas be examined (jaws, submandibular space), as these are often excluded on routine imaging.

The indications for advanced neuroimaging are shown in Box 1-2. For individual patients with pronounced anxiety, imaging may be indicated to alleviate emotional distress. The number of studies comparing CT with MRI is limited, but they suggest that MRI may be more sensitive than CT for identifying clinically insignificant abnormalities. However, MRI may not be more sensitive for identifying clinically significant pathology that is relevant to the cause of headache.[63] Thus, the choice of modality and the region to be scanned need to be based on a differential diagnosis.

Choosing wisely

The use of CT increased threefold from 1993 to 2007, and concerns have been raised over the negative health effects of CT.[64] The authors of a risk-assessment study estimated that approximately 29,000 future cancers could be related to CT scans performed in the United States in 2007. The largest contributions were from scans of the abdomen and pelvis (n = 14,000), chest (n = 4,100), and head (n = 4,000).[64] One-third of the projected cancers were due to

scans performed at the ages of 35 to 54 years. These data indicate that risk-reduction efforts are warranted.

Additionally, overtesting adds a large economic burden to the health care system. To help reduce such waste in the United States and promote physician and patient conversations on choosing treatments and tests wisely, nine medical specialty societies have joined the American Board of Internal Medicine Foundation and Consumer Reports in the first phase of the Choosing Wisely campaign.[65] These nine organizations were asked to pick five tests or treatments within their purview that they believed are overused. The Choosing Wisely website (www.choosingwisely.org) lists 45 such tests and treatments, and eight organizations list at least one imaging test.[66] The American Headache Society's board of directors recently made clear recommendations about not performing neuroimaging studies in patients with stable headaches that meet criteria for migraine and not performing CT imaging for headache when MRI is available, except in emergency settings.[67]

Clearly, organizations that bring together orofacial pain experts need to formulate similar recommendations. Meanwhile, clinicians are advised to carefully consider the use of confirmatory tests and the cost (monetary and healthwise) to benefit ratio of such tests.

Establishing a Diagnosis

Routines in medicine are very effective in that they add confidence, especially to the inexperienced; sometimes save time; and ensure a comprehensive gathering of clinical information. In principle, the diagnosis should follow the history, physical examination, and ancillary tests. Clinical information gathering is a back-and-forth process, mainly dictated by the diagnostic process and the possible differential diagnoses considered.

Indeed, an experienced clinician often formulates initial diagnostic hypotheses very early on in the clinical setting. At a certain point, and usually quite early, we start to depart from the routine and to consider diagnostic hypotheses. We start to test these hypotheses by asking specific questions. The difference is that while routine questions expect an open-ended answer to such questions as "Where do you feel your pain?" most hypothesis-generated questions aim at a closed-ended yes or no answer. For example, asking "Does bending your head aggravate pain?" is useful when a patient is suspected to have sinusitis. "Does the tooth react painfully to a cold stimulus?" may be asked when a caries lesion is suspected in a vital tooth. The answer expected to such questions is yes or no. If the answer, whether to an oral question or a physical test, satisfies the hypothesis, the examiner usually proceeds with another hypothesis-generated question. If the answer leads to a dead end, however, clinicians often return to the routine methodology. Ultimately, we cluster enough positive pieces of information to confirm our hypothesis (diagnosis) and usually some negative pieces of information that enable us to refute other possible diagnoses.

Clustering of information is a useful tool in the decision-making process in that it reduces the number of fragments of information and facilitates the process. The specific clustering of signs, symptoms, and other information leads to a diagnosis based on classification systems, as discussed earlier.

However, gathering information on its own does not make a diagnosis. For the beginner or inexperienced clinician, the question of what to do with all of this information is real. Often, connecting the collected information with a diagnosis or a set of criteria in a classification is difficult.

Diagnosis for beginners

Over the years, the authors have developed a clustering system for diagnostic entities that is useful for the more difficult diagnostic process of chronic orofacial pain and thus useful for trainees and students. The system divides chronic orofacial pain into three main symptomatic classes: musculoskeletal, neurovascular, and neuropathic (detailed in Fig 1-3 and Box 1-3). The authors advise the beginner to examine these entities and the cluster of signs and symptoms relevant for each class of these diagnostic entities. Then proceed to Table 1-4 for a description of the diagnostic process generated by hypotheses based on pain location, and then go to Table 1-5 for the diagnostic process based on the temporal behavior and characteristics of the pain. This system proceeds from signs and symptoms presented by the patient to the disease process hypothesized by the clinician (ie, diagnostic hypothesis). This allows the beginner to get an initial feel for the diagnosis and see which family of entities it belongs to.

After considering a diagnosis, it is legitimate to keep testing it by gathering further information. In reference to points addressed in the "Information critical for hypothesis testing" column of Tables 1-4 and 1-5, further specific information is requested at all levels: history, physical examination, and ancillary tests. The ability to start the diagnostic process from pain location (see Table 1-4) or from pain characteristics (see Table 1-5) demonstrates the versatility of the interview method and allows the clinician to cross-check the hypothesis generation in more than one way. The authors recommend that the reader refer back to this method of diagnosing chronic orofacial pain when reading subsequent chapters, especially the chapters dealing with chronic orofacial pain of musculoskeletal, neurovascular, or neuropathic origin.

Box 1-3	Typical clusters of signs and symptoms in the main chronic orofacial pain entities

1. Musculoskeletal orofacial pain

Temporomandibular joint (TMJ) pain
- Pain fairly localized to TMJ area
- Click/crepitating of TMJ
- Deviation of mouth opening toward affected joint
- TMJ painful on palpation
- Pain on function (biting on contralateral side to affected TMJ)

Masticatory myofascial pain
- Pain, mostly unilateral, at angle of mandible and front of ear (diffuse)
- Masticatory muscle tenderness on palpation, mostly on affected side
- Jaw dysfunction (limited opening, tiredness on chewing)
- Pain on function (eg, yawning, chewing, talking)

Tension-type headache
- Bilateral pain at temples and occipital areas
- Pain is pressing and annoying
- Pain is periodic or chronic
- Anorexia
- Nausea

2. Neurovascular craniofacial pain

Migraine
- Strong, unilateral headache
- Pain is throbbing
- Pain is periodic (lasting a day or two, a couple of times a month)
- Occasional waking from sleep toward morning (REM locked)
- Photophobia/phonophobia
- Nausea and vomiting
- Occasional tearing
- Patient seeks rest in a dark quiet place

Cluster headache
- Periorbital, unilateral, very strong, throbbing pain
- Clusters of active periods of pain (6–10 weeks) mostly once a year
- At active period, 1 to 2 attacks per 24 hours, with clockwise regularity
- Typical attack lasts 45–60 minutes
- Occasional waking from sleep (REM locked)
- Tearing, one eye on affected side
- Rhinorrhea, one nostril on affected side
- Redness, ptosis, and miosis of eye on affected side (possible)
- Patient paces around restlessly

Chronic paroxysmal hemicrania
- Periorbital and temporal, unilateral, strong pain
- Short (lasting only minutes) paroxysmal pain attacks
- Occasional waking from sleep
- Tearing, conjunctival injection, one eye on affected side
- Rhinorrhea, one nostril on affected side
- Head movement may trigger pain

SUNCT (short-lasting unilateral neuralgiform headache attacks with conjunctival injection and tearing)
- Periorbital, unilateral, severe pain
- Paroxysmal, short (lasting seconds) attacks
- Pain precipitated by touch of eyebrow
- Conjunctival injection, tearing

Neurovascular orofacial pain
- Midface, perioral, and intraoral pain
- Spontaneous or evoked pain (mostly by cold food ingestion)
- Occasional swelling or redness of cheek
- Waking from sleep
- Nausea
- Tearing, one eye on affected side (possible)
- Pain mostly periodic but may be chronic

Hemicrania continua
- Unilateral, moderate-intensity headache with no side shifts
- Chronic (lasting more than 3 months), daily nonremitting
- Rare waking from sleep
- Mild tearing, one eye on affected side
- Mild rhinorrhea, one nostril on affected side
- Occasional eye redness, ptosis, and miosis on affected side

3. **Neuropathic orofacial pain**
   Trigeminal neuralgia
   - Unilateral pain in the trigeminal nerve area (mostly 2nd and 3rd divisions)
   - Paroxysmal, electriclike, very short (lasting seconds), strong pain
   - Pain attack accompanied by facial tic
   - Pain triggered by light touch, vibration, and other nonpainful stimuli
   - After triggering, there is a refractory period
   - No sensory deficit

   Traumatic neuropathies (CRPS-I/II)
   - Pain location associated with history of trauma
   - Pain continuous, mostly burning quality
   - Allodynia
   - Edema/redness
   - Trophic changes (mostly in CRPS II)
   - Sensory deficit (in CRPS II)
   - Dysesthesia (in CRPS II)

REM, rapid eye movement; CRPS, complex regional pain syndrome.

234

*

* ipsilateral Autonomic Signs

Table 1-4	**Diagnostic process and hypothesis generation based on pain location**	
Location (unilateral)	**Diagnostic hypothesis**	**Information critical for hypothesis testing**
Frontotemporal*	Migraine Hemicrania continua	Pain attack duration Patterns of periodicity Photo- and/or phonophobia Nausea
Orbital and periorbital	Cluster headache Paroxysmal hemicrania SUNCT	Pain attack duration Attacks/day Periodicity Tearing, rhinorrhea SUNCT triggered by touch
Preauricular, angle of mandible	Temporomandibular joint (TMJ) pain Masticatory muscle pain	Aggravated by chewing Mouth opening dysfunction TMJ tenderness, click Masticatory muscle tenderness
Midface, perioral, or intraoral	Trigeminal neuralgia Neurovascular orofacial pain (NVOP)	Attack duration Triggered by touch, vibration Evoked by cold/hot foods Tearing, rhinorrhea

*If the pain is bilateral, consider tension-type headache.
SUNCT, short-lasting unilateral neuralgiform headache attacks with conjunctival injection and tearing.

Table 1-5	**Diagnostic process and hypothesis generation based on temporal pain behavior and characteristics**	
Temporal pain behavior and characteristics	**Diagnostic hypothesis**	**Information critical for hypothesis testing**
Short, paroxysmal	Trigeminal neuralgia Paroxysmal hemicrania SUNCT	Pain location Duration of pain attack Triggering/evoking stimuli Autonomic signs Wakes from sleep
Periodic, throbbing	Migraine Cluster headache Neurovascular orofacial pain	Pain location Duration of pain attack Periodicity Autonomic signs Nausea
Continuous, pressing	Tension-type headache (TMJ) Temporomandibular joint pain Masticatory muscle pain Hemicrania continua Complex regional pain syndrome (type I or II)	Pain location, laterality Aggravates by chewing Mouth opening dysfunction TMJ tenderness, click Masticatory muscle tenderness History of trauma Sensory abnormality

SUNCT, short-lasting unilateral neuralgiform headache attacks with conjunctival injection and tearing.

The Patient with Pain

Patients with undiagnosed pain may worry that they have cancer or some other threatening disease. Prospective studies suggest a relationship between psychologic distress and pain, which may operate both ways (see chapter 4). A high level of psychologic distress is often a predictor of the onset of future pain or the development of chronic pain. Conversely, ongoing orofacial pain is often associated with psychologic distress.[68] Research shows that patients with chronic craniofacial pain suffer from psychologic distress, increased depression, impaired social performance, and decreased quality of life (see chapters 7 and 9 to 12). Thus, patients with chronic orofacial pain develop maladaptive or illness behavior patterns[68] that are important factors affecting their management and prognosis.

Patients differ in many respects that influence diagnostic considerations, such as responses to pain medications, attitudes toward health care, and behavioral responses to chronic pain. In the sections that follow, the effects of three important factors—genetics, sex, and culture and ethnicity—are discussed.

Genetics and epigenetics

The sequencing of the human genome has elucidated the presence of 30,000 to 40,000 human genes. Some of these genes and protein end-products will emerge as new therapeutic targets for chronic pain. For some pain syndromes, information is available on genetic polymorphisms that may affect disease occurrence; this area is covered in chapters 7, 9, 10, and 11. Information concerning genetically controlled drug toxicity and common adverse drug reactions is available on an individual basis. Genetically governed interindividual differences are found in drug-transport proteins and drug targets (receptors), which may alter the pharmacokinetics and pharmacodynamics of a variety of drugs. For example, the analgesic potency of morphine is partly dictated by variations in the expression of μ-opioid receptors. Polymorphisms in this receptor lead to interindividual differences in responses to pain and its relief by opioid drugs.[69] Pain modulation is impaired in certain ethnic groups, and some of this effect may be related to increased stress.[70]

Gene regulation depends on the function of regulatory elements that turn genes on and off at the right time. Regulatory elements are specific DNA sequences in the vicinity of the gene to be regulated; others may be DNA-binding proteins or micro-RNA molecules that use base-pair specificity to modulate gene expression after transcription. Alterations to the structure of chromatin will modify gene expression and subsequently the phenotype. These changes, which are independent of alterations to the DNA sequence, are called *epigenetic changes*, which include DNA methylation, histone methylation, repressive protein complexes, and RNA interference. Covalent modification of DNA by methylation is a critical epigenetic mechanism that regulates gene expression. Increased methylation will inhibit gene expression, and decreased methylation will increase it. Significant evidence supports the role of epigenetic modification after injury and its involvement in the onset of chronic pain.[71–73] Clearly, genetic considerations will become integral to diagnostic and therapeutic approaches to chronic pain.

Sex

Extensive, and often inconsistent, reports have examined the effects of sex on the epidemiology of pain syndromes, pain thresholds, and analgesic responses.[74,75] Additionally, the menstrual phase may affect the efficacy of the endogenous pain modulatory system.[76] Women suffer significantly more from migraines, TTHs, facial pains, fibromyalgia, and TMDs.[77–81] In general, women do not seek treatment for orofacial pain significantly more frequently than men do.[82] However, for TMDs, women usually demand more care than men do,[83] probably because they have more severe symptoms. Both hormone replacement therapy and use of oral contraceptives have been associated with increased risk of TMD[84,85] (see chapter 8). The use of oral contraceptives has been shown to both improve and worsen headaches, depending on the hormones used, duration of treatment, and dosages.[86] Preliminary data indicate that menopause can affect pain, depending on the painful condition experienced.[87]

Under experimental conditions, women consistently demonstrate a lower pain threshold, often affected by the stage of the menstrual cycle and by exogenous hormones such as oral contraceptives.[88] Injection of capsaicin into the forehead induced trigeminal sensitization and evoked sex-specific sensory and vasomotor responses; menstruating women generally showed the strongest manifestations.[89] Postextraction pain and pain under experimental conditions in women responds better to opioid therapy than it does in men.[90] However, men and women may differ in their response to nonsteroidal anti-inflammatory drugs, and women enjoy less analgesia with ibuprofen than men do.[91] Other studies found no sex-based differences related to ibuprofen use or the level of induced placebo analgesia after tooth extraction.[92,93]

The practical applications of sex differences include menstrual-related changes in pain sensitivity that may be associated with increased analgesic use. Epidemiologic data continue to accumulate concerning pain syndromes in women and pharmacologic traits particular to each sex; clearly, these are areas that will aid pain physicians.

Culture and ethnicity

In 1969, Mark Zborowski highlighted the role of ethnicity in a person's reaction to pain in the classic book *People in Pain*,[94] which deals with the attitudes and reaction to pain in three American ethnic groups and points to striking differences. More recent research examines racial and ethnic variability affecting the pain experience.[95,96]

The terms *culture*, *ethnicity*, and *race* are often used interchangeably, probably because it is difficult to accurately define them. Because of the massive population migration, intermarriage, and genetic polymorphisms, populations such as Africans, whites, and Asians are more genetically heterogenous within than across groups. Indeed, anthropologists and biologists are increasingly defining race as a social construct and not a scientific category.[96] This is not to say that genetically distinct physiologic or medical traits in ethnic populations (eg, Tay-Sachs or drug metabolism conditions such as glucose-6-phosphate dehydrogenase enzyme deficiency) do not exist, but these traits cannot solely define ethnicity.

Cultural and social factors are the foundation for the expression and management of pain.[95] They affect patients' experience of pain as well as their behavioral responses, seeking of health care, and adherence to treatment.[97] In a multiracial environment, we as clinicians must understand these factors and attempt to positively modify the way we practice pain medicine. Examples that highlight the influence of culture and beliefs on the experience and interpretation of pain include the reliance on religion to cope with pain in some ethnic groups[95,96] and differences in the use of local anesthetic for dental treatment.[98] Pain sensitivity, secondary hyperalgesic area, and pressure pain thresholds after capsaicin injection to the forehead were assessed in South Indians and whites.[99] South Indians showed significantly greater pain responses compared with whites. Ethnic differences in pain tolerance reflect traits in the affective dimension of pain; these differences are not innate but learned and may even be modified by the environment at later stages.[96] However, no difference has been observed between ethnic groups in the amounts of self-administered analgesia for acute pain.[100] After consultation for pain management, patients reported significant pain relief, regardless of race or ethnicity.[101] Despite these pain decreases, Latinos were 62% more likely than whites to report pain at discharge and follow-up.[101]

Treatment

The initial aim of the diagnostic process is to initiate the patient on a treatment plan; the ultimate, but elusive, aim is the eradication of pain, which may involve multiple modalities. Patients with acute pain are usually alarmed and anxious by this sudden, mostly unexpected, change in their state of well-being and need a lot of reassurance. An accurate diagnosis, empathetic explanation, and effective treatment are important to reassure patients and obtain their confidence. Treatment of acute pain often includes physical intervention, such as tooth pulp extirpation or use of analgesics (see chapters 6, 7, and 15). Dentists do this almost every day, and the vast majority of patients enjoy rapid and complete relief from acute dental pain within a short time.

Chronic pain, as its name implies, is long standing and many times associated with co-morbidities such as negative changes in function, drug abuse, psychosocial dysfunction, and depression (see chapters 4 and 8 to 12). Consequently, the aims of therapy in chronic or recurrent pain cannot be limited to the alleviation of pain but must include the restoration of quality of life and function as well as the prevention or elimination of drug abuse. Chronic oro-facial pain is difficult to eradicate, particularly in certain syndromes such as traumatic neuropathies, which is why we refer to the *management* of chronic orofacial pain rather than its *treatment*. The goal of pain management, which is often defined as more than a 50% reduction in pain intensity or frequency, must be explained to patients, as this level of improvement is likely way below the patient's initial expectations. Furthermore, results may not be obtained as quickly as patients would wish; multiple lengthy drug trials, prolonged physiotherapy, and psychologic interventions are often needed before a reasonable, successful result can be attained.

Provider Characteristics and Analgesic Prescription

Increasingly, researchers are recognizing the importance of identifying factors that influence health care workers in their decision-making process. Significant differences were shown to occur between the amounts of analgesia prescribed to ethnic subgroups.[100] Among veterans younger than 65 years who reported moderate to high levels of chronic, non–cancer-related pain, blacks were less likely to be prescribed opioids than whites.[102] Eliminating racial differences in pain treatment therefore remains a challenge. Clearly, ethnocultural background may influence a clinician's assessment of pain intensity in patients, and minorities remain at risk for inadequate pain control.[95]

A recent review highlights further factors involved in analgesic prescription by health care providers.[103] These effects include medical specialty, age, experience, and sex interplays.[103] Cultural and demographic factors affect the way patients respond to pain and its management, and we must therefore understand how clinicians and patients interact to influence health care delivery. As clinicians, we should be aware that we tend to have more empathy for the pain suffered by persons of our own race than for those of another race.[104]

Outcomes

How do we define success in the treatment of pain? Pain is an individual experience, so a successful outcome is also an individual, highly personalized result. Some patients with a reduction of more than 50% in pain intensity after permanent ingestion of psychotropic drugs may be dissatisfied, unhappy, and incapable of maintaining normal employment. On the other hand, a patient may be able to function normally after achieving less than 50% reduction in pain intensity obtained with physiotherapy and cognitive behavioral therapy (see chapters 4 and 8). Just as we have come to appreciate that pain is a complex and individual experience, therapeutic outcome needs to assess a broader spectrum, including such factors as restoration of function and psychosocial status. In a highly simplified paradigm, we need to balance the patient's expectations with the physician's possibilities. A more realistic model appreciates that the patient's expectations are a complex result of a painful experience within a context of cultural and ethnic influences, current employment, views on health and disease, and other variables.

Follow-Up

The use of pain diaries is very useful for follow-up, for assessing treatment results, and often for confirming a diagnosis. To ensure compliance, the authors keep their pain diary as simple as possible (see Form 1-3), but this can be modified to meet individual needs. The patient records pain intensity and its effect on quality of life on a numeric scale from 0 to 10 at different times of the day (including night if the pain wakes the patient from sleep). The diary also records dosages of prescribed drugs, escape drugs if used, and adverse pharmacologic effects. A 28-day diary is sufficient to allow the authors to adjust treatment according to pain response and side effects. Patients' reaction to the pain diary is usually very positive; they believe their pain symptoms are taken seriously and are reassured by the attention given to their response to therapy.

The pain diary is also essential in controlling drug abuse. Patients with chronic pain often abuse many drugs, some prescribed and some obtained over the counter. Often drugs prescribed in the past are still taken and added to those currently used; unless specifically instructed, patients may not stop taking previously prescribed medications. The recording of escape drugs in the diary (usually analgesics used to control breakthrough pain), in addition to the prescribed medications, facilitates the detection of drug abuse. Drug consumption in response to breakthrough pain is a learned response that may lead to dependence. Reviewing the pattern and amount of escape drug used allows the authors to advise patients on adequate scheduling and helps break the habit of taking additional medications. This is achieved by shifting the patient from on-demand to per-schedule consumption of the escape drug and gradually decreasing the amount consumed. As a rule, for chronic pain it is always advisable to prescribe medications per schedule rather than per demand, because the latter usually leads to more drug abuse and dependence.

Prognosis and Long-Term Management

Although we as clinicians aim to eradicate or alleviate all pain, we are a long way from optimal patient care. Some of the best drugs offer substantial relief to some patients, but not all patients will be pain free despite our treatment (see clinical chapters and chapter 16). For many patients, particularly those who do not respond well to therapy, we must offer means for better coping with their agony and despair. We can help the patient to increase adaptive skills in order to minimize pain-related stress and avoid unnecessary illness behavior by means of cognitive behavioral therapy and other psychologic pain management approaches. This approach,

discussed in detail in chapter 4, offers an effective mode for improving coping skills. Of special concern are patients with trauma-related pain, who often suffer from post-traumatic stress disorder and need early psychologic intervention.

The Pain Clinic

Pain is one of the prime reasons people seek medical attention. In most instances of orofacial pain, the patient's main route is to look for help at a dental clinic or see the family physician. In most cases, especially for those with acute pain, patient management and treatment results are easily attained. However, when the situation is complicated, especially given the anatomical density of the orofacial region, a visit to an orofacial pain clinic becomes a necessity. Physicians and staff at a pain clinic approach chronic pain as a disease and offer expertise on the pathophysiology of pain, pain medication for acute and chronic pain, and alternative treatment options (see chapters 6, 13, and 15 to 17). An additional strength of the pain clinic is its ability to use a multidisciplinary team approach that involves other professionals, such as psychologists and physiotherapists. The concept of the pain clinic is not new and has developed over the years from a center offering management alternatives for prediagnosed patients (eg, intrathecal injections, regional blocks, surgical interventions) to a center that diagnoses, manages, and follows up patients in pain.

An orofacial pain clinic is therefore involved in the diagnostic process and management of craniofacial pain. Although pain clinics rely heavily on pharmacotherapy, other modalities are performed as appropriate, including muscle trigger-point injection, arthrocentesis of the temporomandibular joint, acupuncture, hypnotherapy, night guards, and physiotherapy. Consultations with neurosurgery, neurology, otolaryngology, and other specialists are common, and patients may be referred for psychiatric evaluation and cognitive behavioral therapy. The intimate relationship between the pain clinic and other members of the medical community has become a two-way channel for patient referral, communication, and constant enrichment of knowledge.

References

1. Sharav Y, Benoliel R. Primary vascular-type craniofacial pain. Compend Contin Educ Dent 2001;22:119–122;124–126;128.

2. Benoliel R, Sharav Y. Accurate diagnosis of facial pain. Cephalalgia 2006;26:902.

3. Benoliel R, Birman N, Eliav E, Sharav Y. The International Classification of Headache Disorders: Accurate diagnosis of orofacial pain? Cephalalgia 2008;28:752–762.

4. Zebenholzer K, Wöber C, Vigl M, Wessely P, Wöber-Bingöl C. Facial pain and the second edition of the International Classification of Headache Disorders. Headache 2006;46:259–263.

5. Zebenholzer K, Wöber C, Vigl M, Wessely P, Wöber-Bingöl C. Facial pain in a neurological tertiary care centre—evaluation of the International Classification of Headache Disorders. Cephalalgia 2005;25:689–699.

6. Headache Classification Subcommittee of the International Headache Society. The international classification of headache disorders, 3rd edition (beta version). Cephalalgia 2013;33:629–808.

7. Gaskin DJ, Richard P. The economic costs of pain in the United States. J Pain 2012;13:715–724.

8. Salter MW. Deepening understanding of the neural substrates of chronic pain. Brain 2014;137:651–653.

9. McMillan AS, Wong MC, Zheng J, Lam CL. Prevalence of orofacial pain and treatment seeking in Hong Kong Chinese. J Orofac Pain 2006;20:218–225.

10. Macfarlane TV, Blinkhorn AS, Davies RM, Kincey J, Worthington HV. Oro-facial pain in the community: Prevalence and associated impact. Community Dent Oral Epidemiol 2002;30:52–60.

11. Ng KF, Tsui SL, Chan WS. Prevalence of common chronic pain in Hong Kong adults. Clin J Pain 2002;18:275–281.

12. Isong U, Gansky SA, Plesh O. Temporomandibular joint and muscle disorder-type pain in U.S. adults: The National Health Interview Survey. J Orofac Pain 2008;22:317–322.

13. Koopman JS, Dieleman JP, Huygen FJ, de Mos M, Martin CG, Sturkenboom MC. Incidence of facial pain in the general population. Pain 2009;147:122–127.

14. Renton T, Durham J, Aggarwal VR. The classification and differential diagnosis of orofacial pain. Expert Rev Neurother 2012;12:569–576.

15. de Leeuw R, Klasser G (eds). Orofacial Pain: Guidelines for Assessment, Diagnosis and Management, ed 5. Chicago: Quintessence, 2013.

16. Schiffman E, Ohrbach R, Truelove E, et al. Diagnostic Criteria for Temporomandibular Disorders (DC/TMD) for clinical and research applications: Recommendations of the International RDC/TMD Consortium Network and Orofacial Pain Special Interest Group. J Oral Facial Pain Headache 2014;28:6–27.

17. Benoliel R, Eliav E, Sharav Y. Classification of chronic orofacial pain: Applicability of chronic headache criteria. Oral Surg Oral Med Oral Pathol Oral Radiol Endod 2010;110:729–737.

18. Silberstein SD. Chronic daily headache. J Am Osteopath Assoc 2005;105:23S–29S.

19. Dodick DW. Indomethacin-responsive headache syndromes. Curr Pain Headache Rep 2004;8:19–26.

20. Anderton LA. Concepts and classification of disease. In: Demeny P, McNicoll G (eds). Encyclopedia of Population. New York: MacMillan Reference, 2003:247–250.

21. Sprenger T, May A. Advanced neuroimaging for the study of migraine pathophysiology. Pain Clinical Updates, vol 6. Seattle: International Association for the Study of Pain, 2012.

22. Pearce JM. Disease, diagnosis or syndrome? Pract Neurol 2011;11:91–97.

23. Aggarwal VR, McBeth J, Zakrzewska JM, Lunt M, Macfarlane GJ. The epidemiology of chronic syndromes that are frequently unexplained: Do they have common associated factors? Int J Epidemiol 2006;35:468–476.

24. Aggarwal VR, McBeth J, Zakrzewska JM, Macfarlane GJ. Unexplained orofacial pain—Is an early diagnosis possible? Br Dent J 2008;205:E6.

25. Olesen J, Lipton RB. Classification of headache. In: Olesen J, Goadsby PJ, Ramadan NM, Tfelt-Hansen P, Welch KMA (eds). The Headaches, ed 2. Philadelphia: Lippincott Williams & Wilkins, 2006:9–25.

26. Nixdorf DR, Drangsholt MT, Ettlin DA, et al. Classifying orofacial pains: A new proposal of taxonomy based on ontology. J Oral Rehabil 2012;39:161–169.

27. Billis E, McCarthy CJ, Gliatis J, Gittins M, Papandreou M, Oldham JA. Inter-tester reliability of discriminatory examination items for sub-classifying non-specific low back pain. J Rehabil Med 2012;44:851–857.

28. Clarke C, Lindsay DR, Pyati S, Buchheit T. Residual limb pain is not a diagnosis: A proposed algorithm to classify postamputation pain. Clin J Pain 2013;29:551-562.

29. Köseoglu E, Naçar M, Talaslioglu A, Cetinkaya F. Epidemiological and clinical characteristics of migraine and tension type headache in 1146 females in Kayseri, Turkey. Cephalalgia 2003;23:381–388.

30. Gupta R, Bhatia MS. Comparison of clinical characteristics of migraine and tension type headache. Indian J Psychiatry 2011;53:134–139.

31. Mongini F, Ciccone G, Deregibus A, Ferrero L, Mongini T. Muscle tenderness in different headache types and its relation to anxiety and depression. Pain 2004;112:59–64.

32. Stuginski-Barbosa J, Macedo HR, Bigal ME, Speciali JG. Signs of temporomandibular disorders in migraine patients: A prospective, controlled study. Clin J Pain 2010;26:418–421.

33. Chabriat H, Danchot J, Michel P, Joire JE, Henry P. Precipitating factors of headache. A prospective study in a national control-matched survey in migraineurs and nonmigraineurs. Headache 1999;39:335–338.

34. Look JO, Schiffman EL, Truelove EL, Ahmad M. Reliability and validity of Axis I of the Research Diagnostic Criteria for Temporomandibular Disorders (RDC/TMD) with proposed revisions. J Oral Rehabil 2010;37:744–759.

35. Dworkin SF, LeResche L. Research diagnostic criteria for temporomandibular disorders: Review, criteria, examinations and specifications, critique. J Craniomandib Disord 1992;6:301–355.

36. Eversole LR, Machado L. Temporomandibular joint internal derangements and associated neuromuscular disorders. J Am Dent Assoc 1985;110:69–79.

37. Fillingim RB, Ohrbach R, Greenspan JD, et al. Potential psychosocial risk factors for chronic TMD: Descriptive data and empirically identified domains from the OPPERA case-control study. J Pain 2011;12(suppl 11):T46–T60.

38. Komiyama O, Obara R, Uchida T, et al. Pain intensity and psychosocial characteristics of patients with burning mouth syndrome and trigeminal neuralgia. J Oral Sci 2012;54:321–327.

39. Porto F, de Leeuw R, Evans DR, et al. Differences in psychosocial functioning and sleep quality between idiopathic continuous orofacial neuropathic pain patients and chronic masticatory muscle pain patients. J Orofac Pain 2011;25:117–124.

40. Dworkin RH, Turk DC, Farrar JT, et al. Core outcome measures for chronic pain clinical trials: IMMPACT recommendations. Pain 2005;113:9–19.

41. Turner JA, Dworkin SF. Screening for psychosocial risk factors in patients with chronic orofacial pain: Recent advances. J Am Dent Assoc 2004;135:1119–1125.

42. Longo DL, Fauci AS, Kasper DL, Hauser SL, Jameson JL, Loscalzo J. The practice of medicine. In: Longo DL, Fauci AS, Kasper DL, Hauser SL, Jameson JL, Loscalzo J (eds). Harrison's Principles of Internal Medicine, ed 18. New York: McGraw Hill Medical, 2012:2–8.

43. Maixner W, Greenspan JD, Dubner R, et al. Potential autonomic risk factors for chronic TMD: Descriptive data and empirically identified domains from the OPPERA case-control study. J Pain 2011;12(suppl 11):T75–T91.

44. Slade GD, Conrad MS, Diatchenko L, et al. Cytokine biomarkers and chronic pain: Association of genes, transcription, and circulating proteins with temporomandibular disorders and widespread palpation tenderness. Pain 2011;152:2802–2812.

45. Smith SB, Maixner DW, Greenspan JD, et al. Potential genetic risk factors for chronic TMD: Genetic associations from the OPPERA case control study. J Pain 2011;12(suppl 11):T92–T101.

46. De Luca GC, Bartleson JD. When and how to investigate the patient with headache. Semin Neurol 2010;30:131–144.

47. Loder E, Rizzoli P. Biomarkers in migraine: Their promise, problems, and practical applications. Headache 2006;46:1046–1058.

48. Montagna P, Cevoli S, Marzocchi N, et al. The genetics of chronic headaches. Neurol Sci 2003;24(2, suppl):S51–S56.

49. Rossi P, Vollono C, Valeriani M, Sandrini G. The contribution of clinical neurophysiology to the comprehension of the tension-type headache mechanisms. Clin Neurophysiol 2011;122:1075–1085.

50. Moldofsky H. Sleep and pain. Sleep Med Rev 2001;5:385–396.

51. Brousseau M, Manzini C, Thie N, Lavigne G. Understanding and managing the interaction between sleep and pain: An update for the dentist. J Can Dent Assoc 2003;69:437–442.

52. Kelman L, Rains JC. Headache and sleep: Examination of sleep patterns and complaints in a large clinical sample of migraineurs. Headache 2005;45:904–910.

53. Nicholson B, Verma S. Comorbidities in chronic neuropathic pain. Pain Med 2004;5(1, suppl):S9–S27.

54. Sabatowski R, Gálvez R, Cherry DA, et al. Pregabalin reduces pain and improves sleep and mood disturbances in patients with post-herpetic neuralgia: Results of a randomised, placebo-controlled clinical trial. Pain 2004;109:26–35.

55. Zelman DC, Brandenburg NA, Gore M. Sleep impairment in patients with painful diabetic peripheral neuropathy. Clin J Pain 2006;22:681–685.

56. Benoliel R, Eliav E, Sharav Y. Self-reports of pain-related awakenings in persistent orofacial pain patients. J Orofac Pain 2009;23:330–338.

57. Sharav Y, Leviner E, Tzukert A, McGrath PA. The spatial distribution, intensity and unpleasantness of acute dental pain. Pain 1984;20:363–370.

58. Moldofsky HK. Disordered sleep in fibromyalgia and related myofascial facial pain conditions. Dent Clin North Am 2001;45:701–713.

59. Rains JC, Poceta JS. Sleep-related headache syndromes. Semin Neurol 2005;25:69–80.

60. Sandrini G, Friberg L, Janig W, et al. Neurophysiological tests and neuroimaging procedures in non-acute headache: Guidelines and recommendations. Eur J Neurol 2004;11:217–224.

61. Lester MS, Liu BP. Imaging in the evaluation of headache. Med Clin North Am 2013;97:243–265.

62. Abrams BM. Factors that cause concern. Med Clin North Am 2013;97:225–242.

63. Frishberg BM, Rosenberg JH, Matchar DB, et al. Evidence-based guidelines in the primary care setting: Neuroimaging in patients with nonacute headache. Am Acad Neurol 2000:3–35.

64. Berrington de González A, Mahesh M, Kim KP, et al. Projected cancer risks from computed tomographic scans performed in the United States in 2007. Arch Intern Med 2009;169:2071–2077.

65. Cassel CK, Guest JA. Choosing wisely: Helping physicians and patients make smart decisions about their care. JAMA 2012;307:1801–1802.

66. Rao VM, Levin DC. The overuse of diagnostic imaging and the Choosing Wisely Initiative. Ann Intern Med 2012;157:574–576.

67. Loder E, Weizenbaum E, Frishberg B, Silberstein S, American Headache Society Choosing Wisely Task Force. Choosing wisely in headache medicine: The American Headache Society's list of five things physicians and patients should question. Headache 2013;53:1651–1659.

68. Macfarlane TV, Kincey J, Worthington HV. The association between psychological factors and oro-facial pain: A community-based study. Eur J Pain 2002;6:427–434.

69. Uhl GR, Sora I, Wang Z. The mu opiate receptor as a candidate gene for pain: Polymorphisms, variations in expression, nociception, and opiate responses. Proc Natl Acad Sci USA 1999;96:7752–7755.

70. Mechlin MB, Maixner W, Light KC, Fisher JM, Girdler SS. African Americans show alterations in endogenous pain regulatory mechanisms and reduced pain tolerance to experimental pain procedures. Psychosom Med 2005;67:948–956.

71. Géranton SM. Targeting epigenetic mechanisms for pain relief. Curr Opin Pharmacol 2012;12:35–41.

72. Denk F, McMahon SB. Chronic pain: Emerging evidence for the involvement of epigenetics. Neuron 2012;73:435–444.

73. Buchheit T, Van de Ven T, Shaw A. Epigenetics and the transition from acute to chronic pain. Pain Med 2012;13:1474–1490.

74. Aloisi AM, Bonifazi M. Sex hormones, central nervous system and pain. Horm Behav 2006;50:1–7.

75. Bartley EJ, Fillingim RB. Sex differences in pain: A brief review of clinical and experimental findings. Br J Anaesth 2013;111:52–58.

76. Rezaii T, Hirschberg AL, Carlström K, Ernberg M. The influence of menstrual phases on pain modulation in healthy women. J Pain 2012;13:646–655.

77. Breslau N, Rasmussen BK. The impact of migraine: Epidemiology, risk factors, and co-morbidities. Neurology 2001;56(1, suppl):S4–S12.

78. Rasmussen BK. Epidemiology of headache. Cephalalgia 1995;15:45–68.

79. Rauhala K, Oikarinen KS, Järvelin MR, Raustia AM. Facial pain and temporomandibular disorders: An epidemiological study of the Northern Finland 1966 Birth Cohort. Cranio 2000;18:40–46.

80. Yunus MB. Gender differences in fibromyalgia and other related syndromes. J Gend Specif Med 2002;5:42–47.

81. Huang GJ, LeResche L, Critchlow CW, Martin MD, Drangsholt MT. Risk factors for diagnostic subgroups of painful temporomandibular disorders (TMD). J Dent Res 2002;81:284–288.

82. Macfarlane TV, Blinkhorn AS, Davies RM, Kincey J, Worthington HV. Factors associated with health care seeking behaviour for orofacial pain in the general population. Community Dent Health 2003;20:20–26.

83. Epker J, Gatchel RJ. Prediction of treatment-seeking behavior in acute TMD patients: Practical application in clinical settings. J Orofac Pain 2000;14:303–309.

84. Dao TT, Knight K, Ton-That V. Modulation of myofascial pain by the reproductive hormones: A preliminary report. J Prosthet Dent 1998;79:663–670.

85. LeResche L, Saunders K, Von Korff MR, Barlow W, Dworkin SF. Use of exogenous hormones and risk of temporomandibular disorder pain. Pain 1997;69:153–160.

86. MacGregor EA. Contraception and headache. Headache 2013;53:247–276.

87. Meriggiola MC, Nanni M, Bachiocco V, Vodo S, Aloisi AM. Menopause affects pain depending on pain type and characteristics. Menopause 2012;19:517–523.

88. Fillingim RB, Ness TJ. Sex-related hormonal influences on pain and analgesic responses. Neurosci Biobehav Rev 2000;24:485–501.

89. Gazerani P, Andersen OK, Arendt-Nielsen L. A human experimental capsaicin model for trigeminal sensitization. Gender-specific differences. Pain 2005;118:155–163.

90. Fillingim RB. Sex differences in analgesic responses: Evidence from experimental pain models. Eur J Anaesthesiol Suppl 2002;26:16–24.

91. Walker JS, Carmody JJ. Experimental pain in healthy human subjects: Gender differences in nociception and in response to ibuprofen. Anesth Analg 1998;86:1257–1262.

92. Averbuch M, Katzper M. A search for sex differences in response to analgesia. Arch Intern Med 2000;160:3424–3428.

93. Averbuch M, Katzper M. Gender and the placebo analgesic effect in acute pain. Clin Pharmacol Ther 2001;70:287–291.

94. Zborowski M. People in Pain. San Francisco: Jossey-Bass, 1969.

95. Green CR, Anderson KO, Baker TA, et al. The unequal burden of pain: Confronting racial and ethnic disparities in pain. Pain Med 2003;4:277–294.

96. Wachholtz AB, Pearce MJ. Does spirituality as a coping mechanism help or hinder coping with chronic pain? Curr Pain Headache Rep 2009;13:127–132.

97. Hobara M. Beliefs about appropriate pain behavior: Cross-cultural and sex differences between Japanese and Euro-Americans. Eur J Pain 2005;9:389–393.

98. Moore R, Brødsgaard I, Mao TK, Miller ML, Dworkin SF. Perceived need for local anesthesia in tooth drilling among Anglo-Americans, Chinese, and Scandinavians. Anesth Prog 1998;45:22–28.

99. Gazerani P, Arendt-Nielsen L. The impact of ethnic differences in response to capsaicin-induced trigeminal sensitization. Pain 2005;117:223–229.

100. Ng B, Dimsdale JE, Rollnik JD, Shapiro H. The effect of ethnicity on prescriptions for patient-controlled analgesia for post-operative pain. Pain 1996;66:9–12.

101. Laguna J, Goldstein R, Braun W, Enguídanos S. Racial and ethnic variation in pain following inpatient palliative care consultations. J Am Geriatr Soc 2014;62:546–552.

102. Burgess DJ, Nelson DB, Gravely AA, et al. Racial differences in prescription of opioid analgesics for chronic non-cancer pain in a national sample of veterans. J Pain 2014;15:447–455.

103. Deepmala D, Franz L, Aponte C, Agrawal M, Jiang W. Identification of provider characteristics influencing prescription of analgesics: A systematic literature review. Pain Pract 2013;13:504–513.

104. Contreras-Huerta LS, Baker KS, Reynolds KJ, Batalha L, Cunnington R. Racial bias in neural empathic responses to pain. PLoS One 2013;8.

Anatomy and Neurophysiology of Orofacial Pain

Michael Tal, DMD, MS
Luis Villanueva, DDS, PhD
Marshall Devor, PhD

2

When it comes to pain, dentists take a bad rap. Going to the dentist universally conjures up fears of painful procedures—the whirring high-speed drill, huge syringes, and blood-curdling extractions. Nothing could be more unfair; dentists are angels of pain relief. A patient who enters a dental clinic with a mind-gouging toothache is almost certain to leave within an hour with the problem resolved and the pain gone. And not only gone, but gone permanently, with very little likelihood of pain recurrence. This happy ending is most unlikely if you visit a rheumatologist with a painful hip or an orthopedist with an aching back. On the other hand, some painful conditions in the trigeminal region are much more difficult to treat than dental caries. Consideration of the anatomy and physiology of craniofacial innervation, compared with innervation at spinal levels, can provide useful insights into what works, what does not work, and why.

Pain in the Orofacial and Cranial Region

All tissues of the body receive sensory innervation, with the sole exception of the brain parenchyma. Although the fundamental patterns of innervation and information processing are similar throughout the body, the orofacial and cranial region has certain peculiarities that motivate a special focus on this region with respect to pain. Most strikingly, the head is functionally unique, mounted as it is on a narrow stalk (the neck), subject to continuous accelerations in all three planes, and containing the vestibule to the digestive system and the lungs, the special sensory organs, and, most important, the brain. The head is also subject to a variety of chronic pain syndromes that do not have obvious parallels in other parts of the body—migraine and trigeminal neuralgia, for example. It is by no means clear why these conditions do not occur in spinal structures. In this chapter, the anatomy and physiology of the pain system that serves the orofacial and cranial region are reviewed, and the features that set this region apart from other somatic tissues are considered.

Nociceptive (Normal), Inflammatory, and Neuropathic Pain

Basic types of pain

Normally, pain is felt when signals originating in thinly myelinated (Aδ) and/or unmyelinated (C) nociceptive afferents reach the conscious brain. The purpose of pain is protective; examples include burning your tongue or biting your lip. The sensation felt (pain) matches the stimulus (noxious). This is nociceptive pain.

Minor tissue injuries, burns, abrasions, and infections often cause ongoing pain and tenderness (hypersensibility). This is inflammatory pain. Current pain nomenclature divides tenderness into two aspects. First, pain in response to a normally painless stimulus is called *allodynia*. In allodynia, the sensation felt in the inflamed tissue (pain) no longer matches the stimulus (non-noxious). Second, excessive pain in response to a stimulus expected to be painful is called *hyperalgesia*.[1] Classically, the allodynia and hyperalgesia caused by everyday injuries have been explained by a putative increase in the responsiveness of nociceptor endings (peripheral sensitization) resulting from chemical inflammatory mediators released in the injured tissue. The resulting sensitized nociceptors respond at a substantially reduced threshold, to lukewarm water, for example, resulting in heat allodynia (ie, pain in response to a normally nonpainful warm stimulus). Some C fibers do not respond to any applied stimulus under normal conditions but begin to respond during inflammation. These are called *silent* or *sleeping nociceptors*.[2]

Peripheral sensitization may well account for thermal allodynia. Evidence is also good that sensitization of normal and silent nociceptors to mechanical forces contributes to pain on movement and bearing weight in joints and other deep tissues where significant mechanical forces are brought to bear. However, it has become increasingly clear that this is not the correct explanation for tactile allodynia in which a light touch to irritated, tender skin and mucous membranes is felt as painful. The reduction in the response threshold of nocicep-

tors to tactile stimuli is much smaller than to heat. Afferent nociceptors in inflamed skin do not generally respond to light brushing of tender skin, even though this brushing is painful.[3,4] Tactile allodynia in the skin has another cause (discussed later).

A third type of pain, neuropathic pain, results from injury or disease of nerves or central nervous system (CNS) structures. This type of pain resembles tissue inflammation in the sense that spontaneous pain and hypersensibility are usually present. However, it differs from inflammatory pain as the injury/disease is in neural tissue. This distinction is not without problems. Pain due to inflammation in a major nerve trunk (neuritis) is generally considered neuropathic.[5] On the other hand, all peripheral tissues are innervated, so minor trauma to skin, muscles, or joints also injures nerve fibers, or at least changes their local chemical milieu. And yet it would be odd to list painful skin abrasions or infections as examples of neuropathic pain. Nomenclature aside, from the point of view of mechanism, there is considerable overlap between neuropathic and inflammatory pain processes. Indeed, at segmental levels, and even more so in the craniofacial area, it is often not known if a particular chronic pain diagnosis is nociceptive, inflammatory, or neuropathic.

Nociceptive pain and inflammatory pain are adaptive design features of the nervous system. They constitute an alarm bell. Temporary hyperresponsiveness to stimuli in inflammatory pain provides a warning and protects against further damage by reducing use of the body part and by suppressing activity in general. Neuropathic pain, in contrast, reflects abnormal (pathophysiologic) functioning of a damaged pain system. This type of pain is maladaptive, the equivalent of a defective alarm system that produces false alarms.

Tactile allodynia and central sensitization

Strong evidence suggests that tenderness to the touch (tactile allodynia) after inflammation and frank nerve injury results from abnormal signal amplification in the CNS rather than from sensitized nociceptors. The process is called *central sensitization*, and it results from a variety of injury-evoked pathophysiologic changes (see following section on neuropathic pain). In the presence of central sensitization, peripheral input entering the CNS along non-nociceptive, thickly myelinated, Aβ touch afferents evokes pain.[6–8] Because mechanical rather than thermal hypersensibility is the most common cause of suffering and disability in patients with chronic pain, pain signaled by Aβ afferents is as important as pain signaled by nociceptors. The concept of Aβ pain constitutes a revolution in the understanding of inflammatory and neuropathic pain.

The paradox of neuropathic pain

Neuropathic pain in the craniofacial area, as elsewhere, is a significant problem for theoretical understanding and clinical management because it is fundamentally paradoxical. Just as cutting a telephone wire leaves the line dead, cutting axons should deaden sensation. Sure enough, complete denervation of a body part does result in numbness, the hallmark negative symptom of neuropathy. Yet nerve trauma and disease are also frequently associated with positive symptoms and signs, some that resemble inflammation and others that are unique. These include (1) spontaneous paresthesias (eg, pins-and-needles sensation), dysesthesias (unpleasant paresthesias), and frank pain; (2) allodynic and hyperalgesic responses to stimuli in the partially denervated regions; (3) pain evoked by deep palpation and by movement of the neck or jaw; and (4) electric shock–like paroxysms and hyperpathia. These pathophysiologic pain states are discussed in the sections that follow.

Sensory and Motor Innervation of Craniofacial Structures

Sensory neurons

Somatovisceral sensation is due to innervation by primary sensory neurons (primary afferents). These neurons reside in the dorsal root ganglia (DRGs) for spinal structures and in the trigeminal ganglia (with a minor contribution of other cranial nerve ganglia) for the head, except for the back of the scalp, which is innervated by sensory cells in the upper cervical DRGs. The bodies of sensory cells have a distinctive pseudounipolar structure unlike any other cell in the nervous system. With rare exceptions (notably MesV, the mesencephalic nucleus of the trigeminal nerve; discussed later), the sensory ganglia are located in a bony cavern between adjacent vertebrae or at the base of the skull and have two axonal processes. One travels from the cell body through a peripheral nerve, usually containing motor and sensory axons, and terminates in one or more sensory endings in innervated tissue. The other runs from the cell body, through the dorsal root or cranial nerve root, and ends in a cluster of synaptic terminals within the CNS. In the trigeminal system, the primary sensory neurons reside in the trigeminal root ganglion (TRG) and terminate as presynaptic terminals on postsynaptic neurons of the brainstem trigeminal complex (Fig 2-1).

Sensory neurons also reside in parasympathetic and enteric ganglia.[10] These ganglia are cell clusters intrinsic to certain tissues, notably the alimentary canal, and can be thought of as evolutionary remnants of a primitive, distributed nervous system. They are capable of carrying out fairly complex functions, such as peristalsis, independent of the brain. A person's conscious sensory experience of the gut and other visceral organs is not due to this autonomic circuitry but rather to pseudounipolar neurons of the DRGs and cranial nerve ganglia. Signals that originate in sensory neurons resident in the parasympathetic or enteric ganglia are unlikely to induce sensory percepts. However, there is tentative evidence that such signals may bypass the spinal cord and reach consciousness via the vagus nerve and brainstem.[11] Parasympathetic ganglia reside in, and serve, some craniofacial structures, but there are no enteric ganglia in the head. The most rostral ones are in the myenteric plexus of the upper esophagus.

Peculiarities of craniofacial sensory innervation

Primary afferent neurons of the trigeminal (and other cranial nerve) ganglia have several anatomical and functional features that distinguish

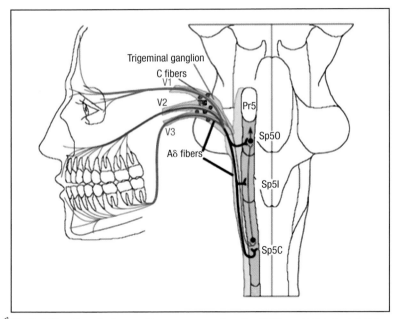

Q # 6

Ⅹ, Ⅶ,
Ⅸ, Ⅹ

Fig 2-1 The trigeminal nerve, its sensory ganglion (the TRG), and trigeminal root terminations within the brainstem trigeminal complex. The territory of distribution of the trigeminal nerve divisions—V1 (ophthalmic), V2 (maxillary), and V3 (mandibular)—are shown on the left. Note that sensory neurons of the facial nerve (VII), glossopharyngeal nerve (IX), and vagus nerve (X) ganglia also innervate craniofacial structures, as do the spinal C1 and C2 DRGs. The divisions of the brainstem trigeminal complex, from caudal to rostral, are Sp5C (nucleus caudalis), SP5I (nucleus interpolaris), SP5O (nucleus oralis), and Pr5 (nucleus principalis). (Drawing modified with permission from Villanueva and Noseda.[9])

See Also p. 46

them from neurons of the spinal DRGs, although the functional significance of these differences is not necessarily obvious. These include fiber types, teeth, trigeminal mesencephalic nucleus, and embryonic origin, which are discussed in the following sections.

Fiber types

The ratio of myelinated (A) to unmyelinated (C) afferent fibers in trigeminal nerve tributaries is higher than in spinal nerves. Cranial nerves have relatively few C fibers.[12,13] Related to this, many of the thermoreceptors that innervate the orofacial area have thinly myelinated Aδ fibers, whereas in other parts of the body most thermoreceptors are C fibers. The tooth pulp chamber is also known to have a high proportion of A-fiber nociceptors compared with the more frequent C-fiber nociceptors at the spinal

level.[14,15] This yields a higher mean conduction velocity for trigeminal versus spinal nociceptive signaling, which is in any event faster because of the shorter propagation distances in the head. The reasons for this emphasis on speed are not clear.

Hoffmann and Matthews[16] reported that peripheral nerves in the head also contain fewer sympathetic efferent axons than somatic peripheral nerves and argued that this may be related to the relative infrequency of sympathetically maintained pain states in the trigeminal region. The hallmark of sympathetically maintained pain is pain relief after sympathetic block or sympatholysis. Interestingly, trigeminal cutaneous and intracerebral blood vessels receive both parasympathetic and sympathetic innervation.[17–19] At segmental levels, parasympathetic innervation of blood vessels is uncommon, if it exists at all.

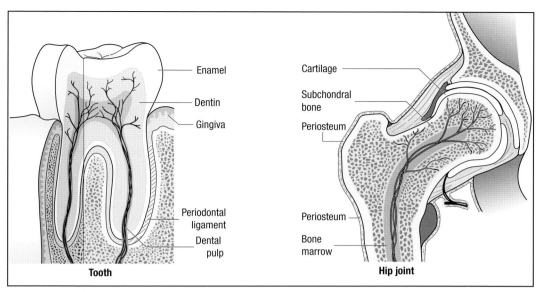

Fig 2-2 The structural analogy between teeth *(left)* and epiphysial bone ends *(right)* may provide useful insights into pain mechanisms in calcified tissues in general. As illustrated in this schematic diagram, tooth enamel is analogous to articular hyaline cartilage (note that neither is innervated), dentin is analogous to subchondral bone, dental pulp is analogous to bone marrow, and the external soft tissues of the tooth (gingiva) are analogous to synovial soft tissue and periosteum of the joint. Important differences are also found between tooth and bone innervation.

Teeth

The teeth are unique structures that have no homologue at spinal levels. A tooth is an open-ended, vital, innervated, calcified box (dentin and cementum) with an internal chamber filled with soft neural tissue (tooth pulp chamber) and coated orally with a relatively nonvital hard tissue that is not innervated (enamel). Teeth have a clear resemblance to the ends of skeletal long bones with the noninnervated (synovial) cartilage being analogous to dental enamel (Fig 2-2).

Trigeminal mesencephalic nucleus

The trigeminal mesencephalic nucleus (MesV), located at the mesopontine junction, is a unique sensory structure that contains cell bodies of primary afferent proprioceptors, Ia afferents that innervate the jaw-closing muscles (masseter, temporalis, and medial pterygoid) and the periodontium. In essence, the MesV is a cranial nerve ganglion displaced into the brain, the only example of this architecture in the CNS. The axons of muscle and periodontal

afferents of MesV neurons travel in the motor rather than the sensory root of the trigeminal nerve. The functional significance of this anomaly is unclear, although there is a hint of special neural processing in the fact that, unlike DRGs and normal cranial nerve ganglia, MesV neurons receive synaptic input. Another hint is that although opposing extensor and flexor muscle blocks are roughly equal in size at spinal levels, in the orofacial motor system there is asymmetry. The jaw-closing muscles, the flexors, are massive and powerful and have rich muscle spindle and Golgi tendon organ innervation. The jaw-opening muscles, the extensors, are small and delicate and lack muscle spindles and Golgi tendon organs.[20]

Embryonic origin

The TRG, the largest of the cranial nerve ganglia, is in essence constructed by fusion of three ganglia associated with the ophthalmic, maxillary, and mandibular branches of the trigeminal complex. All DRG neurons at spinal levels originate in the embryonic neural crest. The TRG, in contrast, contains many neurons of

Mes V - p. 43, Also

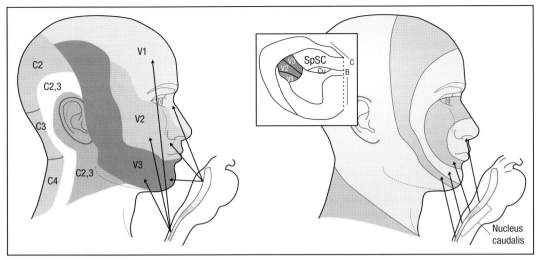

Fig 2-3 Craniofacial input to the brainstem trigeminal complex forms a continuous somatotopic map. Over much of its length, the map follows a segmental pattern with the ophthalmic division (V1) represented laterally (ventral) and the mandibular division (V3) medially (dorsally, *left*, including inset). Within the nucleus caudalis, the map follows an onion-bulb pattern with the nose and lips represented rostrally and the forehead, jaw, and scalp caudally (*right*).

ectodermal (placodal) origin as well as neurons of neural crest origin.[21]

Innervation of the head

Overview

The cranial nerves that support pain sensation are mixed nerves, which means they also contain somatic and autonomic motor axons. This should not matter much as, normally, axons that share a nerve trunk are functionally independent. However, in the event of nerve injury, adjacent axons may interact, and this could contribute to pain pathophysiology. Interactions can be electrical (ephaptic) or chemically mediated. A suspected example of the latter is sympathetically maintained pain (see the section titled "Cellular mechanisms" on page 64).

Somatic and visceral sensory innervation. Somatic and visceral sensory innervation of the orofacial region is provided mainly by the trigeminal nerve (cranial nerve V); partly by the glossopharyngeal nerve (IX), vagus nerve (X), and spinal accessory nerve (XI); and by a very

minor contribution from the facial nerve (VII). The back of the scalp, the angle of the mandible, and parts of the ear and throat are innervated primarily by dorsal roots of the C1 and C2 spinal segments (Fig 2-3). With the exception of MesV, the relevant primary sensory neurons are all located in the corresponding cranial nerve ganglia or DRGs. The special senses (smell, vision, taste, hearing) and the vestibular sense are served by cranial nerves I, II, VII, and VIII. The trigeminal nerve (V) is by far the most important cranial nerve for pain.

Voluntary motor innervation (including somatic and branchial divisions). External ocular muscles are innervated by the oculomotor (III), trochlear (IV), and abducens (VI) nerves. The facial muscles of expression are innervated by the facial nerve (VII). The muscles of mastication are served mostly by the motor branch of the trigeminal nerve (Vm). The muscles that control swallowing and the larynx are served by the glossopharyngeal (IX) and the vagus (X) nerves. The spinal accessory nerve (XI) innervates certain muscles of the neck and shoulder, the hypoglossal nerve (XII) supplies motor innervation to the muscles of the tongue (other than the palatoglossus CN X), and the C1 and C2 ventral roots supply muscles underlying the scalp.

Autonomic innervation. Autonomic innervation is all motor and in the trigeminal region includes both sympathetic and parasympathetic components. Sensory fibers that follow peripheral autonomic pathways, which often carry visceral sensory information, are not part of the autonomic nervous system. The entire sympathetic supply to smooth muscles and glands of the head above the neck, including cranial vasculature, is from motor neurons of the superior cervical sympathetic ganglion. These are driven, in turn, by preganglionic sympathetic neurons of the upper part of the spinal intermediolateral column. The parasympathetic ganglia, including the ciliary, pterygopalatine, submandibular, and otic ganglia, are located within or near the cranial structures that they innervate (juxtamural), and they are driven by preganglionic motor neurons that reside in the brainstem parasympathetic motor nuclei. The axons of the preganglionic motor neurons reach their target juxtamural ganglia via the oculomotor (III), facial (VII), glossopharyngeal (IX), and vagus (X) cranial nerves. The motor neurons of the parasympathetic ganglia in turn have short axons that innervate nearby smooth muscle and glands in the trigeminal distribution, including blood vessels.[17,19]

The trigeminal nerve

The trigeminal nerve (V) is the largest of the cranial nerves, named because it branches into three major peripheral divisions: the ophthalmic (V1), the maxillary (V2), and the mandibular (V3) nerves. These map the face from forehead to jaw (see Figs 2-1 and 2-3). All three divisions contribute sensory fibers to the meninges and the intracranial blood vessels and venous sinuses via a small nerve branch (equivalent to the spinal dorsal ramus) that leaves the nerve just distal to the TRG. The brain parenchyma, including the retina, does not receive any nociceptive innervation.

Except for MesV, the primary sensory neurons of all three divisions reside in the TRG, also termed the *Gasserian* or *semilunar ganglion*. Although merged within a single perineural/dural capsule, the three divisions of this fused ganglion are preserved; cells of V1, V2, and V3 do not intermingle much in the TRG. The topographic layout of the TRG is largely preserved as axons leave the ganglion and pass into the trigeminal root on their way to the brain. This permits a neurosurgeon to target trigeminal pain sources regionally by selectively lesioning parts of the TRG or selectively sectioning fibers in the trigeminal root (see chapter 13). Trigeminal motor fibers originate in pontine trigeminal motor nuclei. They exit the brain as a coherent bundle in the trigeminal root, bypass the TRG, and then follow mandibular nerve (V3) tributaries into the masseter, temporalis, pterygoid, and digastric (anterior belly) muscles and into some small muscles in the soft palate and middle ear.

Ophthalmic division. The ophthalmic division (V1) is the smallest of the three trigeminal nerve tributaries. After entering the orbit through the superior orbital fissure, the ophthalmic nerve splits into the frontal, nasociliary, and lacrimal nerves. These supply the upper eyelid, forehead, and scalp; the sphenoid, ethmoid, and nasal sinus cavities; the orbital contents; and the upper part of the nose (see Fig 2-1).

Maxillary division. The maxillary division (V2) exits the cranium through the foramen rotundum and enters the pterygopalatine fossa. Preganglionic secretomotor fibers that exit the brain in the facial nerve (VII) join V2 en route to the parasympathetic sphenopalatine ganglion (also known as the pterygopalatine ganglion). This large ganglion is an important target for pain control, not so much because of its autonomic role but because of its location. Sphenopalatine ganglion blocks also block the adjacent maxillary nerve trunk, and it is for this reason that they provide at least temporary relief in sphenopalatine neuralgia, certain persistent headaches, herpes zoster pain of the face, and some painful traumatic trigeminal neuropathies.[22,23] The maxillary nerve provides innervation of facial bones and then continues anteriorly, exiting the skull via the infraorbital foramen to enter the orbit through the inferior orbital fissure. At this point it is called the *infraorbital nerve*. This nerve provides postganglionic parasympathetic innervation to the lacrimal

p.183, p.396

① LINGUAL NERVE

and salivary glands and to the mucosal glands of the maxilla (the hard and soft palate, gingiva, maxillary sinuses). The nerve also provides sensory innervation to the teeth of the maxilla and the skin of the middle part of the face, including the lower part of the nose (see Fig 2-1).

Mandibular division. The mandibular division (V3) is the largest of the trigeminal nerves and the only one that carries voluntary motor fibers. This nerve exits the cranium through the foramen ovale and divides into four tributaries in the infratemporal fossa: the auriculotemporal, inferior alveolar, lingual, and buccal nerves. The auriculotemporal nerve provides sensory innervation to the skin of the temporal region, including the ear lobe, and to the temporomandibular joint (TMJ). It also carries postganglionic parasympathetic motor axons from the otic ganglion that serve the parotid gland. The inferior alveolar nerve enters the mandibular canal and supplies the teeth of the mandible. Its mental nerve branch emerges through the mental foramen to supply the skin of the cheek, the mucous membrane of the lower lip, and the vestibular gingiva of the mandibular teeth from the foramen anteriorly to the midline. The lingual nerve innervates the anterior two-thirds of the tongue, the floor of the oral cavity, and the lingual periodontium. The buccal nerve (also called the *long buccal* to distinguish it from the motor buccal branch of VII) innervates the mucous membrane, the vestibular gingiva, and the gingiva posterior to the mental foramen. The chorda tympani nerve, a branch of the facial nerve (VII), joins the lingual nerve in the infratemporal fossa, carrying taste fibers from the anterior two-thirds of the tongue as well as the parasympathetic supply to the submandibular and sublingual salivary glands (see Fig 2-1).

Pain and specific craniofacial structures

Skin

The skin of the face and scalp, including its innervation, is fundamentally the same as the skin in other parts of the body. It is served by a variety of thickly myelinated low-threshold mechanoreceptive afferents (Aβ fibers); thinly myelinated afferents, including Aδ nociceptors; and unmyelinated C fibers, many of which are

nociceptors. Researchers have established that many cutaneous C fibers in the limbs respond to light touch. Such C-tactile afferents also occur in the trigeminal system. A role in pleasant touch (eg, kiss) sensation has been proposed.[24] Among the C nociceptors, a substantial fraction are silent and cannot be activated by any natural stimulus except when they are sensitized by inflammation. Many nonhuman mammals have giant motile facial hairs, that is, vibrissae, with follicles richly innervated by nociceptors and low-threshold Aβ afferents that are sensitive to the direction and dynamics of vibrissal bending. The vibrissae are actively whisked back and forth and, like fingertips, provide the animal with essential detailed touch information.

Nasal and oral cavities

The surface of the nasal and oral cavities, including the cranial air sinuses, is covered with a mucus-secreting epithelial membrane. A special keratinized mucosa covers the dorsal surface of the tongue. This tissue is served by the same families of trigeminal primary afferent neurons that serve the skin, including a rich contribution by C polymodal nociceptors. However, the lack of the tough, poorly penetrable, external corium layer of skin provides mechanical, chemical, and thermal stimuli with much easier access to sensory receptor endings in mucosal tissues. It also permits enhanced access to drugs, such as local anesthetics, and allows a route of delivery of drugs to capillary beds and the circulatory system. The oral cavity is richly invested with receptors for touch and cold sensation, but many areas have little sensitivity to heat. This is why the anterior part of the hard palate is prone to burns; there is only minimal feeling there that food items are too hot.[25] Ongoing pain in conditions such as burning mouth syndrome is very likely due to abnormal activity of intraoral thermal afferents. Inflammation is not obvious in burning mouth syndrome. This has led to the hypothesis that the abnormal neural activity underlying this type of pain may be neuropathic in origin (see chapter 12).

Nasal cavity and smell. The olfactory epithelium on the upper nasal turbinate bones has the same trigeminal innervation as all other nasal and oral mucosas. The intense burning sensa-

p. 46

P. 268

See p. 62!

Afferent vs. Efferent: *A beforE*

Afferent = to the CNS   *Efferent = Away FROM the CNS*

tion that follows sniffing of irritating substances, such as ammonia or spicy horseradish, is thought to be due to the activation of trigeminal C-fiber chemonociceptors, not olfactory receptors. The situation is similar for the sneezing reflex. Trigeminal chemonociception must be distinguished from olfactory chemosensation. The latter is based on an entirely different physiology and functional architecture and a different cranial nerve, the olfactory nerve (I) (and in nonhuman mammals also the vomeronasal nerve). The sensory cell bodies of trigeminal chemonociceptors are located in the TRG. Their axons enter the CNS in the pons and terminate in the brainstem trigeminal complex. Olfactory chemoreceptor neurons do not reside in a ganglion but rather within the nasal olfactory epithelium itself. They are ciliated bipolar neurons with axons that enter the brain along the olfactory nerve (I) to synapse in the olfactory bulbs.

Oral cavity and the tongue, taste, and flavor. The same distinction must be made between chemonociception in the oral cavity and the sense of taste. Taste chemoreceptors are specialized nonneural transduction cells that are present in the taste buds of the tongue and pharynx. The taste receptor cells activate axonal endings of myelinated visceral primary afferents of the chorda tympani nerve, whose cell bodies reside in the geniculate ganglion of the facial nerve (VII). They do not belong to the trigeminal nerve (V) and are not thought to be associated with pain in the oral cavity. An interesting example is the tingling, almost painful sensation in the back of the throat caused by drinking carbonated fizzy drinks. This sensation is due to the response of trigeminal acid-sensing chemonociceptors (V) activated by carbonic acid in the drink, while the flavor of the drink is sensed by taste buds (VII).[26]

Tastants are molecules that activate taste chemoreceptors and give rise to the five basic taste modalities: sweet, sour, salty, bitter, and umami (the taste of monosodium glutamate). Olfactants are the much larger family of molecules that activate olfactory receptor neurons and give rise to a sensation of smell. Olfactants can access the olfactory epithelium via the nostrils and the oral cavity via the pharynx. The flavor of food is due at least as much to olfactory stimulation via these two routes

as it is to taste buds on the tongue. The taste of piquant food items, such as garlic and hot peppers (capsaicin), is due to neither taste nor olfactory receptors but to activation of trigeminal chemonociceptor endings in the tongue, palate, gingiva, and nasal cavity that carry corresponding sensory transduction molecules (eg, TRPA1, TRPV1). Trigeminal innervation is likewise responsible for all other (nonchemical) somatosensory discrimination in the oral cavity, such as heat, cold, and pinprick. Finally, low-threshold mechanoreceptors (LTMs) of the oral mucosa and tongue, together with periodontal and jaw muscle proprioceptors, provide a sense of the texture of food. These various sources of sensory input, taste, olfaction, oral mechanosensation, and proprioception are integrated in the cerebral cortex to provide the final complex sensory experience that people associate with eating a fine meal.

Interestingly, there are occasional reports in which food items, not painful in themselves, are reported to trigger pain. The most common example is migraine, which is said to be sometimes triggered by eating yellow cheese and chocolate or by drinking coffee or red wine. Whether this is due to the taste/smell of these foods or to some chemical absorbed into the circulation is not clear. Headache can also be triggered by drinking orange juice or by eating pineapple, pickled onions, or food items that contain monosodium glutamate, tyramine, or sucrose (see chapter 10). Various gustatory stimuli to the tongue, such as sweet, can induce sweating in the trigeminal nerve distribution. In some patients, taste and smell induce paroxysmal pain attacks resembling trigeminal neuralgia.[27–29] The triggering mechanism is unknown.

Pharynx and larynx. As noted, the lack of the cornified outer layer of skin in the oral mucosa permits easy access of stimulants (mechanical, thermal, and chemical) to mucosal sensory receptor endings and easy access of applied drugs to the underlying vasculature. However, this poses special problems in preventing viral and bacterial infection via the nasal and oral cavities. Protective enzymes are present in the saliva to help manage this problem. Nonetheless, infection, irritation, and consequent painful inflammation in this area are common.

LTM
p 411

To Muscles

The mucosae of the larynx, including the laryngeal surface of the epiglottis, the false and true vocal folds, and the arytenoid region, contain one of the densest concentrations of sensory nerve endings in the human body.[30–32] This provides a sensory basis for coughing, gagging, and other reflexes that protect the lungs. Even brief loss of these functions may lead to life-threatening conditions, such as entry of food into the lungs, and to infections, such as pneumonia. The internal superior and recurrent laryngeal nerves, branches of the vagus nerve (X), supply the sensory innervation to this area.

Cornea and conjunctiva

Like skin and mucosa, the outer surface of the eye, the transparent cornea and the opaque white conjunctiva, has a specialized epithelial outer layer that is innervated by sensitive mechanoreceptor and nociceptor endings. Both low- and high-threshold afferents contribute to the eye-blink reflex. This defensive (protective) reflex is homologous to the flexion reflex at spinal levels; however, it is unique in the body for being triggered not just by noxious stimuli but also by weak stimuli, such as dust particles and air puffs. Tearing, another important protective reflex of the cornea and conjunctiva, is activated mainly by chemical irritation and results in parasympathetic activation of the main and accessory lacrimal glands (see also chapter 11). Mechanical trauma (scratched cornea) and radiant heat injury provoke pain originating in the cornea. Destruction of corneal innervation by radial keratectomy causes pain coupled with reduced response to stimuli in a fraction of patients, probably because of microneuromas. This pain, which sometimes persists, falls into the category of neuropathic pain.[33]

The iris also has nociceptive innervation, although the lens and retina do not. When surgeons lightly touch the iris in the absence of adequate local anesthesia, patients report pain sensation. Reflex hyperconstriction of the iris can evoke pain, which is relieved by mydriatic agents. As lens disruption in cataract surgery and laser tacking of a detached retina are not painful, it is unlikely that pain can originate in the lens or retina.

Muscles

Musculoskeletal pain, after excessive physical exercise, for example, is a common event. Overuse of the masticatory (jaw) and other orofacial muscles is no exception. Some researchers have suggested that the main cause of deep-tissue pain during exercise is reduced blood flow and reduced tissue oxygenation (see chapter 9). This compromises the metabolic status of nociceptive sensory endings and causes depolarization, firing, and pain.[34] An additional potential mechanism is accumulation of various substances in the exercised muscle that excite and/or sensitize muscle nociceptors, increasing responses to muscle contractions that are not normally painful.[35–37] In experimental studies involving intramuscular injection of algesic substances, some of which might be present in exercised muscle, pain is induced. These include low pH (acidic) buffer, hypertonic saline, adenosine triphosphate, glutamate, potassium chloride, capsaicin, bradykinin, serotonin, and l-ascorbic acid. In pathologic conditions characterized by ongoing muscle pain and tenderness, such as masticatory myofascial pain, it is not unlikely that endogenous algesic substances accumulate in abnormally high concentrations, activating muscle nociceptors, and/or that these nociceptors become abnormally sensitized.[35] Building on this idea, it has been postulated that chronic tension-type headache may be caused by abnormal and excessive activity of jaw, head, and neck muscles. However, experimental support for this model is equivocal[38] (see also chapter 8).

Dentition

Extrinsic and intrinsic innervation. Teeth are a source of pain and low-threshold mechanosensation. Like other hard tissues, they have two quite different types of nociceptive innervation (see Fig 2-2). One is extrinsic, the innervation of the periodontium and gingiva at the base of teeth as well as the periosteum of bones. The second is the intrinsic (internal) pain-associated innervation within the tooth pulp and bone marrow. Many pulpal afferents end in fine dentinal tubules in teeth, the equivalent of Haversian canals in porous bone (see also chapter 6). The enamel of teeth, like the epiphyseal cartilage of long bones, is not innervated. The intrinsic innervation of teeth and bones is not known to provide a conscious sensory experience in health. Because of enamel (and cartilage), these nerve endings are isolated from sensory stimuli. Rather, the intrinsic innervation reports on damage, such as a broken tooth or dental caries. When people complain about toothache, the source of the pain may be extrinsic or intrinsic. The associated sensations, however, are subtly different, so they provide clinicians with a hint of the real source. Teeth also have low-threshold touch and proprioceptive input, which originates from the periodontium and associated gingival soft tissues. This contributes to the fine control of mastication (discussed later). Like the fine hand flexor control that is required to pick up an egg without cracking the shell, the forces applied during jaw closure in mastication must be finely controlled to permit effective biting and chewing without breaking teeth.

Algoneurons: Nonclassic pain-related afferents of the tooth pulp. A widely held belief is that pain is the only sensation that can be elicited by stimulation of the intrinsic (pulpal) innervation of teeth.[39,40] However, application of noxious stimuli or peripheral sensitization by inflammatory mediators does not need to occur in order to elicit pain from dentin. Weak stimuli, such as an air puff or a water jet, even when applied to healthy exposed dentin, evoke sharp tooth pain. This paradoxical situation, pain evoked by weak stimuli applied to healthy tissue in healthy people, appears to be unique to teeth. The unusual properties of tooth pulp afferents provide a potential explanation. Within the tooth pulp, sensory axon endings are of a fine diameter and conduct in the Aδ and C fiber range. As they exit the tooth, however, many of these axons have the properties of large-diameter, fast-conducting Aβ fibers.[41] Moreover, retrograde labeling shows that the cell soma of most pulpal afferents within the TRG are of medium and large diameter and express corresponding neurochemical markers (eg, RT97, NF200). Likewise, they are not killed by neonatal capsaicin treatment like most small-diameter TRG neurons.[42] Overall, the structure and response properties of these neurons correspond to low-threshold mecha-

nosensitive afferents, not nociceptors. On the other hand, many (although not all) of these large afferent neurons terminate in the superficial layers of the trigeminal dorsal horn,[43] and many express peptides and neurotrophin receptors normally associated with C-fiber nociceptors. These include calcitonin gene-related peptide (CGRP), substance P, RET (the glial cell line–derived neurotrophic factor receptor), and trkA.[44] Substance P levels are highly increased in inflamed teeth (100-fold) and irreversible pulpitis (1,000-fold) compared with normal conditions.[45] A role for CGRP in inflammatory dental pain is suggested by reduced c-Fos expression in the trigeminal brainstem after treatment with a CGRP-blocking monoclonal antibody.[46] Thus, tooth pulp afferents show some properties of nociceptors and others of LTMs. – P. 39

This observation has led to the hypothesis that the LTM characteristics of tooth pulp afferents allow them to respond to weak stimuli, while their nociceptor connectivity and peptide neurotransmitter release in the trigeminal brainstem cause them to evoke pain. The term *algoneuron* was coined to describe such a neuron. Classically, afferent neurons are classified on the basis of the stimuli they respond to, that is, their receptive field. Thus, the term *nociceptor* derives from the neuron's selective response to noxious stimuli and its ability to encode in the noxious range. True, activity in such neurons typically evokes pain, but this is not a part of the definition of nociceptor. A tooth pulp afferent that responds to weak stimuli but evokes pain sensation is not a nociceptor; it does not respond selectively to noxious stimuli. Formally, it is an LTM. But it clearly is not a normal LTM because activating it evokes pain. The term *algoneuron* shifts the emphasis from the receptive field properties of a neuron to the sensation evoked when the neuron is activated. An algoneuron is a neuron that, when activated, evokes a sensation of pain, irrespective of its receptive field properties.[47] Low-threshold Aβ tooth pulp afferents that signal pain are not nociceptors because they are not activated selectively by noxious stimuli. They are low-threshold algoneurons; their activity evokes pain sensation. The tooth pulp also contains a population of small-diameter afferents that have the characteristics typical of Aδ and C nociceptors. Assuming that selective activation of these neurons also evokes pain, they are high-threshold algoneurons.

The only obvious exception to tooth pulp stimulation evoking pain seems to be the non-painful tingling sensation that is felt during electrical stimulation of the tooth using threshold currents. This is called *pre-pain*.[48,49] Apparently, the tooth pulp also contains some conventional low-threshold Aβ axons that signal nonpainful sensation to the brain. With large numbers of low-threshold pain-provoking algoneurons in the tooth pulp, it is hard to imagine under what natural circumstances such low-threshold touch afferents might be activated selectively. Numerous sympathetic efferents are also present in the tooth pulp. These presumably serve pulpal vasculature.[39,41,50–54]

Stimulus transduction in tooth pulp endings. The sensory endings of intrapulpal afferents have an unusual anatomy. Many end within fine tubules in the dentin. Specifically, about 40% of dentinal tubules contain free nerve endings that extend about 100 μm, and sometimes as far as 200 μm, from the pulp, across the odontoblastic layer, and into the dentin.[55] But this still leaves them about 1 to 3 mm from the dentinoenamel junction. Given the considerable distance of the nerve endings from the outer layer of the dentin, it is not clear how gentle dentinal stimulation activates these endings and causes pain. For chemical stimuli, the gap is presumably crossed by diffusion, and for thermal stimuli, by conduction. For mechanical stimuli, the popular hydrodynamic theory posits that stimuli such as air puff to the dentin cause movement of fluid within the tubules. The fluid pressure then mechanically displaces the membrane of the nerve ending, depolarizing and activating it. Inflammation of dentinal endings may increase their sensitivity to applied stimuli, but it is clear that such sensitization is not required because healthy dentin exposed in dental procedures is sensitive.

The nature of the mechanical transducer molecules in dentinal afferent endings remains unknown. From time to time, some researchers have suggested that the axon ending is not the transducer at all, but rather odontoblasts within dentinal tubules. These would then secondarily drive afferent endings, much as hair cells in the cochlea.[56] Arguing against this idea, there is sparse evidence of synapses or gap junctions between the nerve fiber endings and odontoblasts. Both dental afferent neurons and odontoblasts have been shown to express various transducer channels that could play a role in dental pain. These include TRPV1, TRPV2, TRPA1, TRPM8, and VGLUT in dental primary afferent neurons and TRPV1, TRPV2, TRPV3, TRPV4, and TRPM3 in odontoblasts.[57,58] For a comprehensive discussion of tooth pulp innervation and function, see Byers and Närhim,[55] Chung et al,[59] and Bleicher.[60]

Low-threshold extrinsic innervation. The periodontal apparatus, which serves as an interface between the tooth and its socket in the alveolar bone, supplies the CNS with mechanoreceptor signals about tooth loads for the neural control of jaw movements. When this information is not available (eg, during dental anesthesia), the control of forces that move the jaw is severely impaired. Low-threshold nerve fibers have been described in all four parts of the apparatus: the periodontal ligament, the adjacent gingiva, the cementum, and the alveolar bone. Ruffini-like nerve endings are located among the collagen fibers in the periodontal ligament that anchor the root of the tooth to the jawbone.[61] The ligament also contains endings that appear to be proprioceptive, although no clear encapsulated receptors have been found here.[55,62,63] In the gingiva, neural endings resembling Meissner and Ruffini corpuscles have been described at the papillary and subpapillary lamina, in addition to free nerve endings. These might provide information about tooth displacement.[64–66] Whether the cementum is innervated is uncertain, but nerve endings have been described in alveolar bone in human specimens.[67] Beyond their role in the control of jaw movement, it is possible that low-threshold periodontal afferents play a role in pain. Specifically, in the presence of central sensitization, they could yield Aβ pain. This could account for the frequent sensitivity of healthy tissue (teeth and gingiva) neighboring an inflamed, painful tooth.

Cranial bones

Less is known about the intrinsic innervation of bones than of teeth. For example, aspiration of marrow from skeletal bone shafts and the pelvis is painful, as are intramedullary tumors in skeletal bones. This is in keeping with a sensory role for intrinsic innervation, as in teeth. Pursuing this analogy, the authors have suggested that erosion of epiphysial cartilage in osteoarthritis may result in pain because of the direct application of weight-bearing forces to exposed, innervated, subchondral bone in the same way that mechanical force applied to exposed dentin, healthy or inflamed, is painful[68] (see Fig 2-2). This mechanism might be relevant to pain associated with dysfunction of the TMJ. However, it is probably restricted to articular joints. Anecdotal reports from neurosurgeons indicate that in awake patients undergoing craniotomy, after the fascia and periosteum have been locally anesthetized, drilling through the marrow chamber of flat bones of the calvarium is not noticeably painful. Likewise, tumors within the mandibular bone tend not to be painful unless they breach the bone and press on nearby nerves, periosteum, or other innervated soft tissues. Interestingly, certain chemotherapeutic agents, such as vincristine, are known to cause decalcifying lesions in bones of the jaw while sparing skeletal bone. These observations suggest a fundamental difference in the sensory role of the intrinsic innervation of cranial versus skeletal bones, perhaps because of differences in embryonic origin. P. 35 ◄

Craniocervical joints and mastication

Temporomandibular joint. The TMJ, the articulation of the condylar process of the mandible in the glenoid fossa of the temporal bone, permits opening and closing of the jaw. The articular surfaces of these bones are covered with fibrous (noncellular, nonvascular) cartilage and sealed with a synovial membrane. The capsule is covered externally by periosteum, which extends over the mandible and the temporal bone. Proprioceptors of the TMJ provide sensory input about jaw position and the force being applied by the masticatory muscles. The joint is also innervated by trigeminal nerve nociceptors, as is the periarticular connective tissue.[69–72] The actual articular surfaces have been thought to lack nerve endings.[73] However, the human articular disc, a unique layer of fibrous cartilage within the synovial space that separates the two articular surfaces of the mandible, does contain sensory nerve endings, many of which are probably low-threshold proprioceptors.[74] The relative paucity of low-threshold sensory endings in the TMJ contrasts with their widespread distribution in the associated muscles, tendons, and periodontal ligaments. This has led to the suggestion that the sensory regulation of mastication is due primarily to these surrounding structures, while the nociceptive innervation of the TMJ contributes to limiting excessive force application and the detection of injury.[75,76] Nociceptors in the articular disc might also contribute to pain in disorders of the TMJ[77] (see chapter 9). Despite the fact that the TMJ is not a weight-bearing joint like the knee or hip, the jaw-closing musculature is capable of generating substantial forces that are applied to the joint.[78] Painful disorders of the TMJ exact a considerable toll of suffering and disability (see chapter 9).

Jaw-closing reflex. Stretching of the jaw-closing muscle (masseter) during jaw opening activates Ia muscle spindle afferents in masseter muscles. The result is reflex masseter contraction and jaw closing. This is a classic monosynaptic stretch (myotactic) reflex that is common to many somatic joints. The cell bodies of the muscle spindle afferents are located in MesV, and they connect monosynaptically with the jaw-closing motoneurons in the trigeminal motor nucleus. When the jaw closes and the opposing teeth make contact, proprioceptors of the masseter are suddenly unloaded, and masseter contraction reflexively stops. This prevents fracture of teeth. The jaw-closing reflex also contributes to stabilization of the jaw, preventing it from bouncing during walking and running by maintaining a fixed open-closed jaw position.[79,80] Evidence for a stretch reflex in the jaw-opening muscles is lacking. This is consistent with the observation that the jaw-opening muscles lack muscle spindles or a Golgi apparatus.[81]

Jaw-opening reflex. Jaw opening is a protective reflex that, combined with unloading of the jaw-closing reflex, prevents breakage of tooth cusps by excessive bite force and protects soft oral tissues from being bitten. It is basically like the spinal flexor reflex. Forceful tooth occlusion activates nociceptive fibers (flexor reflex afferents) in the periodontium and in any soft tissue that might be caught between the teeth (gingiva, tongue), triggering reflex contraction of jaw-opening muscles and inhibition of jaw-closing muscles. This occurs rapidly, within about 15 milliseconds. As in limb flexion, it is a bisynaptic protective reflex. But unlike the limbs, it acts bilaterally.

Mastication. Early in the 20th century, Sherrington[82] proposed that reciprocating activities of jaw-opening and jaw-closing reflexes might constitute the basic motor synergy of mastication. In this scheme, food stimuli to the lips or mouth initiate jaw opening. The resulting stretch of the masseter triggers the jaw-closing response. This stretches jaw-opening muscles, once again triggering jaw opening, and so forth. Although this heuristic concept held for years, it has since been replaced in light of more recent neurophysiologic evidence. Problems with the old model included the observation that lesions in the proprioceptors of MesV, which thus eliminate the jaw-closing reflex, do not totally abolish the masticatory rhythm.[83] Likewise, paralysis of the jaw muscles did not eliminate rhythmic masticatory patterns in the brainstem or the motor nerves.[84–86] Masticatory rhythm is now known to be produced by brainstem central pattern generator circuitry, like running, flying, and breathing.[87] The masticatory central pattern generator is located within the rostral medullary reticular formation.[88,89]

Neck joints. Neck pain, though not as common as low back pain, is encountered frequently and is considered one of the most common chronic pain conditions and a major problem in modern society.[90] Nociceptive innervation of various structures in the cervical spine, including facets, intervertebral discs, muscles, and ligaments is capable of causing neck pain, shoulder pain, and headache (see chapter 14). In the presence of cartilage erosion, intrinsic bone innervation might also play a role.[68] The same is true of neuropathy associated with injury to the upper cervical DRGs, spinal roots, and spinal nerves. Because the structural components of and innervation of neck vertebrae are spinal, neck pain is normally managed within the framework of orthopedics, despite the frequent reference of pain to the head.

Intracranial structures (brain, dura, vasculature)

The brain parenchyma is not innervated by sensory axons. For this reason, insertion of intracranial probes and neurosurgical excisions can be carried out in awake patients without pain. However, two intracranial structures do have a sensory innervation: the meninges and the large- and medium-diameter blood vessels. The dura, including the sinuses and tentorium, is innervated primarily by Aδ and C nociceptors, as documented by the presence of histologic markers (eg, substance P and CGRP) and by the electrophysiologic responses of afferent fibers to noxious stimuli. The density of innervation is highest near major dural blood vessels and sinuses. Opening the dura and cauterizing dural blood vessels in an awake patient requires the use of local anesthesia. In the presence of meningeal inflammation, even modest mechanical stimulation of the dura can evoke pain. This is usually described as dull and poorly localized, consistent with the proposal that sensitized dural afferents contribute to headache pain, including migraine.[91,92] Pain is said to be the only sensation evoked by stimulation of the intracranial meninges, regardless of whether the stimulus is electrical, mechanical, thermal, or chemical.[93,94]

The larger intracranial blood vessels, arterial and venous, also have nociceptive Aδ- and C-fiber innervation based on immunolabeling. However, clamping or cauterizing such vessels in awake patients is usually not accompanied by reports of pain. An exception is the rich vascular bed overlying the insular cortex and the temporal operculum. Stimulation of blood vessels and arachnoid in awake patients during open dissection of this region for the removal of tumors is a source of intense pain.[95]

Pain associated with strong stimulation of special sense organs

Unpleasant sensations and frank pain can be evoked by irritating chemical stimulation of the tongue and the olfactory epithelium. Although some of these chemicals can activate taste buds and olfactory receptors, the result is taste and smell sensation. As noted earlier, evoked pain sensations are due to activation of trigem-

MesV — p.35

inal chemonociceptors rather that to impulses generated in taste or smell afferents. However, stimulation of the retina with intense blinding light is usually considered to be unpleasant, if not frankly painful, and intense noise is sometimes described as painful, not just unpleasant on esthetic grounds. Interestingly, these sensations are often enhanced during migraine and other neurovascular headaches (eg, phonophobia and photophobia; see chapters 10 and 11).

Autonomic innervation of trigeminal structures

Sympathetic and parasympathetic efferents

The cranial autonomic nervous system has two components: sympathetic and parasympathetic. The enteric system is not represented in the head. Both autonomic components are purely motor (efferent), although sensory axons of DRG and TRG neurons may run in nerves that are primarily autonomic. The sympathetic and parasympathetic systems differ in a number of ways, including the location of their preganglionic and ganglionic neurons as well as the circuitry that drives their activity.[10] Despite the fact that sympathetic ganglia contain no sensory neurons, sympathetic nerve fibers are nonetheless thought to play an important indirect role in a number of painful conditions. They do this by regulating regional blood flow and temperature and by interacting directly with sensory nerve fibers, particularly in the event of nerve injury (sympathetically maintained pain; see the section titled "Cellular mechanisms" on page 64). Whether parasympathetic efferents also play a role in pain is not known, although this prospect deserves consideration, particularly in light of the evidence for parasympathetic innervation of craniofacial vasculature noted in later sections.

Sympathetic and parasympathetic nerve fibers end on and control smooth muscles and glands. In the orofacial area, autonomic innervation controls salivation, lacrimation, mucosal secretion, vascular smooth muscle tone, intraocular smooth muscles, thermoregulation (vasomotor and pilomotor fibers), and sweating (sudomotor fibers). Evidence also suggests that sympathetic endings affect hard tissue re-

modeling.[96] In structures with parasympathetic innervation, such as the iris, control is through a balance between sympathetic and parasympathetic tone. In other structures, only sympathetic innervation is present. In somatic blood vessels, for example, constriction and dilation are served by different types of sympathetic efferents: vasoconstrictors and vasodilators.[10] In the head, however, the cutaneous vasculature and probably also intracranial blood vessels have extensive parasympathetic innervation, a rarity at spinal levels.[17,19] A role for this innervation in migraine has been proposed.[23] Moreover, these fibers begin to sprout after partial nerve injury, like sympathetic endings. Based on this observation, it has been proposed that parasympathetic activity may contribute to trigeminal neuropathic pain.[19,97]

The sympathetic innervation of the head originates in the most rostral intermediolateral horn cells, located in the upper thoracic and lower cervical segments of the spinal cord. Axons exit the cord via the segmental ventral roots, ascend in connectives of the sympathetic chain, and end synaptically on neurons in the superior cervical sympathetic ganglion. Postganglionic axons of superior cervical sympathetic ganglion neurons ascend into the head as the superior cervical sympathetic nerve trunk and plexus, which parallels the carotid artery. They then distribute to their smooth muscle (eg, vascular) and glandular end targets.

The parasympathetic outflow to the orofacial area originates in parasympathetic brainstem nuclei associated with cranial nerves III, VII, IX, and X, which constitutes the cranial part of the craniosacral parasympathetic outflow. Preganglionic parasympathetic fibers of the oculomotor nerve (III) originate in motor neurons in the midbrain Edinger-Westphal nucleus and end in the ciliary ganglion. The postganglionic axons innervate the iris (papillary sphincter) and ciliary muscles of the eye. Preganglionic parasympathetic fibers of the facial nerve (VII) originate in motor neurons of the upper medullary lacrimal and salivary nuclei and end in ganglia associated with the lacrimal glands, the submandibular and sublingual salivary glands, and the nasal mucous glands. Motor neurons in these ganglia send short postganglionic axons into these glands. Preganglionic parasympathetic fibers of the glossopharyngeal nerve (IX) originate in the inferior salivary nucleus and end in the otic ganglion. The postganglionic axons innervate the parotid salivary gland. Preganglionic parasympathetic fibers of the vagus nerve (X) originate in the medullary dorsal motor nucleus of the vagus nerve. A minority serve structures in the neck, but the large majority leave the head to supply thoracic and abdominal organs.[10] This innervation supports numerous trigeminoparasympathetic reflexes, such as tearing upon irritation of the cornea and mucus secretion in the presence of allergens (see chapter 12).

CNS Processing of Trigeminal Inputs

Orofacial and cranial nociceptive inputs

The brainstem trigeminal complex

Basic organization of the trigeminal brainstem. Orofacial input to the brainstem trigeminal nuclear complex is in some ways analogous to input into the spinal cord from DRGs. This is particularly so caudally, where there is a continuous transition from the cervical spinal dorsal horn to the trigeminal nucleus caudalis. Further rostrally, the spinal trigeminal nucleus (Sp5) shows ever less resemblance to the spinal cord. The continuum of gray matter that receives trigeminal primary afferent input is designated, from caudal to rostral, the nucleus caudalis (Sp5C), nucleus interpolaris (Sp5I), nucleus oralis (Sp5O), and principal (or main) sensory trigeminal nucleus (Pr5). Orofacial Aδ and C primary afferent fibers terminate somatotopically in a pattern that changes somewhat when one moves from rostral to caudal within the complex.[98,99] Rostrally, afferents terminate in a dorsoventral (mediolateral) fashion, with mandibular afferents ending dorsally (medially), maxillary fibers projecting centrally, and ophthalmic fibers innervating the ventralmost (lateralmost) aspect of the complex (see Fig 2-3, left and inset). Moving caudally into the Sp5C, this pattern changes somewhat and begins to resemble an onion-skin arrangement, with inputs from the nose and lips ending rostrally and more posterior craniofacial areas (forehead, jaw, and scalp)

terminating at progressively more caudal levels (see Fig 2-3, right).

The Sp5C is the only portion of the brainstem trigeminal complex that has a laminated structure and a morphologic and functional organization comparable with that of the spinal dorsal horn. For this reason, the caudal extent of the Sp5C is often called the *trigeminal medullary dorsal horn*. The great majority of nociceptive primary afferents terminate in its superficial layers (laminae I and II), although some Aδ fibers terminate in lamina V of the Sp5C. After entering the trigeminal tract at the level of the pons, most nociceptive afferents pass caudally while giving off collaterals that terminate on and activate second-order neurons in the subdivisions of the Sp5 and then the upper cervical spinal cord (see Fig 2-1). Because entry is at the level of the pons, just caudal to Sp5O, the fibers of the trigeminal tract that descend to the Sp5C are much longer than the ones that ascend to the Sp5O.[100,101]

Afferent input. The primary afferents that respond to natural noxious and non-noxious stimuli innervate facial skin, muscles and other external structures, the oral and nasal cavities, and the intracranial tissues. The resulting sensory impulses are carried into the brain almost exclusively along the three branches of the trigeminal nerve: the ophthalmic (V1), maxillary (V2), and mandibular (V3) divisions. Exceptions are much of the scalp and some other caudal parts of the head, which receive their sensory innervation from branches of the upper cervical nerves, as well as the pinna and the auditory meatus, which are innervated by cranial nerves IX and XI. Each trigeminal branch supplies one of the three dermatomes of the face and the underlying deeper tissues. In all mammals, the ophthalmic branch supplies the cornea, neighboring conjunctiva, skin of the dorsum and tip of the nose, intranasal mucosa, upper eyelid, and supraorbital skin. Trigeminal afferents from the ophthalmic branch also supply the supratentorial meninges, whereas the upper cervical nerves innervate the corresponding infratentorial structures. The maxillary branch includes the infraorbital and postorbital skin, upper lip, lateral portion of the nose, intraoral maxillary mucosa, and maxillary teeth. The mandibular branch supplies the TMJ, lower lip skin, intraoral mandibular mucosa, mandibular teeth, and anterior two-thirds of the tongue.

A number of clinical and preclinical findings support the involvement of Sp5 neurons in orofacial and craniofacial nociceptive processing. Neurosurgical transection of the trigeminal descending tract at the rostral pole of the Sp5C produces analgesia and loss of heat sensation on the face without significantly affecting tactile sensation. Painful sensation from the oral cavity, however, is partially preserved after such a neurosurgical lesion, suggesting that intraoral noxious sensations are conveyed also by Sp5 neurons located upstream to Sp5C. Animal studies have confirmed that orofacial tissues have multiple representations in the Sp5C, in the transition zone between Sp5C and Sp5I, and in Sp5O. In addition, neurons of the Sp5C secondarily project rostrally to the ipsilateral Sp5C/Sp5I junction, the Sp5O, and the Pr5 nuclei; therefore, they can carry nociceptive signals to the whole caudal-rostral extent of the brainstem trigeminal complex.[102–106] These intratrigeminal connections are somatotopically organized in both animals[107] and humans.[108] However, their functional significance is not fully understood. One possibility is that they augment the supramedullary effects of the direct noxious inputs to Sp5C and, hence, amplify nociceptive signaling.[109,110]

#1

Neuronal response to afferent input

Numerous electrophysiologic studies have shown that the Sp5C contains neurons activated specifically by nociceptive inputs (nociceptive specific). These are found mainly in laminae I and II. However, this area also contains wide dynamic range (WDR) neurons and neurons that respond specifically to cooling or light touch.[111,112] The restricted cutaneous receptive fields and the somatotopic organization of the nociceptive-specific and WDR neurons of the Sp5C suggest that they are capable of signaling spatial and temporal features of nociceptive information. Many nociceptive-specific and WDR cells with relatively small cutaneous receptive fields are also activated by noxious input originating in deep tissues, thus integrating exteroceptive (cutaneous) and interoceptive (meningeal, muscle, dental pulp) inputs.[102,106,113,114] As in the spinal cord, many such convergent Sp5C WDR cells are found in lamina V and

have a gradient of receptive field sizes and locations, with the lateralmost WDR cells having the smallest receptive fields.[115,116] An additional population of convergent neurons, most with large receptive fields, is found in the subjacent reticular formation.

Studies in anesthetized and awake animals have shown that WDR neurons have a greater ability to encode noxious stimuli and have a wider range of responses than nociceptive-specific neurons.[117,118] WDR neurons receive Aβ-, Aδ-, and C-fiber inputs, and they respond to a large range of mechanical stimuli, from innocuous to strong nociceptive stimuli. They also respond to a variety of other stimuli, including noxious and innocuous thermal and chemical stimuli, and show cutaneous and deep tissue convergence.[104] Although WDR neurons usually have excitatory peripheral fields larger than those of nociceptive-specific cells, their properties are still compatible with a role in stimulus location.

As in the spinal cord, glutamatergic transmission is very important in nociceptive processing in the Sp5C. The local application of glutamate activates nociceptive neurons,[119] and the systemic or local application of antagonists to N-methyl-D-aspartate–type glutamate receptors (NMDA-Rs) in the Sp5C inhibits their activation.[120] Evidence is also strong that the polysynaptic nociceptive signaling of neurons in the rostral trigeminal nuclei, especially Sp5O, conveys extraoral and intraoral inputs that are dependent on glutamatergic inputs from Sp5C.[105,121]

The WDR neurons of the trigeminal Sp5C that convey noxious messages to more rostral CNS structures show a gradient of responsiveness in their excitatory receptive fields. The center responds to both innocuous and noxious stimuli and the periphery responds only to strong stimuli. This receptive field structure, also seen in WDR neurons of the spinal cord, has interesting consequences. Consider a localized innocuous stimulus. This excites only the few neurons with a low-threshold excitatory center at the stimulation site, resulting in localized touch sensation. A noxious stimulus applied at the same location, on the other hand, would excite these neurons (to higher firing rates) and would also excite the much larger number of WDR neurons with a nociresponsive excitatory zone overlapping the stimulus site. The result is a much larger ascending signal and, presumably, a more intense pain sensation. One might argue that weak stimulation over a large area would likewise activate a large number of WDR neurons, evoking pain. Likewise, one might argue that progressively broadening the area of noxious stimulation would increase the intensity of pain without limit. Indeed, spatial summation does occur. However, in addition to their excitatory receptive field, WDR neurons also have a broad surrounding inhibitory receptive field distinct from the excitatory one. Mechanical stimuli applied to this inhibitory field inhibit WDR cell activity, and this limits the degree of excitation—and pain—that can be achieved. The fact that even weak stimulation in areas far outside the excitatory receptive field center of WDR neurons can inhibit their activity contributed to the formulation of the gate control theory of pain. This theory proposed that segmental inhibitions are elicited by activity in large-diameter, Aβ cutaneous afferent fibers and can be activated naturally by innocuous mechanical stimuli[122] (see also Le Bars et al[117]).

p.53, 56

Fiber type–specific input

Q#7

As already noted, most nociceptive afferents terminate in superficial layers of the Sp5C, although some Aδ fibers terminate more deeply. Recent studies have revealed alternative patterns of termination as follows: *(1)* In addition to contacting local interneurons, some Aδ and C peptidergic fibers contact lamina I and outer lamina II neurons that give rise to ascending projections; and *(2)* some nonpeptidergic nociceptive primary afferents terminate in the inner part of lamina II. In contrast, large myelinated Aβ fibers that convey innocuous inputs primarily contact lamina V projection neurons, although they also contact local PKCγ-containing interneurons in inner lamina II.[123] After intense noxious stimulation or nerve injury, fine primary afferents release glutamate and several other peptides and neuromodulators onto lamina I neurons. Normally silent NMDA-Rs become activated by the glutamate released. This leads to a cascade of calcium-dependent and second messenger–dependent signaling that increases the sensitivity of target neurons and the number responding, thus facilitating the transmission of noxious messages to the brain. Under these circumstances, lamina I nociceptive selective neurons could also begin to be activated by Aβ non-nociceptive primary afferents. This might drive tactile allodynia (pain in response to light touch). Similarly, after injury, Aβ fibers could activate PKCγ-expressing interneurons in inner lamina II, which would further enhance the activation of lamina I neurons.[123–125]

Ascending trigeminal pathways

The trigeminal brainstem

The superficial spinal and trigeminal medullary dorsal horn. Lamina I trigeminal neurons, which receive nociceptive-selective signals from the periphery, have ascending axons that terminate in several areas of the brain that are important for processing pain (Figs 2-4 and 2-5). Among the densest projection areas is the lateral parabrachial area (PB), which is a target of more than 50% of the global population of lamina I projection neurons. A second major target is the ventrolateral periaqueductal gray (PAG) matter, which receives nearly 25% of lamina I projections. As a result, many PB and PAG neurons are driven by Aδ and C afferent fibers and respond to thermal and mechanical stimuli in the noxious range. A smaller proportion of these neurons are also responsive to cooling. The nociceptive (lateral) PB area, in turn, projects densely to the central nucleus of the amygdala and the bed nucleus of the stria terminalis, areas thought to be involved in anxiety and fear reactions. PB neurons also project to the hypothalamic ventromedial nucleus, where cellular activation suppresses food intake.[126]

Researchers have suggested that loss of appetite during migraine could be mediated by trigemino-PB circuits, because noxious dural stimulation increases the number of c-Fos positive neurons (a measure of neural activation) in the Sp5C, PB, and hypothalamic ventromedial nucleus. In addition, the activated PB and hypothalamic neurons express the anorectic peptide cholecystokinin.[127] Both effects are expected to reduce appetite. The lateral and ventrolateral columns of the PAG, areas that receive plentiful lamina I projections, contain groups of neurons that, when activated, produce antinociception. In addition, they produce well-defined cardiovascular and defensive reactions, including

CCK

PKC gamma · protein Kinase C - enzyme
[only found in the — serine + threonine-specific
BRAIN + SPINAL cord]

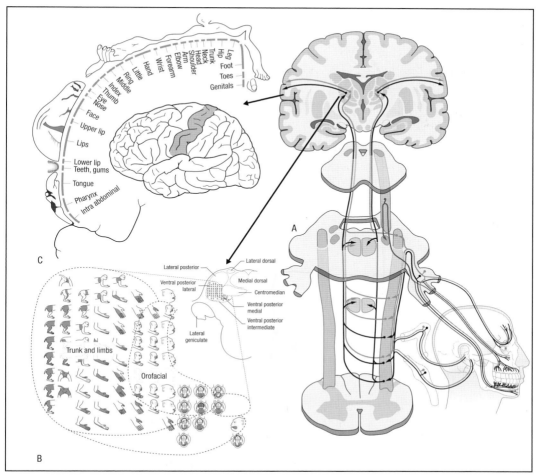

Fig 2-4 The somatotopic mapping of primary sensory input in the brainstem trigeminal complex is reflected in somatotopic representations at higher way stations in the trigeminal pathway. The somatotopic relationship of receptive fields representing craniofacial and spinal-somatic structures in the ventrobasal complex (nuclei VPM and ventral postero-lateral, respectively) is illustrated *(lower left)*. The somatotopic map of craniofacial and spinal-somatic structures in the primary somatosensory cortex (S1) is also shown *(upper left)*.

decreases in blood pressure, hyporeactive immobility, avoidance behavior and vocalization, and a generally emotional state of fear and anxiety.[128] This lamina I-PAG pathway could participate in feedback mechanisms involved in autonomic, aversive, and antinociceptive responses to strong noxious stimulation.

The deep trigeminal medullary dorsal horn. The precise sites of projection of nociceptive neurons in laminae V and VI of the trigeminal complex are still largely unknown because, except for a few anterograde tracer studies,[129,130] most of the available data are based on retrograde tracing. Laminae V and VI neurons project most densely to brainstem reticular areas (see Fig 2-5). As most nociceptive reticular units recorded in older studies showed irregular responses, changes in excitability, and some degree of heterosensory convergence, it was concluded that the reticular formation does not play a specific role in pain processing.

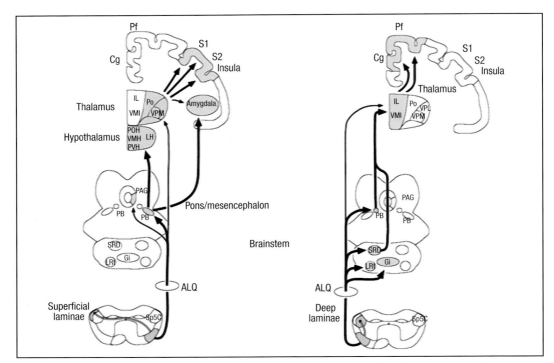

Fig 2-5 The main ascending projections of the brainstem trigeminal complex. *(left)* The lateral ascending system, of which the key forebrain targets are the hypothalamus, contralateral lateral thalamus, amygdala, primary somatosensory cortex (S1), and dorsal operculum (secondary somatosensory cortex [S2] and the insula). *(right)* The medial ascending system, of which the key forebrain targets are the contralateral medial thalamus, the prefrontal cortex (Pf), and the anterior cingulate cortex (Cg). Sp5C, nucleus caudalis; SRD, LRt, and Gi, subdivisions of the brainstem reticular formation; ALQ, anterolateral quadrant; PB, subdivision of the parabrachial nucleus; PAG, periaqueductal gray; POH, VMH, PVH, and LH, subdivisions of the hypothalamus; IL, VMl, Po, and VPM, subdivisions of the thalamus. (Drawing modified with permission from Villanueva and Noseda.[9])

PAG

However, more recently, a key role has been suggested for the medullary reticular formation as a relay for nociceptive signals because most anterolateral quadrant ascending axons, in both animals and humans, terminate within this area (see Villanueva and Nathan[131]). Moreover, numerous other findings indicate that nociceptive inputs are relayed to the thalamus by the caudal medullary reticular formation and not only by the spinothalamic pathway.[116,132] For example, observations in rats revealed neurons within the medullary subnucleus reticularis dorsalis (SRD, also known as RTd) that respond selectively to the activation of peripheral Aδ and C fibers from the whole body surface. They encode the intensity of natural noxious stimuli and

are activated via spinal pathways ascending in the anterolateral quadrant.[133] Neurons with similar properties have also been recorded in the SRD of monkeys.[134]

Forebrain processing

The trigeminal thalamus. The ventral, medial, and posterior aspects of the rat thalamus are innervated by trigeminal lamina I neurons (around 15% of the total population of lamina I–projecting neurons; see Fig 2-5). Thalamic targets of lamina I trigeminal neurons include the posterior complex (Po) and the ventral posteromedial (VPM) nucleus.[129,130] Labeled terminals were also observed in the posterior trian-

SRD definition

gular nucleus, a caudal thalamic nucleus that conveys nociceptive inputs to the secondary somatosensory cortex and tactile and nociceptive inputs to the insular cortex and amygdala. More rostrally, labeled terminals were distributed mainly in the dorsal aspect of the Po and the VPM thalamic nuclei. These two regions convey tactile and nociceptive inputs to the primary and secondary somatosensory cortices and could participate in the sensory-discriminative aspect of pain. Accordingly, recent studies showed that neurons located mainly in the dorsal aspect of the VPM and Po nuclei are activated by electrical, mechanical, and chemical stimulation of the dura[135–137] or chemical stimulation of the tooth pulp in rats.[138] Interestingly, individual trigeminovascular neurons responding to noxious stimulation of meninges and the face have also been recorded outside the VPM/Po thalamic nuclei. These neurons project to multiple cortical areas involved in sensory, motor, associative, and cognitive functions, suggesting that trigeminothalamocortical nociceptive signals are processed in a more widely distributed fashion than previously thought.[137] These data are also in agreement with human functional imaging studies that showed activation of the VPM and dorsal thalamic areas after noxious thermal stimulation of the face[108] and during spontaneous migraine.[135]

In monkeys, the thalamic regions that receive trigeminal inputs include an area within the suprageniculate/Po named the posterior part of the ventromedial nucleus (VMpo), the ventral caudal part of the medial dorsal nucleus/parafascicular (MDvc/Pf), and the VPM nuclei.[139,140] Although lateral, medial, and posterior thalamic areas receive lamina I projections and precisely encode different intensities of noxious stimuli, recordings in anesthetized and awake monkeys have revealed important differences between these areas. A great number of neurons in the MDvc/Pf and ventromedial thalamus are modality specific, showing either nociceptive or thermal responses. The receptive fields of VMpo cells in monkeys are relatively small,[141] whereas those from MDvc/Pf cells are often very large. The receptive field borders and the magnitudes of evoked responses of both cell types change with the monkey's behavioral state.[142–145] This feature makes MDvc/Pf cells well suited to mediate behavioral reactions, hence strongly implicating the region in the affective-emotional aspects of pain. This suggestion is supported by their cortical connectivity and by functional imaging studies. The VMpo cells project to the insular cortex, an area that, when stimulated, may elicit pain in humans[146] and that has been implicated in the affective components of pain on the basis of its projections to various limbic structures, such as the amygdala and perirhinal cortex. However, clinical data have shown that other ventral posterior areas, not necessarily including the VMpo, play a key role in relaying pain-related spinothalamic activity to the cortex.[147] The MDvc/Pf cells project to area 24 of the cingulate cortex, the activity of which appears to be modulated by noxious stimuli. In fact, this is a functionally heterogenous area made up of adjacent zones implicated in attentional, motor, and autonomic reactions. This might allow it to participate in a variety of behavioral reactions.[132]

By contrast, in ventroposterior thalamic areas, most neurons are WDR, have receptive fields that are not modified by the animal's behavioral state, and are smaller than those of spinal or medullary dorsal horn projecting neurons.[142,145] This suggests that ventral posterior areas may subserve spatial discrimination. These regions project to the primary somatosensory cortex. Functional imaging studies have shown that noxious and innocuous stimuli also activate the contralateral primary somatosensory cortex (S1), indicating potential coexistence of pain and tactile representation in this area.[148] Furthermore, single-unit recordings from a caudal ventral region of the thalamus in humans have revealed neurons that could be activated by noxious stimuli. Stimulation of this region induces thermal and/or painful sensations.[149]

Projections from deep laminae are relayed by SRD neurons to the parafascicular and ventromedial thalamus, which, in turn, conveys encoded nociceptive inputs from the entire body surface to layer I of the whole dorsolateral neocortex.[150,151] Ventromedial thalamus neurons cannot be clearly assigned to either the medial or lateral pain system. Their receptive fields have fine discriminative properties as shown by their selective responsiveness to noxious stimuli, their ability to precisely encode

ACC -p.54, Fig2

different kinds of cutaneous stimuli within noxious ranges, and the fact that their activation by innocuous stimuli occurs only under conditions of experimental allodynia. However, they lack topographic discrimination, as illustrated by their whole-body receptive fields and their ability to respond to widespread noxious inputs of cutaneous, muscular, or visceral origins. The ventromedial thalamus, therefore, may constitute an important thalamic nociceptive branch of what was originally termed the *ascending reticular activating system*[152] and, as such, play a role in cortical arousal.

This reticulothalamocortical network could allow painful stimuli anywhere in the body to modify cortical activity in a widespread manner. Because thalamocortical interactions in layer I are assumed to be a key substrate for the synchronization of large ensembles of neurons across extensive cortical territories, they have been associated with changes in states of consciousness. In this respect, layer I inputs may act as a mode switch. By activating a spatially restricted low-threshold zone in the apical dendrites of layer V pyramidal neurons and evoking regenerative potentials that propagate toward the cell soma, these inputs could switch layer V neurons into a burst firing mode.[153] This hypothesis fits with the facts that painful stimuli can elicit widespread cortical activation in humans and that increasing stimulus intensity increases the number of brain regions activated, including the ventral posteromedial thalamic regions and the prefrontal, premotor, and motor cortices.[154,155]

Thalamocortical interactions and pain perception. The findings described earlier show that the labeled-lines concept with regard to pain, that is, the concept that pain is fully accounted for by the thalamic regions that receive direct trigeminothalamic inputs from lamina I neurons, is unlikely to be the complete story. In addition to devoted spinal/trigeminal pathways that carry nociceptive information to the cortex via the thalamus, such information is also relayed to the thalamus and to additional forebrain structures by the caudal brainstem. Indeed, most ascending axons located in the anterolateral quadrant of the spinal white matter that carry ascending pain signals in humans terminate within the medullary reticular formation

and the PB complex.[126,131] The ability to encode noxious inputs is shared by all regions implicated in pain processing: trigeminothalamic and trigeminal brainstem pathways. Moreover, lamina I neurons do not hold a monopoly on the receipt of noxious information from the periphery. Thalamic and extrathalamic areas that do not receive direct trigeminal nociceptive projections from lamina I neurons also participate in pain processing. Although the terms *pain tracts* and *pain system* are common concepts in textbook presentations of the subject, they are an oversimplification. The idea of a specialized chain of neurons from the periphery to the cortex, or of separated unidirectional pathways that convey the information that inevitably produces the sensory experience of pain, paints an inaccurate picture of a much more complex network.

The results of noninvasive functional imaging in humans have shown altered activity in widespread cortical areas after brief noxious stimulation. The areas with the most prominent and reliable responses are the S1, the secondary somatosensory cortex (S2)/insula, the anterior cingulate cortex (ACC), and the dorsolateral prefrontal cortex.[155,156] These cortical regions, as a group, constitute the core of the "pain matrix," the collection of cortical areas whose activity constitutes the cerebral signature of pain perception. This concept, or at least the identity of its specific core constituents, has been contested recently on the grounds that most of the complex functional magnetic resonance imaging response elicited by phasic nociceptive stimuli is common to the processing of virtually all salient sensory stimuli (visual, auditory, etc).[157] They are not specific to pain. Many subcortical regions are also consistently activated by transient painful stimuli and may participate in pain perception. Examples include the cerebellum and the dorsal midbrain.[156]

Perhaps the most compelling reason to be suspicious of the idea that pain perception amounts to activation of the particular areas included in the pain matrix lies in the fact that pain is intrinsically a conscious experience, and cerebral substrates of consciousness are not specifically captured in current imaging studies. Indeed, destruction of individual elements or clusters of elements of the pain matrix does not dull consciousness or pain perception: it frequently induces pain (post-stroke pain). Likewise, direct stimulation of these areas, alone or altogether, does not evoke pain in awake humans and, with rare exceptions,[158] pain is not reported as an aura of epileptic seizures despite the fact that the core pain matrix components are commonly involved in seizure activity. Currently, the only viable candidate for a primary pain cortex is the posterior insula/dorsal operculum, where pain has been reported in response to direct electrical stimulation in a small fraction of persons tested.[158,159] Key aspects of the neural correlates of pain perception continue to evade understanding.

Trigeminal pain is subject to descending control

Gate control: Modulation by peripheral input

The most important contribution of Melzack and Wall's[122] gate control theory of pain was the concept that pain sensation is subject to modulation by innocuous and noxious inputs from the periphery as well as by signals that derive from the brain itself. As originally formulated, low-threshold Aβ input inhibits pain signaling whereas nociceptive input augments it. New information has revised the details, but the principle of modulation has stood the test of time. For example, it is now clear that under some circumstances (central sensitization) Aβ input evokes, rather than inhibits, pain (tactile allodynia). Likewise, beyond simply eliciting pain, the activation of fine-diameter fibers can engage both segmental, heterosegmental, and brainstem pain-inhibitory mechanisms. The latter have functional components beyond the dorsal horn, as originally proposed in the gate control hypothesis. Thus, for example, percutaneous electrical stimuli can elicit both segmental (spinal) and extrasegmental (heterosegmental and supraspinal) postsynaptic inhibitory processes that affect trigeminal WDR neurons. Both effects are triggered exclusively by Aδ-fiber input or by both Aδ-fiber and C-fiber input.[160] Although transcutaneous electrical nerve stimulation (TENS) can be effective when applied at frequencies and intensities that activate mainly Aβ fibers, the resulting pain relief is localized and often limited to the stimulated segment.[161] Stronger and more widespread analgesic effects can be obtained with TENS by using a stimulation intensity that produces an unpleasant, if not quite painful, sensation.[161,162] In summary, a substantial amount of data has implicated the activation of fine-diameter fibers in analgesic procedures based on segmental, percutaneous electrical stimulation. This conclusion is supported by studies showing that the intensity of stimulation is a critical parameter for obtaining greater analgesia using segmental TENS.[163,164]

Descending modulation from the brainstem

Diffuse noxious inhibitory controls. In contrast to segmental controls, heterosegmental controls are elicited mainly by noxious stimuli. Often these inhibitions are mediated by a supraspinal loop with signals that ascend to the brainstem and then descend again to effect inhibition in the spinal cord (Fig 2-6). Such processes are termed *diffuse noxious inhibitory controls* (DNICs) and, more recently in clinical contexts, *conditioned pain modulation* (CPM). Since the pioneering work of Le Bars et al,[165] which demonstrated that DNIC could induce widespread inhibitory controls on rat dorsal horn and medullary trigeminal neurons,[166,167] a number of studies have showed that these controls have common anatomical and functional features in animals and humans. The supraspinal structures responsible for DNIC include the rat SRD in the caudal-dorsal medulla, which contains a homogenous population of neurons that have properties mirroring the functional characteristics of DNIC. They are activated exclusively by noxious stimuli (applied to any region of the body) and precisely encode the intensity of these stimuli.[116,133] Moreover, lesions of the caudal medulla reduce DNIC in both animals[168] and humans.[169] These caudal medullary networks have been proposed to facilitate the extraction of nociceptive information by increasing the signal-to-noise ratio between the pools of dorsal horn neurons that are activated by peripheral noxious drive and adjacent neurons that are simultaneously inhibited. Accordingly, the spatial summation of nociceptive peripheral inputs results in an initial increase in the

ANTERIOR CINGULATE CORTEX (ACC) – p. 52

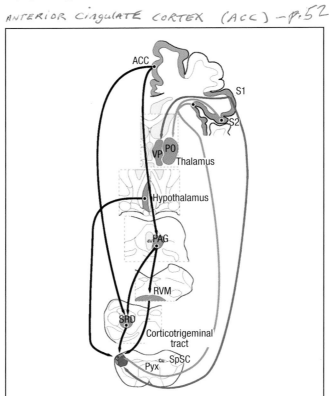

Fig 2-6 The main descending pathways that modulate neural activity in the CNS processing centers of the trigeminal system. Cortical regions (S1, S2, and insular cortex) project ipsilaterally to the thalamic nuclei posterior (Po) and ventralis posterior (VP) and contralaterally to the brainstem trigeminal complex, especially the nucleus caudalis (Sp5C). Modulation of trigeminal nociception from the ACC is relayed by direct projections onto periaqueductal gray (PAG) or by medullary subnucleus reticularis dorsalis (SRD) cells. The hypothalamus and the PAG also project to the Sp5C, the latter via relays in the rostral ventromedial medulla (RVM) and the SRD. (Drawing modified with permission from Villanueva and Noseda.[9])

Anterior cingulate cortex ?

number of neurons activated. But beyond a critical level of surface covered by the stimulus, activation is followed by a decrease in the responses of these neurons.[170] In humans, similar antagonistic processes elicited by interactions of spatial summation and DNIC have been reported.[171] In addition, DNIC is also modulated by the brainstem PAG. This exerts a broader modulatory influence because the PAG also modulates the rostral ventromedial medulla (RVM; see later sections). Thus, noxious inputs can modulate spinal outflow via these brainstem structures bidirectionally, in a widespread fashion.[172]

DNIC-CPM, counterstimulation, and chronic pain. DNIC appears to mediate noxious counterstimulation phenomena ("pain inhibits pain"). In these there is mutual inhibition between (1) pathways that generate sensation and (2) nocifensive responses, in the event that painful stimuli are applied simultaneously at two separate loci. For example, pain due to an injury on the foot is usually suppressed when the hand is immersed in ice-cold water (see Villanueva and Le Bars[173]). Likewise, DNIC reduces spinal[174] and trigeminal reflexes.[175] The DNIC circuitry involves spinobulbospinal loops. In addition, human brain-imaging studies, combined with psychophysics and electrophysiology, have shown an important contribution of cortical regions belonging to the pain matrix in the regulation of pain inhibition by counterstimulation.[176,177] Studies in patients with chronic pain suggest that such higher CNS mechanisms, in addition to the brainstem loops associated with DNIC/CPM, could also be implicated in counterstimulation phenomena. For example, the effects of counterstimulation are altered in patients with neuropathic pain, suggesting that DNIC mechanisms differ in health and disease[178] (see chapter 3).

Light pressure applied to an area of allodynia can inhibit the nocifensive spinal RIII reflex and concomitant painful sensation. In contrast, whereas eliciting a similar level of pain by brushing the allodynic area suppresses the painful sensation, it does not modify the RIII reflex. One can conclude that in the latter situation dynamic mechanoallodynia elicited a counterstimulation effect involving supraspinal but not spinal circuitry. Furthermore, the effects of DNIC on temporally and spatially summated pain are reduced from normal in dysfunctional pain states, such as fibromyalgia and low back pain,[179] and in painful trigeminal conditions, such as temporomandibular disorders and trigeminal neuropathic pain.[180,181] Indeed, these observations suggest that the reduced ability of counterstimulation to inhibit pain in patients with chronic pain could be due in part to dysfunction of the DNIC/CPM system itself.[182–184]

The rostral ventromedial medulla. Early systematic studies of stimulation-produced analgesia in animals showed that localized electrical microstimulation of the ventrolateral PAG and the RVM elicits strong behavioral antinociceptive effects, for example, the inhibition of jaw-opening reflexes elicited by tooth pulp stimulation.[185,186] The PAG projects only minimally to the spinal and trigeminal dorsal horns. However, it projects densely to the RVM, which constitutes a relay for the descending pain modulation observed upon PAG stimulation (see Fig 2-6). The RVM sends dense descending projections to superficial dorsal horn neurons, and these neurons in turn modulate the activity of deep dorsal horn cells at the origin of spinal ascending nociceptive pathways.[187,188] In contrast to the caudal SRD-medullary system

that preferentially modulates deep dorsal horn neurons, RVM cells modulate both deep dorsal horn and lamina I neurons. The RVM is therefore positioned to control the relay of a broad range of nociceptive inputs to supraspinal processing areas and hence to play a particularly broad modulatory role. In this respect, it was proposed that under appropriate environmental circumstances, RVM neurons also integrate sensation with activity from the somatomotor and autonomic systems. In this way, the RVM could contribute not only to the modulation of pain, that is, nocifensive and arousal reactions, but also to homeostatic vasomotor regulation, temperature control, and sexual function, all in a manner appropriate to the behavior.[112,189,190]

Electrophysiologic studies in anesthetized rats have provided a more detailed picture of the role of RVM neurons in the descending control of nociception. The three classes of RVM neurons are (1) off cells, which pause just before withdrawal reflexes; (2) on cells, which show a burst of activity before such reflexes; and (3) neutral cells, which have no reflex-related activity. On and off cells project directly to dorsal horn laminae I, II, and V. Off cells are activated by local infusions of μ-opioid agonists or gamma aminobutyric acid type A receptor (GABA$_A$-R) antagonists, and their activity is correlated with inhibition of nociceptive transmission. In contrast, on cells, whose activity correlates with enhanced nociceptive transmission, are inhibited by local or systemic opioids.[191] Electrophysiologic studies in unanesthetized rats are also illuminating in this regard because they demonstrate powerful state-dependent changes in the activity of RVM neurons. For example, RVM off cells are only intermittently active during waking but become continuously active when animals transition to slow-wave sleep[192] or when they are exposed to barbiturate anesthesia[193] or morphine.[194] On cells show the reciprocal pattern of changes, becoming much less active during slow-wave sleep. Interestingly, compared with the anesthetized and sleeping state, in awake rats both on and off cells are responsive to a variety of innocuous stimuli.

As a whole, the studies described earlier show that several ascending and bulbospinal/trigeminal descending modulatory pain pathways are simultaneously activated when a noxious stimulus occurs. Such networks are

Corticofugal

not somatotopically organized.[188] Rather, they constitute widespread negative and positive spino (trigemino)–bulbospinal feedback loops by which nociceptive signals may attenuate or increase their own magnitudes.

Descending modulation: Inhibition and facilitation. Descending modulation involves facilitation as well as inhibition. Attempts to relate the activity of facilitatory or inhibitory modulatory systems with behavioral analgesia have been hampered by the fact that net effects cannot be attributed exclusively to any single network. Facilitation and inhibition always maintain a dynamic equilibrium. Most of the available data come from studies at spinal levels, but it is likely that processing in the trigeminal complex is similar. Both types of modulatory systems, facilitatory and inhibitory, are triggered by noxious stimuli and are under the direct control of neurons located in the PAG (see Fig 2-6), which projects to both the RVM and the SRD (alternatively named the RTd[195] [medullary dorsal reticular nucleus]). Under certain circumstances, SRD neurons can also facilitate nociceptive responses, as suggested by the reduction of withdrawal reactions in the formalin test after SRD lesions.[196] Accordingly, like PAG-RVM circuits, SRD cells can also exert either inhibitory or excitatory influences on dorsal horn nociceptive processing. Bidirectional control is revealed in experiments on morphine analgesia. Microinjection of morphine into the PAG elicits either activations or inhibitions of dorsal horn nociceptive activities and strongly reduces DNIC.[197] The existence of opioidergic links in the brainstem led to the proposal that noxious stimuli release opioid peptides and, via descending bulbospinal controls relayed in the RVM, elicit endogenous analgesia.[191] An alternative mechanism is DNIC-mediated blockade of the amplification of nociceptive spinal outputs.[117] In fact, it is likely that morphine produces analgesia by interacting with several CNS modulatory systems in addition to its effects on bulbospinal descending controls. Functional imaging studies showed that the CNS structures activated by the endogenous μ-opioid system after sustained pain in humans include widespread areas, such as cingulate, prefrontal, and insular cortices, and subcortical areas, such as the PAG, hypothalamus, amygdala, and ventrolateral thalamus.[198,199] Perhaps the main difficulty in attempting to correlate the activity of bulbospinal modulatory systems with behavioral analgesia is that several descending modulation networks operate in parallel, under the control of CNS regions located upstream, so the net effect cannot be attributed exclusively to activity in any single network.

The ability of PAG and SRD neurons to regulate spinal, and presumably also trigeminal, nociceptive processing bidirectionally probably originates in upstream corticofugal drivers. Both nuclei receive strong, direct influences from numerous cortical regions.[200] Facilitation of spinal nociception from the ACC, for example, is relayed by direct influences onto SRD cells[201] or direct projections from ACC to the PAG[202] (see Fig 2-6). These in turn modify SRD and RVM activities. The possibility of ACC influences on pain processing via the PAG has also been raised by human imaging studies showing that the activity in the ACC covaried with activity in areas close to the PAG during opioid and placebo analgesia.[203,204] In general, the brainstem modulatory networks do not appear to be somatotopically organized.[188] Some other corticospinal modulatory circuitry needs to be invoked to explain topographically specific modulatory phenomena, such as the ability of placebo analgesia to be directed to the right hand and not the left.[205]

The cortex as a widespread source of top-down modulation

The importance of behavioral context and its effects on pain perception, including effects of distraction, hypnosis, catastrophizing, and anticipation/placebo, suggest that powerful endogenous control of nociception originates in the cortex, and not just in afferent input from the periphery.[206–208] This is one of the central messages of the gate control theory of pain. Indeed, most nociceptive relays at lower levels of the CNS are subject to descending corticofugal modulation. This includes downstream networks involved in segmental and heterosegmental modulation, including the RVM and the spinal and trigeminal dorsal horns (see Fig 2-6). In contrast to segmental and brainstem-trigeminal descending controls, corticofugal modulation is not necessarily driven by painful stimulation. For example, the insular cortex is thought to contribute to the processing of paradoxical pain elicited by the concurrent application of innocuous cold and warm stimuli.[209] Likewise, prefrontal, frontal, and primary somatosensory cortical areas may selectively alter the unpleasantness of noxious perception in association with manipulation of attention, expectation, and empathy. The detailed mechanisms underlying modulations from higher cerebral levels remain poorly understood. Modulatory networks that operate entirely within the forebrain are likely at least as important as forebrain control over brainstem modulatory pathways.

Corticofugal modulation of trigeminal nuclear and medullary dorsal horn activities.

Early electrophysiologic studies showed that stimulation of the primary somatosensory cortex inhibits the evoked responses of a proportion of medullary nociceptive neurons in the Sp5C.[210] The specific mediating pathways were not identified. On a functional level, the seminal work of Dubner et al,[118] as noted earlier, has shown that corticofugal controls are likely involved in the modulation of neurons in the trigeminal nucleus caudalis by behaviorally significant stimuli in trained monkeys. This type of task-related modulation may produce a greater neuronal response than that produced by equivalent stimuli in the absence of the relevant behavioral state.[211] In this regard, thermally responsive cells in the Sp5C exhibit an added task-related response to visual or motor cues when those are involved in the behavioral task, but not to similar stimuli that are not relevant to the task.[212] The fact that many of these task-related responses exhibit a preferential association with the visual stimulus or the motor response (hand movement) indicates that the mechanism of the behavioral modulation is mediated by distinct networks involved in sensory anticipation or motor preparation. Interestingly, neither the detection of the visual stimulus nor the movement of the hand was related to the functions normally ascribed to the Sp5C. This indicates that relevant information regarding the environment is disseminated to parts of the nervous system that may be involved directly or indirectly in the animal's ongoing behavior. Thus, neuronal

responsiveness may bear no relationship to the features of stimuli that a sensory nucleus is capable of processing; rather, they appear to be dependent on the behavioral context within which a sensory signal is received. As similar task-related responses have been demonstrated in several cortical areas, the task-related changes in trigeminal neuronal activity could represent a corticofugal reiteration of the task instructions.

Corticofugal modulation of thalamic activity.

Cortical modulation of pain is likely to be highly dependent on reciprocal interactions with thalamic-cortical relays, because there are nearly 10 times as many fibers projecting back from the cortex to the thalamus as there are in the forward direction, from thalamus to cortex.[213] The function of the massive feedback from S1 to the VPM thalamic nucleus in the organization of whisker-barrel and limb tactile receptive fields in the ventral posterolateral has been clearly established. The rat ventrobasal thalamus contains only excitatory neurons that project mainly to layer IV of the S1 cortex. Descending projections in the thalamocortical loop originate primarily in layer VI of the S1 cortex. Distal dendrites of ventrobasal neurons are densely innervated by these projections, which activate ionotropic and metabotropic glutamate receptors. As in the visual and auditory systems, cortical feedback from S1 serves to amplify the effects of sensory stimulation to the classic center-surround receptive fields and helps to sharpen and adjust the profile of thalamic receptive fields[214] (egocentric selection). Krupa et al[215] have shown that inactivation of the S1 cortex results not only in rapid changes in the receptive field properties of VPM cells driven by facial whisker pads but also in a significant reduction in their ability to reorganize their receptive fields after reversible deafferentation of trigeminal primary afferents.

In addition to these electrophysiologic studies, anatomofunctional studies also indicate that the capability to discriminate noxious inputs by S1 cannot be explained exclusively by the projections or the response properties of ventrobasal thalamocortical afferents. Simultaneous thalamic and cortical recording, as well as pharmacologic manipulation of corticothalam-

SSN

ic feedback, has shown that stimulus-driven, modality-specific influences from the S1 cortex are required to discriminate between innocuous and noxious cutaneous inputs. Corticothalamic feedback results in either an enhancement of responses to innocuous cutaneous stimuli or a reduction of noxious-evoked responses. S1 produces such a selective, top-down modulation of thalamic ventrobasal responses to somatosensory inputs by engaging specific, $GABA_A$-R-mediated, corticothalamic modulation.[216] S1 neuronal activity can be related to a specific movement and may be suppressed during that movement by modulatory influences arising in the motor cortex.[217] Speculating that such mechanisms could be involved in pain relief after electrical or repetitive transcranial magnetic stimulation (rTMS) of the motor cortex is tempting. Selective analgesia can be obtained by rTMS of the motor or the dorsolateral prefrontal cortex. Such effects are not topographically distributed and probably occur at supraspinal levels because rTMS does not affect spinal nociceptive processing as assessed with the RIII reflex.[218]

Autonomic, visceral, and neuroendocrine control

P-184

Brainstem. Brainstem, diencephalic, and cortical circuitry provide executive control of the sympathetic and parasympathetic compartments of the autonomic nervous system. Because there are no preganglionic sympathetic motoneurons in the brain (all are in the spinal cord), all sympathetic commands pass along descending spinal tracts to preganglionic spinal cord motoneurons and then back up to effector targets in the head via the sympathetic chain. Most sympathetic and parasympathetic function is organized as spinal and brainstem reflexes that, in turn, are modulated by the forebrain structures noted. Examples of brainstem autonomic reflexes are parasympathetic salivation triggered by the taste of a good meal or the nasal congestion (vasodilation) associated with hay fever. The iris is dually innervated by sympathetic and parasympathetic efferents. Bright light induces pupillary constriction (myosis, parasympathetic); dim light induces pupillary dilation (mydriasis, sympathetic). Both responses are driven via retinal projections to the upper brainstem. Sympathetic and parasympathetic outflow can also be initiated by forebrain regulatory circuits as psychomotor events. For example, sadness on notification of the death of a loved one may initiate parasympathetically driven tearing, and sudden fear from a thunderclap may initiate sympathetically driven vasoconstriction (paling).

Diencephalon. A recent study showed that the paraventricular hypothalamic nucleus (PVN), a key link of neurohormonal and autonomic integration of stress responses (hypothalamic-pituitary-adrenal axis) likely acts as a hub, simultaneously coordinating and regulating trigeminal pain and parasympathetic mechanisms.[219] Descending projections from the PVN are confined to laminae I and II of the trigeminal nucleus caudalis (Sp5C), the ventrolateral PAG matter, and the rostral part of the superior salivatory nucleus (SSN). Caudal SSN neurons regulate the salivatory function of the submandibular and sublingual salivary glands via the submandibular ganglion, whereas the rostral SSN neurons regulate the lacrimal glands, the mucosa of the nose, and the cerebral vasculature via the pterygopalatine ganglion.[220]

During migraine and cluster headache attacks, pterygopalatine ganglion cells may reflexively stimulate lacrimation and mucous secretion in the nasal and oral cavities and induce vasodilation and local release of inflammatory molecules in various intracranial structures. This, in turn, could activate meningeal nociceptors and drive Sp5C neurons, contributing to headache. Cranial autonomic reactions activated by Sp5C neurons are inhibited by drugs effective in treating trigeminal autonomic cephalalgias and migraine.[221] Interestingly, the cluster of PVN neurons that project to Sp5C/SSN cells are densely supplied with corticotropin-releasing hormone.[222] These same neurons also project to sympathetic and parasympathetic preganglionic neurons in the brainstem and spinal cord and are implicated in the autonomic aspect of the stress response.[223] Correspondingly, experimental depression of PVN cells using the $GABA_A$-receptor agonist muscimol inhibits the basal activity of Sp5C neurons and activity evoked by nociceptive input from the meninges.

The hypothesis that hypothalamic-pituitary-adrenal and trigeminovascular activities are

forebrain

iris

processed in parallel by the PVN is further supported by data indicating that $GABA_A$-R–mediated inhibition of the excitatory output of PVN cells onto Sp5C neurons is significantly reduced in a model of acute restraint stress.[219] Interestingly, acute stress reduces the potency of $GABA_A$-R inhibitory synapses impinging on parvocellular PVN neurons by downregulating the transmembrane anion transporter KCC2, which maintains low intracellular chloride concentration, a prerequisite for the generation of chloride-hyperpolarizing $GABA_A$-mediated responses.[224] Loss of inhibition due to changes in the expression of KCC2 could constitute a major maladaptive mechanism by which some primary headaches, and probably other dysfunctional pains as well, may be generated primarily within the hypothalamus.

Cerebral cortex. Behavioral responses associated with endogenous feeling states (interoception), including pain and emotions, are thought to be modulated in a hierarchic manner at multiple forebrain levels. A first level of regulation occurs within the hypothalamus, somatosensory cortices, and insula. A second level involves prefrontal and cingulate cortices.[10,225–228] An interesting speculation holds that cortical processing of autonomic inputs related to homeostatic regulation of energy consumption is organized in an asymmetric fashion. Specifically, energy enrichment is associated with the left hemisphere, whereas energy expenditure is associated with the right hemisphere. This is analogous to the complementary roles played by the parasympathetic and sympathetic efferent systems. Thus, left vagus nerve stimulation primarily activates the left anterior insula, as do cardiorespiratory manipulations, including the Valsalva maneuver, isometric contractions, and dynamic exercise. Gustatory activities subserved by glossopharyngeal and vagal afferents also lateralize to the left insula, consistent with a role in energy acquisition. Conversely, various modalities conveyed by homeostatic afferents associated with sympathetic efferents produce activity in the right insula. Thus, innocuous thermal sensations (warm, cool), hot and cold pain, muscle and visceral pain, sensual touch, and sexual arousal all activate the right anterior insula.[227]

Sensory Dysfunction in Chronic Orofacial Pain States

Overview

Normal (nociceptive) pain and associated nocifensive reflexes, such as tearing, blinking, sneezing, and reflex withdrawal, are designed to minimize tissue damage. In the event of pathology or disease, increased ascending pain signals augment this protection and help to minimize further damage. Baseline pain sensibility also fosters learning of avoidance strategies. However, a variety of chronic craniofacial and orofacial pain states do not appear to have adaptive value, and some are not even clearly related to injury. Specific pain diagnoses of this sort include myofascial pain, primary headache, some trigeminal and other cranial nerve neuralgias, burning mouth syndrome, and painful traumatic trigeminal neuropathy, for example.[229] These and related conditions, which constitute a major burden for patient and therapist alike, are discussed in considerable detail in chapters 7 through 12. Here, some maladaptive pathophysiologic processes of neural plasticity that could be involved in these problematic chronic pain syndromes are considered (see also chapter 12).

Abnormalities of sensation in chronic orofacial diagnoses include two categories of positive phenomena: (1) spontaneous paresthesias, dysesthesias, and pain, and (2) abnormal sensation and pain evoked by natural stimuli. Spontaneous and evoked pain may also include distortions in perceived body image and bizarre sensory abnormalities of sensation in space and time, such as electric shocks and aftersensation. The latter come under the umbrella heading of hyperpathia.

Spontaneous (ongoing) pain

Spontaneous pain is pain present at rest, when no (intentional) stimulus is applied. Accumulating evidence indicates that ongoing sensations, including pain, are related to ongoing neuronal activity generated at one level or another of the somatosensory system. Whether the pain is truly stimulus independent or is actually associated with occult stimuli related to body posture, blood chemistry, tumors, adhesions, autonomic nervous system activity, hormones, or other internal physiologic factors is often unknown. Thus, it is a bad habit to refer to ongoing pain simply as pain.

Stimulus-evoked pain

Activation of nociceptive sensory endings in healthy tissue by noxious stimuli usually evokes pain sensation. In dentin, and perhaps in subchondral bone, pain may be evoked by weak stimulation of "algoneurons" (see previous section on dentition). Exceptionally, pain may be absent despite pain-provoking input from the periphery if central inhibitions are active. Pathophysiologic alterations of this norm include pain in response to normally painless stimuli (allodynia) as well as exaggerated pain from stimuli that are normally only mildly painful (hyperalgesia). Amplified sensation may affect the skin, oral or nasal mucosa, vaculature, or meninges, among other structures. Pain may also be evoked by jaw movement and flexion of the neck or by focal pressure to deep-tissue tender or trigger points in muscle, tendons, and joints. Tissue tenderness has many potential causes, but they all ultimately boil down to the question of neural signals generated by the stimulus. For example, exaggerated sensation may be due to trivial peripheral factors, such as the thickness of the cornified layer of the skin (callous) and other altered viscoelastic or thermal conductive properties of the tissue intervening between the stimulus and the nociceptive nerve endings. Changes in these properties may cause the same stimulus to generate a larger or smaller afferent pain signal. Still, in the periphery, nociceptive sensory endings may be sensitized by inflammation or neuropathology. An example of the latter is the development of local hypersensitivity at a site where a small nerve branch has been pinched as it crossed a fascial plane (microneuroma). Finally, augmented pain sensation may be due to changes in CNS signal processing. In general, when the source of pain is not at the surface, it is inherently difficult to analyze the root cause and even to determine whether the problem is nociceptive, inflammatory, or neuropathic. This uncertainty is common in craniofacial pain syndromes.

Altered sensory quality

The words people with chronic pain use to describe their sensory experience, particularly chronic pain associated with neural damage or disease, can be informative. Some words are generic and common to nociceptive, inflammatory, and neuropathic pain. But some are characteristic of neuropathy in general, or even of particular neuropathic pain syndromes.[230] For example, spontaneous burning pain occurs in postherpetic neuralgia, a neuropathic pain condition, but it also occurs after an acute burn, which is an example of normal nociceptive pain. However, patients with nerve injuries often describe spontaneous and evoked shooting pains and electric shock–like paroxysms, sensations uncommon except in neuropathy. The closest (presumably) nociceptive equivalent occurs when the radial nerve is percussed against bone at the elbow (hitting your funny bone). Another abnormal sensation specific to neuropathy is hyperpathia, a constellation of pain descriptors that do not occur normally or in inflamed tissue. In hyperpathia, for example, a gentle tap on the back of the hand may feel dull, as if felt through a boxing glove. But with repeated tapping, say once or twice a second for 10 to 20 seconds, the sensation winds up, becoming stronger and stronger until it reaches a painful crescendo. Hyperpathic sensations also spread in space; localized touch may trigger a stinging sensation that spreads up the arm.[231–233] Several chronic pain conditions are specific to the craniofacial area and have distinctive sensory characteristics. These include trigeminal neuralgia and migraine.

Distortions in the perception of body image

Modulatory networks might have effects beyond pain amplification and suppression. In principle, under pathologic conditions, corticofugal projections might actually be able to generate activity in networks located downstream, even in the absence of peripheral noxious inputs. That is, they could act as central drivers of spontaneous paradoxical somatic sensations and pain. Injury of a nerve, or nerve block using local anesthetics, reduces or eliminates the ability to evoke sensation by stimuli applied distal to the block. However, in a clinical setting, complete elimination of spontaneous pain is often difficult to achieve. For example, local anesthetic block of the mandibular nerve, as carried out in routine dental practice, eliminates the sensation of stimuli applied to the lip. However, it does not erase the feeling of the existence of the lip; blocks do not leave the impression that there is a hole in the face. Rather, mandibular blocks lead to a sensation of numbness, described by most people as the sensation of a tingling and swollen lip, although a quick look in the mirror is enough to confirm that the lip itself is not in fact swollen. A swollen lip and absence of a lip are two qualitatively different sensations. A dental patient's sensation of a swollen lip is actually phantom limb sensation. Likewise, when all nerves of a limb are blocked, subjects report feeling a (nonpainful) phantom limb[234] rather than absence of the limb. Lesions of the parietal cortex sometimes lead to true erasure of the limb from the patient's perceptual body schema and the patient's denial that the limb belongs to him or her.

Neuropathic pain

Neuropathic pain is chronic pain that results from injury or disease of peripheral nerves (or ganglia) or CNS structures. The former is termed *peripheral neuropathic pain* and the latter *central pain*.

CNS processes

Central neuropathic pain. Central pain is chronic pain associated with CNS injury or disease. Examples are pain in multiple sclerosis and post-stroke pain. Surprisingly little research has been devoted to pain mechanisms in these conditions, especially in the trigeminal region. Likely causes, however, can be intuited from fundamental principles and fall into two large categories: *(1)* intrinsic neuronal hyperexcitability and *(2)* abnormalities in network functioning, with a focus on synaptic connectivity. Pain in multiple sclerosis is likely of the first category. Loss of myelin on CNS fiber tracts permits excess incorporation of voltage-gated Na$^+$ channels into the axon membrane.[235] This sets the stage for abnormal spontaneous impulse

discharge and hypersensitivity to mechanical forces as manifest, for example, in the sign of L'Hermitte (pain on neck flexion[236]). Pain is rarely reported as an aura of epileptic seizures,[237] which suggests that even if cortical neurons developed endogenous hyperexcitability after trauma or disease, it is unlikely that this would cause pain. This is not so, however, for pathologies affecting subcortical structures, including the spinal cord. The second likely cause of central pain is a dysfunction in one or more of the CNS modulatory systems discussed earlier. Inhibitory and facilitatory networks are thought to operate in dynamic equilibrium, and it is easy to imagine this equilibrium being disrupted by CNS injury or disease.

Phantom limb pain in the trigeminal region. The mechanism underlying the sensation of phantom body parts, most notably phantom limb pain (PLP) in amputees, is an enduring puzzle. In the trigeminal region, phantom ear and nose are occasionally reported after amputation. The amputated structure is felt as if it still exists. PLP is felt in an absent limb and needs to be distinguished from pain felt in the residual stump of the amputated limb. This is called *stump pain* and needs to be understood in the context of painful traumatic neuropathy in general (discussed later). Phantom limb sensation, including pain, may occur when sensory input from the limb is eliminated by massive denervation. Complete denervation of the ear or nose, sometimes associated with pain (or itch), may occur in Hansen's disease (leprosy). Often, patients scratch at their numb ear or nose, removing it entirely (self-mutilation). The tissue does not degenerate spontaneously. The unpleasant sensation that provokes the scratching behavior is phantom limb sensation/pain. Many patients with PLP report exacerbating factors, such as emotional upset or cold weather, and indicate that temporary relief may be provided by massage or warming. Distortions in body schema reported by amputees with phantom limbs (eg, telescoping) are not common in the orofacial region. Marbach and Raphael claimed that PLP occurs after tooth extraction,[238] but this pain is better understood in the context of iatrogenic, traumatic neuropathic pain of peripheral nerve origin.

Phantom limb sensation and pain also occur after destruction of several adjacent DRGs or dorsal roots, even when the limb itself has not been amputated. This may occur after brachial plexus avulsion injuries in which the dorsal roots of the limb are physically torn from the spinal cord.[239] Such avulsion injuries do not occur in the head, but complete deafferentation can occur as a complication of overextensive surgical damage to the TRG in the treatment of trigeminal neuralgia. Such deafferentation may lead to an intense, unremitting pain known as *anesthesia dolorosa* (literally, pain in an insensate body structure). The distinction between denervation-induced pain and deafferentation pain is discussed later.

Maladaptive cortical plasticity. A widely held hypothesis is that PLP is attributable to maladaptive cortical plasticity.[240] The key evidence is the observation of a correlation between the extent of PLP felt by individual patients and the amount of amputation-induced distortion observed in the body-surface representation of their limb in S1 cortex. This account has been disputed with evidence that PLP originates primarily in axotomized DRG neurons in amputees.[241] Remapping of cortical topography has also been proposed as the basis for the classic observation that light touch on an amputee's face sometimes evokes referred sensations to a precise area on the phantom hand.[242,243] Presumed silencing of the region of the somatosensory cortex that formerly received inputs from the (amputated) arm induces synapses from neighboring regions (shoulder and face) to become active. These synapses had formerly been subliminal. In this way, stimuli to the face are felt in the (phantom) hand. Somatotopic remapping of this sort is known from animal studies to occur in all mapped structures in the somatosensory system, from the spinal cord and trigeminal complex to the cerebral cortex.[244–246]

Corticofugal changes occurring after amputation can be rapid and idiosyncratic. For example, a facial-map representation may appear in the region of the phantom hand almost immediately after amputation surgery.[247] Psychophysical studies showed that, in healthy subjects, complete local anesthesia of the thumb does not affect the perception of the adjacent finger (or digits on the contralateral side), whereas the perceived size of the unanesthetized lips increased by approximately 50%.[248] Harris[249] proposed that pain in the absence of an organic lesion, and focal hand dystonias in writers, musicians, or keyboard operators, could be due to a mismatch between motor intention, awareness of movement, and visual feedback. This would elicit plastic changes in the sensorimotor cortex leading to inappropriate cortical control of proprioception, a false match between intended and actual movement, and, so Harris speculated, chronic pain. This idea is analogous to the mismatch between vestibular and visual sensations that often results in motion sickness. Putative support for this sensory-sensory mismatch hypothesis includes the fact that watching a virtual phantom limb (a mirror image of the intact hand) move in synchrony with motor commands may relieve PLP, at least transiently.[243,250]

Neuropathic pain: Peripheral nervous system processes

On the face of it, spontaneous pain and amplified evoked sensation after disruption of nerve conduction pathways are paradoxical. Severing a nerve, like severing a telephone line, should eliminate pain, not cause it. The mystery, however, is rooted in the misconception. Nerves are not like copper telephone cables. True, primary afferents convey electrical signals from the periphery to the CNS, but the analogy does not go much beyond that. Axons are not wires but live, protoplasmic extensions of specialized cells. The biology of these cells needs to be taken seriously.[251] New knowledge of how they respond to demyelination and axonopathy and how they interact with adjacent cells and molecules in their peripheral nervous system (PNS) and CNS environment provides a rational account of most peripheral neuropathic pain conditions.

Deafferentation versus denervation. Explanations of persistent pain after loss of normal sensory input, those based on dysfunctional cortical plasticity and those based on sensory-sensory mismatch, stand in contrast to models that posit persistent afferent drive from peripheral tissues. Pain that follows peripheral nerve injury, distal to the sensory ganglion,

p. 3?

Afferent

is often mistakenly called *deafferentation pain*. This is an unfortunate term because it implies a specific pain mechanism residing in the CNS that is related to the loss of afferent input. In fact, as explained later, far from eliminating afferent input, nerve injury may actually augment such input by generating ectopic discharge. The term *deafferentation pain* should be reserved for cases in which there has been nerve root injury central to the ganglion or removal of the ganglion itself. *Peripheral neuropathic pain is the appropriate term for pain due to orofacial peripheral nerve injury.* Incorrect use of the diagnostic term *deafferentation pain* may actually distract from the true pain mechanism and delay effective treatment. Clinicians must realize that pain after neural injury peripheral and central to the trigeminal ganglion is likely to have different causes.

PNS events that precipitate neuropathic pain. Any type of neural damage or disease—physical, chemical, or metabolic—that has the effect of inducing pathology in a peripheral nerve (neuropathy), sensory or autonomic ganglion (ganglionopathy), or cranial nerve root (or dorsal root; radiculopathy) may precipitate peripheral neuropathic pain. Typical precipitating events are trauma (frequently iatrogenic), infection, inflammation, tumors, metabolic abnormalities, malnutrition, ischemia, vascular abnormalities, neurotoxins (including chemotherapeutic agents), radiation, inherited mutations, and autoimmune attack. If damage occurs suddenly, injury discharge may cause acute pain sensation. But, in general, peripheral neuropathic pain results from secondary pathophysiologic changes that develop over time in the PNS and CNS.

The two basic forms of pathologic change are demyelination (or dysmyelination) and various degrees of axonopathy. Disruption of the ability of peripheral axons to conduct nerve impulses causes negative sensory abnormalities, such as hypoesthesia and anesthesia. Understanding positive sensory symptoms and signs such as pain, and why they are common in some diagnoses and not in others, is challenging. A related challenge is understanding the notorious variability in pain from patient to patient, even when the precipitating neuropathy is essentially identical. Environmental

and psychosocial factors play a role. However, there is accumulating evidence for the existence of genetic polymorphisms that affect susceptibility to pain given a fixed neural pathology. Such pain-susceptibility genes must be distinguished from disease-susceptibility genes, mutations that predispose a person to acquiring particular types of nerve pathology that may be painful.[252]

Because the link between pathologic changes in nerve and sensory symptoms is not trivial, interpretation of an objective indicator of neuropathology as necessarily the cause of pain is risky. Significant neuropathic pain may occur without structurally obvious pathology (eg, painful channelopathies), and significant nerve pathology may occur without pain (eg, intervertebral disc herniation or painless phantom limbs). There are also limits on the use of certain diagnostic tools in the orofacial area. For example, electrophysiologic parameters used in the limbs, such as nerve conduction studies, are not available in the orofacial region because of short conduction distances. Histologic methods, such as nerve and skin-punch biopsies, have not been applied much to trigeminal structures and are unlikely to be acceptable in exposed areas of the face. However, these methods can provide useful information in some circumstances (eg, intraoral punch biopsies).

Spontaneous firing and pain in neuropathy. When a peripheral nerve is damaged, the severed or demyelinated axons can no longer pass impulses efficiently from the periphery to the center. This is the cause of negative sensory symptoms, such as numbness, and negative motor symptoms, such as weakness (eg, Bell's palsy). However, severed or demyelinated axons may also undergo changes in their functional properties (their phenotype) that cause positive symptoms. The most important of these is the emergence of electrical hyperexcitability and the consequent generation of abnormal impulse discharge at ectopic locations in the neuron.[251,253–255] For the most part, nerve injury does not cause the death of sensory cell bodies in the TRG or loss of afferent connections in the trigeminal brainstem. The ectopically generated impulses are therefore able to pass from the periphery into the CNS, where they evoke paresthesias, dysesthesias, and pain. Abnormal discharge generated in nearby uninjured neurons may augment this pain. In addition, both sources of abnormal discharge may trigger central sensitization. This amplifies the sensory effects of both the abnormal spontaneous discharge and the signals evoked in residual surviving afferents by natural tactile stimulation.[7,256]

One would expect that the quality of sensation evoked by spontaneous (and evoked) ectopic discharge should be related to the type of afferent involved. Sensibility to heat and cold stimuli, for example, is normally due to the activation of specific thermosensitive C-fiber and Aδ afferents. Correspondingly, spontaneous burning pain, a common symptom in patients with peripheral neuropathy (eg, burning mouth syndrome or postherpetic neuralgia; see chapter 11), is likely due to activity in peripheral thermal nociceptors and/or CNS pathways normally involved in heat sensation. A key difference between normal sensation and burning neuropathic pain is that, in neuropathy, sensory pathways that convey heat sensation can become active at normal body temperature.

Hyperpathia. Mechanisms of hyperpathic sensory peculiarities and their underlying causes have attracted relatively little attention, particularly as they manifest in the trigeminal region. Pathophysiologic behavior of injured sensory neurons, however, coupled with central sensitization, echo and are probably responsible for the bizarre symptoms of hyperpathia.[251] For example, repeated stimulation may result in an incremental buildup of discharge in axotomized DRG and, hence, in postsynaptic spinal neurons, recalling the windup of sensation in hyperpathia. Researchers have also demonstrated that injured sensory neurons communicate with one another through ephaptic (electrical) coupling and through a novel nonsynaptic, paracrine, neurotransmitter-mediated mechanism called axonal and DRG *cross-excitation*.[257] Neuron-to-neuron crosstalk of this sort could account for windup and for the hyperpathic spread of sensation from the site of stimulation. This form of crosstalk is also thought to underly paroxysmal pains in trigeminal neuralgia (the ignition hypothesis[258]; see chapter 11).

Cellular mechanisms

Cellular substrates of ectopic neural discharge. The cascade of events that leads to spontaneous ectopic discharge and spontaneous pain in severed (and perhaps also in demyelinated) afferents begins with blockade of the normal flow of neurotrophic signaling molecules between the periphery and the sensory cell body. This triggers a change in the quantity of various proteins synthesized (expressed) by the cell body and exported to the peripheral and central axon endings.[259] Some proteins start to be expressed in excess (upregulation of gene expression), while the synthesis of others is reduced (downregulation). Upregulation of Na^+ channel types, combined with downregulation of K^+ channel types, is probably the immediate cause of hyperexcitability.[235,251,260] Disrupted delivery (trafficking) of transported molecules, notably the accumulation of Na^+ channels at sites of axonal injury, including zones of demyelination, also contributes to hyperexcitability.[235,261,262] The biophysical process whereby changes in the density of specific ion channels lead to membrane resonance, repetitive firing capability, and ectopic discharge is rapidly coming into focus.[251,263]

Evoked pain in neuropathy. Gentle percussion over sites of nerve injury, areas of entrapment, tumor infiltration, and neuromas typically evokes an intense stabbing or electric shock–like sensation. This pain, called the *Tinel sign*, is thought to be due to the development of ectopic neuropathic mechanosensitivity at these sites. In the event of injuries that leave a nerve in continuity, a second Tinel sign may be evoked further distally, at the farthest position reached by regenerating axon sprouts. Pain may also occur on tapping along the trajectory of an injured nerve (eg, in diabetic polyneuropathy). This activates freely outgrowing sprouts or sprouts that have become trapped along the course of the nerve. Pain evoked by jaw opening sometimes has this paroxysmal neuropathic quality, suggesting that traction on a mandibular nerve branch might activate local ectopic mechanosensitive trigger sites. A tooth may be tender to percussion for years after root canal therapy despite the absence of radiologic or clinical evidence of periapical pathology (see chapter 12). Pain in this situation may be due to the transmission of force to the underlying nerve with consequent generation of ectopic impulses originating in the partly injured nerve trunk. In these cases, destruction of the tooth pulp or tooth extraction has probably left a small neuroma-in-continuity in the nerve at the base of the tooth.

Ectopic mechanosensitivity is also a feature of spinal roots locally demyelinated by stenosis in the spinal canal, entrapped in the constricted space of root foraminae (eg, in the neck), or damaged by continuous percussion by an arterial loop. The latter is thought to underlie pain in trigeminal neuralgia (see later sections and chapter 11). Interestingly, momentary mechanical probing of ectopic pacemaker sites frequently evokes discharge that long outlasts the stimulus itself. Such afterdischarge is the likely explanation of aftersensations, trigger points, and triggered pain paroxysms that may be evoked by pressure applied at nerve loci that have been injured.[233,251]

Exacerbating factors. Spontaneous and pressure-evoked pain may be exacerbated by a variety of additional factors that tend to depolarize and excite sensory axons and neuronal somata that have become hyperexcitable due to injury or disease. Notable among these are ectopic responses to circulating catecholamines and noradrenaline released from nearby postganglionic sympathetic axons. Sympathetic-sensory coupling may account for painful flare-ups at times of emotional upset. Injured sympathetic axon ends sprout and proliferate in the skin and other peripheral tissue as well as at nerve injury sites and neuromas. In addition, intact sympathetic endings associated with blood vessels may sprout within sensory ganglia and engulf neuronal cell bodies, causing excitation and pain.[97,264,265] However, there is some uncertainty as to whether sympathetic sprouting occurs as readily in the cranial TRG as it does in sensory ganglia at spinal levels.[266–268] Sympathetic-sensory coupling may be an important substrate for sympathetically maintained chronic pain states.[269] Afferent response to local and circulating inflammatory mediators is a second example of ectopic chemosensitivity. Proinflammatory cytokines, such as interleukin-1β, interleukin-6, and tumor

necrosis factor α, are candidate mediators of the generalized aching feeling associated with many disease states.[270] They are also generated locally, in inflamed tissue, neuromas, sensory ganglia, and the spinal cord, particularly in the event of neuropathy. Cytokines released from activated glial cells are thought to further enhance the hyperexcitability of axotomized afferent neurons. This process blurs the distinction between neuropathy and inflammation.

Abnormal discharge may also arise from temperature changes, ischemia, hypoxia, hypoglycemia, and most any additional condition capable of locally depolarizing afferent neurons at sites at which they have developed local resonance and ectopic pacemaker capability.[251] Although sensory endings of specialized nociceptive neurons may be sensitive to this chemical and physical stimulation, it is important to recall that the intact nervous system, nerve trunks, and sensory ganglia do not normally respond to it. The key change in neuropathic pain is not the appearance of excitatory physical and chemical stimuli at ectopic pacemaker sites but rather the emergence of abnormal sensitivity to such stimuli.

Central sensitization

Allodynia and Aβ pain. Pain in response to light touch of the skin—tactile allodynia—is a common symptom in craniofacial neuropathy. The simplest explanation is reduced response threshold in nociceptive afferents, that is, the classic excitable nociceptor hypothesis. However, as noted earlier, there is precious little evidence that fibers that were originally nociceptors ever come to respond to the very weak tactile stimuli that typically evoke allodynia in neuropathy or even in inflamed tissues.[44,256,271] Rather, tactile allodynia appears to be a sensory response to impulse activity in low-threshold mechanosensitive Aβ afferents. This touch signal is abnormally amplified in the CNS by one or more CNS changes triggered by nerve injury and collectively called *central sensitization*. Aβ afferents normally signal touch and vibration sense, but in the event of neuropathy (and inflammation), they can evoke Aβ pain.[6,8,272] A proposed example is tenderness of the scalp during migraine. Aβ afferents activated by touching skin or brushing hair are amplified centrally and rendered painful.[273] The discovery that tactile allodynia is primarily or exclusively signaled by low-threshold mechanoreceptive afferents overturns the classic dogma that pain is due exclusively to activity in Aδ and C nociceptors.

Neuropathic Aβ pain is relatively easy to recognize when it occurs in the skin; light touch is painful. However, it is likely that low-threshold afferent innervation of deep structures can also induce Aβ pain. If so, pain evoked by deep palpation or jaw movements may be due to activity of Aβ afferents in the presence of central sensitization, rather than to peripherally sensitized deep nociceptors as is generally presumed. Proprioceptive input could possibly contribute in this way to muscle ache. One must assume that central sensitization also causes ectopic spontaneous activity in Aβ fibers to be felt as painful, and likewise for Aβ fiber activity evoked at ectopic sites by mechanical and other applied stimuli. Central sensitization also amplifies afferent input of nociceptors, rendering painful stimuli more painful than normal (hyperalgesia).

The relation of PNS injury to central sensitization. The term *central sensitization* deserves special comment. Although postulated as far back as the 1950s,[274] the phenomenon was first described experimentally in rats in which nociceptors were activated by tissue injury or electrical stimulation.[272] This caused transiently enhanced response of dorsal horn neurons to touch stimuli as well as tactile allodynia in awake animals. Some authors limit use of the term *central sensitization* to functional changes that are dependent on nociceptive afferent activity and reverse rapidly when the impulse activity is blocked.[7,8,275] The best documented mechanism of this sort involves the recruitment of NMDA-Rs on postsynaptic dorsal horn pain-signaling neurons.[276] These neurons normally receive effective glutamatergic nociceptive input but also receive low-threshold input that is relatively ineffective because it is delivered to NMDA-Rs, which are inactive at normal resting potential because of Mg^{2+} block of their central ion pore. Depolarization due to afferent nociceptor activity displaces this Mg^{2+} block and enables enhanced NMDA-R response to glutamate released from the Aβ touch afferents (hence, Aβ pain). In this way, the effectiveness of the low-threshold input is enhanced. Initially, ineffective synaptic input from touch afferents drives the central pain-signaling neurons at higher rates, resulting in pain sensation from light touch stimuli, that is, tactile allodynia.

Beyond the recruitment of blocked NMDA-Rs, many other potential central sensitizing mechanisms have been revealed in recent years.[251] This has led to a broader definition of *central sensitization* that encompasses all of the central changes that tend to increase spinal gain (amplification) whether or not they are labile and whether or not they are closely linked to impulse traffic in afferent nociceptors. Such changes include altered expression and release of neuromodulatory peptides from primary afferent terminals (eg, downregulation of the inhibitory neuropeptide galanin); spinal disinhibition by selective loss of inhibitory interneurons containing GABA, glycine, taurine, and/or endogenous opiates; altered gene expression and consequent hyperexcitability of intrinsic spinal neurons; denervation supersensitivity; release by activated microglia and astrocytes of proinflammatory compounds; upregulation of postsynaptic transcription factors and other transmembrane signaling molecules (eg, pERK, CREB); suppression of brainstem descending inhibition; and augmentation of brainstem descending facilitation.

All of these changes can apparently be triggered by nerve injury (and some by peripheral inflammation), although in most instances little is known about the relation of the injury to the central change. The three fundamental possibilities are *(1)* tonic depolarization due to sustained background impulse traffic per se, *(2)* the action of neuroactive substances released within the spinal cord by impulse traffic, and *(3)* trophic interactions between primary afferents and postsynaptic neurons in the dorsal horn that may or may not be directly related to impulse traffic.[277] Interestingly, there is evidence that in the presence of chronic inflammation or neuropathy, Aβ afferents begin to synthesize and release the very peptides (eg, substance P and CGRP) that are normally present only in nociceptors and are thought to trigger central sensitization when released in the CNS.[278–282] Through this mechanism, Aβ afferents may acquire the ability not only to signal pain but also to trigger and maintain central sensitization.

Pain Mechanisms and Craniofacial Pain Diagnoses

This chapter has considered the variety of physiologic and pathophysiologic mechanisms that underlie pain in the craniofacial area. In some conditions, precipitating factors, signs, symptoms, and response to treatment are strongly suggestive of a particular pain mechanism. In others, causes of pain may be ambiguous or multiple. As a prelude to the comprehensive discussion of specific pain diagnoses presented in the rest of the book, this chapter closes by considering how some of these diagnoses are related to the pain mechanisms discussed earlier.

Nociceptive (normal) pain

The hallmark of nociceptive pain is a response that is appropriate in terms of intensity and quality to the stimulus applied. Pain in response to an acute trauma or burn, pinprick, sniffing of a strong irritant chemical, accidental biting of the lip, or a grain of sand on the cornea are all examples of nociceptive pain. Note that, if repeated, pain from such acute noxious stimuli might well be considered chronic, but it would remain nociceptive. Only if such repeated stimuli begin to cause tissue injury, with associated pathophysiologic changes, would the process change from nociceptive to inflammatory. Spontaneous pain in the absence of a defined stimulus and pain in response to a non-noxious stimulus are not normal. They indicate an inflammatory or a neuropathic process.

Inflammatory pain

Inflammation is a near-universal response to tissue injury or disease, and it is usually signaled by the clinical quadruple response of heat, reddening, swelling, and pain (calor, rubor, tumor, and dolor) and the expression of a variety of cellular mediators and markers. However, inflammation is not always accompanied by pain, and its presence with pain does not necessarily exclude the possibility that the accompanying pain is actually due to a neuropathic process or even to normal nociception. Simple inflammatory pain due to peripheral sensitization of nociceptors is the likely mechanism when there is excessive pain on strong pressure and abnormal sensitivity to heat or cold (hyperalgesia). Examples include painful cutaneous or mucosal ulcerations or periapical disease. Spontaneous burning pain may be present, indicating that heat-sensitized nociceptors are firing at normal body temperature. When there is tenderness to light touch or other weak mechanical stimuli (eg, swallowing in the presence of a sore throat or tonsillitis), a different mechanism is likely. Specifically, such tenderness is likely due to central sensitization of LTM input. That is, it is likely to be Aβ pain.   'P 39'

Interestingly, some conditions show a clear inflammatory response without spontaneous pain or even noticeable tenderness. This may occur with an intact epithelium/mucosa (eg, in candidiasis and nonerosive lichen planus; see chapter 6), but it may also occur in the presence of open ulcers. Examples of the latter are facial leishmaniasis, a parasitic infection common in the underdeveloped world; chronic periodontal disease; and some chronic periapical radiolucencies. It is not clear why ulceration from leishmaniasis infection is basically painless while ulceration from herpes zoster infection, for example, is typically intensely painful. Research on inflammation with respect to pain has typically stressed the large variety of mediator substances present (inflammatory soup). Little attention has been given to the possibility that different lesions may be characterized by different mediators, of which only some induce sensitization and pain.

Even if an inflammatory lesion does not generate pain-provoking mediators, it may nonetheless cause intense pain if present in an enclosed space. Pressure buildup within the tooth pulp chamber in pulpitis or periapical abscess may be enough to activate normal nociceptive endings, even if they have not been mechanosensitized by inflammatory mediators. Release of the pressure in these conditions causes instant pain relief even though the mediator substances are still present. This is an example of normal (nociceptive) pain caused secondarily by inflammation. Painful osteomyelitis due to infection in the mandibular bone marrow may have a similar source, as may tumors within the medullary bone canal, such as in multiple myeloma. Elevated intracranial pressure can cause headache, likely by activating mechanonociceptors in the meninges, particularly the dura, and perhaps blood vessels. This effect is no doubt exacerbated when the nociceptive endings are sensitized by inflammatory mediators, as in meningitis. A leading hypothesis holds that ongoing activity of meningeal endings sensitized by an as-yet unknown mechanism, perhaps associated with abnormal cortical activity, is the primary pain source in migraine headache. This activity also triggers and maintains central sensitization, amplifying the pain and rendering Aβ input from intracranial and extracranial sources (eg, skin and hair afferents in migraine[273]; see chapter 10).

Neuropathic pain

Trigeminal neuralgia (tic douloureux) and other cranial nerve neuralgias are the most recognizable neuropathic pains of the head. Nothing quite like trigeminal neuralgia, with its intense, recurring, lightning pains, occurs at axial levels. The widely held belief is that trigeminal neuralgia results from a demyelinating lesion in the trigeminal root or, less frequently, in the descending trigeminal tract, where the demyelination is thought to be due to microvascular compression, tumor, or multiple sclerosis (see chapter 11). The distinctive characteristics of this condition can be explained in terms of known pathophysiologic properties of injured sensory axons.[258] Why these symptoms rarely take such dramatic form at spinal levels is not clear. Likewise, it is not clear why pain develops in only a tiny fraction of people who have the underlying neural pathology.[283] A genetic predisposition is suspected.

Trigeminal neuropathic pain, where the lesion is within the TRG or distal to it, must be distinguished from trigeminal neuralgia in which the lesion is proximal to the TRG. For example, herpes zoster and consequent postherpetic neuralgia is a neuropathic pain condition that affects the trigeminal area much more frequently than trigeminal neuralgia. Well known also at spinal levels, pain in this condition is likely due to ectopic hyperexcitability of virus-infected TRG (and DRG) neurons. Interestingly, another common source of neuropathic pain in the limbs and trunk—diabetic neuropathy—has only minimal effects in the head. This is prob-ably because metabolically compromised sensory neurons of the TRG are nonetheless able to support their distal axon ends given the short length of the axons and the rich blood supply typical of the head and neck. These factors also appear to protect cranial innervation from a variety of inherited dying-back neuropathies. Like segmental nerves, cranial nerves are subject to neuropathy due to focal injury. Trauma to trigeminal nerve tributaries, for example, due to mandibular fracture, nerve compression, and iatrogenic causes, frequently generates neuropathic pain, as do tumors and local infections. Previously classified as atypical facial pain, such cases are better termed *painful trigeminal neuropathy*, which is akin to neuropathic pain elsewhere in the body.

A major mystery is why destruction of dental nerves by tooth extraction and root canal treatment so rarely causes pain due to neuroma formation. Perhaps these neurons are less likely than others to develop ectopic excitability.[267,284] Another possible explanation is enhanced retrograde degeneration of the cell body due to the proximity of the lesion to the ganglion. If many of the TRG neurons that innervate the pulp chamber of a particular tooth die back, then they will not be present to generate ectopic firing and to cause neuroma pain. Loss of these neurons, however, would result in only minor brainstem deafferentation and would therefore not be expected to trigger true deafferentation pain.

When inflammation affects sensory endings in innervated tissue, causing pain, the pain is inflammatory. However, inflammation sometimes occurs along the course of a nerve trunk, in the presence of infection or in the early stages of malignancy. Resulting injury (eg, demyelination) may induce ectopic firing in the injured axons, and the resulting neuropathic pain may be exacerbated by local inflammatory mediators.[5,285,286] Neuropathic changes secondary to trauma, compression, and in-continuity inflammation, for example, may be important causes of painful trigeminal neuropathy, referred pain, and altered sensation in rhinosinusitis.[287] Finally, as noted, nerve injury may also cause the release of inflammatory mediators from activated glia in the DRG and CNS, and injury or disease of the CNS itself may trigger central neuropathic pain.

The understanding of pain remains limited to the generation of nerve impulses, their transmission centrally, and their activation of neuronal networks in the brain. A satisfactory answer to the hard problem—how neural activity gives rise to subjective experience and conscious perception—remains as far off as it ever was. Pain management is typically empiric. Clinicians learn diagnoses and treatments that may be effective, but the ability to go beyond the routine, to solve problems that are atypical, can be greatly facilitated by an understanding of the underlying pain process. The key question to ask is "Where are the neural impulses coming from that are causing this patient's pain?"

Acknowledgments

We thank Kaj Fried, Rami Burstein, Jimmy Hu, Margaret Byers, and the volume editors for helpful comments on the manuscript. Our research on trigeminal pain mechanisms is supported, among other sources, by the Hebrew University Center for Research on Pain (MT and MD), the Israel Science Foundation (MD), and INSERM Université Paris Descartes, Institut UPSA de la Douleur, and Association Gliaxone (LV).

References

1. Mersky H, Bogduk N (eds). Classification of Chronic Pain: Descriptions of Chronic Pain Syndromes and Definitions of PainTerms. Seattle: IASP, 1994.
2. Schmidt R, Schmelz M, Forster C, Ringkamp M, Torebjörk E, Handwerker H. Novel classes of responsive and unresponsive C nociceptors in human skin. J Neurosci 1995;15:333–341.
3. Schmelz M, Schmidt R, Ringkamp M, Forster C, Handwerker HO, Torebjörk HE. Limitation of sensitization to injured parts of receptive fields in human skin C-nociceptors. Exp Brain Res 1996;109:141–147.
4. Banik RK, Brennan TJ. Spontaneous discharge and increased heat sensitivity of rat C-fiber nociceptors are present in vitro after plantar incision. Pain 2004;112:204–213.
5. Eliav E, Herzberg U, Ruda MA, Bennett GJ. Neuropathic pain from an experimental neuritis of the rat sciatic nerve. Pain 1999;83:169–182.
6. Campbell JN, Raja SN, Meyer RA, Mackinnon SE. Myelinated afferents signal the hyperalgesia associated with nerve injury. Pain 1988;32:89–94.
7. Gracely RH, Lynch SA, Bennett GJ. Painful neuropathy: Altered central processing maintained dynamically by peripheral input. Pain 1992;51:175–194.
8. Torebjörk HE, Lundberg LE, LaMotte RH. Central changes in processing of mechanoreceptive input in capsaicin-induced secondary hyperalgesia in humans. J Physiol 1992;448:765–780.
9. Villanueva L, Noseda R. Trigeminal mechanisms of nociception. In: McMahon SL, Koltzenburg M, Tracey I, Turk DC (eds). Wall and Melzack's Textbook of Pain, ed 6. Philadelphia: Elsevier-Saunders, 2013:793–802.
10. Janig W. Integrative Action of the Autonomic Nervous System: Neurobiology of Homeostasis. Cambridge: Cambridge University, 2006.
11. Komisaruk BR, Whipple B, Crawford A, Liu WC, Kalnin A, Mosier K. Brain activation during vaginocervical self-stimulation and orgasm in women with complete spinal cord injury: FMRI evidence of mediation by the vagus nerves. Brain Res 2004;1024:77–88.
12. Darian-Smith I. Neural mechanisms of facial sensation. Int Rev Neurobiol 1966;9:301–395.
13. Young RF, King RB. Fiber spectrum of the trigeminal sensory root of the baboon determined by electron microscopy. J Neurosurg 1973;38:65–72.
14. Jyväsjärvi E, Kniffki KD. Afferent C fibers innervation of cat tooth pulp: Confirmation by electrophysiological methods. J Physiol 1989;411:663–675.
15. Mengel MK, Jyväsjärvi E, Kniffki KD. Evidence for slowly conducting afferent fibres innervating both tooth pulp and periodontal ligament in the cat. Pain 1996;65:181–188.
16. Hoffmann KD, Matthews MA. Comparison of sympathetic neurons in orofacial and upper extremity nerves: Implications for causalgia. J Oral Maxillofac Surg 1990;48:720–726.
17. Kaji A, Maeda T, Watanabe S. Parasympathetic innervation of cutaneous blood vessels examined by retrograde tracing in the rat lower lip. J Auton Nerv Syst 1991;32:153–158.
18. Uddman R, Tajti J, Möller S, Sundler F, Edvinsson L. Neuronal messengers and peptide receptors in the human sphenopalatine and otic ganglia. Brain Res 1999;826:193–199.
19. Ramien M, Ruocco I, Cuello AC, St Louis M, Ribeiro-da-Silva A. Parasympathetic nerve fibers invade the upper dermis following sensory denervation of the rat lower lip skin. J Comp Neurol 2004;469:83–95.
20. Lennartsson B. Number and distribution of muscle spindles in the masticatory muscles of the rat. J Anat 1980;130:279–288.
21. Le Douarin NM, Kalcheim C. The Neural Crest. Cambridge: Cambridge University, 1999.
22. Klein RN, Burk DT, Chase PF. Anatomically and physiologically based guidelines for use of the sphenopalatine ganglion block versus the stellate ganglion block to reduce atypical facial pain. Cranio 2001;19:48–55.
23. Yarnitsky D, Goor-Aryeh I, Bajwa ZH, et al. 2003 Wolff Award: Possible parasympathetic contributions to peripheral and central sensitization during migraine. Headache 2003;43:704–714.
24. Olausson H, Lamarre Y, Backlund H, et al. Unmyelinated tactile afferents signal touch and project to insular cortex. Nat Neurosci 2002;5:900–904.

25. Junge D. Oral Sensorimotor Function. St. Louis: Medico Dental Media International, 1998.

26. Simons C, Dessirier JM, Carstens M, O'Mahony M, Carstens E. The tingling sensation of carbonated drinks is mediated by a carbonic anhydrase-dependent excitation of trigeminal nociceptive neurons. In: Devor M, Rowbotham MC, Wiesenfeld-Hallin Z (eds). Progress in Pain Research and Management Series, vol 16 [Proceedings of the 9th World Congress on Pain, 22–27 Aug 1999, Vienna, Austria]. Seattle: IASP, 2000:225–232.

27. Sharav Y, Benoliel R, Schnarch A, Greenberg L. Idiopathic trigeminal pain associated with gustatory stimuli. Pain 1991;44:171–174.

28. Helcer M, Schnarch A, Benoliel R, Sharav Y. Trigeminal neuralgic-type pain and vascular-type headache due to gustatory stimulus. Headache 1998;38:129–131.

29. Goldstein DS, Pechnik S, Moak J, Eldadah B. Painful sweating. Neurology 2004;63:1471–1475.

30. Villaverde R, Pastor LM, Calvo A, Ferrán A, Sprekelsen C. Nerve endings in the epithelium and submucosa of human epiglottis. Acta Otolaryngol 1994;114:453–457.

31. Mu L, Sanders I. Sensory nerve supply of the human oro- and laryngopharynx: A preliminary study. Anat Rec 2000;258:406–420.

32. Yoshida Y, Tanaka Y, Hirano M, Nakashima T. Sensory innervation of the pharynx and larynx. Am J Med 2000;108(4, suppl):51S–61S.

33. Belmonte C, Tervo TT. Pain in and around the eye. In: McMahon SL, Koltzenburg M (eds). Wall and Melzack's Textbook of Pain, ed 5. London: Churchill Livingstone, 2006:887–901.

34. Martens MA, Moeyersoons JP. Acute and recurrent effort-related compartment syndrome in sports. Sports Med 1990;9:62–68.

35. Graven-Nielsen T, Mense S. The peripheral apparatus of muscle pain: Evidence from animal and human studies. Clin J Pain 2001;17:2–10.

36. Graven-Nielsen T, Jansson Y, Segerdahl M, et al. Experimental pain by ischaemic contractions compared with pain by intramuscular infusions of adenosine and hypertonic saline. Eur J Pain 2003;7:93–102.

37. Hoheisel U, Reinöhl J, Unger T, Mense S. Acidic pH and capsaicin activate mechanosensitive group IV muscle receptors in the rat. Pain 2004;110:149–157.

38. Stohler CS, Zhang X, Lund JP. The effect of experimental jaw muscle pain on postural muscle activity. Pain 1996;66:215–221.

39. Byers MR. Dental sensory receptors. Int Rev Neurobiol 1984;25:39–94.

40. Brännström M. Etiology of dentin hypersensitivity. Proc Finn Dent Soc 1992;88(1, suppl):7–13.

41. Cadden SW, Lisney SJ, Matthews B. Thresholds to electrical stimulation of nerves in cat canine tooth-pulp with A beta-, A delta- and C-fibre conduction velocities. Brain Res 1983;261:31–41.

42. Fried K, Aldskogius H, Hildebrand C. Proportion of unmyelinated axons in rat molar and incisor tooth pulps following neonatal capsaicin treatment and/or sympathectomy. Brain Res 1988;463:118–123.

43. Marfurt CF, Turner DF. The central projections of tooth pulp afferent neurons in the rat as determined by the transganglionic transport of horseradish peroxidase. J Comp Neurol 1984;223:535–547.

44. Fehrenbacher JC, Sun XX, Locke EE, Henry MA, Hargreaves KM. Capsaicin-evoked iCGRP release from human dental pulp: A model system for the study of peripheral neuropeptide secretion in normal healthy tissue. Pain 2009;144:253–261.

45. Sacerdote P, Levrini L. Peripheral mechanisms of dental pain: The role of substance P. Mediators Inflamm 2012;2012.

46. Bowler KE, Worsley MA, Broad L, et al. Evidence for anti-inflammatory and putative analgesic effects of a monoclonal antibody to calcitonin gene-related peptide. Neuroscience 2013;228:271–282.

47. Fried K, Sessle BJ, Devor M. The paradox of pain from tooth pulp: Low-threshold "algoneurons"? Pain 2011;152:2685–2689.

48. McGrath PA, Gracely RH, Dubner R, Heft MW. Non-pain and pain sensations evoked by tooth pulp stimulation. Pain 1983;15:377–388.

49. Virtanen AS, Huopaniemi T, Närhi MV, Pertovaara A, Wallgren K. The effect of temporal parameters on subjective sensations evoked by electrical tooth stimulation. Pain 1987;30:361–371.

50. Matthews B. Nerve impulses recorded from dentine in the cat. Arch Oral Biol 1970;15:523–530.

51. Dong WK, Chudler EH, Martin RF. Physiological properties of intradental mechanoreceptors. Brain Res 1985;334:389–395.

52. Holland GR, Matthews B, Robinson PP. An electrophysiological and morphological study of the innervation and reinnervation of cat dentine. J Physiol 1987;386:31–43.

53. Jyväsjärvi E, Kniffki KD, Mengel MK. Functional characteristics of afferent C fibres from tooth pulp and periodontal ligament. Prog Brain Res 1988;74:237–245.

54. Dong WK, Shiwaku T, Kawakami Y, Chudler EH. Static and dynamic responses of periodontal ligament mechanoreceptors and intradental mechanoreceptors. J Neurophysiol 1993;69:1567–1582.

55. Byers MR, Närhi MV. Dental injury models: Experimental tools for understanding neuroinflammatory interactions and polymodal nociceptor functions. Crit Rev Oral Biol Med 1999;10:4–39.

56. Magloire H, Couble ML, Thivichon-Prince B, Maurin JC, Bleicher F. Odontoblast: A mechano-sensory cell. J Exp Zool Part B Mol Dev Evol 2009;312:416–424.

57. Paik SK, Kim SK, Choi SJ, Yang ES, Ahn SH, Bae YC. Vesicular glutamate transporters in axons that innervate the human dental pulp. J Endod 2012;38:470–474.

58. Chung G, Oh S. TRP Channels in Dental Pain. Open Pain J 2013;6(suppl M5):31–36.

59. Chung G, Jung SJ, Oh SB. Cellular and molecular mechanisms of dental nociception. J Dent Res 2013;92:948–955.

60. Bleicher F. Odontoblast physiology. Exp Cell Res 2014;325(2):65–71.

61. Byers MR. Sensory innervation of periodontal ligament of rat molars consists of unencapsulated Ruffini-like mechanoreceptors and free nerve endings. J Comp Neurol 1985;231:500–518.
62. Biemesderfer D, Munger BL, Binck J, Dubner R. The pilo-Ruffini complex: A non-sinus hair and associated slowly-adapting mechanoreceptor in primate facial skin. Brain Res 1978;142:197–222.
63. Byers MR, Dong WK. Comparison of trigeminal receptor location and structure in the periodontal ligament of different types of teeth from the rat, cat, and monkey. J Comp Neurol 1989;279:117–127.
64. Johnsen SE, Trulsson M. Receptive field properties of human periodontal afferents responding to loading of premolar and molar teeth. J Neurophysiol 2003;89:1478–1487.
65. Johnsen SE, Trulsson M. Encoding of amplitude and rate of tooth loads by human periodontal afferents from premolar and molar teeth. J Neurophysiol 2005;93:1889–1897.
66. Macefield VG. Physiological characteristics of low-threshold mechanoreceptors in joints, muscle and skin in human subjects. Clin Exp Pharmacol Physiol 2005;32:135–144.
67. Abarca M, Van Steenberghe D, Malevez C, Jacobs R. The neurophysiology of osseointegrated oral implants. A clinically underestimated aspect. J Oral Rehabil 2006;33:161–169.
68. Niv D, Gofeld M, Devor M. Causes of pain in degenerative bone and joint disease: A lesson from vertebroplasty. Pain 2003;105:387–392.
69. Hutchins B, Spears R, Hinton RJ, Harper RP. Calcitonin gene-related peptide and substance P immunoreactivity in rat trigeminal ganglia and brainstem following adjuvant-induced inflammation of the temporomandibular joint. Arch Oral Biol 2000;45:335–345.
70. Kyrkanides S, Tallents RH, Macher DJ, Olschowka JA, Stevens SY. Temporomandibular joint nociception: Effects of capsaicin on substance P-like immunoreactivity in the rabbit brain stem. J Orofac Pain 2002;16:229–236.
71. Ichikawa H, Fukunaga T, Jin HW, Fujita M, Takano-Yamamoto T, Sugimoto T. VR1-, VRL-1- and P2X3 receptor-immunoreactive innervation of the rat temporomandibular joint. Brain Res 2004;1008:131–136.
72. Oliveira MC, Parada CA, Veiga MC, Rodrigues LR, Barros SP, Tambeli CH. Evidence for the involvement of endogenous ATP and P2X receptors in TMJ pain. Eur J Pain 2005;9:87–93.
73. Davidson JA, Metzinger SE, Tufaro AP, Dellon AL. Clinical implications of the innervation of the temporomandibular joint. J Craniofac Surg 2003;14:235–239.
74. Asaki S, Sekikawa M, Kim YT. Sensory innervation of temporomandibular joint disk. J Orthop Surg (Hong Kong) 2006;14:3–8.
75. Capra NF. Localization and central projections of primary afferent neurons that innervate the temporomandibular joint in cats. Somatosens Res 1987;4:201–213.
76. Andoh S, Uemura-Sumi M, Kawagishi S, Yoshino K, Matsuoka H, Amano N. An HRP study of primary afferent and postganglionic sympathetic neurons which innervate the temporomandibular joint in the cat. Japanese J Oral Biol 1988;30:772–785.
77. Broton JG, Hu JW, Sessle BJ. Effects of temporomandibular joint stimulation on nociceptive and nonnociceptive neurons of the cat's trigeminal subnucleus caudalis (medullary dorsal horn). J Neurophysiol 1988;59:1575–1589.
78. Tanaka E, Yamano E, Dalla-Bona DA, et al. Dynamic compressive properties of the mandibular condylar cartilage. J Dent Res 2006;85:571–575.
79. Lund JP, Drew T, Rossignol S. A study of jaw reflexes of the awake cat during mastication and locomotion. Brain Behav Evol 1984;25:146–156.
80. Miles TS, Flavel SC, Nordstrom MA. Control of human mandibular posture during locomotion. J Physiol 2004;554:216–226.
81. Abbink JH, van der Bilt A, Bosman F, van der Glas HW. A comparison of jaw-opener and jaw-closer muscle activity in humans to overcome an external force counteracting jaw movement. Exp Brain Res 1998;118:269–278.
82. Sherrington CS. The Integrative Action of the Nervous System. New Haven: Yale University, 1906.
83. Goodwin GM, Luschei ES. Effects of destroying spindle afferents from jaw muscles on mastication in monkeys. J Neurophysiol 1974;37:967–981.
84. Dellow PG, Lund JP. Evidence for central timing of rhythmical mastication. J Physiol 1971;215:1–13.
85. Goldberg LJ, Tal M. Intracellular recording in trigeminal motoneurons of the anesthetized guinea pig during rhythmic jaw movements. Exp Neurol 1978;58:102–110.
86. Goldberg LJ, Chandler SH. Evidence for pattern generator control of the effects of spindle afferent input during rhythmical jaw movements. Can J Physiol Pharmacol 1981;59:707–712.
87. Camhi JM. Neuroethology: Nerve Cells and the Natural Behavior of Animals. Sunderland: Sinauer Associates, 1984.
88. Chandler SH, Tal M. The effects of brain stem transections on the neuronal networks responsible for rhythmical jaw muscle activity in the guinea pig. J Neurosci 1986;6:1831–1842.
89. Nakamura Y, Katakura N. Generation of masticatory rhythm in the brainstem. Neurosci Res 1995;23:1–19.
90. Manchikanti L, Singh V, Rivera J, Pampati V. Prevalence of cervical facet joint pain in chronic neck pain. Pain Physician 2002;5:243–249.
91. Pietrobon D, Striessnig J. Neurological diseases: Neurobiology of migraine. Nat Rev Neurosci 2003;4:386–398.
92. Strassman AM, Weissner W, Williams M, Ali S, Levy D. Axon diameters and intradural trajectories of the dural innervation in the rat. J Comp Neurol 2004;473:364–376.
93. Ray BS, Wolff HG. Experimental studies on headache. Pain sensitive structures of the head and their significance in headache. Arch Surg 1940;41:813–856.
94. Penfield W, Rasmussen T. The Cerebral Cortex of Man. New York: MacMillan, 1955.

95. Pereira LC, Modesto AM, Sugai R, da Mota LA. Pain sensitive cerebral areas and intracranial structures revealed at fully awake craniotomies for primary intracranial tumor resection. In: Abstracts IASP 11th World Congress on Pain. Seattle: IASP, 2005:1517–1520.

96. Haug SR, Heyeraas KJ. Modulation of dental inflammation by the sympathetic nervous system. J Dent Res 2006;85:488–495.

97. Grelik C, Bennett GJ, Ribeiro-da-Silva A. Autonomic fibre sprouting and changes in nociceptive sensory innervation in the rat lower lip skin following chronic constriction injury. Eur J Neurosci 2005;21:2475–2487.

98. Waite PM, Tracey DJ. Trigeminal sensory system. In: Paxinos G (ed). The Rat Nervous System, ed 2. San Diego: Academic, 1995:705–724.

99. Waite PM, Ashwell KW. Trigeminal sensory system. In: Paxinos G, Mai JK (eds). The Human Nervous System, 2 ed. Amsterdam: Elsevier Academic, 2004:1093–1124.

100. O'Connor TP, van der Kooy D. Pattern of intracranial and extracranial projections of trigeminal ganglion cells. J Neurosci 1986;6:2200–2207.

101. Li YQ, Takada M, Ohishi H, Shinonaga Y, Mizuno N. Collateral projections of trigeminal ganglion neurons to both the principal sensory trigeminal and the spinal trigeminal nuclei in the rat. Exp Brain Res 1993;93:205–212.

102. Sessle BJ, Hu JW, Amano N, Zhong G. Convergence of cutaneous, tooth pulp, visceral, neck and muscle afferents onto nociceptive and non-nociceptive neurones in trigeminal subnucleus caudalis (medullary dorsal horn) and its implications for referred pain. Pain 1986;27:219–235.

103. Bereiter DA, Hirata H, Hu JW. Trigeminal subnucleus caudalis: Beyond homologies with the spinal dorsal horn. Pain 2000;88:221–224.

104. Sessle BJ. Acute and chronic craniofacial pain: Brainstem mechanisms of nociceptive transmission and neuroplasticity, and their clinical correlates. Crit Rev Oral Biol Med 2000;11:57–91.

105. Woda A, Molat JL, Luccarini P. Low doses of N-methyl-D-aspartate antagonists in superficial laminae of medulla oblongata facilitate wind-up of convergent neurones. Neuroscience 2001;107:317–327.

106. Shimizu K, Guo W, Wang H, et al. Differential involvement of trigeminal transition zone and laminated subnucleus caudalis in orofacial deep and cutaneous hyperalgesia: The effects of interleukin-10 and glial inhibitors. Mol Pain 2009;5:75.

107. Jacquin MF, Chiaia NL, Haring JH, Rhoades RW. Intersubnuclear connections within the rat trigeminal brainstem complex. Somatosens Mot Res 1990;7:399–420.

108. da Silva AF, Becerra L, Makris N, et al. Somatotopic activation in the human trigeminal pain pathway. J Neurosci 2002;22:8183–8192.

109. Peschanski M. Trigeminal afferents to the diencephalon in the rat. Neuroscience 1984;12:465–487.

110. Jacquin MF, Barcia M, Rhoades RW. Structure-function relationships in rat brainstem subnucleus interpolaris: IV. Projection neurons. J Comp Neurol 1989;282:45–62.

111. Dostrovsky JO, Craig AD. Cooling-specific spinothalamic neurons in the monkey. J Neurophysiol 1996;76:3656–3665.

112. Craig AD. A new view of pain as a homeostatic emotion. Trends Neurosci 2003;26:303–307.

113. Burstein R, Yamamura H, Malick A, Strassman AM. Chemical stimulation of the intracranial dura induces enhanced responses to facial stimulation in brain stem trigeminal neurons. J Neurophysiol 1998;79:964–982.

114. Noseda R, Constandil L, Bourgeais L, Chalus M, Villanueva L. Changes of meningeal excitability mediated by corticotrigeminal networks: A link for the endogenous modulation of migraine pain. J Neurosci 2010;30:14420–14429.

115. Devor M, Wall PD. Dorsal horn cells with proximal cutaneous receptive fields. Brain Res 1976;118:325–328.

116. Villanueva L, Bouhassira D, Bing Z, Le Bars D. Convergence of heterotopic nociceptive information onto subnucleus reticularis dorsalis neurons in the rat medulla. J Neurophysiol 1988;60:980–1009.

117. Le Bars D, Dickenson AH, Besson JM, Villanueva L. Aspects of sensory processing through convergent neurons. In: Yaksh TL (ed). Spinal Afferent Processing. New York: Plenum, 1986:467–504.

118. Dubner R, Kenshalo DR, Maixner W, Bushnell MC, Oliveras JL. The correlation of monkey medullary dorsal horn neuronal activity and the perceived intensity of noxious heat stimuli. J Neurophysiol 1989;62:450–457.

119. Henry JL, Sessle BJ, Lucier GE, Hu JW. Effects of substance P on nociceptive and non-nociceptive trigeminal brain stem neurons. Pain 1980;8:33–45.

120. Bereiter DA, Bereiter DF. N-methyl-D-aspartate and non-N-methyl-D-aspartate receptor antagonism reduces Fos-like immunoreactivity in central trigeminal neurons after corneal stimulation in the rat. Neuroscience 1996;73:249–258.

121. Parada CA, Luccarini P, Woda A. Effect of an NMDA receptor antagonist on the wind-up of neurons in the trigeminal oralis subnucleus. Brain Res 1997;761:313–320.

122. Melzack R, Wall PD. Pain mechanisms: A new theory. Science 1965;150:971–979.

123. Basbaum AI, Bautista DM, Scherrer G, Julius D. Cellular and molecular mechanisms of pain. Cell 2009;139:267–284.

124. Miraucourt LS, Dallel R, Voisin DL. Glycine inhibitory dysfunction turns touch into pain through PKCgamma interneurons. PLoS One 2007;2:e1116.

125. Nakajima A, Tsuboi Y, Suzuki I, et al. PKCgamma in Vc and C1/C2 is involved in trigeminal neuropathic pain. J Dent Res 2011;90:777–781.

126. Bernard JF, Bester H, Besson JM. The spinoparabrachio-amygdaloid and hypothalamic nociceptive pathways. In: Besson JM, Guilbaud G, Ollat H (eds). Forebrain Areas Involved in Pain Processing. Paris: John Libbey Eurotext, 1995:27–48.

127. Malick A, Jakubowski M, Elmquist JK, Saper CB, Burstein R. A neurohistochemical blueprint for pain-induced loss of appetite. Proc Natl Acad Sci USA 2001;98:9930–9935.

128. Bandler R, Depaulis A. Midbrain periaqueductal gray control of defensive behavior in the cat and the rat. In: Depaulis A, Bandler R (eds). The Midbrain Periaqueductal Gray Matter: Functional, Anatomical and Neurochemical Organization. New York: Plenum, 1991:175–198.

129. Gauriau C, Bernard JF. Posterior triangular thalamic neurons convey nociceptive messages to the secondary somatosensory and insular cortices in the rat. J Neurosci 2004;24:752–761.

130. Noseda R, Monconduit L, Constandil L, Chalus M, Villanueva L. Central nervous system networks involved in the processing of meningeal and cutaneous inputs from the ophthalmic branch of the trigeminal nerve in the rat. Cephalalgia 2008;28:813–824.

131. Villanueva L, Nathan P. Multiple pain pathways. In: Devor M, Rowbotham MC, Wiesendfeld-Hallin Z (eds). Progress in Pain Research and Management Series, vol 16 [Proceedings of the 9th World Congress on Pain 22–27 Aug 1999, Vienna, Austria]. Seattle, WA: IASP, 2000:371–386.

132. Vogt BA. Pain and emotion interactions in subregions of the cingulate gyrus. Nat Rev Neurosci 2005;6:533–544.

133. Villanueva L, Bouhassira D, Le Bars D. The medullary subnucleus reticularis dorsalis (SRD) as a key link in both the transmission and modulation of pain signals. Pain 1996;67:231–240.

134. Villanueva L, Cliffer KD, Sorkin LS, Le Bars D, Willis WD. Convergence of heterotopic nociceptive information onto neurons of caudal medullary reticular formation in monkey (macaca fascicularis). J Neurophysiol 1990;63:1118–1127.

135. Burstein R, Jakubowski M, García-Nicas E, et al. Thalamic sensitization transforms localized pain into widespread allodynia. Ann Neurol 2010;68:81–91.

136. Noseda R, Kainz V, Jakubowski M, Burstein R. Mapping cortical projections of dura-sensitive thalamic neurons completes the anatomical description of the trigeminovascular pathway. Presented at Neuroscience 2010, the 40th Annual Meeting of the Society for Neuroscience, San Diego, 15 Nov 2010.

137. Noseda R, Kainz V, Jakubowski M, et al. A neural mechanism for exacerbation of headache by light. Nat Neurosci 2010;13:239–245.

138. Zhang S, Chiang CY, Xie YF, et al. Central sensitization in thalamic nociceptive neurons induced by mustard oil application to rat molar tooth pulp. Neuroscience 2006;142:833–842.

139. Ralston HJ, Ralston DD. The primate dorsal spinothalamic tract: Evidence for a specific termination in the posterior nuclei (Po/SG) of the thalamus. Pain 1992;48:107–118.

140. Craig AD. Distribution of trigeminothalamic and spinothalamic lamina I terminations in the macaque monkey. J Comp Neurol 2004;477:119–148.

141. Craig AD, Bushnell MC, Zhang ET, Blomqvist A. A thalamic nucleus specific for pain and temperature sensation. Nature 1994;372(6508):770–773.

142. Bushnell MC. Thalamic processing of sensory-discriminative and affective-motivational dimensions of pain. In: Besson JM, Guilbaud G, Ollat H (eds). Forebrain Areas Involved in Pain Processing. Paris: John Libbey Eurotext, 1995:63–77.

143. Bushnell MC, Duncan GH. Mechanical response properties of ventroposterior medial thalamic neurons in the alert monkey. Exp Brain Res 1987;67:603–614.

144. Bushnell MC, Duncan GH. Sensory and affective aspects of pain perception: Is medial thalamus restricted to emotional issues? Exp Brain Res 1989;78:415–418.

145. Bushnell MC, Duncan GH, Tremblay N. Thalamic VPM nucleus in the behaving monkey. I. Multimodal and discriminative properties of thermosensitive neurons. J Neurophysiol 1993;69:739–752.

146. Ostrowsky K, Magnin M, Ryvlin P, Isnard J, Guenot M, Mauguière F. Representation of pain and somatic sensation in the human insula: A study of responses to direct electrical cortical stimulation. Cereb Cortex 2002;12:376–385.

147. Montes C, Magnin M, Maarrawi J, et al. Thalamic thermo-algesic transmission: Ventral posterior (VP) complex versus VMpo in the light of a thalamic infarct with central pain. Pain 2005;113:223–232.

148. Chen JI, Ha B, Bushnell MC, Pike B, Duncan GH. Differentiating noxious- and innocuous-related activation of human somatosensory cortices using temporal analysis of fMRI. J Neurophysiol 2002;88:464–474.

149. Mandir AS, Rowland LH, Dougherty PM, Lenz FA. Microelectrode recording and stimulation techniques during stereotactic procedures in the thalamus and pallidum. Adv Neurol 1997;74:159–165.

150. Monconduit L, Bourgeais L, Bernard JF, Le Bars D, Villanueva L. Ventromedial thalamic neurons convey nociceptive signals from the whole body surface to the dorsolateral neocortex. J Neurosci 1999;19:9063–9072.

151. Desbois C, Villanueva L. The organization of lateral ventromedial thalamic connections in the rat: A link for the distribution of nociceptive signals to widespread cortical regions. Neuroscience 2001;102:885–898.

152. Herkenham M. New perspectives on the organization and evolution of nonspecific thalamocortical projections. In: Jones EG, Peters A (eds). Cerebral cortex: Sensory-motor Areas and Aspects of Cortical Connectivity, vol 5. New York: Plenum, 1986:403–445.

153. Larkum ME, Zhu JJ. Signaling of layer 1 and whisker-evoked Ca2+ and Na+ action potentials in distal and terminal dendrites of rat neocortical pyramidal neurons in vitro and in vivo. J Neurosci 2002;22:6991–7005.

154. Derbyshire SW, Jones AK, Gyulai F, Clark S, Townsend D, Firestone LL. Pain processing during three levels of noxious stimulation produces differential patterns of central activity. Pain 1997;73:431–445.

155. Apkarian AV, Baliki MN, Geha PY. Towards a theory of chronic pain. Prog Neurobiol 2009;87(2):81–97.

156. Peyron R, Laurent B, García-Larrea L. Functional imaging of brain responses to pain. A review and meta-analysis (2000). Neurophysiol Clin 2000;30:263–288.

157. Mouraux A, Diukova A, Lee MC, Wise RG, Iannetti GD. A multisensory investigation of the functional significance of the "pain matrix". Neuroimage 2011;54:2237–2249.

158. Isnard J, Magnin M, Jung J, Mauguire F, García-Larrea L. Does the insula tell our brain that we are in pain? Pain 2011;152:946–951.

159. García-Larrea L. The posterior insular-opercular region and the search for a primary cortex for pain. Neurophysiol Clin 2012;42:299–313.

160. Bouhassira D, Le Bars D, Villanueva L. Heterotopic activation of A delta and C fibres triggers inhibition of trigeminal and spinal convergent neurones in the rat. J Physiol 1987;389:301–317.

161. Andersson SA. Pain control by sensory stimulation. In: Bonica J, Liebeskind JC, Albe-Fessard D (eds). Advances in Pain Research and Therapy, vol 3. Seattle: IASP, 1979:569–585.

162. Melzack R. Acupuncture and related forms of folk medicine. In: Wall PD, Melzack R (eds). Textbook of Pain. Edinburgh: Churchill Livingstone, 1984:691–701.

163. Delisle D, Plaghki L. La neuro-stimulation électrique transcutanée est-elle capable d'influencer la perception de douleur? Une méta-analyse. Doul et Analg 1990;3:115–122.

164. Chesterton LS, Foster NE, Wright CC, Baxter GD, Barlas P. Effects of TENS frequency, intensity and stimulation site parameter manipulation on pressure pain thresholds in healthy human subjects. Pain 2003;106:73–80.

165. Le Bars D, Dickenson AH, Besson JM. Diffuse noxious inhibitory controls (DNIC). I. Effects on dorsal horn convergent neurones in the rat. Pain 1979;6:283–304.

166. Dickenson AH, Le Bars D, Besson JM. Diffuse noxious inhibitory controls (DNIC). Effects on trigeminal nucleus caudalis neurones in the rat. Brain Res 1980;200:293–305.

167. Villanueva L, Cadden SW, Le Bars D. Diffuse noxious inhibitory controls (DNIC): Evidence for post-synaptic inhibition of trigeminal nucleus caudalis convergent neurones. Brain Res 1984;321:165–168.

168. Bouhassira D, Villanueva L, Bing Z, Le Bars D. Involvement of the subnucleus reticularis dorsalis in diffuse noxious inhibitory controls in the rat. Brain Res 1992;595:353–357.

169. De Broucker T, Cesaro P, Willer JC, Le Bars D. Diffuse noxious inhibitory controls in man. Involvement of the spinoreticular tract. Brain 1990;113:1223–1234.

170. Le Bars D. The whole body receptive field of dorsal horn multireceptive neurones. Brain Res Brain Res Rev 2002;40:29–44.

171. Defrin R, Tsedek I, Lugasi I, Moriles I, Urca G. The interactions between spatial summation and DNIC: Effect of the distance between two painful stimuli and attentional factors on pain perception. Pain 2010;151:489–95.

172. Villanueva L, Fields HL. Endogenous central mechanisms of pain modulation. In: Villanueva L, Dickenson AH, Ollat H (eds). The Pain System in Normal and Pathological States: A Primer for Clinicians. Seattle: IASP, 2004:223–246.

173. Villanueva L, Le Bars D. The activation of bulbo-spinal controls by peripheral nociceptive inputs: Diffuse noxious inhibitory controls. Biol Res 1995;28:113–125.

174. Roby-Brami A, Bussel B, Willer JC, Le Bars D. An electrophysiological investigation into the pain-relieving effects of heterotopic nociceptive stimuli. Probable involvement of a supraspinal loop. Brain 1987;110:1497–1508.

175. Maillou P, Cadden SW. Effects of remote deep somatic noxious stimuli on a jaw reflex in man. Arch Oral Biol 1997;42:323–327.

176. Piché M, Arsenault M, Rainville P. Cerebral and cerebrospinal processes underlying counterirritation analgesia. J Neurosci 2009;29:14236–14246.

177. Sprenger C, Bingel U, Büchel C. Treating pain with pain: Supraspinal mechanisms of endogenous analgesia elicited by heterotopic noxious conditioning stimulation. Pain 2011;152:428–439.

178. Bouhassira D, Danziger N, Atta N, Guirimand F. Comparison of the pain suppressive effects of clinical and experimental painful conditioning stimuli. Brain 2003;126:1068–1078.

179. Staud R. Evidence for shared pain mechanisms in osteoarthritis, low back pain, and fibromyalgia. Curr Rheumatol Rep 2011;13:513–520.

180. King CD, Wong F, Currie T, Mauderli AP, Fillingim RB, Riley JL 3rd. Deficiency in endogenous modulation of prolonged heat pain in patients with irritable bowel syndrome and temporomandibular disorder. Pain 2009;143:172–178.

181. Leonard G, Goffaux P, Mathieu D, Blanchard J, Kenny B, Marchand S. Evidence of descending inhibition deficits in atypical but not classical trigeminal neuralgia. Pain 2009;147:217–223.

182. Yarnitsky D. Conditioned pain modulation (the diffuse noxious inhibitory control-like effect): Its relevance for acute and chronic pain states. Curr Opin Anaesthesiol 2010;23:611–615.

183. Lewis GN, Rice DA, McNair PJ. Conditioned pain modulation in populations with chronic pain: A systematic review and meta-analysis. J Pain 2012;13:936–944.

184. Granovsky Y. Conditioned pain modulation: A predictor for development and treatment of neuropathic pain. Curr Pain Headache Rep 2013;17:361.

185. Oliveras JL, Besson JM. Stimulation-produced analgesia in animals: Behavioural investigations. In: Fields HL, Besson JM (eds). Pain modulation, Progress in Brain Research. Amsterdam: Elsevier, 1988:141–157.

186. Tal M, Sharav Y, Devor M. Modulation of the jaw-opening reflex by peripheral electrical stimulation. Exp Neurol 1981;74:907–919.

187. Suzuki R, Morcuende S, Webber M, Hunt SP, Dickenson AH. Superficial NK1-expressing neurons control spinal excitability through activation of descending pathways. Nat Neurosci 2002;5:1319–1326.

188. Lefler Y, Arzi A, Reiner K, Sukhotinsky I, Devor M. Bulbospinal neurons of the rat rostromedial medulla are highly collateralized. J Comp Neurol 2008;506:960–978.

189. Lovick TA. The medullary raphe nuclei: A system for integration and gain control in autonomic and somatomotor responsiveness? Exp Physiol 1997;82:31–41.

190. Mason P. Contributions of the medullary raphe and ventromedial reticular region to pain modulation and other homeostatic functions. Annu Rev Neurosci 2001;24:737–777.

191. Fields HL, Heinricher MM, Mason P. Neurotransmitters in nociceptive modulatory circuits. Annu Rev Neurosci 1991;14:219–245.

192. Leung CG, Mason P. Physiological properties of raphe magnus neurons during sleep and waking. J Neurophysiol 1999;81:584–595.

193. Olivéras JL, Martin G, Montagne-Clavel J. Drastic changes of ventromedial medulla neuronal properties induced by barbiturate anesthesia. II. Modifications of the single-unit activity produced by Brevital, a short-acting barbiturate in the awake, freely moving rat. Brain Res 1991;563:251–260.

194. McGaraughty S, Reinis S, Tsoukatos J. Two distinct unit activity responses to morphine in the rostral ventromedial medulla of awake rats. Brain Res 1993;604:331–333.

195. Almeida A, Cobos A, Tavares I, Lima D. Brain afferents to the medullary dorsal reticular nucleus: A retrograde and anterograde tracing study in the rat. Eur J Neurosci 2002;16:81–95.

196. Almeida A. The medullary dorsal reticular nucleus facilitates pain behaviour induced by formalin in the rat. Eur J Neurosci 1999;11:110–122.

197. Dickenson AH, Le Bars D. Supraspinal morphine and descending inhibitions acting on the dorsal horn of the rat. J Physiol 1987;384:81–107.

198. Zubieta JK, Smith YR, Bueller JA, et al. Regional mu opioid receptor regulation of sensory and affective dimensions of pain. Science 2001;293(5528):311–315.

199. Petrovic P, Kalso E, Petersson KM, Ingvar M. Placebo and opioid analgesia—Imaging a shared neuronal network. Science 2002;295(5560):1737–1740.

200. Desbois C, Le Bars D, Villanueva L. Organization of cortical projections to the medullary subnucleus reticularis dorsalis: A retrograde and anterograde tracing study in the rat. J Comp Neurol 1999;410:178–196.

201. Zhang L, Zhang Y, Zhao ZQ. Anterior cingulate cortex contributes to the descending facilitatory modulation of pain via dorsal reticular nucleus. Eur J Neurosci 2005;22:1141–1148.

202. Kobayashi S. Organization of neural systems for aversive information processing: Pain, error, and punishment. Front Neurosci 2012;6:136.

203. Scott DJ, Stohler CS, Egnatuk CM, Wang H, Koeppe RA, Zubieta JK. Placebo and nocebo effects are defined by opposite opioid and dopaminergic responses. Arch Gen Psychiatry 2008;65:220–231.

204. Colloca L, Klinger R, Flor H, Bingel U. Placebo analgesia: Psychological and neurobiological mechanisms. Pain 2013;154:511–514.

205. Benedetti F, Arduino C, Amanzio M. Somatotopic activation of opioid systems by target-directed expectations of analgesia. J Neurosci 1999;19:3639–3648.

206. Apkarian AV, Bushnell MC, Treede RD, Zubieta JK. Human brain mechanisms of pain perception and regulation in health and disease. Eur J Pain 2005;9:463–484.

207. Colloca L, Benedetti F. Placebos and painkillers: Is mind as real as matter? Nat Rev Neurosci 2005;6:545–552.

208. Tracey I, Mantyh PW. The cerebral signature for pain perception and its modulation. Neuron 2007;55:377–391.

209. Craig AD, Bushnell MC. The thermal grill illusion: Unmasking the burn of cold pain. Science 1994;265(5169):252–255.

210. Sessle BJ, Hu JW, Dubner R, Lucier GE. Functional properties of neurons in cat trigeminal subnucleus caudalis (medullary dorsal horn). II. Modulation of responses to noxious and nonnoxious stimuli by periaqueductal gray, nucleus raphe magnus, cerebral cortex, and afferent influences, and effect of naloxone. J Neurophysiol 1981;45:193–207.

211. Bushnell MC, Duncan GH, Dubner R, He LF. Activity of trigeminothalamic neurons in medullary dorsal horn of awake monkeys trained in a thermal discrimination task. J Neurophysiol 1984;52:170–187.

212. Duncan GH, Bushnell MC, Bates R, Dubner R. Task-related responses of monkey medullary dorsal horn neurons. J Neurophysiol 1987;57:289–310.

213. Deschênes M, Veinante P, Zhang ZW. The organization of corticothalamic projections: Reciprocity versus parity. Brain Res Rev 1998;28:286–308.

214. Rauschecker JP. Cortical control of the thalamus: Top-down processing and plasticity. Nat Neurosci 1998;1:179–180.

215. Krupa DJ, Ghazanfar AA, Nicolelis MA. Immediate thalamic sensory plasticity depends on corticothalamic feedback. Proc Natl Acad Sci USA 1999;96:8200–8205.

216. Monconduit L, López-Avila A, Molat JL, Chalus M, Villanueva L. Corticofugal output from the primary somatosensory cortex selectively modulates innocuous and noxious inputs in the rat spinothalamic system. J Neurosci 2006;26:8441–8450.

217. Avivi-Arber L, Martin R, Lee JC, Sessle BJ. Face sensorimotor cortex and its neuroplasticity related to orofacial sensorimotor functions. Arch Oral Biol 2011;56:1440–1465.

218. Nahmias F, Debes C, de Andrade DC, Mhalla A, Bouhassira D. Diffuse analgesic effects of unilateral repetitive transcranial magnetic stimulation (rTMS) in healthy volunteers. Pain 2009;147:224–232.

219. Robert C, Bourgeais L, Arreto CD, et al. Paraventricular hypothalamic regulation of trigeminovascular mechanisms involved in headaches. J Neurosci 2013;33:8827–8840.

220. Spencer SE, Sawyer WB, Wada H, Platt KB, Loewy AD. CNS projections to the pterygopalatine parasympathetic preganglionic neurons in the rat: A retrograde transneuronal viral cell body labeling study. Brain Res 1990;534:149–169.

221. Akerman S, Holland PR, Summ O, Lasalandra MP, Goadsby PJ. A translational in vivo model of trigeminal autonomic cephalalgias: Therapeutic characterization. Brain 2012;135:3664–3675.

222. Simmons DM, Swanson LW. Comparison of the spatial distribution of seven types of neuroendocrine neurons in the rat paraventricular nucleus: Toward a global 3D model. J Comp Neurol 2009;516:423–441.

223. Swanson LW, Sawchenko PE. Paraventricular nucleus: A site for the integration of neuroendocrine and autonomic mechanisms. Neuroendocrinology 1980;31:410–417.

224. Hewitt SA, Wamsteeker JI, Kurz EU, Bains JS. Altered chloride homeostasis removes synaptic inhibitory constraint of the stress axis. Nat Neurosci 2009;12:438–443.

225. Critchley HD, Mathias CJ, Dolan RJ. Neuroanatomical basis for first- and second-order representations of bodily states. Nat Neurosci 2001;4:207–212.

226. Critchley HD, Wiens S, Rotshtein P, Ohman A, Dolan RJ. Neural systems supporting interoceptive awareness. Nat Neurosci 2004;7:189–195.

227. Craig AD. Forebrain emotional asymmetry: A neuroanatomical basis? Trends Cogn Sci 2005;9:566–571.

228. Geerling JC, Shin JW, Chimenti PC, Loewy AD. Paraventricular hypothalamic nucleus: Axonal projections to the brainstem. J Comp Neurol 2010;518:1460–1499.

229. Benoliel R, Birenboim R, Regev E, Eliav E. Neurosensory changes in the infraorbital nerve following zygomatic fractures. Oral Surg Oral Med Oral Pathol Oral Radiol Endod 2005;99:657–665.

230. Bouhassira D, Attal N, Alchaar H, et al. Comparison of pain syndromes associated with nervous or somatic lesions and development of a new neuropathic pain diagnostic questionnaire (DN4). Pain 2005;114:29–36.

231. Kugelberg E, Lindblom U. The mechanism of the pain in trigeminal neuralgia. J Neurol Neurosurg Psychiatry 1959;22:36–43.

232. Noordenbos W. Pain. Amsterdam: Elsevier, 1959.

233. Gottrup H, Kristensen AD, Bach FW, Jensen TS. Aftersensations in experimental and clinical hypersensitivity. Pain 2003;103:57–64.

234. Melzack R, Bromage PR. Experimental phantom limbs. Exp Neurol 1973;39:261–269.

235. Waxman SG (ed). Sodium Channels and Neuronal Hyperexcitability: Novartis Foundation Symposium 241. West Sussex: Wiley, 2002.

236. Nordin M, Nystrom B, Wallin U, Hagbarth KE. Ectopic sensory discharges and paresthesiae in patients with disorders of peripheral nerves, dorsal roots and dorsal columns. Pain 1984;20:231–245.

237. Nair DR, Najm I, Bulacio J, Lüders H. Painful auras in focal epilepsy. Neurology 2001;57:700–702.

238. Marbach JJ, Raphael KG. Phantom tooth pain: A new look at an old dilemma. Pain Med 2000;1:68–77.

239. White JC, Sweet WH. Pain and the neurosurgeon: A forty-year experience. Springfield: Charles C Thomas, 1969.

240. Flor H. Remapping somatosensory cortex after injury. Adv Neurol 2003;93:195–204.

241. Vaso A, Adahan H-M, Gjika A, et al. Peripheral nervous system origin of phantom limb pain. Pain 2014;155:1384–1391.

242. Cronholm B. Phantom limbs in amputees; A study of changes in the integration of centripetal impulses with special reference to referred sensations. Acta Psychiatr Neurol Scand Suppl 1951;72:1–310.

243. Ramachandran VS, Altschuler EL. The use of visual feedback, in particular mirror visual feedback, in restoring brain function. Brain 2009;132:1693–1710.

244. Devor M, Wall PD. Reorganisation of spinal cord sensory map after peripheral nerve injury. Nature 1978;276(5683):75–76.

245. Wall PD, Fitzgerald M, Nussbaumer JC, Van der Loos H, Devor M. Somatotopic maps are disorganized in adult rodents treated neonatally with capsaicin. Nature 1982;295(5851):691–693.

246. Kaas JH, Merzenich MM, Killackey HP. The reorganization of somatosensory cortex following peripheral nerve damage in adult and developing mammals. Annu Rev Neurosci 1983;6:325–356.

247. Borsook D, Becerra L, Fishman S, et al. Acute plasticity in the human somatosensory cortex following amputation. Neuroreport 1998;9:1013–1017.

248. Gandevia SC, Phegan CM. Perceptual distortions of the human body image produced by local anaesthesia, pain and cutaneous stimulation. J Physiol 1999;514:609–616.

249. Harris AJ. Cortical origin of pathological pain. Lancet 1999;354(9188):1464–1466.

250. Giraux P, Sirigu A. Illusory movements of the paralyzed limb restore motor cortex activity. Neuroimage 2003;20(suppl 1):S107–S111.

251. Devor M. Neuropathic pain: Pathophysiological response of nerves to injury. In: Mcmahon SL, Koltzenburg M, Tracey I, Turk DC (eds). Wall and Melzack's Textbook of Pain, ed 6. Philadelphia: Elsevier-Saunders, 2013:861–888.

252. Devor M. How do pain genes affect pain experience? In: Belfer I, Diatchenko L (eds). Pain Genetics: Basic to Translational Science. Hoboken:Wiley Blackwell, 2014:1–14.

253. Burchiel KJ, Wyler AR. Ectopic action potential generation in peripheral trigeminal axons. Exp Neurol 1978;62:269–281.

254. Bongenhielm U, Robinson PP. Spontaneous and mechanically evoked afferent activity originating from myelinated fibres in ferret inferior alveolar nerve neuromas. Pain 1996;67:399–406.

255. Bongenhielm U, Robinson PP. Afferent activity from myelinated inferior alveolar nerve fibres in ferrets after constriction or section and regeneration. Pain 1998;74:123–132.

256. Tsuboi Y, Takeda M, Tanimoto T, et al. Alteration of the second branch of the trigeminal nerve activity following inferior alveolar nerve transection in rats. Pain 2004;111:323–334.

257. Amir R, Devor M. Functional cross-excitation between afferent A- and C-neurons in dorsal root ganglia. Neuroscience 2000;95:189–195.

258. Devor M, Amir R, Rappaport ZH. Pathophysiology of trigeminal neuralgia: The ignition hypothesis. Clin J Pain 2002;18:4–13.

259. Boucher TJ, McMahon SB. Neurotrophic factors and neuropathic pain. Curr Opin Pharmacol 2001;1:66–72.

260. Kocsis JD, Devor M. Altered excitability of large-diameter cutaneous afferents following nerve injury: Consequences for chronic pain. In: Devor M, Rowbotham M, Wiesenfeld-Hallin Z (eds). Progress in Pain Research and Management Series, vol 17 [Proceedings of the 9th World Congress on Pain, 22–27 Aug 1999, Vienna, Austria]. Seattle, WA: IASP, 2000:119–136.

261. Devor M, Keller CH, Deerinck TJ, Levinson SR, Ellisman MH. Na+ channel accumulation on axolemma of afferent endings in nerve end neuromas in *Apteronotus*. Neurosci Lett 1989;102:149–154.

262. Devor M. Sodium channels and mechanisms of neuropathic pain. J Pain 2006;7(suppl 1):S3–S12.

263. Amir R, Liu CN, Kocsis JD, Devor M. Oscillatory mechanism in primary sensory neurones. Brain 2002;125:421–435.

264. McLachlan EM, Jänig W, Devor M, Michaelis M. Peripheral nerve injury triggers noradrenergic sprouting within dorsal root ganglia. Nature 1993;363(6429):543–546.

265. Shinder V, Govrin-Lippmann R, Cohen S, et al. Structural basis of sympathetic-sensory coupling in rat and human dorsal root ganglia following peripheral nerve injury. J Neurocytol 1999;28:743–761.

266. Davis BM, Albers KM, Seroogy KB, Katz DM. Overexpression of nerve growth factor in transgenic mice induces novel sympathetic projections to primary sensory neurons. J Comp Neurol 1994;349:464–474.

267. Bongenhielm U, Boissonade FM, Westermark A, Robinson PP, Fried K. Sympathetic nerve sprouting fails to occur in the trigeminal ganglion after peripheral nerve injury in the rat. Pain 1999;82:283–288.

268. Benoliel R, Eliav E, Tal M. No sympathetic nerve sprouting in rat trigeminal ganglion following painful and non-painful infraorbital nerve neuropathy. Neurosci Lett 2001;297:151–154.

269. Harden RN, Baron R, Janig W. Complex Regional Pain Syndrome, Progress in Pain Research and Management, vol 22. Seattle: IASP, 2001.

270. Yirmiya R, Pollak Y, Morag M, et al. Illness, cytokines, and depression. Ann NY Acad Sci 2000;917:478–487.

271. Shim B, Kim DW, Kim BH, Nam TS, Leem JW, Chung JM. Mechanical and heat sensitization of cutaneous nociceptors in rats with experimental peripheral neuropathy. Neuroscience 2005;132:193–201.

272. Woolf CJ. Evidence for a central component of post-injury pain hypersensitivity. Nature 1983;306(5944):686–688.

273. Burstein R, Yarnitsky D, Goor-Aryeh I, Ransil BJ, Bajwa ZH. An association between migraine and cutaneous allodynia. Ann Neurol 2000;47:614–624.

274. Hardy JD, Wolf HG, Goodell H. Pain Sensations and Reactions. New York: William & Wilkins, 1952.

275. Ji RR, Kohno T, Moore KA, Woolf CJ. Central sensitization and LTP: Do pain and memory share similar mechanisms? Trends Neurosci 2003;26:696–705.

276. Willis W (ed). Hyperalgesia and Allodynia. New York: Raven, 1992.

277. Devor M. Central changes after peripheral nerve injury. In: Willis WD, Schmidt R (eds). Encyclopedia of Pain. Berlin: Springer-Verlag, 2007:306–311.

278. Molander C, Hongpaisan J, Persson JK. Distribution of c-fos expressing dorsal horn neurons after electrical stimulation of low threshold sensory fibers in the chronically injured sciatic nerve. Brain Res 1994;644:74–82.

279. Noguchi K, Kawai Y, Fukuoka T, Senba E, Miki K. Substance P induced by peripheral nerve injury in primary afferent sensory neurons and its effect on dorsal column nucleus neurons. J Neurosci 1995;15:7633–7643.

280. Neumann S, Doubell TP, Leslie T, Woolf CJ. Inflammatory pain hypersensitivity mediated by phenotypic switch in myelinated primary sensory neurons. Nature 1996;384(6607):360–364.

281. Weissner W, Winterson BJ, Stuart-Tilley A, Devor M, Bove GM. Time course of substance P expression in dorsal root ganglia following complete spinal nerve transection. J Comp Neurol 2006;497:78–87.

282. Nitzan-Luques A, Devor M, Tal M. Genotype-selective phenotypic switch in primary afferent neurons contributes to neuropathic pain. Pain 2011;152:2413–2426.

283. Miller JP, Acar F, Hamilton BE, Burchiel KJ. Radiographic evaluation of trigeminal neurovascular compression in patients with and without trigeminal neuralgia. J Neurosurg 2009;110:627–632.

284. Tal M, Devor M. Ectopic discharge in injured nerves: Comparison of trigeminal and somatic afferents. Brain Res 1992;579:148–151.

285. Eliav E, Benoliel R, Tal M. Inflammation with no axonal damage of the rat saphenous nerve trunk induces ectopic discharge and mechanosensitivity in myelinated axons. Neurosci Lett 2001;311:49–52.

286. Benoliel R, Wilensky A, Tal M, Eliav E. Application of a pro-inflammatory agent to the orbital portion of the rat infraorbital nerve induces changes indicative of ongoing trigeminal pain. Pain 2002;99:567–578.

287. Benoliel R, Biron A, Quek SY, Nahlieli O, Eliav E. Trigeminal neurosensory changes following acute and chronic paranasal sinusitis. Quintessence Int 2006;37:437–443.

Measuring and Assessing Pain

Eli Eliav, DMD, MSc, PhD
Richard H. Gracely, MS, PhD

P. 79-96

Pain measurement is an essential element in any medical assessment, including diagnosis, monitoring of disease progress, and evaluation of treatment effectiveness. Unfortunately, there is no single common or easy method of pain measurement. Because pain is a personal and private experience that cannot be seen or felt by others, the methods that must be used for pain assessment include indirect, self-report, physiologic, and behavioral methods. The target of these pain assessments should be multidimensional; pain is both a somatic sensation and an emotional state that evokes behaviors that minimize bodily harm and promote healing.[1] In this chapter, current techniques used in the assessment of pain are reviewed.

Pain experience and intensity may vary among different populations and are affected by a broad range of factors. Emotional states may have divergent effects on the pain experience. Fear, exercise, or additional painful stimuli can reduce pain. Anxiety and stress can aggravate pain (see also chapter 4), particularly in chronic conditions, and exercise may induce analgesia.[2,3] The duration of pain is an important variable in pain assessment; long-lasting or frequent pain episodes can induce processes in the central nervous system that extend the normal duration of pain secondary to injury (see posttraumatic neuropathy in chapter 12). The character of pain onset will also substantially affect the experience; pain that develops gradually may be quite different from pain that develops abruptly. Pain can occur at different periods of the day, and it may be invalid to compare intensity of pain on awakening from sleep to pain occurring during the day or during function. Moreover, major variations in pain intensity can occur during the day, the week (weekend headaches), and the month (menstrually related headaches). Pain localization may affect the pain experience. Similar pathologic processes in different sites can produce different pain experiences. For example, pain induced by inflammation within a tooth pulp (pulpitis) or in the hip joint cannot be compared with inflammatory-related temporomandibular joint pain (capsulitis or osteoarthritis) despite a common mechanism (inflammatory process).

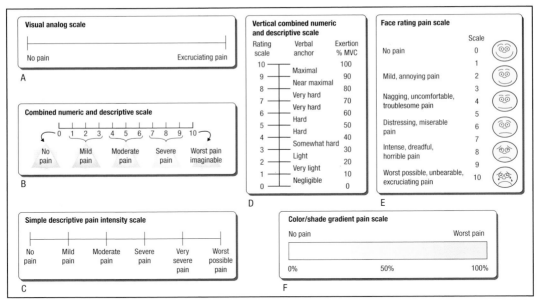

Fig 3-1 Scales commonly used to assess pain severity. The choice of which scale to adopt is dictated by the setting (eg, clinic, research project) and by the study population (eg, children, adults).

The word *pain* embraces many conditions and qualities. Pain can be throbbing, burning, aching, diffuse, tingling, stabbing, cramping, and pressing. Some qualities are more specific to certain conditions. For example, migraine has a throbbing quality, whereas myofascial pain is pressing and dull. Electric shock–like pain has been frequently associated with trigeminal neuralgia, whereas other neuropathic conditions are characterized by burning pain. However, it is not clear if clinicians and patients use the same terms to describe the same sensations.

Pain intensity and frequency are probably the most important features measured to assess a patient's well being. However, pain quality, onset, duration, localization and other factors that modify the condition (alleviating or aggravating), occurrence of pain elsewhere in the body, and associated psychosocial problems must also be assessed.

Accurate measurement of the pain experience can be performed only with the assistance of several tools and methods. Drawing the painful area on a body map and maintaining a pain diary may provide necessary information for pain location, duration, frequency, and modifying factors. These methods should be standardized and used consistently with each patient. Chapters 8 through 12 and 14, which deal with the major clinical pain syndromes, contain extensive examples of the use of pain diaries as well as methods for drawing and mapping pain to aid in diagnosis and follow-up.

Methods for Pain Assessment

Pain scales

Visual analog scale

The visual analog scale (VAS) is the most frequently used method to assess pain intensity. The scale is usually a horizontal[4,5] or vertical 10-cm line[6] labeled at each end by descriptors such as "no pain" and "worst pain ever" (Fig 3-1). The patient marks the line to indicate pain severity, which is quantified by measuring the distance in centimeters from zero (no pain) to the patient's marked rating. This method was validated in a number of studies[7] but was found to be insufficient in others.[8] However, this method is simple and easy to use in a clinical situation; it also aids in monitoring treatment efficacy. A popular variation of the VAS that was designed for children or for patients who do not have the verbal skills to describe their symptoms is the Faces Pain Rating Scale[9,10] (see Fig 3-1). This scale consists of a series of faces with different expressions. The facial expressions vary in a continuum from a happy face for no pain to a very sad face for intense pain; a written description often accompanies each face. The patient is asked to choose the face that best describes his or her pain.[11,12]

Numeric and verbal rating scales

In a numeric rating scale, patients are asked to rate their pain on a scale from 0 to 10 or 0 to 100, in which "0" is no pain and the other end of the scale represents the worst possible pain.[13] Alternatively, verbal descriptive scales incorporate specific words organized to express the increasing and progressive intensity of pain. A category scale is a simple form of a verbal scale; in clinical trials it is usually composed of four pain descriptions, such as none, mild, moderate, or severe. Simple category scales can be used for rough comparisons or in addition to other pain scales, and the number of categories can be increased to achieve greater resolution. Hybrid scales combine verbal scales with graphic rating or with numeric scales; the descriptors are placed in appropriate locations on the analog scale.[14,15] Nominal verbal scales include a list of qualitative descriptive words, such as burning, cramping, or pricking. This scale supplements pain-intensity scales with additional clinically useful information.

No simple guide is available to help clinicians select a pain scale. Numeric, visual, and verbal scales have been validated in numerous studies, and the choice must be specifically established considering the individual patient or research project in question. For example, it has been shown that elderly patients make fewer mistakes with verbal scales than with VASs.[16,17] Using a numeric or verbal scale eliminates the task of marking a line and therefore may be useful for patients with motor disability.

VASs have been integrated in computerized systems that can calculate and measure pain over time.[18,19] Adding a time element to the assessment of intensity can provide important information concerning pain pattern over time, prolonged stimulus-evoked pain sensations, and spontaneous or specific factors that aggravate pain intensity. Computerized systems can also assess pain for longer periods using personal electronic devices. This method has been validated in patients who are pain free and has been shown to be sensitive in a clinical trial.[20,21]

Most visual analog, numeric, or verbal pain scales rate pain as a unidimensional experience. More sophisticated questionnaires have been developed that address the multidimensional experience that pain induces.

Pain questionnaires

The McGill Pain Questionnaire

The McGill Pain Questionnaire (MPQ)[22] is the most frequently used questionnaire for the multidimensional assessment of pain. The MPQ assesses three separate components of the pain experience: sensory intensity, emotional impact, and cognitive evaluation of pain. Patients are presented with 78 adjectives in 20 groups and are instructed to select one from each group for the particular groups that most closely match their own pain experience. An overall score for each major dimension is obtained from the sum of weighted scores or from the ranks of the chosen word within each group.

Once the MPQ was translated into many languages, it was shown that people from different ethnic and educational backgrounds use similar adjectives to describe the same pain conditions.[23] In certain specific pain disorders that are characterized with typical adjectives, the questionnaire may also help clinicians make a diagnosis.[24] Moreover, the MPQ has been found to be sensitive to pain interventions and, therefore, can evaluate treatment efficacy.[25–27] In the orofacial pain region, the MPQ has

Short-form McGill Pain Questionnaire and pain diagram
(Reproduced with permission of author © Dr Ron Melzack, for publication and distribution)

Date: _____

Name: _____

Check the column to indicate the level of your pain for each word, or leave blank if it does not apply to you.

	Mild	Moderate	Severe
1. Throbbing	____	____	____
2. Shooting	____	____	____
3. Stabbing	____	____	____
4. Sharp	____	____	____
5. Cramping	____	____	____
6. Gnawing	____	____	____
7. Hot-burning	____	____	____
8. Aching	____	____	____
9. Heavy	____	____	____
10. Tender	____	____	____
11. Splitting	____	____	____
12. Tiring-Exhausting	____	____	____
13. Sickening	____	____	____
14. Fearful	____	____	____
15. Cruel-Punishing	____	____	____

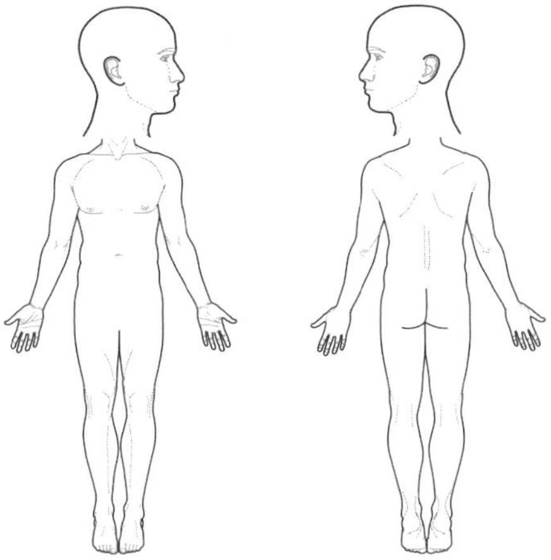

Mark or comment on the above figure where you have your pain or problems

Indicate on this line how bad your pain is — at the left end of line means no pain at all, at right end means worst pain possible

No pain		Worst possible pain

S	/33	A	/12	VAS	/10

Fig 3-2 McGill Pain Questionnaire Short Form. The questionnaire includes a VAS, a map to define location, and a short list of descriptive terms.

been validated in trigeminal neuralgia, atypical odontalgia, toothache, and burning mouth syndrome.[24,28] A short-form MPQ is available that consists of 15 selected adjectives that patients score on a four-point scale and a VAS that is used for measurement of pain intensity[16,29–31] (Fig 3-2).

Other multidimensional questionnaires have found common psychologic patterns for patients in pain, regardless of etiology, location, treatment, and the medical or dental diagnosis.[32,33]

The Research Diagnostic Criteria for Temporomandibular Disorders

The Research Diagnostic Criteria for Temporomandibular Disorders (RDC-TMD) is an example of a multidimensional questionnaire designed for temporomandibular disorders (TMDs) (see chapters 8 and 9) that was developed by Dworkin and LeResche[34] and revised recently by the International RDC/TMD Consortium Network of the International Association for Dental Research and the Orofacial Pain

Special Interest Group of the International Association for the Study of Pain.[35] This classification and assessment system includes two axes: Axis I comprises clinical and physical examination items, and Axis II consists of pain-related and psychosocial disability ratings. The RDC-TMD can be used for diagnostic evaluation of TMDs, making it a useful tool for both clinical and research purposes. Multicenter studies confirmed the reliability of the RDC-TMD for the most common TMD diagnoses,[36–40] and a validated questionnaire is available in various languages (http://www.rdc-tmdinternational. org/). Other diagnostic criteria and tools, such as those outlined by the American Academy of Orofacial Pain,[41] the International Headache Society,[42] or the International Association for the Study of Pain,[43] can be used for the diagnosis and assessment of neuropathic (chapters 12 and 14) and neurovascular (chapters 10 and 11) orofacial pain conditions.

Spontaneous and behavioral responses

Single or multidimensional pain scales are not useful for patients with language deficits or for children of preverbal age, and in these cases pain assessment relies on observation. Facial expressions related to pain may serve as a limited tool for pain evaluation in infants or disabled patients.[44,45] At present, this is not a validated method; however, experienced clinicians can gather valuable information about a patient's pain experience from his or her facial expressions. In addition, observations of altered orofacial functions, such as avoidance or altered biting or chewing patterns, can signify the presence of orofacial pain (see chapters 8 and 9).

Physiologic measurements

Autonomic responses, such as heart rate, blood pressure, skin conductivity, pupil size, or hormone release, intensify during painful conditions.[46,47] Unfortunately, these signs tend to diminish (habituate) over time. In addition, autonomic responses are not specific to pain but are influenced by other factors, such as startle response, anger, or fear. Specific autonomic signs are common in neurovascular headaches, particularly trigeminal autonomic cephalalgias (see chapter 11). Autonomic signs are also observed in complex regional pain syndrome, which is considered to be rare in the orofacial region (see chapter 12). In these specific syndromes, physiologic measurements as indicators of pain severity are complex and best avoided.

Electromyography

Electromyography measures action potential from muscles as an indication of muscle activity. However, the correlation between muscle activity and orofacial pain conditions is debatable[48–50] (this is discussed in depth in chapter 7). Orofacial pain conditions can alter trigeminal reflex activities, suggesting a connection between the nociceptive pathways and trigeminal reflexes.[51–53] However, this extensively studied method has never been validated as a clinical tool for pain assessment.

Microneurography

In animal studies, neurophysiologic recording from peripheral nerve fibers has been shown to provide valuable information on neuronal function and pain mechanisms. A similar method has been developed for use in humans to explore the characteristics of nociceptors, mainly different populations of C fibers,[54–56] and this method has been used to assess function in the trigeminal system.[57] Microneurography is an excellent research tool that directly evaluates primary afferent function. However, the invasive nature of the method and the significant requirements for subject compliance limit its clinical utility.

Imaging

Standard imaging techniques are very useful for diagnosis but not for pain assessment. No correlation has been found between the extent of a lesion or tissue damage established by imaging and the magnitude of pain severity.

Functional magnetic resonance imaging and positron emission tomography are used in research laboratories to assess brain activity associated with pain. These studies and earlier electroencephalogram studies mapped the areas in the brain that appear to be involved in

p. 236

pain perception.[58–60] Recent findings suggest the presence of brain-augmented pain processing in patients suffering from fibromyalgia.[61] However, these promising techniques are not clinically applicable to pain measurement as yet. Similar to most other pain studies using brain-imaging methods, the studies average group data to investigate pain-processing mechanisms. Therefore, these studies have not examined the ability of these methods to provide clinically useful information about single subjects or their possible utility in clinical decision-making.[62]

Quantitative Sensory Testing

The term *quantitative sensory testing* (QST) encompasses several methods used to quantify sensory nerve function. QST uses noninvasive assessment and quantification of sensory nerve function in patients with suspected neurologic damage or disease. The common concepts in QST methods are that the assessment of normal and abnormal responses to various stimuli provides information about the functioning of the peripheral and central nervous system and that these responses can be quantified by the amount of physical stimuli required to evoke specific levels of sensory perception. External stimuli are usually mechanical, thermal, or electrical. The response to gross external stimuli has been part of the formal neurologic evaluation since the late 19th century. The concept is still valid, and years of research and development of new tools have improved the benefit gained from such tests.

The establishment of clinically normal QST ranges is complicated by numerous variables, including probe or electrode size, stimulus frequency, site, rate of stimulus change, clinical environment, sex, age, and ethnicity. Furthermore, data from one assessment system cannot be easily transferred to or compared with another. This variance can be reduced to some extent by routinely using the same methods and devices. For localized unilateral pathologies, expressing thresholds as the ratio between the ipsilateral (affected) and the contralateral (unaffected, control) sides improves consistency.[63]

Bilateral pathologies may be compared with adjacent dermatomes (see Case 3-1).

QST methods

In general, QST methods can be divided into two broad classes. The first is based on a fixed set of stimuli and requires a response indicating the magnitude of the sensation evoked by each stimulus. This class is used for suprathreshold pain sensations. The response intensity can be measured with visual analog, numeric, or verbal scales as described earlier. In the second class, the response is fixed, and the stimulus varies; this is usually used to measure pain or sensory thresholds. These methods have been referred to as response dependent and stimulus dependent, respectively, and may be further classified on the basis of the type of data collected (eg, modality used, units, test).

In both classes, the test accuracy is largely dependent on the patient response. The patient's response can be biased by delayed responses or by a range of expectations. These biases are controlled to some extent by more time-consuming psychophysical methods that deliver numerous stimuli but are less controlled in typical fast assessments performed in a clinical setting. In many cases, the features, such as hyperalgesia, are quite evident and appropriately assessed by the fast methods. Cases of more subtle sensory abnormalities may require more extensive procedures.

Stimulus-dependent methods express results in terms of physical units of stimulus intensity, which avoids the use of subjective scaling units and provides a convenient measure for comparison between persons and within persons over time. Two main stimulus-dependent protocols are used: methods of limits and methods of levels.

In *methods of limits,* the subject is required to indicate detection of an increasing stimulus or the disappearance of a decreasing stimulus. In pain studies, this method is usually modified to present only ascending series to avoid excessively painful stimulation at the beginning of a descending series. This modification tends to be less accurate, mainly because the method is sensitive to patient reaction time and errors of anticipation.[8,64] Yet, this is a simple, fast method that can be very useful in situations in which

CASE 3-1

Bilateral mental neuropathy in a 45-year-old woman.

This rare case of bilateral mental numbness after insertion of dental implants demonstrates the use of QST in an orofacial pain clinic.

Present complaint: Bilateral numbness in the mental nerve territory. The area of paresthesia on the right side is larger and accompanied by an intermittent, mild burning sensation.

History of present complaint: Five days ago, the patient underwent insertion of mandibular dental implants bilaterally (three on the left side and four on the right). Immediately after resolution of the local anesthesia, the patient indicated that the right side felt "different," a sensation that developed into numbness within 24 hours. Two days after the procedure, left-side mental paresthesia and numbness developed. For the past 24 hours, the right-side paresthesia has been accompanied by a mild burning sensation.

Examination: Excluding the mental nerve territories, head and neck examination was unremarkable. QST using electrical and thermal stimuli was performed in the mental and infraorbital nerve dermatomes, respectively. Testing revealed that relative to the infraorbital dermatomes, the mental dermatomes expressed elevated heat-detection and electrical detection thresholds in the right side and a reduced electrical detection threshold in the left side (see Fig 3-3).

Relevant medical history: None.

Diagnosis: The history and findings indicated right-side nerve damage and left-side perineural inflammation. A computed tomography (CT) scan (see Fig 3-4) clearly showed impingement of a right implant in the inferior alveolar (mandibular) canal.

Treatment: Immediately, 60 mg of prednisone was initiated; the dose was reduced by 10 mg each subsequent day for 5 days. Three days later, the aberrant sensation on the left side disappeared, but the right side had only improved slightly. A few days later, the misplaced implant on the right side was surgically removed. Right-side pain was dramatically improved within 3 weeks, though sensory function returned only after 3 months. Compare this case to Case 12-2, where removal of the implants resulted in no change in pain or sensory disturbance. In Case 3-1, the amount of nerve damage may have been less than that in the case depicted in Fig 12-9.

Conclusions: The left-side numbness was the result of perineural inflammation, and the left-side aberrant sensation was related to direct nerve damage. Early intervention and radiographic identification of an intact left inferior dental canal were good prognostic factors for the neural recovery of the left side.

the expected abnormalities are obvious or as a means of determining the range of stimuli for further tests.

In *methods of levels* a specific stimulus intensity is delivered, and the subject signals whether the stimulus is detected or is painful. In adaptive methods, such as the staircase procedure, the response is used to modify the intensity of future stimulation to track a specific subjective level, such as pain threshold of moderate pain.[65] Usually this method requires longer examination times; however, it is more accurate and reliable.

Additional QST methods assess a subject's ability to discriminate in space rather than by sensory intensity. The *two-point discrimination test* assesses the differentiation between two mechanical punctuate stimuli placed at variable distances on the skin. The recorded variable is the distance between stimuli while the stimulus intensity is fixed. This test has been used to evaluate nerve repair after surgery.[66,67] The two-point discrimination values on the face, lips (5 mm), and fingers (2 or 3 mm) are lower (more sensitive) than on the back (39 mm) or abdomen (30 mm).

A quantitative sensory examination usually must assess sensitivity at a number of locations. At the very least, the painful, neighboring, and contralateral sites should be systematically mapped for pain and detection thresholds (Case 3-1; Figs 3-3 and 3-4). Sensory alterations beyond the primary site may indicate systemic disease or centrally mediat-

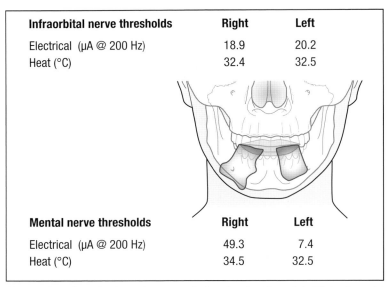

Infraorbital nerve thresholds	Right	Left
Electrical (µA @ 200 Hz)	18.9	20.2
Heat (°C)	32.4	32.5

Mental nerve thresholds	Right	Left
Electrical (µA @ 200 Hz)	49.3	7.4
Heat (°C)	34.5	32.5

Fig 3-3 Location of pain and sensory dysfunction for Case 3-1. Bilateral mental paresthesia (*gray areas*) 3 days after insertion of dental implants. Sensory testing was performed with electrical and thermal stimuli. The right side demonstrated elevated heat-detection and electrical detection thresholds, indicating nerve damage. The left side demonstrated a normal heat-detection threshold and a reduced electrical detection threshold, indicating neuritis (inflammation).

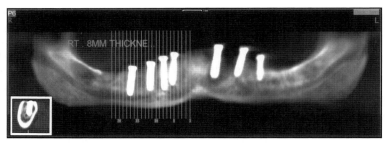

Fig 3-4 CT scan of the patient's mandible in Case 3-1. The CT scan demonstrates the inserted implants and the proximity of the most distal implant on the right side to the inferior alveolar canal. Inset is a section through this area confirming that the implant had penetrated the canal.

ed conditions requiring further tests. Case 3-1 demonstrates the diagnostic and therapeutic applicability of QST techniques in a patient complaining of bilateral numbness in the area of the mental nerve.

Levels of sensation

An increasing stimulus can be described by three simple levels of sensation: detection threshold, pain threshold, and pain tolerance. The threshold value describes the transition be-

tween the presence and qualities of sensation; in simple terms, these describe the lowest stimulus level that is detected, produces pain, or is unbearably painful. More complete descriptions include a level of probability. For example, the detection threshold can be described as a level that is sensed 50% or 75% of the time. Pain tolerance is defined as the highest stimulus level that a subject will willingly tolerate for stimuli with controllable magnitudes or, in the case of stimuli that are uncontrolled, such as tourniquet ischemia, the length of time the stimulus is endured. This latter class of stimuli is rarely used in QST but is occasionally used in studies examining the recruitment of endogenous inhibitory controls in response to pain.[68,69] In the presence of pathologic states, both the pain and detection thresholds can be reduced or elevated.

Modalities and nerve fibers

Specific QST modalities selectively activate different sensory nerve fibers that fall into four major groups. Aα fibers are characterized by a thick coat of myelin (12 to 22 mm in diameter, conduction velocity of 70 to 120 m/s) and conduct stimuli from neuromuscular spindles and Golgi tendon organs. Aβ fibers have a slightly thinner myelin coat (6 to 12 mm in diameter, conduction velocity of 35 to 70 m/s) and mediate touch and vibratory sensations. Aβ fibers are preferentially activated by pulsed electrical stimuli at the threshold for detection.

Nociceptive and thermal stimuli are transmitted by thinner fibers. Aδ fibers possess a thin myelinated sheath (1 to 5 mm in diameter, conduction velocity of 4 to 30 m/s) and are activated mainly by cold stimuli, fast-onset mechanical stimuli, radiant (including laser) heat, and punctuate mechanical stimulation, such as a sharp pin. C fibers are unmyelinated (0.3 to 1.5 mm in diameter, conduction velocity of 0.4 to 2.0 m/s) and make up 60% to 90% of the cutaneous nerve fibers that are activated by heat stimuli. The polymodal nociceptors are an important subclass of C fibers that respond to chemical, mechanical, and thermal nociceptive stimuli.

The most commonly used stimulus modalities for QST are mechanical, thermal, electrical, and chemical. Each stimulus modality has unique characteristics and clinical relevance.

Mechanical stimuli

Mechanical stimuli evoke sensations of prickle, vibration, pressure, or touch. The tools used to evoke mechanical sensations include calibrated von Frey (or Semmes-Weinstein) monofilaments for punctuate stimulation or electronic devices for quantitative punctuate or vibration stimulation. A blunt needle (eg, safety pin) or dental explorer can be used to test for sharp pain or a pricking sensation (pinprick). Pressure algometers provide quantitative values of blunt-pressure sensitivity and are used mainly to assess the pressure pain threshold. A cotton swab can assess light touch over a larger area and, along with other stimuli, such as an artist's brush or gauze, can provide a moving stimulus that is particularly effective for demonstrating dynamic mechanical allodynia.

Mechanical stimuli are translated to neural activity by several types of receptors. These receptors can be classified as fast adapting or slow adapting and are defined by the rate of decline in neural activity during stimulation. Fast-adapting receptors are made of Meissner corpuscles, hair receptors, and Pacinian corpuscles. Slow-adapting receptors are made of Merkel cell–neurite complexes, touch pads, and Ruffini endings. Proprioception is mediated by muscle spindles located in muscle and by Golgi tendon organs, which attach the muscles to bone and joint capsules and contain a group of endings similar in structure to the tactile receptors. Sensations evoked by vibration and light mechanical stimuli are conducted via the large Aβ myelinated nerve fibers described earlier.

Altered response to vibration has been found in diabetic neuropathy[70] (though not as severe and not as common as the altered response to heat) and in toxic and chemotherapy-related neuropathies.[71] Uremic neuropathy and chronic inflammatory demyelinating polyradiculoneuropathies predominantly affect large myelinated fibers.[72,73] Allodynia to pressure has been observed over an inflamed joint; however, long-term arthritic conditions (> 5 years) have been associated with hyposensitivity to light touch.[74]

In orofacial evaluations, practitioners assess mechanical allodynia by tapping a tooth to diagnose periapical, periodontal, or other dental pathologies (see chapter 6). Prolonged hyperalgesia to cold stimuli on the tooth crown is pathognomonic of irreversible pulpitis. Elevated mechanical detection thresholds have been observed in an experimental model of muscular orofacial pain,[75] and an elevated vibrotactile threshold has been observed on the cheek skin in patients with TMDs.[76] Increased sensitivity (allodynia) has been evaluated in the gingivae of patients diagnosed with atypical odontalgia,[77] and hyperalgesia (reduced pain thresh-

Peltier effect

old) was found up to 30 days after extraction of third molars.[78] Reduced detection thresholds to electrical and mechanical stimuli have been demonstrated in the lingual and mental dermatomes 2 days after simple third molar extractions, normalizing to baseline levels 8 days after the procedure.[79] Muscle and generalized hypersensitivity are also consistently found in patients with fibromyalgia.[61,80–82]

Thermal stimuli

Thermoreceptors are histologically described as having free, nonspecialized nerve endings. In general, thermoreceptors are divided into low- and high-threshold receptors. Low-threshold receptors are activated by temperatures between 15°C and 45°C; they are usually not painful, and the brief stimulus durations usually used for assessment do not damage tissue. High-threshold receptors respond mainly to temperatures higher than 45°C and lower than 15°C. The warm sensation is conducted mostly via the slowly conducting unmyelinated C fibers, whereas the thinly myelinated Aδ fibers largely mediate cold sensation and are also responsible for the sensation of pricking heat pain.

The receptor channels that are involved in thermal sensation are the vanilloid receptor subtype 1, which is activated by temperatures above 41°C; the vanilloid receptor–like type 1, which is activated by temperatures above 50°C; and the cold menthol receptor type 1, which is activated by a temperature range of 2°C to 7°C. Interestingly, these receptors are activated by chemical compounds such as capsaicin (the active component in hot chili pepper), which reduces the channel-opening temperature significantly in vanilloid receptor subtype 1 and vanilloid receptor–like type 1, whereas the menthol-related compounds increase the sensitivity to cold via cold menthol receptor type 1.

For both cold and warm sensations, the range of temperatures between 29°C and 37°C is an adaptation zone. Application of an experimental stimulus or natural object within this temperature zone is initially felt as warm or cold on the skin or mucosa but becomes neutral within minutes. This phenomenon of thermal adaptation must be considered while assessing the detection threshold; continuous or prolonged application may lead to erroneous values.

The temperatures people report as painful vary, although temperatures above 45°C and below 15°C are generally considered to be painful. Of importance to note is that temperatures above 50°C and below 0°C can cause notable tissue damage. Thermal stimuli can be applied by heated objects, water, coolant sprays, or more modern devices based on electrical, radiant, or laser heat, whereas thermal stimuli based on the Peltier effect or circulating fluids can be used for both heat and cold stimulation.

Stimulus assessment can be affected by skin temperature. Under normal conditions, the temperature of the face skin is slightly elevated compared with that of the rest of the body (33°C to 34°C versus 30°C to 33°C),[83] and the temperatures of the mucosa and tongue are higher still (34°C to 35°C and 36°C to 37°C, respectively).[84] Heat stimuli applied within the oral cavity are affected by mucosal thickness and the presence and quantity of saliva. In the dental office, simple cold and heat sensory tests are commonly used to assess tooth pathology, as described earlier (see also chapter 5). Prolonged and intense thermally evoked pain suggests pulpitis, but a lack of response may indicate a nonvital tooth.

Thermal tests provide information about the function of unmyelinated (C fibers) and thinly myelinated (Aδ fibers) fibers. Heat stimuli can provide a fast initial Aδ response, but slow onset rates or repeated stimulation of the same location evoke C-fiber–mediated sensations (Gracely, unpublished data). Aδ fibers are also tested by cold stimulation. Altered thermal pain and detection thresholds have been reported in diabetic neuropathy,[64,85,86] postherpetic neuralgia,[87] fibromyalgia,[81,88,89] chronic pelvic pain syndrome,[90] and small-fiber sensory polyneuropathy.[91]

In the orofacial area, the results of studies applying thermal stimuli to assess patients with burning mouth syndrome have been less conclusive (see chapter 12). Thermal detection thresholds were similar in patients with burning mouth syndrome and healthy volunteers, but thermal pain tolerance was significantly lower in patients with burning mouth syndrome.[92–94] Studies in patients with trigeminal neuralgia (see chapter 11) have found increased thresholds to warm and cold that are resolved after neurosurgical decompression of the trigeminal nerve root.[95,96] The thermal detection threshold has been found to be elevated in patients suffering from chronic sinusitis or after acute facial trauma.[97,98] Patients suffering from posttraumatic trigeminal neuropathy demonstrated a longer duration of aftersensation with cold stimulus applied to the affected gingivae.[99]

Chemical stimulation

As stated earlier, chemical compounds such as capsaicin and menthol can alter the performance of thermal receptors. Capsaicin, bee venom, or mustard oil are used to induce experimental dermal, mucosal (nasal, gastric), muscular, or tooth pain.[100–102] Intramuscular infusion of hypertonic saline is used to induce experimental muscular orofacial pain,[75,103] as discussed in chapter 7.

The pain induced by chemical compounds may be specific, but there is poor control of stimulus magnitude and resultant pain sensations and minimal, if any, application for clinical pain assessment. Various chemical compounds are useful for evaluating taste and smell, and in dental practice, pain induced by sweet compounds can be an important sign for exposed dentin and deep caries.

Electrical stimulation

Electrical nerve stimulation evokes a nonnatural sensation that is used extensively for sensory testing, sometimes with conflicting and inconsistent results.[104,105] However, electrical stimulation provides unique and useful properties for sensory assessment. Unlike other methods that naturally stimulate nerve receptors, electrical stimuli bypass the receptor to stimulate the primary afferent axon. As a result, primary neurons activated by electrical stimulation do not show the same temporal profile regarding sensitization, suppression, or fatigue. In addition, at the threshold for detection, electrical stimuli exclusively activate the thickly myelinated fibers (Aβ fibers). Thus, a comparison of the detection threshold for both mechanical and electrical stimuli can provide a differential method that isolates receptor and postreceptor processes in Aβ fibers. Changes in both thresholds, or

in only the electrical detection threshold, indicate a postreceptor process, whereas isolated changes in mechanical stimulation indicate a receptor process.

As previously stated, interpatient variability is a common problem in QST, particularly with electrical sensory assessment. This inconsistency can be reduced by expressing the electrical detection thresholds as the ratio between the pathologic and the contralateral control side.[63] A study assessing sensory changes in patients with diabetic neuropathy showed that the electrical perception threshold to a high-frequency stimulus (2,000 Hz) correlated best with vibratory thresholds (large myelinated fibers), and the low-frequency stimulus (5 Hz) correlated with thresholds to warm sensations.[106]

In dentistry, electrical stimulation is used to assess tooth vitality; however, stimulus, or response intensity, does not correlate with tooth pathology. Electrical stimulation is used to assess taste and function of the chorda tympani nerve.[107,108] An elevated taste threshold has been found in the chorda tympani nerve of patients with burning mouth syndrome.[109,110] The electrical detection threshold is reduced (hypersensitivity) in joint-related TMDs,[111] in early oral malignancy,[112] in the first days after extraction of the third molars,[79] and in patients suffering from acute sinusitis.[97] An elevated detection threshold (hyposensitivity) is found in muscle-related TMDs,[111] in chronic sinusitis, and in the delayed phase after facial trauma.[98]

Dynamic psychophysical testing

A growing body of evidence suggests that a new generation of dynamic pain psychophysical testing is able to evaluate modulation processes in addition to the thresholds or suprathreshold magnitudes that can be evaluated with static pain psychophysical testing. Dynamic testing relies on the fact that pain perception is the result of data generated from the peripheral nervous system and then modulated in the central nervous system before it arrives in the cortex and the consciousness. Similar external stimuli may evoke different perceptions among different people, depending on their modulation processes. Two modulation components are routinely tested in the laboratory: (1) temporal summation, which is thought to be the psy-

Chronic pain after root canal treatment, associated with altered pain modulation.

Present complaint: Persistent, mild, spontaneous pain as well as sensitivity to cold and light touch in the gingiva apical to the maxillary left second premolar.

History of present complaint: Eleven months ago, the patient underwent root canal treatment in the maxillary left second premolar. The tooth was asymptomatic and nonvital before treatment. In the first days after treatment, the patient experienced severe pain in the tooth area (8/10 on the VAS) that subsided to mild pain (4/10 on the VAS) a couple of weeks after the procedure and remained at this intensity.

Examination: The head and neck examination was unremarkable. QST using thermal and mechanical stimuli was performed extraorally in the mental and infraorbital nerve dermatomes and intraorally in the gingivae apical to the second premolars. Testing revealed that response to cold stimulation in the painful area (the area apical to the second left premolar) was prolonged; the cold pain sensation continued for almost a minute after removal of the cold stimulus compared with 5 to 10 seconds after a similar stimulus in any other tested area (see Fig 3-5). Response to 26 g and 2 g of mechanical stimulation was significantly more painful in the affected area than in all the other tested areas.

The patient's pain-modulation system (CPM) was assessed by immersion of the nondominant hand to the wrist level in a hot water bath serving as the conditioning stimulus and repeated mechanical stimulation with a 26-g filament as the test stimulus. The subject was asked to report a number reflecting the level of stimulus intensity on a VAS of 1 through 100. Normally, pain intensity induced by a mechanical stimulus in the presence of a conditioning stimulus (a hand in a hot water bath in this case) is significantly lower than the response when there is no other stimulus. In this case, there was no difference between the pain intensity with or without a conditioning stimulus.

Relevant medical history: None.

Diagnosis: The history and findings indicated posttraumatic trigeminal neuropathic pain induced by root canal treatment. A faulty pain-modulation system may support the development and/or maintenance of this condition.

Treatment: Any further dental treatments in the area have been stopped. The patient was treated with a topical combination of ketoprofen, duloxetine, and pregabalin delivered by a neurostent (see Fig 3-5). A significant reduction in pain levels was achieved within 2 weeks.

---

chophysical correlate of second- or third-order neuron windup, probably reflecting central sensitization, and *(2)* conditioned pain modulation (CPM), which is the human psychophysical equivalent of diffuse noxious inhibitory control.

Temporal summation is associated with excessive activation of *N*-methyl-D-aspartate receptors in response to extensive nociceptive input. The clinical manifestation may be allodynia and hyperalgesia.[113–115] Temporal summation is tested by applying identical repetitive stimuli and determining whether an increase in pain scores is documented along or at the end of the stimuli. CPM represents the endogenous analgesia system, where descending pathways induce modulatory effects on incoming painful stimuli. This phenomenon is based on a spinal-bulbar-spinal loop under cerebral control, which is at least partially opioid mediated.[116] Animal studies demonstrated the role of spinal serotonin and noradrenaline in mediation of pain inhibition and CPM.[117–119] CPM is tested by using two remote noxious stimuli, with one (the conditioning pain) inhibiting the other (the test pain). In recent years, many reports used both temporal summation and CPM to demonstrate altered pain modulation in patients with chronic pain. Enhanced temporal summation was found in such chronic pain conditions as fibromyalgia,[120–123] tension headache and musculoskeletal pain,[124,125] migraine,[126] chronic low back pain,[127] and TMDs.[128–132] Similarly, a less efficient CPM response was found in many idiopathic pain syndromes, such as TMDs,[69] fibromyalgia,[89,123,133,134] tension headache,[135] and irritable bowel syndrome.[136] Among healthy subjects, reduced pain-modulatory capacity was demonstrated in older subjects[137] and was more frequent among females compared with males.[138] A combination of reduced CPM and temporal summation was found among patients with chronic pain after endodontic treatment (Case 3-2; Fig 3-5) (Nasri-Heir et al, unpublished data, 2015).

Researchers have suggested that the pain-modulatory system can define susceptibility to the development of chronic pain disorders.[139–142] Patients who presented with altered pain modulation were found to be more prone to develop postoperative (thoracotomy) chronic pain.[143] Moreover, a recent study showed that patients with painful diabetic neuropathy and less efficient CPM benefited from treatment with duloxetine,[144] which has the potential to enhance the descending pain inhibition by inhibiting reuptake of spinal noradrenaline and serotonin.[144–146]

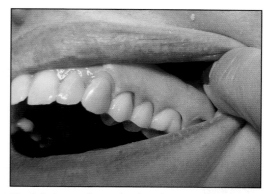

Fig 3-5 An acrylic overlay (stent) to the area affected by neuropathic pain in Case 3-2. The surface facing the gingival tissues is concave, forming a "bath" for the topical medication.

Clinical relevance of QST

QST is an accepted tool for assessing diabetic neuropathies[147] and other sensory abnormalities.[148] Although it is an important tool, however, currently QST cannot be used alone to diagnose neuropathies.[147] The results of thermal and electrical QST offer insight as to the pathologic processes in the peripheral nerves (see Case 3-1).

Mechanical nerve damage, or total nerve transection, is characterized by myelinated and unmyelinated nerve fiber hyposensitivity that can be clinically translated to elevated detection thresholds to heat, electrical, and mechanical stimulation.[149] Partial damage may be followed by hyposensitivity or hypersensitivity accompanied by ongoing neuropathic pain.[98,150,151] In contrast to the neuropathic process of mechanical nerve damage, other specific nociceptive processes may provide a different, identifiable sensory signature. For example, early perineural inflammation produces short-lasting hypersensitivity of large, myelinated nerve fibers that is clinically revealed by reduced detection to electrical and mechanical stimuli. This increased sensitivity has been demonstrated in clinical and animal spinal nerve models[79,112,152–155] and reproduced in a model of inflammatory trigeminal nerve neuropathy.[151]

QST can add a further dimension to pain evaluation. For example, *allodynia* is defined as pain due to a stimulus that normally does not evoke pain. By using QST, a practitioner can distinguish between several allodynic conditions. By definition, the pain threshold is reduced in all cases of allodynia; however, the detection threshold and pain tolerance can decrease, increase, or remain unchanged. Measurements such as the interval between detection and pain thresholds and the detection to pain ratio can be useful in these conditions. These features have been shown to have clinical significance in the assessment of centrally mediated pain conditions.[156]

Hyperalgesia is defined as an increased response to a stimulus that is normally painful. Pain intensity can be measured with one of the tools described previously (most commonly, the VAS). However, similar to allodynia, there are several types of hyperalgesic conditions. Heat hyperalgesia, for example, is related to thin unmyelinated nerve fibers, whereas tactile hyperalgesia may suggest involvement of myelinated fibers (see chapter 12). Moreover, any stimulus applied can vary in intensity, frequency, or rate change (increasing or decreasing rate).

A notable attempt at QST standardization was made by the German Research Network on Neuropathic Pain.[157] Systematic sequences of thermal and mechanical QST were used on patients suffering from various neuropathic pain conditions. The findings were categorized as gain and loss of sensation. Of the patients, 92% presented at least one sensory abnormality, and a sensory profile was suggested for each neurologic syndrome. However, combinations of gain and loss sensations were found to be shared across the syndromes.

The use of QST in the trigeminal system or other orofacial areas requires further research before being adopted in routine clinical practice; however, the field is sufficiently developed to aid in the diagnosis and evaluation of treatment.[158]

References

1. Wall PD. On the relation of injury to pain. The John J. Bonica lecture. Pain 1979;6:253–264.
2. Ortiz JP, Close LN, Heinricher MM, Selden NR. Alpha(2)-noradrenergic antagonist administration into the central nucleus of the amygdala blocks stress-induced hypoalgesia in awake behaving rats. Neuroscience 2008;157:223–228.
3. Ragan AR, Lesniak A, Bochynska-Czyz M, et al. Chronic mild stress facilitates melanoma tumor growth in mouse lines selected for high and low stress-induced analgesia. Stress 2013;16:571–580.
4. Huskisson EC, Sturrock RD, Tugwell P. Measurement of patient outcome. Br J Rheumatol 1983;22(suppl 3):86–89.
5. Joyce CR, Zutshi DW, Hrubes V, Mason RM. Comparison of fixed interval and visual analogue scales for rating chronic pain. Eur J Clin Pharmacol 1975;8:415–420.
6. Sriwatanakul K, Kelvie W, Lasagna L, Calimlim JF, Weis OF, Mehta G. Studies with different types of visual analog scales for measurement of pain. Clin Pharmacol Ther 1983;34:234–239.
7. Rosier EM, Iadarola MJ, Coghill RC. Reproducibility of pain measurement and pain perception. Pain 2002;98:205–216.
8. Yarnitsky D, Sprecher E. Thermal testing: Normative data and repeatability for various test algorithms. J Neurol Sci 1994;125:39–45.
9. Bieri D, Reeve RA, Champion GD, Addicoat L, Ziegler JB. The Faces Pain Scale for the self-assessment of the severity of pain experienced by children: Development, initial validation, and preliminary investigation for ratio scale properties. Pain 1990;41:139–150.
10. Wong DL, Baker CM. Smiling faces as anchor for pain intensity scales. Pain 2001;89:295–300.
11. Chang J, Versloot J, Fashler SR, McCrystal KN, Craig KD. Pain assessment in children: Validity of facial expression items in observational pain scales. Clin J Pain 2015;31:189–197.
12. Quinn BL, Sheldon LK, Cooley ME. Pediatric pain assessment by drawn faces scales: A review. Pain Manag Nurs 2014;15:909–918.
13. Jensen MP, Karoly P, Huger R. The development and preliminary validation of an instrument to assess patients' attitudes toward pain. J Psychosom Res 1987;31:393–400.
14. Naliboff BD, Munakata J, Fullerton S, et al. Evidence for two distinct perceptual alterations in irritable bowel syndrome. Gut 1997;41:505–512.
15. Sternberg WF, Bokat C, Kass L, Alboyadjian A, Gracely RH. Sex-dependent components of the analgesia produced by athletic competition. J Pain 2001;2:65–74.
16. Gagliese L, Melzack R. Chronic pain in elderly people. Pain 1997;70:3–14.
17. Herr KA, Spratt K, Mobily PR, Richardson G. Pain intensity assessment in older adults: Use of experimental pain to compare psychometric properties and usability of selected pain scales with younger adults. Clin J Pain 2004;20:207–219.
18. Gracely RH. Measuring pain in the clinic. Anesth Prog 1990;37:88–92.
19. Graven-Nielsen T, McArdle A, Phoenix J, et al. In vivo model of muscle pain: Quantification of intramuscular chemical, electrical, and pressure changes associated with saline-induced muscle pain in humans. Pain 1997;69:137–143.
20. Gendreau M, Hufford MR, Stone AA. Measuring clinical pain in chronic widespread pain: Selected methodological issues. Best Pract Res Clin Rheumatol 2003;17:575–592.
21. Jamison RN, Gracely RH, Raymond SA, et al. Comparative study of electronic vs. paper VAS ratings: A randomized, crossover trial using healthy volunteers. Pain 2002;99:341–347.
22. Melzack R. The McGill Pain Questionnaire: Major properties and scoring methods. Pain 1975;1:277–299.
23. Gaston-Johansson F, Albert M, Fagan E, Zimmerman L. Similarities in pain descriptions of four different ethnic-culture groups. J Pain Symptom Manage 1990;5:94–100.
24. Melzack R, Terrence C, Fromm G, Amsel R. Trigeminal neuralgia and atypical facial pain: Use of the McGill Pain Questionnaire for discrimination and diagnosis. Pain 1986;27:297–302.
25. Burchiel KJ, Anderson VC, Brown FD, et al. Prospective, multicenter study of spinal cord stimulation for relief of chronic back and extremity pain. Spine 1996;21:2786–2794.
26. Nikolajsen L, Hansen CL, Nielsen J, Keller J, Arendt-Nielsen L, Jensen TS. The effect of ketamine on phantom pain: A central neuropathic disorder maintained by peripheral input. Pain 1996;67:69–77.
27. Tesfaye S, Watt J, Benbow SJ, Pang KA, Miles J, MacFarlane IA. Electrical spinal-cord stimulation for painful diabetic peripheral neuropathy. Lancet 1996;348:1698–1701.
28. Grushka M, Sessle BJ. Applicability of the McGill Pain Questionnaire to the differentiation of 'toothache' pain. Pain 1984;19:49–57.

29. Grönblad M, Lukinmaa A, Konttinen YT. Chronic low-back pain: Intercorrelation of repeated measures for pain and disability. Scand J Rehabil Med 1990;22:73–77.

30. Harden RN, Carter TD, Gilman CS, Gross AJ, Peters JR. Ketorolac in acute headache management. Headache 1991;31:463–464.

31. McGuire DB, Altomonte V, Peterson DE, Wingard JR, Jones RJ, Grochow LB. Patterns of mucositis and pain in patients receiving preparative chemotherapy and bone marrow transplantation. Oncol Nurs Forum 1993;20:1493–1502.

32. Turk DC, Rudy TE. Toward an empirically derived taxonomy of chronic pain patients: Integration of psychological assessment data. J Consult Clin Psychol 1988;56:233–238.

33. Turk DC, Rudy TE. The robustness of an empirically derived taxonomy of chronic pain patients. Pain 1990;43:27–35.

34. Dworkin SF, LeResche L. Research diagnostic criteria for temporomandibular disorders: Review, criteria, examinations and specifications, critique. J Craniomandib Disord 1992;6:301–355.

35. Schiffman E, Ohrbach R, Truelove E, et al. Diagnostic Criteria for Temporomandibular Disorders (DC/TMD) for clinical and research applications: Recommendations of the International RDC/TMD Consortium Network and Orofacial Pain Special Interest Group. J Oral Facial Pain Headache 2014;28:6–27.

36. John MT, Dworkin SF, Mancl LA. Reliability of clinical temporomandibular disorder diagnoses. Pain 2005;118:61–69.

37. Schiffman EL, Ohrbach R, Truelove EL, et al. The Research Diagnostic Criteria for Temporomandibular Disorders. V: Methods used to establish and validate revised Axis I diagnostic algorithms. J Orofac Pain 2010;24:63–78.

38. Schiffman EL, Truelove EL, Ohrbach R, et al. The Research Diagnostic Criteria for Temporomandibular Disorders. I: Overview and methodology for assessment of validity. J Orofac Pain 2010;24:7–24.

39. Steenks MH, de Wijer A. Validity of the Research Diagnostic Criteria for Temporomandibular Disorders Axis I in clinical and research settings. J Orofac Pain 2009;23:9–16.

40. Truelove E, Pan W, Look JO, et al. The Research Diagnostic Criteria for Temporomandibular Disorders. III: Validity of Axis I diagnoses. J Orofac Pain 2010;24:35–47.

41. de Leeuw R, Klasser GD. Orofacial Pain: Guidelines for Assessment, Diagnosis, and Management, ed 5. Chicago: Quintessence, 2013.

42. Headache Classification Committee of the International Headache Society. The International Classification of Headache Disorders, 3rd edition (beta version). Cephalalgia 2013;33:629–808.

43. Merskey H, Bogduk N. Classification of Chronic Pain: Descriptions of Chronic Pain Syndromes and Definition of Pain Terms. Seattle: IASP Press, 1994.

44. LeResche L, Dworkin SF. Facial expression accompanying pain. Soc Sci Med 1984;19:1325–1330.

45. Carroll JM, Russell JA. Do facial expressions signal specific emotions? Judging emotion from the face in context. J Pers Soc Psychol 1996;70:205–218.

46. Drummond PD. Noradrenaline increases hyperalgesia to heat in skin sensitized by capsaicin. Pain 1995;60:311–315.

47. Drummond PD. Lacrimation and cutaneous vasodilatation in the face induced by painful stimulation of the nasal ala and upper lip. J Auton Nerv Syst 1995;51:109–116.

48. Glaros AG, Glass EG, Brockman D. Electromyographic data from TMD patients with myofascial pain and from matched control subjects: Evidence for statistical, not clinical, significance. J Orofac Pain 1997;11:125–129.

49. Gramling SE, Grayson RL, Sullivan TN, Schwartz S. Schedule-induced masseter EMG in facial pain subjects vs. no-pain controls. Physiol Behav 1997;61:301–309.

50. Liu ZJ, Yamagata K, Kasahara Y, Ito G. Electromyographic examination of jaw muscles in relation to symptoms and occlusion of patients with temporomandibular joint disorders. J Oral Rehabil 1999;26:33–47.

51. Sharav Y, Tal M. Hypnotic analgesia and reflex activity. Pain 1995;63:391–392.

52. Tal M, Sharav Y. Development of sensory and reflex responses to tooth-pulp stimulation in children. Arch Oral Biol 1985;30:467–470.

53. Tal M. The threshold for eliciting the jaw opening reflex in rats is not increased by neonatal capsaicin. Behav Brain Res 1984;13:197–200.

54. Weidner C, Schmelz M, Schmidt R, et al. Neural signal processing: The underestimated contribution of peripheral human C-fibers. J Neurosci 2002;22:6704–6712.

55. Weidner C, Schmidt R, Schmelz M, Hilliges M, Handwerker HO, Torebjork HE. Time course of post-excitatory effects separates afferent human C fibre classes. J Physiol 2000;527:185–191.

56. Weidner C, Schmidt R, Schmelz M, Torebjork HE, Handwerker HO. Action potential conduction in the terminal arborisation of nociceptive C-fibre afferents. J Physiol 2003;547:931–940.

57. Jääskeläinen SK, Teerijoki-Oksa T, Forssell H. Neurophysiologic and quantitative sensory testing in the diagnosis of trigeminal neuropathy and neuropathic pain. Pain 2005;117:349–357.

58. Bentley DE, Derbyshire SW, Youell PD, Jones AK. Caudal cingulate cortex involvement in pain processing: An inter-individual laser evoked potential source localisation study using realistic head models. Pain 2003;102:265–271.

59. Frot M, Mauguière F. Dual representation of pain in the operculo-insular cortex in humans. Brain 2003;126:438–450.

60. Coghill RC, Gilron I, Iadarola MJ. Hemispheric lateralization of somatosensory processing. J Neurophysiol 2001;85:2602–2612.

61. Gracely RH, Grant MA, Giesecke T. Evoked pain measures in fibromyalgia. Best Pract Res Clin Rheumatol 2003;17:593–609.

62. Davis KD, Racine E, Collett B. Neuroethical issues related to the use of brain imaging: Can we and should we use brain imaging as a biomarker to diagnose chronic pain? Pain 2012;153:1555–1559.

63. Kemler MA, Schouten HJ, Gracely RH. Diagnosing sensory abnormalities with either normal values or values from contralateral skin: Comparison of two approaches in complex regional pain syndrome I. Anesthesiology 2000;93:718–727.

64. Dyck PJ, Karnes JL, Gillen DA, O'Brien PC, Zimmerman IR, Johnson DM. Comparison of algorithms of testing for use in automated evaluation of sensation. Neurology 1990;40:1607–1613.

65. Gracely RH, Lota L, Walter DJ, Dubner R. A multiple random staircase method of psychophysical pain assessment. Pain 1988;32:55–63.

66. Ziccardi VB, Dragoo J, Eliav E, Benoliel R. Comparison of current perception threshold electrical testing to clinical sensory testing for lingual nerve injuries. J Oral Maxillofac Surg 2012;70:289–294.

67. Ziccardi VB, Steinberg MJ. Timing of trigeminal nerve microsurgery: A review of the literature. J Oral Maxillofac Surg 2007;65:1341–1345.

68. Oono Y, Baad-Hansen L, Wang K, Arendt-Nielsen L, Svensson P. Effect of conditioned pain modulation on trigeminal somatosensory function evaluated by quantitative sensory testing. Pain 2013;154:2684–2690.

69. Maixner W, Fillingim R, Booker D, Sigurdsson A. Sensitivity of patients with painful temporomandibular disorders to experimentally evoked pain. Pain 1995;63:341–351.

70. Guy RJ, Clark CA, Malcolm PN, Watkins PJ. Evaluation of thermal and vibration sensation in diabetic neuropathy. Diabetologia 1985;28:131–137.

71. Chaudhry V, Rowinsky EK, Sartorius SE, Donehower RC, Cornblath DR. Peripheral neuropathy from taxol and cisplatin combination chemotherapy: Clinical and electrophysiological studies. Ann Neurol 1994;35:304–311.

72. Tegnér R, Lindholm B. Vibratory perception threshold compared with nerve conduction velocity in the evaluation of uremic neuropathy. Acta Neurol Scand 1985;71:284–289.

73. Krajewski KM, Lewis RA, Fuerst DR, et al. Neurological dysfunction and axonal degeneration in Charcot-Marie-Tooth disease type 1A. Brain 2000;123(Pt 7):1516–1527.

74. Leffler AS, Hansson P, Kosek E. Somatosensory perception in a remote pain-free area and function of diffuse noxious inhibitory controls in patients suffering from long-term trapezius myalgia. Eur J Pain 2002;6:149–159.

75. Stohler CS, Kowalski CJ, Lund JP. Muscle pain inhibits cutaneous touch perception. Pain 2001;92:327–333.

76. Hollins M, Sigurdsson A, Fillingim L, Goble AK. Vibrotactile threshold is elevated in temporomandibular disorders. Pain 1996;67:89–96.

77. List T, Leijon G, Helkimo M, Oster A, Svensson P. Effect of local anesthesia on atypical odontalgia—A randomized controlled trial. Pain 2006;122:306–314.

78. Juhl GI, Svensson P, Norholt SE, Jensen TS. Long-lasting mechanical sensitization following third molar surgery. J Orofac Pain 2006;20:59–73.

79. Eliav E, Gracely RH. Sensory changes in the territory of the lingual and inferior alveolar nerves following lower third molar extraction. Pain 1998;77:191–199.

80. Giesecke T, Williams DA, Harris RE, et al. Subgrouping of fibromyalgia patients on the basis of pressure-pain thresholds and psychological factors. Arthritis Rheum 2003;48:2916–2922.

81. Petzke F, Clauw DJ, Ambrose K, Khine A, Gracely RH. Increased pain sensitivity in fibromyalgia: Effects of stimulus type and mode of presentation. Pain 2003;105:403–413.

82. Alonso-Blanco C, Fernández-de-las-Peñas C, Morales-Cabezas M, Zarco-Moreno P, Ge HY, Florez-García M. Multiple active myofascial trigger points reproduce the overall spontaneous pain pattern in women with fibromyalgia and are related to widespread mechanical hypersensitivity. Clin J Pain 2011;27:405–413.

83. Verdugo RJ, Bell LA, Campero M, et al. Spectrum of cutaneous hyperalgesias/allodynias in neuropathic pain patients. Acta Neurol Scand 2004;110:368–376.

84. Green BG, Gelhard B. Perception of temperature on oral and facial skin. Somatosens Res 1987;4:191–200.

85. Report and recommendations of the San Antonio conference on diabetic neuropathy. Consensus statement [editorial]. Diabetes 1988;37:1000–1004.

86. Navarro X, Kennedy WR. Evaluation of thermal and pain sensitivity in type I diabetic patients. J Neurol Neurosurg Psychiatry 1991;54:60–64.

87. Rowbotham MC, Fields HL. The relationship of pain, allodynia and thermal sensation in post-herpetic neuralgia. Brain 1996;119(Pt 2):347–354.

88. Geisser ME, Casey KL, Brucksch CB, Ribbens CM, Appleton BB, Crofford LJ. Perception of noxious and innocuous heat stimulation among healthy women and women with fibromyalgia: Association with mood, somatic focus, and catastrophizing. Pain 2003;102:243–250.

89. Lautenbacher S, Rollman GB. Possible deficiencies of pain modulation in fibromyalgia. Clin J Pain 1997;13:189–196.

90. Lee JC, Yang CC, Kromm BG, Berger RE. Neurophysiologic testing in chronic pelvic pain syndrome: A pilot study. Urology 2001;58:246–250.

91. Holland NR, Crawford TO, Hauer P, Cornblath DR, Griffin JW, McArthur JC. Small-fiber sensory neuropathies: Clinical course and neuropathology of idiopathic cases. Ann Neurol 1998;44:47–59.

92. Grushka M, Sessle BJ, Howley TP. Psychophysical assessment of tactile, pain and thermal sensory functions in burning mouth syndrome. Pain 1987;28:169–184.

93. Lamey PJ. Burning mouth syndrome. Dermatol Clin 1996;14:339–354.

94. Lamey PJ, Hobson RS, Orchardson R. Perception of stimulus size in patients with burning mouth syndrome. J Oral Pathol Med 1996;25:420–423.

95. Bowsher D, Miles JB, Haggett CE, Eldridge PR. Trigeminal neuralgia: A quantitative sensory perception threshold study in patients who had not undergone previous invasive procedures. J Neurosurg 1997;86:190–192.

96. Miles JB, Eldridge PR, Haggett CE, Bowsher D. Sensory effects of microvascular decompression in trigeminal neuralgia. J Neurosurg 1997;86:193–196.

97. Benoliel R, Biron A, Quek SY, Nahlieli O, Eliav E. Trigeminal neurosensory changes following acute and chronic paranasal sinusitis. Quintessence Int 2006;37:437–443.

98. Benoliel R, Birenboim R, Regev E, Eliav E. Neurosensory changes in the infraorbital nerve following zygomatic fractures. Oral Surg Oral Med Oral Pathol Oral Radiol Endod 2005;99:657–665.

99. Zagury JG, Eliav E, Heir GM, et al. Prolonged gingival cold allodynia: A novel finding in patients with atypical odontalgia. Oral Surg Oral Med Oral Pathol Oral Radiol Endod 2011;111:312–319.

100. Khalili N, Wendelschafer-Crabb G, Kennedy WR, Simone DA. Influence of thermode size for detecting heat pain dysfunction in a capsaicin model of epidermal nerve fiber loss. Pain 2001;91:241–250.

101. Coghill RC, Sang CN, Berman KF, Bennett GJ, Ladarola MJ. Global cerebral blood flow decreases during pain. J Cereb Blood Flow Metab 1998;18:141–147.

102. Sang CN, Hostetter MP, Gracely RH, et al. AMPA/kainate antagonist LY293558 reduces capsaicin-evoked hyperalgesia but not pain in normal skin in humans. Anesthesiology 1998;89:1060–1067.

103. Svensson P, Miles TS, Graven-Nielsen T, Arendt-Nielsen L. Modulation of stretch-evoked reflexes in single motor units in human masseter muscle by experimental pain. Exp Brain Res 2000;132:65–71.

104. Bendtsen L, Jensen RA, Olesen J. Decreased pain threshold and tolerance in patients with chronic tension headache [in Danish]. Ugeskr Laeger 1997;159:4521–4525.

105. Vecchiet L, Giamberardino MA, Saggini R. Myofascial pain syndromes: Clinical and pathophysiological aspects. Clin J Pain 1991;7(1, suppl):S16–S22.

106. Masson EA, Veves A, Fernando D, Boulton AJ. Current perception thresholds: A new, quick, and reproducible method for the assessment of peripheral neuropathy in diabetes mellitus. Diabetologia 1989;32:724–728.

107. Murphy C, Quinoñez C, Nordin S. Reliability and validity of electrogustometry and its application to young and elderly persons. Chem Senses 1995;20:499–503.

108. Yamada Y, Tomita H. Influences on taste in the area of chorda tympani nerve after transtympanic injection of local anesthetic (4% lidocaine). Auris Nasus Larynx 1989;16(1, suppl):S41–S46.

109. Eliav E, Kamran B, Schaham R, Czerninski R, Gracely RH, Benoliel R. Evidence of chorda tympani dysfunction in patients with burning mouth syndrome. J Am Dent Assoc 2007;138:628–633.

110. Nasri-Heir C, Gomes J, Heir GM, et al. The role of sensory input of the chorda tympani nerve and the number of fungiform papillae in burning mouth syndrome. Oral Surg Oral Med Oral Pathol Oral Radiol Endod 2011;112:65–72.

111. Eliav E, Teich S, Nitzan D, et al. Facial arthralgia and myalgia: Can they be differentiated by trigeminal sensory assessment? Pain 2003;104:481–490.

112. Eliav E, Teich S, Benoliel R, et al. Large myelinated nerve fiber hypersensitivity in oral malignancy. Oral Surg Oral Med Oral Pathol Oral Radiol Endod 2002;94:45–50.

113. Woolf CJ, Thompson SW. The induction and maintenance of central sensitization is dependent on N-methyl-D-aspartic acid receptor activation; implications for the treatment of post-injury pain hypersensitivity states. Pain 1991;44:293–299.

114. Arendt-Nielsen L, Petersen-Felix S, Fischer M, Bak P, Bjerring P, Zbinden AM. The effect of N-methyl-D-aspartate antagonist (ketamine) on single and repeated nociceptive stimuli: A placebo-controlled experimental human study. Anesth Analg 1995;81:63–68.

115. Eide PK. Wind-up and the NMDA receptor complex from a clinical perspective. Eur J Pain 2000;4:5–15.

116. Yaksh TL, Elde RP. Factors governing release of methionine enkephalin-like immunoreactivity from mesencephalon and spinal cord of the cat in vivo. J Neurophysiol 1981;46:1056–1075.

117. Lu Y, Perl ER. Selective action of noradrenaline and serotonin on neurones of the spinal superficial dorsal horn in the rat. J Physiol 2007;582:127–136.

118. Pedersen LH, Scheel-Krüger J, Blackburn-Munro G. Amygdala GABA-A receptor involvement in mediating sensory-discriminative and affective-motivational pain responses in a rat model of peripheral nerve injury. Pain 2007;127:17–26.

119. Pedersen LH, Nielsen AN, Blackburn-Munro G. Anti-nociception is selectively enhanced by parallel inhibition of multiple subtypes of monoamine transporters in rat models of persistent and neuropathic pain. Psychopharmacology (Berl) 2005;182:551–561.

120. Graven-Nielsen T, Aspegren Kendall S, Henriksson KG, et al. Ketamine reduces muscle pain, temporal summation, and referred pain in fibromyalgia patients. Pain 2000;85:483–491.

121. Staud R, Vierck CJ, Cannon RL, Mauderli AP, Price DD. Abnormal sensitization and temporal summation of second pain (wind-up) in patients with fibromyalgia syndrome. Pain 2001;91:165–175.

122. Price DD, Staud R, Robinson ME, Mauderli AP, Cannon R, Vierck CJ. Enhanced temporal summation of second pain and its central modulation in fibromyalgia patients. Pain 2002;99:49–59.

123. Staud R, Robinson ME, Vierck CJ Jr, Price DD. Diffuse noxious inhibitory controls (DNIC) attenuate temporal summation of second pain in normal males but not in normal females or fibromyalgia patients. Pain 2003;101:167–174.

124. Kleinböhl D, Hölzl R, Möltner A, Rommel C, Weber C, Osswald PM. Psychophysical measures of sensitization to tonic heat discriminate chronic pain patients. Pain 1999;81:35–43.

125. Ashina S, Bendtsen L, Ashina M, Magerl W, Jensen R. Generalized hyperalgesia in patients with chronic tension-type headache. Cephalalgia 2006;26:940–948.

126. Weissman-Fogel I, Sprecher E, Granovsky Y, Yarnitsky D. Repeated noxious stimulation of the skin enhances cutaneous pain perception of migraine patients in-between attacks: Clinical evidence for continuous sub-threshold increase in membrane excitability of central trigeminovascular neurons. Pain 2003;104:693–700.

127. Kleinböhl D, Görtelmeyer R, Bender HJ, Hölzl R. Amantadine sulfate reduces experimental sensitization and pain in chronic back pain patients. Anesth Analg 2006;102:840–847.

128. Sarlani E, Greenspan JD. Why look in the brain for answers to temporomandibular disorder pain? Cells Tissues Organs 2005;180:69–75.

129. Maixner W, Fillingim R, Sigurdsson A, Kincaid S, Silva S. Sensitivity of patients with painful temporomandibular disorders to experimentally evoked pain: Evidence for altered temporal summation of pain. Pain 1998;76:71–81.

130. Sarlani E, Grace EG, Reynolds MA, Greenspan JD. Sex differences in temporal summation of pain and aftersensations following repetitive noxious mechanical stimulation. Pain 2004;109:115–123.

131. Sarlani E, Grace EG, Reynolds MA, Greenspan JD. Evidence for up-regulated central nociceptive processing in patients with masticatory myofascial pain. J Orofac Pain 2004;18:41–55.

132. Raphael KG, Janal MN, Anathan S, Cook DB, Staud R. Temporal summation of heat pain in temporomandibular disorder patients. J Orofac Pain 2009;23:54–64.

133. Julien N, Goffaux P, Arsenault P, Marchand S. Widespread pain in fibromyalgia is related to a deficit of endogenous pain inhibition. Pain 2005;114:295–302.

134. Kosek E, Hansson P. Modulatory influence on somatosensory perception from vibration and heterotopic noxious conditioning stimulation (HNCS) in fibromyalgia patients and healthy subjects. Pain 1997;70:41–51.

135. Pielsticker A, Haag G, Zaudig M, Lautenbacher S. Impairment of pain inhibition in chronic tension-type headache. Pain 2005;118:215–223.

136. King CD, Wong F, Currie T, Mauderli AP, Fillingim RB, Riley JL 3rd. Deficiency in endogenous modulation of prolonged heat pain in patients with irritable bowel syndrome and temporomandibular disorder. Pain 2009;143:172–178.

137. Edwards RR, Fillingim RB, Ness TJ. Age-related differences in endogenous pain modulation: A comparison of diffuse noxious inhibitory controls in healthy older and younger adults. Pain 2003;101:155–165.

138. Fillingim RB, King CD, Ribeiro-Dasilva MC, Rahim-Williams B, Riley JL 3rd. Sex, gender, and pain: A review of recent clinical and experimental findings. J Pain 2009;10:447–485.

139. Pud D, Granovsky Y, Yarnitsky D. The methodology of experimentally induced diffuse noxious inhibitory control (DNIC)-like effect in humans. Pain 2009;144:16–19.

140. van Wijk G, Veldhuijzen DS. Perspective on diffuse noxious inhibitory controls as a model of endogenous pain modulation in clinical pain syndromes. J Pain 2010;11:408–419.

141. Yarnitsky D. Conditioned pain modulation (the diffuse noxious inhibitory control-like effect): Its relevance for acute and chronic pain states. Curr Opin Anaesthesiol 2010;23:611–615.

142. Staud R. Abnormal endogenous pain modulation is a shared characteristic of many chronic pain conditions. Expert Rev Neurother 2012;12:577–585.

143. Yarnitsky D, Crispel Y, Eisenberg E, et al. Prediction of chronic post-operative pain: Pre-operative DNIC testing identifies patients at risk. Pain 2008;138:22–28.

144. Yarnitsky D, Granot M, Nahman-Averbuch H, Khamaisi M, Granovsky Y. Conditioned pain modulation predicts duloxetine efficacy in painful diabetic neuropathy. Pain 2012;153:1193–1198.

145. Smith T, Nicholson RA. Review of duloxetine in the management of diabetic peripheral neuropathic pain. Vasc Health Risk Manag 2007;3:833–844.

146. Iyengar S, Webster AA, Hemrick-Luecke SK, Xu JY, Simmons RM. Efficacy of duloxetine, a potent and balanced serotonin-norepinephrine reuptake inhibitor in persistent pain models in rats. J Pharmacol Exp Ther 2004;311:576–584.

147. Shy ME, Frohman EM, So YT, et al. Quantitative sensory testing: Report of the Therapeutics and Technology Assessment Subcommittee of the American Academy of Neurology. Neurology 2003;60:898–904.

148. Eliav E, Gracely RH, Nahlieli O, Benoliel R. Quantitative sensory testing in trigeminal nerve damage assessment. J Orofac Pain 2004;18:339–344.

149. Dao TT, Mellor A. Sensory disturbances associated with implant surgery. Int J Prosthodont 1998;11:462–469.

150. Benoliel R, Eliav E, Iadarola MJ. Neuropeptide Y in trigeminal ganglion following chronic constriction injury of the rat infraorbital nerve: Is there correlation to somatosensory parameters? Pain 2001;91:111–121.

151. Benoliel R, Wilensky A, Tal M, Eliav E. Application of a pro-inflammatory agent to the orbital portion of the rat infraorbital nerve induces changes indicative of ongoing trigeminal pain. Pain 2002;99:567–578.

152. Chacur M, Milligan ED, Gazda LS, et al. A new model of sciatic inflammatory neuritis (SIN): Induction of unilateral and bilateral mechanical allodynia following acute unilateral peri-sciatic immune activation in rats. Pain 2001;94:231–244.

153. Gazda LS, Milligan ED, Hansen MK, et al. Sciatic inflammatory neuritis (SIN): Behavioral allodynia is paralleled by peri-sciatic proinflammatory cytokine and superoxide production. J Peripher Nerv Syst 2001;6:111–129.

154. Eliav E, Benoliel R, Tal M. Inflammation with no axonal damage of the rat saphenous nerve trunk induces ectopic discharge and mechanosensitivity in myelinated axons. Neurosci Lett 2001;311:49–52.

155. Eliav E, Herzberg U, Ruda MA, Bennett GJ. Neuropathic pain from an experimental neuritis of the rat sciatic nerve. Pain 1999;83:169–182.

156. Sang CN, Max MB, Gracely RH. Stability and reliability of detection thresholds for human A-Beta and A-delta sensory afferents determined by cutaneous electrical stimulation. J Pain Symptom Manage 2003;25:64–73.

157. Maier C, Baron R, Tölle TR, et al. Quantitative sensory testing in the German Research Network on Neuropathic Pain (DFNS): Somatosensory abnormalities in 1236 patients with different neuropathic pain syndromes. Pain 2010;150:439–450.

158. Svensson P, Baad-Hansen L, Pigg M, et al. Guidelines and recommendations for assessment of somatosensory function in oro-facial pain conditions—A taskforce report. J Oral Rehabil 2011;38:366–394.

Psychologic Aspects of Chronic Orofacial Pain

Karen Raphael, PhD
Donald S. Ciccone, PhD

4

p. 97-122

As many as 12% of patients who are seen in dental practices are estimated to have pain that cannot be ascribed to a known physiologic cause.[1] A more recent population-based study in Britain[2] suggested that 4.3% of the general population suffer from idiopathic orofacial pain. This same study[2] commented that conditions such as temporomandibular disorders (TMDs) often have no underlying pathology, suggesting that the prevalence of unexplained orofacial pain is underestimated by their own research. Burning mouth syndrome (BMS) was recently described as a nonorganic orofacial pain.[3] The terms *idiopathic* and *atypical* facial pain become wastebasket diagnoses when clinicians cannot identify the specific etiology,[4] reflecting our limited knowledge of pathogenesis. Such diagnoses of exclusion are often inherently difficult to treat[5] without knowledge of symptom mechanism.

When organic factors appear insufficient to explain a complaint of pain, and when patients are difficult to treat, it may be tempting to assume that psychiatric and psychologic factors must be involved. The goals of this chapter are, first, to review the evidence for this common assumption and, second, to introduce the reader to selected methods that have proven effective in managing psychologic complications when present. The first part of the chapter addresses the potentially separate effects of psychologic factors on pain onset and etiology and on pain course. Models of how psychologic factors can affect orofacial pain are also reviewed and evaluated. The second part presents a theoretic framework for psychologic intervention, describes psychologic methods shown to be effective in randomized controlled trials, and concludes with a discussion of psychologic screening and referral.

Comorbidity of Psychiatric and Chronic Orofacial Pain Conditions

Multiple reviews have noted that patients with various types of orofacial pain appear to be at risk of psychiatric disorders and psychologic symptoms. In particular, migraineurs (see chapter 10) have been shown to present with increased risk of depression, anxiety, panic attacks, and other psychiatric disorders[6–39] in diverse samples. BMS (see chapter 13) appears to be comorbid with personality disorders[40] as well as depression and anxiety disorders[41,42] and symptoms.[43–45]

Patients with TMDs (see chapters 8 and 9) have an increased risk of depression,[46,47] particularly when the masticatory muscles rather than the joint are involved[48–51] and even when the disorder is considered acute rather than chronic.[52] Patients with masticatory muscle pain are also more likely to present with psychologic symptoms than patients with neuropathic orofacial pain.[53] A diverse group of patients with orofacial pain,[54] and patients with TMDs in particular,[55] are reported to have elevated rates of posttraumatic stress disorder (PTSD). A more recent twin study confirmed these findings[56] in a community sample, suggesting that the concordance was partially explained by genetic factors.

These patterns reflect, in part, the fact that psychiatric disorders and psychologic symptoms are common among pain patients in general, not solely among patients with orofacial pain. In fact, it has been argued that psychiatric comorbidity, especially depression, is more marked among a diverse group of patients with chronic pain conditions than among those with serious medical conditions, such as cardiac disease or cancer.[57]

Thus, it is likely that a large subset of patients presenting for orofacial treatment will have a comorbid psychiatric disorder. Establishing comorbidity between orofacial pain and psychiatric disorders does not provide an understanding of the nature of the conditions or the mechanisms through which they are linked, however. Indeed, their comorbidity provokes important questions about the relation of psychiatric disorders or subthreshold psychologic symptoms to the etiology and course of orofacial pain.

Psychologic Factors and Orofacial Pain: An Overview of Explanatory Models

As other chapters in this text discuss, the cause of certain orofacial pain conditions is controversial or elusive. The danger for orofacial pain specialists is in assuming that medically unexplained orofacial pain is therefore psychologically explained. The contribution of psychologic factors to symptom presentation must be distinguished from their role as primary cause.

The psychogenic model

A purely psychological or psychogenic model of orofacial pain, in which the patient presents symptoms in the absence of demonstrable pathology, derives in part from a half-century-old view of psychogenic pain[58,59] that has roots in psychoanalytic theory. In one of George Engel's early works,[59] "atypical facial neuralgia" was posed as a model hysterical conversion syndrome. Engel notes that several of Sigmund Freud's monographs from the late 19th and early 20th centuries describe facial neuralgias that "proved to be hysterical." The model of purely psychologic orofacial pain continued to gain advocates in the 1960s and 1970s,[60–63] and concepts of atypical facial pain as "masked depression" were introduced.[62,64,65] One publication even proposed that atypical facial pain can develop as "a defense against psychosis."[66]

Moving into more recent approaches to the purely psychologic model, the bible for classification of psychiatric disorder, the Diagnostic and Statistical Manual of Mental Disorders (DSM), made some important changes in the classification of pain disorders as it moved from the fourth (DSM-IV)[67] to the fifth (DSM-5)[68] edition. The DSM-IV included a classification of somatoform disorder labeled "pain

p. 4/52
Burning Mouth Syndrome

disorder" (or "pain disorder associated with psychological factors" in the text revision of DSM-IV). A subtype of pain disorder was postulated to exist in which, in the absence of a general medical condition, psychologic factors were considered the primary cause of onset, severity, exacerbation, or pain maintenance. This category no longer exists. The DSM-5 now recognizes that the distinction among pain caused solely by psychologic factors, solely by medical factors, or some combination of both cannot be made with sufficient reliability or validity. In the DSM-5, some people might still be classified as having somatic symptom disorder with pain as a predominant feature. Others may be classified as having psychologic factors that affect other medical conditions or an adjustment disorder.

Aside from the theoretic support offered from a psychoanalytic perspective, the concept of psychogenic pain is supported by several sources of data. First is the striking comorbidity of several orofacial pain disorders with psychiatric disorders, as described earlier in this chapter. Second, the efficacy of tricyclic antidepressants in the treatment of orofacial pain may be viewed as support for a psychologic etiology. However, compelling evidence indicates that their mechanism of pain relief is independent of their antidepressant effect.[69-71]

Many of the orofacial pain conditions that are sometimes considered to have primary psychologic causes show an epidemiologic preponderance in women. The striking preponderance of women with TMDs,[72-74] BMS,[75,76] tension-type headache (TTH),[77] and migraine[8,78] parallels the preponderance of women with anxiety disorders[79,80] and mood disorders,[79,81] especially depression with somatic features, including pain.[82,83] Clinicians may tend to view women as having more psychosomatic illness, more emotional liability, and more symptoms due to emotional factors.[84]

Adding to the belief that orofacial pain can be due primarily to psychologic factors, over and above comorbidity with specific psychiatric disorders, is the fact that some patients with chronic orofacial pain may present with distinct cognitive styles and personality characteristics. Clinicians who note the presence of such dysfunctional personality characteristics in their patients with orofacial pain may be further encouraged to assume that pain is primarily due to psychologic factors. For example, patients with TMDs may show affective inhibition and somatosensory amplification.[85,86] One large study of patients with BMS found that they had elevated rates of psychiatrically assessed personality disorder,[40] and another[45] showed that patients with BMS had higher scores than control subjects on scales of neuroticism but lower scores on such measures as openness and extraversion.

Refutation of the concept of psychogenic pain comes from several sources. First, although a female preponderance is common to several psychiatric conditions and several orofacial pain disorders, there are numerous other disorders with a high female-to-male ratio for which no psychologic risk factors have been firmly identified. These include dermatologic conditions,[87] sexually transmitted diseases,[88] and autoimmune diseases,[89] among many others. Tertiary factors that link orofacial pain and psychiatric disorder and are associated with female sex, such as estrogenic hormones,[90-92] may eventually be identified. Second, elevated rates of psychiatric disorder in treatment-seeking patients may reflect the fact that psychiatric comorbidity increases the probability that a person will seek treatment for any disorder[93]; whether these psychiatric comorbidities would indeed be detected in more representative community samples of people with various orofacial pain conditions has yet to be examined. Additionally, psychiatric comorbidity may well develop as a consequence of the stress of living with chronic pain. Indeed, one family study supported this explanation for masticatory muscle pain; it found that patients with depression had low rates of depression in their families, indicating that their depression was likely reactive to the stress of living with chronic orofacial pain.[94] Although the implications of this pattern of familial aggregation was not interpreted as reflecting reactive depression in pain patients, a similar observation was made decades earlier regarding the absence of family history of depression in patients with atypical facial pain who had depression themselves.[63]

Patient follow-up studies also provide evidence that psychologic symptoms can develop in reaction to the stress of living with orofacial pain. A study of patients undergoing arthroscopy for temporomandibular joint pain[95] found that after arthroscopy, some psychosocial variables did improve at a 3-month postoperative visit, specifically, a dysfunctional index from the Multidimensional Pain Inventory[96] consisting of high pain, high life interference, high affective distress, and low perceived life control. Similarly, a 5-year outcome study of patients with TMDs[97] found that those with high levels of psychologic distress whose pain improved also showed improvement in psychologic distress, suggesting that at least part of the distress for some patients with TMDs represents a reaction to their pain. The stigma of living with chronic orofacial pain[98] could indeed induce a psychologically defensive response style.[86] Indeed, patients' self-reports suggest that dysfunctional personality characteristics were not evident before the onset of orofacial pain but manifested later.[99]

Feinmann and Newton-John describe this shift in patient personality and consequent shift in clinician attitude toward the patient:

> Failure to identify the cause of pain or to effect a cure is then interpreted as a sign that either the examination or test used was faulty ... or that the clinician was less than capable (so a different one is sought, often many times). As the patient becomes increasingly frustrated and despondent with the inability of the medical system to cure him or her, there may also be a change in the attitudes of the treating professionals toward the patient. The persistence of pain over time despite the application of multiple tests and multiple treatment approaches is interpreted as a sign of an underlying psychopathology, which only causes the patient further distress.[100p361]

The major logical fallacy for the purely psychologic model of orofacial pain is that it assumes that failure to find a biologic marker for a particular orofacial pain condition implies that psychologic factors must be primary. However, pain researchers increasingly recognize that the association between observable tissue damage or another identifiable pathologic process and the presence or extent of pain is weak at best.[101] Multiple factors, including genetic susceptibility to pain and neuronal plasticity, can at least partially explain the continuation of pain beyond localized healing and the lack of correlation between injury and pain.

Psychosocial stress as the link between orofacial pain and psychologic symptoms

Another model would suggest that the link between orofacial pain and psychologic factors may also be due to their shared association with psychosocial stress. In theory, stress might seem to be important in the genesis of orofacial pain, as experimental stress can modulate jaw reflexes.[102] Nevertheless, although stress may be associated with pain modulation and impaired coping, muscle hyperactivity is no longer considered a risk factor for muscle pain (see chapter 8).

Note that one should differentiate between psychosocial stress due to major life events (eg, death of a loved one), hassles (eg, more common, daily, small events such as a fight with a spouse), and chronic environmental burdens (eg, financial problems, chronic medical illness) and the harmful consequences of stress, that is, distress.[103] This distinction is important, because research often fails to differentiate the two. Thus, patients with orofacial pain may have elevated levels of distress, but this does not necessarily mean that they were exposed to high levels of specific psychosocial sources of stress over and above the stressful experience of living with pain.

Psychosocial stress and TMDs

The role of psychosocial stress has been particularly implicated for TMDs. In shifting from earlier mechanistic theories of TMD etiology,[104] the psychophysiologic model of masticatory muscle pain etiology was first proposed by Laszlo Schwartz in the 1950s[105,106] and expanded later by Daniel Laskin.[107] The model focused on the muscle rather than the joint as a primary source of pain and integrated psychosocial factors as a cause. The foundation of the psychophysiologic model of TMDs is that psychosocial stress initiates a distress response or tension in a person, causing dysfunctional oral habits such as tooth grinding and clenching. These oral habits are presumed to promote muscle contraction and hyperactivity and subsequent facial pain (see chapter 8 for further discussion). Recently,[108] research has shown that levels of grinding and clenching at night are identical among a large sample of patients with TMDs and matched control subjects.

Nevertheless, this model has been widely adopted by members of the dental community. A 1993 survey in the Seattle, Washington, area[109] found that stress was identified as a major factor by 92% of general dentists and specialists and by 85% of "TMD experts" who were selected for their extensive contributions to the peer-reviewed literature on TMDs. Supporting these endorsements are research studies that find patients with TMDs, especially those with a myogenous disorder, to have an increased likelihood of reporting selective types of major life stressors[110,111] but not necessarily hassles.[112] An uncontrolled study[113] also suggested that patients with TMDs have high exposure to traumatic stress, but lack of a control group makes interpretation of these findings difficult. What is particularly clear is that subjective distress, often mislabeled as stress, is elevated in patients with TMDs,[110,114–118] but, as discussed earlier, this may be a consequence of living with pain rather than represent a reaction to other psychosocial stressors. Chronic pain is a powerful stressor.

Thus, compared with the widespread belief in the role of stress as a major factor in TMDs, the body of evidence for psychosocial stress in TMD onset is relatively limited. Prospective research offers more promise. Although a recent prospective study of new TMD onsets detected more stressful events in the year before initial interview,[119] retrospective reports of frequent stressful life events in patients with TMDs must be viewed with some degree of skepticism, given the unreliability of self-reported life-event exposure,[120] even over periods as short as 6 months. Moreover, there is a possibility that high levels of distress in patients with TMDs may bias recall of prior life events in mood-congruent ways.[121] Of note, in this particular study,[119] the authors comment that respondents misunderstood instructions and sometimes endorsed sex-inappropriate events.

Psychosocial stress and other orofacial pain conditions

Although the role of psychosocial stress has been most often implicated for TMDs, research has also examined its role in other orofacial pain conditions. For example, although patients with BMS were more likely to report psychologic symptoms, psychiatric hospitalization, and outpatient psychologic treatment than control subjects with no pain, they did not report more recent life events.[122] The support for major life stress in BMS is confined to an uncontrolled study of 18 patients with BMS who frequently reported acute stressors before pain onset.[123] A similar uncontrolled study points to stress as a migraine precipitant (see chapter 10 for a discussion on migraine triggers).[124] A larger study[125] suggests that although stress is mentioned as a common precipitant for both migraine and TTH, it is cited more often among migraineurs. In contrast, patients with typical and atypical trigeminal neuralgia rarely implicate psychologic factors as precipitants.[126]

Although neither BMS nor trigeminal neuralgia has been clearly linked to psychosocial stress, headache may have some relationship. The 1985 Nuprin Pain Report[127] found that self-reported stress and daily hassles were more often reported by a community sample of people who had experienced at least one headache in the prior year. Although major life events do not appear to be associated with diverse types of headache,[128] perceived stress, a possible indicator of distress or daily hassles, has been associated with it. Similarly, Smitherman et al[12] found an association between PTSD but not traumatic event exposure per se in migraine. The role of major life events in headache was also discounted in another study, which still found daily hassles to be elevated in patients with chronic headache, particularly among those with TTH or mixed headache rather than migraine.[129] Another study[130] reported no relation between headache frequency and major life events but a modest relationship between headache frequency and daily hassles. A small relationship has been detected between more frequent headache and major life events in several large-sample studies,[130–132] though the relationship was restricted to younger people. Thus, although there may be some relationship between headache and psychosocial stress, most likely centered on daily hassles and headache frequency, its role in BMS and trigeminal neuralgia is not supported.

Psychosocial characteristics as risk factors for pain onset

Distinct from the reductionistic and deterministic model of psychosocial characteristics as a primary cause of orofacial pain is the more integrative model of psychosocial characteristics as risk factors for pain onset, in which they are considered part of a constellation of other factors affecting pain onset. A classic example is provided by Von Korff et al,[133] who examined depression as a risk factor for onset of five common pain symptoms, including TMD pain, when studying a large sample of adults at baseline and at a 3-year follow-up. They found that depression severity and chronicity increased the risk of new onset of severe headache and chest pain, but the relationship between baseline depression and later TMD pain onset was not significant. Nevertheless, the nonsignificant trend was in the predicted direction, in which new-onset rates for TMD pain were 6% for those with clinically normal scores on a depression symptom index but 12% for those with severe depressive symptoms or more chronic symptoms. In contrast, new onset of severe headache was significantly associated with more severe and more chronic depressive symptoms. New-onset probabilities for severe headache were 3% for those with normal scores on a depression index but more than 9% for those with severe depressive symptoms.

Newer prospective studies have added to our understanding of psychosocial factors in the development of new TMD onsets or TMD chronicity. Health anxiety was found to be a stronger predictor of self-reported chronic orofacial pain in a community study than a simple measure of mechanical factors.[134] Results from an initial prospective cohort study of TMD-free young women were reported.[135] Depression, perceived stress, and mood were associated with baseline pain sensitivity and were predictive of a two- to threefold increase in risk of TMD symptoms at the 3-year follow-up. A recent German population-based study[136] concluded

that depressive symptoms predicted new onset of temporomandibular joint pain on palpation, whereas anxiety symptoms were stronger predictors of new onset of masticatory muscle pain on palpation than depressive symptoms. A US-based community study[137] found that both depressive symptoms and catastrophizing predicted the progression of TMD pain and disability. In the large and unprecedented prospective OPPERA (Orofacial Pain Prospective Evaluation and Risk Assessment) study of initially TMD-free community residents, premorbid global psychologic factors were among the most robust predictors of new TMD onset when examining psychologic factors in isolation from other factors.[138] A community study in Finland reported that depressive symptoms predicted onset or persistence of self-reported facial pain 3 years later. However, after accounting for widespread pain, depressive symptoms were no longer significant predictors. This type of analysis shows the importance of considering the biopsychosocial spectrum of potential risk factors when trying to understand the importance of psychosocial factors in onset of facial pain.

A critical example is provided when comparing results reported by the OPPERA group for psychologic factors alone[138] versus psychologic factors in combination with other domains. Examined alone, nearly all psychologic factors associated with depression and anxiety predicted new-onset TMDs. However, when examined in combination with other domains of premorbid status,[139] of the 30 most important predictors of first-onset TMD, the psychologic factor bearing the most importance in predicting incident TMD—high somatic awareness—was ranked 10th. It is debatable whether this is a psychosocial factor at all. Catastrophizing ranked 30th and was the only other psychosocial measure in the top 30. Clearly more important were measures of health status, that is, the number of comorbid conditions, nonspecific orofacial symptoms, and bodily pain. Thus, although psychosocial factors are part of the biopsychosocial montage that is involved in the pathogenesis of TMDs, concepts that psychologic factors play an important role in the etiopathogenesis of TMDs[140] confuse prominence of psychologic factors in patient presentation with their reduced prominence as risk factors for TMD onset.

SLADE

Q #I

But NOT estrogen levels

diathesis - AN UNUSUAL CONSTITUTIONAL OR predisposition to A disease (PARTICULAR DISEASE)

Consideration of psychologic and psychosocial factors as one of many factors increasing risk of pain is consistent with a general biopsychosocial model of orofacial pain. Sherman and Turk summarize this model:

> The model presumes physical pathology, or at least physical changes in muscle, joints, and nerves that generate pain signals, but also presumes that psychological and social processes interact with pathology to result in overt expression of pain such as functional impairment, disability, and distress.[141p423]

Although a variety of specifications of the biopsychosocial model of orofacial pain exist,[142–144] it has been argued that, despite the important heuristic value of these models, they tend to be neglected because they fail to specify testable hypotheses.[145] A specific form of the biopsychosocial model, the *vulnerability-diathesis-stress model*,[145] proposes an interaction between a physiologic predisposition (ie, a diathesis from genetic vulnerability or acquired vulnerability from prior exposures such as disease or injury) and psychosocial stress leading to development of a pain disorder. According to this view, psychosocial stress is pathogenic only for persons who are constitutionally susceptible. Advances in psychiatric research support the interaction of genes and environment. For example, psychosocial stress affects risk of developing depression[146] or psychosis,[147] particularly for those with genetic or familial vulnerability.

Attempts to test a stress vulnerability model in pain disorders in general and orofacial pain specifically are limited to date, despite the heuristic appeal of the model. An example is provided by Janke et al,[148] who found that depression was a risk factor for the development of TTHs during and after a laboratory stress task, at least among those with a history of prior TTHs. A series of studies on TMD pain[149–154] suggests that patients with TMDs have an increased risk of reacting to experimental stressors with increased electromyography (EMG) activity. Although these stress reactivity studies have sometimes been interpreted to suggest that those with chronic TMDs have a specific vulnerability to stress, whether such patterns were evident before the establishment of a pain disorder is unknown. In fact, numerous studies contradict the role of muscle hyperactivity in pain onset (see chapter 8).

Psychosocial characteristics as risk factors for course and outcome of orofacial pain

Although a review of the literature suggests that the concept of psychogenic orofacial pain is misguided, limited available data support the idea that psychosocial factors can influence the risk of onset of at least some orofacial pain conditions. Where psychologic and psychosocial factors become more prominent is in explaining the course of and disability associated with pain conditions. For example, why do some patients who have a TMD experience it as a minor inconvenience, while others with the same disorder become disabled? Why do some patients have symptoms for only a couple of weeks, while others have a lifelong pattern of facial pain exacerbations and remissions?

Psychosocial characteristics as risk factors for TMD outcome

Once again, the bulk of the research literature on the role of psychologic factors in the course of chronic orofacial pain focuses on TMDs. One study examined the relation between clinical and psychologic variables and 5-year outcome for persons with TMDs.[97] The researchers found that changes in depression and anxiety over 5 years were not consistently related to degree of improvement in pain intensity but that baseline depression and anxiety tended to be highest in the group whose symptoms were considered to be worse at the 5-year follow-up. Notably, changes in physical measures were not consistently related to changes in pain at follow-up, suggesting "at best only an indirect relationship between TMD pain report and clinical status for both the physical and psychologic domains."[97p322] Mixed findings were also reported by Rammelsberg et al.[155] They found that patients with myofascial TMDs whose symptoms had remitted at the 5-year follow-up were more likely than those with persistent or recurrent pain to be depressed at baseline. However, patients whose pain had remitted at follow-up were the only group of subjects whose depression also significantly decreased at follow-up. The authors interpret this finding as suggesting that baseline depression was actually caused by their baseline pain severity. Another study[156] examined physical and psychologic variables that determined whether acute TMD pain was considered to be chronic at a 6-month follow-up. Although higher levels of depression and nonspecific physical symptoms at baseline predicted chronic pain status at 6 months, neither factor was significant in a multivariate model that controlled for type of TMD (with myogenous TMD most likely to be chronic) or characteristic pain intensity at baseline. A similar study[157] found that in patients with TMDs, satisfaction with improvement and subjective pain relief at 8 months after initial evaluation for treatment was predicted by initial symptoms of anxiety but not depression. They also found that patients who engaged in pretreatment use of cognitive coping strategies, including distancing from pain, coping self-statements, and ignoring pain, had more satisfactory status at follow-up. These findings also suggest the potential utility of cognitive-behavioral therapy (CBT) (discussed later) in patients with TMDs.

Other studies have found baseline psychologic factors to predict pain severity at a later point. Auerbach et al[51] reported that TMD pain severity at a variable follow-up period was associated with baseline depression severity. Similarly, Epker et al[158] found that patients with TMDs who continued to have TMD pain at a 6-month follow-up differed from those whose pain had remitted in that they had more baseline depression. In a related publication,[159] patients who were classified on a prior algorithm as being at high risk of progressing from acute to chronic TMD pain[158] were further characterized as having elevated scores on self-reported measures of depression and coping, as well as interview-based measures of major psychiatric disorder and personality disorders. A study by Fricton and Olsen[160] found that various factors associated with depression, including low self-esteem and worried feelings, were associated with posttreatment symptom improve-

ment among patients with chronic TMDs. Most recently, evidence[161] indicated that psychosocial factors even predicted treatment outcome after a cycle of five weekly hyaluronic acid injections immediately following anthrocentesis.

In contrast to studies supporting some role of psychologic factors as predictors of TMD course, one study[162] found that none of the baseline psychologic measures examined, including affective disturbance and anxiety, predicted rapid versus slow response to conservative treatment of TMDs. In another study, baseline depressive symptoms showed a nonsignificant trend toward prediction of treatment response after 6 months of conservative treatment for TMDs.[163] Negative findings were also reported by Steed,[164] who found that a general scale assessing anxiety, depression, and frustration and another scale assessing chronic and recent stress showed elevated responses among patients with TMDs at initial symptoms, but neither scale related to symptoms at time of "maximum medical improvement," as judged by the treating clinician. Of course, the subjectivity in determining the time of maximum medical improvement creates interpretive problems. A well-cited article by Rudy et al[165] concluded that "dysfunctional" patients with TMDs and the highest degree of psychologic distress showed greater improvement in pain than other patients with TMDs who received conservative, standardized treatment, but a careful review of their findings suggests that this pattern was found for only a self-reported measure of pain symptoms and not muscle pain on palpation.

Review of the relatively large body of literature on psychologic factors in the course of TMDs leads to the conclusion that results are mixed. Differences in defining a successful outcome, assessing psychologic symptoms, and sample size are among the factors likely to explain this inconsistent pattern. Regardless of the explanation, psychologic factors have not been able to consistently forecast the outcome of treatment or the clinical course of TMD symptoms. Nevertheless, psychologic treatment studies of TMDs have yielded promising results (discussed later), suggesting that such factors may yet prove to be clinically significant.

Psychosocial characteristics as risk factors for outcome in other orofacial pain disorders

The smaller body of literature on psychologic factors as predictors of the course of other orofacial pain conditions is also inconsistent. For example, in a mixed group of patients with "psychogenic" facial pain,[70] treatment outcome at 12 months was predicted by a history of an adverse major life event before pain onset. In a later 4-year follow-up[166] of the same group of patients (later labeled by the author as having "chronic idiopathic facial pain"), presence of a baseline psychiatric diagnosis did not predict pain status at the 4-year follow-up. Finally, in an 8-year follow-up of juvenile-onset migraine or TTH,[167] presence of baseline psychiatric co-morbidity predicted a worse outcome.

Shared pathogenesis for psychiatric disorders and orofacial pain

Finally, another model of the relation between psychiatric conditions (or less severe psychologic symptoms) and orofacial pain posits that they have a shared pathogenesis. This model has been suggested as explaining the general pain-depression relationship,[168] the general pain-PTSD relationship,[169] and, more specifically, the orofacial pain–depression relationship.[170] For example, at the neurobiologic level, neurotransmitters such as serotonin and norepinephrine have been implicated in pain modulation and psychiatric disorders.[171,172] Stress vulnerability may be implicated in depression and facial pain, probably involving dysregulation of the hypothalamic-pituitary-adrenal axis.[170] At a psychologic level, vulnerability to negative affectivity or dysphoric states[173,174] may link psychologic symptoms with somatic symptoms, including orofacial pain. In addition, Krueger et al[175] proposed that chronic pain is linked to psychiatric disorders such as depression and anxiety through a specific tendency of certain persons to express distress inward ("internalizing disorders") rather than outward through antisocial behavior, substance abuse, and impulsivity ("externalizing disorders").

Several studies have established that fibromyalgia, a condition that is itself comorbid with myofascial TMDs,[176,177] and depression share familially mediated risk factors.[178,179] Specifically, these studies established that having a family member with fibromyalgia places a person at increased risk for depression, and having a family member with depression places a person at increased risk for fibromyalgia. A shared-vulnerability explanation has been proposed specifically for migraine and depression,[180,181] with evidence of bidirectional influences, so that persons with depression have an increased risk of migraine and persons with migraine have an increased risk of developing depression. Additional studies suggest that the bidirectional relationship applies to migraine but not to other severe headaches.[182]

Psychologic factors and illness behavior

Despite a long history of speculation, the evidence for psychosocial factors as a primary cause of orofacial pain is weak. On the other hand, consistent with a biopsychosocial perspective on chronic orofacial pain, psychosocial factors may trigger an episode of pain in susceptible persons, may cause pain exacerbation, and may lead to a more chronic course of pain. On these last points, however, the literature is inconsistent. A limited explanation is that psychologic factors have small and inconsistent effects on orofacial pain symptoms. However, inconsistent prediction from psychologic factors does not mean primary prediction from physical factors: As Ohrbach and Dworkin[97] have shown, prediction of 5-year outcomes of TMD pain from either physical or psychologic measures is weak.

To understand the juncture at which psychologic factors become critical, it is first necessary to distinguish between disease and illness (see Fig 4-1). *Disease* refers to the objective evidence of a pathologic state. In the case of chronic pain syndromes, including but not limited to orofacial pain, externally verifiable evidence of an underlying pathologic state causing and maintaining the pain may often be lacking or only tentatively present. *Illness* refers to patients' beliefs and views of their ill health and is inferred from symptom reports and behavior. The traditional biomedical model views psychologic factors as secondary, influencing the transition from disease and illness to clinical outcome; it assumes that biologic processes are sufficient to cause disease and illness. In contrast, the biopsychosocial model[183] views psychologic factors as contributing to the expression of disease and illness. Although psychologic factors are again viewed as affecting ultimate clinical outcome, they are thought to have the potential to exert influences on illness and disease, even at a biologic level.

Empiric data clearly support the importance of psychologic and psychosocial factors as affecting illness behavior. Although the focus in this chapter is on the sparse literature examining these factors for patients with orofacial pain specifically, a much broader literature is available that addresses the relation between psychosocial factors and adjustment to diverse pain conditions.[184] Particularly relevant is the concept of catastrophizing (discussed later). Pain-related catastrophizing is characterized by an extreme focus on pain, exaggeration of the threat associated with the pain, and feelings of helplessness related to the control of pain. Although catastrophizing has been related to pain severity in diverse conditions, even during dental hygiene treatment,[185] it may be particularly relevant as a predictor of illness behavior after the onset of orofacial pain. For example, Turner et al[186] reported that catastrophizing was associated with pain severity, activity interference, and number of health care visits among patients with TMDs.

The nature of the specific psychosocial factors predicting health care–seeking behavior may differ depending on the specific orofacial pain diagnosis. One study[187] reported that affective distress predicted treatment-seeking behavior for patients with a myofascial TMD, but treatment-seeking for patients with temporomandibular joint conditions was better predicted by other factors, such as psychologic introversion.

Despite the small body of literature specifically examining illness behavior in orofacial pain, it cannot be overemphasized that the broader body of literature on psychologic factors in all types of chronic pain is relevant. Dworkin[188] concluded that TMDs are chronic pain conditions that share many important features with other common chronic pain conditions. This perspective therefore "places TMDs within the same biopsychosocial model currently used to study and manage all illness, including common chronic pain conditions."[188p862] Although these issues have been explored relatively more often for TMDs, the application of a biopsychosocial model for understanding and treating all orofacial pain conditions is strongly advocated.

Despite the cautious interpretation of the literature presented in this chapter, which suggests that psychologic factors do not cause orofacial pain or may not reliably predict the outcome of traditional orofacial pain therapy, nevertheless psychologic factors are likely to be important in clinical practice. This belief stems from the fact that orofacial pain is clearly associated with increased risk of psychiatric disorder and increased likelihood of subthreshold psychologic symptoms. When present, these factors can amplify or distort the perception of pain and thus compromise the accuracy of symptom reporting. In the behavioral realm, psychologic factors can undermine motivation to comply with therapeutic instruction and impede efforts to correct maladaptive illness behavior. Psychologic factors may not be an issue for many (or even most) patients with orofacial pain, but, when present, they may threaten the outcome of an otherwise effective treatment. Moreover, the presence of psychiatric disorder, or even psychologic distress in the absence of full-fledged disorder, may be sufficient to significantly diminish quality of life. Therefore, it merits clinical attention from orofacial pain practitioners. The following section examines selected psychologic methods used to treat such patients and argues for the value of routine psychologic screening.

Psychologic Management of Chronic Orofacial Pain

Patients with chronic orofacial pain are confronted with the prospect of living with pain that cannot be relieved by conventional medical or dental treatment. Although psychologic factors may not cause orofacial pain, they can nevertheless determine its impact on emotional and behavioral well-being. Depending on the patient's coping skills, for example, he or she may respond to painful injury or illness by either minimizing or maximizing pain-related suffering.[189] The psychologic consequences of orofacial pain, whether adaptive or maladaptive, are not dictated by pathophysiology alone. As described in the following sections, the goals of psychologic treatment are to minimize pain-related distress and, to the extent possible, avoid unnecessary illness behavior.

Before discussing the psychologic techniques used to achieve these aims, it may be helpful to present an overview of cognitive theory because it provides a framework for understanding the causes of pain-related emotion and behavior.[190] In the next section, a version of this theory is used to explain how changes in cognition may lead to corresponding changes in pain-related affect and coping behavior. It should be acknowledged, however, that important components of the theory have yet to undergo scientific testing. The goal here is to familiarize nonspecialists with a treatment approach that has produced promising results in patients with chronic orofacial pain[191,192] and that, at the same time, has been widely used to treat psychiatric disorders in the general population.[193] Specifically, the reader will be introduced to cognitive psychotherapy,[194,195] followed by a brief discussion of adjunctive techniques, including biofeedback and relaxation training.[196] Finally, descriptions are provided of screening procedures that permit dental practitioners to identify patients most likely to profit from mental health services along with a rationale for referral that may facilitate communication with difficult patients.

Cognitive-behavioral theory (CBT) of illness behavior

The core assumption of the cognitive model is that people do not respond directly to a stimulus event but rather to a cognitive interpretation of that event.[197] A person's emotional and behavioral responses to orofacial pain, for example, depend on whether it is perceived as a threat or simply an inconvenience. According to the cognitive model, threat perception triggers a response from the sympathetic nervous system as well as action tendencies that govern overt responses in the form of illness behavior. An examination of the assumptions underlying a cognitive-relational theory of human behavior is not within the scope of this discussion.[190] Nevertheless, it may be useful to illustrate the central role of cognition in regulating emotional and behavioral responses to pain. An early demonstration of this role was provided by Beecher,[198] who interviewed soldiers about wounds they had received in battle. He was struck by the fact that some of the soldiers expressed an "optimistic, even cheerful, state of mind" despite having sustained an objectively painful injury. This emotional reaction to pain was explained by the fact that serious injury required relocation to the relative safety of a field hospital. He concluded that the personal significance of an injury and not its objective severity was primarily responsible for the ensuing emotional response. Therefore, it may be important to understand what the patient thinks about orofacial pain if the goal is to mitigate its effects on emotional and physical functioning.

Figure 4-1 provides an overview of human information processing; the diagram shows that sensory events, including pain, are subject to routine cognitive appraisal. A fundamental tenet of the model is that virtually all transactions with the environment are subject to cognitive interpretation and evaluation. Persistent face pain, for example, may be perceived as a symptom of disease or, alternatively, as an uncomfortable but benign sensation. The interpretation of somatosensory information is made in accordance with preexisting knowledge about causes of facial pain and the likelihood of disease (among other factors). After deciding how to categorize this event, the person is faced with the task of evaluating its personal significance. If pain sensation is judged to be a threat (labeled "unbearable" or "awful"), a corresponding affective response is mobilized and the person is biologically prepared for fight or flight. Unfortunately, in the case of chronic pain, such a response is not only unnecessary but also counterproductive. Advantages and disadvantages of various behavioral options may be weighed as the person decides how to cope with the problem at hand. Behavioral options are selected from an existing repertoire of skills and reflect efficacy expectations or beliefs about personal coping ability.

The presence of social and economic disincentives in the environment may further influ-

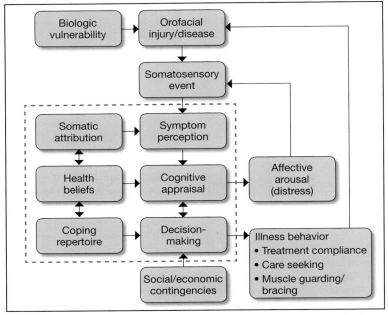

Fig 4-1 A cognitive-behavioral model of affective arousal and illness behavior in patients with chronic orofacial pain.

ence the choice of coping options. The patient may know, for example, that expressions of pain and suffering are met with increased social support or that treatment-seeking enables him or her to avoid social (or work) obligations.[199] The consequences of faulty cognitive appraisal and ineffective coping may exacerbate pain, compromise the outcome of dental therapy, and lead to emotional and behavioral problems requiring mental health intervention.

In sum, the model portrayed in Fig 4-1 conveys a dynamic process in which pain-related affect and coping behavior interact with orofacial pain symptoms. The processes of interpretation and evaluation are iterative and subject to modification as new information or experiences are acquired. The model does not suggest that cognitive processing entails conscious reflection and/or deliberation. In fact, automaticity is more likely the norm as thinking habits and perceptual bias become overlearned. To efficiently interpret the meaning of a rapidly changing environment, humans may necessarily rely on a set of perceptual rules and unconscious assumptions that can be deployed quickly and effortlessly.[200]

Psychologic management of chronic orofacial pain

Even though a dental practitioner may never conduct psychotherapy, he or she may wish to integrate dental treatment within a comprehensive plan that includes a mental health component. This is sufficient justification for a nonspecialist to consider the methods used to treat pain-related psychologic dysfunction. Before describing these methods, however, it is useful to distinguish between the goals of the psychotherapist and those of the orofacial pain specialist. Although a dentist is appropriately focused on symptom reduction or even alleviation, a psychotherapist is focused on ameliorating stress, minimizing dysfunctional illness behavior, and treating comorbid psychiatric disorder, when present. Although some patients have reported a reduction in pain after psychologic treatment,[192,201] the primary justification for referral should be to reduce emotional distress and/or minimize pain-related impairment. The goal(s) of psychologic treatment remain the same whether the distress developed in response to chronic pain or existed before onset. In either case, psychologic dysfunction undermines quality of life and may compromise the outcome of dental therapy.[189,191] The most popular psychologic treatment for patients with chronic orofacial pain and the one described in this chapter is called cognitive-behavioral therapy (CBT). Other psychologic techniques, such as psychodynamic therapy, may also be appropriate and effective but, as yet, have not been tested in rigorous clinical trials.

Evidence-based psychologic treatment

Controlled trials of CBT for patients with chronic orofacial pain have yielded promising results. Unfortunately, almost all of these clinical trials have focused on TMDs to the exclusion of other, less prevalent, orofacial pain conditions. Nevertheless, the results of these studies may be generalized beyond the treatment of TMDs. This is likely because CBT is known to be effective in patients with chronic pain regardless of pain location and irrespective of whether pain is explained or unexplained.[202–205] A relatively recent trial involving TMDs was reported by Turner et al[192]; they compared four sessions of CBT administered over 8 weeks to a usual-care control group that received an equivalent amount of therapist attention but no active psychologic treatment. The CBT group received the same usual care supplemented by instruction in cognitive coping and relaxation training. When assessed 12 months later, the researchers found that CBT-treated patients reported a significant reduction in jaw pain and improved masticatory function compared with control patients. An earlier study by the same group compared six sessions of CBT plus conservative care to conservative care only for patients with TMDs "who demonstrated poor psychosocial adaptation."[191] When assessed 4 months after enrollment, patients in the CBT group reported significantly less pain and an improved ability to control self-rated TMD symptoms. Similar results have also been reported by Gardea et al,[206] who administered 12 sessions of CBT to patients with TMDs. When compared with a no-treatment control group 1 year later, CBT-treated patients reported significant reductions in pain severity and pain-related disability as well as improved mandibular func-

tion. Finally, Turk et al[207] compared two treatment protocols for TMDs: one included CBT and the other provided "nondirective, supportive counseling." The group that received CBT "demonstrated significantly greater reductions in pain, depression, and medication use." In addition, only the CBT group showed continued improvements in terms of pain associated with muscle palpation and self-reported pain severity. Similar results have been reported for other orofacial pain disorders, including chronic TTH[208] and migraine without aura.[209] Although the preceding clinical trials provide a strong evidence base from which to recommend CBT for patients with chronic orofacial pain, it is perhaps more impressive to consider the larger body of evidence showing that CBT is effective for the most common forms of psychiatric disorder,[210] including depression[211] and generalized anxiety disorder.[212,213] Because our primary justification for psychologic referral is to treat emotional distress and behavioral dysfunction rather than pain sensation, this larger body of evidence is equally relevant to the choice of treatment modality. At present, the consensus appears to favor CBT as the preferred mode of psychologic intervention for patients with chronic pain.[214,215]

The next section provides a brief introduction to cognitive therapy, a core component of CBT, originally developed by Albert Ellis[197,216] and Aaron Beck.[194] This is followed by a description of the use of biofeedback and related relaxation training to improve self-control over dysfunctional muscle activity in patients with myofascial TMDs[196] and reduce autonomic hyperarousal in patients with TTH or migraine headache.[208,209]

Cognitive therapy

As suggested by the model in Fig 4-1, the goal of cognitive therapy is to produce a philosophic shift in the way patients think about negative events or, more specifically, the way they think about orofacial pain. The process of achieving cognitive change, sometimes called cognitive restructuring, has been described in detail by Walen et al,[217] among others. The limited goal of this section is to provide an overview of this treatment using the ABC framework originally proposed by Albert Ellis.[195,197] The three components of the model are designated as follows: *A* is an antecedent event that may occur inside or outside a person, *B* is a belief or belief system that serves as a subjective interpretation of the event, and *C* refers to the emotional and behavioral consequences of the belief. After a stimulus is detected at A, a person immediately interprets its personal significance or meaning at B, which in turn elicits an emotional response and illness behavior at point C. For the purposes of this discussion, the cognitive process used to construct a mental representation of the stimulus is called an *inference*. This type of activity occurs whenever a person recognizes a stimulus as functionally equivalent to one encountered in the past. Using prior knowledge to infer the meaning of new events allows a person to unconsciously access properties or attributes of stimuli that were not directly observed or perceived.[218] At least two types of inference are required to interpret the significance of events in the environment.[217] The first is descriptive and serves to identify or categorize the event in question. For example, hearing a loud noise may be perceived as a car backfiring or as a gunshot. After categorizing the event (inferring the source of the noise), the person is left with the task of appraising its significance. The same event may be appraised as threatening or irrelevant depending on prior knowledge of similar auditory events and expectations of coping ability. If a person is standing next to a window and perceives gunshots coming from the street, he or she might decide to seek cover in anticipation of danger. On the other hand, if a person perceives car noises instead of gunshots, he or she may not react at all. Identical stimuli can thus give rise to vastly different emotional and behavioral responses, depending on a person's cognitive interpretation. Despite the central role of cognition in regulating human behavior, the inference process is notoriously fallible. Humans often rely on faulty logic (jumping to conclusions) as they strive to decipher the personal significance of their changing environment. This leads to the second assumption underlying cognitive therapy, namely that faulty inference and mistaken appraisal are responsible for eliciting maladaptive emotion and self-defeating illness behavior. In cognitive therapy, the goal is to dispute these erroneous inferences or thinking

mistakes and replace them with beliefs that are logical or more consistent with empiric observation. Persistent depression, anxiety, and anger are said to be unhealthy emotions and thus products of irrational belief, whereas sadness, concern, and annoyance are considered healthy or adaptive emotions and products of rational belief.

One of the most common of all thinking mistakes and the frequent subject of therapeutic intervention is called *catastrophizing*. As the name suggests, this refers to the mistaken belief that difficult or unpleasant events are literally unbearable or catastrophic. Patients with chronic orofacial pain, for example, often use melodramatic language to describe their symptoms as "devastating" or "awful." This type of exaggerated appraisal, according to cognitive theory, elicits an intense affective and behavioral response out of proportion to the sensory event. By definition, chronic pain is unpleasant but not unbearable because patients actually bear or tolerate the sensation for months or even years. An alternative (rational) belief might be as follows: "My dental problem is exceptionally painful at times, but it is hardly unbearable or more than I can stand." Another common thinking error occurs when patients insist that they must or should have what they want or deserve. For example, a cure for chronic pain is highly advantageous and thus preferable but hardly necessary. When patients confuse what they need with what they prefer (by demanding a cure), they unwittingly increase their emotional discomfort. Demanding pain relief may also lead to dysfunctional coping by motivating patients to go doctor shopping, use medication excessively, or engage in unnecessary medical visitation. These emotional and behavioral consequences are maladaptive because they compromise quality of life and, under certain circumstances, exacerbate pain severity.

The process by which a therapist challenges and hopefully modifies a patient's irrational belief is called *cognitive disputing*. This is achieved by asking patients to explain or defend their logical fallacies or unproven assumptions. Typical examples of disputing include the following: "Where is the evidence that it would be awful?" or "Why do things have to be the way you want them to be?" As noted earlier, the aim is not to correct grammatical or linguistic errors but to produce profound changes in the way patients evaluate the consequences of a negative life event. In the case of patients who catastrophize, for example, the therapist explains that chronic pain, unlike acute pain, does not signal the onset of physical injury (or tissue damage). The patient is advised that habitual use of a word such as "unbearable" to describe pain sensation is understandable but likely to prove self-defeating. Cognitive therapists believe catastrophic thought causes self-inflicted stress, which they refer to as *emotional pain*. This is above and beyond the physical pain caused by an orofacial pain disorder. In the language of the therapeutic cover story, a patient who is catastrophizing is said to be confronted with two types of pain instead of one. According to the cognitive model, catastrophizing is a form of *evaluative inference* or *misappraisal* leading to an unnecessary fight-or-flight response. Once the patient expresses a willingness to correct this thinking habit, the therapist may begin disputing by asking for proof that the pain is actually unbearable as opposed to extremely uncomfortable. Therapeutic benefits are contingent upon the patient's believing and not simply understanding that pain exacerbations are tolerable despite being unpleasant. The shift from irrational to rational thought is accomplished gradually through repeated disputation during the session and frequent practice outside the clinic in the form of weekly homework assignments. For example, the patient might be encouraged to resist the natural temptation to label an exacerbation as "awful" and instead substitute the rational belief that pain is bad at times but all the evidence shows that a person can certainly stand it.

Aside from catastrophic appraisal, other common thinking mistakes may compromise psychologic adjustment. For example, patients (and nonpatients) have been known to engage in any or all of the following:

- *Demandingness:* "Life should not be so difficult or unfair" or "doctors should do more to relieve my pain."
- *Fortune-telling:* "Since I haven't gotten better up to now, I never will" or "I'll never be able to enjoy myself or look forward to anything."
- *Self-downing:* "Since losing my job, I feel like a complete failure" or "now that I have to de-

pend on others for help, I feel like less of a person."
- *All or none:* "If I can't enjoy my life the way I did before I got hurt, then I can't enjoy anything" or "in order for the treatment to be successful, I have to be completely pain free."

Cognitive therapists have an extensive repertoire of philosophic and empiric disputing strategies available to address each of these erroneous beliefs. Describing these strategies in more detail, however, is beyond the scope of this chapter. Interested readers are referred to comprehensive manuals prepared by Walen et al[217] and Beck et al.[219] Although the vast majority of pain practitioners will not practice psychotherapy, it is possible to collaborate with a psychotherapist by reinforcing a rational acceptance of chronic pain and offering a realistic appraisal of pain severity. In particular, it may be useful for practitioners to refrain from catastrophic or absolutistic language when describing pain symptoms or past treatment failures (eg, "I know the pain can be unbearable at times" or "there has to be a solution for your problem"). Practitioners may also wish to shift the focus of treatment away from pain alleviation in favor of pain management and restoration of functional capacity. This allows the patient to expect waxing and waning of symptoms without a promise of symptom remission. Despite the presence of pain and physical restrictions, the patient can be encouraged to maintain an adequate activity level, avoid excessive rest, correct defective posture and poor body mechanics, and, when physically possible, resume domestic and work-related chores.

Adjunctive modalities: Biofeedback and relaxation training

The aim of biofeedback training is to provide patients with information or feedback about physiologic activity for the purpose of bringing that activity under voluntary control. The biofeedback device usually includes a sensor that detects and records information about bodily functions (eg, skin temperature, blood pressure, or muscle tension) and an electronic amplifier that converts this information into an auditory or visual display that can be monitored by the patient in near real time. In most clinical applications, the device allows patients to access physiologic events that may otherwise go unnoticed or that lie outside the boundaries of human proprioception. The assumption is that with the aid of biofeedback, patients may be able to bring physiologic activity under voluntary (cognitive) control. One of the first clinical demonstrations of this technique was reported by Budzynski et al,[220] who trained patients with TTH headache to lower muscle activity using surface electromyography (sEMG) related feedback.

A number of studies have evaluated the clinical efficacy of sEMG training for patients with myofascial TMDs.[196] The usual aim of this training is to reduce hypertonicity and/or hyperactivity of the masseter and anterior temporalis muscles. Training may target elevated tension in the muscle at rest or, more realistically, provide patients with an opportunity to reduce hyperactivity during or after a routine motor task (eg, chewing). Aside from re-educating the muscles of mastication, biofeedback may also be used to facilitate generalized relaxation.[206] In this case, the biofeedback device provides information about one or more parameters of the autonomic nervous system, such as skin temperature or electrodermal activity. By providing access to hand temperature during thermal biofeedback, for example, patients may acquire a hand-warming response and thereby reduce sympathetically mediated arousal. At present, there is insufficient evidence to show that specialized sEMG biofeedback to correct abnormal muscle function in the face is any more or less effective than biofeedback-assisted relaxation to lower physiologic arousal. A direct comparison of relaxation training with and without biofeedback for patients with myofascial TMDs found that both were effective, producing improvement in 70% and 71% of patients, respectively.[221] Reduced arousal was apparently sufficient to reduce TMD symptoms without explicit sEMG training. These findings strongly suggest that reduced tension in the masseter muscle may not be necessary to achieve a good clinical outcome and are consistent with a large body of literature (see earlier in this chapter and chapter 8) critiquing the role of muscle hyperactivity in pain.

Although the underlying mechanism may not be known, the efficacy of biofeedback for myofascial TMDs is less in doubt. Crider et al[196] identified six randomized controlled trials, five of which yielded significant "evidence for the efficacy of biofeedback-based treatments of TMD compared to appropriate control conditions." The clinical utility of biofeedback when used alongside (or instead of) other conservative modalities, such as physical rehabilitation or oral splint therapy, has not been established. Finally, note that the preceding trials were limited to patients who reported pain upon palpation of masticatory muscles and cannot be generalized to patients with TMD pain primarily related to joint problems.

Biofeedback has played a limited role in the treatment of myofascial TMDs but is widely accepted as a frontline therapy for patients with TTH or migraine headache. Behavioral treatments for headache have been recognized by, among others, the National Institutes of Health (1996) and the World Health Organization.[222,223] A meta-analysis by Goslin et al[209] examined the efficacy of behavioral therapy, including biofeedback, for migraine without aura. Biofeedback alone, or in combination with CBT and relaxation training, produced dramatic (32% to 49%) reductions in migraine activity compared with results for untreated control subjects (5%). Thermal and EMG modalities were equally effective, but neither was superior to relaxation training without biofeedback. A similar meta-analysis of behavioral treatments for TTH reached similar conclusions.[208] Relatively few studies have compared the efficacy of biofeedback or other behavioral modalities to pharmacotherapy, but the few that have suggest that these techniques are equally efficacious. Holroyd et al,[224] for example, compared tricyclic antidepressant therapy with stress management for TTH. The latter included instruction in cognitive coping and relaxation but no biofeedback. When delivered alone, medication and stress management produced clinically significant improvement in headache activity for 35% and 38% of patients, respectively. When delivered together in a combined treatment group, they produced improvement in 64% of patients.

As noted earlier, the theoretic rationale used to justify biofeedback for patients with myofascial TMDs has been called into question. Similar doubts have been raised about the mechanism underlying thermal biofeedback for migraine[225] and about the mechanism underlying EMG biofeedback for TTH.[226] In an effort to test the muscle-tension hypothesis, Holroyd et al[227] trained one group of patients to decrease muscle tension (as per the hypothesis) while training another to increase muscle tension. This was achieved by altering the feedback contingency so that decreased EMG activity was fed back as increased and vice versa. All patients were led to believe that training would lead to decreased muscle tension. At the same time, the researchers manipulated outcome expectations by informing one group that they were "highly successful" while informing others that they were only "moderately successful." Headache activity improved regardless of whether participants were trained to increase or decrease muscle tension. Moreover, those with the best outcomes were those led to believe they were highly successful at the biofeedback task. Whereas changes in muscle tension could not account for observed reductions in headache activity, the investigators showed that changes in cognition, specifically in self-efficacy beliefs, were correlated with clinical outcomes. This study does not rule out the muscle-tension hypothesis, but it does raise questions about whether other factors, such as cognitive expectations, might be more important determinants of headache activity. It remains to be seen whether other psychologic treatments, aside from biofeedback, can effect similar changes in self-efficacy leading to similar improvements in headache symptoms.

Screening patients for psychiatric disorder or psychologic dysfunction

Although orofacial pain specialists may play a supportive role, psychologic intervention is ideally provided by a mental health clinician (psychologist or psychiatrist) with specialized training in behavioral medicine and chronic pain. This section addresses two fundamental questions facing orofacial pain practitioners: *(1)* When should I request a psychologic evaluation or consultation? *(2)* How do I explain the referral to my patient?

Given the prevalence of psychiatric disorders in this population (see earlier sections) and the possibility that subclinical psychologic dysfunction can undermine even the most appropriate intervention, the authors and others[191,228] believe that routine psychologic screening of patients with orofacial pain is justified. The decision to screen, however, is not without consequences as pain practitioners incur a professional obligation to refer once they become aware that a patient is suffering from psychologic dysfunction. Thus, it is advisable to identify low-cost or subsidized mental health services in the community before deciding whether to implement screening procedures. Once the decision is made to proceed, it is advisable to screen all patients who receive a diagnosis of chronic orofacial pain without exception, rather than limiting the assessment to those suspected of psychologic involvement. This allows the orofacial pain clinician to inform patients that screening is routine and not reserved for special cases. In addition, the detection of psychiatric disorder or psychologic dysfunction can be subtle, and medical practitioners are notoriously poor at this task.[229]

Screening instruments

Patients at risk of psychiatric disorder or those who are suffering from psychologic distress may be identified by one or more screening questionnaires administered at enrollment. One of the most comprehensive instruments available for this purpose is the Patient Health Questionnaire (PHQ).Originally intended for primary care settings, the PHQ is self-administered and provides algorithmic diagnoses based on DSM-IV criteria for eight psychiatric disorders: major depression; other depressive disorder; panic; other anxiety disorder; binge eating; bulimia nervosa; somatoform disorder; and alcohol use or dependence. Patients are instructed to code each symptom based on how often it bothered them over the preceding 2 weeks on a scale ranging from *not at all to several days, more than half the days, or nearly every day*. Aside from a psychiatric diagnosis, these ratings also yield a continuous measure of syndrome severity. The section on symptom reporting contains 15 ailments that account for more than 90% of physical complaints report-

Box 4-1   **Tool developed by Weathers et al[235] to screen for PTSD**

In your lifetime, have you ever had any experience that was so frightening, horrible, or upsetting that, in the *past month*, you . . . *(Circle Y for yes or N for no)*

1. Had nightmares about it or thought about it when you did not want to?   Y   N

2. Tried hard not to think about it or went out of your way to avoid situations that reminded you of it?   Y   N

3. Were constantly on guard, watchful, or easily startled?   Y   N

4. Felt numb or detached from others, activities, or your surroundings?   Y   N

ed by outpatients in primary care.[230] Patients rate each of these symptoms as *not bothered, bothered a little, or bothered a lot.* Spitzer et al[231,232] conducted two separate validity studies involving 6,000 adults attending primary care and obstetrics-gynecology clinics, respectively. Both found adequate levels of agreement between PHQ diagnoses and those derived from clinical interviews by independent mental health clinicians. According to them,[231] most completed questionnaires (85%) could be reviewed by a physician in under 3 minutes. The PHQ is currently available as a free download for clinical (noncommercial) purposes at www. pdhealth.mil/guidelines/downloads/appendix2. pdf. A Spanish-language version has also been developed and is equally well validated.[233]

The PHQ is sufficiently sensitive to identify most cases of psychiatric disorder and/or psychologic dysfunction. It does not, however, explicitly screen for PTSD, which may be prevalent in patients with orofacial pain (see earlier sections). One recent study estimates that as many as 23% of these patients may screen positive for this disorder.[54] This is potentially important for pain practitioners because PTSD is known to be associated with increased pain and is highly treatable in the acute stage.[234] Left undetected, it may compromise the efficacy of otherwise appropriate therapy. Fortunately, a brief screening instrument developed by Weathers et al[235] is available with known diagnostic sensitivity and specificity (91% and 72%, respectively).[236] The tool consists of four items that are answered with either yes or no (Box 4-1). Patients with two or more yes responses are at risk of PTSD and should be referred for psycho-

logic evaluation, if they are not already under the care of a mental health provider.

Referral to a mental health provider

Before making a mental health referral, pain practitioners may wish to offer patients a rationale for combining mental health services with existing physical and pharmacologic approaches. One approach is to suggest that there are two types of pain, one of physical or biologic origin (even if unknown) and the other of emotional origin. Use of this cover story is not intended to suggest an actual dualism. Instead, the goal is to introduce the concept of coping by drawing a distinction between physical versus emotional problems. Although patients often have little or no control over pain sensation (the physical problem), they have (or can acquire) control over their emotional distress (the emotional problem). The unfortunate choice often confronting a patient with chronic orofacial pain is to *(1)* make a difficult situation more unpleasant by disturbing himself or herself about it or *(2)* make the best of a difficult situation by minimizing emotional distress. The pain practitioner may wish to explain this dilemma and, at the same time, refer the patient to a mental health provider by paraphrasing the following narrative:

> Chronic or long-lasting pain, like the kind you have, sometimes forces people to make changes in the way they live. Sometimes you have to cut back on activities at home or at work, and sometimes you even have to give up

activities you enjoy. When this happens, it's normal for most of us to get upset or feel stressed out. The problem is that the added stress can aggravate the pain problem, making it worse than it already is. When this happens, we wind up with two problems for the price of one. In order to manage the pain in the most effective way possible, it is important for you to learn how to live with this problem without getting yourself overly stressed or upset. This means you have to develop an unusual coping ability that most people never have to think about. But when you have chronic pain it's something you have to take seriously. That's why I want you to see a colleague of mine who specializes in helping patients with [TMDs, headache, etc]. My colleague can help you minimize your pain-related stress and give us the best chance possible for a good treatment outcome. How do you feel about this suggestion? Do you have any questions about what I'm suggesting?

In summary, when referring a patient to a mental health provider, the pain practitioner ideally treats the pain as real (ie, not of psychogenic origin) while shifting the emphasis of treatment away from symptom alleviation and toward the restoration of function and the acquisition of enhanced coping ability.

Conclusion

Psychiatric disorders and subthreshold symptoms of distress are prevalent in patients with chronic orofacial pain. Left untreated, these psychologic factors may undermine quality of life, despite appropriate conservative or surgical intervention. The critical review of the literature in this chapter strongly refutes a psychogenic explanation, but there is evidence showing that psychologic factors can affect the course of orofacial pain symptoms. Although not present in all cases, these factors play an important role for some patients and deserve the attention of orofacial pain practitioners. The preceding evidence-based review of psychologic methods and suggestions for routine psychologic screening may help nonspecialists identify patients likely to profit from a collaborative care or interdisciplinary approach that includes mental health consultation.

References

1. Horowitz LG, Kehoe L, Jacobe E. Multidisciplinary patient care in preventive dentistry: Idiopathic dental pain reconsidered. Clin Prevent Dent 1991;13:23–29.
2. Aggarwal VR, McBeth J, Lunt M, Zakrzewska JM, Macfarlane GJ. Development and validation of classification criteria for idiopathic orofacial pain for use in population-based studies. J Orofac Pain 2007;21:203–215.
3. Nagashima W, Kimura H, Ito M, et al. Effectiveness of duloxetine for the treatment of chronic nonorganic orofacial pain. Clin Neuropharmacol 2012;35:273–277.
4. Graff-Radford SB. Facial pain. Neurologist 2009;15:171–177.
5. Obermann M, Holle D, Katsarava Z. Trigeminal neuralgia and persistent idiopathic facial pain. Expert Rev Neurother 2011;11:1619–1629.
6. Scher AI, Bigal ME, Lipton RB. Comorbidity of migraine. Curr Opin Neurol 2005;18:305–310.
7. Low NC, Merikangas KR. The comorbidity of migraine. CNS Spectr 2003;8:433–434.
8. Patel NV, Bigal ME, Kolodner KB, Leotta C, Lafata JE, Lipton RB. Prevalence and impact of migraine and probable migraine in a health plan. Neurology 2004;63:1432–1438.
9. Stewart W, Breslau N, Keck PE Jr. Comorbidity of migraine and panic disorder. Neurology 1994;44(7, suppl):S23–S27.
10. Breslau N, Merikangas K, Bowden CL. Comorbidity of migraine and major affective disorders. Neurology 1994;44(7, suppl):S17–S22.
11. Jiménez-Sánchez S, Fernández-de-las-Peñas C, Jiménez-García R, et al. Prevalence of migraine headaches in the Romany population in Spain: Sociodemographic factors, lifestyle and co-morbidity. J Transcult Nurs 2013;24:6–13.
12. Smitherman TA, Kolivas ED, Bailey JR. Panic disorder and migraine: Comorbidity, mechanisms, and clinical implications. Headache 2013;53:23–45.
13. Buse DC, Silberstein SD, Manack AN, Papapetropoulos S, Lipton RB. Psychiatric comorbidities of episodic and chronic migraine. J Neurol 2013;260:1960–1969.
14. Gelaye B, Peterlin BL, Lemma S, Tesfaye M, Berhane Y, Williams MA. Migraine and psychiatric comorbidities among sub-Saharan African adults. Headache 2013;53:310–321.
15. Nguyen TV, Low NC. Comorbidity of migraine and mood episodes in a nationally representative population-based sample. Headache 2013;53:498–506.
16. Ligthart L, Gerrits MM, Boomsma DI, Penninx BW. Anxiety and depression are associated with migraine and pain in general: An investigation of the interrelationships. J Pain 2013;14:363–370.

17. Lucchetti G, Peres MF, Lucchetti AL, Mercante JP, Guendler VZ, Zukerman E. Generalized anxiety disorder, subthreshold anxiety and anxiety symptoms in primary headache. Psychiatry Clin Neurosci 2013;67:41–49.

18. Balottin U, Poli PF, Termine C, Molteni S, Galli F. Psychopathological symptoms in child and adolescent migraine and tension-type headache: A meta-analysis. Cephalalgia 2013;33:112–122.

19. Ashina S, Serrano D, Lipton RB, et al. Depression and risk of transformation of episodic to chronic migraine. J Headache Pain 2012;13:615–624.

20. Teixeira AL, Costa EA, da Silva AA Jr, et al. Psychiatric comorbidities of chronic migraine in community and tertiary care clinic samples. J Headache Pain 2012;13:551–555.

21. Baptista T, Uzcátegui E, Arapé Y, et al. Migraine lifetime prevalence in mental disorders: Concurrent comparisons with first-degree relatives and the general population. Invest Clin 2012;53:38–51.

22. Modgill G, Jette N, Wang JL, Becker WJ, Patten SB. A population-based longitudinal community study of major depression and migraine. Headache 2012;52:422–432.

23. Moschiano F, D'Amico D, Canavero I, Pan I, Micieli G, Bussone G. Migraine and depression: Common pathogenetic and therapeutic ground? Neurol Sci 2011;32(1, suppl):S85–S88.

24. Antonaci F, Nappi G, Galli F, Manzoni GC, Calabresi P, Costa A. Migraine and psychiatric comorbidity: A review of clinical findings. J Headache Pain 2011;12:115–125.

25. Peterlin BL, Rosso AL, Sheftell FD, Libon DJ, Mossey JM, Merikangas KR. Post-traumatic stress disorder, drug abuse and migraine: New findings from the National Comorbidity Survey Replication (NCS-R). Cephalalgia 2011;31:235–244.

26. Ligthart L, Nyholt DR, Penninx BW, Boomsma DI. The shared genetics of migraine and anxious depression. Headache 2010;50:1549–1560.

27. Ligthart L, Penninx BW, Nyholt DR, et al. Migraine symptomatology and major depressive disorder. Cephalalgia 2010;30:1073–1081.

28. Senaratne R, Van Ameringen M, Mancini C, Patterson B, Bennett M. The prevalence of migraine headaches in an anxiety disorders clinic sample. CNS Neurosci Ther 2010;16:76–82.

29. Beghi E, Bussone G, D'Amico D, et al. Headache, anxiety and depressive disorders: The HADAS study. J Headache Pain 2010;11:141–150.

30. Smitherman TA, Rains JC, Penzien DB. Psychiatric comorbidities and migraine chronification. Curr Pain Headache Rep 2009;13:326–331.

31. Peterlin BL, Katsnelson MJ, Calhoun AH. The associations between migraine, unipolar psychiatric comorbidities, and stress-related disorders and the role of estrogen. Curr Pain Headache Rep 2009;13:404–412.

32. Baskin SM, Smitherman TA. Migraine and psychiatric disorders: Comorbidities, mechanisms, and clinical applications. Neurol Sci 2009;30(1, suppl):S61–S65.

33. Smitherman TA, Penzien DB, Maizels M. Anxiety disorders and migraine intractability and progression. Curr Pain Headache Rep 2008;12:224–229.

34. Kalaydjian A, Merikangas K. Physical and mental comorbidity of headache in a nationally representative sample of US adults. Psychosom Med 2008;70:773–780.

35. Jette N, Patten S, Williams J, Becker W, Wiebe S. Comorbidity of migraine and psychiatric disorders—A national population-based study. Headache 2008;48:501–516.

36. Tietjen GE, Herial NA, Hardgrove J, Utley C, White L. Migraine comorbidity constellations. Headache 2007;47:857–865.

37. Hamelsky SW, Lipton RB. Psychiatric comorbidity of migraine. Headache 2006;46:1327–1333.

38. Mongini F, Rota E, Deregibus A, et al. Accompanying symptoms and psychiatric comorbidity in migraine and tension-type headache patients. J Psychosom Res 2006;61:447–451.

39. Samaan Z, Farmer A, Craddock N, et al. Migraine in recurrent depression: Case-control study. Br J Psychiatry 2009;194:350–354.

40. Maina G, Albert U, Gandolfo S, Vitalucci A, Bogetto F. Personality disorders in patients with burning mouth syndrome. J Personal Disord 2005;19:84–93.

41. Bogetto F, Maina G, Ferro G, Carbone M, Gandolfo S. Psychiatric comorbidity in patients with burning mouth syndrome. Psychosom Med 1998;60:378–385.

42. de Souza FT, Teixeira AL, Amaral TM, et al. Psychiatric disorders in burning mouth syndrome. J Psychosom Res 2012;72:142–146.

43. Schiavone V, Adamo D, Ventrella G, et al. Anxiety, depression, and pain in burning mouth syndrome: First chicken or egg? Headache 2012;52:1019–1025.

44. Gao J, Chen L, Zhou J, Peng J. A case-control study on etiological factors involved in patients with burning mouth syndrome. J Oral Pathol Med 2009;38:24–28.

45. Al Quran FA. Psychological profile in burning mouth syndrome. Oral Surg Oral Med Oral Pathol Oral Radiol Endod 2004;97:339–344.

46. Korszun A, Hinderstein B, Wong M. Comorbidity of depression with chronic facial pain and temporomandibular disorders. Oral Surg Oral Med Oral Pathol Oral Radiol Endod 1996;82:496–500.

47. Gallagher RM, Marbach JJ, Raphael KG, Dohrenwend BP, Cloitre M. Is major depression comorbid with temporomandibular pain and dysfunction syndrome? A pilot study. Clin J Pain 1991;7:219–225.

48. Yap AU, Tan KB, Chua EK, Tan HH. Depression and somatization in patients with temporomandibular disorders. J Prosthet Dent 2002;88:479–484.

49. Huang GJ, LeResche L, Critchlow CW, Martin MD, Drangsholt MT. Risk factors for diagnostic subgroups of painful temporomandibular disorders (TMD). J Dent Res 2002;81:284–288.

50. Kight M, Gatchel RJ, Wesley L. Temporomandibular disorders: Evidence for significant overlap with psychopathology. Health Psychol 1999;18:177–182.

51. Auerbach SM, Laskin DM, Frantsve LM, Orr T. Depression, pain, exposure to stressful life events, and long-term outcomes in temporomandibular disorder patients. J Oral Maxillofac Surg 2001;59:628–633.

52. Dougall AL, Jimenez CA, Haggard RA, Stowell AW, Riggs RR, Gatchel RJ. Biopsychosocial factors associated with the subcategories of acute temporomandibular joint disorders. J Orofac Pain 2012;26:7–16.

53. Porto F, De Leeuw R, Evans DR, et al. Differences in psychosocial functioning and sleep quality between idiopathic continuous orofacial neuropathic pain patients and chronic masticatory muscle pain patients. J Orofac Pain 2011;25:117–124.

54. Sherman JJ, Carlson CR, Wilson JF, Okeson JP, McCubbin JA. Post-traumatic stress disorder among patients with orofacial pain. J Orofac Pain 2005;19:309–317.

55. De Leeuw R, Bertoli E, Schmidt JE, Carlson CR. Prevalence of post-traumatic stress disorder symptoms in orofacial pain patients. Oral Surg Oral Med Oral Pathol Oral Radiol Endod 2005;99:558–568.

56. Afari N, Wen Y, Buchwald D, Goldberg J, Plesh O. Are post-traumatic stress disorder symptoms and temporomandibular pain associated? Findings from a community-based twin registry. J Orofac Pain 2008;22:41–49.

57. Banks SM, Kerns RD. Explaining high rates of depression in chronic pain: A diathesis-stress framework. Psychol Bull 1996;119:95–110.

58. Engel GL. "Psychogenic" pain and the pain-prone patient. Am J Med 1959;26:899–918.

59. Engel GL. Primary atypical facial neuralgia: An hysterical conversion symptom. Psychosom Med 1951;13:375–396.

60. Lefer L. A psychoanalytic view of a dental phenomenon: Psychosomatics of the temporomandibular joint pain dysfunction syndrome. Contemporary psychoanalysis 1966;2:135–150.

61. Moulton RE. Emotional factors in non-organic temporomandibular joint pain. Dent Clin North Am 1966:609–620.

62. Lesse S. Atypical facial pain of psychogenic origin: A masked depression syndrome. In: Lesse S (ed). Masked Depression. New York: Jason Aronson; 1974:302–317.

63. Lascelles RG. Atypical facial pain and depression. Br J Psychiatry 1966;112:651–659.

64. Lehmann HJ, Buchholz G. Atypical facial neuralgia or depressive facial pain. Diagnostic aspects of a well-demarcated form of masked depression [in German]. Fortschr Neurol Psychiatr 1986;54:154–157.

65. Violon A. The onset of facial pain. A psychological study. Psychother Psychosom 1980;34:11–16.

66. Delaney JF. Atypical facial pain as a defense against psychosis. Am J Psychiatry 1976;133:1151–1154.

67. Diagnostic and Statistical Manual of Mental Disorders, ed 4. Washington, DC: American Psychiatric Association, 1994.

68. Diagnostic and Statistical Manual of Mental Disorders, ed 5. Washington, DC: American Psychiatric Association , 2013.

69. Sharav Y, Singer E, Schmidt E, Dionne RA, Dubner R. The analgesic effect of amitriptyline on chronic facial pain. Pain 1987;31:199–209.

70. Feinmann C, Harris M, Cawley R. Psychogenic facial pain: Presentation and treatment. Br Med J (Clin Res Ed) 1984;288:436–438.

71. Cohen SP, Abdi S. New developments in the use of tricyclic antidepressants for the management of pain. Curr Opin Anaesthesiol 2001;14:505–511.

72. Dworkin SF, Huggins KH, LeResche L, et al. Epidemiology of signs and symptoms in temporomandibular disorders: Clinical signs in cases and controls. J Am Dent Assoc 1990;120:273–281.

73. LeResche L. Epidemiology of temporomandibular disorders: Implications for the investigation of etiologic factors. Crit Rev Oral Biol Med 1997;8:291–305.

74. Marbach JJ, Ballard GT, Frankel MR, Raphael KG. Patterns of TMJ surgery: Evidence of sex differences. J Am Dent Assoc 1997;128:609–614.

75. Bergdahl M, Bergdahl J. Burning mouth syndrome: Prevalence and associated factors. J Oral Pathol Med 1999;28:350–354.

76. Tammiala-Salonen T, Hiidenkari T, Parvinen T. Burning mouth in a Finnish adult population. Community Dent Oral Epidemiol 1993;21:67–71.

77. Russell MB. Tension-type headache in 40-year-olds: A Danish population-based sample of 4000. J Headache Pain 2005;6:441–447.

78. Lipton RB, Bigal ME. The epidemiology of migraine. Am J Medicine 2005;118(suppl 1):3–10.

79. Kessler RC, McGonagle KA, Zhao S, et al. Lifetime and 12-month prevalence of DSM-III-R psychiatric disorders in the United States. Results from the National Comorbidity Survey. Arch Gen Psychiatry 1994;51:8–19.

80. Regier DA, Narrow WE, Rae DS. The epidemiology of anxiety disorders: The Epidemiologic Catchment Area (ECA) experience. J Psychiatr Res 1990;24(2, suppl):3S–14S.

81. Weissman MM, Bland RC, Canino GJ, et al. Cross-national epidemiology of major depression and bipolar disorder. JAMA 1996;276:293–299.

82. Silverstein B. Gender differences in the prevalence of somatic versus pure depression: A replication. Am J Psychiatry 2002;159:1051–1052.

83. Silverstein B. Gender difference in the prevalence of clinical depression: The role played by depression associated with somatic symptoms. Am J Psychiatry 1999;156:480–482.

84. Unruh AM. Gender variations in clinical pain experience. Pain 1996;65:123–167.

85. Speculand B, Goss AN, Spence ND, Pilowsky I. Intractable facial pain and illness behaviour. Pain 1981;11:213–219.

86. Raphael KG, Marbach JJ, Gallagher RM. Somatosensory amplification and affective inhibition are elevated in myofascial face pain. Pain Med 2000;1:247–253.

87. Robinson JK. Anatomical and hormonal influences on women's dermatologic health. JAMA 2006;295:1443–1445.

88. Madkan VK, Giancola AA, Sra KK, Tyring SK. Sex differences in the transmission, prevention, and disease manifestations of sexually transmitted diseases. Arch Dermatol 2006;142:365–370.

89. Lockshin MD. Sex ratio and rheumatic disease: Excerpts from an Institute of Medicine report. Lupus 2002;11:662–666.

90. LeResche L, Saunders K, Von Korff MR, Barlow W, Dworkin SF. Use of exogenous hormones and risk of temporomandibular disorder pain. Pain 1997;69:153–160.

91. Dao TT, Knight K, Ton-That V. Modulation of myofascial pain by the reproductive hormones: A preliminary report. J Prosthet Dent 1998;79:663–670.

92. Macfarlane TV, Blinkhorn AS, Davies RM, Kincey J, Worthington HV. Association between female hormonal factors and oro-facial pain: Study in the community. Pain 2002;97:5–10.

93. Galbaud du Fort G, Newman SC, Bland RC. Psychiatric comorbidity and treatment seeking. Sources of selection bias in the study of clinical populations. J Nerv Ment Dis 1993;181:467–474.

94. Dohrenwend BP, Raphael KG, Marbach JJ, Gallagher RM. Why is depression comorbid with chronic myofascial face pain? A family study test of alternative hypotheses. Pain 1999;83:183–192.

95. Dahlström L, Widmark G, Carlsson SG. Changes in function and in pain-related and cognitive-behavioral variables after arthroscopy of temporomandibular joints. Eur J Oral Sci 2000;108:14–21.

96. Kerns RD, Turk DC, Rudy TE. The West Haven-Yale Multidimensional Pain Inventory (WHYMPI). Pain 1985;23:345–356.

97. Ohrbach R, Dworkin SF. Five-year outcomes in TMD: Relationship of changes in pain to changes in physical and psychological variables. Pain 1998;74:315–326.

98. Marbach JJ, Lennon MC, Link BG, Dohrenwend BP. Losing face: Sources of stigma as perceived by chronic facial pain patients. J Behav Med 1990;13:583–604.

99. Vickers ER, Boocock H. Chronic orofacial pain is associated with psychological morbidity and negative personality changes: A comparison to the general population. Aust Dent J 2005;50:21–30.

100. Feinmann C, Newton-John T. Psychiatric and psychological management considerations associated with nerve damage and neuropathic trigeminal pain. J Orofac Pain 2004;18:360–365.

101. Melzack R, Wall PD. The Challenge of Pain, ed 2. Harmondsworth: Penguin Global, 1996.

102. Lobbezoo F, Trulsson M, Jacobs R, Svensson P, Cadden SW, van Steenberghe D. Topical review: Modulation of trigeminal sensory input in humans: Mechanisms and clinical implications. J Orofac Pain 2002;16:9–21.

103. Selye H. Stress Without Distress. Philadelphia: Lippincott, 1974.

104. Costen J. A syndrome of ear and sinus symptoms dependent upon disturbed function of the temporomandibular joint. Ann Otol Rhinol Laryngol 1934;43:1–15.

105. Schwartz LL. A temporomandibular joint pain-dysfunction syndrome. J Chronic Dis 1956;3:284–293.

106. Marbach JJ. Laszlo Schwartz and the origins of clinical research in TMJ disorders. N Y State Dent J 1991;57:38–41.

107. Laskin DM. Etiology of the pain-dysfunction syndrome. J Am Dent Assoc 1969;79:147–153.

108. Raphael KG, Sirois DA, Janal MN, et al. Sleep bruxism and myofascial temporomandibular disorders: A laboratory-based polysomnographic investigation. J Am Dent Assoc 2012;143:1223–1231.

109. LeResche L, Truelove EL, Dworkin SF. Temporomandibular disorders: A survey of dentists' knowledge and beliefs. J Am Dent Assoc 1993;124:90–94, 97–106.

110. Marbach JJ, Lennon MC, Dohrenwend BP. Candidate risk factors for temporomandibular pain and dysfunction syndrome: Psychosocial, health behavior, physical illness and injury. Pain 1988;34:139–151.

111. Speculand B, Hughes AO, Goss AN. Role of recent stressful life events experience in the onset of TMJ dysfunction pain. Community Dent Oral Epidemiol 1984;12:197–202.

112. Wright J, Deary IJ, Geissler PR. Depression, hassles and somatic symptoms in mandibular dysfunction syndrome patients. J Dent 1991;19:352–356.

113. De Leeuw R, Bertoli E, Schmidt JE, Carlson CR. Prevalence of traumatic stressors in patients with temporomandibular disorders. J Oral Maxillofac Surg 2005;63:42–50.

114. Beaton RD, Egan KJ, Nakagawa-Kogan H, Morrison KN. Self-reported symptoms of stress with temporomandibular disorders: Comparisons to healthy men and women. J Prosthet Dent 1991;65:289–293.

115. Pallegama RW, Ranasinghe AW, Weerasinghe VS, Sitheeque MA. Anxiety and personality traits in patients with muscle related temporomandibular disorders. J Oral Rehabil 2005;32:701–707.

116. Glaros AG, Williams K, Lausten L. The role of parafunctions, emotions and stress in predicting facial pain. J Am Dent Assoc 2005;136:451–458.

117. Ferrando M, Andreu Y, Galdón MJ, Durá E, Poveda R, Bagán JV. Psychological variables and temporomandibular disorders: distress, coping, and personality. Oral Surg Oral Med Oral Pathol Oral Radiol Endod 2004;98:153–160.

118. Macfarlane TV, Gray RJM, Kincey J, Worthington HV. Factors associated with the temporomandibular disorder, pain dysfunction syndrome (PDS): Manchester case-control study. Oral Dis 2001;7:321–330.

119. Smith SB, Mir E, Bair E, et al. Genetic variants associated with development of TMD and its intermediate phenotypes: The genetic architecture of TMD in the OPPERA prospective cohort study. J Pain 2013;14(suppl 12):T91–T101.

120. Raphael KG, Cloitre M, Dohrenwend BP. Problems of recall and misclassification with checklist methods of measuring stressful life events. Health Psychol 1991;10:62–74.

121. Raphael KG, Cloitre M. Does mood-congruence or causal search govern recall bias? A test of life event recall. J Clin Epidemiol 1994;47:555–564.

122. Eli I, Kleinhauz M, Baht R, Littner M. Antecedents of burning mouth syndrome (glossodynia)—Recent life events vs. psychopathologic aspects. J Dent Res 1994;73:567–572.

123. Hakeberg M, Hallberg LR, Berggren U. Burning mouth syndrome: Experiences from the perspective of female patients. Eur J Oral Sci 2003;111:305–311.

124. Deniz O, Aygül R, Koçak N, Ohran A, Kaya MD. Precipitating factors of migraine attacks in patients with migraine with and without aura. The Pain Clinic 2004;16:451–456.

125. Zivadinov R, Willheim K, Sepic-Grahovac D, et al. Migraine and tension-type headache in Croatia: A population-based survey of precipitating factors. Cephalalgia 2003;23:336–343.

126. Rasmussen P. Facial pain. IV. A prospective study of 1052 patients with a view of: precipitating factors, associated symptoms, objective psychiatric and neurological symptoms. Acta Neurochir (Wien) 1991;108:100–109.

127. Sternbach RA. Pain and 'hassles' in the United States: Findings of the Nuprin pain report. Pain 1986;27:69–80.

128. Martin PR, Theunissen C. The role of life event stress, coping and social support in chronic headaches. Headache 1993;33:301–306.

129. De Benedittis G, Lorenzetti A. The role of stressful life events in the persistence of primary headache: Major events vs. daily hassles. Pain 1992;51:35–42.

130. Fernandez E, Sheffield J. Relative contributions of life events versus daily hassles to the frequency and intensity of headaches. Headache 1996;36:595–602.

131. Passchier J, Schouten J, van der Donk J, van Romunde LK. The association of frequent headaches with personality and life events. Headache 1991;31:116–121.

132. Reynolds DJ, Hovanitz CA. Life event stress and headache frequency revisited. Headache 2000;40:111–118.

133. Von Korff M, LeResche L, Dworkin SF. First onset of common pain symptoms: A prospective study of depression as a risk factor. Pain 1993;55:251–258.

134. Aggarwal VR, Macfarlane GJ, Farragher TM, McBeth J. Risk factors for onset of chronic oro-facial pain—Results of the North Cheshire oro-facial pain prospective population study. Pain 2010;149:354–359.

135. Slade GD, Diatchenko L, Bhalang K, et al. Influence of psychological factors on risk of temporomandibular disorders. J Dent Res 2007;86:1120–1125.

136. Kindler S, Samietz S, Houshmand M, et al. Depressive and anxiety symptoms as risk factors for temporomandibular joint pain: A prospective cohort study in the general population. J Pain 2012;13:1188–1197.

137. Velly AM, Look JO, Carlson C, et al. The effect of catastrophizing and depression on chronic pain—A prospective cohort study of temporomandibular muscle and joint pain disorders. Pain 2011;152:2377–2383.

138. Fillingim RB, Ohrbach R, Greenspan JD, et al. Psychological factors associated with development of TMD: The OPPERA prospective cohort study. J Pain 2013;14(suppl 12):T75–T90.

139. Bair E, Ohrbach R, Fillingim RB, et al. Multivariable modeling of phenotypic risk factors for first-onset TMD: The OPPERA prospective cohort study. J Pain 2013;14(suppl 12):T102–T105.

140. Manfredini D, Bandettini di Poggio A, Cantini E, Dell'Osso L, Bosco M. Mood and anxiety psychopathology and temporomandibular disorder: A spectrum approach. J Oral Rehabil 2004;31:933–940.

141. Sherman JJ, Turk DC. Nonpharmacologic approaches to the management of myofascial temporomandibular disorders. Curr Pain Headache Rep 2001;5:421–431.

142. Dworkin SF, Massoth DL. Temporomandibular disorders and chronic pain: Disease or illness? J Prosthet Dent 1994;72:29–38.

143. Suvinen TI, Reade PC, Kemppainen P, Könönen M, Dworkin SF. Review of aetiological concepts of temporomandibular pain disorders: Towards a biopsychosocial model for integration of physical disorder factors with psychological and psychosocial illness impact factors. Eur J Pain 2005;9:613–633.

144. Andrasik F, Flor H, Turk DC. An expanded view of psychological aspects in head pain: The biopsychosocial model. Neurol Sci 2005;26(suppl 2):S87–S91.

145. Dworkin RH, Hetzel RD, Banks SM. Toward a model of the pathogenesis of chronic pain. Semin Clin Neuropsychiatry 1999;4:176–185.

146. Caspi A, Sugden K, Moffitt TE, et al. Influence of life stress on depression: Moderation by a polymorphism in the 5-HTT gene. Science 2003;301:386–389.

147. van Os J, Hanssen M, Bak M, Bijl RV, Vollebergh W. Do urbanicity and familial liability coparticipate in causing psychosis? Am J Psychiatry 2003;160:477–482.

148. Janke EA, Holroyd KA, Romanek K. Depression increases onset of tension-type headache following laboratory stress. Pain 2004;111:230–238.

149. Nicholson RA, Townsend DR, Gramling SE. Influence of a scheduled-waiting task on EMG reactivity and oral habits among facial pain patients and no-pain controls. Appl Psychophysiol Biofeedback 2000;25:203–219.

150. Kapel L, Glaros AG, McGlynn FD. Psychophysiological responses to stress in patients with myofascial pain-dysfunction syndrome. J Behav Med 1989;12:397–406.

151. Mercuri LG, Olson RE, Laskin DM. The specificity of response to experimental stress in patients with myofascial pain dysfunction syndrome. J Dent Res 1979;58:1866–1871.

152. Yemm R. Comparison of the activity of left and right masseter muscles of normal individuals and patients with mandibular dysfunction during experimental stress. J Dent Res 1971;50:1320–1323.

153. Yemm R. A comparison of the electrical activity of masseter and temporal muscles of human subjects during experimental stress. Arch Oral Biol 1971;16:269–273.

154. Flor H, Birbaumer N, Schulte W, Roos R. Stress-related electromyographic responses in patients with chronic temporomandibular pain. Pain 1991;46:145–152.

155. Rammelsberg P, LeResche L, Dworkin S, Mancl L. Longitudinal outcome of temporomandibular disorders: A 5-year epidemiologic study of muscle disorders defined by research diagnostic criteria for temporomandibular disorders. J Orofac Pain 2003;17:9–20.

156. Garofalo JP, Gatchel RJ, Wesley AL, Ellis E 3rd. Predicting chronicity in acute temporomandibular joint disorders using the research diagnostic criteria. J Am Dent Assoc 1998;129:438–447.

157. Riley JL 3rd, Myers CD, Robinson ME, Bulcourf B, Gremillion HA. Factors predicting orofacial pain patient satisfaction with improvement. J Orofac Pain 2001;15:29–35.

158. Epker J, Gatchel RJ, Ellis E 3rd. A model for predicting chronic TMD: Practical application in clinical settings. J Am Dent Assoc 1999;130:1470–1475.

159. Wright AR, Gatchel RJ, Wildenstein L, Riggs R, Buschang P, Ellis E 3rd. Biopsychosocial differences between high-risk and low-risk patients with acute TMD-related pain. J Am Dent Assoc 2004;135:474–483.

160. Fricton JR, Olsen T. Predictors of outcome for treatment of temporomandibular disorders. J Orofac Pain 1996;10:54–65.

161. Manfredini D, Favero L, Del Giudice A, Masiero S, Stellini E, Guarda-Nardini L. Axis II psychosocial findings predict effectiveness of TMJ hyaluronic acid injections. Int J Oral Maxillofac Surg 2013;42:364–368.

162. Suvinen TI, Hanes KR, Reade PC. Outcome of therapy in the conservative management of temporomandibular pain dysfunction disorder. J Oral Rehabil 1997;24:718–724.

163. Grossi ML, Goldberg MB, Locker D, Tenenbaum HC. Reduced neuropsychologic measures as predictors of treatment outcome in patients with temporomandibular disorders. J Orofac Pain 2001;15:329–339.

164. Steed PA. TMD treatment outcomes: A statistical assessment of the effects of psychological variables. Cranio 1998;16:138–142.

165. Rudy TE, Turk DC, Kubinski JA, Zaki HS. Differential treatment responses of TMD patients as a function of psychological characteristics. Pain 1995;61:103–112.

166. Feinmann C. The long-term outcome of facial pain treatment. J Psychosom Res 1993;37:381–387.

167. Guidetti V, Galli F, Fabrizi P, et al. Headache and psychiatric comorbidity: Clinical aspects and outcome in an 8-year follow-up study. Cephalalgia 1998;18:455–462.

168. Bair MJ, Robinson RL, Katon W, Kroenke K. Depression and pain comorbidity: A literature review. Arch Intern Med 2003;163:2433–2445.

169. Asmundson GJ, Coons MJ, Taylor S, Katz J. PTSD and the experience of pain: Research and clinical implications of shared vulnerability and mutual maintenance models. Can J Psychiatry 2002;47:930–937.

170. Korszun A. Facial pain, depression and stress—Connections and directions. J Oral Pathol Med 2002;31:615–619.

171. Stahl S, Briley M. Understanding pain in depression. Hum Psychopharmacol 2004;19(suppl 1):S9–S13.

172. Ward NG, Bloom VL, Dworkin S, Fawcett J, Narasimhachari N, Friedel RO. Psychobiological markers in coexisting pain and depression: Toward a unified theory. J Clin Psychiatry 1982;43(8 Pt 2):32–41.

173. Von Korff M, Simon G. The relationship between pain and depression. Br J Psychiatry Suppl 1996;(30):101–108.

174. Kirmayer LJ, Robbins JM, Paris J. Somatoform disorders: Personality and the social matrix of somatic distress. J Abnorm Psychol 1994;103:125–136.

175. Krueger RF, Tackett JL, Markon KE. Structural models of comorbidity among common mental disorders: Connections to chronic pain. Adv Psychosom Med 2004;25:63–77.

176. Aaron LA, Burke MM, Buchwald D. Overlapping conditions among patients with chronic fatigue syndrome, fibromyalgia, and temporomandibular disorder. Arch Intern Med 2000;160:221–227.

177. Plesh O, Wolfe F, Lane N. The relationship between fibromyalgia and temporomandibular disorders: Prevalence and symptom severity. J Rheumatol 1996;23:1948–1952.

178. Arnold LM, Hudson JI, Hess EV, et al. Family study of fibromyalgia. Arthritis Rheum 2004;50:944–952.

179. Raphael KG, Janal MN, Nayak S, Gallagher RM, Schwartz JE. Familial aggregation of depression in fibromyalgia: A community-based test of alternate hypotheses. Pain 2004;110:449–460.

180. Breslau N, Davis GC, Schultz LR, Peterson EL. Joint 1994 Wolff Award Presentation. Migraine and major depression: A longitudinal study. Headache 1994;34:387–393.

181. Breslau N, Lipton RB, Stewart WF, Schultz LR, Welch KM. Comorbidity of migraine and depression: Investigating potential etiology and prognosis. Neurology 2003;60:1308–1312.

182. Breslau N, Schultz LR, Stewart WF, Lipton RB, Lucia VC, Welch KM. Headache and major depression: Is the association specific to migraine? Neurology 2000;54:308–313.

183. Drossman DA. Presidential address: Gastrointestinal illness and the biopsychosocial model. Psychosom Med 1998;60:258–267.

184. Keefe FJ, Rumble ME, Scipio CD, Giordano LA, Perri LM. Psychological aspects of persistent pain: Current state of the science. J Pain 2004;5:195–211.

185. Sullivan MJ, Neish NR. Catastrophizing, anxiety and pain during dental hygiene treatment. Community Dent Oral Epidemiol 1998;26:344–349.

186. Turner JA, Brister H, Huggins K, Mancl L, Aaron LA, Truelove EL. Catastrophizing is associated with clinical examination findings, activity interference, and health care use among patients with temporomandibular disorders. J Orofac Pain 2005;19:291–300.

187. Epker J, Gatchel RJ. Prediction of treatment-seeking behavior in acute TMD patients: Practical application in clinical settings. J Orofac Pain 2000;14:303–309.

188. Dworkin SF. Perspectives on the interaction of biological, psychological and social factors in TMD. J Am Dent Assoc 1994;125:856–863.

189. Turner JA, Dworkin SF, Mancl L, Huggins KH, Truelove EL. The roles of beliefs, catastrophizing, and coping in the functioning of patients with temporomandibular disorders. Pain 2001;92:41–51.

190. Lazarus RS. Emotion and Adaptation. New York: Oxford University, 1991.

191. Dworkin SF, Turner JA, Mancl L, et al. A randomized clinical trial of a tailored comprehensive care treatment program for temporomandibular disorders. J Orofac Pain 2002;16:259–276.

192. Turner JA, Mancl L, Aaron LA. Short- and long-term efficacy of brief cognitive-behavioral therapy for patients with chronic temporomandibular disorder pain: A randomized, controlled trial. Pain 2006;121:181–194.

193. Beck AT. The current state of cognitive therapy: A 40-year retrospective. Arch Gen Psychiatry 2005;62:953–959.

194. Beck AT. Cognitive Therapy and the Emotional Disorders. New York: International Universities, 1976.

195. Ellis A. Reason and Emotion in Psychotherapy. New York: Birch Lane, 1994.

196. Crider A, Glaros AG, Gevirtz RN. Efficacy of biofeedback-based treatments for temporomandibular disorders. Appl Psychophysiol Biofeedback 2005;30:333–345.

197. Ellis A. Reason and Emotion in Psychotherapy. Secaucus: Citadel, 1962.

198. Beecher HK. Relationship of significance of wound to the pain experienced. JAMA 1956;161:1609–1613.

199. Ciccone DS, Just N, Bandilla EB. A comparison of economic and social reward in patients with chronic nonmalignant back pain. Psychosom Med 1999;61:552–563.

200. Glaser J, Kihlstrom JF. Compensatory automaticity: Unconscious volition is not an oxymoron. In: Hassin RR, Uleman JS, Bargh JA (eds). The New Unconscious. New York: Oxford University, 2005:171–195.

201. Morishige E, Ishigaki S, Yatani H, Hirokawa M. Clinical effectiveness of cognitive behavior therapy in the management of TMD. Int J Prosthodont 2006;19:31–33.

202. McCracken LM, Turk DC. Behavioral and cognitive-behavioral treatment for chronic pain: Outcome, predictors of outcome, and treatment process. Spine 2002;27:2564–2573.

203. Morley S, Eccleston C, Williams A. Systematic review and meta-analysis of randomized controlled trials of cognitive behaviour therapy and behaviour therapy for chronic pain in adults, excluding headache. Pain 1999;80:1–13.

204. Sharpe L, Sensky T, Timberlake N, Ryan B, Brewin CR, Allard S. A blind, randomized, controlled trial of cognitive-behavioural intervention for patients with recent onset rheumatoid arthritis: Preventing psychological and physical morbidity. Pain 2001;89:275–283.

205. Turk DC. Cognitive-behavioral approach to the treatment of chronic pain patients. Reg Anesth Pain Med 2003;28:573–579.

206. Gardea MA, Gatchel RJ, Mishra KD. Long-term efficacy of biobehavioral treatment of temporomandibular disorders. J Behav Med 2001;24:341–359.

207. Turk DC, Rudy TE, Kubinski JA, Zaki HS, Greco CM. Dysfunctional patients with temporomandibular disorders: Evaluating the efficacy of a tailored treatment protocol. J Consult Clin Psychol 1996;64:139–146.

208. McCrory DC, Penzien DB, Hasselblad V, Gray RN. Evidence Report: Behavioral and Physical Treatments for Tension-Type and Cervicogenic Headache. Des Moines, IA: Foundation for Chiropractic Education and Research, 2001.

209. Goslin RE, Gray RN, McCrory DC, Penzien D, Rains J, Hasselblad V. Behavioral and Physical Treatments for Migraine Headache. Technical Review 2.2. Rockville, MD: Agency for Health Care Policy and Research, 1999.

210. Butler AC, Chapman JE, Forman EM, Beck AT. The empirical status of cognitive-behavioral therapy: A review of meta-analyses. Clin Psychol Rev 2006;26:17–31.

211. Scott J. Cognitive therapy for depression. Br Med Bull 2001;57:101–113.

212. Durham RC, Murphy T, Allan T, Richard K, Treliving LR, Fenton GW. Cognitive therapy, analytic psychotherapy and anxiety management training for generalised anxiety disorder. Br J Psychiatry 1994;165:315–323.

213. Linden M, Zubraegel D, Baer T, Franke U, Schlattmann P. Efficacy of cognitive behaviour therapy in generalized anxiety disorders. Results of a controlled clinical trial (Berlin CBT-GAD Study). Psychother Psychosom 2005;74:36–42.

214. Aggarwal VR, Tickle M, Javidi H, Peters S. Reviewing the evidence: Can cognitive behavioral therapy improve outcomes for patients with chronic orofacial pain? J Orofac Pain 2010;24:163–171.

215. Aggarwal VR, Lovell K, Peters S, Javidi H, Joughin A, Goldthorpe J. Psychosocial interventions for the management of chronic orofacial pain. Cochrane Database Syst Rev 2011;(11).

216. Ellis A. New approaches to psychotherapy techniques. J Clinl Psychol 1955;11:207–260.

217. Walen SR, DiGiuseppe R, Dryden W. A Practitioner's Guide to Rational-Emotive Therapy, ed 2. New York: Oxford University, 1992.

218. Hommel B, Müsseler J, Aschersleben G, Prinz W. The Theory of Event Coding (TEC): A framework for perception and action planning. Behav Brain Sci 2001;24:849–878.

219. Beck AT, Rush AJ, Shaw BF, Emery G. Cognitive Therapy of Depression. New York: Guilford, 1979.

220. Budzynski TH, Stoyva JM. An instrument for producing deep muscle relaxation by means of analog information feedback. J Appl Behav Anal 1969;2:231–237.

221. Brooke RI, Stenn PG. Myofascial pain dysfunction syndrome—How effective is biofeedback-assisted relaxation training? Adv Pain Res Ther 1983;5:809–812.

222. National Institutes of Health. Management of temporomandibular disorders. NIH Technology Assessment Statement. Kensington, MD: 1996.

223. Holroyd KA, Penzien DB. Self-Management of Recurrent Headache. Geneva: World Health Organization, 1993.

224. Holroyd KA, O'Donnell FJ, Stensland M, Lipchik GL, Cordingley GE, Carlson BW. Management of chronic tension-type headache with tricyclic antidepressant medication, stress management therapy, and their combination: A randomized controlled trial. JAMA 2001;285:2208–2215.

225. Mullinix JM, Norton BJ, Hack S, Fishman MA. Skin temperature biofeedback and migraine. Headache 1978;17:242–244.

226. Andrasik F, Holroyd KA. A test of specific and nonspecific effects in the biofeedback treatment of tension headache. J Consult Clin Psychol 1980;48:575–586.

227. Holroyd KA, Penzien DB, Hursey KG, et al. Change mechanisms in EMG biofeedback training: Cognitive changes underlying improvements in tension headache. J Consult Clin Psychol 1984;52:1039–1053.

228. McCreary CP, Clark GT, Oakley ME, Flack V. Predicting response to treatment for temporomandibular disorders. J Craniomandib Disord 1992;6:161–169.

229. Cassano P, Fava M. Depression and public health: An overview. J Psychosom Res 2002;53:849–857.

230. Kroenke K, Arrington ME, Mangelsdorff AD. The prevalence of symptoms in medical outpatients and the adequacy of therapy. Arch Intern Med 1990;150:1685–1689.

231. Spitzer RL, Kroenke K, Williams JB. Validation and utility of a self-report version of PRIME-MD: The PHQ primary care study. Primary care evaluation of mental disorders. Patient health questionnaire. JAMA 1999;282:1737–1744.

232. Spitzer RL, Williams JB, Kroenke K, Hornyak R, Mc-Murray J. Validity and utility of the PRIME-MD patient health questionnaire in assessment of 3000 obstetric-gynecologic patients: The PRIME-MD Patient Health Questionnaire Obstetrics-Gynecology Study. Am J Obstet Gynecol 2000;183:759–769.

233. Diez-Quevedo C, Rangil T, Sanchez-Planell L, Kroenke K, Spitzer RL. Validation and utility of the Patient Health Questionnaire in diagnosing mental disorders in 1003 general hospital Spanish inpatients. Psychosom Med 2001;63:679–686.

234. Foa EB, Keane TM, Friedman MJ (eds). Effective Treatments for PTSD: Practice Guidelines from the International Society for Traumatic Stress Studies. New York: Guilford, 2000.

235. Weathers FW, Litz BT, Herman DS, Huska JA, Keane TM. The PTSD Checklist (PCL): Reliability, Validity, and Diagnostic Utility [Proceedings of the Annual Conference of the International Society for Traumatic Stress Studies, 25 Oct 1993, San Antonio]. San Antonio: National Center for PTSD, 1993.

236. Prins A, Ouimette P, Kimerling R, et al. The primary care PTSD screen (PC-PTSD): Development and operating characteristics. Primary Care Psychiatry 2003;9:9–14.

Orofacial Pain, Headache, and Sleep

Rachel E. Salas, MD
Charlene E. Gamaldo, MD
Bonnie Kaas, MD
B. Lee Peterlin, DO
Michael T. Smith, PhD

More than 100 million Americans suffer from chronic pain,[1] and it is estimated that 60% of all persons with a chronic pain disorder also report poor sleep.[2–4] Pain in the region above the neck, in front of the ears and below the orbitomeatal line, and within the oral cavity constitutes orofacial pain. Orofacial pain includes pain of dental origin and temporomandibular disorders (TMDs), is associated with significant morbidity and increased health care utilization,[5] and can negatively affect daily life.[6] Sleep disruption has a direct effect on pain processing and tolerance in persons suffering from chronic headache and pain disorders in the orofacial region. This chapter reviews the mechanisms and contributors surrounding this interrelationship between orofacial pain/headache and sleep. The chapter opens with a discussion of the basic fundamentals of sleep physiology as the backdrop for discussing the evidence supporting the neurobiologic mechanisms that tie sleep function to pain processing. Next, the relationship between sleep disorders and disruption is discussed in the context of the specific pain syndromes of the face and neck. The chapter concludes with a discussion of behavioral and pharmacotherapeutic strategies for treating patients suffering from both sleep disruption and chronic head/neck pain disorders.

Sleep Basics

Sleep is a basic human need. Normal human sleep comprises rapid eye movement (REM) and non-REM sleep.[7] Over the course of a normal sleep period, REM and non-REM sleep alternate cyclically.[8] Sleep naturally begins with the transition from wake into non-REM sleep, which is further characterized into three stages (N1, N2, and N3), each of which is progressively deeper from a neurophys-

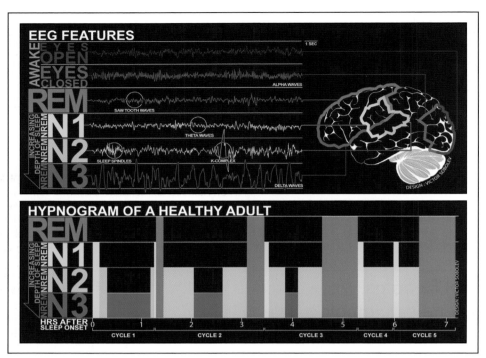

Fig 5-1 *(top)* Typical EEG pattern rhythms from each sleep stage and with eyes open and closed at rest as well as the dominant corresponding areas of origin in the brain. *(bottom)* A typical hypnogram of a healthy individual within five cycles of sleep and sleep stages depicted within each cycle. (Courtesy of Victor Sobolev.)

iologic and behavioral perspective (ie, electro-encephalogram [EEG] rhythms become slower and arousal thresholds increase) (Fig 5-1). REM sleep appears typically 90 to 120 minutes after sleep initiation and is classified into two domains: the *(1)* tonic (parasympathetically driven) stage and the *(2)* phasic (sympathetically driven) stage. Tonic REM is characterized by a low amplitude, a variable and relatively fast EEG pattern, suppression of muscle tone, and loss of thermoregulation. Phasic REM is characterized by irregular, relatively brief bursts of eye movements, cardiorespiratory activity, and muscle contractions (ie, brief muscle twitches) that break through normal muscle atonia, a physiologic feature unique to REM sleep. Typically, over the course of the night, a normal, healthy person will have four or five distinct REM periods. Each successive REM period is slightly longer, and a larger portion demonstrates phasic REM stages in each cycle. For this reason,

REM sleep primarily occupies the final third of the overall sleep period, whereas N3 sleep primarily occupies the first third.

Over the past 20 years, the average nightly sleep duration has been decreasing among US adults and children.[9] In short, sleep deprivation occurs when a person fails to get enough sleep, either willingly (insufficient sleep syndrome) or because of an undiagnosed and/or an untreated sleep disorder. Sleep disorders are medical conditions that prevent a person from getting restful sleep, resulting in daytime sleepiness and dysfunction. Approximately 80 different types of sleep disorders exist, and more than 50 million Americans are affected by a chronic sleep disorder.[10,11] The most common sleep disorders are shown in Box 5-1. Many patients with the sleep disorders identified in Box 5-1 also have a pain syndrome in parallel, such as orofacial pain, which may promote or exacerbate sleep disruption.

PSG

Box 5-1	Sleep disorders*

- Insomnia
- Sleep-related breathing disorders
- Hypersomnias of central origin
- Circadian rhythm sleep-wake disorders
- Parasomnias
- Sleep-related movement disorders

*According to the ICSD-3.[10]

Sleep Disturbance and Pain

Sleep disturbance and chronic pain

The comorbidity of sleep disruption and chronic pain conditions is well described in the literature. Persons with chronic pain have a higher prevalence of insomnia and other sleep disorders compared with the general population.[12,13] One meta-analysis that evaluated 13 studies of patients with chronic low back pain found that 60% of these persons also suffered from sleep disturbance,[14] and another large population-based study found that approximately two-thirds of persons with chronic pain reported poor or unrefreshing sleep.[15] Conversely, almost half of patients with insomnia report chronic pain.[12,16] Disrupted sleep and poor sleep quality have been correlated with polysomnography (PSG) findings of increased sleep latency, increased awakenings, and a relatively reduced ratio of overall slow wave (ie, non-REM or N3) sleep in patients with chronic pain.[17-19] Because pain can negatively affect sleep, it is crucial for treating clinicians to recognize the high prevalence of sleep disturbance in this population. Further, once a person experiences poor sleep due to nocturnal pain or other causes, he or she is likely to experience more severe pain on the subsequent day, therefore setting up a vicious cycle of poor sleep begetting more pain and more pain begetting poor sleep.[20]

Sleep disturbance and pain perception measured by quantitative sensory testing

A growing body of research in healthy participants suggests that the relationship between pain and sleep is causally reciprocal; sleep deprivation causes increased pain sensitivity and vice versa. Not surprisingly, the application of noxious stimulation during sleep has been shown to induce arousals. Although early studies[21,22] evaluating the effects of sleep deprivation on laboratory measures of pain threshold yielded somewhat mixed results and were criticized for small sample sizes and lack of control conditions,[23-28] newer, more well-controlled studies have consistently found that various forms of partial and total sleep deprivation induce hyperalgesia to thermal and pressure stimulation.[27,29,30]

To date, however, even fewer studies have sought to establish the potential mechanisms of sleep loss–induced hyperalgesia. Interestingly, animal studies have described descending circuits involving the rostral ventral medulla and periaqueductal gray regions that dampen ascending nociception at the level of the spinal cord dorsal horn cells. The authors' group, using a psychophysiologic test of descending pain inhibitory capacity, found that sleep disruption impairs conditioned pain modulation (CPM) in humans.[31] These study findings may be particularly relevant to chronic pain associated with TMDs and tension headache disorder, as deficient CPM has been found in both disorders.[32,33] Furthermore, several other studies have also found impaired CPM to be linked with sleep disturbance in patients with TMDs and fibromyalgia.[34,35] Alterations in CPM suggest that poor sleep may contribute to pain amplification by impairing opioidergic descending pain modulatory circuits in the medullary brainstem.[36]

Sleep disturbance, proinflammatory substances, and pain perception

In addition to impaired descending pain modulation, other sleep factors are likely to be involved in pain perception. For example, some

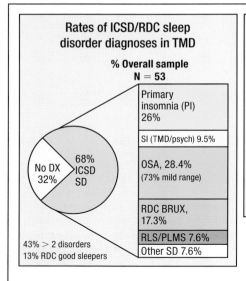

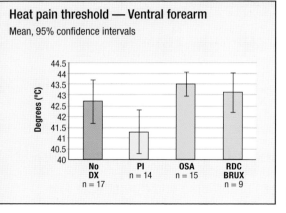

Fig 5-2 Sleep disorders in chronic jaw pain (TMD) and their association with pain sensitivity. ICSD, International Classification of Sleep Disorders; RDC, research diagnostic criteria; DX, diagnosis; SI, secondary insomnia; OSA, obstructive sleep apnea; RLS, restless leg syndrome; PLMS, periodic limb movement syndrome; SD, sleep disorder; BPI, brief pain inventory.

investigators have found that sleep deprivation–induced inflammation may be another promising mechanism by which sleep loss amplifies pain.[37,38] Additionally, several proinflammatory cytokines have been identified to have sleep regulatory actions.[39] As with other pain disorders (eg, migraine), sleep restriction is associated with an increase in inflammatory markers (tumor necrosis factor alpha [TNF-α], interleukin [IL]-1, and IL-6).[37,40,41] Some of these same cytokines have also been shown to contribute to peripheral sensitization of neurons, and TNF-α likely has a role in pain mediation in the central nervous system.[42] Haack et al[37] reported that sleep restriction induces elevations in IL-6, which may exacerbate or induce pain.

Currently, very few studies have sought to determine the extent to which experimental sleep loss in patients with chronic pain aggravates laboratory and/or clinical pain. Irwin et al,[43] however, reported that experimental sleep restriction (4 hours/night) increased self-reported rheumatoid arthritis pain as well as clinician-assessed joint involvement. Alternatively, patients with chronic somatoform pain have been shown to demonstrate increased pain complaints after sleep deprivation but no change in objective pain threshold measurements.[44]

Sleep and Temporomandibular Disorders

Comorbidity with sleep disorders

TMDs are a diverse group of pain disorders affecting the masticatory muscles and temporomandibular joint. TMDs are more prevalent in women of child-bearing age, and most patients with TMDs have disturbed sleep; up to 70% meet criteria for at least one sleep disorder, and 43% meet criteria for two or more[45,46] (Fig 5-2). Self-reported poor sleep quality has been shown to be associated with higher subjective ratings of pain and psychologic distress among persons with TMDs.[46–48] One of the few investigations to include a formal clinical sleep assessment and diagnostic PSG sleep studies to diagnose sleep disorders in TMDs found that insomnia and mild obstructive sleep apnea (OSA) were the two most prevalent sleep disorders in this population.[47] These comorbid sleep disorders may also affect pain thresholds; patients suffering from primary insomnia are more likely to demonstrate thermal hyperalgesia than

---

Box 5-2 **When a patient should be referred for a formal sleep evaluation**

- Persistent daytime sleepiness or fatigue despite adequate quantity of sleep
- Loud snoring accompanied by pauses in breathing
- Difficulty falling asleep or staying asleep
- Unrefreshing sleep despite adequate quantity
- Frequent morning headaches

- Uncomfortable sensations in legs that occur at bedtime but improve with movement and/or walking
- Inability to move while falling asleep or waking up
- Physically acting out dreams during sleep
- Falling asleep at inappropriate times

---

good sleepers.[47] Thus, clinicians treating persons with TMDs should be aware of the high prevalence of sleep disorders, such as insomnia and sleep apnea, in this population, particularly given their association with self-reported pain and objective pain thresholds. Clinicians should be aware that any reports of poor sleep quality warrant further investigation (Box 5-2; see also Box 5-1).

Insomnia disorder and TMDs

Based on existing, albeit limited, data, insomnia is likely the most common sleep disorder in patients with TMDs. Thus, it is particularly important to solicit a sleep history in patients with TMDs and other types of orofacial pain because insomnia is known to aggravate pain. In particular, spontaneous changes in insomnia symptom severity have been shown to predict prospective increases in clinical TMD pain.[49] Moreover, insomnia is also a robust predictor of new-onset major depression,[50] which is known to contribute substantially to disability in chronic pain and TMDs.[51–53] The use of brief screening tools, such as the Insomnia Severity Index[54] used in the aforementioned study, may be particularly useful to orofacial pain specialists seeking to screen and monitor insomnia symptom severity in their patient population.[50]

Insomnia is defined by the *Diagnostic and Statistical Manual of Mental Disorders, Fifth Edition*[55] and the *International Classification of Sleep Disorders – Third Edition* (ICSD-3)[10] as a persistent difficulty with sleep initiation, duration, consolidation, or quality that occurs de-

spite adequate opportunity and circumstances for sleep and that results in some form of daytime impairment (ie, fatigue, decreased memory and concentration, daytime distress). Chronic insomnia, now defined in the ICSD-3 as insomnia symptoms lasting longer than 3 months, has a prevalence of up to 15% in the general population and is a major public health problem that negatively affects morbidity and mortality.[56] Women have a 1.5 to 2 times higher incidence of insomnia than men do; however, the incidence increases with age for both men and women.[57] The mechanisms underlying chronic insomnia remain uncertain, but chronic insomnia is believed to result from a dysregulation of autonomic and central nervous system arousal networks that leads to sleep-interfering hyperarousal.[58–60] Chronic insomnia often presents in association with primary medical illnesses, mental disorders, other sleep disorders, and exposure to, use of, and abuse of certain substances.[10,58] For example, chronic insomnia is a common feature of anxiety, depression, and posttraumatic stress disorder.[61] Thus, predisposing factors such as comorbid psychiatric or medical illnesses should prompt evaluation of sleep disruption, particularly insomnia.[62] Although the relationship between insomnia and pain requires more investigation, the combination of these two disorders may predispose a patient to more complicated presentations, which makes management of both disorders difficult. For example, substance abuse occurs at double the rate in persons with insomnia, potentially negatively affecting pain management in these patients.[62] Interestingly, current and/or past stimulant abusers may be especially vulnerable to the development of insomnia, chronic pain, and depression, which further complicates treatment of patients with pain.[63] Finally, the combination of high pain intensity and insomnia has been shown to further increase the already doubled suicide risk found in patients suffering from chronic pain.[64–66] Given that insomnia is often associated with, and in many cases is the initial symptom of, other underlying and undiagnosed sleep disorders, it is important for clinicians to evaluate for other potential sleep disorders or refer patients for a formal sleep evaluation (see Box 5-2).

Obstructive sleep apnea and TMDs

The health repercussions of OSA are increasingly recognized as its associations with hypertension and other cardiovascular and metabolic complications have been well elucidated. Nonetheless, potential associations with chronic pain disorders in general and TMDs in particular have largely been neglected. Recent studies, however, suggest a possible association. Pain-free adults reporting two or more common symptoms of sleep apnea, that is, loud snoring, excessive daytime sleepiness, witnessed apnea, and hypertension, were found to be 75% more likely to develop new-onset TMDs than adults without these symptoms, after adjusting for many potential confounders.[67] This same study, using a screening questionnaire, found that patients with TMDs had a threefold greater odds of having OSA symptoms.[67] Conversely, another study in patients with sleep apnea found that more than 50% reported comorbid TMDs.[68] The authors' group found that nearly 30% of patients with TMDs demonstrated polysomnographically diagnosed sleep apnea and that the respiratory disturbance index was associated with greater clinical pain but no alterations in heat pain threshold.[47] A more recent case-control study found that patients with myofascial TMDs demonstrated heightened sleep fragmentation due to respiratory-related events compared with controls.[69] Conservative management of OSA includes weight loss, change in sleeping position, and avoidance of alcohol. If these measures fail, institution of continuous positive airway pressure (CPAP), use of oral appliances (OAs), or surgical intervention

can be considered. The American Academy of Sleep Medicine recommends use of OAs for primary snorers, persons with mild to moderate OSA who prefer OAs to CPAP therapy, and persons with severe OSA in whom CPAP was unsuccessful.[70] Although many types of OAs are available, the general concept behind them all is to mechanically advance the mandible and tongue to improve upper airway caliber.[71] Candidates for OAs must have adequate jaw range of motion and no preexisting TMDs.[72] Healthy dentition is also ideal because it allows for more options in terms of different types of OAs. Studies using radiographic and magnetic resonance imaging analysis of the dentition and the temporomandibular joint have demonstrated changes in mandibular position and dentition associated with long-term nocturnal use of mandibular advancement devices, although the clinical consequences of these changes have not been well defined.[73–76] A 2006 systematic review of 85 studies concluded that OAs are associated with frequent associated minor and temporary adverse effects, though significant and persistent temporomandibular joint problems are rare.[77] Jaw discomfort in the early stages of OA use is not generally considered to be a reason to discontinue treatment, and studies demonstrate that these symptoms are generally mild and improve with time.[71,78–81] Close dental follow-up is advised because long-term use of OAs in rare instances can be associated with considerable long-term dental and orofacial discomfort.[71]

Sleep bruxism

The diagnosis of sleep bruxism is considered to be closely related to TMDs. In dentistry, *bruxism* traditionally refers to an involuntary grinding and clenching of the teeth. The American Academy of Sleep Medicine classifies sleep bruxism as a sleep-related movement disorder.[10] In sleep bruxism, the characteristic electromyography pattern is that of episodes of rhythmic masticatory muscle activity of the masseter and temporalis muscles that are recurrent and often associated with sleep arousals.[82] Although many studies have focused on whether sleep bruxism contributes to the development of TMDs, the resulting body of evidence is inconclusive.[82–87] However, sleep bruxism does appear to be associated with the presence of signs and symptoms of TMDs, and it has been suggested to be a risk factor for painful TMDs, possibly through peripheral sensitization.[88] A relationship between sleep bruxism and primary headache has also been suggested, although there are concerns about confounding overlap with TMD-associated headache as well as with the diagnoses of insomnia and sleep-disordered breathing that commonly afflict patients with TMDs.[82,89,90] TMDs themselves have been shown to be associated with primary headaches, particularly migraine, further confounding the assessment of the contribution of sleep bruxism.[91,92]

Sleep and Primary Headache Disorders

The association between sleep and primary headache disorders has long been recognized. Headache pain, like other chronic pain conditions, may contribute to sleep fragmentation and other disorders of sleep. On the other hand, poor sleep may also contribute to the pathogenesis or triggering of primary headaches. Although the interdependence of these two broad pathologic entities has not yet been fully characterized, several possibilities have been suggested: (1) the headache may be the result of disrupted sleep or the process that resulted in the disruption (eg, sleep-disordered breathing); (2) the headache may itself cause sleep disruption; or (3) the headache and sleep are intrinsically linked by anatomy/physiology.[93,94] Although some studies support an association between several primary headache disorders and sleep disturbances, the best studied are migraine and cluster headaches, which are described in detail in the sections that follow.[95–97]

Migraine

Whereas tension-type headache is generally described as a mild, pressure-like pain, typically bilateral in nature, migraine-associated features typically involve unilateral pounding or throbbing pain that is moderate to severe in intensity, exacerbated by activity, and associated with one of the following: nausea and/or vomiting or photophobia and phonophobia.[98]

Migraine may also be associated with aura or focal neurologic symptoms that precede or accompany the headache. Persons in whom headaches occur less than 15 days per month are classified as episodic migraineurs, whereas those with headaches at least 15 days per month for more than 3 months are chronic migraineurs.[98] Although not present in all migraineurs, several migraine triggers have been described, including stress, menstruation, fasting, strong odors, alcohol, weather, specific foods, and, notably, oversleeping or undersleeping.[99] More recent functional brain imaging supports activation of the hypothalamus during acute migraine attacks. Interestingly, morning and evening chronotypes (rather than intermediate chronotypes) are more highly represented among migraineurs and are associated with poorer reported sleep quality.[100] Sleep complaints are prevalent among migraineurs, many of whom report insomnia-like symptoms, shortened sleep periods, and poor sleep quality, which are associated with a worse symptom profile and increased disability.[101,102] Insomnia-like symptoms (eg, difficulty initiating or maintaining sleep, chronically shortened sleep duration) and poor sleep quality are reported commonly by migraine sufferers, up to three times more often than the general population.[101,103,104] PSG studies confirm increased sleep latency and disrupted sleep architecture in migraineurs.[105,106] Evidence also suggests that baseline insomnia increases the risk of subsequently developing migraine or tension-type headache.[107] Persons who experience both episodic and chronic migraine have been shown to suffer from increased rates of excessive daytime sleepiness compared with control subjects, although this may represent a symptom of migraine rather than evidence of an underlying sleep disorder.[108–110] Sleep is known as a terminator of migraine, and the transition between sleep and awakening may lower the threshold for a migraine to occur. Migraine associated with insomnia may occur with circadian timing that is different from that of attacks not related to insomnia.[111] Understanding the factors that determine periodic susceptibility to migraine (ie, sleep and circadian rhythm) may allow clinicians to better predict attacks and provide more insightful patient education to reduce migraines.

In addition to insomnia, restless legs syndrome (RLS), parasomnias, and excessive daytime sleepiness have also been linked to migraine. RLS is a condition characterized by an irresistible urge to move due to uncomfortable sensations in the lower extremities and that is relieved primarily with movement. Sleep disruption commonly results, as the RLS symptoms primarily peak in the evening.[112,113] RLS is more common among migraineurs, and migraineurs with this comorbidity suffer increased sleep disruption and have a worse symptom profile than those without RLS.[114–117] Furthermore, RLS is more common with migraine than with tension-type and cluster headache.[115,118] Migraine has also been associated with other sleep disorders, such as bruxism, somnambulism, night terrors, sleep talking, and sleep-disordered breathing.[119] Thus, patients with migraine should undergo a formal sleep evaluation if they report any sleep disruption to help identify the source of their sleep complaints and to subsequently target therapy to address the etiology.

Cluster headache

Cluster headaches occur as attacks of severe unilateral pain, typically in the distribution of the first division of the trigeminal nerve. Ipsilateral autonomic activation is also characteristic and manifested by lacrimation, rhinorrhea or nasal congestion, conjunctiva injection, ptosis, meiosis, or periorbital edema.[98] These headaches are so named because they tend to occur with variable frequency (every other day to eight times daily) in bouts (ie, clusters) lasting several weeks at a time, with periods of remission in between.[98] Acute attacks are generally responsive to high-flow oxygen and parenteral triptans, and verapamil is generally the preventive agent of choice.[120–122] Cluster headaches have been shown to have a strong circadian component, meaning that attacks generally occur during nocturnal sleep, frequently awakening the patient, and have been shown to be associated

with irregularity of the sleep-wake cycle.[123–125] Early studies suggested an association between episodic cluster headaches and REM sleep, although this has not been consistently demonstrated and remains controversial.[123,124,126–129] Given the responsiveness of cluster headaches to oxygen therapy and the frequent nocturnal occurrence of attacks, association with OSA has also been explored. Patients with cluster headache seem to be more likely to suffer from OSA, although it is unclear whether there is a causal association.[126,130–132] Nocturnal desaturation may act as a trigger or be related to the pathogenesis of cluster headache.[126] Experimentally induced hypoxemic states have been shown to trigger cluster headache attacks for patients in the active cluster period.[133] Several cases have been described where treatment of OSA with noninvasive positive pressure ventilation (CPAP or bilevel positive airway pressure), and, in one case, with an OA, resulted in improvement in cluster headache symptoms, although there have been no larger or randomized follow-up studies exploring this interrelationship further.[126,134–136] The hypothalamus has been implicated in the occurrence of cluster headache, and positron emission tomography has demonstrated increased ipsilateral activation in patients suffering an acute attack.[137] This hypothalamic dysfunction may trigger carotid body activity, resulting in autonomic symptoms of cluster headache. A role for the hypothalamus has also been proposed in OSA, suggesting that the association between OSA and cluster headache may be parallel processes mediated by the hypothalamus.[138] Regardless of the mechanism, it is important for clinicians to be aware of the increased prevalence of OSA in this patient population, and patients with risk factors for sleep apnea (obesity, family history of sleep apnea, male sex, postmenopausal state, and a thick, short neck) with symptoms of apnea (snoring, witnessed apnea, excessive daytime sleepiness, gastroesophageal reflux disease, and increased headaches) should be referred for a formal sleep evaluation.

p. 39

VERAPAMIL

Sleep and Secondary Headache

Obstructive sleep apnea as a cause of headache

Headache associated with sleep apnea is a separate diagnostic entity in the International Classification of Headache Disorders classification system.[98] Morning headache is generally considered to be part of the clinical presentation for OSA, though headache characteristics vary widely among persons.[139] Studies have estimated that a third to half of persons with OSA experience morning headaches, and headache prevalence increases with OSA severity.[139–141] Although more common in OSA, morning headache is also associated with habitual snoring independent of a diagnosis of OSA by PSG.[142] The apnea-hypopnea index, a combined measure of sleep disruption and desaturation events, is higher in patients who have morning headache.[141] Several studies have found that morning headaches respond to institution of CPAP or other OSA treatment, suggesting a causal relationship.[140–143] Presumed mechanisms have included increased intracranial pressure due to apnea-related carbon dioxide retention. Neither migraine nor tension-type headache seems to be specifically associated with OSA, although the presence of OSA increases the risk of general chronic headache severalfold, especially for cluster headache (as previously described).[144–146]

Other Topics

Trigeminal neuralgia

Trigeminal neuralgia (TGN) is a rare, debilitating neuropathic pain disorder characterized by episodes of unilateral, severe, stabbing pain in the distribution of the fifth cranial nerve. The paroxysms of pain associated with TGN occur during the night and during the day, although interestingly most patients report that these episodic and debilitating pain episodes rarely occur while sleeping.[147] Patients with chronic orofacial pain (including TGN) not only report pain-related awakenings (correlated with pain intensity) but also other sleep disturbances.[148,149] These patients are frequently prescribed sedative or hypnotic medications to address the sleep disturbance.[150] Comorbidity of TGN with specific sleep disorders has not been studied. Nonetheless, these patients should be referred for a formal sleep evaluation if sleep disturbance continues or if the patient is at risk for a sleep disorder (eg, sleep apnea, insomnia).

Treatment of sleep disorders in patients with chronic pain

Undiagnosed and untreated sleep disorders contribute to poor sleep quality, often affecting other health domains. Thus, identifying those at risk for sleep disorders is the first step in managing patients with chronic pain, followed by identification and treatment of their sleep disorder. Because many patients with chronic pain experience insomnia and have poor sleep practices, behavioral modification is critical and may be combined with therapies being implemented for other comorbid sleep disorders, such as sleep apnea. Cognitive behavioral therapy for insomnia demonstrates sustained long-term outcomes relative to pharmacotherapies and has the advantage of minimal side effects and drug interactions.[151]

Behavioral sleep modification

Cognitive behavioral therapy (CBT) has long been shown to be effective for treatment of insomnia (CBT-I) occurring in the context of comorbid medical and psychiatric disorders.[152,153] CBT-I is a short-term, collaborative, data-driven therapy that involves multiple intervention components that are tailored to individual needs. Typically, CBT-I is conducted by a sleep psychologist or other behavioral sleep medicine specialist. Sleep is self-monitored via diaries and typical interventions, including (1) stimulus control therapy to reestablish the sleep environment as a contingency for sleep,[154] (2) sleep restriction therapy to consolidate sleep,[155] (3) cognitive therapy to address maladaptive sleep-related beliefs and sleep-interfering ruminative processes,[156] (4) relaxation therapies, and (5) light therapy to regulate the circadian rhythm.[157] Several randomized controlled trials (RCTs) have also demonstrated its effectiveness in persons suffering from chronic pain. CBT-I has been shown to result in superior sleep-related symptom reduction and improvements in sleep parameters compared with sleep hygiene education and attention-control conditions in patients with fibromyalgia, mixed chronic pain conditions, back pain, and arthritis.[158–164]

CBT-I may also result in improvement in chronic pain in some patients, though this is only beginning to be explored. A secondary analysis of an RCT demonstrated improvement in some self-reported pain symptoms, but not others, in patients with osteoarthritis pain who underwent CBT-I.[165] A recent clinical trial comparing CBT for pain, CBT for pain plus CBT-I, and an education control failed to demonstrate a differential effect of the combined treatment on pain over 9 months in older adults with knee osteoarthritis. However, the combined intervention demonstrated superior sleep-related outcomes. Post hoc analyses found that patients with greater pain severity and insomnia at baseline had significant reduction in pain after 18 months when undergoing CBT focused on both pain and insomnia compared with CBT for pain alone. This suggests that patients with a higher burden of comorbid pain and sleep disturbance may have more clinically meaningful long-term improvement with inclusion of insomnia treatment in their CBT regimen.[166] However, this study failed to find an overall reduction in pain or sleep disturbance at 18 months, suggesting that some ongoing maintenance interventions may be recommended. Several other smaller studies of CBT in chronic pain also suggest mixed results with respect to pain reduction, although pain-related outcomes that include interference of pain in daily function appear to be more promising.[158–160] More work using placebo-controlled studies, laboratory measures of pain sensitivity, and efforts to optimize the sequence of behavioral components is necessary.[167]

Although CBT is an effective therapy for insomnia, lack of availability can be a challenge to its utilization. A study that examined use of a self-help book containing CBT-based strategies in patients with insomnia found that bibliotherapy (ie, reading therapy) alone resulted in significant symptomatic improvement. Thus, self-help[168] may represent a more affordable

and readily accessible option to CBT in certain patients suffering from sleep disruption, particularly if CBT is unavailable. However, although it is unclear which patients may be most appropriate for self-help options, clinicians may want discuss this option with patients who are open to this treatment. In recent years, there has been a proliferation in RCTs testing interactive, Internet-based self-help treatments for insomnia. In general, studies using alternative CBT delivery modes demonstrate more modest (small to moderate), but nonetheless significant, effects on some, but not all, sleep continuity measures, compared with the moderate to large effects consistently demonstrated with standard face-to-face treatment.[169] Additional major caveats related to the burgeoning self-help literature is that it exclusively relies on self-reported outcomes, and only two studies have evaluated and demonstrated potential long-term effects.[170,171] Moreover, most of the self-help studies recruited subjects exclusively online and excluded subjects with poor physical or mental health. One study that involved clinical patients found high dropout rates, particularly among patients referred by physicians.[172] The extent to which these interventions may be useful to patients with clinical orofacial pain is therefore unclear. More research is needed to identify which patients might benefit from self-help options and which require face-to-face traditional treatments.

To date, CBT-I has yet to be applied to the treatment of chronic orofacial pain and headache disorders. The general literature for CBTs for orofacial pain has been somewhat limited. A Cochrane review from 2011 concluded that there is weak evidence to support the use of psychosocial interventions for chronic orofacial pain alone.[173] This was primarily due to a paucity of studies and the high risk of bias in existing studies. However, the authors advocated for the use of these noninvasive interventions over more invasive therapies that have also been demonstrated to have limited efficacy.[173] A later systematic review specifically considering the use of CBT for TMDs was also limited by the lack of available controlled studies.[174] Despite these limitations, existing RCTs demonstrate compelling results. For example, CBT approaches for pain management in headache disorders have improved relief.[175] Subjective and objective assessments of pain and psychologic distress were significantly improved for 9 months after intervention in patients with TMDs randomized to undergo CBT, including hypnosis in addition to standard therapy. Currently,[176] cognitive-behavioral interventions for pain do not typically include CBT-I as a treatment component. Given the more promising efficacy data for CBT-I collectively targeting pain and insomnia in other chronic pain syndromes, perhaps hybrid therapies that combine elements for sleep and pain may be a particularly promising approach for chronic orofacial pain syndromes. For CBT to be effective, such complicating factors as medication overuse, psychiatric comorbidity, stress, poor coping skills, and sleep disturbance must all be addressed.[175]

Pharmacologic management of insomnia associated with chronic pain

Many studies of disrupted sleep in chronic pain have been performed in patients with fibromyalgia[177–179] and TMDs.[180] Amitriptyline and other tricyclic antidepressants have long been used in the treatment of fibromyalgia and may provide long-term benefits for improving sleep, although more rigorous trials are needed.[181,182] A Cochrane review concluded that although serotonin–norepinephrine reuptake inhibitors (eg, duloxetine and milnacipran) produced a small improvement in pain symptoms, they were no more effective than a placebo at addressing sleep symptoms in patients with fibromyalgia, and, in fact, insomnia was disclosed as a frequently reported side effect.[183] On the other hand, another systematic review concluded that pregabalin demonstrates a significant benefit in the treatment of sleep disturbance and pain symptoms in patients with fibromyalgia.[184,185] A recent double-blinded crossover trial with pregabalin in patients with fibromyalgia also demonstrated significant improvements in sleep parameters measured by PSG.[186]

Studies specifically addressing pharmacologic treatment for patients with orofacial pain and coexisting sleep disorders are lacking. A recent, small RCT studied the effect of melatonin on pain and sleep symptoms in women with myofascial TMDs.[160] Subjects taking melatonin demonstrated increased pressure pain thresholds and improved sleep quality.[187] Although further studies are needed, melatonin has the benefit of being a well-tolerated medication with few side effects. More investigation of the potential benefits of melatonin or melatonin receptor agonists is necessary.

Conclusion

The relationship between pain and sleep is causally reciprocal. As with many chronic pain conditions, chronic orofacial pain of various etiologies has been demonstrated to be strongly associated with sleep disruption. The presence of a coexisting, often undiagnosed and untreated, sleep disorder is often associated with increased symptom burden. Health care providers treating these patients should be aware of the ways poor quality sleep (particularly in the context of a potentially undiagnosed comorbid sleep disorder) affects management of patients with chronic pain. For many patients, treating sleep disorders could improve pain symptoms and likely quality of life. Performing a basic screening for sleep disorders in patients with orofacial pain disorders provides an opportunity for improved care and should be part of the formal evaluation in this patient population.

References

1. Institute of Medicine. Relieving pain in America: A Blueprint for Transforming Prevention, Care, Education, and Research. Washington, DC: The National Academies, 2011.
2. Morin CM, Bootzin RR, Buysse DJ, Edinger JD, Espie CA, Lichstein KL. Psychological and behavioral treatment of insomnia: Update of the recent evidence (1998–2004). Sleep 2006;29:1398–1414.
3. Smith BH, Elliott AM, Chambers WA, Smith WC, Hannaford PC, Penny K. The impact of chronic pain in the community. Fam Pract 2001;18:292–299.
4. Mundal I, Gråwe RW, Bjørngaard JH, Linaker OM, Fors EA. Prevalence and long-term predictors of persistent chronic widespread pain in the general population in an 11-year prospective study: The HUNT study. BMC Musculoskelet Disord 2014;15:213.
5. Aggarwal VR, McBeth J, Zakrzewska JM, Lunt M, Macfarlane GJ. The epidemiology of chronic syndromes that are frequently unexplained: Do they have common associated factors? Int J Epidemiol 2006;35:468–476.
6. Cioffi I, Perrotta S, Ammendola L, Cimino R, Vollaro S, Paduano S, Michelotti A. Social impairment of persons suffering from different types of chronic orofacial pain. Prog Orthod 2014;15:27.

7. Collop NA, Salas RE, Delayo M, Gamaldo C. Normal sleep and circadian processes. Crit Care Clin 2008;24:449–460.

8. Carskadon MA, Dement WC. Monitoring and staging human sleep. In: Kryger MH, Roth T, Dement WC (eds). Principles and Practice of Sleep Medicine, ed 5. St Louis: Elsevier Saunders:16–26.

9. Ursin R, Bjorvatn B, Holsten F. Sleep duration, subjective sleep need, and sleep habits of 40- to 45-year-olds in the Hordaland Health Study. Sleep 2005;28:1260–1269.

10. The International Classification of Sleep Disorders (ICSD-3). Darien, IL: The American Academy of Sleep Medicine, 2014.

11. Colton HR, Altevogt BM (eds). Sleep Disorders and Sleep Deprivation: An Unmet Public Health Problem. Washington, DC: National Academies Press, 2006.

12. Ohayon MM. Relationship between chronic painful physical condition and insomnia. J Psychiatr Res 2005;39:151–159.

13. Ancoli-Israel S. The impact and prevalence of chronic insomnia and other sleep disturbances associated with chronic illness. Am J Manag Care 2006;12(suppl 8):S221–S229.

14. Alsaadi SM, McAuley JH, Hush JM, Maher CG. Prevalence of sleep disturbance in patients with low back pain. Eur Spine J 2011;20:737–743.

15. National Sleep Foundation. Women and Sleep. http://sleepfoundation.org/sleep-topics/women-and-sleep. Accessed 3 November 2014.

16. Roth T. Comorbid insomnia: Current directions and future challenges. Am J Manag Care 2009;15(Suppl):S6–S13.

17. Wittig RM, Zorick FJ, Blumer D, Heilbronn M, Roth T. Disturbed sleep in patients complaining of chronic pain. J Nerv Ment Dis 1982;170:429–431.

18. Palermo TM, Toliver-Sokol M, Fonareva I, Koh JL. Objective and subjective assessment of sleep in adolescents with chronic pain compared to healthy adolescents. Clin J Pain 2007;23:812–820.

19. Blågestad T, Pallesen S, Lunde LH, Sivertsen B, Nordhus IH, Grønli J. Sleep in older chronic pain patients: A comparative polysomnographic study. Clin J Pain 2012;28:277–283.

20. Affleck G, Urrows S, Tennen H, Higgins P, Abeles M. Sequential daily relations of sleep, pain intensity, and attention to pain among women with fibromyalgia. Pain 1996;68:363–368.

21. Lavigne G, Zucconi M, Castronovo C, Manzini C, Marchettini P, Smirne S. Sleep arousal response to experimental thermal stimulation during sleep in human subjects free of pain and sleep problems. Pain 2000;84:283–290.

22. Bentley AJ, Newton S, Zio CD. Sensitivity of sleep stages to painful thermal stimuli. J Sleep Res 2003;12:143–147.

23. Smith MT, Haythornthwaite JA. How do sleep disturbance and chronic pain inter-relate? Insights from the longitudinal and cognitive-behavioral clinical trials literature. Sleep Med Rev 2004;8:119–132.

24. Drewes AM, Rössel P, Arendt-Nielsen L, et al. Sleepiness does not modulate experimental joint pain in healthy volunteers. Scand J Rheumatol 1997;26:399–400.

25. Older SA, Battafarano DF, Danning CL, et al. The effects of delta wave sleep interruption on pain thresholds and fibromyalgia-like symptoms in healthy subjects; correlations with insulin-like growth factor I. J Rheumatol 1998;25:1180–1186.

26. Lentz MJ, Landis CA, Rothermel J, Shaver JL. Effects of selective slow wave sleep disruption on musculoskeletal pain and fatigue in middle aged women. J Rheumatol 1999;26:1586–1592.

27. Onen SH, Alloui A, Gross A, Eschallier A, Dubray C. The effects of total sleep deprivation, selective sleep interruption and sleep recovery on pain tolerance thresholds in healthy subjects. J Sleep Res 2001;10:35–42.

28. Arima T, Svensson P, Rasmussen C, Nielsen KD, Drewes AM, Arendt-Nielsen L. The relationship between selective sleep deprivation, nocturnal jaw-muscle activity and pain in healthy men. J Oral Rehabil 2001;28:140–148.

29. Kundermann B, Hemmeter-Spernal J, Huber MT, Krieg JC, Lautenbacher S. Effects of total sleep deprivation in major depression: Overnight improvement of mood is accompanied by increased pain sensitivity and augmented pain complaints. Psychosom Med 2008;70:92–101.

30. Roehrs TA, Harris E, Randall S, Roth T. Pain sensitivity and recovery from mild chronic sleep loss. Sleep 2012;35:1667–1672.

31. Smith MT, Edwards RR, McCann UD, Haythornthwaite JA. The effects of sleep deprivation on pain inhibition and spontaneous pain in women. Sleep 2007;30:494–505.

32. Maixner W, Fillingim R, Booker D, Sigurdsson A. Sensitivity of patients with painful temporomandibular disorders to experimentally evoked pain. Pain 1995;63:341–351.

33. Pielsticker A, Haag G, Zaudig M, Lautenbacher S. Impairment of pain inhibition in chronic tension-type headache. Pain 2005;118:215–223.

34. Edwards RR, Almeida DM, Klick B, Haythornthwaite JA, Smith MT. Duration of sleep contributes to next-day pain report in the general population. Pain 2008;137:202–207.

35. Paul-Savoie E, Marchand S, Morin M, et al. Is the deficit in pain inhibition in fibromyalgia influenced by sleep impairments? Open Rheumatol J 2012;6:296–302.

36. Basbaum AI, Fields HL. Endogenous pain control systems: Brainstem spinal pathways and endorphin circuitry. Annu Rev Neurosci 1984;7:309–338.

37. Haack M, Sanchez E, Mullington JM. Elevated inflammatory markers in response to prolonged sleep restriction are associated with increased pain experience in healthy volunteers. Sleep 2007;30:1145–1152.

38. Irwin M, McClintick J, Costlow C, Fortner M, White J, Gillin JC. Partial night sleep deprivation reduces natural killer and cellular immune responses in humans. FASEB J 1996;10:643–653.

39. Gamaldo CE, Shaikh AK, McArthur JC. The sleep-immunity relationship. Neurol Clin 2012;30:1313–1343.

40. Vgontzas AN, Zoumakis E, Bixler EO, et al. Adverse effects of modest sleep restriction on sleepiness, performance, and inflammatory cytokines. J Clin Endocrinol Metab 2004;89:2119–2126.

41. Sarchielli P, Alberti A, Baldi A, et al. Proinflammatory cytokines, adhesion molecules, and lymphocyte integrin expression in the internal jugular blood of migraine patients without aura assessed ictally. Headache 2006;46:200–207.

42. McMahon SB, Cafferty WB, Marchand F. Immune and glial cell factors as pain mediators and modulators. Exp Neurol 2005;192:444–462.

43. Irwin MR, Olmstead R, Carrillo C, et al. Sleep loss exacerbates fatigue, depression, and pain in rheumatoid arthritis. Sleep 2012;35:537–543.

44. Busch V, Haas J, Crönlein T, et al. Sleep deprivation in chronic somatoform pain-effects on mood and pain regulation. Psychiatry Res 2012;195:134–143.

45. Smith SL. Mood and the menstrual cycle. In: Sachar EJ (ed). Topics in Psychoendocrinology. New York: Grune & Stratton, 1975:19–58.

46. Riley JL 3rd, Benson MB, Gremillion HA, et al. Sleep disturbance in orofacial pain patients: Pain-related or emotional distress? Cranio 2001;19:106–113.

47. Smith MT, Wickwire EM, Grace EG, et al. Sleep disorders and their association with laboratory pain sensitivity in temporomandibular joint disorder. Sleep 2009;32:779–790.

48. Yatani H, Studts J, Cordova M, Carlson CR, Okeson JP. Comparison of sleep quality and clinical and psychologic characteristics in patients with temporomandibular disorders. J Orofac Pain 2002;16:221–228.

49. Quartana PJ, Wickwire EM, Klick B, Grace E, Smith MT. Naturalistic changes in insomnia symptoms and pain in temporomandibular joint disorder: A cross-lagged panel analysis. Pain 2010;149:325–331.

50. Breslau N, Roth T, Rosenthal L, Andreski P. Sleep disturbance and psychiatric disorders: A longitudinal epidemiological study of young adults. Biol Psychiatry 1996;39:411–418.

51. Hooley JM, Franklin JC, Nock MK. Chronic pain and suicide: Understanding the association. Curr Pain Headache Rep 2014;18:435.

52. Björnsdottir S, Jónsson S, Valdimarsdóttir U. Mental health indicators and quality of life among individuals with musculoskeletal chronic pain: A nationwide study in Iceland. Scand J Rheumatol 2014:1–15.

53. Kindler S, Samietz S, Houshmand M, et al. Depressive and anxiety symptoms as risk factors for temporomandibular joint pain: A prospective cohort study in the general population. J Pain 2012;13:1188–1197.

54. Bastien CH, Vallières A, Morin CM. Validation of the insomnia severity index as an outcome measure for insomnia research. Sleep Med 2001;2:297–307.

55. Diagnostic and Statistical Manual of Mental Disorders (DSM-5). Arlington: American Psychiatric Association, 2013.

56. Bastien CH. Insomnia: Neurophysiological and neuropsychological approaches. Neuropsychol Rev 2011;21:22–40.

57. Wilson SJ, Nutt DJ, Alford C, et al. British Association for Psychopharmacology consensus statement on evidence-based treatment of insomnia, parasomnias and circadian rhythm disorders. J Psychopharmacol 2010;24:1577–1601.

58. Monroe LJ. Psychological and physiological differences between good and poor sleepers. J Abnorm Psychol 1967;72:255–264.

59. Perlis ML, Giles DE, Mendelson WB, Bootzin RR, Wyatt JK. Psychophysiological insomnia: The behavioural model and a neurocognitive perspective. J Sleep Res 1997;6:179–188.

60. Nofzinger EA, Buysse DJ, Germain A, Price JC, Miewald JM, Kupfer DJ. Functional neuroimaging evidence for hyperarousal in insomnia. Am J Psychiatry 2004;161:2126–2128.

61. Pigeon WR. Diagnosis, prevalence, pathways, consequences & treatment of insomnia. Indian J Med Res 2010;131:321–332.

62. Passarella S, Duong MT. Diagnosis and treatment of insomnia. Am J Health Syst Pharm 2008;65:927–934.

63. Finan PH, Smith MT. The comorbidity of insomnia, chronic pain, and depression: Dopamine as a putative mechanism. Sleep Med Rev 2013;17:173–183.

64. Smith MT, Perlis ML, Haythornthwaite JA. Suicidal ideation in outpatients with chronic musculoskeletal pain: An exploratory study of the role of sleep onset insomnia and pain intensity. Clin J Pain 2004;20:111–118.

65. Tang NK, Crane C. Suicidality in chronic pain: A review of the prevalence, risk factors and psychological links. Psychol Med 2006;36:575–586.

66. Roth T, Franklin M, Bramley TJ. The state of insomnia and emerging trends. Am J Manag Care 2007;13(suppl 5):S117–S120.

67. Sanders AE, Essick GK, Fillingim R, et al. Sleep apnea symptoms and risk of temporomandibular disorder: OPPERA cohort. J Dent Res 2013;92(7, suppl):70S–77S.

68. Cunali PA, Almeida FR, Santos CD, et al. Prevalence of temporomandibular disorders in obstructive sleep apnea patients referred for oral appliance therapy. J Orofac Pain 2009;23:339–344.

69. Dubrovsky B, Raphael KG, Lavigne GJ, et al. Polysomnographic investigation of sleep and respiratory parameters in women with temporomandibular pain disorders. J Clin Sleep Med 2014;10:195–201.

70. Kushida CA, Morgenthaler TI, Littner MR, et al. Practice parameters for the treatment of snoring and obstructive sleep apnea with oral appliances: An update for 2005. Sleep 2006;29:240–243.

71. Chen H, Lowe AA. Updates in oral appliance therapy for snoring and obstructive sleep apnea. Sleep Breath 2013;17:473–486.

72. Epstein LJ, Kristo D, Strollo PJ Jr, et al. Clinical guideline for the evaluation, management and long-term care of obstructive sleep apnea in adults. J Clin Sleep Med 2009;5:263–276.

73. Bondemark L. Does 2 years› nocturnal treatment with a mandibular advancement splint in adult patients with snoring and OSAS cause a change in the posture of the mandible? Am J Orthod Dentofacial Orthop 1999;116:621–628.

74. Bondemark L, Lindman R. Craniomandibular status and function in patients with habitual snoring and obstructive sleep apnoea after nocturnal treatment with a mandibular advancement splint: A 2-year follow-up. Eur J Orthod 2000;22:53–60.

75. Almeida FR, Lowe AA, Sung JO, Tsuiki S, Otsuka R. Long-term sequellae of oral appliance therapy in obstructive sleep apnea patients: Part 1. Cephalometric analysis. Am J Orthod Dentofacial Orthop 2006;129:195–204.

76. Almeida FR, Lowe AA, Otsuka R, Fastlicht S, Farbood M, Tsuiki S. Long-term sequellae of oral appliance therapy in obstructive sleep apnea patients: Part 2. Study-model analysis. Am J Orthod Dentofacial Orthop 2006;129:205–213.

77. Ferguson KA, Cartwright R, Rogers R, Schmidt-Nowara W. Oral appliances for snoring and obstructive sleep apnea: A review. Sleep 2006;29:244–262.

78. de Almeida FR, Bittencourt LR, de Almeida CI, Tsuiki S, Lowe AA, Tufik S. Effects of mandibular posture on obstructive sleep apnea severity and the temporomandibular joint in patients fitted with an oral appliance. Sleep 2002;25:507–513.

79. Gindre L, Gagnadoux F, Meslier N, Gustin JM, Racineux JL. Mandibular advancement for obstructive sleep apnea: Dose effect on apnea, long-term use and tolerance. Respiration 2008;76:386–392.

80. Giannasi LC, Almeida FR, Magini M, et al. Systematic assessment of the impact of oral appliance therapy on the temporomandibular joint during treatment of obstructive sleep apnea: Long-term evaluation. Sleep Breath 2009;13:375–381.

81. Doff MH, Veldhuis SK, Hoekema A, et al. Long-term oral appliance therapy in obstructive sleep apnea syndrome: A controlled study on temporomandibular side effects. Clin Oral Investig 2012;16:689–697.

82. Carra MC, Huynh N, Lavigne G. Sleep bruxism: A comprehensive overview for the dental clinician interested in sleep medicine. Dent Clin North Am 2012;56:387–413.

83. Rompré PH, Daigle-Landry D, Guitard F, Montplaisir JY, Lavigne GJ. Identification of a sleep bruxism subgroup with a higher risk of pain. J Dent Res 2007;86:837–842.

84. Rossetti LM, Pereira de Araujo Cdos R, Rossetti PH, Conti PC. Association between rhythmic masticatory muscle activity during sleep and masticatory myofascial pain: A polysomnographic study. J Orofac Pain 2008;22:190–200.

85. van Selms MK, Lobbezoo F, Visscher CM, Naeije M. Myofascial temporomandibular disorder pain, parafunctions and psychological stress. J Oral Rehabil 2008;35:45–52.

86. Svensson P, Jadidi F, Arima T, Baad-Hansen L, Sessle BJ. Relationships between craniofacial pain and bruxism. J Oral Rehabil 2008;35:524–547.

87. Yachida W, Castrillon EE, Baad-Hansen L, et al. Craniofacial pain and jaw-muscle activity during sleep. J Dent Res 2012;91:562–567.

88. Fernandes G, Franco AL, Siqueira JT, Gonçalves DA, Camparis CM. Sleep bruxism increases the risk for painful temporomandibular disorder, depression and non-specific physical symptoms. J Oral Rehabil 2012;39:538–544.

89. Lavigne G, Palla S. Transient morning headache: Recognizing the role of sleep bruxism and sleep-disordered breathing. J Am Dent Assoc 2010;141:297–299.

90. Fernandes G, Franco AL, Gonçalves DA, Speciali JG, Bigal ME, Camparis CM. Temporomandibular disorders, sleep bruxism, and primary headaches are mutually associated. J Orofac Pain 2013;27:14–20.

91. Franco L, Rompre PH, de Grandmont P, Abe S, Lavigne GJ. A mandibular advancement appliance reduces pain and rhythmic masticatory muscle activity in patients with morning headache. J Orofac Pain 2011;25:240–249.

92. Gonçalves DA, Camparis CM, Speciali JG, Franco AL, Castanharo SM, Bigal ME. Temporomandibular disorders are differentially associated with headache diagnoses: A controlled study. Clin J Pain 2011;27:611–615.

93. Dodick DW, Eross EJ, Parish JM, Silber M. Clinical, anatomical, and physiologic relationship between sleep and headache. Headache 2003;43:282–292.

94. Aguggia M, Cavallini M, Divito N, et al. Sleep and primary headaches. Neurol Sci 2011;32(suppl 1):S51–S54.

95. Rasmussen BK. Migraine and tension-type headache in a general population: Precipitating factors, female hormones, sleep pattern and relation to lifestyle. Pain 1993;53:65–72.

96. Boardman HF, Thomas E, Millson DS, Croft PR. Psychological, sleep, lifestyle, and comorbid associations with headache. Headache 2005;45:657–669.

97. Epstein LJ, Kristo D, Strollo PJ Jr, et al. Clinical guideline for the evaluation, management and long-term care of obstructive sleep apnea in adults. J Clin Sleep Med 2009;5:263–276.

98. Headache Classification Committee of the International Headache Society. The International Classification of Headache Disorders, 3rd edition (beta version). Cephalalgia 2013;33:629–808.

99. Martin PR. Behavioral management of migraine headache triggers: Learning to cope with triggers. Curr Pain Headache Rep 2010;14:221–227.

100. Gori S, Morelli N, Maestri M, Fabbrini M, Bonanni E, Murri L. Sleep quality, chronotypes and preferential timing of attacks in migraine without aura. J Headache Pain 2005;6:258–260.

101. Kelman L, Rains JC. Headache and sleep: Examination of sleep patterns and complaints in a large clinical sample of migraineurs. Headache 2005;45:904–910.

102. Walters AB, Hamer JD, Smitherman TA. Sleep disturbance and affective comorbidity among episodic migraineurs. Headache 2014;54:116–124.

103. Maizels M, Burchette R. Somatic symptoms in headache patients: The influence of headache diagnosis, frequency, and comorbidity. Headache 2004;44:983–993.

104. Lateef T, Swanson S, Cui L, Nelson K, Nakamura E, Merikangas K. Headaches and sleep problems among adults in the United States: Findings from the National Comorbidity Survey-Replication Study. Cephalalgia 2011;31:648–653.

105. Vendrame M, Kaleyias J, Valencia I, Legido A, Kothare SV. Polysomnographic findings in children with headaches. Pediatr Neurol 2008;39:6–11.

106. Karthik N, Kulkarni GB, Taly AB, Rao S, Sinha S. Sleep disturbances in migraine without aura—A questionnaire based study. J Neurol Sci 2012;321:73–76.

107. Ødegård SS, Sand T, Engstrøm M, Stovner LJ, Zwart JA, Hagen K. The long-term effect of insomnia on primary headaches: A prospective population-based cohort study (HUNT-2 and HUNT-3). Headache 2011;51:570–580.

108. Barbanti P, Fabbrini G, Aurilia C, Vanacore N, Cruccu G. A case-control study on excessive daytime sleepiness in episodic migraine. Cephalalgia 2007;27:1115–1119.

109. Ødegård SS, Engstrøm M, Sand T, Stovner LJ, Zwart JA, Hagen K. Associations between sleep disturbance and primary headaches: The third Nord-Trøndelag Health Study. J Headache Pain 2010;11:197–206.

110. Barbanti P, Aurilia C, Egeo G, Fofi L, Vanacore N. A case-control study on excessive daytime sleepiness in chronic migraine. Sleep Med 2013;14:278–281.

111. Alstadhaug K, Salvesen R, Bekkelund S. Insomnia and circadian variation of attacks in episodic migraine. Headache 2007;47:1184–1188.

112. Ekbom KA. Restless legs syndrome. Neurology 1960;10:868–873.

113. García-Borreguero D, Allen RP, Kohnen R, et al. Diagnostic standards for dopaminergic augmentation of restless legs syndrome: Report from a World Association of Sleep Medicine-International Restless Legs Syndrome Study Group consensus conference at the Max Planck Institute. Sleep Med 2007;8:520–530.

114. Rhode AM, Hösing VG, Happe S, Biehl K, Young P, Evers S. Comorbidity of migraine and restless legs syndrome—A case-control study. Cephalalgia 2007;27:1255–1260.

115. Chen PK, Fuh JL, Chen SP, Wang SJ. Association between restless legs syndrome and migraine. J Neurol Neurosurg Psychiatry 2010;81:524–528.

116. Cannon PR, Larner AJ. Migraine and restless legs syndrome: Is there an association? J Headache Pain 2011;12:405–409.

117. Suzuki S, Suzuki K, Miyamoto M, et al. Evaluation of contributing factors to restless legs syndrome in migraine patients. J Neurol 2011;258:2026–2035.

118. d'Onofrio F, Bussone G, Cologno D, et al. Restless legs syndrome and primary headaches: A clinical study. Neurol Sci 2008;29(suppl 1):S169–S172.

119. Cevoli S, Giannini G, Favoni V, Pierangeli G, Cortelli P. Migraine and sleep disorders. Neurol Sci 2012;33(suppl 1):S43–S46.

120. Francis GJ, Becker WJ, Pringsheim TM. Acute and preventive pharmacologic treatment of cluster headache. Neurology 2010;75:463–473.

121. Peterlin BL, Purdy RA, Rapoport AM, et al. Acute and preventive pharmacologic treatment of cluster headache. Neurology 2011;77:921–922.

122. Nesbitt AD, Goadsby PJ. Cluster headache. BMJ 2012;344:e2407.

123. Pfaffenrath V, Pöllmann W, Rüther E, Lund R, Hajak G. Onset of nocturnal attacks of chronic cluster headache in relation to sleep stages. Acta Neurol Scand 1986;73:403–407.

124. Russell D. Cluster headache: Severity and temporal profiles of attacks and patient activity prior to and during attacks. Cephalalgia 1981;1:209–216.

125. Della Marca G, Vollono C, Rubino M, Capuano A, Di Trapani G, Mariotti P. A sleep study in cluster headache. Cephalalgia 2006;26:290–294.

126. Nobre ME, Leal AJ, Filho PM. Investigation into sleep disturbance of patients suffering from cluster headache. Cephalalgia 2005;25:488–492.

127. Terzaghi M, Ghiotto N, Sances G, Rustioni V, Nappi G, Manni R. Episodic cluster headache: NREM prevalence of nocturnal attacks. Time to look beyond macrostructural analysis? Headache 2010;50:1050–1054.

128. Barloese M, Jennum P, Knudsen S, Jensen R. Cluster headache and sleep, is there a connection? A review. Cephalalgia 2012;32:481–491.

129. Zaremba S, Holle D, Wessendorf TE, Diener HC, Katsarava Z, Obermann M. Cluster headache shows no association with rapid eye movement sleep. Cephalalgia 2012;32:289–296.

130. Kudrow L, McGinty DJ, Phillips ER, Stevenson M. Sleep apnea in cluster headache. Cephalalgia 1984;4:33–38.

131. Chervin RD, Zallek SN, Lin X, Hall JM, Sharma N, Hedger KM. Timing patterns of cluster headaches and association with symptoms of obstructive sleep apnea. Sleep Res Online 2000;3:107–112.

132. Graff-Radford SB, Teruel A. Cluster headache and obstructive sleep apnea: Are they related disorders? Curr Pain Headache Rep 2009;13:160–163.

133. Kudrow L, Kudrow DB. Association of sustained oxyhemoglobin desaturation and onset of cluster headache attacks. Headache 1990;30:474–480.

134. Buckle P, Kerr P, Kryger M. Nocturnal cluster headache associated with sleep apnea. A case report. Sleep 1993;16:487–489.

135. Nath Zallek S, Chervin RD. Improvement in cluster headache after treatment for obstructive sleep apnea. Sleep Med 2000;1:135–138.

136. Ranieri AL, Tufik S, de Siqueira JT. Refractory cluster headache in a patient with bruxism and obstructive sleep apnea: A case report. Sleep Breath 2009;13:429–433.

137. May A, Bahra A, Büchel C, Frackowiak RS, Goadsby PJ. Hypothalamic activation in cluster headache attacks. Lancet 1998;352(9124):275–278.

138. Graff-Radford SB, Newman A. Obstructive sleep apnea and cluster headache. Headache 2004;44:607–610.

139. Alberti A, Mazzotta G, Gallinella E, Sarchielli P. Headache characteristics in obstructive sleep apnea syndrome and insomnia. Acta Neurol Scand 2005;111:309–316.

140. Loh NK, Dinner DS, Foldvary N, Skobieranda F, Yew WW. Do patients with obstructive sleep apnea wake up with headaches? Arch Intern Med 1999;159:1765–1768.

141. Goksan B, Gunduz A, Karadeniz D, et al. Morning headache in sleep apnoea: Clinical and polysomnographic evaluation and response to nasal continuous positive airway pressure. Cephalalgia 2009;29:635–641.

142. Chen PK, Fuh JL, Lane HY, Chiu PY, Tien HC, Wang SJ. Morning headache in habitual snorers: Frequency, characteristics, predictors and impacts. Cephalalgia 2011;31:829–836.

143. Johnson KG, Ziemba AM, Garb JL. Improvement in headaches with continuous positive airway pressure for obstructive sleep apnea: A retrospective analysis. Headache 2013;53:333–343.

144. Kristiansen HA, Kværner KJ, Akre H, Overland B, Russell MB. Tension-type headache and sleep apnea in the general population. J Headache Pain 2011;12:63–69.

145. Kristiansen HA, Kværner KJ, Akre H, Overland B, Russell MB. Migraine and sleep apnea in the general population. J Headache Pain 2011;12:55–61.

146. Rains JC, Poceta JS. Sleep-related headaches. Neurol Clin 2012;30:1285–1298.

147. Devor M, Wood I, Sharav Y, Zakrzewska JM. Trigeminal neuralgia during sleep. Pain Pract 2008;8:263–268.

148. Benoliel R, Eliav E, Sharav Y. Self-reports of pain-related awakenings in persistent orofacial pain patients. J Orofac Pain 2009;23:330–338.

149. Pérez C, Navarro A, Saldaña MT, Martínez S, Rejas J. Patient-reported outcomes in subjects with painful trigeminal neuralgia receiving pregabalin: Evidence from medical practice in primary care settings. Cephalalgia 2009;29:781–790.

150. Tölle T, Dukes E, Sadosky A. Patient burden of trigeminal neuralgia: Results from a cross-sectional survey of health state impairment and treatment patterns in six European countries. Pain Pract 2006;6:153–160.

151. Morin CM, Colecchi C, Stone J, Sood R, Brink D. Behavioral and pharmacological therapies for late-life insomnia: A randomized controlled trial. JAMA 1999;281:991–999.

152. Smith MT, Huang MI, Manber R. Cognitive behavior therapy for chronic insomnia occurring within the context of medical and psychiatric disorders. Clin Psychol Rev 2005;25:559–592.

153. Hofmann SG, Asnaani A, Vonk IJ, Sawyer AT, Fang A. The efficacy of cognitive behavioral therapy: A review of meta-analyses. Cognit Ther Res 2012;36:427–440.

154. Bootzin RR, Epstein D, Ward JM. Stimulus control instructions. In: Hauri P (ed). Case Studies in Insomnia. New York: Plenum, 1991:19–28.

155. Spielman AJ, Saskin P, Thorpy MJ. Treatment of chronic insomnia by restriction of time in bed. Sleep 1987;10:45–56.

156. Morin CM. Insomnia: Psychological Assessment and Management. New York: Guilford, 1993.

157. Smith MT, Neubauer DN. Cognitive behavior therapy for chronic insomnia. Clin Cornerstone 2003;5(3):28–40.

158. Currie SR, Wilson KG, Pontefract AJ, deLaplante L. Cognitive-behavioral treatment of insomnia secondary to chronic pain. J Consult Clin Psychol 2000;68:407–416.

159. Edinger JD, Wohlgemuth WK, Krystal AD, Rice JR. Behavioral insomnia therapy for fibromyalgia patients: A randomized clinical trial. Arch Intern Med 2005;165:2527–2535.

160. Jungquist CR, O'Brien C, Matteson-Rusby S, et al. The efficacy of cognitive-behavioral therapy for insomnia in patients with chronic pain. Sleep Med 2010;11:302–309.

161. Miró E, Lupiáñez J, Martínez MP, Sanchez AI, et al. Cognitive-behavioral therapy for insomnia improves attentional function in fibromyalgia syndrome: A pilot, randomized controlled trial. J Health Psychol 2011;16:770–782.

162. Jungquist CR, Tra Y, Smith MT, et al. The durability of cognitive behavioral therapy for insomnia in patients with chronic pain. Sleep Disord 2012;1–8.

163. Martínez MP, Miró E, Sánchez AI, et al. Cognitive-behavioral therapy for insomnia and sleep hygiene in fibromyalgia: A randomized controlled trial. J Behav Med 2013;37:683–697.

164. Pigeon WR, Moynihan J, Matteson-Rusby S, et al. Comparative effectiveness of CBT interventions for co-morbid chronic pain & insomnia: A pilot study. Behav Res Ther 2012;50:685–689.

165. Vitiello MV, Rybarczyk B, Von Korff M, Stepanski EJ. Cognitive behavioral therapy for insomnia improves sleep and decreases pain in older adults with co-morbid insomnia and osteoarthritis. J Clin Sleep Med 2009;5:355–362.

166. McCurry SM, Shortreed SM, Von Korff M, et al. Who benefits from CBT for insomnia in primary care? Important patient selection and trial design lessons from longitudinal results of the Lifestyles trial. Sleep 2014;37:299–308.

167. Finan PH, Goodin BR, Smith MT. The association of sleep and pain: An update and a path forward. J Pain 2013;14:1539–1552.

168. Jernelöv S, Lekander M, Blom K, et al. Efficacy of a behavioral self-help treatment with or without therapist guidance for co-morbid and primary insomnia—A randomized controlled trial. BMC Psychiatry 2012;12:5.

169. Cheng SK, Dizon J. Computerised cognitive behavioural therapy for insomnia: A systematic review and meta-analysis. Psychother Psychosom 2012;81:206–216.

170. Ritterband LM, Thorndike FP, Gonder-Frederick LA, et al. Efficacy of an Internet-based behavioral intervention for adults with insomnia. Arch Gen Psychiatry 2009;66:692–698.

171. Lancee J, van den Bout J, Sorbi MJ, van Straten A. Motivational support provided via email improves the effectiveness of Internet-delivered self-help treatment for insomnia: A randomized trial. Behav Res Ther 2013;51:797–805.

172. Vincent N, Lewycky S. Logging on for better sleep: RCT of the effectiveness of online treatment for insomnia. Sleep 2009;32:807–815.

173. Aggarwal VR, Lovell K, Peters S, Javidi H, Joughin A, Goldthorpe J. Psychosocial interventions for the management of chronic orofacial pain. Cochrane Database Syst Rev 2011;(11).

174. Liu HX, Liang QJ, Xiao P, Jiao HX, Gao Y, Ahmetjiang A. The effectiveness of cognitive-behavioural therapy for temporomandibular disorders: A systematic review. J Oral Rehabil 2012;39:55–62.

175. Lipchik GL, Nash JM. Cognitive-behavioral issues in the treatment and management of chronic daily headache. Curr Pain Headache Rep 2002;6:473–479.

176. Ferrando M, Galdón MJ, Durá E, Andreu Y, Jiménez Y, Poveda R. Enhancing the efficacy of treatment for temporomandibular patients with muscular diagnosis through cognitive-behavioral intervention, including hypnosis: A randomized study. Oral Surg Oral Med Oral Pathol Oral Radiol 2012;113:81–89.

177. Mork PJ, Nilsen TI. Sleep problems and risk of fibromyalgia: Longitudinal data on an adult female population in Norway. Arthritis Rheum 2012;64:281–284.

178. McBeth J, Lacey RJ, Wilkie R. Predictors of new-onset widespread pain in older adults: Results from a population-based prospective cohort study in the UK. Arthritis Rheumatol 2014;66:757–767.

179. Frange C, Hirotsu C, Hachul H, Araujo P, Tufik S, Andersen ML. Fibromyalgia and sleep in animal models: A current overview and future directions. Curr Pain Headache Rep 2014;18:434.

180. Edwards RR, Grace E, Peterson S, Klick B, Haythornthwaite JA, Smith MT. Sleep continuity and architecture: Associations with pain-inhibitory processes in patients with temporomandibular joint disorder. Eur J Pain 2009;13:1043–1047.

181. Roizenblatt S, Neto NS, Tufik S. Sleep disorders and fibromyalgia. Curr Pain Headache Rep 2011;15:347–357.

182. Häuser W, Petzke F, Üçeyler N, Sommer C. Comparative efficacy and acceptability of amitriptyline, duloxetine and milnacipran in fibromyalgia syndrome: A systematic review with meta-analysis. Rheumatology (Oxford) 2011;50:532–543.

183. Häuser W, Urrútia G, Tort S, Üçeyler N, Walitt B. Serotonin and noradrenaline reuptake inhibitors (SNRIs) for fibromyalgia syndrome. Cochrane Database Syst Rev 2013;(1).

184. Straube S, Derry S, Moore RA, Paine J, McQuay HJ. Pregabalin in fibromyalgia—Responder analysis from individual patient data. BMC Musculoskelet Disord 2010;11:150.

185. Smith MT, Moore BJ. Pregabalin for the treatment of fibromyalgia. Expert Opin Pharmacother 2012;13:1527–1533.

186. Roth T, Lankford DA, Bhadra P, Whalen E, Resnick EM. Effect of pregabalin on sleep in patients with fibromyalgia and sleep maintenance disturbance: A randomized, placebo-controlled, 2-way crossover polysomnography study. Arthritis Care Res (Hoboken) 2012;64:597–606.

187. Vidor LP, Torres IL, Custódio de Souza IC, Fregni F, Caumo W. Analgesic and sedative effects of melatonin in temporomandibular disorders: A double-blind, randomized, parallel-group, placebo-controlled study. J Pain Symptom Manage 2013;46:422–432.

Acute Orofacial Pain

Yair Sharav, DMD, MS
Rafael Benoliel, BDS

6

Acute orofacial pain is most frequently dental in origin, associated with the teeth and their support-ing structures—the periodontium. Dental pain is primarily due to dental caries. Other oral pains are periodontal or gingival in origin. Acute dental and periodontal pain is moderate to severe in intensity or ranges from 60 to 100 on a 100-mm visual analog scale.[1] In about 60% of patients, pain is not localized but spreads into remote areas of the head and face and is reported in sites that differ from the pain source.[1,2] Pain-referral patterns for maxillary and mandibular sources have considerable overlap, and the source of pain cannot be predicted from the pain location. Consequently, maps of facial pain-spread patterns are of no use diagnostically. Pain spread is correlated with pain intensity, and stronger pain tends to spread more (Fig 6-1), but neither duration nor quality of pain influences the incidence of referred pain.[3] Pain spread is not dependent on the tissue affected by the patho-logic process, for example, dental or periodontal structures.[1] The mechanisms responsible for pain spread are of central origin, resulting from interactions between primary nociceptive afferents and trigeminothalamic neurons. Factors that may be important for the extensive pain-spread patterns in the facial area include convergence of primary afferents from different areas, such as cutaneous, tooth pulp, visceral, neck, and muscle afferents, onto nociceptive and non-nociceptive neurons in the trigeminal subnucleus caudalis on common dorsal horn neurons; the large receptive fields of the wide dynamic range neurons; and the somatotopic organization.[4,5] As pain intensity increases, neu-rons whose receptive field center lies within the source of pain would increase their activity, thereby activating a larger receptive field and somatotopically adjacent neurons.[5]

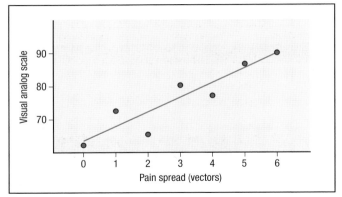

Fig 6-1 Spread of acute dental pain as a function of pain intensity. Pain intensity is described on a 0- to 100-mm visual analog scale. Pain spread denotes the number of locations on the face to which the pain spreads (vectors). Pain spread is clearly a function of pain intensity. (Modified from Sharav et al[1] with permission.)

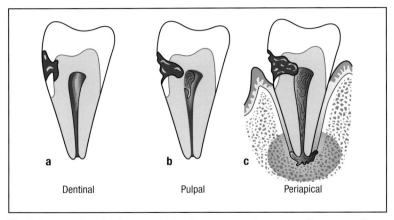

Fig 6-2 Acute dental pain presented at three progressive consecutive stages of caries penetration: *(a)* Dentinal pain is associated with caries penetrating into the dentin; *(b)* pulpal pain is associated with deep caries penetration approaching the dental pulp; *(c)* periapical periodontitis occurs when the inflammatory process invades the periapical area.

Caries and Symptom Progression

No pain is associated with caries confined to the enamel. As caries progresses to the superficial layer of the dentin, however, pain is evoked by various stimuli, such as change in temperature and sweet substances. As the lesion penetrates deeper into the tooth, the pain from these stimuli becomes stronger and

lasts longer. Finally, when the caries lesion approaches the tooth pulp, a strong, spontaneous, paroxysmal pain develops, which is usually intermittent in nature. Microorganisms and products of tissue disintegration invade the area around the root apex, and the tooth becomes very sensitive to chewing, touch, and percussion. Usually at that stage the paroxysmal, intermittent pain has a continuous dull nature, and the tooth is no longer sensitive to changes in temperature. The development of

ANAMNESTIC

Table 6-1	Anamnestic details of dental and periodontal pain			
Pain origin	**Localization**	**Character**	**Intensity**	**Aggravated by**
Dental				
Dentinal	Poor	Evoked, does not outlast stimulus	Mild to moderate	Hot, cold, sweet, or sour foods
Pulpal	Very poor	Spontaneous, paroxysmal, intermittent	Moderate to severe	Hot, cold, sometimes chewing
Periodontal				
Periapical/lateral	Good	Continues for hours, deep, boring	Moderate to severe	Chewing

Table 6-2	Physical and radiographic signs of dental and periodontal pain		
Pain origin	**Associated signs**	**Diagnostic findings**	**Radiography**
Dental			
Dentinal	Caries, exposed dentin, defective restorations	Sensitive to cold application, pain moderate, no overshoot	Proximal caries, defective restorations
Pulpal	Deep caries, extensive restorations	Strong pain to cold application with overshoot, may be tender to percussion	Deep caries or restorations, pulp exposure
Periodontal			
Periapical	Periapical tenderness, redness and swelling, vertical tooth mobility	Very tender to percussion, nonvital tooth pulp	Usually no periapical changes at acute stage
Lateral	Periodontal tenderness, redness and swelling, tooth mobility	Tender to percussion, deep pockets on probing	Alveolar bone resorption

symptoms follows the progression of pathology and the dental structures involved: initially dentin, followed by pulp, and ultimately the periodontal tissues (Fig 6-2). In clinical practice, the demarcation between these various stages is sometimes indistinct; the tooth may be sensitive simultaneously to temperature changes and to chewing.

Pain arising from the oral mucosa may be localized and associated with a detectable erosive or ulcerative lesion or may be of a diffuse nature. Pain descriptors on their own are not sufficient for diagnosis, and orofacial diseases must be validated by other diagnostic procedures, such as physical examination and radiographs. The anamnestic details of dental and periodontal pain are described in Table 6-1, and the physical and radiographic signs are described in Table 6-2.

Epidemiology

Epidemiologic data on dental pain are sparse and of poor quality. The reported prevalence of dental pain in community-dwelling adults ranges from 12% to 40%, depending on the description used for dental pain.[6–9]

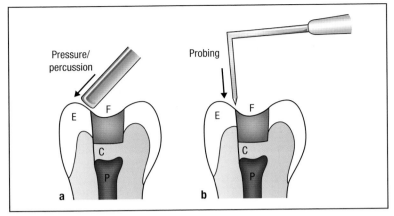

Fig 6-3 Detecting a crack in dentin by *(a)* oblique percussion or pressure on one cusp or *(b)* firm probing between filling and tooth with a sharp explorer to widen the crack. This will activate dentinal and/or pulpal nociceptive mechanisms. C, crack; E, enamel; F, filling; P, pulp chamber.

Dental Pain

Dentinal pain

Symptoms

The pain originating in dentin is a sharp, deep sensation evoked by external stimuli that subsides within a few seconds. Hot, cold, and sweet are among the external stimuli that may produce pain. Pain is poorly localized, often only to an approximate area within two or three teeth adjacent to the affected tooth. Frequently, the patient is unable to distinguish whether the pain originates from the mandible or the maxilla.

Physical and radiographic signs

Common pathologies associated with dentinal pain are early dental caries, defective restorations, and areas of exposed dentin (due to abrasion or erosion of the enamel) and exposed roots (due to gingival recession or periodontal therapy).[10] Duplication of pain produced by controlled application of cold or hot stimuli to various teeth in the suspected area as well as direct observation and examination with a sharp dental probe are useful in locating the affected tooth. Areas of exposed dentin, for example, are scratched with a sharp dental probe

to evoke pain and locate its source. Not all areas of exposed dentin are sensitive, and therefore not all areas are a source of pain.

A bitewing dental radiograph (see Fig 6-4a) is a useful diagnostic aid in these cases, especially when the caries lesion is situated on a proximal tooth surface that is not easily visualized by direct observation or probing. A periapical dental radiograph is useful for assessing processes affecting the tooth root (see Fig 6-4b).

Cracked tooth syndrome

Symptoms. In addition to the symptoms typical for dentinal pain, a patient may also complain of a sharp pain, elicited by biting, that resolves immediately. Localization of the source of pain is not precise but aided by the biting location. Typically, the patient also complains of pain and discomfort associated with cold and hot foods. These complaints indicate a crack in the dentin, known as *cracked tooth syndrome*.[11,12] These incompletely fractured teeth may be associated with long-lasting diffuse orofacial pain and are difficult to diagnose.[13]

Physical and radiographic signs. The main diagnostic challenge is localizing the affected tooth, especially because the crack is not readily detected and radiographs are not helpful. Localization can be achieved by causing the crack to widen, and thus duplicating the pain, by the following techniques:

- Using percussion or pressure on the cusps of the suspected teeth at different angles (Fig 6-3a)
- Asking the patient to bite on individual cusps using a fine wooden stick or a predesigned bite stick (available commercially)
- Probing firmly around the margins of fillings and in suspected fissures (Fig 6-3b)

The bite test was found to be the most reliable for reproducing symptoms.[12] A similar but distinct entity, a vertical root fracture, may produce similar symptomatology and is discussed under the periodontal pain section.

Treatment of dentinal pain

Dentinal pain due to caries is best treated by removing the caries lesion and restoring the tooth. Sensitivity usually disappears within a day or two, although when the caries lesion is deep the tooth may remain sensitive to cold stimulation for a week or two. Treatment of the cracked tooth depends on the state of the tooth (existing restorations, periodontal condition) and the extent of the fracture. Often, removal of an existing restoration allows the fracture to be localized and its extent determined. Isolated fractures of single cusps may be treated by their removal and subsequent tooth restoration. In some cases, restoring the tooth is inevitable, but root canal treatment is usually not indicated. Of 127 teeth that were restored because of a crack and specifically diagnosed with reversible pulpitis, 100 did not require root canal treatment within 6 years of follow-up. The researchers concluded, however, that about 20% of the patients would need root canal treatment within 6 months.[14]

Hypersensitive (exposed) dentin can be treated by interventions that reduce dentinal tubule permeability. Desensitizing toothpastes with ingredients such as stannous fluoride or potassium nitrate will improve symptoms for most patients.[15,16] Other tubule-blocking agents include resins; glass-ionomer cements and bonding agents; strontium chloride or acetate; aluminum, potassium, or ferric oxalates; silica- or calcium-containing materials; and protein precipitants.[16,17] The use of CO_2 and Nd:YAG lasers for cervical hypersensitivity were also found to be effective, as no damage to the tooth pulp was recorded.[18] A recent systematic review and network meta-analysis concluded that most active treatment options had a significantly better treatment outcome than the placebo.[19]

Pulpal pain

Symptoms

Pulpal pain is spontaneous, strong, often throbbing, and exacerbated by changes in temperature and pressure on the caries lesion. When evoked, pain outlasts the stimulus (unlike stimulus-induced dentinal pain) and can be excruciating for many minutes (see Table 6-1). Similar to dentinal pain, localization is poor and becomes even poorer when pain is more intense. Pain tends to radiate or refer to the ear, temple, and cheek, but there are no definitive pain-radiation patterns, and there is considerable overlap in pain reference locations of maxillary and mandibular teeth.[1,3] Pain does not usually cross the midline. Patients may describe pain as a continuous dull ache that is periodically exacerbated (by stimulation or spontaneously) for short (minutes) or long (hours) periods.[20]

Pain may increase and throb when the patient lies down, and, in many instances, it wakes the patient from sleep.[1] Many believe that this throbbing is associated with arterial pulsations. However, contrary to this accepted view, it was found that the throbbing rate (44 ± 3 beats per minute [mean ± SEM]) was much slower than the arterial pulsation rate (73 ± 2 beats per minute [mean ± SEM]; $P < .001$) and that the two rhythms exhibited no underlying synchrony.[21] Pain originating from the pulp is frequently not continuous and abates spontaneously; the precise explanation for such abatement is unclear. This episodic, sharp, paroxysmal, non-localized pain may lead to the misdiagnosis of other conditions that mimic pain of pulpal origin (eg, cluster headache, trigeminal neuralgia; see chapters 10 and 11).

Although pain is the most common symptom of a diseased pulp, no correlation exists between specific pain characteristics and the histopathologic status of the pulp.[22] Further-

Table 6-3	Clinical characteristics to consider when deciding whether to preserve (reversible) or extirpate (irreversible) the tooth pulp in cases of painful pulpitis	
Characteristics	**Reversible**	**Irreversible**
Pain intensity	Mild	Severe
History of spontaneous pain	No	Yes
Pain duration	Short	Prolonged, recurrent
Temperature sensitivity	Mild, short-lasting	Strong, overshoot
Percussion	Usually not tender	Tender
Caries removal	Usually no exposure	Very often clear pulp exposure
Radiographs	Early caries or shallow restoration, recent tooth preparation	Deep caries or restoration with no secondary dentin

more, despite the fact that pain associated with pulpitis is severe, there are instances when a diseased tooth pulp can progress directly to pulp necrosis without pain. Approximately 40% of 2,202 teeth that were treated endodontically had no history of spontaneous pain or of prolonged pain to thermal stimulation.[23]

Physical and radiographic signs

Localization of the affected tooth is the initial aim of the diagnostic process, and it is achieved through the same methods detailed for dentinal pain (see Table 6-2). The application of heat or cold to the teeth should be done carefully because it can cause unbearable pain. In reversible pulpitis, pain response outlasts the stimulus, usually by less than 10 seconds. In irreversible pulpitis, cold application results in excruciating pain that outlasts the stimulus for well beyond 10 seconds. Vital teeth requiring endodontic treatment and painful on percussion are common.[24] Therefore, percussion is a quick test for localizing the affected tooth, as about 80% of teeth with painful pulpitis are tender to percussion. The state of the pulp cannot be judged from a single symptom, however; diagnosis should be based on the combination of several signs and symptoms[20] (Table 6-3).

Treatment

Depending on the diagnosis, treatment may aim at conserving the pulp (reversible pulpitis), extirpating the pulp (irreversible pulpitis),

or extracting the tooth. When pain is mild or moderate and there is normal pulpal vitality, no previous history of pain, and no pain on percussion, the pulp is in the reversible category, and the tooth pulp should be preserved by caries removal and indirect pulp capping.[25] The success rate of a calcium hydroxide–based direct capping agent in permanent teeth was 80.1% after 1 year, 68.0% after 5 years, and 58.7% after 9 years.[26] Spontaneous, severe pain with a history of previous pain and prolonged pain on cold stimuli was significantly more frequent in patients with irreversible pulpitis.[27] One should be aware, however, that these indications are under debate and some controversies exist.[28] Pulpal pain normally disappears immediately after treatment. Persistent pain, regardless of etiology, lasting 6 months or longer after endodontic treatment was estimated to be 5.3%, though higher-quality studies suggested that it is greater than 7%,[29] of which about half was thought to have a nonodontogenic origin.[30] Systemic penicillin administration clearly has no effect on pain amelioration or prognosis of irreversible pulpitis.[31,32] The anesthetic efficacy of inferior alveolar nerve blocks in patients with irreversible pulpitis ranges between 26% and 56%. The rate of success can be improved by doubling the volume of anesthetics[33] or, even better, by combining it with buccal infiltration.[34–36] The clinical characteristics that dictate treatment indications for teeth with painful pulpitis are summarized in Table 6-3. Case 6-1 demonstrates a patient with irreversible pulpitis (Fig 6-4).

CASE 6-1

A 22-year-old woman with acute pulpitis.

Primary complaint: For the past 2 days, the patient has suffered from strong, paroxysmal pain in the lower mandible. Pain radiates to the ear and wakes the patient from sleep.

Findings: The bitewing radiograph (Fig 6-4a) exhibits more than one deep carious location and therefore presents difficulty in locating the source of the spontaneous pain. The source of pain is detected by means of a physical examination. A periapical radiograph of the mandibular left first molar (Fig 6-4b) demonstrates periapical radiolucency. Note that periapical radiolucency and tenderness to percussion coexist with strong pain to cold stimulation.

Diagnosis and treatment: The diagnosis was irreversible pulpitis. The tooth pulp was extirpated, resulting in complete subsequent pain relief.

Comments: The history and type of pain indicate the diagnosis of acute pulpitis. Although the type of pain was typical for acute pulpitis, locating the affected tooth was somewhat problematic because there was more than one possible source. The source of the acute, spontaneous, severe pain was evident from the signs of the physical examination. Although the maxillary left second premolar and the mandibular left first molar both responded with strong pain to cold application, only the first molar exhibited overshoot and tenderness to percussion. Note that periapical radiolucency and tenderness to percussion coexisted with strong pain to cold stimulation.

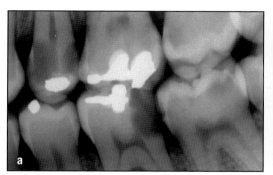 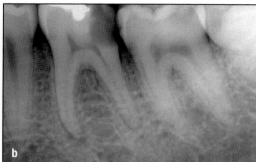

Fig 6-4 Case 6-1. *(a)* Bitewing radiograph of the left side demonstrating multiple locations with deep caries, especially the maxillary second premolar and mandibular first molar. *(b)* Periapical radiograph of the mandibular left first molar demonstrating deep caries, widening of the periodontal ligament, and periapical radiolucency (especially at the mesial root).

Mechanisms of dental pain

Dentinal sensitivity

The mechanisms of dentinal sensitivity and pain have been extensively reviewed.[37–40] Morphologically, nerve fibers may penetrate into the dentin about halfway into the odontoblastic process but certainly do not reach the dentinoenamel junction[37,41] (Fig 6-5). Furthermore, the concept that the odontoblast has a role as a sensory receptor of the dentin has not been substantiated.[42] Experimental pain may be induced by applying various stimuli to exposed dentin, that is, drying by application of absorbent paper or a stream of air; mechanical stimulation (eg, cutting, scratching, probing); and changes in osmotic pressure, pH, or temperature. However, the application of well-established algesic substances, such as potassium chloride, acetylcholine, 5-hydroxytryptamine, bradykinin, and histamine, to exposed dentin does not evoke pain.[43,44] All of these substances can produce pain, however, when placed on a skin blister base.[45] The limited distribution of nerve fibers in dentin and the fact that neuroactive chemicals

Algesic

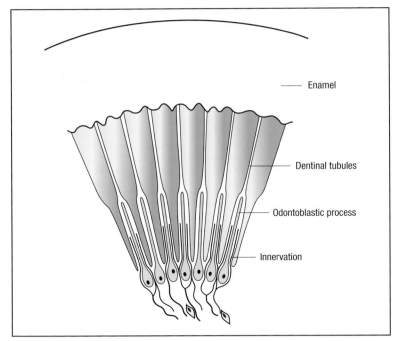

Fig 6-5 Diagram of dentinal innervation. Note that the intratubular odontoblastic process penetrates only about half of the dentinal tubule. Also, not all dentinal tubules are innervated. The percentage of innervated tubules decreases from the tip of the crown toward the root. (Modified with permission from Byers and Närhi.[37])

fail to stimulate or anesthetize dentin led Brannstrom[46] to propose a hydrodynamic mechanism. According to Brannstrom's hypothesis, the movement of extracellular fluid that fills the dentinal tubules will distort the pain-sensitive nervous structure in the pulp and predentinal area and activate mechanoreceptors to produce pain. Several other theories have been proposed, such as the so-called neural theory and odontoblast transduction theory, but most of the evidence supports the hydrodynamic theory.[47] The dentinal tubules seem to act as passive hydraulic links between the site of stimulation and nerve endings sensitive to pressure at the pulpal end in the underlying pulp. Analysis of thermal-induced dentinal fluid flow and its implications in dental thermal pain were examined by using a mathematic model to simulate the temperature and thermal stress distribution in a tooth undergoing thermal stimulation.[39] The researchers concluded that rapid fluid flow caused by thermal deformation of den-

tinal tubules may account for the short latency (< 1 second) activation of mechanosensitive receptors after cooling. Long latency (> 10 seconds) neural responses could be associated with the activation of thermosensitive receptors.[39] Facts and hypotheses regarding dental pain and odontoblasts are further discussed in a recent topical review.[38] Immunohistochemical observation showed localization of transient receptor potential vanilloid subfamily member 1 (TRPV1) channel immunoreactions on the distal regions of odontoblast membranes, suggesting that odontoblasts may directly respond to noxious stimuli such as a thermal-heat stimulus.[48] The expression of TRPV1 (heat) and TRPV2 (heat/mechanical) channels in the cell bodies and terminal arborizations of neurons that innervate the dental pulp and periodontal tissues were recently evaluated.[49] The TRPV1 receptor was more extensively expressed in neurons innervating the periodontal ligament (26%), and about 50% of trigeminal ganglion neurons retrogradely labeled from the dental pulp expressed TRPV2.[49] The cellular and molecular mechanisms of dental nociception were recently reviewed[40] in a study that discussed three hypotheses proposed to explain dentinal hypersensitivity: The first hypothesis emphasizes the direct transduction of noxious temperature-sensitive transient receptor potential by dental primary afferent neurons. The second, known as the *hydrodynamic theory*, attributes dental pain to fluid movement within dentinal tubules. The third focuses on the potential sensory function of odontoblasts in the detection of thermal or mechanical stimuli.[40]

Pulpal pain

Pain mechanisms underlying pulpal pain are related to inflammation and include a host of mediators found in the pulp, such as cholinergic and adrenergic neurotransmitters, prostaglandins, and cyclic adenosine monophosphate.[17,50] Some substances, such as prostaglandins (particularly prostaglandin E_2 [PGE_2]), serotonin, and bradykinin contribute to tooth-pulp nerve excitability, and PGE_2 enhances bradykinin-evoked calcitonin gene-related peptide release in bovine dental pulp.[51] Bradykinin released during inflammation may contribute to the initiation of neurogenic inflammation in dental pulp and may regulate pulpal response to injury or inflammation. The expression of substance P, a neuropeptide with a major role in nociception, significantly increases with caries progression. Of clinical significance was the fact that this increase in substance P was significantly greater in carious specimens that were painful than in asymptomatic carious specimens.[52] Substance P increases microvascular permeability, edema formation, and subsequent plasma protein extravasation, which underlie its powerful proinflammatory properties.[53] In endodontically affected teeth, higher levels of endotoxin were detected in teeth with exudation, whereas elevated levels of PGE_2 were found in teeth with tenderness to percussion and pain on palpation.[54] Irreversible pulpitis (but not reversible pulpitis) is associated with upregulation of tumor necrosis factor alpha (TNF-α) gene expression in human pulp, and this gene expression in inflamed human dental pulp tissue is positively associated with the severity of clinical symptoms.[55] Researchers suspect that, unlike pulpal C fibers, A fibers are relatively insensitive to inflammatory mediators.[56] On the other hand, it was found that leukotriene B4 (LTB4) can sensitize pulpal Aδ fibers and may be a long-lasting hyperalgesic factor that contributes to pain of pulpal origin.[57] Pulpal C nociceptors, however, seem to have a predominant role in transmitting pain from inflamed pulp tissue.[17]

Neurophysiologic and neurochemical central nervous system reactions occur as a result of local inflammatory changes in the dental pulp, some of which have been recorded in trigeminal nuclei. These responses include significant changes in mechanoreceptive fields, altered response properties of brainstem neurons in the trigeminal nucleus, and neuroplastic changes involving *N*-methyl-D-aspartate receptor mechanisms.[4]

Differential diagnosis of odontalgia

Diagnosis of toothache is challenging because teeth often refer pain to other teeth and to other craniofacial locations.[1,2] Other craniofacial pain disorders may refer pain to teeth and be expressed as toothache, including pretrigeminal neuralgia, neurovascular orofacial pain, or atypical pains associated with gustatory stimuli[58–61] (see chapters 10 and 12). One should consider that about half of all cases of persistent tooth pain after root canal therapy were thought to have a nonodontogenic origin.[30] In this respect, neurovascular orofacial pain is of great diagnostic importance[62,63]; it is discussed in more detail in chapter 10. Other conditions mimicking odontalgia may refer from the maxillary sinus or the ear (see chapter 6). Pain may also be referred from more remote structures, such as the carotid artery or heart and mimic the symptoms of a toothache[64,65] (see chapter 14). Of particular importance is pain referred to the oral cavity that is associated with intracranial tumors[66,67] (see chapter 12).

Periodontal Pain

Periodontal pain is usually experienced in response to localized acute inflammation. Pain originating in the structures surrounding the teeth is easily localized; the affected teeth are very tender on chewing and are readily localized by percussion. Etiologically, three clinical conditions are possible: *(1)* acute periapical inflammation as a result of pulp infection and pulp necrosis, *(2)* acute periodontal infection associated with deep pocket formation, and *(3)* acute gingival bacterial or viral inflammation.

Although the pain characteristics, ability to localize, and pain-producing situations are similar for acute periapical and lateral periodontal abscess (see Table 6-1), the physical and radiographic signs differ (see Table 6-2). Treatment modalities are based on the etiology of each condition and are entirely different.

Acute periapical periodontitis

Symptoms

Pain associated with acute periapical inflammation is spontaneous, of moderate to severe intensity, and long lasting (hours). Pain is exacerbated by biting on the affected tooth and, in more advanced cases, even by closing the mouth and bringing the tooth into contact with the opposing teeth.

Localization is usually precise, and the patient is able to indicate the affected tooth. In this respect, periodontal pain differs from the poorly localized dentinal or pulpal pain. The improved localization of pain may be attributed to the proprioceptive and mechanoreceptive sensibility of the periodontium that is lacking in the pulp.[68,69] Although localized, in approximately 50% of patients the pain is diffuse and spreads into the jaw on the affected side of the face.[1]

Physical and radiographic signs

The affected tooth is readily located by means of gentle tooth percussion, and the periapical vestibular area may be tender to palpation. The pulp of the affected tooth is nonvital. However, in clinical practice pulpal and periapical pain could occur at the same time. In these cases, it is thought that algesic substances, endogenous from pulp tissue damage or neurogenic inflammation and exogenous from bacterial toxins, invade the periapical area in spite of the fact that the pulp has not completely degenerated and can still react to stimuli such as

temperature changes.[53] Regression analysis revealed that a closed pulp chamber and caries were highly associated with pulpal pain, and, conversely, an open pulp chamber was associated with periapical pain ($P < .001$).[70]

In more severe, purulent cases, swelling of the face associated with cellulitis is sometimes present and can be associated with fever and malaise. The affected tooth may be extruded and mobile, both vertically and horizontally. When facial swelling appears, pain usually diminishes in intensity, probably because of rupture of the local periosteum and the decrease in tissue pressure caused by pus accumulation. These cases are diagnosed as dentoalveolar abscess. Case 6-2 depicts a patient with periapical periodontitis that developed into a dentoalveolar abscess (Fig 6-6).

Radiographs are of limited use in diagnosing acute periapical periodontitis because no periapical radiographic changes are detectable in the early stages. If a radiographic periapical rarefying osteitis is noticed in a tooth that is sensitive to touch and percussion, the condition is then classified as re-acutization of chronic periapical periodontitis (as in Case 6-2). Many times, however, such a rarefying osteitis lesion is present in an otherwise asymptomatic situation. Furthermore, there is a lack of correlation between the radiographic picture and the microbiology or histology of the periapical lesion.[71,72]

Pathophysiology

The recent discovery of a new class of protease-activated receptors has shed light on enzyme-mediated sensory nerve activation, especially on the important role of protease-activated receptor-2 in disease states associated with inflammation.[73] Substance P immunoreactive nerve fibers have been found in the vicinity of tryptase-positive mast cells (tryptase constitutes the major protein released during mast cell degranulation) in human periapical granulomas.[74] Of special interest is the fact that the gingival crevicular fluid around teeth with acute pain of pulpal origin demonstrated increased levels of substance P and neurokinin-A compared with healthy teeth, and these levels decreased significantly 1 week after pulpectomy.[75] Painful stimulation of the

CASE 6-2

A 20-year-old man with periapical periodontitis and acute dentoalveolar abscess.

Primary complaint: The patient has experienced strong continuous pain on the left side of the face for the past 3 days. The maxillary left second premolar is very sensitive to chewing. Swelling of the left side of the face has developed rapidly since yesterday accompanied by marked relief in pain intensity.

Findings: The left side of the face is swollen (Fig 6-6a). The maxillary left second premolar is sensitive to percussion, does not respond to cold application, and is slightly mobile; no periodontal pockets can be detected. A periapical radiograph (Fig 6-6b) demonstrates a deep disto-occlusal cavity in the maxillary left second premolar with a temporary filling and a periapical radiolucency with concentric condensing osteitis.

Past history: Three months ago, the patient complained of discomfort on chewing and a sensitivity to cold foods on the left side of his mouth. A temporary filling of the maxillary left second premolar was performed. At first the tooth was very sensitive to cold foods, but then it became comfortable until 3 days ago, when the strong pain started.

Comments: This is a classic case that starts with discomfort and pain due to caries associated with dentinal allodynia and food impaction. Pulp irritation develops subsequent to cavity preparation and placement of the temporary filling, which eventually leads to pulp necrosis. A periapical lesion develops asymptomatically, and some 3 months later an acute exacerbation with strong pain occurs because of acute periapical periodontitis.

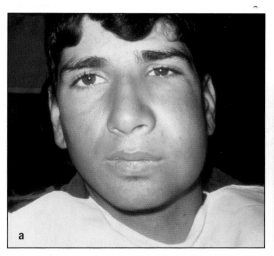
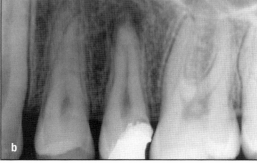

Fig 6-6 Case 6-2. *(a)* Note the acute swelling of the left side of the face (cellulitis) due to acute dentoalveolar abscess of the maxillary left second premolar. Note also the swelling of the left cheek, the left lower eyelid closing the eye, and the disappearance of the left nasolabial fold due to swelling. The left nostril and left upper lip are swollen, too. *(b)* Periapical radiograph demonstrating a deep disto-occlusal cavity in the maxillary left second premolar with a temporary filling and a periapical radiolucency with concentric condensing osteitis.

maxillary central incisor also caused significant elevations of substance P levels in the gingival crevicular fluid of the stimulated tooth; this supports the possibility of a local neurogenic spread of inflammatory reactions from intrapulpal to surrounding periodontal tissues.[76]

Treatment

Although pain originates from the periodontal periapical tissues, the source of insult and infection usually lies within the pulp chamber and the root canal. To eliminate this source, the pulp

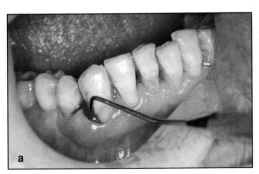
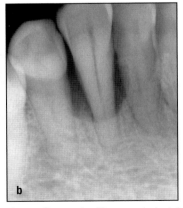

Fig 6-7 *(a)* Lateral periodontal abscess associated with pain, swelling, and a 10-mm periodontal pocket. *(b)* Intrabony periodontal pocket.

chamber is opened and the root canal cleansed and dressed in accordance with current endodontic practice. Localized periapical pain or swelling generally recovers quickly with local treatment, and there is no demonstrable benefit from penicillin supplementation[77] or amoxicillin plus clavulanic acid.[78] However, if cellulitis, fever, and malaise are present, systemic administration of antibiotics is recommended in addition to abscess drainage and tooth debridement. Amoxicillin, metronidazole, and clindamycin are the antibiotics most widely used and are recommended for patients suffering from acute dentoalveolar infections who have become systemically unwell as a result of their infection or for patients who are significantly immunocompromised.[79] Grinding the tooth to prevent contact with the opposing teeth helps to relieve pain.

Lateral periodontal abscess

Symptoms

Pain characteristics of a lateral periodontal abscess are similar to those of acute periapical periodontitis (see Tables 6-1 and 6-2). The pain is continuous, moderate to severe in intensity, well localized, and exacerbated by biting on the affected tooth.

Physical and radiographic signs

Swelling and redness of the gingiva may be noticed and are located more frequently in coronal than in acute periapical lesions. The swelling is tender to palpation, and the affected tooth is sensitive to percussion and may be mobile and slightly extruded. In more severe cases, cellulitis, fever, and malaise may occur. A deep periodontal pocket is usually located around the tooth (Fig 6-7a); once probed, pus exudation may occur, bringing occasional pain relief. Frequently, probing is quite painful and has been correlated to the degree of the inflammatory process.[80] The tooth pulp is usually vital but may occasionally be slightly hyperalgesic. In a sample of 29 patients,[81] more than 75% of the abscesses demonstrated edema, redness, and swelling, and 90% of the patients reported pain. Bleeding occurred in all abscesses, and suppuration on sampling was detected in 66%. Mean associated pocket depth was 7.28 mm, and 79% of teeth presented some degree of mobility. Cervical lymphadenopathy was seen in 10% of patients, and elevated leukocyte counts were observed in 32%. Abscess formation usually results from a blockage of drainage from a deep periodontal pocket, and it is frequently associated with a deep intrabony pocket and teeth with root furcation involvement. A deep intra-

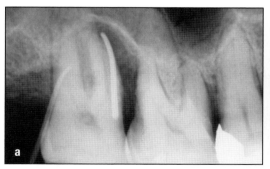 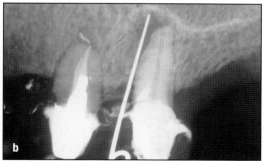

Fig 6-8 *(a)* A perio-endo lesion in which the mesial pocket is demonstrated with a gutta-percha point that approaches the apex of the mesiobuccal root of the maxillary second molar. In this case, the tooth pulp was vital. The patient complained of strong pain with hot and cold foods and sometimes strong spontaneous pain that lasted 10 to 15 minutes. *(b)* A perio-endo lesion in which a silver point was inserted into the pocket and a well-demarcated periapical radiolucent lesion was also demonstrated. The tooth pulp was nonvital and could be approached by drilling through the temporary acrylic crown without using any local anesthesia.

bony pocket may be present on the radiograph (Fig 6-7b). Acute periodontal abscesses may also be associated with dental implants.[82,83]

Pathophysiology

A high prevalence of putative periodontal pathogens were found, including *Fusobacterium nucleatum*, *Peptostreptococcus micros*, *Porphyromonas gingivalis*, *Prevotella intermedia*, and *Bacteroides forsythus*.[81]

Significant differences in the levels of PGE_2 and LTB4 were found in patients with and without periodontitis. The levels of PGE_2 and LTB4 were correlated with clinical parameters and decreased markedly after phase one of periodontal treatment.[84] Levels of PGE_2 correlated with the severity of the periodontal status, and levels of LTB4 correlated with gingival inflammation.

↘ p. 149

Treatment

Gentle irrigation and curettage of the pocket should be performed. A vertical incision for drainage is recommended when the abscess is fluctuant but cannot be adequately approached through the pocket. Acute lateral periodontal abscess causes rapid alveolar bone destruction (see Fig 6-7b), hence the need for early and prompt intervention. Selective grinding of the tooth should be performed to avoid contact with the opposing teeth, reduce pain, and restore tooth stability. When cellulitis, fever,

and malaise are present, systemic antibiotic administration may be recommended. As with periapical periodontitis, the need for antibiotic supplementation in addition to local treatment is unclear.[85] Pain usually subsides within 24 hours of treatment.

Interrelationships between pulpal and periodontal diseases: The "perio-endo" lesion

The interrelationship between periodontal and endodontic disease may cause diagnostic confusion and difficulty. A symptomatic tooth may have pain of periodontal and/or pulpal origin. The nature of that pain is often the first clue in determining the etiology, assisted by radiographic and clinical evaluation. In some cases, pulpal pathology may create periodontal participation. In others, periodontal pathology may create pulpal involvement.[86] Deep periodontal pockets sometimes involve accessory canals (in the furcation or laterally) and in extensive lesions may reach the root apex of the tooth and cause retrograde pulp inflammation (Fig 6-8a). The major initial symptom is sensitivity to temperature changes, a situation that may progress to irreversible pulpitis. A second possibility is an apical abscess that exudates through a periodontal pocket (Fig 6-8b). In this case, pain can be minimal due to the release of pressure through the pocket, or sometimes it may exac-

[handwritten: "TRUE" endo - perio]

erbate into an acute dentoalveolar abscess. Finally, the co-occurrence of symptomatic active periodontal disease together with independent endodontic pathology is a possibility that is termed a "true" combined lesion.

Treatment

Treatment for all these situations is initially endodontic, followed by conventional periodontal treatment. The prognosis of endodontic lesions causing periodontal symptomatology is better than in periodontal-initiated or combined lesions.

Vertical root fracture

A fracture of the tooth that involves most of the root will induce pain on biting. Root fractures are more common in endodontically treated teeth that have been restored with a post and core. Pain on biting in such cases is therefore of periodontal origin. Initially, there may be no clinical or radiographic signs. An isolated periodontal pocket in the area of the fracture is often found. Disease progression usually leads to a typical radiographic picture of a lengthwise rarefying osteitis. If left untreated, infection and abscess may develop. Currently, the only treatment option for vertical root fractures is extraction.

Gingival pain

Gingival pain may occur as a result of mechanical irritation, such as food impaction, acute inflammation associated with a partially erupted tooth (pericoronitis), or acute inflammation as a result of an acute bacterial or viral infection.

Food impaction

Symptoms. The patient typically complains of a localized pain that develops between two teeth after meals, especially when food is fibrous. The pain is associated with a feeling of pressure and discomfort that is annoying and sometimes severe.[1] The patient may report that pain gradually diminishes until evoked again at the next meal, or the pain may be relieved immediately by removing the food impacted between the teeth with a toothpick or dental floss. Food impaction usually results from a loss in interdental contacts and may cause periodontal disease.[87] Remarkably, this loss of contact is highly prevalent (43%) between fixed implant prostheses and adjacent teeth, especially when the implant is distal to the adjacent tooth.[88]

Physical and radiographic signs. A faulty contact between two adjacent teeth is noticed so that food is usually trapped between these teeth; the gingival papilla is tender to touch and bleeds easily. Food impaction should be treated promptly because it may cause cervical caries and interdental alveolar bone resorption.[89]

Treatment. The cause of the faulty contact between the teeth is often a caries lesion, and restoring the tooth will eliminate pain. In some cases, though the contacts are tight, food impaction may occur, so creating anatomical escape grooves adjacent to the marginal ridge may eliminate food impaction.[90]

Pericoronitis

Symptoms. Pain, which may be severe, is usually located at the distal end of the arch of teeth in the mandible. Pain is spontaneous and may be exacerbated by closing the mouth. In more severe cases, pain is aggravated by swallowing, and trismus may occur. Acute pericoronal infections are common in teeth that are incompletely erupted and are partially covered by a flap or operculum of gingival tissue.

Physical and radiographic signs. The operculum is acutely inflamed (red, edematous), and an indentation of the opposing tooth is frequently seen on the swollen gingival flap. Occasionally, there is fever, malaise, and restricted mouth opening (trismus).

Pathophysiology. Ten patients with pericoronitis and 10 healthy control subjects were investigated for the presence of TNF-α.[91] TNF receptors 1 and 2 were found in macrophage-like and fibroblast-like cells, vascular endothelial cells in postcapillary venules, and basal epithelial cells in pericoronitis, but they were only weakly expressed in control subjects. The researchers concluded that the potent proinflammatory cytokine TNF-α plays a role in the pain and inflammation associated with pericoronitis.[91] A study of 2,151 patients with pericoronitis found that the peak age of occurrence was from 21 to 25 years, and the most frequent predisposing factors were upper respiratory infection (38%) and stress (22%).[90]

Treatment. Irrigate debris between the operculum and the affected tooth with saline or antibacterial agent (eg, chlorhexidine 0.5%), and eliminate trauma by grinding or extracting the opposing tooth. Removal of the third molar, the affected tooth, positively influenced quality-of-life outcomes in patients with minor symptoms of pericoronitis.[92] The risk of seeding the infection into deeper spaces by performing immediate extraction is low. Systemic antibiotic administration is recommended when trismus occurs or when the patient is febrile. Microbiologic cultures from 26 patients with pericoronitis demonstrated that 9 of 26 samples contained beta-lactamase-producing strains.[93] The infection in pericoronitis is multimicrobial, predominantly caused strictly by beta-lactamase-producing anaerobic microorganisms; the suggested first-line treatment is amoxicillin with clavulanic acid.[94,95]

Augmentin

Acute necrotizing ulcerative gingivitis

Symptoms. Soreness and pain are characteristically felt at the margin of the gingiva and are fairly well localized to the affected areas. Pain is intensified by eating and tooth brushing, and both activities are usually accompanied by gingival bleeding. A metallic taste is sometimes experienced, and there is usually a fetid odor from the mouth.

Physical and radiographic signs. Necrosis and ulceration are present on the marginal gingiva accompanied by different degrees of gingival papillary destruction. This is an ulcerative gingival disease characterized by pain, bleeding, and papillary necrosis.[96] An adherent grayish slough represents the so-called pseudomembrane that is present in the acute stage (Fig 6-9). Acute herpetic infection of the gingiva (herpetic gingivostomatitis) can sometimes resemble acute necrotizing ulcerative gingivitis (ANUG), but the clinical appearance and associated signs and symptoms are different. The papillary necrosis typical for ANUG (see Fig 6-9)

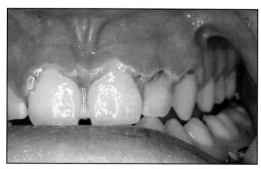

Fig 6-9 Acute necrotizing ulcerative gingivitis. Note the destruction of the gingival papillae and pseudomembrane at the marginal border.

is absent with herpetic infection, in which the herpetic lesions typically create a punched-out appearance at the gingival margin.

Relatively little is known about the epidemiology of ANUG in healthy adolescent populations. Most studies have focused on special target groups, such as military recruits, patients with human immunodeficiency virus, or subjects who are severely malnourished.[97] In 9,203 students aged 12 to 21 years in Santiago, Chile, the estimated prevalence of ANUG was 6.7%.[98] Of 19,944 patients examined at a periodontal clinic in Cape Town, South Africa, less than 0.5% were found to have ANUG, and the study demonstrated significant seasonal variation in the occurrence of the disease.[99] On the other hand, ANUG was found to be very prevalent (up to 37%) among boarding-school children in a poor, developing country.[100]

Pathophysiology. ANUG is considered to be an acute opportunistic gingival infection caused by bacterial plaque. The condition appears more frequently in undernourished children and young adults as well as in patients with immunodeficiency.[101] The pathogenesis involves factors related to the oral microbiology and its invasive ability as well as factors associated with the host, including capillary and immunologic disorders.

Treatment. Treatment includes swabbing and gently irrigating the ulcerative lesions, preferably with chlorhexidine or an oxidizing agent (hydrogen peroxide), and then scaling and

diclofenac

cleaning the teeth. Systemic antibiotics are recommended, especially when fever and malaise are present.[102]

Mucosal Pain

Pain originating from the oral mucosa can be localized or have a more generalized, diffuse nature. Detailed descriptions of the various lesions of the oral mucosa are beyond the scope of this chapter, and only the most common lesions—recurrent aphthous stomatitis and acute herpetic gingivostomatitis—are briefly discussed here.

Localized mucosal pain

Localized pain is usually associated with a detectable erosive or ulcerative lesion that results from physical, chemical, or thermal trauma; viral infection; or lesions of unknown origin. Pain is usually mild to moderate but may become quite severe and last for some minutes when irritated, whether mechanically or by sour, spicy, or hot foods.[103] Pain is burning in quality and characterized by a higher degree of discomfort than pain intensity. Additionally, the pain is more visceral than cutaneous. In about 50% of patients, the pain wakes them from sleep, a feature that is correlated with the female sex and pain intensity. Pain intensity or unpleasantness is not related to the size or number of the lesions.[103]

Aphthous lesions

Recurrent aphthous stomatitis is characterized by a prodromal burning sensation 2 to 48 hours before an ulcer appears. Although small in diameter (0.3 to 1.0 cm), this type of lesion may be quite painful and induces a painful regional lymphadenopathy. In up to 80% of patients, the pain is described as burning in quality followed by stabbing (33%) and throbbing (11%).[103] In the mild form, healing occurs within 10 days, and pain is usually mild to moderate in severity.

Recurrent aphthous ulcers represent a very common but poorly understood mucosal disorder. They occur in men and women of all ages, races, and geographic regions. An estimated one in five persons has been afflicted with aphthous ulcers at least once.[104] The condition is classified as minor, major, or herpetiform on the basis of ulcer size and number.

Local and systemic conditions, as well as genetic, immunologic, or microbial factors, may all play a role in the pathogenesis of recurrent aphthous ulceration. No principal cause has been discovered, but an autoimmune pathophysiology is suspected. Because the etiology is unknown, diagnosis is entirely based on history and clinical criteria; there are no laboratory procedures to confirm the diagnosis.[105]

Treatment. Treatment for localized mucosal pain is mostly symptomatic and includes the application of a topical protective emollient for the mild form and the use of topical corticosteroids and tetracycline to decrease healing time for the more severe form.[106,107] Cyanoacrylate has been used as an effective tissue adhesive for steroids and tetracycline.[107] The use of diclofenac, a topical nonsteroidal anti-inflammatory drug, was also found to be effective.[108] Patients who underwent a single, low-intensity, nonthermal session of CO_2 laser irradiation had significantly reduced pain from minor aphthous stomatitis compared with the placebo group and had no visible side effects.[109]

Acute herpetic gingivostomatitis

Oral infections caused by herpes simplex type 1 are widespread, even among otherwise healthy people.[110] Although most of these herpetic infections are mildly symptomatic, young children are at risk for developing extensive oropharyngeal vesicular eruptions when first infected with the virus. This initial outbreak is known as *primary herpetic gingivostomatitis*. The mean age of patients with acute herpetic stomatitis has shown a general trend to increase, and, currently, most (> 50%) patients suffer their first attack during their third decade.[111,112] Diagnosis can be performed clinically and confirmed by laboratory tests. Symptoms may persist for 2 weeks, causing significant mouth discomfort, fever, lymphadenopathy, and difficulty eating and drinking. Pain is described by 71% of subjects as burning, followed by stabbing or throbbing (28% each). More than half (57%) of patients are awakened from sleep by the pain. No correlation has been found between pain and the size or number of lesions.[103] The incidence of oral herpes simplex infection is particularly high in immunocompromised patients, and it occurs in up to 50% of hospitalized patients with acute leukemia.[113] Cytology (Tzanck testing) may serve as a useful adjunct in diagnosis, but rapid and highly specific detection of human herpes simplex type 1 in saliva is possible by in vitro amplification using polymerase chain reaction.[114]

Treatment. Antiviral agents such as acyclovir and famciclovir should be considered part of early management of primary herpetic gingivostomatitis.[115,116] A soft, bland diet preceded by a local anesthetic mouthrinse is recommended. Oral hygiene may be maintained by rinsing with a mild bicarbonate or saline solution or a non-alcoholic solution of 0.2% chlorhexidine. Providing supportive care and educating parents about transmission of the virus are important.[112]

Diffuse mucosal pain

When generalized diffuse pain is felt in the oral mucosa, it usually has a burning nature and may be accompanied by a dysgeusia, predominantly of a bitter metallic quality. This pain may result from a direct insult to the tissues due to bacterial, viral, or fungal infection, which can be identified by the characteristic appearance of the oral mucosa. Diagnosis is aided by microbiologic and other laboratory examinations. In cases of chronic fungal infection (candidiasis), possible underlying etiologic factors such as prolonged broad-spectrum antibiotic therapy, immunodeficiencies, and other debilitating factors should be investigated.[117] Radiation therapy to the head and neck region may result in acute mucositis with severe generalized mucosal pain.[118] Burning sensation of the oral mucosa, particularly the tongue, may result from systemic diseases, such as chronic iron-deficiency anemia, and may be associated with atrophic glossitis.[117] Atrophic glossitis and burning mouth sensations have also been associated with *Helicobacter pylori* colonization of tongue mucosa and nutritional deficiency.[119] Mucosal pain associated with underlying systemic factors is detailed in chapter 14.

A large proportion of patients, mostly women between the ages of 50 and 70 years, complain of a burning sensation in the mouth and the tongue, though there are no observable changes in the oral mucosa and no detectable underlying systemic changes. This group of patients is usually diagnosed with burning mouth syndrome, which is discussed in chapter 11.

Pain from Salivary Glands

Pain from salivary glands is localized to the affected gland, is of moderate to severe intensity, and is usually associated with blockage of the salivary gland duct. The salivary gland is swollen and very tender to palpation, and salivary flow is reduced and sometimes completely abolished. Pain is intensified by increased saliva production on starting meals or by applying an acidic stimulant (citric acid is the standard stimulant) to the tongue. Pus may secrete from the salivary duct when the gland is infected, and the condition may be associated with fever and malaise.

Calcified calculus may block the salivary duct and is often identifiable on a radiograph. Ultrasound or sialography can aid in diagnosis.[120,121] The incidence of salivary calculi is 60 cases/million/year, and most stones are situated in the middle or proximal portion of the duct.[122]

In children, the most common blockage occurs with mumps and acute recurrent parotitis. Recurrent parotitis of childhood is a rare condition of unknown etiology, though it is probably immunologically mediated. A clinical diagnosis can often be confirmed by ultrasound.[123] Recently, a new method that includes a salivary intraductal endoscopic technique was introduced for diagnosis and treatment of these conditions.[124]

Treatment

When a blockage is diagnosed, surgical or endoscopic approaches are indicated.[125] A combined external lithotripsy/sialoendoscopy method for advanced salivary gland sialolithiasis was recently developed.[126] In the acute stage of bacterial infection, antibiotic therapy is recommended. No antibiotics are recommended for mumps or recurrent parotitis, however.[123]

Conclusion

Diagnosis and treatment of acute orofacial pain is usually encountered in a first-aid situation. The task is complex, similar to that of any emergency treatment; the patient is anxious and seeks immediate relief, so the diagnosis has to be reached under time pressure. Getting a precise and full story is of utmost importance, as the pain history is usually the main lead for a diagnosis. As with most cases of acute pain, the pain results from an acute inflammatory process that must be treated. Keep in mind, however, the possibility of misdiagnosis due to nonodontogenic and, frequently, noninflammatory causes. About half of all cases of persistent tooth pain after root canal therapy were thought to have a nonodontogenic origin. Other craniofacial pain disorders, mimicking odontalgia, may refer from the maxillary sinus or the ear. Pain may also be referred from more remote structures, such as the carotid artery or heart, and may resemble the symptoms of toothache. Pretrigeminal neuralgia may be very misleading and hard to diagnose.

Diagnosis and treatment of orofacial pain is a complex process compounded by the density of anatomical structures. Because of this dense anatomy, management of orofacial pain calls for the services of clinicians from various specialties, such as dentistry, otolaryngology, ophthalmology, and neurology to name a few. It has been the authors' experience that patients without a diagnosis are referred from one specialist to another, trying to find help "somewhere else." Teamwork seems to be the ideal solution, but ideals rarely exist. The right solution is to have clinicians who specialize in the diagnosis and treatment of orofacial pain and headache and can cross all specialties.

References

1. Sharav Y, Leviner E, Tzukert A, McGrath PA. The spatial distribution, intensity and unpleasantness of acute dental pain. Pain 1984;20:363–370.
2. Hashemipour MA, Borna R. Incidence and characteristics of acute referred orofacial pain caused by a posterior single tooth pulpitis in an Iranian population. Pain Pract 2014;14:151–157.
3. Falace DA, Reid K, Rayens MK. The influence of deep (odontogenic) pain intensity, quality, and duration on the incidence and characteristics of referred orofacial pain. J Orofac Pain 1996;10:232–239.
4. Sessle BJ. Peripheral and central mechanisms of orofacial pain and their clinical correlates. Minerva Anestesiol 2005;71:117–136.
5. Sessle BJ, Hu JW, Amano N, Zhong G. Convergence of cutaneous, tooth pulp, visceral, neck and muscle afferents onto nociceptive and non-nociceptive neurones in trigeminal subnucleus caudalis (medullary dorsal horn) and its implications for referred pain. Pain 1986;27:219–235.
6. Locker D, Grushka M. Prevalence of oral and facial pain and discomfort: Preliminary results of a mail survey. Community Dent Oral Epidemiol 1987;15:169–172.
7. Lipton JA, Ship JA, Larach-Robinson D. Estimated prevalence and distribution of reported orofacial pain in the United States. J Am Dent Assoc 1993;124(10):115–121.
8. Pau AK, Croucher R, Marcenes W. Prevalence estimates and associated factors for dental pain: A review. Oral Health Prev Dent 2003;1:209–220.
9. Goes PS, Watt R, Hardy RG, Sheiham A. The prevalence and severity of dental pain in 14-15 year old Brazilian schoolchildren. Community Dent Health 2007;24:217–224.
10. von Troil B, Needleman I, Sanz M. A systematic review of the prevalence of root sensitivity following periodontal therapy. J Clin Periodontol 2002;29(3, suppl):173–177.
11. Goose DH. Cracked tooth syndrome. Br Dent J 1981;150:224–225.
12. Seo DG, Yi YA, Shin SJ, Park JW. Analysis of factors associated with cracked teeth. J Endod 2012;38:288–292.
13. Brynjulfsen A, Fristad I, Grevstad T, Hals-Kvinnsland I. Incompletely fractured teeth associated with diffuse longstanding orofacial pain: Diagnosis and treatment outcome. Int Endod J 2002;35:461–466.
14. Krell KV, Rivera EM. A six year evaluation of cracked teeth diagnosed with reversible pulpitis: Treatment and prognosis. J Endod 2007;33:1405–1407.
15. Poulsen S, Errboe M, Hovgaard O, Worthington HW. Potassium nitrate toothpaste for dentine hypersensitivity. Cochrane Database Syst Rev 2001;(2).
16. Brookfield JR, Addy M, Alexander DC, et al. Consensus-based recommendations for the diagnosis and management of dentin hypersensitivity. J Can Dent Assoc 2003;69:221–226.
17. Hargreaves KM, Seltzer S. Pharmacologic control of dental pain. In: Hargreaves KM, Goodis HE (eds). Seltzer and Bender's Dental Pulp. Chicago: Quintessence, 2002:205–225.
18. Kimura Y, Wilder-Smith P, Yonaga K, Matsumoto K. Treatment of dentine hypersensitivity by lasers: A review. J Clin Periodontol 2000;27:715–721.
19. Lin PY, Cheng YW, Chu CY, Chien KL, Lin CP, Tu YK. In-office treatment for dentin hypersensitivity: A systematic review and network meta-analysis. J Clin Periodontol 2013;40:53–64.
20. Bender IB. Pulpal pain diagnosis–A review. J Endod 2000;26:175–179.

21. Mirza AF, Mo J, Holt JL, et al. Is there a relationship between throbbing pain and arterial pulsations? J Neurosci 2012;32:7572–7576.

22. Tyldesley WR, Mumford JM. Dental pain and the histological condition of the pulp. Dent Pract Dent Rec 1970;20:333–336.

23. Michaelson PL, Holland GR. Is pulpitis painful? Int Endod J 2002;35:829–832.

24. Parirokh M, Rekabi AR, Ashouri R, Nakhaee N, Abbott PV, Gorjestani H. Effect of occlusal reduction on postoperative pain in teeth with irreversible pulpitis and mild tenderness to percussion. J Endod 2013;39:1–5.

25. Bender IB. Reversible and irreversible painful pulpitides: Diagnosis and treatment. Aust Endod J 2000;26:10–14.

26. Willershausen B, Willershausen I, Ross A, Velikonja S, Kasaj A, Blettner M. Retrospective study on direct pulp capping with calcium hydroxide. Quintessence Int 2011;42:165–171.

27. Cisneros-Cabello R, Segura-Egea JJ. Relationship of patient complaints and signs to histopathologic diagnosis of pulpal condition. Aust Endod J 2005;31:24–27.

28. Bergenholtz G, Spångberg L. Controversies in endodontics. Crit Rev Oral Biol Med 2004;15:99–114.

29. Nixdorf DR, Moana-Filho EJ, Law AS, McGuire LA, Hodges JS, John MT. Frequency of persistent tooth pain after root canal therapy: A systematic review and meta-analysis. J Endod 2010;36:224–230.

30. Nixdorf DR, Moana-Filho EJ, Law AS, McGuire LA, Hodges JS, John MT. Frequency of nonodontogenic pain after endodontic therapy: A systematic review and meta-analysis. J Endod 2010;36:1494-1498.

31. Nagle D, Reader A, Beck M, Weaver J. Effect of systemic penicillin on pain in untreated irreversible pulpitis. Oral Surg Oral Med Oral Pathol Oral Radiol Endod 2000;90:636–640.

32. Fedorowicz Z, van Zuuren EJ, Farman AG, Agnihotry A, Al-Langawi JH. Antibiotic use for irreversible pulpitis. Cochrane Database Syst Rev 2013;12.

33. Aggarwal V, Singla M, Miglani S, Kohli S, Singh S. Comparative evaluation of 1.8 mL and 3.6 mL of 2% lidocaine with 1:200,000 epinephrine for inferior alveolar nerve block in patients with irreversible pulpitis: A prospective, randomized single-blind study. J Endod 2012;38:753–756.

34. Poorni S, Veniashok B, Senthilkumar AD, Indira R, Ramachandran S. Anesthetic efficacy of four percent articaine for pulpal anesthesia by using inferior alveolar nerve block and buccal infiltration techniques in patients with irreversible pulpitis: A prospective randomized double-blind clinical trial. J Endod 2011;37:1603–1607.

35. Parirokh M, Satvati SA, Sharifi R, et al. Efficacy of combining a buccal infiltration with an inferior alveolar nerve block for mandibular molars with irreversible pulpitis. Oral Surg Oral Med Oral Pathol Oral Radiol Endod 2010;109:468–473.

36. Kanaa MD, Whitworth JM, Meechan JG. A prospective randomized trial of different supplementary local anesthetic techniques after failure of inferior alveolar nerve block in patients with irreversible pulpitis in mandibular teeth. J Endod 2012;38:421–425.

37. Byers MR, Närhi MV. Dental injury models: Experimental tools for understanding neuroinflammatory interactions and polymodal nociceptor functions. Crit Rev Oral Biol Med 1999;10:4–39.

38. Magloire H, Maurin JC, Couble ML, et al. Topical review. Dental pain and odontoblasts: Facts and hypotheses. J Orofac Pain 2010;24:335–349.

39. Lin M, Liu S, Niu L, Xu F, Lu TJ. Analysis of thermal-induced dentinal fluid flow and its implications in dental thermal pain. Arch Oral Biol 2011;56:846–854.

40. Chung G, Jung SJ, Oh SB. Cellular and molecular mechanisms of dental nociception. J Dent Res 2013;92:948–955.

41. Byers MR, Kish SJ. Delineation of somatic nerve endings in rat teeth by radioautography of axon-transported protein. J Dent Res 1976;55:419–425.

42. Byers MR, Neuhaus SJ, Gehrig JD. Dental sensory receptor structure in human teeth. Pain 1982;13:221–235.

43. Anderson DJ, Naylor MN. Chemical excitants of pain in human dentine and dental pulp. Arch Oral Biol 1962;7:413–415.

44. Brannstrom M. The elicitation of pain in human dentine and pulp by chemical stimuli. Arch Oral Biol 1962;7:59–62.

45. Armstrong D, Dry RM, Keele CA, Markham JW. Observations on chemical excitants of cutaneous pain in man. J Physiol 1953;120:326–351.

46. Brannstrom M. Dentin sensitivity and aspiration of odontoblasts. J Am Dent Assoc 1963;66:366–370.

47. Matthews B, Sessle BJ. Peripheral mechanisms of orofacial pain. In: Lund JP, Lavinge G, Dubner R, Sessle BJ (eds). Orofacial Pain from Basic Science to Clinical Management. Chicago: Quintessence, 2000:37–46.

48. Okumura R, Shima K, Muramatsu T, et al. The odontoblast as a sensory receptor cell? The expression of TRPV1 (VR-1) channels. Arch Histol Cytol 2005;68:251–257.

49. Gibbs JL, Melnyk JL, Basbaum AI. Differential TRPV1 and TRPV2 channel expression in dental pulp. J Dent Res 2011;90:765–770.

50. Byers MR, Narhi MVO. Nerve supply of the pulpodentin complex and response to injury. In: Hargreaves KM, Goodis HE (eds). Seltzer and Bender's Dental Pulp. Chicago: Quintessence, 2002:151–179.

51. Goodis HE, Bowles WR, Hargreaves KM. Prostaglandin E2 enhances bradykinin-evoked iCGRP release in bovine dental pulp. J Dent Res 2000;79:1604–1607.

52. Rodd HD, Boissonade FM. Substance P expression in human tooth pulp in relation to caries and pain experience. Eur J Oral Sci 2000;108:467–474.

53. Lundy FT, Linden GJ. Neuropeptides and neurogenic mechanisms in oral and periodontal inflammation. Crit Rev Oral Biol Med 2004;15:82–98.

54. Martinho FC, Chiesa WM, Leite FR, Cirelli JA, Gomes BP. Antigenicity of primary endodontic infection against macrophages by the levels of PGE(2) production. J Endod 2011;37:602–607.

55. Kokkas AB, Goulas A, Varsamidis K, Mirtsou V, Tziafas D. Irreversible but not reversible pulpitis is associated with up-regulation of tumour necrosis factor-alpha gene expression in human pulp. Int Endod J 2007;40:198–203.

56. Olgart LM. The role of local factors in dentin and pulp in intradental pain mechanisms. J Dent Res 1985;64 (special issue):572–578.

57. Madison S, Whitsel EA, Suarez-Roca H, Maixner W. Sensitizing effects of leukotriene B4 on intradental primary afferents. Pain 1992;49:99–104.

58. Helcer M, Schnarch A, Benoliel R, Sharav Y. Trigeminal neuralgic-type pain and vascular-type headache due to gustatory stimulus. Headache 1998;38:129–131.

59. Fromm GH, Graff-Radford SB, Terrence CF, Sweet WH. Pre-trigeminal neuralgia. Neurology 1990;40:1493–1495.

60. Sharav Y, Benoliel R, Schnarch A, Greenberg L. Idiopathic trigeminal pain associated with gustatory stimuli. Pain 1991;44:171–174.

61. Sharav Y. Orofacial pain: How much is it a local phenomenon? J Am Dent Assoc 2005;136:432, 434, 436.

62. Benoliel R, Elishoov H, Sharav Y. Orofacial pain with vascular-type features. Oral Surg Oral Med Oral Pathol Oral Radiol Endod 1997;84:506–512.

63. Czerninsky R, Benoliel R, Sharav Y. Odontalgia in vascular orofacial pain. J Orofac Pain 1999;13:196–200.

64. Tzukert A, Hasin Y, Sharav Y. Orofacial pain of cardiac origin. Oral Surg Oral Med Oral Pathol 1981;51:484–486.

65. Roz TM, Schiffman LE, Schlossberg S. Spontaneous dissection of the internal carotid artery manifesting as pain in an endodontically treated molar. J Am Dent Assoc 2005;136:1556–1559.

66. Aiken A. Facial pain—toothache or tumour? Int J Oral Surg 1981;10(suppl 1):187–190.

67. Bullitt E, Tew JM, Boyd J. Intracranial tumors in patients with facial pain. J Neurosurg 1986;64:865–871.

68. Griffin CJ, Harris R. Innervation of human periodontium. I. Classification of periodontal receptors. Aust Dent J 1974;19:51–56.

69. van Steenberghe D. The structure and function of periodontal innervation. A review of the literature. J Periodontal Res 1979;14:185–203.

70. Estrela C, Guedes OA, Silva JA, Leles CR, Estrela CR, Pécora JD. Diagnostic and clinical factors associated with pulpal and periapical pain. Braz Dent J 2011;22:306–311.

71. Block RM, Bushell A, Rodrigues H, Langeland K. A histopathologic, histobacteriologic, and radiographic study of periapical endodontic surgical specimens. Oral Surg Oral Med Oral Pathol 1976;42:656–678.

72. Langeland K, Block RM, Grossman LI. A histopathologic and histobacteriologic study of 35 periapical endodontic surgical specimens. J Endod 1977;3:8–23.

73. Vergnolle N, Hollenberg MD, Sharkey KA, Wallace JL. Characterization of the inflammatory response to proteinase-activated receptor-2 (PAR2)-activating peptides in the rat paw. Br J Pharmacol 1999;127:1083–1090.

74. Kabashima H, Nagata K, Maeda K, Iijima T. Involvement of substance P, mast cells, TNF-alpha and ICAM-1 in the infiltration of inflammatory cells in human periapical granulomas. J Oral Pathol Med 2002;31:175–180.

75. Awawdeh LA, Lundy FT, Linden GJ, Shaw C, Kennedy JG, Lamey PJ. Quantitative analysis of substance P, neurokinin A and calcitonin gene-related peptide in gingival crevicular fluid associated with painful human teeth. Eur J Oral Sci 2002;110:185–191.

76. Avellán NL, Sorsa T, Tervahartiala T, Forster C, Kemppainen P. Experimental tooth pain elevates substance P and matrix metalloproteinase-8 levels in human gingival crevice fluid. Acta Odontol Scand 2008;66:18–22.

77. Fouad AF, Rivera EM, Walton RE. Penicillin as a supplement in resolving the localized acute apical abscess. Oral Surg Oral Med Oral Pathol Oral Radiol Endod 1996;81:590–595.

78. Lewis MA, Carmichael F, MacFarlane TW, Milligan SG. A randomised trial of co-amoxiclav (Augmentin) versus penicillin V in the treatment of acute dentoalveolar abscess. Br Dent J 1993;175:169–174.

79. Ellison SJ. The role of phenoxymethylpenicillin, amoxicillin, metronidazole and clindamycin in the management of acute dentoalveolar abscesses—A review. Br Dent J 2009;206:357–362.

80. Heft MW, Perelmuter SH, Cooper BY, Magnusson I, Clark WB. Relationship between gingival inflammation and painfulness of periodontal probing. J Clin Periodontol 1991;18:213–215.

81. Herrera D, Roldán S, González I, Sanz M. The periodontal abscess (I). Clinical and microbiological findings. J Clin Periodontol 2000;27:387–394.

82. Takeshita F, Iyama S, Ayukawa Y, Suetsugu T, Oishi M. Abscess formation around a hydroxyapatite-coated implant placed into the extraction socket with autogenous bone graft. A histological study using light microscopy, image processing, and confocal laser scanning microscopy. J Periodontol 1997;68:299–305.

83. Serino G, Ström C. Peri-implantitis in partially edentulous patients: Association with inadequate plaque control. Clin Oral Implants Res 2009;20:169–174.

84. Tsai CC, Hong YC, Chen CC, Wu YM. Measurement of prostaglandin E2 and leukotriene B4 in the gingival crevicular fluid. J Dent 1998;26:97–103.

85. Herrera D, Roldán S, Sanz M. The periodontal abscess: A review. J Clin Periodontol 2000;27:377–386.

86. Shenoy N, Shenoy A. Endo-perio lesions: Diagnosis and clinical considerations. Indian J Dent Res 2010;21:579–585.

87. Hancock EB, Mayo CV, Schwab RR, Wirthlin MR. Influence of interdental contacts on periodontal status. J Periodontol 1980;51:445–449.

88. Koori H, Morimoto K, Tsukiyama Y, Koyano K. Statistical analysis of the diachronic loss of interproximal contact between fixed implant prostheses and adjacent teeth. Int J Prosthodont 2010;23:535–540.

89. Jernberg GR, Bakdash MB, Keenan KM. Relationship between proximal tooth open contacts and periodontal disease. J Periodontol 1983;54:529–533.

90. Newell DH, John V, Kim SJ. A technique of occlusal adjustment for food impaction in the presence of tight proximal contacts. Oper Dent 2002;27:95–100.

91. Beklen A, Laine M, Ventä I, Hyrkäs T, Konttinen YT. Role of TNF-alpha and its receptors in pericoronitis. J Dent Res 2005;84:1178–1182.

92. Bradshaw S, Faulk J, Blakey GH, Phillips C, Phero JA, White RP Jr. Quality of life outcomes after third molar removal in subjects with minor symptoms of pericoronitis. J Oral Maxillofac Surg 2012;70:2494–2500.

93. Sixou JL, Magaud C, Jolivet-Gougeon A, Cormier M, Bonnaure-Mallet M. Microbiology of mandibular third molar pericoronitis: Incidence of beta-lactamase-producing bacteria. Oral Surg Oral Med Oral Pathol Oral Radiol Endod 2003;95:655–659.

94. Gutiérrez-Pérez JL. Third molar infections [in Spanish]. Med Oral Patol Oral Cir Bucal 2004;9(suppl 1):122–125.

95. Brescó-Salinas M, Costa-Riu N, Berini-Aytés L, Gay-Escoda C. Antibiotic susceptibility of the bacteria causing odontogenic infections [in Spanish]. Med Oral Patol Oral Cir Bucal 2006;11:70–75.

96. Bermejo-Fenoll A, Sánchez-Pérez A. Necrotising periodontal diseases [in Spanish]. Med Oral Patol Oral Cir Bucal 2004;9(suppl 1):114–119.

97. Jiménez LM, Duque FL, Baer PN, Jiménez SB. Necrotizing ulcerative periodontal diseases in children and young adults in Medellin, Colombia, 1965–2000. J Int Acad Periodontol 2005;7:55–63.

98. Lopez R, Fernandez O, Jara G, Baelum V. Epidemiology of necrotizing ulcerative gingival lesions in adolescents. J Periodontal Res 2002;37:439–444.

99. Arendorf TM, Bredekamp B, Cloete CA, Joshipura K. Seasonal variation of acute necrotising ulcerative gingivitis in South Africans. Oral Dis 2001;7:150–154.

100. Diouf M, Cisse D, Faye A, et al. Prevalence of necrotizing ulcerative gingivitis and associated factors in Koranic boarding schools in Senegal. Community Dent Health 2012;29:184–187.

101. Folayan MO. The epidemiology, etiology, and pathophysiology of acute necrotizing ulcerative gingivitis associated with malnutrition. J Contemp Dent Pract 2004;5(3):28–41.

102. Brook I. Microbiology and management of periodontal infections. Gen Dent 2003;51:424–428.

103. Abdalla-Aslan R, Benoliel R, Sharav Y, Czerninski R. Oral mucosal pain characteristics: A prospective study. Poster, European Association of Oral Medicine, September 2014, Antalya, Turkey.

104. Kovac-Kovacic M, Skaleric U. The prevalence of oral mucosal lesions in a population in Ljubljana, Slovenia. J Oral Pathol Med 2000;29:331–335.

105. Natah SS, Konttinen YT, Enattah NS, Ashammakhi N, Sharkey KA, Häyrinen-Immonen R. Recurrent aphthous ulcers today: A review of the growing knowledge. Int J Oral Maxillofac Surg 2004;33:221–234.

106. Lo Muzio L, della Valle A, Mignogna MD, et al. The treatment of oral aphthous ulceration or erosive lichen planus with topical clobetasol propionate in three preparations: A clinical and pilot study on 54 patients. J Oral Pathol Med 2001;30:611–617.

107. Ylikontiola L, Sorsa T, Häyrinen-Immonen R, Salo T. Doxymycine-cyanoacrylate treatment of recurrent aphthous ulcers. Oral Surg Oral Med Oral Pathol Oral Radiol Endod 1997;83:329–333.

108. Saxen MA, Ambrosius WT, Rehemtula al-KF, Russell AL, Eckert GJ. Sustained relief of oral aphthous ulcer pain from topical diclofenac in hyaluronan: a randomized, double-blind clinical trial. Oral Surg Oral Med Oral Pathol Oral Radiol Endod 1997;84:356–361.

109. Zand N, Ataie-Fashtami L, Djavid GE, et al. Relieving pain in minor aphthous stomatitis by a single session of non-thermal carbon dioxide laser irradiation. Lasers Med Sci 2009;24:515–520.

110. Chayavichitsilp P, Buckwalter JV, Krakowski AC, Friedlander SF. Herpes simplex. Pediatr Rev 2009;30:119–129.

111. Main DM. Acute herpetic stomatitis: Referrals to Leeds Dental Hospital 1978–1987. Br Dent J 1989;166:14–16.

112. Chauvin PJ, Ajar AH. Acute herpetic gingivostomatitis in adults: A review of 13 cases, including diagnosis and management. J Can Dent Assoc 2002;68:247–251.

113. Greenberg MS, Cohen SG, Boosz B, Friedman H. Oral herpes simplex infections in patients with leukemia. J Am Dent Assoc 1987;114:483–486.

114. Robinson PA, High AS, Hume WJ. Rapid detection of human herpes simplex virus type 1 in saliva. Arch Oral Biol 1992;37:797–806.

115. Schiffer JT, Magaret A, Selke S, Corey L, Wald A. Detailed analysis of mucosal herpes simplex virus-2 replication kinetics with and without antiviral therapy. J Antimicrob Chemother 2011;66:2593–2600.

116. Field HJ, Vere Hodge RA. Recent developments in anti-herpesvirus drugs. Br Med Bull 2013;106:213–249.

117. Terai H, Shimahara M. Atrophic tongue associated with Candida. J Oral Pathol Med 2005;34:397–400.

118. Kolbinson DA, Schubert MM, Flournoy N, Truelove EL. Early oral changes following bone marrow transplantation. Oral Surg Oral Med Oral Pathol 1988;66:130–138.

119. Gall-Troselj K, Mravak-Stipetić M, Jurak I, Ragland WL, Pavelić J. Helicobacter pylori colonization of tongue mucosa—Increased incidence in atrophic glossitis and burning mouth syndrome (BMS). J Oral Pathol Med 2001;30:560–563.

120. Haring JI. Diagnosing salivary stones. J Am Dent Assoc 1991;122(5):75–76.

121. Murray ME, Buckenham TM, Joseph AE. The role of ultrasound in screening patients referred for sialography: A possible protocol. Clin Otolaryngol Allied Sci 1996;21:21–23.

122. Iro H, Zenk J, Escudier MP, et al. Outcome of minimally invasive management of salivary calculi in 4,691 patients. Laryngoscope 2009;119:263–268.

123. Leerdam CM, Martin HC, Isaacs D. Recurrent parotitis of childhood. J Paediatr Child Health 2005;41:631–634.

124. Nahlieli O, Shacham R, Shlesinger M, Eliav E. Juvenile recurrent parotitis: A new method of diagnosis and treatment. Pediatrics 2004;114:9–12.

125. Nahlieli O, Shacham R, Bar T, Eliav E. Endoscopic mechanical retrieval of sialoliths. Oral Surg Oral Med Oral Pathol Oral Radiol Endod 2003;95:396–402.

126. Nahlieli O, Shacham R, Zaguri A. Combined external lithotripsy and endoscopic techniques for advanced sialolithiasis cases. J Oral Maxillofac Surg 2010;68:347–353.

Otolaryngologic Aspects of Orofacial Pain

Menachem Gross, MD
Ron Eliashar, MD

7

p. 163 - p. 194

Orofacial pain is a relatively common complaint in general medical and dental practice. The diagnosis and management of orofacial pain originating from the ear, sinonasal area, oropharyngeal region, facial area, and neck has been a subject of great controversy over the years, and the controversy continues to date. This situation is unfortunate because there have been great advances in our understanding of these conditions based on solid research over the past 25 years. Otolaryngologists are often involved when primary disorders of the ear, nose, and throat or the head and neck are the source of pain. This chapter deals with the differential diagnosis and management of common painful disorders affecting these areas.

Different pitfalls may lead to misdiagnosis of orofacial pain. Therefore, it is important for clinicians to understand the following factors that can lead to misdiagnosis[1]:

- The complex regional anatomy of the head and neck often results in disparity between the site and the source of pain.
- Symptoms of pain, limitation of mandibular movement, joint noise, tinnitus, and altered occlusion are not specific for the pathologic condition. Thus, these symptoms can be caused by local otologic and temporomandibular joint disorders or by infectious, neoplastic, neurologic, and systemic conditions.
- Chronic tissue damage from trauma and/or multiple surgical procedures can lead to central sensitization of sensory nerve pathways, leading to neuropathic pain, allodynia (pain response to non-painful stimuli), and hyperalgesia (excessive pain response to mildly painful stimuli). The presence of neuropathic pain can make accurate diagnosis extremely difficult because clinicians can be easily misled into believing that the source of the pain is localized when, in fact, there is a central nervous system–mediated component.

Handwritten note at top: Q# 8 Referred pain to the ear CN V, VII, IX, X — 5, 7, 9, 10

Ear Pain (Otalgia)

Earache, or *otalgia*, is quite common among children and adults. The pain can vary from mild to excruciating, severe, dull, aching, or lancinating. Otalgia may be associated with such sensations as a sense of fullness in the ear, burning, throbbing, tenderness, or itching. The exact incidence of otalgia is not known. Adults tend to suffer from fewer ear problems and otalgia than children. Children are mostly affected because acute otitis media (AOM), which is the most common cause of otalgia, occurs mainly in young people.[2,3]

According to the *International Classification of Headache Disorders, third edition* (ICHD-3), headache attributed to disorder of the ears is headache caused by an inflammatory, neoplastic, or other disorder of one or both ears and associated with other symptoms and/or clinical signs of the disorder.[4] The ICHD-3 criteria are described in Table 7-1. Because of nociceptive field overlap and convergence in the nociceptive pathways of the head and neck, it seems clear that a painful disorder or lesion of the ear may lead to headache. It is highly unlikely that headache in such conditions can occur in the absence of ear pain, the typical manifestation of otologic pathology.

Otalgia may be caused by several different medical conditions. Detailed history and physical examination, with directed studies as indicated, can clarify the source of the pain. Based on the resultant findings, the disease is classified as primary (Table 7-2) or secondary (referred) otalgia (Table 7-3).

Primary otalgia is caused by a disease in the ear itself (a direct cause of earache), and the most serious problems are usually caused by infection (see Table 7-2). The areas most commonly involved in causing pain, or becoming infected, are the external ear and the middle ear. Pain in the external ear radiates most often to the vertex and to the temple, but it sometimes spreads toward other areas of the head. Often patients cannot differentiate between pain originating in the inner ear and pain originating in the external or middle ear.[5]

Secondary or referred otalgia (see Table 7-3) is pain stemming from another region or location in the body and radiating to the ear (an indirect cause of earache). Because of the nature of the ear's sensory innervation, a wide variety of disorders can produce referred otalgia. Branches of the trigeminal, facial, glossopharyngeal, and vagus cranial nerves all participate, as do the lesser occipital and the great auricular cervical nerve roots. The ear thus shares its sensory innervation with other head and neck structures, including the face, eyes, jaws, teeth, pharynx, and larynx.

The incidence of referred otalgia increases with age. About half of otalgia cases are caused by referred pain from non–ear-related problems, and half these cases of referred otalgia are caused by dental disorders.[1,6,7] Diseased molars are the most common dental cause of secondary otalgia, which results in severe unremitting pain that often worsens when cold fluids enter the oral cavity (see chapter 6).

Muscular pain originating in the muscles, tendons, or fascia of the head or neck, such as myofascial pain and tension-type headache (see chapter 8), can also produce ear pain.[1] The pain is constant, dull, and aching and is usually not throbbing.[8] Movement of the jaw or the head worsens the pain. Prolonged clenching of the teeth, abnormal jaw movements, and dental disease may cause a type of muscle spasm known as *protective muscle splinting* (see chapter 8).

Pharyngeal and laryngeal diseases cause referred otalgia via the glossopharyngeal nerve. Associated symptoms may include dysphagia, throat pain, and breathing difficulty. After tonsillectomy, patients almost always complain of postoperative otalgia.[3,8] The pathologies of cervical vertebrae have also been identified as causing referred otalgia.[9]

Persistent earache with a normal ear examination increases the suspicion of carcinoma, especially when associated with hemoptysis, weight loss, tooth pain, or difficulty in swallowing. Otalgia is one of the earliest symptoms of carcinoma of the pyriform sinus, although neoplasia producing otalgia may also be located in the larynx, esophagus, nasopharynx, lungs, tonsils, or tongue.[5,8,10,11] In patients suffering from carcinoma of the base of the tongue, the incidence of otalgia was found to be 33%.[12] Amundson[13] stressed that unilateral ear pain in an adult who is a heavy smoker or a heavy drinker is most likely a sign of cancer until ruled out.

Table 7-1	Diagnostic criteria for headache attributed to disorder of the ears*

Diagnostic criteria

A. Any headache fulfilling criterion C

B. Clinical, laboratory, and/or imaging evidence of an infectious, neoplastic, or other irritative disorder or lesion of one or both ears, known to be able to cause headache

C. Evidence of causation demonstrated by at least two of the following:
    1. Headache has developed in temporal relation to the onset of the ear disorder or appearance of the ear lesion
    2. Either or both of the following:
        a. Headache has significantly worsened in parallel with worsening or progression of the ear disorder or lesion
        b. Headache has significantly improved or resolved in parallel with improvement in or resolution of the ear disorder or lesion
    3. Headache is exacerbated by pressure applied to the affected ear(s) or periauricular structures
    4. In the case of a unilateral ear disorder or lesion, headache is localized ipsilateral to it

D. Not better accounted for by another ICHD-3 diagnosis

*Reproduced with permission from the International Headache Society.

Table 7-2	Causes of primary otalgia	

Classification	Condition	Comments for entities not covered in this chapter
Auricular disorders	Auricular cellulitis	
	Auricular trauma	Injury to the ear may cause hyperemia, abrasions, lacerations, and auricular hematoma in cases of blunt trauma. The hematoma should be drained to relieve pain and to prevent abscess formation and such auricular deformities as "cauliflower ear."
	Relapsing polychondritis	
Disorders of the external ear	Impacted cerumen	Wax may obstruct the ear canal and may cause pain, itching, and temporary hearing loss. Wax is removed by irrigation or by rolling it by a blunt curette or loop.
	Foreign object in the external ear	Children often insert foreign bodies such as beads, erasers, and beans into the ear. Foreign bodies should be removed by raking them out with a blunt hook.
	Furuncle of the external ear canal	
	Otitis externa	
	Necrotizing otitis externa	
	Ramsay Hunt syndrome (herpes zoster oticus)	
Disorders of the middle ear	Otitis media	
	Myringitis bullosa	
	Traumatic tympanic membrane rupture	The tympanic membrane may be perforated by objects placed in the external canal; by sudden overpressure, such as an explosion, a slap, or diving; or by sudden negative pressure. This results in sudden severe pain followed by bleeding from the ear. Spontaneous closure of the perforation is usual. Persistent perforation is indication for myringoplasty.
	Eustachian tube dysfunction	
	Barotrauma	

Ⓐ Ramsay Hunt Syndrome p.168, p.450, p.425

Table 7-3	Causes of secondary otalgia	
Classification	**Condition**	**Comments**
Dental problems	Infant teething, pain of tooth eruption, impacted third molars (wisdom teeth), dental infections in the maxillary molars, fractured tooth, dry socket after dental extraction, gingivitis and other periodontal disease	See chapter 6.
Infections	Upper respiratory tract infection	An acute, usually viral infection of the respiratory tract with inflammation in the nose, throat, larynx, and trachea that is associated with watery nasal secretions, sore throat, cough, and referred otalgia through the glossopharyngeal nerve.
	Sinusitis	See the Facial Pain section in this chapter.
	Infection of the throat: tonsillitis, pharyngitis, and peritonsillary abscess	These conditions are covered in the Throat Pain section in this chapter.
	Laryngitis	An acute viral inflammation of the larynx that is associated with unnatural change of voice, throat pain, and referred otalgia through the vagus nerve.
	Salivary gland infection	See chapter 6.
Diseases of the joints and muscles of the mandible	Masticatory muscle disorders	See chapter 8.
	Temporomandibular joint dysfunction	See chapter 8.
Head and neck muscle spasms		See chapter 8.
Removal of tonsils	Post-tonsillectomy pain	After tonsillectomy, patients have throat pain and may feel a referred pain in one or both ears through the glossopharyngeal nerve. The pain vanishes within a few weeks.
Cervical spine problems		See chapter 14.
Inflammation of the blood vessels in the temple	Temporal arteritis	See chapter 14.
Neuralgic disorders	Trigeminal neuralgia	See chapter 11.
	Glossopharyngeal neuralgia	See chapter 12.
	Arnold's nerve cough syndrome	Reflex cough, caused by chronic irritation of auricular branch of the vagus (X) nerve. It is associated with an attack of suboccipital stabbing or burning pain and auricular pain.
Cancer of the head or neck		See chapter 14.

Common diseases causing primary otalgia

Auricular cellulitis

Auricular cellulitis is a diffuse, spreading, acute infection of the auricular skin or subcutaneous structures that is characterized by hyperemia and edema with no cellular necrosis or suppuration. The most common pathogen is *Streptococcus pyogenes* (group A beta-hemolytic streptococci [GABHS]). *Staphylococcus aureus* occasionally causes superficial auricular cellulitis, which is less extensive than that of streptococcal origin. The infective process involves the entire auricle, including the auricular lobule. The infection can occur spontaneously or after acute external otitis, chronic auricular dermatitis, or trauma (such as auricular piercing). Primary treatment includes parenteral antibiotic therapy, such as oxacillin or cefazolin, with topical antibiotic therapy.

Relapsing polychondritis

Relapsing polychondritis is an episodic inflammatory condition of the cartilaginous and non-cartilaginous tissues that causes progressive destruction of the head and neck cartilages, predominantly those of the ear, nose, and laryngotracheobronchial tree.[14,15] Other affected structures may include the eye, the cardiovascular system, small and large peripheral joints, and the middle and inner ear.[14-16] The etiology is unknown; however, the pathogenesis of relapsing polychondritis involves an autoimmune response to as yet unidentified cartilage antigens, followed by cartilage matrix destruction by proteolytic enzymes.[15] Signs and symptoms of relapsing polychondritis of the auricle include auricular cellulitis, typically with a sudden onset of unilateral or bilateral auricular pain; tenderness; swelling; and redness with sparing of the lobules. The pain and redness usually disappear within 2 to 4 weeks but may recur. Auricular chondritis is specific to relapsing polychondritis once a local disease or infection has been ruled out. Auricular chondritis is found in 20% of patients at presentation and in 90% of patients at some point during the course of the disease.[15] A definitive diagnosis of relapsing polychondritis is made by biopsy of the affected cartilaginous tissue in which infiltration of the cartilage and perichondrial tissues with neutrophils and lymphocytes as well as loss of cartilaginous matrix are demonstrated. Michet et al[17] developed criteria for diagnosing relapsing polychondritis. An advantage of their criteria is that a biopsy does not need to be obtained routinely. Although not validated, these criteria are useful in clinical practice.

Mild cases may respond to symptomatic treatment with aspirin, indomethacin, or other nonsteroidal anti-inflammatory drugs. Patients with severe cases are initially treated with systemic corticosteroids, and the dose is tapered in accordance with the clinical response. In very severe cases, an immunosuppressive agent, such as cyclophosphamide, is also required.

Furuncle of the external ear canal

Furuncle of the external ear canal is an acute, tender, perifollicular inflammatory nodule resulting from an *S aureus* infection. The initial nodule evolves into a pustule with central necrosis, which later discharges a sanguineous purulent exudate. A furuncle causes localized pain within the external auditory meatus, which is intensified by local pressure. Treatment includes surgical drainage of the furuncle; systemic antibiotic therapy with oxacillin or cefazolin may be added when required.

Acute otitis externa

Acute otitis externa, an infective condition involving the external ear canal, is usually caused by a gram-negative rod such as *Pseudomonas aeruginosa* or *Escherichia coli*; however, *S aureus* or, rarely, a fungus, may also be a causative agent.[18] This infection is often caused by moisture in the external ear canal, such as in warm, moist climates or after bathing. Injury caused by attempts to clean or to scratch an itching ear, as in patients suffering from contact dermatitis (from earrings or earphones), allergic dermatitis, or seborrheic dermatitis, is another common cause.[19] A variant of acute otitis externa is swimmer's ear, a condition caused by a combination of external ear canal trauma and humidity during the swimming

Vestibulo cochlear Nerve VIII — textbook error!

herpes virus 3 ~ HHV VZV - p.425

Genicul Gangli

season. Signs and symptoms of acute otitis externa include mild to severe otalgia associated with purulent discharge from the external ear canal. Auricular movement or pressure on the tragus intensifies the pain. The otalgia can become extreme as the canal swells and becomes blocked.

Appropriate treatment includes topical application of a combination of antibiotic and corticosteroid eardrops instilled directly into the ear canal. Irrigation of the ear canal with hydrogen peroxide or 70% alcohol can temporarily stop the pain and itching.

Necrotizing otitis externa

Necrotizing external otitis usually starts as an external otitis caused by *P aeruginosa* and progresses into an osteomyelitis of the temporal bone.[18] This disease commonly occurs in elderly patients with diabetes and occasionally in patients who are immunocompromised.[20] The disease spreads outside the external ear canal through the fissures of Santorini (two slits located at the anterior cartilaginous external canal wall and the osseocartilaginous junction) into the skull base. Necrotizing external otitis is characterized by persistent severe otalgia, purulent otorrhea, and granulation tissue in the external ear canal.[20] Preauricular and temporomandibular joint pain, intensified by opening the mouth or by chewing, may be present. Severe headache in the temporal or occipital areas may accompany the earache. The severity of the pain can give a clue to the diagnosis. In severe cases, facial nerve involvement may occur, indicating an invasive infection. Other cranial nerve palsies, for example, in nerves IX, X, XI, and XII, may also occur. Imaging evaluation by computed tomography (CT) usually demonstrates soft tissue infiltration and bone destruction. Technetium-99 bone scan is usually positive and is highly sensitive to necrotizing external otitis.

Treatment includes good control of diabetes and prolonged therapy with an antipseudomonal antibiotic such as ciprofloxacin for at least 6 weeks, in addition to local therapy for the otitis externa. Surgical debridement through a mastoidectomy approach is occasionally required to control the spread of the infection.

Ramsay Hunt syndrome (herpes zoster oticus)

- p.450

Ramsay Hunt syndrome, also called *herpes zoster oticus*, is a herpesvirus 3 infection (varicella zoster virus infection, which causes chickenpox and shingles) of the geniculate ganglion (facial nerve ganglion). The virus spreads from the geniculate ganglion to the facial nerve and to the adjacent vestibulocochlear (XIII) nerve. The syndrome consists of unilateral facial paralysis, severe ear pain on the same side of the infection, tinnitus, vertigo, and herpetic blistering rash or vesicles on the pinna, external canal, and sometimes the roof of the mouth, in the distribution of the sensory branches of the facial nerve.[21,22] Other cranial nerves may be involved, and some degree of meningeal inflammation may occur.[23] Ramsay Hunt syndrome is usually more painful than Bell's palsy. The condition is rare in healthy people and occurs more commonly in people with a weakened immune system, such as the elderly and immunocompromised persons.[24] Diagnosis of Ramsay Hunt syndrome is based on the clinical symptoms and signs.

(NOT XI)

Prompt treatment with corticosteroids and antiviral medications, such as acyclovir and famcyclovir, reduces the symptoms and improves recovery.[25,26] A recent report recommends antiviral medication in combination with corticosteroids to improve the outcome for patients with Ramsay Hunt syndrome.[27] Overall, chances of recovery are better if treatment is started within 3 days of the onset of symptoms. Certain degrees of hearing loss or facial paralysis may become permanent.[26] Recovery may be complicated if the nerve grows back to the wrong areas (synkinesis). This may cause inappropriate responses, such as tearing when laughing or chewing (crocodile tears). Some patients may start blinking when talking or eating.

Acute otitis media

AOM is an infection of the middle ear cavity that occurs most frequently in infants and children, particularly between the ages of 3 months and 3 years, although it may occur at any age. AOM usually follows or accompanies an upper respiratory infection (URI) or a reduced immune response with no special reason.[28] AOM is the second most common childhood disease after

URI

● RAMSAY HUNT Syndrome - p.165, p.450

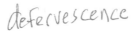
defervescence

URI. The first complaint is usually persistent, severe otalgia, which is often caused by an accumulation of fluid and pressure behind the tympanic membrane (TM). Other symptoms include hearing loss, fever, chills, irritability, and a feeling of fullness and pressure in the affected ear. Spontaneous drainage of pus or a clear or bloody fluid from the middle ear is common and may indicate perforation of the TM.[29] Rupture of the eardrum usually results in a sudden, marked decrease in pain and defervescence of fever.

Otoscopic examination reveals abnormal findings of the TM, including an erythematous and bulging TM, middle ear effusion, nondistinct anatomical middle ear landmarks, displaced or absent TM light reflex, and decreased TM mobility on pneumatic otoscopy. The most common bacterial pathogen in AOM is *streptococcus pneumoniae*, followed by *Haemophilus influenzae* and *Moraxella catarrhalis*.[29] These three organisms are responsible for more than 95% of all AOM cases with a bacterial etiology. The most important factors in the pathogenesis of a middle ear infection are eustachian tube dysfunction and direct extension of infectious processes from the nasopharynx into the middle ear cleft.[29]

AOM is treated with painkillers and oral amoxicillin systemic antibiotics.[28] Topical analgesics, such as tetracaine applied by eardrops, and oral decongestants, such as xylometazoline, may be helpful. Antibiotic therapy relieves the symptoms, hastens resolution of the infection, and reduces the chance for developing complications (eg, mastoiditis or meningitis). However, the Cochrane Review of antibiotics for AOM in children, representing a more cosmopolitan perspective, notes that antibiotic treatment slightly decreases pain at 24 hours and for a few days and that delayed antibiotic prescribing works as well as immediately prescribed antibiotics.[30] The Cochrane Review also notes that antibiotics make no difference in recurrence or in preventing more severe complications, such as temporary deafness, rupture of the TM, or mastoiditis. However, complications from the antibiotic treatment (vomiting, diarrhea, and rash) were common (37%). The Cochrane Review concludes that antibiotics should not be used for most cases of AOM, and they are appropriate only if there is bilateral AOM or AOM with otorrhea (discharge from

the ear). Myringotomy (small incision of the TM) should be considered in cases of a bulging TM or a persistent earache.

Myringitis bullosa

Myringitis bullosa is an inflammatory infection of the TM caused by a viral or bacterial infection. *Mycoplasma pneumoniae* and *S pneumoniae* are the most common bacteria responsible for myringitis bullosa. The disease is characterized by very painful vesicles on the TM, which may be full of serous or hemorrhagic fluid. A URI can precede the ear manifestations. Pain is severe, starts suddenly, persists for 24 to 72 hours, and is caused by the TM blisters, which appear between the richly innervated outer epithelium and the middle fibrous layers of the TM. Bullae involving the TM may also extend toward portions of the external auditory canal immediately adjacent to the TM. Objective cochlear and vestibular involvement manifested by sensorineural or mixed-type hearing loss and vertigo have been reported in patients suffering from myringitis bullosa.[31,32] Treatment includes analgesic and antibiotic therapy, such as azithromycin, which is applied against the major known pathogens causing myringitis bullosa.

Eustachian tube dysfunction

The middle ear is connected to the nasopharynx by the eustachian tube, which enables normal fluids to drain from the middle ear and has an important role in equalizing the pressure in the middle ear when the atmospheric pressure of ambient air shifts. Acute obstruction of the eustachian tube, mainly in cases of URI, may cause otalgia. This is especially common in small children, in whom the eustachian tube is naturally shorter and more horizontal. Eustachian tube dysfunction (ETD) in adults also occurs when there is an increase of postnasal drainage, allergy, rhinosinusitis, nasopharyngeal mass, and adenoidal hypertrophy.[33]

Brunworth et al[34] showed that ETD was more likely to be associated with a higher number of nasopharyngeal acid reflux events and a higher acid reflux finding score. He concluded that nasopharyngeal acid reflux may have a role in the pathogenesis of ETD. As the postnasal secretions drain posteriorly, or as acid refluxes into the nasopharynx around the opening of the eustachian tube, the eustachian tube gets irritated and swollen and eventually becomes blocked on one or both sides. When this happens, surrounding tissue absorbs the air in the affected tube, creating a vacuum, which causes the differences in pressure to pull the TM inward, the result being a sensation of fullness and pain. Hearing can be slightly impaired, and the ears can feel blocked or stuffed.

In isolated ETD, otoscopic examination will show a normal or retracted TM or, in more severe cases, middle ear effusion. Neck examination and fiber-optic nasopharyngoscopy are important parts of the physical examination in patients with ETD to exclude cervical lymphadenopathy or a nasopharyngeal mass, which may be associated with nasopharyngeal carcinoma.

One-third of patients with ETD show spontaneous improvement at the 6-month follow-up.[35] Intranasal medications have no proven benefit for symptomatic relief of ETD, although studies are limited in number.[35] However, topical nasal decongestants may be used, but only for a maximum of 7 days because of the risk of a rebound rhinitis medicamentosa associated with long-term use. Intranasal steroids are safe for use on a longer-term basis than decongestants, although the lowest possible dose should be prescribed, and the patient should be warned of local side effects, such as nasal crusting and dryness. Intranasal antihistamines may be used when an allergic cause of rhinitis is thought to have precipitated the ETD. Evidence suggests a benefit of autoinflation devices (eg, Otovent, Abigo; Ear Popper, Summit Medical), which apply positive pressure through the nose during swallowing and improve tympanogram and audiometry results at follow-up.[36] These devices can be bought over the counter and are recommended for use two or three times a day for at least 2 weeks initially. Eustachain tuboplasty, which is a balloon catheter used to dilate the eustachian tube, is relatively novel and was assessed by the National Institute for Health and Care Excellence in 2011.[37] Early data indicate that this technique is thought to be safe, has the advantage over tympanostomy of being relatively noninvasive, and may have greater longevity of results.

Ear barotrauma

Barotitis media, also known as *aerotitis*, represents damage to the middle ear and TM due to ambient pressure changes. When ambient pressure suddenly increases, air must move from the nasopharynx into the middle ear to maintain equilibrium on both sides of the TM. In cases of ETD, the pressure in the middle ear is below the ambient pressure, and the relative negative pressure in the middle ear results in retraction of the TM and transudation of blood from vessels. Very severe and sudden pressure differences may rupture the TM, causing bleeding in the middle ear with severe earache and conductive hearing loss. A perilymphatic fistula through the oval or round windows can occur, causing sensorineural hearing loss and vertigo. Barotrauma commonly occurs with altitude changes, such as in the descent of an airplane, deep sea diving, scuba diving, or driving in the mountains.[38,39]

Otalgia is the most common complaint of scuba divers and is experienced at some point by almost every diver. Some divers call it the *ear squeeze*. A person with an acute URI or allergic rhinitis should be advised to abstain from diving. Topical application of a nasal vasoconstrictor, such as xylometazoline, before any activity associated with descent and pressure changes can prevent barotrauma.

Facial Pain

Sinus-related headaches are located in the forehead, behind the eye, or in the occiput. Occasionally, they may radiate to the ears or to the temporal region. Headache related to the paranasal sinuses is often associated with facial pain. Facial pain complaints are commonly encountered and treated by primary care physicians. However, persistent or severe facial pain should be referred to otolaryngology, dental, ophthalmology, or neurology clinics because the condition often requires multidisciplinary evaluation and management.[40]

Facial pain is located in the area between or below the eyebrows, or the supraorbital rim, extending along the course of one or more trigeminal dermatomes. Facial pain may be caused by local disease of any of the major facial structures

Table 7-4	Differential diagnosis of facial pain from an otolaryngologist's viewpoint	
Classification	**Entity**	**Comments for entities not covered in this chapter**
Sinonasal pain	Rhinosinusitis	
	Mucosal contact point headache	
	Intranasal tumor	Nasal obstruction and local nasal pain may occur as the intranasal tumor enlarges, especially is it invades nerves.
	Granulomatous diseases of the nose	Granulomatosis with polyangiitis (Wegener granulomatosis) and sarcoidosis may affect the nasal cavity, causing congestion, nasal secretions, and local pain due to destructive lesions of soft tissue cartilage and bone.
Midfacial segment pain		
Persistent idiopathic facial pain	Formerly called *atypical facial pain*	See also chapter 12.
Scuba diving– caused pain	Sinus pain	
	Tension-type headache or muscle pain	
	Carbon dioxide toxicity	
	Decompression sickness headache	
Neuralgias	Trigeminal	See chapter 11.
	Sphenopalatine	
Primary headaches	Tension headache	See chapter 8.
	Migraine	See chapter 10.
	Cluster headache	See chapter 11.
	Chronic paroxysmal hemicrania	See chapter 11.

WG
P. 496

(eg, rhinosinusitis) or by a condition affecting their innervation (eg, neuralgia) (Table 7-4). The latter can occur anywhere between the posterior cranial fossa and the distal ends of the trigeminal nerve. The most common acute causes of pain are dental. The most common nondental pains are temporomandibular disorders, especially musculoskeletal disorders involving the muscles of mastication.[40] The prevalence of facial pain of paranasal sinus origin has probably been overestimated. Patients' expectations are often tempered by a prior diagnosis of sinusitis, guided by their knowledge of the location of the sinuses or by their primary care physician.

However, many patients suffering from this so-called sinusitis have no evidence of a sinonasal disease. Awareness is increasing among primary care physicians and otolaryngologists that other, non–sinus-related causes may be responsible for most of the suffering experienced by patients with facial pain or headache. The gold standard in establishing a sinonasal etiology for facial pain or headache is a diagnosis made by obtaining a thorough personal history and conducting a careful physical examination. Imaging studies, response to medical and surgical treatment, and an extended follow-up period may help establish the diagnosis.[41]

> ### Box 7-1 — Proposed International Headache Society diagnostic criteria for mucosal contact point headache
>
> A. Any headache fulfilling criterion C
> B. Clinical, nasal endoscopic, and/or imaging evidence of a hypertrophic or inflammatory process within the nasal cavity
> C. Evidence of causation demonstrated by at least two of the following:
>   1. Headache has developed in temporal relation to the onset of the intranasal lesion
>   2. Headache has significantly improved or significantly worsened in parallel with improvement in (with or without treatment) or worsening of the nasal lesion
>   3. Headache has significantly improved following local anesthesia of the mucosa in the region of the lesion
>   4. Headache is ipsilateral to the site of the lesion
> D. Not better accounted for by another ICHD-3 diagnosis

Common diseases causing facial pain

Sinonasal disorders causing pain: The neurobiology of primary sinonasal pain

The trigeminal nerve is the main facial sensory supply. The ophthalmic (V1) and maxillary (V2) divisions of the trigeminal nerve provide sensation to the mucosa of the sinonasal cavity. These nerve branches terminate as extensive uncovered nerve terminal endings next to the basal cells of the nasal epithelium.[42]

Nasal pain is mediated by Aδ fibers, the fast-responding, primarily mechanoreceptive pain fibers, and by C fibers, the slower, unmyelinated fibers associated with a duller pain from mechanothermal and chemosensory stimulation.[42]

Theories of sinonasal pain from contact points or pressure from sinus inflammation are based on substance P release from trigeminal sensory neurons located in the nasal mucosa.[43–46] This may be accompanied by the release of various other neuropeptides, such as calcitonin gene-related peptide and vasoactive intestinal peptide, which appear to be involved in the inflammatory cascade.[42] The local stimulation of the trigeminal fibers leads to a painful orthodromic and an antidromic response typified by vasodilation and hypersecretion.[42,43] Despite this cited mechanism for contact-point sinonasal pain, it is poorly documented and highly controversial.[47–49] A systematic review aiming to analyze the evidence that intranasal mucosal contact points cause facial pain or headache, and that their removal is therapeutic, concluded that most people with contact points experience no facial pain, the presence of a contact point is not a good predictor of facial pain, and the removal of a contact point rarely results in the total elimination of facial pain, making the theory that a contact point is responsible unlikely[50] (Box 7-1).

According to the ICHD-3, headache attributed to disorder of the nose or sinuses is headache caused by a disorder of the nose and/or paranasal sinuses and associated with other symptoms and/or clinical signs of the disorder.[4] The term *sinus headache* is considered outmoded by the ICHD-3, because it has been applied both to primary headaches and to headache supposedly attributed to various conditions involving the nasal or sinus structures.

Rhinosinusitis

Rhinosinusitis is a group of disorders characterized by inflammation of the mucosa of the nose and paranasal sinuses. The term *rhinosinusitis* is used instead of *sinusitis* because the latter is almost always accompanied by concurrent nasal airway inflammation, and, in many cases, sinusitis is preceded by rhinitis. Rhinosinusitis has been estimated to affect approximately 24 million patients in the United States each year.[51] Total direct health care costs related to recurrent acute rhinosinusitis (ARS), which affects approximately 1 in 3,000 adults per year, average around $1,100/patient each year, and oral antibiotic and nasal prescriptions cost an average of $210 and $450 per year, respectively. Thus, rhinosinusitis has a significant direct health care cost.[52]

Rhinosinusitis may be classified by duration as acute (less than 4 weeks), subacute (4 to 12 weeks), or chronic (more than 12 weeks, with or without acute exacerbations).

ARS may be classified further by symptom pattern into viral rhinosinusitis or acute bacterial rhinosinusitis (ABRS). Recurrent ARS is when a patient has four or more acute episodes of ABRS per year without persistent symptoms between episodes.[53]

A common presenting symptom of ARS is facial pain or headache. The pain is usually accompanied by other symptoms, such as nasal congestion, anterior and posterior purulent nasal drainage, and hyposmia or anosmia. The pain is a subjective complaint; however, tenderness on percussion is a function of spinal cord pain processing (hyperalgesia). People with ARS had a significantly lower pain and sensory detection threshold in their sinus regions compared with a healthy control group.[54,55] Sinus pain caused by inflammation induced by infection (bacterial or viral) or allergic rhinosinusitis occurs when exudate blocks the sinus ostium and exerts pressure stimulating local trigeminal nerve fibers. The local release of proinflammatory and proalgesic mediators is an early mechanism (this is probably as important as the pressure).

The development of rhinosinusitis depends on a variety of environmental and host factors, and rhinosinusitis is considered to be a disease with multifactorial causes. Host factors include genetic or congenital conditions (eg., cystic fibrosis, immotile cilia syndrome), allergic rhinitis, sinonasal anatomical abnormalities, and systemic diseases. Environmental factors include infectious agents, trauma, noxious chemicals, and iatrogenic causes.

Three major systems are used for classification of and for establishing diagnostic criteria relating to headaches and sinus disease: the working definitions recommended by the American Academy of Otolaryngology-Head and Neck Surgery (AAO-HNS), the ICHD-3 criteria, and the European Position Paper on Rhinosinusitis and Nasal Polyps (EPOS).[4,53,55–58] As

expected, the ICHD-3 classification relates to diseases that may induce facial pain or headache, whereas the AAO-HNS and EPOS classifications are concerned primarily with the disease process of sinusitis itself.

Rhinosinusitis may be diagnosed clinically in most patients based on history and physical examination. Physical examination includes otoscopy, anterior rhinoscopy, percussion over the areas of the paranasal sinuses, and oropharyngeal and neck examination. Nasal endoscopy and imaging are usually not required for an initial diagnosis of any form of rhinosinusitis. However, these modalities may be very helpful in obtaining a definitive diagnosis of rhinosinusitis. Patients with recurrent or complicated sinus disease may require imaging. CT is superior to radiography because plain radiographs are imprecise at determining the extent of the disease and the patency of the sinus ostium.[53,56,58,59] CT scanning of the sinonasal region has two major roles in rhinosinusitis:

1. To define the anatomy of the sinuses before surgery
2. To aid in the diagnosis and management of chronic rhinosinusitis (CRS), complicated ARS, or recurrent rhinosinusitis

Acute rhinosinusitis. ARS is an acute inflammatory condition involving the paranasal sinuses and the lining of the nasal passages. The most recent US classification defines ARS when there is up to 4 weeks of purulent nasal drainage (anterior, posterior, or both) accompanied by nasal obstruction, facial pain/pressure/fullness, or both.

ABRS is distinguished from ARS caused by viral URIs and noninfectious conditions. ABRS is diagnosed when (1) symptoms or signs of ARS are present 10 days or more beyond the onset of upper respiratory symptoms or (2) symptoms or signs of ARS worsen within 10 days after an initial improvement (double worsening).[53] The EPOS classification defines ARS in adults as sudden onset of two or more symptoms, one of which should be nasal blockage/obstruction/congestion or nasal discharge (anterior/posterior nasal drip) with or without facial pain/pressure and with or without reduction or loss of smell for less than 12 weeks, with symptom-free intervals if the problem is recur-

PROAlgesic

Box 7-2   **Clinical criteria for the diagnosis of acute rhinosinusitis (ARS)**

Major factors
- Purulent anterior nasal discharge
- Purulent, discolored posterior nasal drainage
- Nasal obstruction or blockage
- Facial pain/pressure/congestion/fullness
- Hyposmia or anosmia
- Fever

Minor factors
- Headache
- Ear pain/pressure/fullness
- Halitosis
- Dental pain
- Cough
- Fever (all nonacute)
- Fatigue

---

rent, and with validation by telephone or by interview. ABRS is suggested by the presence of at least three of the following symptoms/signs: discolored discharge (with unilateral predominance) and purulent nasal secretions, severe local pain (with unilateral predominance), fever (> 38°C), elevated erythrocyte sedimentation rate/C-reactive protein, or "double worsening" (ie, deterioration after an initial milder phase of illness).[58]

The most common cause of ARS is a community-acquired viral infection leading to a self-limiting period of upper respiratory symptoms.[55] Viral ARS is characterized by cough, sneezing, rhinorrhea, sore throat, and nasal congestion. Antibiotics are not recommended for treating ARS because they are ineffective for viral illness and do not relieve symptoms directly.[53] Human rhinovirus is the most common cause of viral ARS. Other viruses include coronavirus, influenza A and B virus, parainfluenza virus, respiratory syncytial virus, and adenovirus. Occasionally, a secondary bacterial infection of the paranasal sinuses occurs and requires specific antimicrobial therapy.[53,58] Allergic rhinitis, nasal polyposis, a foreign body in the nasal cavity, trauma, dental infection, and other factors leading to inflammation of the nose and paranasal sinuses can also predispose people to develop ARS.

Commonly isolated bacteria in patients with ABRS include *S pneumoniae*, nontypeable *H influenzae*, *S pyogenes*, *M catarrhalis*, *S aureus*, and occasionally anaerobes.[53,58] Nosocomial rhinosinusitis often occurs in patients who require extended periods of intensive care and involves such risk factors as nasogastric

tubes, mechanical ventilation, failure of defense mechanisms, and pronged supine posture. Isolates from hospitalized patients usually contain gram-negative enterics such as *P aeruginosa*, *Klebsiella pneumoniae*, *Enterobacter* sp, *Proteus mirabilis*, *Serratia marcescens*, and *coagulase-negative S aureus*.[55]

The diagnosis of ARS focuses on clinical history and physical examination findings. Imaging, hematologic and microbiologic investigations, and endoscopy are not routinely required in the diagnosis of ARS or ABRS but may be needed in particular settings, such as in research studies or in high-risk patients.[53,58]

The clinical diagnostic criteria for ARS, as defined previously by the Task Force on Rhinosinusitis of the AAO-HNS, included major and minor symptoms or signs and disease duration of less than 4 weeks (Box 7-2). According to this classification, facial pain or pressure is regarded as a major symptom, whereas headache is considered to be a minor symptom.[55,56] This classification was designed to be used by primary care physicians and specialists. A diagnosis of rhinosinusitis is possible if two or more major symptoms or one major symptom and two or more minor symptoms are present. However, nasal purulence is a strong indicator of an accurate diagnosis. Facial pain or pressure alone does not constitute a suggestive history in the absence of another major nasal symptom or sign. Fever in itself does not constitute a strongly suggestive history in the absence of another major nasal symptom or sign.

Rosenfeld et al[53] define the clinical criteria for ARS as up to 4 weeks of purulent nasal drainage (anterior, posterior, or both) accompa-

Table 7-5	Diagnostic criteria for headache attributed to acute rhinosinusitis*

Diagnostic criteria

A. Any headache fulfilling criterion C

B. Clinical, nasal endoscopic, and/or imaging evidence of acute rhinosinusitis

C. Evidence of causation demonstrated by at least two of the following:
1. Headache has developed in temporal relation to the onset of the rhinosinusitis
2. Either or both of the following:
   a. Headache has significantly worsened in parallel with worsening of the rhinosinusitis
   b. Headache has significantly improved or resolved in parallel with improvement in or resolution of the rhinosinusitis
3. Headache is exacerbated by pressure applied over the paranasal sinuses
4. In the case of a unilateral rhinosinusitis, headache is localized ipsilateral to it

D. Not better accounted for by another ICHD-3 diagnosis

*Reproduced with permission from the International Headache Society.

nied by nasal obstruction, facial pain/pressure/fullness, or both, in which (1) purulent nasal discharge is cloudy or colored, in contrast to the clear secretions that typically accompany viral URI, and may be reported by the patient or observed on physical examination; (2) nasal obstruction may be reported by the patient as nasal obstruction, congestion, blockage, or stuffiness, or may be diagnosed by physical examination; and (3) facial pain/pressure/fullness may involve the anterior face or periorbital region or may manifest with headache that is localized or diffuse. As discussed previously, they then divide ARS into viral ARS, in which symptoms or signs of ARS are present less than 10 days and the symptoms are not worsening, and ABRS, in which (1) symptoms or signs of ARS are present 10 days or more beyond the onset of upper respiratory symptoms or (2) symptoms or signs of ARS worsen within 10 days after an initial improvement (double worsening). Note that Rosenfeld et al[53] *recommend against* radiographic imaging for patients who clinically meet the diagnostic criteria for ARS.

The EPOS[58] combines these two clinical classification schemes and includes the possibility of both endoscopy and imaging when the treating physician is an otolaryngologist. The EPOS defines the clinical criteria of ARS as inflammation of the nose and the paranasal sinuses characterized by two or more symptoms, one of which should be either nasal blockage/obstruction/congestion or nasal discharge (anterior/posterior nasal drip) with or without facial pain/pressure, with or without reduction or loss of smell, and the other of which should be either endoscopic signs of nasal polyps and/or mucopurulent discharge, primarily from the middle meatus, and/or edema/mucosal obstruction primarily in the middle meatus, and/or CT changes, including mucosal changes within the ostiomeatal complex and/or sinuses. The EPOS further defines common cold/ARS as duration of symptoms for less than 10 days; acute postviral rhinosinusitis as increase of symptoms after 5 days or persistent symptoms after 10 days with less than 12 weeks duration; and ABRS in the presence of at least three of the following symptoms/signs: (1) discolored discharge (with unilateral predominance) and purulent secretion in the cavum nasi, (2) severe local pain (with unilateral predominance), (3) fever (> 38°C), (4) elevated erythrocyte sedimentation rate/C-reactive protein, and (5) "double worsening."[58]

The ICHD-3 diagnostic criteria for headache attributed to ARS are presented in Table 7-5.[4]

In an immunocompetent person living in the general community, ARS is typically believed to be induced by viruses. Only about 0.5% to 2.0% of ARS episodes are complicated by a bacterial infection.[53] Therefore, antibiotics are not recommended when the treating physician did not specifically diagnose ABRS. Initial treatment depends on the severity of the disease[58]:

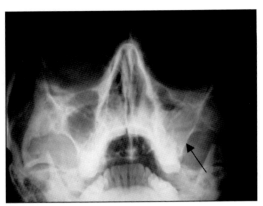

Fig 7-1 Radiographic image demonstrating left acute maxillary rhinosinusitis with air-fluid level in the left maxillary sinus *(arrow)*.

- *Mild symptoms (viral, common cold):* Start with symptomatic relief, such as analgesics (eg, oral acetaminophen), saline irrigation, decongestants (eg, xylometazoline), herbal compounds
- *Moderate symptoms:* Add topical steroids
- *Severe symptoms (including ABRS):* Add topical steroids and consider antibiotics

If the physician decides to treat ABRS with an antibiotic agent, a short-course treatment, particularly for patients without severe disease and complicating factors, might lead to fewer adverse events, better patient compliance, a lower rate of resistance development, and fewer costs.[58] No significant differences have been found in clinical outcomes for ABRS treated with different antibiotic agents. Clinicians should therefore prescribe amoxicillin as first-line therapy for most adults. Amoxicillin increases rates of clinical cure or improvement compared with placebo. The justification for amoxicillin as first-line therapy for most patients with ABRS relates to its safety, efficacy, low cost, and narrow microbiologic spectrum. For penicillin-allergic patients, folate inhibitors (trimethoprim-sulfamethoxazole) are a cost-effective alternative to amoxicillin. The macrolide class of antibiotics may also be used for patients with penicillin allergy.[53]

Acute maxillary rhinosinusitis. Acute maxillary rhinosinusitis is the most common sinus

disease causing facial pain (Fig 7-1). The pain is usually related to the affected maxillary antrum but is often referred to the maxillary teeth (in which the roots are embedded in the maxilla and are intimately related to the floor of the maxillary sinus) or to the forehead. Purulent nasal discharge in the middle nasal meatus and sensitivity to percussion over the cheek or teeth confirm the diagnosis.

Sinonasal toothache. Diseases in the maxillary sinus mucosa may refer pain to the maxillary teeth. The pain is usually felt in several teeth as dull, aching, or throbbing. Occasionally, the pain is associated with pressure below the eyes, which increases when bending the head, applying pressure over the sinuses, coughing, or sneezing. Tests performed on the teeth, such as applying ice, chewing, and percussion, may increase pain from a sinonasal origin. History of URI, nasal congestion, or other sinus problem is suspicious for a sinus toothache. A thorough dental examination (clinical and radiographic) excludes a primary dental cause.

Acute ethmoiditis. Acute ethmoiditis causes pain at the root of the nose or behind the eye. Seldom does ethmoiditis occur as an isolated infection. More often it is part of an acute pansinusitis involving the maxillary and frontal sinuses as well, because all of these sinuses drain into the osteomeatal complex in the middle nasal meatus. Purulent anterior and posterior nasal discharge and tenderness over the inner canthus of the eye are characteristic. The pain may spread laterally into the orbit or radiate to the temporal region. Occasionally, an orbital complication (eg, periorbital cellulitis or abscess) may occur when the infection spreads into the orbit through the thin lamina papyracea or the venous system.

Acute frontal rhinosinusitis. Acute suppurative frontal rhinosinusitis is not very common, apparently because of the vertical nature of the frontal sinus and its natural advantage of dependent drainage through the nasofrontal duct (Fig 7-2). Thus, the common forehead pain is seldom due to an underlying frontal rhinosinusitis. The characteristic pain is over the affected sinus and often along the upper orbital rim. The pain may radiate to the vertex and behind

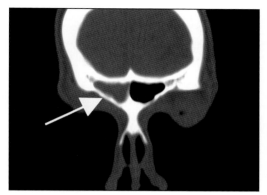

Fig 7-2 Coronal CT scan demonstrating right acute frontal rhinosinusitis with opacification of the right frontal sinus *(arrow)*.

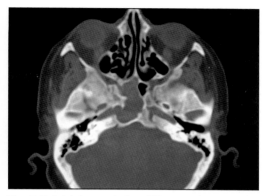

Fig 7-3 Axial bone-window CT scan demonstrating opacification of the right sphenoid sinus compatible with sinusitis. Note the dehiscence of the right internal carotid artery.

the eye. Tenderness is usually felt in the frontal sinus or along its floor. When frontal sinusitis is complicated by osteomyelitis of the frontal bone, the pain is prominent, diffuse, and intense, and it often worsens at night and keeps the patient awake.

Acute sphenoiditis. Acute sphenoiditis is rare and is characterized by a wide variety of types and distributions of pain. These include severe occipital headache, retro-orbital dull and aching pain, and a stabbing pain at the vertex. Definitive diagnosis is made by a CT scan (Fig 7-3).

Pain assessment of ABRS. Pain relief is a major goal in managing ABRS, and it is often the main reason patients with ABRS seek medical assistance. Ongoing assessment of the severity of pain is essential for proper management. Severity may be assessed using a faces pain scale or a simple visual analog scale (VAS), or by asking the patient to qualitatively rate the discomfort as "mild" versus "moderate/severe."[53] When using a VAS, the disease can be divided into mild, moderate, or severe based on the total score on a scale of 0 to 10[58]:

- Mild = VAS score of 0 to 3
- Moderate = VAS score > 3 to 7
- Severe = VAS score > 7 to 10

Frequent use of analgesics is often necessary. Orally administered analgesics are the preferred route of administration. When frequent dosing is required to maintain adequate pain relief, administering analgesics at fixed intervals may be more effective than a pro re nata (as-needed) basis.[53]

Subacute rhinosinusitis. Subacute rhinosinusitis may represent a continuum of the natural progression of ARS that has not resolved completely. According to the US classification, subacute rhinosinusitis is diagnosed after 4 weeks' duration of symptoms or signs of rhinosinusitis and lasts up to 12 weeks.[53] However, the European group thought a separate term to describe patients with prolonged ARS was not necessary because the number of patients who have such a prolonged course is small, and there are very few data on which to base evidence-based recommendations on how to manage these patients. They therefore define ARS as an infection lasting up to 12 weeks and do not use the term *subacute rhinosinusitis* at all.[58]

Recurrent acute rhinosinusitis. Recurrent ARS is also classified only in the US literature as a situation in which four or more episodes of ABRS occur per year, without signs or symptoms of rhinosinusitis between the episodes. Although recognized as a distinct form of rhinosinusitis, only a few cohort studies have documented the characteristics and clinical impact of recurrent ARS. The proper

---

Box 7-3   **Clinical criteria for the diagnosis of chronic rhinosinusitis (CRS)***

Major factors
- Nasal obstruction
- Facial congestion
- Facial pain/pressure/fullness
- Nasal discharge (anterior/posterior purulent discharge)
- Loss of smell

Minor factors
- Fatigue
- Headache
- Ear pain/pressure
- Cough
- Halitosis
- Dental pain
- Fever

*Symptoms of CRS are milder than in the acute form, and CRS may present with only one symptom. However, according to the International Headache Society, CRS has not been validated as a cause of headache/facial pain.[53]

---

diagnosis of recurrent ARS requires that each episode meet the criteria for ABRS. Culture is most useful during an acute episode, and imaging is most useful between episodes to identify anatomical changes that may predispose a patient to recurrent disease. An allergy-immunology evaluation may be considered to detect coexisting allergic rhinitis or an underlying immunologic deficiency. Surgical intervention, which is not appropriate for uncomplicated ABRS, may have a role in managing recurrent ARS.[53]

Chronic rhinosinusitis

The US classification defines CRS as 12 weeks or longer of two or more of the following signs and symptoms—mucopurulent drainage (anterior, posterior, or both), nasal obstruction (congestion), facial pain/pressure/fullness, or decreased sense of smell—accompanied by the presence of inflammation documented by one or more of the following findings: purulent (not clear) mucus or edema in the middle meatus or ethmoid region, polyps in the nasal cavity or the middle meatus, and/or radiographic imaging showing inflammation of the paranasal sinuses[53] (Box 7-3 and Table 7-6).

The Europeans classify CRS (with or without nasal polyps) in adults as[58] presence of two or more symptoms, one of which should be nasal blockage/obstruction/congestion or nasal discharge (anterior/posterior nasal drip); with or without facial pain/pressure; with or without reduction or loss of smell; and lasting at least 12 weeks. This should be supported by demonstrable disease by either endoscopic signs of nasal polyps; and/or mucopurulent discharge, primarily from the middle meatus; and/or edema/mucosal obstruction, primarily in the middle meatus; and/or CT changes consisting of mucosal changes within the ostiomeatal complex and/or sinuses.

CRS may be divided into two major categories: CRS with nasal polyposis (CRSwNP) and CRS without nasal polyposis (CRSsNP). This subclassification is more pronounced in the European classification than in the US one.[53,58] Recently, there has been discussion among rhinologists regarding the possibility that CRSsNP and CRSwNP are two distinct entities and not a spectrum of the same disease process; however, more research is required. In any case, there is a paucity of accurate information on the epidemiology and course of CRSsNP and CRSwNP.

Symptoms of CRS vary in severity and prevalence. Nasal obstruction is most common (81% to 95%), followed by facial congestion/pressure/fullness (70% to 85%), discolored nasal discharge (51% to 83%), and hyposmia (61% to 69%).[53] Facial pain or headache alone is not suggestive of CRS in the absence of other nasal symptoms or signs.[53,58] Other causes of

Table 7-6	Diagnostic criteria for headache attributed to chronic rhinosinusitis*

Diagnostic criteria

A. Any headache fulfilling criterion C

B. Clinical, nasal endoscopic, and/or imaging evidence of current or past infection or other inflammatory process within the paranasal sinuses

C. Evidence of causation demonstrated by at least two of the following:
　1. Headache has developed in temporal relation to the onset of chronic rhinosinusitis
　2. Headache waxes and wanes in parallel with the degree of sinus congestion, drainage, and other symptoms of chronic rhinosinusitis
　3. Headache is exacerbated by pressure applied over the paranasal sinuses
　4. In the case of a unilateral rhinosinusitis, headache is localized ipsilateral to it

D. Not better accounted for by another ICHD-3 diagnosis

*Reproduced with permission from the International Headache Society.

headache or facial pain should be considered in the differential diagnosis of such cases. According to the authors' experience, headache and facial pressure are much more prominent in CRSsNP and are rare in CRSwNP.

The pathogenesis of CRS is described as multifactorial, and there is no clearly delineated single molecular pathway. An emerging consensus, however, posits that the persistent inflammation defining CRS results from a dysfunctional host-environment interaction involving various exogenous agents and changes in the sinonasal mucosa. In accordance with the definition of CRS as an inflammatory disorder, there has been movement away from pathogen-driven hypotheses.[58]

CRS has four basic clinical courses: resolution, persistence, development of adverse sequelae, and progression to generalized airway reactivity. CRS is predominately a medical condition where surgery can relieve symptoms and sometimes bring about a reversal in the course of the disease. Endoscopic sinus surgery has become the gold standard approach to sinonasal pathologies requiring surgical intervention. Current indications for endoscopic sinus surgery include CRS, recurrent ARS, complications of rhinosinusitis, nasal polyposis, mucocele, epistaxis, cerebrospinal fluid leakage, fungal balls, allergic fungal rhinosinusitis, invasive fungal rhinosinusitis, removal of foreign bodies, repair of choanal atresia, tumors, and, finally,

approach to the skull base and orbit.[60] In patients with CRS or recurrent ARS, the purpose of surgery is to restore the normal function of the sinuses; therefore, it is termed *functional endoscopic sinus surgery*.

Chronic frontal rhinosinusitis. Pain is seldom a symptom of CRS of the frontal sinus. This condition is usually part of chronic pansinusitis, which also involves the ethmoid and maxillary sinuses. The most common symptom is chronic purulent nasal discharge.

Chronic maxillary rhinosinusitis. The most characteristic symptom of this condition is persistent purulent rhinorrhea with localization of pus in the middle meatus (Fig 7-4). CRS in the maxillary sinus seldom gives rise to facial pain or headache, except during an episode of acute exacerbation or with progression toward maxillary pyocele or maxillary osteomyelitis.

Rhinosinusitis of dental origin: Odontogenic rhinosinusitis

The close association of the maxillary teeth and gingiva to the maxillary sinus floor may explain the common finding of acute or chronic maxillary sinusitis caused by a dental disease, which is responsible for about 20% of maxillary sinus-

Pyocele

itis cases.[61] The causes of odontogenic sinusitis may include:

- Endodontic disease
- Periodontal disease (Fig 7-5)
- Complication of tooth extraction
- Dental material in the antrum (Fig 7-6)
- Infected dental cysts/tumors (Fig 7-7)
- Oroantral communication/fistula (Fig 7-8)
- Complications of dental implants/sinus elevation (Fig 7-9)

A prospective study on refractory acute maxillary sinusitis found that intrusion of teeth into the maxillary sinus antrum is a common finding (in about 50% of patients) and is not necessarily associated with the formation of sinusitis. Yet, refractory cases should be examined by a dentist because a dental infection may be the source of the resistant infection.[62]

Sinusitis caused by complications of sinus elevation and/or dental implants

Use of dental implants to replace missing teeth is thought to date back to the time of the ancient Egyptians. Since the first titanium implantation in 1965, dental implants have become extremely popular. Sinus elevation is a procedure for increasing bone height in the posterosuperior alveolar region to allow oral rehabilitation and to restore masticatory function by means of insertion of a dental implant, even in an atrophic maxilla (Fig 7-10). This procedure has also gained popularity among dentists in recent years.[63] Both procedures may cause acute or chronic maxillary sinusitis when performed improperly or in patients with a preoperative maxillary sinus disease, even when they are asymptomatic.[64]

Midfacial segment pain

Midfacial segment pain (MSP) may have all the same pain characteristics as tension headache, but it affects the face and may involve the nasion, the area under the bridge of the nose,

either side of the nose, the periorbital region, the retro-orbital region, or the cheeks.[49] The forehead is often affected as well. The pain is described as a dull ache, a feeling of pressure, or tightness. Some patients may feel that their nose is blocked, although they have no nasal airway obstruction. The forehead and the occipital region are affected simultaneously in approximately 60% of patients.[49] No consistent exacerbating or relieving factor is found. The pain may be chronic or episodic, and the skin and soft tissues over the forehead or cheek may be sensitive to palpation. Nasal endoscopy and CT scan of the paranasal sinuses are typically clinically normal. MSP is the most common cause of non-rhinologic facial pain seen in otolaryngologic practice.

The etiology of MSP is uncertain, and it may be myofascial or neurovascular in origin. However, Olesen's theory, which integrates the effects of myofascial afferents, the activation of peripheral nociceptors, and their convergence on the caudal nucleus of the trigeminal nerve, along with qualitative changes in the central nervous system, provides one of the best models.[65,66]

Leong et al[67] characterized pretreatment MSP patients using the Sino-Nasal Outcome Test (SNOT-22). Average SNOT-22 scores of patients with MSP were higher than those of healthy volunteers. They concluded that MSP has an adverse effect on physical and psychologic well-being and proposed that the SNOT-22 may be used in MSP to document disease severity and to measure response to treatment. The treatment of choice in this condition is amitriptyline for 6 months.[49]

Persistent idiopathic facial pain *Or fem*

Persistent idiopathic facial pain (PIFP) is most common in women over the age of 40 years. The prevalence rates of PIFP are 0.03% to 1.0% in the general population and 3.0% to 12% in patients who have undergone endodontic procedures (nonsurgical and/or surgical root canal treatments).[68]

Q # C
D

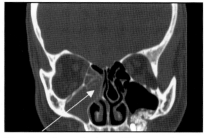

Fig 7-4 Coronal sinus CT scan demonstrating right chronic maxillary and ethmoid rhinosinusitis with complete opacification of the right maxillary sinus and obstruction of the sinus osteomeatal complex *(arrow)*.

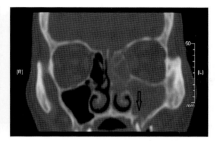

Fig 7-5 Coronal sinus CT scan showing opacification of the left maxillary and ethmoid sinuses secondary to severe periodontal disease *(arrow)*.

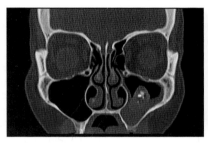

Fig 7-6 Coronal sinus CT scan demonstrating dental material in the left maxillary sinus antrum.

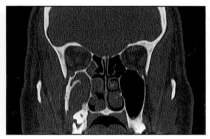

Fig 7-7 Coronal sinus CT scan showing an infected dental cyst in the right maxillary sinus antrum.

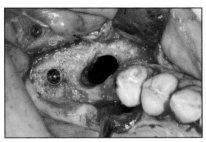

Fig 7-8 Oroantral fistula during surgical closure. Note the dental implants.

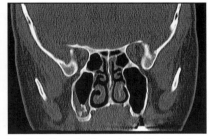

Fig 7-9 Complication of a right-sided dental implantation with rupture of the mucosa during a sinus elevation procedure.

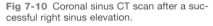

Fig 7-10 Coronal sinus CT scan after a successful right sinus elevation.

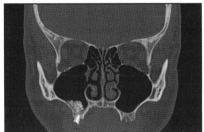

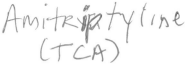

Table 7-7	Diagnostic criteria for persistent idiopathic facial pain*

Diagnostic criteria

A. Facial and/or oral pain fulfilling criteria B and C

B. Recurring daily for > 2 hours per day for > 3 months

C. Pain has both of the following characteristics:
   1. Poorly localized and not following the distribution of a peripheral nerve
   2. Dull, aching, or nagging quality

D. Clinical neurological examination is normal

E. A dental cause has been excluded by appropriate investigations

F. Not better accounted for by another ICHD-3 diagnosis

*Reproduced with permission from the International Headache Society.

PIFP is characterized by deep, achy, ill-defined, pulling or crushing pain involving diffuse areas of the face in the territory of the trigeminal nerve. The pain fluctuates in intensity and severity. Occasionally, patients use such terms as *sharp* or *knifelike* to describe the pain. The pain often worsens at night and can be aggravated by activity or stress. In most cases, only one side of the face is affected, but pain on both sides is possible. The pain may move from one part of the face to another and may be accompanied by such complaints as mucus moving in the sinuses.[49] Interestingly, the pain often crosses the recognized neurologic dermatomes. PIFP may be comorbid with other pain conditions, such as chronic widespread pain and irritable bowel syndrome.[4] Many patients suffering from PIFP show a significant psychosocial disability or psychiatric comorbidity, such as depression, and are unable to function normally as a result of the pain.[4,49]

According to the ICHD-3, PIFP is a persistent facial and/or oral pain that has varying presentations but recurs daily for more than 2 hours per day over more than 3 months in the absence of clinical neurologic deficit.[4] The ICHD-3 criteria are described in Table 7-7. In some patients with PIFP, the symptoms may initially appear to be similar to trigeminal neuralgia, but then they progress toward a PIFP pattern. Whereas trigeminal neuralgia is characterized by quick episodes of jabbing or lancinating pain, PIFP attacks always last longer than a few seconds, usually minutes or hours (see chapter 12). Moreover, no trigger points on the face are detected in PIFP.

PIFP usually has no specific cause. PIFP may originate from a minor operation or injury to the face, maxillae, teeth, or gingiva (any peripheral or proximal branch of the trigeminal nerve) but typically persists after the initial noxious event has healed and has no demonstrable local cause. However, psychophysical or neurophysiologic tests may demonstrate sensory abnormalities.[4]

Medical treatment of PIFP is often difficult and less satisfactory than treatment of trigeminal neuralgia. The treatment of choice is amitriptyline for 6 months (see chapters 12 and 16). Conventional analgesic drugs, including opioids, can also be effective in some patients, often accompanied by a comprehensive pain-management program. Behavioral medicine approaches are also recommended to complement cognitive-behavioral therapy, coping strategies, relaxation techniques, biofeedback, or psychotherapy.[68]

Scuba diving and facial pain

Orofacial pain and headache occasionally occur during or after scuba diving.[69] Although it is often benign, headache may signal a serious neurologic disorder in some circumstances. Jagger et al[70] evaluated the prevalence of orofacial complications associated with scuba diving in 125 divers by questionnaires. The prevalence of reported orofacial pain was 44%; 21% of the respondents reported toothache, 27% sinus pain, 16% jaw pain, and 12% other types of pain.

Several causes have been associated with pain and diving:

- *Sinus pain:* Sinus barotrauma, also known as *sinus squeeze*, is caused by failure to equalize pressure during descent. Pressurized air cannot be forced into the sinuses. The air within the sinus contracts and causes the walls of the sinus to bleed. This is accompanied by intense, sharp pain. Common causes of sinus barotrauma include allergic rhinitis, vasomotor rhinitis, nasal deformity, nasal polyposis, acute URI, and chronic irritation (eg, smoking, diesel fumes, chemicals, and prolonged use of decongestant nasal drops). Symptoms include pain in the area of the affected sinus or in the maxillary teeth (when the maxillary sinus is involved), and nose bleeding. The frontal sinuses are the most frequently affected because the nasofrontal duct draining the frontal sinus is longer and more tortuous. A reverse squeeze occurs during ascent, when air in the sinus expands without any ability to escape. This is extremely painful. The situation is self-limiting, however, because air is gradually absorbed into the mucosa lining the sinuses. When a sinus squeeze occurs, a slow ascent to the surface generally alleviates most of the pain. Because the sinus may be filled with blood, the patient is at high risk of developing consequent sinusitis. Antibiotic therapy is recommended, along with oral and nasal topical decongestants to promote drainage. Persistence of severe pain with no signs of ARS may be treated by a short course of steroids. Diving is not recommended for patients with URI.

- *Tension-type headache*: Symptoms of a tension-type headache include headache and pain in the nape (see chapter 8). Tension headaches may be caused by muscle strain due to anxiety and muscular rigidity. To prevent the development of muscle strain and, consequently, a tension headache, divers must learn to adopt a proper posture and relax in the water.
- *Carbon dioxide toxicity*: A dull throbbing headache after diving is usually caused by carbon dioxide toxicity. This type of pain is common in divers and is caused by an accumulation of carbon dioxide in the body. Hypoventilation happens when a scuba diver does not inhale long, deep breaths from the air tank or does not do this often enough. The best therapy for this type of headache is taking slow, deep breaths to reduce the carbon dioxide retention. Carbon dioxide–induced headaches do not respond well to pain relievers.
- *Decompression sickness headache*: Headaches can be a symptom of decompression sickness, which is caused by the formation of bubbles when dissolved nitrogen is discharged from the tissues on ascent. Associated symptoms include joint pain and swelling, skin rash, itching, dizziness, nausea, vomiting, tinnitus (ringing inside the ears), and extreme exhaustion. Scuba divers are at a higher risk of decompression sickness when they do not decompress after a long or deep dive or before surfacing, or when they ascend too quickly or make a panic ascent.

Other causes of pain are otic barotrauma, hyperbaric-triggered migraine, cervical and temporomandibular joint strain, supraorbital neuralgia, carotid artery dissection, and exertional and cold-stimulus headache syndromes.[71]

Focal neurologic symptoms should not be ignored but rather treated with 100% oxygen acutely. The patient should be referred without delay to a facility with a hyperbaric chamber.

Sphenopalatine neuralgia

Sphenopalatine neuralgia, also known as *Sluder's neuralgia*, is characterized by a unilateral headache behind the eyes with pain in the maxilla or soft palate.[72–74] Pain in the back of the nose, teeth, temple, occiput, or neck may also occur. The pain is associated with sinonasal congestion, swelling of the nasal mucous membranes, tearing, and redness of the face.[74] Sphenopalatine neuralgia is more common in women (2:1 ratio). The condition should be distinguished from a cluster headache, although both are characterized by similar symptoms. However, sphenopalatine neuralgia pain lasts longer and is associated with inflamed nasal mucosa on the involved side.[75] Sphenopalatine neuralgia is evidently caused by an irritation of the sphenopalatine ganglion from intranasal infection, deformity, or scarring. *p. 37*

A topical decongestant may occasionally alleviate the nasal symptoms. Ganglion blocks (by intranasal application or direct injection) are effective for controlling the pain.[76,77] Sumatriptan, which is effective in the treatment of cluster headache, has given satisfactory results in patients with Sluder's neuralgia; the outcomes are equivalent to those obtained by applying Bonain's liquid (eg, lidocaine, menthol, phenol) below and behind the tail of the middle turbinate.[75]

Migraine and sinus headache

The ICHD-3 lists operational diagnostic criteria for migraine (see chapter 10). Migraine and tension-type headache are often confused with true sinus headache because of their similar locations.[4,78] Publications have stated that patients with sinus headache, at least those with no obvious signs of infection, have a 58% to 88% incidence of a migraine-type headache.[79,80] Migraine can cause symptoms similar to those of rhinosinusitis, such as facial pain, nasal congestion, and rhinorrhea. This form of migraine has been termed *facial migraine* and is discussed in chapter 10.

A certain proportion of patients seeking treatment at an ear, nose, and throat clinic suffer from some facial pain resulting from migraine. A prospective evaluation of 100 sequential patients who complained of "sinus headaches" demonstrated that 86% had migraine or "probable migraine," while only 3% had actual sinus-related headaches.[81] Eross et al[82] evaluated 100 consecutive patients with a self-diagnosed sinus headache. The actual diagnoses were migraine (52%), probable migraine (23%), chronic migraine (11%), other unclassifiable headaches (9%), cluster headache (1%), and hemicrania continua (1%). Only 3% of the patients were accurately diagnosed with headache attributable to rhinosinusitis. Nasal congestion was present in 73% of patients and postnasal drip in 56%. Most patients reported pain triggered by changes in weather or season, and many noted changes with allergies or altitude, which are common migraine triggers.

The reason for the high rate of patients misdiagnosed with sinus headache by their physicians is related to the pathophysiology of migraine and the nature of nasal pain. The neurovascular theory of migraine implicates the nervous system as being the initiator of the process, and the blood vessel involvement occurs as a consequence of the neuronal process. This migraine model identifies the starting point in the central nervous system followed by sensitization of the peripheral neurons of the trigeminal nerve, including those supplying sensation to the meninges. When the peripheral early phase is not treated, central sensitization at the level of the caudal nucleus of the trigeminal nerve occurs, with concomitant repetitive firing of the involved neurons and pain in the distribution of the ophthalmic (V1) and/or maxillary (V2) branches of the trigeminal nerve. These nerves also provide sensation to the mucosa of the sinonasal cavity and are involved in the neurobiology of primary sinonasal pain. The early sensitization phase is accompanied by cutaneous allodynia (pain induced by stimulation that is normally nonpainful) in most patients (80%), and it often occurs in the distribution of V1 and V2.[83] This may include stimulation of the nose, such as while breathing cold air. A migraine attack may include secondary nasal symptoms, which are probably mediated by stimulation of the parasympathetic nervous system via the superior salivary nucleus of the facial nerve (VII). This reflex activation is extensively discussed in chapters 10 and 11. A report on patients with sinus headaches fulfilling the migraine criteria demonstrated that 84% reported sinus pressure, 82% sinus pain, 63% nasal congestion, 40% rhinorrhea, 38% watery eyes, and 27% itchy nose.[79] Occasionally, sinonasal disease or nasal allergy can play a role in triggering migraine, which may respond to nasal steroids or leukotriene antagonists.[83] The appearance of neurogenic rhinitis along with a sinus headache in patients with migraine is often misunderstood and contributes to misdiagnosis.

The duration of sinus headache and sinus symptoms is important for differentiating rhinosinusitis from a migraine attack. In contrast to rhinosinusitis, migraine headache typically resolves within 72 hours. ARS pain typically worsens after 5 to 7 days and is usually associated with hyposmia or anosmia, fever, cough, maxillary dental pain, and ear fullness or pressure. The diagnostic features of facial migraine are primarily based on the patient's history and the features reminiscent of typical migraine headaches as defined in the ICHD-3 (see chapter 10).

Box 7-4	Causes of throat pain

- Acute pharyngitis
- Tonsillitis
  - Acute
  - Chronic
- Peritonsillar cellulitis and abscess
- Lingual tonsillitis
- Pharyngeal space infections
  - Parapharyngeal space
  - Retropharyngeal space
- Ludwig's angina

Throat Pain

Throat pain, or a sore throat, is a common symptom described as pain, discomfort, or raw feeling of the throat, especially while swallowing. The vast majority of sore throats are caused by viral infections of the pharynx or tonsils. Many people experience a mild sore throat at the beginning of a common cold. The differential diagnosis of sore throat also includes various diseases of the oropharyx (Box 7-4).

Acute pharyngitis

Acute pharyngitis is an infection of the pharynx, which may involve the tonsils. The condition may be part of a generalized URI or may be a specific localized infection inside the pharynx. The most common cause of acute pharyngitis is a viral infection, but it can also be caused by a bacterial infection, such as group A streptococci, *M pneumoniae*, and *Chlamydia pneumoniae*. The viruses causing viral pharyngitis are highly contagious and tend to spread quickly, especially during the winter. Throat symptoms include soreness, scratchiness, or irritation. Associated symptoms include fever and discomfort while swallowing, or odynophagia. Fever is more prominent in young children than in adults. Most viral pharyngitis cases are accompanied by a flu or cold, along with a stuffy, runny nose; sneezing; and generalized aches, such as arthralgia and muscle pain. Nonproductive cough and hoarseness may also be present. Edema and erythema of the pharyngeal walls are the typical findings on physical examination. Pharyngeal exudation occurs infrequently and is generally less effusive than in patients suffering from bacterial pharyngitis.

The most common viruses causing viral pharyngitis are rhinovirus and adenovirus. Other less common viruses include Epstein-Barr virus, herpes simplex virus, influenza virus, parainfluenza virus, coronavirus, coxsackievirus, echovirus, respiratory syncial virus, and cytomegalovirus.

Rhinovirus, which is responsible for the common cold, is one of the most common causes of viral pharyngitis. The virus does not invade the pharyngeal mucosa but causes edema and hyperemia of the mucous membranes and increases the secretory activity of the mucous glands. Bradykinin and lysyl-bradykinin are generated in the nasal mucous membranes and stimulate pain nerve endings.

Adenovirus pharyngitis is common among young children and military recruits. The most common adenovirus types causing pharyngitis are adenovirus types 1 through 3 and type 5, which directly invade the pharyngeal mucosa. Specific symptoms include fever, sore throat (more intense than that of the common cold), and conjunctivitis.

Epstein-Barr virus pharyngitis is usually associated with infectious mononucleosis. Edema and hyperemia of the pharyngeal mucosa and uvula, with enlargement of the tonsils, are characteristic signs. Approximately half of patients with infectious mononucleosis have gray-white thick patches of exudates distributed over the tonsils and pharyngeal walls, thus mimicking streptococcal pharyngitis. Palatal petechiae associated with infectious mononucleosis tend to be confined to the soft palate. An inflammatory exudate and nasopharyngeal lymphoid hyperplasia (adenoiditis) may also develop. Body temperature is usually high and may reach up to 104°F (40°C). Generalized lymphadenopathy is common and is usually prominent in the anterior and posterior cervical triangles. Splenomegaly is present in approximately 50% of patients and hepatomegaly in 10% to 15%. Patients treated with ampicillin may develop a diffuse, pruritic maculopapular eruption.

Herpetic pharyngitis is caused by herpes simplex virus types 1 and 2. This infection is commonly observed in children and young adults. Herpes simplex virus may cause gingivitis or stomatitis. A sore throat with associated gingivostomatitis is the typical presenting symptom. Other associated symptoms include fever, odynophagia, myalgia, and malaise.

Enteroviral pharyngitis is usually caused by coxsackievirus or echovirus. Enteroviral lesions in the oropharyngeal mucosa are usually a result of a secondary infection of small mucosal vessels' endothelial cells and occur during viremia. Coxsackievirus infection is common in the late summer and early fall and may cause the following pathologies:

- Herpangina is usually caused by group A coxsackieviruses and tends to occur in epidemics, most commonly in infants and children. The condition is characterized by multiple, small (1 to 2 mm), grayish papulovesicular lesions on the tonsils, tonsillar pillars, uvula, or soft palate. The lesions may occasionally grow up to 4 mm or have an erythematous ring as large as 10 mm. The vesicles become shallow ulcers in about 3 days and heal after a few days. The pharynx is usually not involved. Associated symptoms include a sudden onset of fever with a sore throat, headache, anorexia, and frequently pain in the neck, abdomen, and extremities.
- Acute lymphonodular pharyngitis is caused by coxsackievirus A10 and is characterized by a distribution of oral and pharyngeal lesions similar to those seen in herpangina. However, the lesions are protruding, whitish to yellowish nodules that do not evolve into vesicles or ulcers. They remain papular and become grayish-white and nodular, secondary to infiltration by lymphocytes.
- Hand-foot-and-mouth disease is usually caused by coxsackievirus A16 and is characterized by 4- to 8-mm ulcers on the tongue, buccal mucosa, and occasionally tonsillar pillars. Vesicular exanthems develop on the hands and feet, and, in infants, occasionally in the diaper area.

Differentiating viral from bacterial pharyngitis solely on the basis of physical examination is not easy. In viral pharyngitis, the total white blood cell count may initially be slightly high, followed by a decrease to fewer than 5,000 cells after 4 to 7 days of illness in about half of patients. Atypical lymphocytosis is frequently associated with viral pharyngitis. In infectious mononucleosis pharyngitis, the peripheral blood smear reveals relative and absolute lymphocytosis, with more than 10% atypical lymphocytes. Liver function test results are abnormal in 90% of infectious mononucleosis cases. A mononucleosis spot test (monospot) is usually positive and allows rapid screening for heterophile antibodies. Immunoglobulin M antibody to Epstein-Barr virus capsid antigen and antibody to early antigen are useful for diagnosing an acute infection, particularly in patients who are heterophile negative. Rapid streptococcal antigen test and bacterial culture of a throat swab are negative. Leukopenia and proteinuria may be seen in influenza virus pharyngitis.

Treatment of viral pharyngitis includes bed rest, saltwater gargling, and drinking. Analgesics and antipyretics are used to relieve pain and fever.

Tonsillitis

Acute tonsillitis is inflammation of the palatine tonsils, usually due to GABHS or, less commonly, to a viral infection. Acute tonsillitis caused by *Streptococcus* sp usually occurs in children ages 5 to 15 years. Approximately 10% to 20% of sore throats in adults are caused by streptococcal infection. Fever, chills, sore throat, foul breath, dysphagia, odynophagia, and tenderness in the angle of the jaw characterize acute tonsillitis. The pain is frequently referred to the ears. Physical examination reveals hyperemic and swollen palatine tonsils, uvula, tongue base, and pharyngeal walls, with irregular, thin, nonconfluent patches of white exudates on the tonsils forming the typical appearance of follicular tonsillitis. Submandibular lymph nodes are often enlarged and tender. Leukocytosis with an increased neutrophil count (shift to the left) is commonly present in bacterial infections. Mere reliance on clinical criteria, such as the presence of follicular exudate, erythema, fever, and lymphadenopathy, is not an accurate means for distinguishing streptococcal from viral tonsillitis. Throat culture is the gold standard for detecting GABHS tonsillitis with a sensitivity of 80% to 95%. Rapid antigen detection test confirms the presence of GABHS cell-wall carbohydrate from swabbed material and is considered less sensitive than throat cultures. However, the rapid antigen detection test has a high specificity and produces results in significantly less time than a throat culture.

Chronic tonsillitis is characterized by chronic sore throat, halitosis, recurrent tonsillitis, and persistent tender cervical lymph nodes. A polymicrobial bacterial population is observed in most cases, with alpha- and beta-hemolytic *streptococcal species*, *S aureus*, *H influenzae*, and *Bacteroides* sp identified.

Complications of GABHS tonsillitis are classified into suppurative and nonsuppurative. Nonsuppurative complications include scarlet fever, acute rheumatic fever, and poststreptococcal glomerulonephritis. Suppurative complications include peritonsillar, parapharyngeal, and retropharyngeal cellulitis and/or abscess.

Treatment of acute streptococcal tonsillitis includes adequate hydration and caloric intake. Analgesics and antipyretics are used to relieve pain and fever. GABHS infection obligates antibiotic therapy, which is directed toward *(1)* preventing acute rheumatic fever, *(2)* preventing suppurative complications, *(3)* abating clinical symptoms and signs, and *(4)* reducing transmission of GABHS to close contacts. Penicillin is the treatment of choice in streptococcal tonsillitis. Cochrane analysis on the benefits of antibiotics for sore throat for patients in primary care settings showed that antibiotic therapy confers relative benefits in treating sore throat.[84] However, the absolute benefits are modest, and the therapy shortens the duration of symptoms by about 16 hours overall.[84]

Analysis of different recommendations from international guidelines for the management of acute pharyngitis in adults and children showed substantial discrepancies.[85] However, all guidelines agree that narrow-spectrum penicillin is the first choice of antibiotic for treating streptococcal pharyngitis and that treatment should last for 10 days to eradicate the microorganism. A systematic review and meta-analysis that evaluated whether systemic corticosteroids improve symptoms of sore throat in adults and children showed that corticosteroids provide symptomatic relief of pain in sore throat, in addition to antibiotic therapy, mainly in participants with severe or exudative sore throat.[86]

Peritonsillar cellulitis and abscess

Peritonsillar infection, also known as *Quincy's angina*, is an infection located between the tonsil and the superior pharyngeal constrictor muscle. The most common pathogen causing peritonsillar cellulites/abscess is GABHS. Anaerobic *Bacteroides* can also cause this type of infection. Occasionally, culture results are positive for multiple common throat bacteria. Presenting symptoms include severe throat pain, especially on swallowing, fever, drooling, foul breath, trismus, "hot potato voice," and unilateral referred otalgia. Limited mouth opening (trismus) is always present in varying severity. The tonsil and uvula are displaced medially by the peritonsillar infection. The soft palate and anterior pillar are swollen and hyperemic. Unilateral enlarged and tender submandibular lymph nodes are present.

Drainage, along with intravenous penicillin, is required in peritonsillar abscess. Peritonsillar cellulitis without pus formation usually responds to intravenous penicillin therapy. Peritonsillar abscess tends to recur when there is history of recurrent tonsillitis, and tonsillectomy is then indicated. A dental source should be ruled out in de novo cases.

Lingual tonsillitis

Lingual tonsillitis is an infection of the lymphatic tissue located in the base of the tongue. Most patients with lingual tonsillitis have undergone palatine tonsillectomy in the past. Lingual tonsillitis presents with fever, sore throat, glossal pain, dysphagia, muffled voice, and pain at the level of the hyoid bone during swallowing. Lingual tonsillitis is visible only by means of a laryngeal mirror or fiber-optic examination. The base of the tongue is enlarged, edematous, and covered by exudates. The pharynx may appear normal or mildly hyperemic. The anterior portion of the neck may be tender at the level of the hyoid bone, and cervical and submandibular adenopathy may be observed. Treatment includes intravenous penicillin.

Parapharyngeal space infection

The parapharyngeal space (PPS) (ie, lateral pharyngeal space, pharyngomaxillary space, pterygomaxillary space, pterygopharyngeal space) occupies an inverted pyramidal area lateral to the superior constrictor muscles and bounded by multiple components of the fascial system. The styloid process divides the PPS into an anterior or prestyloid compartment and a neurovascular or poststyloid compartment.

PPS infections may follow an infection in the pharynx, tonsils, adenoids, teeth, parotid gland, peritonsillar area, submandibular space, retropharyngeal space, Bezold abscess (mastoid abscess on the inner aspect of the mastoid tip along the digastric ridge), and adjacent lymph nodes. Despite the multitude of well-defined potential sources, in nearly half of the cases, the etiology cannot be defined. Signs and symptoms of PPS infection differ depending on whether the prestyloid or poststyloid compartment is involved. Anterior PPS infection is characterized by pain in the angle of the jaw, preauricular area, ear, and adjacent upper neck. Rotating the head and neck to the contralateral side intensifies the pain. Other symptoms include dysphagia, odynophagia, drooling, trismus (due to medial pterygoid muscle irritation), fever, chills, and malaise. Edema and medial displacement or bulging of the lateral pharyngeal wall and tonsil is a hallmark of PPS infection. Swelling, induration, and tenderness at the angle of the mandible are also commonly observed. Dyspnea and other symptoms of airway obstruction may occur in severe cases. Posterior PPS infection is not associated with trismus or tonsillar displacement and may have no localizing signs on examination. Despite this, the patients appear to be toxic with parotid space swelling. Involvement of the neurovascular structures may lead to complications such as cranial neuropathies, Horner syndrome, septic internal jugular thrombosis, and carotid artery rupture.

CT scan of the neck (with contrast medium) facilitates the diagnosis and assessment of the extent of PPS infection. Sichel et al[87] redefined PPS infection into two different disorders that are clinically and therapeutically relevant:

1. *Parapharyngeal lymphadenitis*: Infection is located in the posterior part of the PPS with no invasion into the parapharyngeal fat and with no extensions into other cervical spaces except the adjacent retropharyngeal space. This condition is relatively benign, and intravenous antibiotics and nonsurgical treatment are recommended.
2. *Parapharyngeal abscess*: With this condition, also known as *deep neck abscess*, infection is located in the anterior part of the PPS and involves the parapharyngeal fat. Diffusion into the mediastinum and other severe complications are frequent. Early diagnosis, aggressive intravenous antibiotics, and urgent surgical drainage are recommended.

Retropharyngeal space infection

The retropharyngeal space (RPS) lies between the visceral division of the middle layer of the deep cervical fascia behind the pharyngeal constrictors and the alar division of the deep layer of the deep cervical fascia posteriorly. RPS infection may follow infection in the nasopharynx, oropharynx, sinonasal region, and rarely mastoiditis. RPS infection may also occur directly after a traumatic perforation of the posterior pharyngeal wall or esophagus, or indirectly from the parapharyngeal space. Most RPS infections in children are secondary to URI, whereas trauma or foreign bodies cause most RPS infections in adults. Retropharyngeal lymph nodes tend to regress by the age of 5 years, so infection in this area is much more common in children than in adults. RPS infection may drain into the prevertebral space and through this space into the chest, thus causing mediastinitis. Symptoms of RPS infection include sore throat, dysphagia, stiff neck, fever, and, rarely, posterior neck and shoulder pain aggravated by swallowing.

Examination reveals anterior displacement or bulging of one or both sides of the posterior pharyngeal wall due to involvement of lymph nodes, which are distributed lateral to the midline fascial raphe. Lateral neck radiograph (demonstrating widening of the retropharyngeal space) and neck CT scan with contrast facilitate diagnosis and assessment of the extent of RPS infection.

Early diagnosis and aggressive intravenous antibiotics are mandatory. Transoral incision and drainage are recommended in cases with abscess formation.

Ludwig's angina

Ludwig's angina is a potentially life-threatening, rapidly expanding and spreading, gangrenous cellulitis of the submandibular space. Swelling of this region can compromise the airway. Most Ludwig's angina infections are odontogenic, usually from the second or third mandibular molar. Other causes include peritonsillar or parapharyngeal abscesses, mandibular fracture, oral lacerations or piercing, and, rarely, submandibular sialadenitis. Predisposing factors include dental caries, recent dental treatment, systemic illnesses (eg, diabetes mellitus), malnutrition, alcoholism, compromised immune system (eg, AIDS), and organ transplantation. The term *Ludwig's angina* is reserved for infections meeting the following five criteria:

P. 233

1. Cellulitis (not an abscess) of the submandibular space
2. Involvement of only the submandibular space, although this might be bilateral and spread into secondary spaces
3. The finding of gangrene with foul serosanguineous fluid on incision but no frank purulence
4. Involvement of the fascia, muscle, and connective tissue, with sparing of the glandular tissue
5. Direct spread of infection rather than spread by lymphatics

The most common microbes involved are *Streptococcus* sp and oral anaerobic bacteria. Symptoms include painful neck swelling, tooth pain, dysphagia, odynophagia, dyspnea, fever, and malaise. Ludwig's angina is characterized by a brawny induration of the mouth floor and suprahyoid region (bilaterally) with elevation or protrusion of the tongue, thus potentially obstructing the airway. Other signs include a tender, firm swelling in the submental and anterior neck without fluctuance, tachypnea, stridor, trismus, muffled or "hot potato" voice, and drooling. The white blood cell count is high with a shift to the left. Airway management is the primary therapeutic concern.

Airway control by endotracheal intubation is mandatory. Therapy includes intravenous broad-spectrum antibiotics and occasionally drainage of the swelling through a cervical incision with placement of drains. Dental treatment may be needed to treat the initiating tooth infection. Complications such as sepsis and descending necrotizing mediastinitis may occur through the retropharyngeal space and carotid sheath.

Vestibular Syndromes Related to Orofacial Pain or Structures

Vestibular migraine

Vertigo is an illusion that the environment is moving or that the patient is moving in relation to the environment. Migraine associated with attacks of vertigo has been repeatedly documented in the medical literature. Various terms have been used to designate vertigo caused by a migraine mechanism, including *migraine-associated vertigo*, *migraine-associated dizziness*, *migraine-related vestibulopathy*, *migrainous vertigo*, *benign recurrent vertigo*, and *basilar migraine*.[88,89] The term *vestibular migraine* has been convincingly advocated as a condition that stresses the particular vestibular manifestation of migraine and thus best avoids confounding it with nonvestibular dizziness associated with migraine.[90] Therefore, the Bárány Society, which represents the international community of vestibular research, and the Migraine Classification Subcommittee of the International Headache Society have opted for vestibular migraine in their joint article on the classification of the disorder.[91] The term *migraine with brainstem aura* (formerly, *basilar-type migraine*) should be restricted to patients who fulfill the respective diagnostic criteria of the ICHD-3.

In 2013, the ICHD-3 listed new operational diagnostic criteria for vestibular migraine (section A1.6.5), as shown in Table 7-8. Transient auditory symptoms, nausea, vomiting, prostra-

Table 7-8   **Diagnostic criteria for vestibular migraine**

Diagnostic criteria	Notes
A. At least five episodes fulfilling criteria C and D	
B. A current or past history of 1.1 Migraine without aura or 1.2 Migraine with aura	Code also for the underlying migraine diagnosis.

C. Vestibular symptoms of moderate or severe intensity, lasting between 5 minutes and 72 hours	Vestibular symptoms, as defined by the Bárány Society's Classification of Vestibular Symptoms and qualifying for a diagnosis of A1.6.5 Vestibular migraine, include:
	  a. Spontaneous vertigo:
	    i. Internal vertigo (a false sensation of self motion)
	    ii. External vertigo (a false sensation that the visual surround is spinning or flowing)
	  b. Positional vertigo, occurring after a change of head position
	  c. Visually induced vertigo, triggered by a complex or large moving visual stimulus
	  d. Head motion–induced vertigo, occurring during head motion
	  e. Head motion–induced dizziness with nausea (dizziness is characterized by a sensation of disturbed spatial orientation; other forms of dizziness are currently not included in the classification of vestibular migraine)
	Vestibular symptoms are rated moderate when they interfere with but do not prevent daily activities and severe when daily activities cannot be continued.
	
	Duration of episodes is highly variable. About 30% of patients have episodes lasting minutes, 30% have attacks for hours, and another 30% have attacks over several days. The remaining 10% have attacks lasting seconds only, which tend to occur repeatedly during head motion, visual stimulation, or after changes of head position. In these patients, episode duration is defined as the total period during which short attacks recur. At the other end of the spectrum, there are patients who may take 4 weeks to recover fully from an episode. However, the core episode rarely exceeds 72 hours.

D. At least 50% of episodes are associated with at least one of the following three migrainous features:
1. Headache with at least two of the following four characteristics:
  a. Unilateral location
  b. Pulsating quality
  c. Moderate or severe intensity
  d. Aggravation by routine physical activity
2. Photophobia and phonophobia
3. Visual aura
	One symptom is sufficient during a single episode. Different symptoms may occur during different episodes. Associated symptoms may occur before, during or after the vestibular symptoms.
	
	Phonophobia is defined as sound-induced discomfort. It is a transient and bilateral phenomenon that must be differentiated from recruitment, which is often unilateral and persistent. Recruitment leads to an enhanced perception and often distortion of loud sounds in an ear with decreased hearing.
	
	Visual auras are characterized by bright scaintillating lights or zigzag lines, often with a scotoma that interferes with reading. Visual auras typically expand over 5–20 minutes and last for less than 60 minutes. They are often, but not always restricted to one hemifield. Other types of migraine aura, for example somatosensory or dysphasic aura, are not included as diagnostic criteria because their phenomenology is less specific and most patients also have visual auras.

E. Not better accounted for by another ICHD-3 diagnosis or by another vestibular disorder	History and physical examinations do not suggest another vestibular disorder or such a disorder has been considered but ruled out by appropriate investigations or such a disorder is present as a comorbid or independent condition, but episodes can be clearly differentiated. Migraine attacks may be induced by vestibular stimulation. Therefore, the differential diagnosis should include other vestibular disorders complicated by superimposed migraine attacks.

tion, and susceptibility to motion sickness may be associated with vestibular migraine. However, they also occur with various other vestibular disorders, so they are not included as diagnostic criteria.

The prevalence of vestibular migraine is variable and probably underdiagnosed, as shown by a study from a dizziness clinic in Switzerland, where vestibular migraine accounted for 20.2% of the diagnoses in young patients but was suspected by the referring physicians in only 1.8%.[92] In a community-based sample of middle-aged women in Taiwan, vestibular migraine was identified in 5%, and in 30% of all women with migraine.[93] Vestibular migraine has a female preponderance, and the reported female-to-male ratio is between 1.5 and 5 to 1.[88] Familial occurrence is not uncommon, probably based on an autosomal-dominant pattern of inheritance with decreased penetrance in men.[94] In most patients, migraine begins earlier in life than vestibular migraine. Not infrequently, migraine headaches are replaced by vertigo attacks in women around menopause.

Patients with vestibular migraine typically report spontaneous or positional vertigo. Some experience a sequence of spontaneous vertigo transforming into positional vertigo after several hours or days. This positional vertigo is distinct from benign paroxysmal positional vertigo with regard to duration of individual attacks (often as long as the head position is maintained in vestibular migraine versus seconds only in benign paroxysmal positional vertigo), duration of symptomatic episodes (minutes to days in vestibular migraine versus weeks in benign paroxysmal positional vertigo), and nystagmus findings. Vertigo can precede headache, as would be typical for an aura; may begin with headache; or may appear late in the headache phase.

Auditory symptoms, including hearing loss, tinnitus, and aural pressure have been reported in up to 38% patients with vestibular migraine.[88]

Genetic and neural mechanisms have been described for vestibular migraine. The only hypothesis that is actually based on a human experimental model of vestibular migraine relates to the known reciprocal connections between the trigeminal and vestibular nuclei. Trigeminal activation by painful electrical stimulation of the forehead produced spontaneous nystagmus in patients with migraine but not in control subjects, indicating that those with migraine have a lowered threshold for crosstalk between these neighboring brainstem structures.[95]

Migraine is more common in patients with Ménière's disease than in healthy control subjects. Many patients with features of both Ménière's disease and vestibular migraine have been reported. In fact, migraine and Ménière's disease can be inherited as a symptom cluster. Fluctuating hearing loss, tinnitus, and aural pressure may occur in vestibular migraine, but hearing loss does not progress to profound levels. Similarly, migraine headaches, photophobia, and even migraine auras are common during attacks of Ménière's disease. The pathophysiologic relationship between vestibular migraine and Ménière's disease remains uncertain. In the first year after onset of symptoms, differentiation between them may be challenging, as Ménière's disease can be monosymptomatic with only vestibular symptoms in the early stages of the disease. When the criteria for Ménière's disease are met, particularly hearing loss as documented by audiometry, Ménière's disease should be diagnosed, even when migraine symptoms occur during the vestibular attacks. Only patients who have two different types of attacks, one fulfilling the criteria for vestibular migraine and the other for Ménière's disease, should be diagnosed with both disorders.

The therapeutic recommendations for vestibular migraine are currently based on the treatment guidelines for migraine (see chapter 10). Zolmitriptan is recommended for acute vestibular migraine.[96] Non-pharmaceutical approaches in the treatment of vestibular migraine should not be neglected and may be even more effective than drugs in individual patients. A thorough explanation of the migraine origin of the attacks can relieve unnecessary fears. Avoidance of identified triggers, regular sleep, regular meals, and exercise have a firm place in migraine prophylaxis. Selected patients, particularly those with persistent symptoms between attacks, may profit from vestibular rehabilitation.[97]

Mastication-induced vertigo and nystagmus

Various maneuvers may trigger vertigo and nystagmus according to the pathology involved.

Although reciprocal connections exist between the trigeminal and vestibular systems, induction of dizziness or oscillopsia by mastication has been reported only as a mechanical or vascular steal phenomenon.[98–100]

Mastication-induced vertigo and nystagmus are rare phenomena. Park et al[101] determined induction or modulation of nystagmus in two index patients with mastication-induced vertigo, 12 healthy control subjects, and 52 additional patients with peripheral or central vestibulopathy during their acute or compensated phase. Both index patients developed mastication-induced vertigo after near-complete resolution of the spontaneous vertigo from presumed acute unilateral peripheral vestibulopathy. The nystagmus and vertigo gradually built up during mastication and dissipated slowly after cessation of mastication. Mastication did not induce nystagmus in healthy control subjects. However, mastication-induced nystagmus appeared in five (24%) of the 21 patients without spontaneous nystagmus who had a previous history of a vestibular syndrome, and mastication either increased (21/31, 68%) or decreased (7/31, 23%) the spontaneous nystagmus in almost all the patients (28/31, 90%) with spontaneous nystagmus. They concluded that mastication may induce significant vertigo and nystagmus in patients with a prior history of acute vestibulopathy. The induction or modulation of nystagmus by mastication in both peripheral and central vestibulopathies supports trigeminal modulation of the vestibular system in humans. The gradual buildup and dissipation suggest a role of the velocity storage mechanism in the generation of mastication-induced vertigo and nystagmus.

References

1. Israel HA, Davila LJ. The essential role of the otolaryngologist in the diagnosis and management of temporomandibular joint and chronic oral, head, and facial pain disorders. Otolaryngol Clin North Am 2014;47:301–331.
2. Murtagh J. The painful ear. Aust Fam Physician 1991;20:1779–1783.
3. Conover K. Earache. Emerg Med Clin North Am 2013;31:413–442.
4. Headache Classification Committee of the International Headache Society. The International Classification of Headache Disorders, 3rd edition (beta version). Cephalalgia 2013;33:629–808.
5. Harvey H. Diagnosing referred otalgia: The ten Ts. Cranio 1992;10:333–334.
6. Yanagisawa K, Kveton JF. Referred otalgia. Am J Otolaryngol 1992;13:323–327.
7. Kim DS, Cheang P, Dover S, Drake-Lee AB. Dental otalgia. J Laryngol Otol 2007;121:1129–1134.
8. Wazen JJ. Referred otalgia. Otolaryngol Clin N Am 1989;22:1205–1215.
9. Jaber JJ, Leonetti JP, Lawrason AE, Feustel PJ. Cervical spine causes for referred Otaligia. Otolaryngol Head Neck Surg 2008;138:479–85.
10. Nestor JJ, Ngo LK. Incidence of facial pain caused by lung cancer. Otolaryngol Head Neck Surg 1994;111(1):155-156.
11. Morgan NJ, Skipper JJ, Allen GM. Referred otalgia: An old lesson. Br J Oral Maxillofac Surg 1995;33:332–333.
12. Mulwafu W, Fagan J, Lentin R. Suprahyoid approach to base-of-tongue squamus cell carcinoma. S Afr J Surg 2006;44:120–124.
13. Amundson LH. Disorders of the external ear. Prim Care 1990;17:213–231.
14. Gergely P Jr, Poór G. Relapsing polychondritis. Best Pract Res Clin Rheumatol 2004;18:723–738.
15. Puéchal X, Terrier B, Mouthon L, Costedoat-Chalumeau N, Guillevin L, Le Jeunne C. Relapsing polychondritis. Joint Bone Spine 2014;81:118–124.
16. Staats BA, Utz JP, Michet CJ Jr. Relapsing polychondritis. Semin Respir Crit Care Med 2002;23:145–154.
17. Michet CJ Jr, McKenna CH, Luthra HS, O'Fallon WM. Relapsing polychondritis. Survival and predictive role of early disease manifestations. Ann Intern Med 1986;104:74–78.
18. Sander R. Otitis externa: A practical guide to treatment and prevention. Am Fam Physician 2001;63:927–36;941–942.
19. Hirsch BE. Infection of the external ear. Am J Otolaryngol 1992;13:145–155.
20. Handzel O, Halperin D. Necrotizing (malignant) external otitis. Am Fam Physician 2003;68:309–312.
21. Kim YH, Chang MY, Jung HH, et al. Prognosis of Ramsay Hunt syndrome presenting as cranial polyneuropathy. Laryngoscope 2010;120:2270–2276.
22. Shim HJ, Jung H, Park DC, Lee JH, Yeo SG. Ramsay Hunt syndrome with multicranial nerve involvement. Acta Otolaryngol 2011;131:210–215.
23. Ko JY, Sheen TS, Hsu MM. Herpes zoster oticus treated with acyclovir and prednisolone: Clinical manifestations and analysis of prognostic factors. Clin Otolaryngol Allied Sci 2000;25:139–142.
24. Goldani LZ, da Silva LF, Dora JM. Ramsay Hunt syndrome in patients infected with human immunodeficiency virus. Clin Exp Dermatol 2009;34:e552–e554.
25. Kinishi M, Amatsu M, Mohri M, Saito M, Hasegawa T, Hasegawa S. Acyclovir improves recovery rate of facial nerve palsy in Ramsay Hunt syndrome. Auris Nasus Larynx 2001;28:223–226.
26. Morrow MJ. Bell's palsy and herpes zoster oticus. Curr Treat Options Neurol 2000;2:407–416.
27. de Ru JA, van Benthem PP. Combination therapy is preferable for patients with Ramsay Hunt syndrome. Otol Neurotol 2011;32:852–855.
28. Harmes KM, Blackwood RA, Burrows HL, Cooke JM, Harrison RV, Passamani PP. Otitis media: Diagnosis and treatment. Am Fam Physician 2013;88:435–440.

29. Qureishi A, Lee Y, Belfield K, Birchall JP, Daniel M. Update on otitis media—Prevention and treatment. Infect Drug Resist 2014;7:15–24.

30. Venekamp RP, Sanders S, Glasziou PP, Del Mar CB, Rovers MM. Antibiotics for acute otitis media in children. Cochrane Database Syst Rev 2013;1.

31. Drendel M, Yakirevitch A, Kerimis P, Migirov L, Wolf M. Hearing loss in bullous myringitis. Auris Nasus Larynx 2012;39:28–30.

32. Eliashar R, Gross M, Saah D, Elidan J. Vestibular involvement in myringitis bullosa. Acta Otolaryngol 2004;124:249–252.

33. Sproat R, Burgess C, Lancaster T, Martinez-Devesa P. Eustachian tube dysfunction in adults. BMJ 2014;348:g1647.

34. Brunworth JD, Mahboubi H, Garg R, Johnson B, Brandon B, Djalilian HR. Nasopharyngeal acid reflux and eustachian tube dysfunction in adults. Ann Otol Rhinol Laryngol 2014;123:415–419.

35. Gluth MB, McDonald DR, Weaver AL, Bauch CD, Beatty CW, Orvidas LJ. Management of eustachian tube dysfunction with nasal steroid spray: A prospective, randomized, placebo-controlled trial. Arch Otolaryngol Head Neck Surg 2011;137:449–455.

36. Perera R, Glasziou PP, Heneghan CJ, McLellan J, Williamson I. Autoinflation for hearing loss associated with otitis media with effusion. Cochrane Database Syst Rev 2013;(5).

37. National Institute for Health and Clinical Excellence. Balloon dilatation of the eustachian tube. (Interventional procedure guidance 409.) 2011. https//www.nice.org.uk/guidance/ipg409. Accessed 20 March 2015.

38. Mirza S, Richardson H. Otic barotrauma from air travel. J Laryngol Otol 2005;119:366–370.

39. Lynch JH, Deaton TG. Barotrauma with extreme pressures in sport: From scuba to skydiving. Curr Sports Med Rep 2014;13:107–112.

40. Zakrzewska JM. Differential diagnosis of facial pain and guidelines for management. Br J Anaesth 2013;111:95–104.

41. Pearlman AN, Conley DB. Review of current guidelines related to the diagnosis and treatment of rhinosinusitis. Curr Opin Otolaryngol Head Neck Surg 2008;16:226–230.

42. Baraniuk JN. Neurogenic mechanisms in rhinosinusitis. Curr Allergy Asthma Rep 2001;1:252–261.

43. Stammberger H, Wolf G. Headaches and sinus disease: The endoscopic approach. Ann Otol Rhinol Laryngol Suppl 1988;134:3–23.

44. Clerico DM. Sinus headaches reconsidered: Referred cephalgia of rhinologic origin masquerading as refractory primary headaches. Headache 1995;35:185–192.

45. Clerico DM. Pneumatized superior turbinate as a cause of referred migraine headache. Laryngoscope 1996;106:874–879.

46. Chow JM. Rhinologic headaches. Otolaryngol Head Neck Surg. 1994;111:211–218.

47. Abu-Bakra M, Jones NS. Does stimulation of nasal mucosa cause referred pain to the face? Clin Otolaryngol Allied Sci 2001;26:430–432.

48. Abu-Bakra M, Jones NS. Prevalence of nasal mucosal contact points in patients with facial pain compared with patients without facial pain. J Laryngol Otol 2001;115:629–632.

49. Jones NS. Midfacial segment pain: Implications for rhinitis and sinusitis. Curr Allergy Asthma Rep 2004;4:187–192.

50. Harrison L, Jones NS. Intranasal contact points as a cause of facial pain or headache: A systematic review. Clin Otolaryngol 2013;38:8–22.

51. Anon JB. Upper respiratory infections. Am J Med 2010;123(4, suppl):S16–S25.

52. Bhattacharyya N, Grebner J, Martinson NG. Recurrent acute rhinosinusitis: Epidemiology and health care cost burden. Otolaryngol Head Neck Surg 2012;146:307–312.

53. Rosenfeld RM, Andes D, Bhattacharyya N, et al. Clinical practice guideline: Adult sinusitis. Otolaryngol Head Neck Surg 2007;137(3, suppl):S1–S31.

54. Benoliel R, Quek S, Biron A, Nahlieli O, Eliav E. Trigeminal neurosensory changes following acute and chronic paranasal sinusitis. Quintessence Int 2006;37:437–443.

55. Meltzer EO, Hamilos DL, Hadley JA, et al. Rhinosinusitis: Establishing definitions for clinical research and patient care. Otolaryngol Head Neck Surg 2004;131(6, suppl):S1–S62.

56. Lanza DC, Kennedy DW. Adult rhinosinusitis defined. Otolaryngol Head Neck Surg 1997;117(3 Pt 2):S1–S7.

57. Benninger MS, Ferguson BJ, Hadley JA, et al. Adult chronic rhinosinusitis: Definitions, diagnosis, epidemiology, and pathophysiology. Otolaryngol Head Neck Surg 2003;129(3, suppl):S1–S32.

58. Fokkens WJ, Lund VJ, Mullol J, et al. European position paper on rhinosinusitis and nasal polyps 2012. Rhinol Suppl 2012;23:1–298.

59. Anon JB, Jacobs MR, Poole MD, et al. Antimicrobial treatment guidelines for acute bacterial rhinosinusitis. Otolaryngol Head Neck Surg 2004;130(1, suppl):S1–S50.

60. Lai D, Stankiewicz JA. Primary sinus surgery. In: Flint PW, Haughey BH, Lund VJ, et al (eds). Cummings Otolaryngology: Head and Neck Surgery, ed 5. Philadelphia: Mosby Elsevier, 2010:739–774.

61. Flynn TR. Complex odontogenic infections. In: Hupp JR, Ellis E, Tucker MR (eds). Contemporary Oal and Maxillofacial Surgery, ed 5. St Louis: Mosby Elsevier, 2008:317–333.

62. Hirshoren N, Hirschenbein A, Eliashar R. Risk stratification of severe acute rhinosinusitis unresponsive to oral antibiotics. Acta Otolaryngol 2010;130:1065–1069.

63. Pignataro L, Mantovani M, Torretta S, Felisati G, Sambataro G. ENT assessment in the integrated management of candidate for (maxillary) sinus lift. Acta Otorhinolaryngol Ital 2008;28:110–119.

64. Anavi Y, Allon DM, Avishai G, Calderon S. Complications of maxillary sinus augmentations in a selective series of patients. Oral Surg Oral Med Oral Pathol Oral Radiol Endod 2008;106:34–38.

65. Olesen J. Clinical and pathophysiological observations in migraine and tension-type headache explained by integration of vascular, supraspinal and myofascial inputs. Pain 1991;46:125–132.

66. Jensen R, Olesen J. Tension-type headache: An update on mechanisms and treatment. Curr Opin Neurol 2000;13:285–289.

67. Leong SC, Tsang HK, Wilkie MD, Banhegyi G. Characterisation of patients with endoscopy-negative, computer tomography-negative midfacial segment pain using the sino-nasal outcome test. Rhinology 2014;52:78–83.

68. Klasser G. Management of persistent idiopathic facial pain. J Can Dent Assoc 2013;79:d71.

69. Zadik Y, Drucker S. Diving dentistry: A review of the dental implications of scuba diving. Aust Dent J 2011;56:265–271.

70. Jagger RG, Shah CA, Weerapperuma ID, Jagger DC. The prevalence of orofacial pain and tooth fracture (odontocrexis) associated with SCUBA diving. Prim Dent Care 2009;16:75–78.

71. Cheshire WP. Headache and facial pain in scuba divers. Curr Pain Headache Rep 2004;8:315–320.

72. Sluder G. The syndrome of sphenopalatine ganglion neurosis. New York Med J 1910;140:868–878.

73. Sluder G. Etiology, diagnosis, prognosis and treatment of sphenopalatine neuralgia. J Am Med Assoc 1913;61:1202–1206.

74. Ahamed SH, Jones NS. What is Sluder's neuralgia? J Laryngol Otol 2003;117:437–443.

75. Farri A, Enrico A, Farri F. Headaches of otolaryngological interest: Current status while awaiting revision of classification. Practical considerations and expectations. Acta Otorhinolaryngol Ital 2012;32:77–86.

76. Puig CM, Driscoll CL, Kern EB. Sluder's sphenopalatine ganglion neuralgia—treatment with 88% phenol. Am J Rhinol 1998;12:113–118.

77. Day M. Sphenopalatine ganglion analgesia. Curr Rev Pain 1999;3:342–347.

78. Marmura MJ, Silberstein SD. Headaches caused by nasal and paranasal sinus disease. Neurol Clin 2014;32:507–523.

79. Schreiber CP, Hutchinson S, Webster CJ, Ames M, Richardson MS, Powers C. Prevalence of migraine in patients with a history of self-reported or physician-diagnosed "sinus" headache. Arch Intern Med 2004;164:1769–1772.

80. Perry BF, Login IS, Kountakis SE. Nonrhinologic headache in a tertiary rhinology practice. Otolaryngol Head Neck Surg 2004;130:449–452.

81. Mudgil SP, Wise SW, Hopper KD, Kasales CJ, Mauger D, Fornadley JA. Correlation between presumed sinusitis-induced pain and paranasal sinus computed tomographic findings. Ann Allergy Asthma Immunol 2002;88:223–226.

82. Eross E, Dodick D, Eross M. The Sinus, Allergy and Migraine Study (SAMS). Headache 2007;47:213–224.

83. Cady RK, Schreiber CP. Sinus headache: A clinical conundrum. Otolaryngol Clin North Am 2004;37:267–288.

84. Spinks A, Glasziou PP, Del Mar CB. Antibiotics for sore throat. Cochrane Database Syst Rev 2013;11.

85. Chiappini E, Regoli M, Bonsignori F, et al. Analysis of different recommendations from international guidelines for the management of acute pharyngitis in adults and children. ClinTher 2011;33:48–58.

86. Hayward G, Thompson M, Heneghan C, Perera R, Del Mar C, Glasziou P. Corticosteroids for pain relief in sore throat: Systematic review and meta-analysis. BMJ 2009;339:b2976.

87. Sichel JY, Attal P, Hocwald E, Eliashar R. Redefining parapharyngeal space infections. Ann Otol Rhinol Laryngol 2006;115:117–123.

88. Lempert T. Vestibular migraine. Semin Neurol 2013;33:212–218.

89. Cherchi M, Hain TC. Migraine-associated vertigo. Otolaryngol Clin North Am 2011;44:367–75.

90. Brandt T, Strupp M. Migraine and vertigo: Classification, clinical features, and special treatment considerations. Headache Curr 2006;3:12–19.

91. Lempert T, Olesen J, Furman J, et al. Vestibular migraine: Diagnostic criteria. J Vestib Res 2012;22:167–172.

92. Geser R, Straumann D. Referral and final diagnoses of patients assessed in an academic vertigo center. Front Neurol 2012;3:169.

93. Hsu LC, Wang SJ, Fuh JL. Prevalence and impact of migrainous vertigo in mid-life women: A community-based study. Cephalalgia 2011;31:77–83.

94. Oh AK, Lee H, Jen JC, Corona S, Jacobson KM, Baloh RW. Familial benign recurrent vertigo. Am J Med Genet 2001;100:287–291.

95. Marano E, Marcelli V, Di Stasio E, et al. Trigeminal stimulation elicits a peripheral vestibular imbalance in migraine patients. Headache 2005;45:325–331.

96. Neuhauser H, Radtke A, von Brevern M, Lempert T. Zolmitriptan for treatment of migrainous vertigo: A pilot randomized placebocontrolled trial. Neurology 2003;60:882–883.

97. Whitney SL, Wrisley DM, Brown KE, Furman JM. Physical therapy for migraine-related vestibulopathy and vestibular dysfunction with history of migraine. Laryngoscope 2000;110:1528–1534.

98. Buisseret-Delmas C, Compoint C, Delfini C, Buisseret P. Organisation of reciprocal connections between trigeminal and vestibular nuclei in the rat. J Comp Neurol 1999;409:153–168.

99. Knight RT, St John JN, Nakada T. Chewing oscillopsia. A case of voluntary visual illusions of movement. Arch Neurol 1984;41:95–96.

100. Fox D, Herron BE, Yonover PM, Baker WH. Mastication steal: An unusual precipitant of cerebrovascular insufficiency. J Vasc Surg 1999;29:734–736.

101. Park SH, Kim HJ, Kim JS, et al. Mastication-induced vertigo and nystagmus. J Neurol 2014;261:480–489.

Myalgia, Myofascial Pain, Tension-Type Headaches, and Fibromyalgia

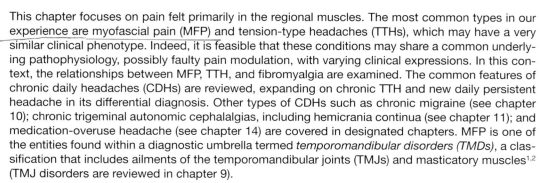

Peter Svensson, DDS, PhD, Dr Odont
Yair Sharav, DMD, MS
Rafael Benoliel, BDS

8

This chapter focuses on pain felt primarily in the regional muscles. The most common types in our experience are myofascial pain (MFP) and tension-type headaches (TTHs), which may have a very similar clinical phenotype. Indeed, it is feasible that these conditions may share a common underlying pathophysiology, possibly faulty pain modulation, with varying clinical expressions. In this context, the relationships between MFP, TTH, and fibromyalgia are examined. The common features of chronic daily headaches (CDHs) are reviewed, expanding on chronic TTH and new daily persistent headache in its differential diagnosis. Other types of CDHs such as chronic migraine (see chapter 10); chronic trigeminal autonomic cephalalgias, including hemicrania continua (see chapter 11); and medication-overuse headache (see chapter 14) are covered in designated chapters. MFP is one of the entities found within a diagnostic umbrella termed *temporomandibular disorders (TMDs)*, a classification that includes ailments of the temporomandibular joints (TMJs) and masticatory muscles[1,2] (TMJ disorders are reviewed in chapter 9).

In its most recent classification, the International Headache Society (IHS) has significantly changed the approach to TMDs as a possible cause of head or facial pain.[3] Disorders of the TMJ and masticatory muscle are now included as possible causes of secondary headache, and reference is made to the Diagnostic Criteria for Temporomandibular Disorders (DC/TMD) (Table 8-1). Nevertheless, for TMDs the IHS classification is limiting, and orofacial pain specialists have tended to use the DC/TMD based on the original Research Diagnostic Criteria for Temporomandibular Disorders (RDC/TMD)[1,2,4] (Table 8-2). In the current classification, muscle pain is subdivided into three categories based on the degree of referred pain: *(1) myalgia*, when pain is only elicited locally; *(2) MFP*, when there is pain referral within the boundaries of the muscle examined; and *(3) MFP with referral*, when pain referral is to a distant site beyond the muscle boundaries. The original RDC/TMD system has been extensively tested and translated into various languages so that it has wide universal acceptance. In addition to the physical diagnosis (Axis I), the RDC/TMD system is unique because it also assesses psychologic, behavioral, and psychosocial factors (Axis II). Axis II parameters

195

Table 8-1	Diagnostic criteria for headache attributed to TMDs*	
Diagnostic criteria		**Notes**
A. Any headache fulfilling criterion C		
B. Clinical and/or imaging evidence of a pathologic process affecting the TMJ, muscles of mastication, and/or associated structures		Clinicians should use the DC/TMD. Most prominent in the preauricular areas of the face, masseter muscles, and/or temporal regions. Some overlap exists between headache attributed to a TMD as a result of muscular tension and TTH. When the diagnosis of a TMD is uncertain, the headache should be coded as TTH, presumably with pericranial muscle tenderness.

C. Evidence of causation demonstrated by at least two of the following:
1. Headache has developed in temporal relation to the onset of the TMD
2. Either or both of the following:
   a. Headache has significantly worsened in parallel with progression of the TMD
   b. Headache has significantly improved or resolved in parallel with improvement in or resolution of the TMD
3. The headache is produced or exacerbated by active jaw movements, passive movements through the range of motion of the jaw, and/or provocative maneuvers applied to temporomandibular structures such as pressure on the TMJ and surrounding muscles of mastication
4. Headache, when unilateral, is ipsilateral to the side of the TMD		

D. Not better accounted for by another *International Classification of Headache Disorders,* third edition diagnosis		

*Reproduced with permission from the International Headache Society.

are further discussed later in this chapter and in chapter 4. The Axis II questionnaires used in the DC/TMD have clinically relevant and acceptable psychometric properties for reliability, validity, and utility as instruments for identifying patients with TMDs who have high levels of distress, pain, and disability that can interfere with treatment response and course of Axis I disorders.[5] Research on TMDs should therefore use the DC/TMD criteria, although for routine situations clinicians can use the screening version of the DC/TMD.

TMDs are among the most common orofacial pain conditions in the general population. TTH is the most common primary headache,[6] and referral of pain to the orofacial region is suspected in some cases. General dentists and orofacial pain specialists are therefore regularly required to diagnose and manage these patients.

Clinical Approach

A thorough pain history must be recorded, including specific questions on masticatory dysfunction. Pain location should be augmented by drawings that outline the extent and referral pattern of pain (Case 8-1; Fig 8-1). The referral patterns are also subject to particular investigations during a clinical examination using the DC/TMD system.

A routine head and neck examination must be performed, including cranial nerve assessment. Specifically, the interincisal mouth opening should be recorded in millimeters and any deviation or accompanying pain adequately described. The DC/TMD system offers operationalized guidelines for the specific examination procedures for the jaw muscles, TMJs, and opening

Table 8-2	DC/TMD diagnostic criteria for myalgia*

**Axis I:
Methodology**
	• Minimum of 2 lb (range 2 to 3 lb) for masseter and temporalis sites
	• Pressure is held for 2 seconds for myalgia and 5 seconds for myofascial pain
	• Pain on palpation in one or more of the following sites, at least one of which is ipsilateral to the pain complaint (right/left muscles count for separate sites):
	  ○ Right/left temporalis anterior
	  ○ Right/left temporalis middle
	  ○ Right/left temporalis posterior
	  ○ Right/left masseter origin
	  ○ Right/left masseter body
	  ○ Right/left masseter insertion

History	1. Pain in the jaw, temple, in front of the ear, or in the ear AND 2. Pain modified with jaw movement, function, or parafunction

Examination	1. Confirmation of pain location(s) in the temporalis or masseter muscle
	AND
	2. Report of familiar pain in the temporalis or masseter muscle with at least one of the following provocation tests:
	  a. Palpation of the temporalis or masseter muscle
	  OR
	  b. Maximum unassisted or assisted opening

Subclassifications
*(additional
examination criteria to
the aforementioned
for specific diagnosis)*
	1. Local myalgia AND:
	  3. Pain with muscle palpation with pain localized to the immediate site of the palpating finger(s)
	2. Myofascial pain AND:
	  3. Pain with muscle palpation with spreading of the pain beyond the location of the palpating finger(s) but within the boundary of the muscle
	3. Myofascial pain with referral AND:
	  3. Pain with muscle palpation beyond the boundary of the muscle

**Axis II:
Psychosocial
comorbidity**
	• Pain intensity and pain-related disability
	  ○ Graded chronic pain scale
	  ○ Jaw disability checklist
	• Depression and somatization
	  ○ Symptom Checklist for Depression and Somatization (SCL-90)

*Adapted from Schiffman et al.[2]

patterns.[7] In all patients seeking musculoskeletal treatment, it is imperative to carefully palpate the regional muscles (masticatory/pericranial, cervical) and TMJs to locate painful areas or trigger points. Muscle trigger points refer pain and are distinct from muscle tenderness, which reflects a generalized sensitivity over the affected muscle. The patient's reaction and assessment of resultant pain or tenderness should be recorded, and it may be important to distinguish between pain and tenderness on palpation. Particularly in MFP, the examination is crucial in diagnosis; it is therefore essential to develop a reliable technique whereby even and consistent pressure is applied across all patients.[7] Clinical signs are difficult to measure with consistency, and interrater reliability is not good for some signs of MFP, so close conformity with accepted classification criteria and thorough self-calibration are essential.[8] Examiner calibration rather than professional experience seems to be the most important factor for reliable measurement of TMD symptoms.[9] The DC/TMD system suggests that pressure application be standardized to 1 kg at the masseter and temporalis muscles and to 0.5 kg and 1 kg at the TMJ.[7] Other intraoral or extraoral sites should be approached with 0.5 kg of pressure. Practicing pressure application on weight scales using the fingers or thumbs is advisable, but recent research has clearly shown a huge variability of manually applied forces, which can almost be eliminated using simple palpometer devices.[10] For neck and shoulder muscles, a somewhat higher force should be applied, aiming at a

Masticatory myofascial pain in a 27-year-old woman.

Present complaint: Pain on the right side of the face, particularly around the angle of the mandible and the preauricular region (Fig 8-1a). The pain is constant, and recently the pain severity became worse, graded around 6 on a 10-cm visual analog scale (VAS). Pain severity fluctuates throughout the days and is worse in the afternoon or after chewing or yawning. Other than mild neck discomfort, the patient reports no generalized symptoms. The patient has no record of absenteeism from work and reports that she sleeps well. Pain has occasionally referred to the teeth, but her dentist has not detected pathology. Descriptors for pain quality are pressure, dull, and annoying.

History of present complaint: Present for the past 4 months but before that has occurred and remitted for some months.

Physical examination: Extraoral examination revealed regional muscle tenderness (Fig 8-1b) bilaterally but more pronounced in the ipsilateral masseter and temporalis muscles. Interincisal mouth opening was 34 mm and accompanied by pain. Examiner-assisted opening was 39 mm with severe pain. No TMJ sounds were detected, and the joints were not tender. Cranial nerve examination was normal. Intraoral examination and full-mouth radiographs revealed no dental problems.

Relevant medical history: The patient was diagnosed with hypothyroidism 4 years ago and has been taking 100 µg of thyroxine daily.

Diagnosis: Masticatory muscle myofascial pain.

Diagnostic and treatment considerations: Conservative treatment options were discussed with the patient, and therapy was initiated with analgesics (ibuprofen 400 mg three times daily for 10 days) and physiotherapy for the jaw and neck muscles (see text). The patient was also referred to her family physician to check on her thyroid status. Over the next 6 weeks, the patient reported no significant improvement and began to complain of disturbed sleep and increased neck discomfort (Fig 8-1c). Thyroid hormone and thyroid-stimulating hormone levels were normal. Amitriptyline (10 mg at bedtime) was therefore initiated, together with continuing physiotherapy. Based on response and side effects, the dose was increased to 20 mg at bedtime, and over a period of 15 weeks the pain severity decreased to a mean VAS score of 1. The patient reported increasingly longer periods during the day when she was pain free. On examination, the masticatory muscles were not significantly tender, and unassisted, pain-free mouth opening was 41 mm. The patient was then lost to follow-up for about 12 weeks and subsequently returned and requested that the amitriptyline be withdrawn. She also commented that pain was aggravated during intensive work at her desk. The amitriptyline was withdrawn, and the patient was instructed to continue physiotherapy and obtain advice regarding ergonomics in her immediate work environment. Over the next 4 or 5 weeks, the patient reported no significant pain and was released.

pressure of about 4 kg.[11] The authors' approach is to begin by applying pressure on unaffected regions (eg, forehead, shoulder) so the patient becomes familiar with the technique. Patient response can be recorded for each muscle or joint and graded on a scale from 0 to 3, where 0 is no pain, 1 is mild, 2 is moderate, and 3 is severe pain.[12] Pain ratings may then be summated to give a total pain score.[11,13] Patients with MFP or fibromyalgia consistently display more pain and have more involved muscles than control subjects, but the findings for TTH are inconsistent and vary among patients. Radiation of pain or referral to particular sites is not a constant feature,

as reflected in the different subgroups of MFP in the new DC/TMD (see Table 8-2). Most masticatory muscles are examined extraorally, except for the lateral pterygoid, which is approached from the maxillary retromolar region. However, palpation of the lateral pterygoid is notoriously associated with false-positive responses (eg, pain due to stimulation of the oral mucosa) and has low inter- and intraexaminer reliability. The temporalis muscle has an insertion to the coronoid process, and the tendon may be palpated intraorally. Patients should be questioned about other body pains and these areas examined if need be.

[Handwritten annotations: "LATERAL pterygoids see P. 202", "PALPATION of LATERAL Pterygoi"]

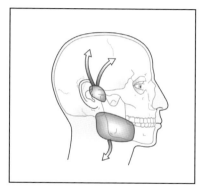

Fig 8-1a Pain location for the patient described in Case 8-1.

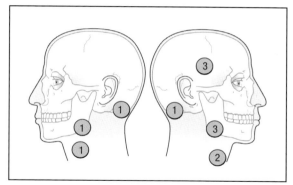

Fig 8-1b Muscle pain in the same patient. Tenderness is graded from 1 to 3 (mild to severe). The ipsilateral masseter and temporal muscles were the most tender (scored 3). The contralateral masseter muscle was also mildly tender. Additionally, the suboccipital and sternocleidomastoid muscles were mild to moderately tender bilaterally.

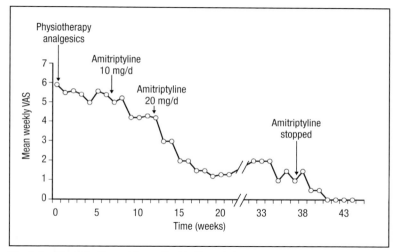

Fig 8-1c The pain diary of the patient in Case 8-1.

In the general population, clicking or popping jaw joints are very common and may occur during opening and/or closing; often, this is an isolated symptom that requires no treatment. The interincisal opening at each click and associated deviation in the mouth opening should be recorded. At times, joint sounds may be pathognomonic of underlying disease; for example, crepitation (a sound or feeling like sand or walking on snow) commonly occurs in degenerative joint disease. Because the mandible connects the TMJs, joint sounds are often transduced to the opposite side, so careful examination is required. Lateral and protrusive movements of the jaw should be examined and irregularities or concomitant pain recorded. Joint pain should also be examined and recorded under ipsilateral and contralateral loading (biting a bite stick). Guidelines, manuals, and clinical examination forms for a systematic and standardized examination may be downloaded from the International RDC-TMD Consortium (www.rdc-tmdinternational.org).

UNIVARIATE

Intraoral examination should rule out dental pathology as the source of pain or referred pain to the musculoskeletal structures. Furthermore, the occlusion/articulation should be checked for gross problems and/or recent changes that may have been associated with or caused by a TMD. The dentition and periodontal tissues should be assessed for possible pathology.

Temporomandibular Disorders

Study design and reliability

Depending on the specific subdiagnosis, the cardinal features of TMDs include muscle and/or joint pain, joint sounds, and masticatory dysfunction. Many studies have therefore focused on the prevalence of TMD signs and symptoms without knowing their clinical significance. Moreover, because studies address a number of symptoms, conclusions about the behavior of any one sign or symptom should be arrived at with care. Other studies have reported on samples of patients seeking treatment or on convenience samples that are misrepresentative of the population, that is, they have selection bias. A major historical problem has been the use of diverse inclusion and exclusion criteria by different groups. This is reflected in the diverse terminology used in the literature: *mandibular dysfunction*, *craniomandibular disorders*, *myofascial pain dysfunction syndrome*, etc. These terms have been substituted with *TMD* throughout this chapter (see Peck et al[1] and Schiffman et al[7]). The universal use of accepted research criteria will no doubt increase practitioners' understanding of the processes and epidemiology involved in TMDs and our diagnostic skills. The use of the term *TMD* is widespread; however, research on epidemiology, treatment response, natural history, and genetic factors must clearly differentiate among the diagnostic subgroups.

When examining the literature, it is important to assess the study design, statistical power, and presence of confounding variables. For example, studies of pain and bruxism often ignore confounding parameters, such as stress and anxiety, and therefore the results may be misrepresentative. The case could be made that instead of performing univariate analyses and looking for specific and dominant risk factors, a more fruitful approach would be to recognize the complex interactions among multiple factors and adopt a multivariate analytic approach. Ascertaining the parameters the study assessed is important, that is, patient report or physical findings of signs and symptoms by examination. The examination usually uncovers more physical findings than the patient is aware of.[14] The physical assessment of patients in TMD studies requires standardization of methods, reliability data, and interrater calibration. The double-blind placebo controlled trial is the gold standard for therapeutic interventions but may be problematic in some physical therapy modalities. Comparative studies of different interventions are needed to identify the more efficacious treatments. Evidence-based therapies in TMDs are rare, and expert opinion or personal preference often replaces a sound scientific approach. Although clinical experience and individual judgment are important in the assessment and treatment of patients, incorporating evidence-based principles is essential.

Epidemiology

TMDs are recognized as the most common chronic orofacial pain condition, and only minor differences are found among racial groups.[15,16] As previously mentioned, TMDs refer to a group of pain conditions and dysfunctions, and not all epidemiologic studies have used the same classification or differentiated between muscle and joint disorders. Indeed, inclusion criteria used in studies before modern classifications grouped a number of disorders into one entity. This raises questions about the current validity of much of the epidemiologic research performed before criteria and diagnoses were standardized.

Signs and symptoms versus treatment need

Studies reveal that 6% to 93% of the general population have or report signs and symptoms of TMDs. Study results show great disparity, however, and prevalences of common signs, such as clicking joints, range from 6% to 48%,

REF. P. 239 240

CONFOUNDING

which suggests that the methodology and definitions account for the observed variability.

Moreover, data are lacking on the significance of these highly prevalent signs and symptoms. Thus, practitioners cannot reliably predict which signs and symptoms will deteriorate and therefore justify early treatment. Clinical judgment alone is relied on to decide which signs and symptoms will be treated, but clinical judgment varies, and in the absence of clear criteria, this alone should not be relied on. Based on available data, clear indications for treatment are pain and/or significant dysfunction.

The data should therefore reflect the severe cases (pain and/or dysfunction) that need treatment. For example, although signs or symptoms of dysfunction are extremely common, only 3% to 11% of patients are assessed as needing treatment.[17] TMD-related facial pain has been found to occur in 4% to 12% of the population,[18,19] and severe symptoms are reported by 10% of subjects. These figures are compatible with the data on the percentage of people who seek treatment (1.4% to 7%).[20] In a large population, masticatory muscle and TMJ tenderness were found in 15% and 5% of patients, respectively,[21] but were self-reported only by about 4% and 6% to 8% of patients, respectively, which suggests that muscular tenderness is less bothersome to patients or that examination techniques are resulting in overdiagnosis.[22,23] Longitudinal studies suggest that symptoms of TMDs fluctuate considerably, particularly in patients with MFP, and progression to severe pain and dysfunction of the masticatory system is rare.[17] MFP has been clearly shown to be a chronic or fluctuating pain condition; over 5 years, 31% of patients suffered continuous MFP, 36% experienced recurrent pain, and 33% remitted.[24] Clinical experience confirms that there is extreme symptom fluctuation, and new symptoms appear as often as old ones disappear. Significant predictors of persistence were high baseline pain frequency, painful palpation sites, and other body sites with pain.[24] First, onset of any painful TMD has recently been reported to be about 4% per annum and is influenced by multiple factors, such as sociodemographic characteristics, health status, clinical orofacial factors, psychologic functioning, pain sensitivity, cardiac autonomic features, and to some extent genetic risk factors.[16,25,26] Taking findings from the Orofacial Pain: Prospective Evaluation and Risk Assessment (OPPERA) study into account, it seems inappropriate to consider TMD solely as a localized orofacial pain condition.[16,25,26]

Age distribution of TMDs

Signs and symptoms of TMDs have been found in all age groups, peaking in 20- to 40-year-olds. Signs of TMDs have been described in children and adolescents but are usually mild.[27] In a group of adolescents, treatment need was assessed at 7%.[28] TMDs may also occur in edentulous patients.[29] Accumulated evidence suggests that symptoms in the elderly may be lower than in the general population, but some studies show a slight elevation in the prevalence of some signs in this age group, including asymptomatic joint sounds (eg, crepitation) and limited mouth opening.[30] In a longitudinal study of elderly patients, signs and symptoms of TMDs tended to decrease over the follow-up period.[31] These data suggest that TMDs are not progressive and most symptoms resolve with increasing age.

Sex

TMD signs and symptoms have a female preponderance, especially those of muscular origin.[17] Most studies also report that the vast majority of patients (up to 80%) who seek treatment are girls or women.[32,33] Back pain, headache, and TMD-related pain were found to increase significantly with increasing pubertal development in girls.[34] Additionally, women with TMDs generally have more severe physical and psychologic symptoms than do men.[35] TMD pain and related symptoms appear to improve over the course of pregnancy and are not paralleled by improvements in psychologic distress.[36] This is most likely associated with the dramatic hormonal changes during pregnancy. Indeed, TMD pain in women is highest at times of lowest estrogen and may also be related to periods of rapid estrogen change.[37] A recent study identified only a slightly greater incidence of first onset of any painful TMDs for women.[16] Sex-related effects are examined further in the section on TMD pathophysiology.

[handwritten: bilAteral Q #3 B]

Personal and societal impact of TMDs

Although progression to severe TMD-related pain and dysfunction is rare, the personal and societal impact of TMDs is significant. Patients with TMDs request sick leave significantly more often, visit a physician more frequently, and use more physical therapy services than control subjects. Disabling TMDs cause an estimated 18 lost workdays annually for every 100 working adults in the United States.[38] During the early 1990s, it was calculated that approximately 3.6 million acrylic splints were constructed yearly in the United States to treat TMDs and bruxism, accounting for an annual expenditure of US $990 million (not adjusted for inflation), or about 3% of the total US dental health care expenditure.[39] Subjects with TMDs use significantly more health care services than control subjects—about 50% more in mean costs for drug utilization, outpatient visits, and specialist services.[33] Most of the increased costs were accounted for by about 10% of those with TMDs, probably the most severely affected.[33]

[handwritten: see p.198]

Myofascial Pain

[handwritten: LATERAL Pterygoids]

Clinical features

[handwritten: p.203]

The masticatory muscles involved in jaw closure include the masseter, temporalis, and medial pterygoids. The lateral pterygoids are involved in opening, in laterotrusive and protrusive movements, and, to some extent, in articular disc/condylar stabilization, whereas the digastric muscles assist in mouth opening. Other pericranial and cervical muscles are concomitantly involved or provide support and stability during mastication, speech, and swallowing. MFP is characterized primarily by pain and tenderness from the jaw-closing muscles. The specialized function of the masticatory muscles, the presence of bilateral joints with occluding teeth, and their important roles in chewing produce specific clinical features, such as significant masticatory dysfunction. In addition, the intimate anatomical relationships produce complex and overlapping referral patterns.

[handwritten: Q #3 Stem of Question]

At present, the diagnosis of MFP is based on the history and clinical examination of the patient; Table 8-2 lists clinical criteria for diagnosis. No classification system is perfect, however, and clinical diagnosis needs to rely on more than just a list of criteria. For example, most clinicians would be comfortable with diagnosing a patient with MFP in the presence of chronic orofacial pain and dysfunction and only two painful muscle sites, whereas the original RDC/TMD criteria required three or more painful muscle sites. This criterion has been revised in the new DC/TMD,[7] demonstrating the need for critical reflections and continuous adjustment of all classification systems guided by high-quality clinical research.

Location and quality

[handwritten: UNILATERAL   RegioNAl PAIN   Q p]

By definition, MFP is characterized by regional, and often unilateral, pain; however, it is important to check for more systemic pain complaints. Patients typically localize the pain to areas around the ear, the angle/body of the mandible, and the temporal region (Fig 8-2).

Referral patterns include intraoral, auriculotemporal, supraorbital, and maxillary areas depending on the muscles involved and the intensity of the pain, and perhaps reflecting individual propensity for pain spread and referral.[11,40–42] Intraoral referral of pain is well documented and may be the prime complaint from the patient.[11] At times the pain refers diffusely throughout one side of the face, compounding diagnosis.[11,40] Although MFP is typically a unilateral pain condition, it may also occur bilaterally, particularly when associated with generalized disorders such as fibromyalgia and trauma.[11,43] Pain quality is dull, heavy, tender, or aching and rarely throbbing.[44] Emotive descriptors, such as "tiring" and "troublesome" are often reported by patients with MFP.[44] Pain severity may fluctuate during the day but is usually about 3 to 5 on a 10-cm visual analog scale (VAS); however, it varies considerably across patients.[44,45] Some patients may report more severe pain (VAS 7), but this is rare.[11] More severe pain in patients with MFP is associated with increased reports of pain-related awakenings.[46]

[handwritten: AWAKeNs Q #3]

Temporal pattern

Some patients experience the most intense pain in the morning (21%) or late afternoon (79%),

[handwritten footer: Opening/closing muscles   Quality of PAIN: Dull Ach. Q # 3, C]

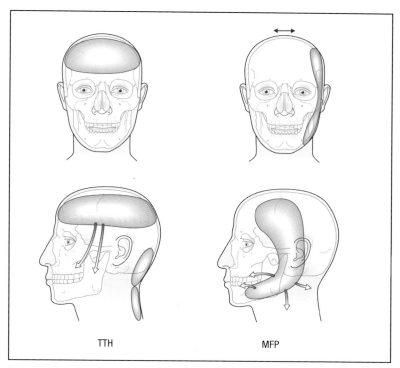

Fig 8-2 Typical pain location in TTH and MFP.

See p. 225 1st column

P. 197 Table 8-2 History 2

though others have no fixed pattern; fortunately, the pain rarely wakes the patient.[45] Pain-free days may be reported, and on a painful day average pain duration ranges from 5.5 to 18 hours.[11,45] Typically and per definition, MFP is characterized by chronicity with reported onset being months to several years previously.[24,44] The temporal pain pattern varies considerably among patients but should be carefully explored during the pain history. Pain occurring on most days of the month is typical of patients with MFP.[11]

Triggers

on Function

Pain may be aggravated during jaw function, with transient spikes of pain occurring spontaneously; indeed, pain on function may be the patient's primary complaint. Nevertheless, a subset of patients may also experience relief of pain during function such as mastication, suggesting different phenotypes of MFP. Note that in the new DC/TMD system, one of the criteria for MFP is that pain is changed (not necessarily increased) during jaw function. Further studies are needed to determine the clinical significance of this apparent dilemma in the clinical examination.

Associated signs

In addition to pain, there may be deviation of the mandible on opening, fullness of the ear, dizziness, and soreness of the neck. Dizziness has been associated with pain in the sternocleidomastoid muscle and ear stuffiness with spasm of the medial pterygoid. Some patients may report tinnitus that is correlated with a number of tender muscles.[47,48] Tinnitus often improves with treatment, together with other TMD signs and symptoms. Interestingly, tinnitus is also associated with depression levels, thus indicating complex and multifactorial relationships.[49]

PAIN ON Function

Physical findings

Examination usually reveals limited mouth opening (< 40 mm, interincisal)[11] with a soft-end feel. The presence of limited mouth opening in a patient with MFP may also indicate TMJ pathology that may be clinically difficult to diagnose.[50] Pain to palpation is usually present in ipsilateral masticatory muscles and is a distinguishing feature of MFP. The masseter is the muscle most commonly involved (> 60%), and the medial pterygoid and temporalis muscles are painful in about 40% to 50% of patients, often unilaterally.[11] The sternocleidomastoid, trapezius, and suboccipital muscles are usually painful in a small number of patients, very often bilaterally.[11]

Typically, there are localized tender sites and trigger points in muscle, tendon, or fascia.[42,51] A so-called hypersensitive bundle or nodule of muscle fiber of harder-than-normal consistency is the physical finding most often associated with a trigger point. Trigger points are traditionally described to be associated with a twitch response when stimulated. Additionally, trigger point palpation may provoke a characteristic pattern of regional referred pain and/or autonomic symptoms. The importance of trigger points remains controversial, and an alternative interpretation is that they may simply be epiphenomena of deep tissue pain. Areas of referred pain may include perioral and intraoral (teeth) structures and may depend on the muscles involved and the intensity of pain.[52,53] Referral to the teeth may be prominent and may often cause misdiagnosis as dental pathology. Referral of pain from trigger points in the deep part of the masseter muscle includes the TMJ and ear, which causes possible misdiagnosis with intra-articular or ear disorders (see chapters 7 and 9). Trigger points may be active (ie, induce clinical symptoms) or latent, in which case they only induce pain on stimulation. Some researchers suggest that muscle overload may activate latent trigger points.[54,55] In the authors' experience, tender or painful points are far more common in patients with MFP than are trigger points; the DC/TMD criteria relate to this by including the diagnosis of myofascial pain with referrals. Indeed, as discussed later, the presence or absence of trigger points seems unnecessary in the diagnosis of chronic musculoskeletal conditions such as fibromyalgia, myofascial pain, and probably MFP.[56] Patients will often have extratrigeminal pain and tenderness, and the presence of widespread body tenderness is associated with more severe TMDs and increased somatic symptoms.[57,58]

Differential diagnosis

MFP needs to be differentiated from other conditions that may affect the masticatory muscles. Inflammation of a muscle and myositis secondary to infection or trauma are commonly seen in dental practice. Myositis is usually associated with a pertinent history or significant clinical findings, such as muscle or regional swelling, redness, and dental or periodontal infection. The affected muscles are tender, located in the vicinity of the inflammation, and accompanied by limitation of mouth opening. Myositis may precede or be associated with a painful contraction or myospasm in the regional muscles that is of acute onset. Treatment of these involves the effective eradication of the initiating cause and analgesics in accordance with pain intensity (see chapters 6 and 16). Active physiotherapy helps restore normal mouth opening. Local muscle pain may occur 24 to 48 hours after acute overuse of the masticatory muscles; this delayed-onset muscle soreness is similar to that observed in patients with TMDs or in other body muscles after exercise.[59] Treatment should be tailored to reported symptomatology and usually includes analgesics and physiotherapy.

Pain referral to intraoral structures has often caused serious misdiagnosis and unwarranted dental treatment, but this can be easily avoided by careful clinical and radiographic examination. The differentiation from painful TMJ disorders may also be complex because of the overlapping symptomatology; regional pain, pain-referral patterns, and pain evoked by mandibular movement are common to both MFP and TMJ disorders (see chapter 9). Careful clinical assessment and follow-up are essential. Clinicians must be alert to the possible contribution of systemic comorbidities. Hypothyroidism, statin use, connective tissue disease, and AIDS may cause a diffuse myalgia and therefore require investigation in relevant situations.

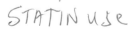

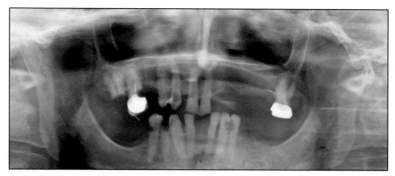

Fig 8-3 Metastatic lesion to the left condyle mimicking a temporomandibular disorder. The condylar anatomy is distorted, and a pathologic fracture is present. The patient had a previous adenocarcinoma of the breast.

The occurrence of regional primary or metastatic tumors may induce TMD-like symptomatology and should be excluded. Although relatively rare, reports in the literature continue to suggest that such misdiagnosis is possible.[60,61] Warning signs include pain of sudden onset or acute worsening of existing pain; focal neurologic findings, such as disturbances in somatosensory function; a lack of response to therapy; and atypical distribution or characteristics of the pain. Particularly, patients with a history of previous malignancy are at risk and should be referred for relevant imaging studies (Fig 8-3). Furthermore, movement disorders such as orofacial dyskinesia and oromandibular dystonia may sometimes be associated with muscle pain symptoms (see Peck et al[1]). Finally, fibromyalgia (discussed later in this chapter) and widespread pain, whiplash-associated disorders, and headaches attributed to TMDs should be considered in the differential diagnosis.

Additional diagnostic tools

The doubtful role of muscle hyperactivity in the pathophysiology of MFP, as discussed later, suggests that the use of electromyography (EMG) measurements is not useful in patient diagnosis and management.[62] Moreover, surface EMG recordings are often contaminated by the muscles of facial expression. Trigeminal reflex recordings are valuable tools for assessing neurologic disorders or pain mechanisms but hold little potential to be easily implemented in routine clinical examination.[63] Pressure algometers attempt to accurately assess pressure pain thresholds but are affected by rate of application, sex, and site.[62] Neurophysiologic methods and quantitative sensory testing offer excellent tools in assessing trigeminal somatosensory function and the contribution of the central nervous system in orofacial pain conditions, which makes them useful for research[64] (see chapter 3). Quantitative sensory testing techniques measure pain and sensory thresholds to electrical, mechanical, and thermal stimuli and are able to distinguish TMJ from MFP cases, but they are time-consuming.[65]

A relatively understudied yet clinically useful and well-known technique is the use of differential analgesic blocks and provocation tests.[66] Application of local anesthetics may help to determine the peripheral nociceptive source, but sensitivity, specificity, and predictive values remain to be established.

Treatment

Treatment of TMDs with a variety of conservative methods consistently results in high (75% to 90%) success rates.[32,67–70] In general, treatment is aimed at palliation and is based on clinical diagnosis; because the etiology is unclear, no treatment is curative. An interesting approach is to identify individual factors in specific patients and attempt to recognize their roles as possible predisposing, initiating, and perpetuating factors. Individual factors may serve any or all of these roles in different patients.

Table 8-3	Treatment aims in masticatory myofascial pain
Aims	**Examples of available therapies**
Reduce pain	Simple analgesics, tricyclic antidepressants, rest
Restore function and range of motion	Physiotherapy, reduced pain
Decrease aggravating or contributing factors	Identify specific variables acting in the individual patient and attempt to eradicate; these may include emotional and physical variables
Increase bite comfort	Occlusal appliances (eg, guards)
Increase muscle strength	Physiotherapy, restored function
Reduce physiologic distress	Empathy, information; referral for counseling, cognitive-behavioral therapy when needed
Prevent drug abuse	Careful monitoring of drug use, efficient and prophylactic pain therapy
Restore social functioning	Cooperation with family physician, family members; referral for social and emotional help/counseling

Extensive research in the field of TMD therapy shows that there are no compelling data to support any intervention as being capable of disease eradication or modification. Moreover, conservative therapies are consistently successful and are in no way inferior to more invasive or irreversible procedures, such as surgery, occlusal adjustment, or prosthetic rehabilitation.[32] The data support a conservative approach to the management of TMDs.[71] This is reinforced by findings that the natural history of MFP includes an extensive number of patients that will substantially fluctuate or remit over time and rarely progress to severe pain.[17,24] A patient's beliefs, medical status, type of employment, and personal preference may often dictate the treatment plan; the patient should therefore be actively involved in the decision-making process.

Therapy for MFP falls into four main categories—physical, pharmacologic, psychologic, or trigger point injection—and is often multidisciplinary.[72,73] Treatment of MFP often combines conservative interventions, and different centers have variable protocols depending on patients' signs, symptoms, and personal preferences. Treatment duration is usually 4 to 6 months but in selected cases may be longer.

Most patients with MFP seek treatment to alleviate pain; thus, significant reduction or eradication of pain must be one of the primary aims. However, treatment aims in MFP patients are usually more complex and ambitious; these are summarized in Table 8-3. The assessment of treatment outcomes should be based on accurate assessment of pain intensity and frequency (see chapter 3) and the evaluation of changes in psychosocial comorbidity (see chapter 4). The Initiative on Methods, Measurement, and Pain Assessment in Clinical Trials (IMMPACT) suggests that the following domains need to be considered in the comprehensive analyses of treatment outcomes: pain intensity, physical functioning, emotional functioning, and participant's rating of overall improvement.[74]

Chronicity in myofascial pain

The transition from acute to chronic MFP is dictated partly by response to initial treatment and is therefore discussed in this section. High characteristic pain intensity, high disability score, higher scores of emotional distress, and being female with myofascial pain (versus TMJ disorders) are the most significant predictors of chronicity. Patients developing chronicity differ significantly in numerous biopsychosocial variables (eg, they suffer from more current anxiety disorders, mood disorders, and somatization disorders). Patients with TMDs who did not respond to treatment were found to suffer from significantly higher rates of fatigue and sleep disturbances.[75] Researchers have suggested that the development of chronicity involves neuroplastic changes in the medullary dorsal horn, including functional and morphologic changes. At the same time, endogenous factors, such as descending inhibition, are working to attenuate these changes and may vary in effect between patients. These findings are consistent with the theory that prolonged and intense nociceptive input is one of the initiating factors for chronicity with decreased biopsychosocial abilities, sex-related variables in pain modulation, and generalized symptomatology possibly acting as perpetuating factors. Recent research also emphasizes the contribution of genetic factors and multisystem dysregulation for persistent pain conditions, including MFP.[76]

Physical and combined modalities

Most pain physicians with experience in the field of MFP will attest to the success of conservative physical therapy, including muscle exercise, thermal packs, and oral splints. However, few, if any, of these therapies have been unequivocally proven in controlled trials. Often, reassurance and education of the patient, combined with simple muscle exercises for masticatory and neck muscles, will result in pain alleviation and restored mandibular function.[67,69] Chewing exercises may be beneficial for some patients with MFP, but there may be increased pain after vigorous exercise.[77] Based on accepted principles,[55] the authors have the patient perform simple, active stretch exercises: two minimal mouth openings followed by a gentle and slow maximal opening (stretch) without causing extreme pain. The patient may use wooden or plastic tongue spatulas as a dynamic record of maximal opening. These exercises are performed three or more times every 1 or 2 hours. Patients with suboccipital and cervical muscle tenderness or chronic pain will benefit from the addition of active neck exercises. Rotation of the head and ear-to-shoulder movements with mild stretching to each side (three times each) are similarly prescribed every 1 or 2 hours. Under normal conditions, patients will rotate the head by about 70 degrees, whereas ear-to-shoulder movements are inherently more limited (40 degrees). Although clinical experience with physiotherapy and exercises is usually good, a recent study challenged this notion by showing no significant differences in outcome between a group receiving physiotherapy and a control group only receiving education.[78] Perhaps the beneficial effects of physiotherapy are closely linked to the more cognitive-behavioral aspects (eg, education and self-awareness) of a management program.

Muscle tenderness and pain may also be treated with vapocoolant sprays and concomitant stretching, known as *spray and stretch*.[55] This usually induces immediate relief and is often used as a diagnostic test, although sensitivity, specificity, and predictive values have not been established (see Table 8-1). Other commonly used techniques, such as ultrasound and thermal packs, have not been rigorously assessed. However, because these are conservative approaches, individual patients who benefit from their use should be encouraged to continue. Some evidence supports the use of low-level laser therapy in patients with TMDs, particularly MFP.[79] When combined with an exercise program, laser therapy significantly improved symptoms more than exercise alone.[80] However, there was no advantage in adding laser therapy when pain intensity was specifically analyzed.[80] Other systematic reviews do not offer much support in terms of clinical efficacy of low-level laser therapy,[71,81] and it may not be appropriate to include this in the first line of treatment options.

A physical self-regulation program consisting of training in breathing, postural relaxation, and proprioceptive re-education has been shown to be superior to conservative therapy (flat-plane intraoral appliance and self-care instructions) at a 6-month follow-up.[82] In a further study, conservative treatment by specialists was compared with a structured self-care program in patients with TMDs and minimal levels of psychosocial dysfunction.[68] The specialist treatments included splints, physiotherapy, analgesics, muscle relaxants, and patient education (diet and parafunctional habits). No limitations were imposed on the combinations of treatments or the number of visits. The self-care program incorporated cognitive-behavioral therapy and self-care techniques, such as relaxation. One year later, both groups showed improvement in all clinical and self-report categories measured.[68] However, the patients in the self-care program showed significantly decreased TMD pain, decreased pain-related interference in activity, and a reduced number of painful masticatory muscles; they also required fewer visits. These studies indicate the importance of education and self-care in the management of TMDs, and these strategies are supported by systematic reviews.[71]

Occlusal adjustments and the management of TMDs

There is no doubt that occlusion is of paramount importance in restorative and prosthetic dentistry (ie, oral rehabilitation). The question remains as to the relationship between TMDs and occlusion/malocclusion. The historical importance of occlusion in the etiology of TMDs, although largely unproven, led to the extensive use of occlusal adjustment. Occlusal adjustment may induce pain relief in some cases, but the irreversible nature of this procedure is problematic. To date, opinions diverge concerning occlusal and skeletal factors in TMDs. A large number of general and specialist dentists still view occlusal factors as important in the pathophysiology and management of TMDs, and many continue to equilibrate the occlusion as therapy for TMDs. Based on published research, comprehensive reviews, and clinical experience, irreversible occlusal adjustment or rehabilitation for the treatment of TMDs is contraindicated.[83–85] Patients with prosthodontic needs will benefit from sound prosthodontic rehabilitation, but that should not be confused with the treatment of TMDs.

The sum results of the studies supporting adjustment are equivocal. Factors not considered in these studies are the irreversible nature of occlusal adjustments and that these adjustments are not stable over time and tend to partially recur.[86] Moreover, occlusal adjustment shows no advantage over any other conservative and reversible therapy.[71] Occlusion plays a minor role, if any, in the etiology and therefore in the treatment of TMDs, including MFP.[87,88]

p. 242

Occlusal splints

Occlusal splints may be soft or hard and may be fabricated with full or partial tooth coverage. A recent example of a new type of partial-coverage bite plate is the nociceptive trigeminal inhibition tension suppression system, which has been advocated for the treatment of headache.[89] Some splints are designed with the aim

of repositioning the mandible in a new maxillomandibular relationship (repositioning splints). Soft appliances are probably as efficacious as hard splints in the management of MFP but are difficult to adjust and repair.[90] Repositioning appliances have been used extensively to treat internal derangements of the TMJ and aim to recapture the disc (see chapter 9). Although these appliances may successfully capture discs in internal derangement and provide reduction in the short term, they fail to do so at all for internal derangement without reduction or osteoarthritis.[91] Moreover, long-term stability of successful treatment is usually not good, and clicks or abnormal disc positions tend to recur.[92,93] Recent studies show that repositioning appliances have no significant benefit over stabilization appliances in the treatment of TMJ sounds.[94] In addition, repositioning splints may induce irreversible occlusal changes and are therefore not recommended. When managing conditions like TMDs, it should be emphasized that the number needed to harm (NNH; that is, the number of patients to be treated before one patient will experience an unwanted or side effect due to the treatment) value should be extremely high. In the management of TMJ disorders, splints are sometimes constructed to reduce TMJ loading by providing occlusal contacts in the posterior region only.[95] This is further discussed in chapter 9.

Flat occlusal splints (relaxation or stabilizing splints) are in widespread use and provide even occlusal contacts; these may be constructed for the maxilla or the mandible. Stabilization splints are effective in managing TMJ arthralgia[96] (see chapter 9). No difference in effect is apparent between flat splints and splints designed to provide canine guidance on lateral excursions of the mandible.[97] The authors are reluctant to use partial-coverage splints because of the inherent potential to cause permanent occlusal changes and the lack of evidence for any advantage over flat splints.[98,99] To avoid occlusal changes, all patients with any appliance must be instructed not to wear it all the time. Additionally, appliances must be regularly checked and repaired if need be. In some cases, the splint has fractured in the area of the most-distal molars (the thinnest part) and has allowed the selective overeruption of these teeth, therefore causing an anterior open bite.

Meta-analyses consistently demonstrate benefit for oral splints in TMDs in general.[71,83,100] The most recent meta-analytic review concluded that "stabilization splint therapy may be beneficial for reducing pain severity at rest and on palpation and depression when compared to no treatment."[101] Several studies have investigated the efficacy of occlusal appliances in the treatment of MFP.[70,102,103] Most have found improvement in the active and placebo arms (nonoccluding splints) of the trial but only marginal superiority of the active splint.[90] Similar effects of nonoccluding splints on TMJ pain and clicking have been observed.[97] The presence of widespread pain reduces the effectiveness of oral splints and suggests that they should only be prescribed for patients with regional myofascial facial pain.[104] The number needed to treat (NNT) for occlusal appliances in the treatment of TMDs has been calculated.[100] The NNT calculates the number of patients that need to be treated to obtain one patient with 50% or greater reduction of the worst pain. For oral splints, an NNT of 6 was obtained for TMJ pain and 4.3 for MFP. The relatively good success rate and generally conservative nature of splints accounts for their extensive use. However, splints entail substantial costs to manufacture and maintain. A recent study suggests that splint therapy, whether high-cost laboratory-processed splints or chairside thermoplastic splints, offer no significant advantage over conservative self-care strategies,[105] including jaw relaxation, reduction of parafunction, thermal packs, physiotherapy, stress reduction, and the use of nonsteroidal anti-inflammatory drugs (NSAIDs).[105]

The exact mode of action of splints is unproven. Splints may reduce sleep bruxism, but both control and placebo splints induce similar reductions in muscle activity.[106] In fact, these effects appear to be temporary because muscle activity reaches baseline levels after about 6 weeks according to another controlled trial.[107] After prolonged wear of splints, bruxing movements tend to recur in spite of the fact that symptoms such as pain remain improved.[108] The aforementioned data and the lack of evidence for the role of muscle hyperactivity in TMDs confirm that reducing bruxism is not the mode of action of splints in the relief of TMDs. Currently, splints are considered to act through nonspecific mechanisms probably involving placebo and anticipation and possibly involving some behavior-modifying properties.

Pharmacologic

Simple analgesics. NSAIDs are used extensively in the management of pain and disability associated with musculoskeletal pain. Although the antiplatelet and gastrointestinal safety profile of selective cyclooxygenase-2 inhibitors is superior, they still have potentially serious side effects on the renal and cardiovascular system (see chapter 15). For the treatment of TMDs, calculations of NNTs for drugs versus placebo reveal encouraging figures of 2.7 to 3.5.[100] Based on current evidence, ibuprofen (400 mg three times daily) or naproxen (250 mg twice daily) is efficacious (see chapter 15). Simple analgesics or combination analgesics (eg, codeine and acetaminophen) may also provide good analgesia and may be safer than NSAIDs. In patients with myofascial pain, ibuprofen combined with diazepam is superior to ibuprofen. The use of benzodiazepines as analgesics is of questionable value, however, and antidepressants, muscle relaxants, and anticonvulsant drugs are more efficacious.

Antidepressants, benzodiazepines, muscle relaxants, and antiepileptic drugs. Amitriptyline at low doses (10 to 30 mg/day) is superior to placebo[109] and has been consistently reported as beneficial for patients with craniofacial myofascial pain, including predominantly muscular TMDs,[110] and posttraumatic myofascial pain.[111] The use of clonazepam, a long-acting benzodiazepine with anticonvulsant properties, has been beneficial,[112] but the muscle relaxant cyclobenzaprine has proven superior to clonazepam in another study on pain upon awakening.[113] More recently, gabapentin, an antiepileptic drug, has been tested for the treatment of MFP in a randomized double-blind study.[114] Gabapentin was found to be clinically and statistically superior to placebo in reducing reported pain, masticatory muscle hyperalgesia, and the impact of MFP on daily functioning. Reduction in muscle tenderness was observed after 8 weeks, but the effects on pain appeared only after 12 weeks of therapy at

How splints (probably) work

a mean dose of about 3,400 mg gabapentin per day.[114] The NNT was calculated at 3.4 for gabapentin in the treatment of MFP. Involvement of the sympathetic nervous system is suspected in MFP, similar to that observed in fibromyalgia (discussed in later sections). Recent findings of genetically based abnormalities in the catecholamine pathophysiology of MFP[115] theoretically support the treatment of MFP with adrenergic blockers; in fact, preliminary evidence from a randomized clinical trial suggests that propranolol can decrease pain scores in patients with painful TMDs, depending on the catechol-O-methyltransferase (*COMT*) haplotype.[116] More quality drug trials in craniofacial, myofascial, and arthralgic pain and in patients with MFP are needed, and treatment remains somewhat empiric.

Biobehavioral therapy

Pain is a subjective experience with important affective, cognitive, behavioral, and sensory components (see chapter 4). Like other longer-lasting pain conditions, MFP is a complex entity associated with changes in mood, behavior, and attitudes to life, in addition to drug abuse and secondary psychologic gains. Therefore, outcomes such as restoration of functional activity, eradication of drug abuse and dependency, and rehabilitation of residual emotional distress need to be addressed. Careful review of such parameters as lost work days, sleep disturbance, and general functioning provide valuable insight as to the emotional well-being of patients in accordance with IMMPACT proposals.[117] Patients reporting a high degree of disability, psychologic distress, and drug or alcohol abuse may suffer from underlying psychosocial distress. Sleep disturbances are often part of emotional disorders and are intimately related to a number of chronic pain conditions.[118] Although experienced clinicians may obtain much information from an interview, it is generally accepted that this is insufficient for a reliable psychosocial assessment. The assessment of psychologic distress in patients with MFP may be performed with the DC/TMD questionnaire or with established alternatives.[7,117,119]

Cognitive-behavioral therapy (CBT) is an option that aims to alter negative overt behavior, thoughts, or feelings in patients with chronic pain and to diminish distress and suffering (see chapter 4). Whether implemented separately or in combination with other pain treatments, CBT produced significantly decreased pain, emotional distress, and disability and is of proven efficacy in patients with TMD.[120] Biofeedback is one such technique that aims to teach patients to control behavior that is possibly part of the pain etiology[121] (see chapter 4). The lack of evidence for muscle hyperactivity in the etiology of MFP raises questions about the validity of this method. Indeed, some studies have shown that headache improves whether patients increase or decrease muscle activity.[122] Biofeedback, however, is efficacious in regulating muscle tension in patients with TMDs and produces good long-term results,[123] and the limited data available support the efficacy of EMG biofeedback treatments for TMDs.[71,121] This may be particularly useful for TMJ disorders associated with overloading (see chapter 9). Combining biofeedback with CBT techniques significantly improves treatment outcomes versus CBT alone.[124,125]

Trigger point injections and needling

Clinical experience suggests that injections of local anesthetics into trigger points induce pain relief that may be prolonged beyond the effect of the anesthetic agent.[55] Few controlled studies have systematically tested this intervention for MFP, but the technique for the head and neck muscles is simple. The presumed trigger point is located and immobilized followed by injection using a standard dental syringe and a 27-gauge needle, though other body areas may require thicker needles (Fig 8-4). Introducing the needle into the trigger point may induce sharp pain, muscle twitching, or an unpleasant sensation. Before injection, the overlying skin should be cleansed with an approved antiseptic. Some suggest that the needle be inserted 1 to 2 cm away from the trigger point and then advanced at an acute angle of 30 degrees to the skin into the trigger point proper. Once an initial injection is performed (about 0.2 mL), the needle may be withdrawn to the level of the subcutaneous tissue, then redirected superiorly, inferiorly, laterally, and medially, repeating the needling and injection process in each direction. All injections should be preceded by aspiration to ensure that the needle is not in a blood vessel. After the injection, the muscle should be gently mobilized. Stretch exercises and analgesics are prescribed postoperatively to ensure that mouth opening and muscle function remain improved. In patients with myofascial pain, bupivacaine (0.5%) is equally efficacious to botulinum toxin in the relief of pain and cost-effectiveness, which would suggest the former's preferential use.[126] Furthermore, botulinum toxin injections have not been found to be superior to placebo injections in patients with MFP.[127,128] The authors suggest that, initially, mepivacaine (3%) should be used to test patient response. If the results are encouraging and the patient needs further injections, bupivacaine (0.5%) may then be used, although there are reports of bupivacaine-induced damage to muscle fibers. However, based on an extensive literature review, direct (or dry) needling of myofascial trigger points appears to be an effective treatment, most likely because of the needle or placebo rather than the injection of saline or active drug.[129] Thus, whether these needling therapies have efficacy beyond placebo is unclear. Dry needling of trigger points is very similar to some acupuncture techniques.

p. 626

Complementary and alternative therapy

Patient interest and demand for complementary or alternative medicine (CAM) is increasing (see chapter 17). Approximately 20% of patients with facial pain in a referral center had previously seen a CAM specialist, and up to 36% of patients with TMDs reported treating their symptoms with CAM techniques (see chapter 17). The existing evidence supports the value of acupuncture for the management of idiopathic headaches and has shown promise in the management of TMDs[71] (see chapter 17). However, well-planned studies are needed to assess the clinical value and cost-effectiveness of acupuncture and other CAM therapies for facial pain.

Treatment: Summary and prognosis

A clinician may choose from a number of conservative therapeutic options that depend on the history, physical findings, and comorbid signs in the individual patient (Fig 8-5).

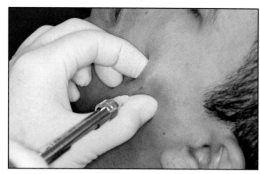

Fig 8-4 Trigger point injection. Identifiable trigger points are immobilized between two fingers, and local anesthetic solution is then injected. Injection should be performed at a number of points around the trigger. The needle should be retracted (but not withdrawn from the skin) and reinserted at each injection point. This technique combines the effects of local anesthetic with the effects of needling.

Chronicity of MFP is manifest by the increased need for long-term treatment of these patients.[130] However, prognosis in most patients with MFP is moderately good, and remission of pain and dysfunction is readily achieved for long periods.

Pathophysiology of MFP

The etiologic theory of TMDs, including MFP, much of which is based on deep-rooted historical concepts, is clouded by controversy and lack of stringent classification schemes. Current evidence supports the belief that the appearance of myofascial pain involves the interplay among a peripheral nociceptive source in muscle, a faulty component of the central nervous system (sensitization), and decreased coping ability.[131] In patients with MFP specifically, it is widely accepted that a complex interaction of variable intrinsic and extrinsic factors induces craniofacial pain and dysfunction. The clinical presentation and symptoms of MFP resemble that of muscular pain disorders elsewhere in the body. Similarly, it is thought that the pathophysiology of MFP may share mechanisms with such entities as regional myofascial pain, TTH, and fibromyalgia. Figure 8-6 presents a conceptual model for understanding the many factors involved in MFP.

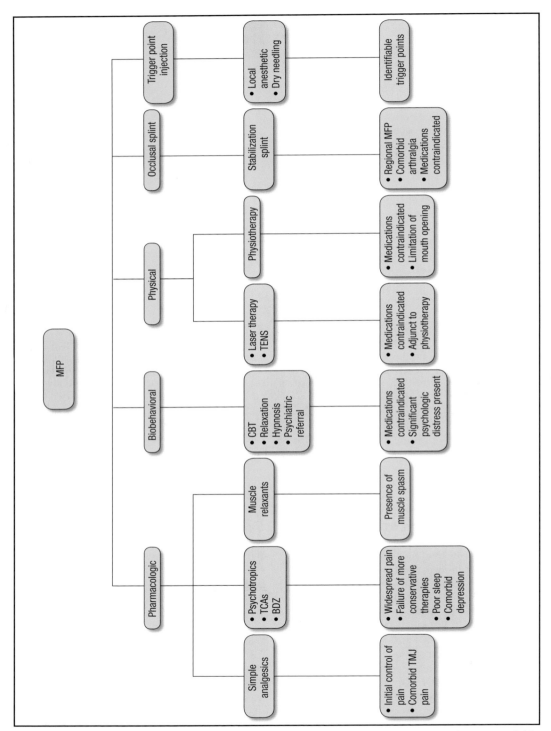

Fig 8-5 Treatment of masticatory myofascial pain. A wide variety of conservative treatment options are available. Symptomatology, comorbid medical or psychologic problems, and physician or patient preference dictate choice. TCA, tricyclic antidepressants; BDZ, benzodiazepine; TENS, transcutaneous electrical nerve stimulation.

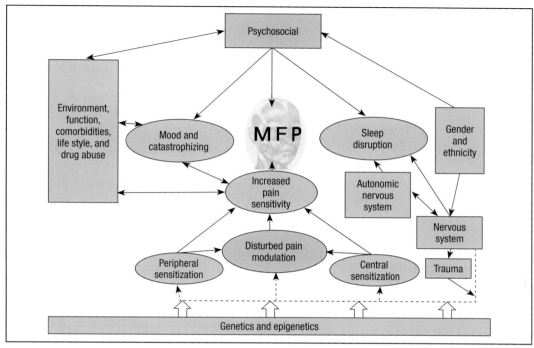

Fig 8-6 Conceptual model of the pathophysiologic factors influencing the development of MFP, which is considered a complex disease and is assumed to share features of other persistent pain conditions. Pain occurs within a framework of nervous system changes initiated by external events and modified by various intrinsic factors (mood, cognitive set, neurodegeneration) on the basis of genetic factors (and epigenetic changes). In essence, this is a gene by pain modulatory circuits by environment interaction. Multiple genes, for example, *COMT*, or α-adrenoreceptor 2, glucocorticoid receptors, protein kinase, muscarinic receptors, transcription coregulators, and phosphorylators of G proteins have been identified that carry an increased risk for higher pain sensitivity. Environmental factors can increase the risk through psychosocial mechanisms, physical factors such as trauma, or epigenetic modifications. The exact pain phenotype is determined by the interplay of several brain factors, such as context, cognition, mood, learning, memory, sleep, and neurodegeneration, that affect inhibitory circuits.[132,133] Biologic sex and ethnicity may influence the balance among factors.

Historical perspective on TMD concepts

The first description of a TMD-like entity emphasized the etiologic importance of tooth loss. This established the concept that regional musculoskeletal pain was invariably associated with dental occlusion and other anatomical factors, such as skeletal relationships. The resultant structural and mechanistic concepts of TMD etiology remain unproven but widely publicized. In view of such concepts, dentists have treated TMDs while other medical specialties have cared for additional chronic musculoskeletal craniofacial pain such as TTH. Unfortunately, this has resulted in a separation of MFP from other chronic regional pain conditions, such as

TTH, regional myofascial pain, or fibromyalgia. However, data expressing common ground between TTH and MFP is available, which suggests that we need to reexamine the present nosologic separation.

Historically, the diagnosis of pain associated with TMDs has been approached under more than a dozen names, including *temporomandibular joint dysfunction syndrome* and *myofascial pain dysfunction syndrome*, which reflects the confusion surrounding its etiology and often its therapy. Research in the late 1950s attempted to shift attention from the TMJ to the muscles of mastication. Early studies also emphasized the contribution of psychologic factors to TMDs, which produced the psychophysiologic

Nosologic — classification of disease

theory. Psychologic components as contributing factors in TMDs were demonstrated by extensive work on large patient populations, and it was hypothesized that parafunctional activities to relieve psychologic stress led to muscle fatigue, spasm, and pain (see chapter 4). Recent research has shown that patients with MFP consistently suffer higher levels of distress than patients with articular TMDs.[134,135] However, some patients with TMDs suffer from complex psychosocial disorders, and the role of such influences as initiating factors remains unclear, particularly in TMJ-related TMDs.[136]

Early theories offered one-cause, one-disease hypotheses (that is, they were overly simplistic and univariate models), but accumulating data indicating a more complex TMD etiology disproved these. Subsequently, new theories proposed a combination of stress and occlusal disharmonies, but the focus remained on occlusal adjustment as the preferred therapy. The most popular current theories are the multifactorial,[137] biopsychosocial,[138] and multisystem vulnerability and dysregulation[76] theories. All of these propose a complex interaction among environmental, emotional, behavioral, genetic, and physical factors in the etiology of TMDs, which strongly suggests the need for multivariate approaches to study and understand these disorders. However, specific risk factors may or may not be active in any given patient and therefore do not answer the question of why an individual patient develops a TMD. Thus, although these concepts are helpful at a population or group level, they may be limited for individual patients.

Some etiologic factors have received wide acceptance. A proportion of patients with acute TMDs report a clear association with trauma. In chronic cases, initiation of pain is often associated with a history of trauma, but whether this is the etiology, a cofactor, or a trigger is unclear. However, the patient's psychologic status and psychosocial functioning have emerged as central in determining the establishment of chronic muscular pain and its treatment response.[139] In support, baseline and longitudinal data from the OPPERA case-control study identify complex multifactorial conditions.[16,140] Unfortunately, the patients in the OPPERA study largely (85%) suffered from both MFP and TMJ disorders,[16,141,142] which limits the conclusions that can be drawn specifically about MFP pathophysiology.

In the following section, possible factors that may be active in the initiation and maintenance of chronic muscle pain are reviewed. These factors act with genetics, proinflammatory states, cardiovascular and neuroendocrine function, trauma, and the social and environmental makeup and may serve to protect or increase a person's risk[132] (see Fig 8-6).

Nervous system alterations and pain modulation

The sensation of muscle pain is usually the result of activation of polymodal muscle nociceptors, groups III and IV, which are functionally and anatomically equivalent to $A\delta$ and C fibers, respectively. These fibers have a high stimulation threshold and, under normal conditions, are therefore not activated to physiologic movement or normal muscle stretch. However, muscle nociceptors may be sensitized by peripherally released neuropeptides that increase their response to suprathreshold stimuli and may induce long-term changes in the central nervous system, such as central sensitization.[131] Damage to individual muscle cells releases sufficient intracellular adenosine triphosphate to activate purinergic receptors and induce pain.

In subgroups of patients with muscle pain, however, such as in fibromyalgia, pain may not be dependent on any peripheral input. Indeed, as discussed later, pain can occur secondary to a dysfunctional descending antinociceptive system, an overactive descending facilitatory system, or loss of central inhibitory neurons (see also chapter 12).

Evidence suggests that multiple mechanisms are involved at the level of the peripheral nervous system and the central nervous system. The complex and heterogenous clinical phenotype of muscle pain (TTH, myofascial pain, fibromyalgia) probably involves different combinations of peripheral and central nervous system mechanisms at different and even changing levels of activity. For example, fibromyalgia may be mainly an expression of central nervous system dysfunction, whereas myofascial pain may initially involve peripheral mechanisms that may over time trigger central nervous system changes. Evidence of central sensitization was shown to be present in patients with MFP and those with mixed MFP and TMJ disorders.[143]

Numerous studies have documented neurophysiologic characteristics of patients with TMDs. Unfortunately, many of these did not differentiate between muscular- versus joint-based etiologies, so their usefulness is extremely limited. Moreover, most of these studies were inconclusive and have largely been replaced by quantitative sensory testing and functional studies of the somatosensory system.

Complex behavioral influences, such as anxiety, depression, belief states, and cognition, can separately influence pain perception and the pain experience. A key system that is able to directly change pain intensity is the brainstem's descending modulatory network with its pro- and antinociceptive components.[133]

Altered pain modulation is suggested by findings of significantly more prevalent generalized body pain (eg, fibromyalgia and back pain) and headache in patients with TMDs,[144,145] whereby most patients suffering from painful joint or muscle pain report pain outside the craniocervical region.[146,147] Patients with MFP display augmented central nervous system processing of pain (central sensitization) and a deficit in endogenous pain inhibition.[148–150] However, in other experiments[151] no generalized hypersensitivity has been shown in patients with MFP. This suggests that there may be two clinical and possibly therapeutic subtypes of MFP: those patients with and those without extracranial muscle involvement.[58] Alternatively, multisite hyperalgesia may be a graded, time-dependent phenomenon[41]; and indeed, experimental studies have shown that somatosensory sensitivity develops gradually in the presence of experimental jaw muscle pain.[152] Additionally, in patients with MFP, widespread pain and tenderness are associated with long-standing MFP.[153]

Quantitative sensory testing studies have been applied to the study of TMDs and frequently reveal evidence for abnormal somatosensory processing in patients with MFP[58,64,65] (see also chapter 3). Patients with TMDs exhibit lower pain thresholds, greater temporal summation of mechanically and thermally evoked pain, stronger aftersensations, and multisite hyperalgesia.[149,150,154–156] These findings indicate faulty nervous system inhibition but also suggest an additional component of enhanced pain facilitation that contributes to the greater pain sensitivity observed in patients with TMDs. In support of this concept, patients with TMDs have repeatedly been shown to be more pain sensitive and to have concomitantly reduced pain inhibition; these findings are similar to what has been demonstrated in patients with other types of chronic pain, such as those with irritable bowel syndrome.[154]

Lowered pressure-pain thresholds in deep tissues have been consistently reported in patients with MFP, which suggests a failure in modulation and peripheral sensitization of muscle nociceptors.[150,157–159] Because pressure-pain thresholds are changed not only in the painful region but also at other sites, these studies suggest that those patients have central sensitization.[42,159,160] Activators of peripheral muscle nociceptors may include peripheral chemical or mechanical agents and trigger point activity (discussed later), in addition to reactive or even primary central mechanisms that can lead to neurogenic inflammation.[41]

The largest effects on experimental pain measures shown in patients with TMDs have been on the pressure-pain thresholds at multiple body sites and on the cutaneous mechanical pain threshold. These results largely confirm previous studies that found that patients with chronic TMDs are more sensitive to many experimental noxious stimuli at extracranial body sites, and they also provide clinicians with the ability to directly compare the case-control effect sizes of a wide range of pain sensitivity measures for the first time.[161] These data indicate generalized hyperexcitability of the central nervous system and generalized upregulation of nociceptive processing, and thus, they suggest that these may be pathophysiologic mechanisms.[156] Moreover, the response of patients with MFP to experimental ischemic pain also depends on their depression and somatization scores.[162] This complex interaction among psychosocial and biologic variables in MFP patients may occur independently or may share a common biologic basis (see the section on psychosocial factors). In any event, this clearly indicates the need for a combined therapeutic approach and for multivariate research approaches. A recent study demonstrated the potential for a multivariate approach by showing that modulation of emotions by negative- or positive-loaded pictures were only able to increase and decrease, respectively, the pain sensitivity in people with high expression of the serotonin transporter protein (this is a demonstration of gene × emotions × pain interactions).[163]

Molecular imaging studies are providing highly novel information regarding faulty pain processing in patients with chronic pain. Although the data are not conclusive regarding causality, they clearly show that in patients suffering chronic pain, the brain is fundamentally disturbed and demonstrates faults and degenerative changes in areas involved in pain modulation.[143] They also show differences among patients with various orofacial pain conditions[164] and volumetric changes in gray and white matter in patients with chronic painful TMDs.[165,166]

Autonomic nervous system and MFP

The role of the autonomic nervous system has been investigated in persistent muscle pain, particularly fibromyalgia. Although the exact pathophysiology of fibromyalgia is unclear, there is evidence of dysautonomia with increased neural sympathetic activation and lack of an adequate sympathetic response to stressor or cardiovascular challenges[167] (see the section on fibromyalgia).

Patients with fibromyalgia suffer dysfunction of the hypothalamic-pituitary-adrenal axis, similar to that found in MFP,[168] and this is thought to partly underlie sleep disorders, some pain symptoms, and autonomic nervous system imbalance.[169–172] Another view is that fibromyalgia may represent a neuroplastic idiopathic pain condition with similar neurobiologic changes but not specifically caused by a distinct lesion or disease of the somatosensory system.

In a similar fashion, these findings indicate statistically significant differences between patients with TMDs and control subjects across multiple autonomic constructs, particularly elevated heart rate, reduced heart rate variability, and reduced baroreflex sensitivity at rest and during physically and psychologically challenging conditions.[173] Patients with MFP demonstrate increased levels of catecholamines[174] and reduced COMT activity.[175] In contrast, later experiments on patients with MFP found that beta-adrenergic sympathomimetic stimulation

did not influence pain-pressure thresholds or EMG activity in the masseter and trapezius muscles.[176] In light of the evidence on the connections among the beta-adrenergic system, COMT, and MFP[177,178] (see the section on genetics), it is reasonable to assume that future research will establish the involvement of sympathetic dysfunction in patients with MFP.[179]

Neuropeptides and MFP

Little is known about pain and inflammatory mediators or neuropeptides in muscle tissue.[131] Serotonin and prostaglandin E_2 are involved in the development of pain and hyperalgesia/allodynia of the masseter muscle in patients with fibromyalgia, whereas local myalgia (myofascial pain) seems to be modulated by other as yet unknown mediators.[180] Injection of neuropeptides into muscle and the resultant changes have provided important insight into the cascade of events that lead to persistent muscle pain. Inclusion of male and female subjects also allows the analysis of sex differences.

Injection of glutamate into muscle is painful[181–184] and, acting through N-methyl-D-aspartate (NMDA) receptors and glutamate receptors (GluR1), it has been shown to be important in producing muscle pain.[185,186] Protein kinase C activation is also required for this effect in craniofacial muscle tissue.[186] Glutamate excites and sensitizes rat masseter muscle afferent fibers through similar activation of peripheral receptors. However, the resultant afferent fiber activity is greater in female than male rats,[181] an effect observed in human subjects as well.[184,187] These studies clearly demonstrate sex-related differences in glutamate-evoked jaw-muscle activity that are dependent on female sex hormones.

Some of the mechanisms of muscle sensitivity to palpation (allodynia) have been elucidated by extensive experiments by Svensson et al,[188–192] particularly the powerful effects of nerve growth factor on muscle sensitization and its sex-selective effects (see below). These experiments indicate that human nerve growth factor–induced sensitization of masseter nociceptors results, in part, from the activation of tyrosine kinase receptors. In contrast to findings from previous experiments on pain, muscle sensitivity does not appear to be mediated through enhanced peripheral NMDA receptor activity.[193,194]

HPA AXIS

In a study examining the levels of serotonin in masseter muscle in a heterogenous group of fibromyalgia and MFP patients, it was found that serotonin is present in the human masseter muscle in a steady state and that it is associated with pain and allodynia. The origin of the serotonin seems to be partly from the blood, but results indicate that peripheral release also occurs.[195]

Although most of these neuropeptide experiments were performed with only one agent, the in vivo milieu includes the interaction among a number of neuropeptides and amines that may act synergistically to increase sensitivity and pain in muscle.[196] Indeed, combined administration of bradykinin, serotonin, histamine, prostaglandin E$_2$, and adenosine triphosphate in healthy subjects produces prolonged moderate levels of pain and tenderness and has been suggested as a useful model to mimic myofascial pain and TTHs.[197,198]

Trauma

Researchers have increasingly recognized that trauma to the craniofacial region can lead to MFP.[199] The exact mechanisms of how this results in MFP are unclear but may include direct/invasive muscle damage, stretch injuries to muscle, or long-term immobilization (eg, with fractured jaws). Indirect injury of brain tissue may also lead to persistent head and facial pain, although there is no correlation between the degree of injury and the incidence or severity of the pain. Shear forces applied to the brain may result in severe damage. After even relatively minor head trauma, progressive and extensive axonal injury can occur, which is commonly known as *diffuse axonal injury*.[200,201] A history of trauma is present in significant numbers of patients with TMDs.[199,202–205] Dental surgery has also been found to increase the prevalence and symptomatology of TMDs.[206,207]

Whether patients with posttraumatic TMDs suffer more severe symptoms or are more resistant to treatment is unclear.[208–210] Indications suggest that early intervention with a conservative approach (physical therapy, tricyclic antidepressants, NSAIDs) significantly improves the prognosis in cases of posttraumatic pain.[111]

Whiplash, a hyperextension-flexion injury to the neck, has been implicated in the etiology of TMDs,[211] but how it can lead to MFP is

unclear.[212] A neurobiologic basis is supported by prospective studies showing that about a third of patients develop TMJ arthralgia after neck injury, despite not showing any structural damage to the TMJ.[213] Patients with whiplash demonstrate changes in thermal sensitivity in facial regions, suggesting cervically driven neuroplastic changes in the trigeminal system.[214]

An increased incidence of facial or jaw pain in patients after whiplash trauma has been shown.[213,215] MFP and neck pain are often comorbid,[216] but they may also be confounders, because one of the features of MFP is neck muscle pain. Moreover, patients with headache and facial pain frequently report concomitant cervical pain and vice versa, probably because of convergence of trigeminal and cervical afferents on second-order neurons in the brainstem trigeminocervical complex.[217] This bidirectionality of pain referral has been experimentally demonstrated.[218] Additionally, masseter pain can alter the strategy for jaw-neck motor control, which further underlines the functional integration between the jaw and neck regions.[219]

Functional findings in the masticatory apparatus in patients after whiplash include decreased range of motion, disturbed coordination, and impaired endurance.[220–223] Although functional impairment may be present in patients with a history of whiplash, long-term follow-up of these patients does not indicate an increased risk for persistent MFP.[224–226]

Many studies have assessed the presence of TMDs (both MFP and TMJ disorders)[227] or have solely assessed the TMJ,[213] making interpretation of the literature difficult. Moreover, it has been suggested that whiplash can lead to widespread body pain and that TMDs may be just one expression rather than a specific outcome of whiplash.[228] Notwithstanding, recent systematic reviews conclude that whiplash trauma is a clear comorbid condition in patients with TMDs but could also be an initiating and/or aggravating factor for TMDs.[229,230] The exact role of whiplash in TMD/MFP remains unclear.[209]

Psychosocial factors

Persistent pain, from whatever source, is associated with psychologic distress and psychosocial disturbances in many patients. These levels of distress may significantly affect patient compliance and treatment outcomes. Several methods have been designed to measure the emotional results of stress or the intensity of environmental stress. These methods are used as secondary end points in the assessment of outcomes in the treatment of chronic pain. The methodologies have recently been reviewed, and the Depression Inventory and the Profile of Mood States questionnaires are recommended for the assessment of treatment outcomes and for research in chronic pain.[117] For TMDs, the RDC/TMD and DC/TMD Axis II criteria have been extensively applied.

The level of psychologic and psychosocial disturbance often predicts treatment demand and outcome in patients with MFP[139,231,232] (see chapter 4). Patients with persistent pain who seek treatment usually have more severe pain and distress and a poorer prognosis. Cognitive coping abilities in response to injury and pain are also thought to be important. Recently, stress, negative affectivity, global psychosocial symptoms, and active and passive pain coping have been significantly associated with TMDs.[233] Two aspects of coping emerge as therapeutically relevant in TMDs: control or adjustment in response to pain and the recruitment of maladaptive coping strategies, such as catastrophizing, in an attempt to control pain.[139] A positive response to TMD treatment has been correlated with increased coping abilities.[234]

Psychologic status and psychosocial functioning of the patient have also been implicated in determining the establishment of MFP.[139] Patients with TMDs will manifest significantly higher levels of psychosocial symptoms, affective distress, somatic awareness, and pain catastrophizing.[233] Patients with MFP are frequently found to suffer from other stress-related disorders, such as migraine headache, backache, nervous stomach, and gastrointestinal ulcers.[235,236] Patients with MFP consistently suffer higher levels of distress than those with articular TMDs.[134,135] Depression and lack of sleep have also been found to be significantly increased in patients with TMDs.[204,237–239] Depression and chronic widespread pain are significant risk factors for the onset of MFP.[240]

Earlier studies suggest that stress-related disorders may underlie or contribute to the development of TMD chronicity and may therefore be viewed as perpetuating rather than initiating factors.[151,204,237,241] More recently, evidence suggests that global psychologic and somatic symptoms emerge as one of the most robust risk factors for incident TMD pain.[242] Dysregulation in terms of enhanced negative feedback suppression of the hypothalamic-pituitary-adrenal axis exists in chronic myogenous facial pain. These results suggest a more central etiology, with dysregulation in the stress- and pain-modulating systems.[168] Indeed, patients with TMDs who have increased self-efficacy measures suffered lower levels of pain, disability, or psychologic distress and reported greater use of an active, adaptive pain-coping strategy.[243] These findings form the justification and basis for biobehavioral interventions.

Occlusion

The relationship between occlusion and MFP is based on the vicious cycle theory in which an occlusal interference is supposed to induce hyperactivity and spasm of the affected muscles, which in turn leads to ischemia secondary to blood vessel compression. According to this rather old theory, the ischemic contractions are painful and activate muscle nociceptors, thereby completing the vicious cycle. Although the extent of the occlusal interference may be minute, it supposedly upsets proprioceptive feedback and triggers bruxism and spasm of the masticatory muscles. These assumptions have been refuted by experiments demonstrating that artificial occlusal discrepancies tend to reduce rather than enhance bruxism[244,245] and by the lack of correlation between oral parafunction and pain intensity in patients with TMDs.[246,247] Clinically, no correlation has been found between bruxism and muscle tenderness.[248] Interestingly, however, the effect of occlusal interferences appears to be dependent on the self-reported levels of oral parafunctions.[244]

Several long-term follow-up studies have also shown no consistent pattern between occlusal variables and TMDs,[249,250] although some show weak associations.[251] In patients awaiting full dentures, no statistically significant correlations were found between signs and symptoms of TMDs and occlusal errors or freeway space.[29] Malocclusion in adolescents is not associated with TMDs.[252] However, some

LACK OF Sleep

rare malocclusions have been associated with signs or symptoms of TMDs, including unilateral open bite, some crossbites, negative overjet, unilateral scissors bite in men, and edge-to-edge bite in women.[253] Some of these malocclusions are more significant in the presence of bruxism.[254] In several large population studies, such malocclusions (and functional occlusion factors) accounted for only a small part of the differences between the control population and the study population with signs or symptoms of TMDs.[255,256] Patients with deep bite, in particular those with retroclined maxillary incisors, frequently reported jaw stiffness and muscle disorders, and this may represent a risk factor for TMDs.[257] However, this is tempered by the fact that somatization scores were significantly higher in the deep bite group compared with the control group and that all patients were referred for treatment.[257] The data indicate that support for a causal relationship is weak. Only bruxism, loss of posterior support, and unilateral posterior crossbite show some consistency across studies, and these may be more important in TMJ disorders than in MFP.[85]

Recent studies have reexamined the effects of acute artificial occlusal interferences on such parameters as facial pain, chewing ability, and jaw fatigue.[258] Acute malocclusions usually cause variable amounts of discomfort in clinically normal subjects. However, this experimental design does not parallel the clinical situation in patients with MFP, where purported malocclusions occur slowly and are accompanied by skeletal growth and adaptation. Other experimental results seem to indicate that patients with MFP have less adaptive capabilities to both active and control interventions, but they leave the precise relationship between TMD pain and occlusion unanswered,[258] and no studies have yet demonstrated a specific effect of occlusal interferences rather than a more generalized hypervigilance response.

In conclusion, studies of this relationship have shown no functional occlusal factors to be consistently associated with TMD onset, and no specific type of malocclusion has been found to be an accurate predictor of TMD incidence.[259–261] Taken together, these data indicate that occlusal factors seem to be of minor, if any, importance in the etiology of TMDs.[85]

Skeletal morphologic features and orthodontics

The association between certain skeletal morphologic features and the prevalence of TMDs has been the focus of some controversy. Most research has focused on derangements and degenerative changes in the TMJ as they relate to skeletal morphology, so few data are available on MFP.[262] Nevertheless, data presented in early reviews and in recent research indicate that the distribution of major skeletal/occlusal categories in patients with TMDs does not differ significantly from the clinically normal population and that no single skeletal/occlusal problem can accurately predict the possibility of myogenous or arthrogenous TMD onset.[263,264]

The possibility that orthodontic treatment in any of its many forms can lead to the initiation or deterioration of TMDs has been a topic of great concern within the orthodontic community.[83] However, research consistently indicates that orthodontic treatment does not entail an increased risk for developing signs or symptoms of a TMD.[256,263–269] Therefore, the relationship of TMDs to occlusion and orthodontic treatment is minor. One review concluded that because signs and symptoms of TMDs occur in healthy people and increase with age, particularly during adolescence, TMDs that originate during various types of dental treatment may not be related to the treatment but may be a naturally occurring phenomenon.[270] Moreover, in two meta-analyses, no study was found indicating that traditional orthodontic treatment increased the prevalence of TMDs.[268,271] An interesting preliminary observation reported that subjects with a pain-sensitive variant of the *COMT* gene who underwent orthodontic treatment were more likely to report subsequent TMD pain,[272] indicating a complex interaction between genetics and environmental factors in accordance with the conceptual model for MFP (see Fig 8-6).

Orthodontic therapy aimed at improving or resolving a symptomatic TMD condition also has largely no supporting data[266,269,273] apart from correction of unilateral open bite, which has a weak association with TMD improvement. However, this finding needs further confirmation.[88]

TMJ disorders

Theoretically, trauma or noxious stimulation of TMJ tissues can produce a sustained excitation of the masticatory muscles, which may serve to protect the masticatory system from potentially damaging stimuli and movements. This has been shown in animal models.[274] Clinically, the frequent comorbidity of arthralgia and myalgia[202] has led to hypotheses linking their etiologies, but these have not been proven.[275] Such comorbidity may reflect sensitization and referral patterns mediated by primary afferents in the TMJ and muscles of mastication co-synapsing on dorsal horn neurons (convergence).[276,277] Moreover, experimental injection of algesic chemicals into the rat TMJ resulted in a sustained reflex increase in EMG activity of the jaw-opening muscles. Excitatory effects were also seen in the jaw-closing muscles, but these were generally weaker.[278] The weak effects in jaw-closing muscles and the stronger effects in the antagonist muscles suggest associations more in keeping with protective, withdrawal-type reflexes, at least in animal models.[274] Based on the present available data, it seems that pain originating in the TMJ contributes minimally to the development of MFP.

Muscle hyperactivity, bruxism, and MFP

A thorough understanding of bruxism is essential to fully appreciate the implications of the ongoing debate relating to its role in the pathophysiology of MFP.[279–283] The etiology of sleep bruxism is probably related to arousal responses and changes in the central/autonomic nervous system that may be modulated by stress[279] (see also chapter 5). The etiology of awake bruxism is unclear and may involve stress in predisposed persons.

Bruxism can cause muscle hypertrophy and severe damage to the dentition. The parafunctional forces applied during bruxism have also been suggested as a cause of dental implant failure, periodontal tissue damage, and tooth fracture. Hypothetically, the repetitive overloading of the TMJ and masticatory muscles by bruxing movements may cause tissue damage leading to TMDs. Muscle overload may also initiate or reactivate trigger points in susceptible persons.

Excessive bruxism with insufficient relaxation, as in jaw clenching, is thought to lead to muscle ischemia and pain. In this context, the most widespread belief is that repetitive tooth clenching, grinding, or abnormal posturing of the jaw induces MFP. However, these habits are extremely common and statistically have not been proven to induce MFP.

Exogenous models of muscle pain involve the injection of algesic substances into muscle. Endogenous models of experimental pain have been studied extensively and involve the persistent contraction or exercise of the masticatory muscles.[41,284–291] These experiments, although not identical to the chronic parafunctional activities that occur in patients, have produced inconsistent, nonspecific, and inconclusive results, raising questions about the role of muscle hyperactivity/overload in the etiology of MFP. A more clinically applicable situation is chronic low-level clenching, which does induce muscle pain but, again, only in a subset of patients.[292] Similarly, self-reported clenching is more consistently associated with MFP than grinding, although no cause-and-effect relationship has been established.[205] In this context, the Cinderella hypothesis, which provides a possible explanation for tissue damage after long-lasting and low-level muscle contractions,[293,294] may be relevant.[295] This hypothesis postulates that some motor units containing type I fibers remain contracted throughout the motor task and lead to localized overload, damage, subsequent inflammation, and muscle nociceptor sensitization. These motor units have been demonstrated in the masseter muscle, but so far no correlation has been found with postexperimental pain.[295] Work is currently underway to attempt to more closely reproduce naturally occurring long-lasting and low-level masticatory muscle activity and relate this to the Cinderella hypothesis.

Population studies suggest that self-reported tooth grinding (bruxism) may cause myalgia.[204,296,297] Investigations based on self-reported bruxism generally show a positive association with TMD pain, but they are characterized by bias and confounders.[298] For example, the reliability of self-reported bruxing habits is problematic; 85% to 90% of the population report that at some time they have ground or clenched their teeth.[282] Many patients who self-report tooth grinding admit that this was first brought to their attention by their dentist. Moreover, the reliability of clinician judgments of bruxism has been found to be extremely poor.[299] Notwithstanding all of these limitations, self-reported clenching and grinding have frequently been associated with MFP.[202,300] In contrast, and raising further questions about the association between bruxism and MFP, studies based on more quantitative and specific methods to diagnose bruxism showed a much lower association with TMD symptoms.[247]

In summary, available data do not support the traditional concept of MFP being induced or maintained by muscle hyperactivity (ie, the vicious cycle theory).[301] Little evidence is available to support sleep bruxism in the etiology of MFP, but the role of bruxing and clenching habits, particularly in the daytime, are as yet unclear.[205,292,295,296] Based on the data, the vicious cycle theory is untenable, and an alternative model—the pain adaptation model—has been proposed to explain motor changes in patients with muscle pain and disorders. *PAM p.230*

Muscle hyperactivity and the pain adaptation model

The pain adaptation model is based on data from persistent musculoskeletal pain conditions (including MFP), and it proposes that the observed changes in motor function are secondary to persistent pain and are mediated at the spinal or brainstem level.[301] Changes in masticatory muscle function secondary to experimental muscle pain, as previously described, support this model and confirm the clinical complaints of dysfunction in patients with MFP.[41] Injection of hypertonic saline into the jaw muscles induces pain with a significant reduction in jaw movements and in EMG activity during the agonist phase; this is accompanied by a small increase in antagonist muscle activity.[302,303] The pain adaptation model suggests that pain will inhibit alpha motor neurons during jaw closing and facilitate them during antagonist (opening) activity.[301] This model accurately fits the currently available data. More recently, a broader model, termed the *integrated pain adaptation model*, has been suggested[304] that includes the existing pain adaptation model as a subset. This new model is based on the prem-

ise that pain acts as a homeostatic emotion that requires a behavioral response. It involves an optimized recruitment of motor units, which represents a person's integrated response to the sensory-discriminative, motivational-affective, and cognitive-evaluative components of the pain. This recruitment strategy aims to minimize pain and maintain homeostasis and puts more emphasis on how patients perceive and cope with their muscle pain.

It is important to appreciate that rhythmic masticatory muscle activity (RMMA) produces positive EMG findings that may occur with no tooth grinding.[283] RMMA is extremely common and occurs in 60% of healthy control subjects and may easily be mistaken for tooth grinding.[305] Yet the number of RMMA episodes in bruxers is three times higher than in control subjects and is associated with tooth grinding in 33% of episodes.[283] However, two recent studies suggested an inverse relationship between sleep bruxism RMMA activity and measures of TMD pain and a positive relationship between background non-RMMA activity and TMD pain.[306,307]

If muscle dysfunction is not the cause of pain, but rather part of the spectrum of a pain adaptation response, then some parafunctions, including some bruxing habits, can no longer be considered primary etiologic mechanisms in MFP.[301] However, the precise association between bruxism and MFP remains unclear at this stage. Further refinement of how bruxism is being assessed and quantified is obviously needed.

Trigger points and the sympathetic nervous system

Myofascial pain, whether in the facial area, head, or other body parts, is often characterized by the presence of painful trigger points.[54,55] Pressure on a trigger point will activate intense pain and induce referral to characteristic sites. The muscle around a trigger point is usually hard and may be nodular or a taut band. Data suggest that trigger points are found in the area of unchecked electrophysiologic activity at the neuromuscular junction in the motor end plate. This results in localized contraction, which, together with the adjacent active motor end plates, contributes to the formation of the taut band or nodule.[54] Continued contraction in the area of trigger points leads to localized hypoxia, lowered pH, and the accumulation of proinflammatory mediators.[55,308] Lowered pH increases the activity of the peripheral receptors, further sensitizing the muscle nociceptors.[131] However, the localized contraction in trigger points is not associated with generalized muscle hyperactivity, so this phenomenon should not be confused with the muscle hyperactivity theory. Furthermore, controlled studies have not been able to identify more spontaneous EMG activity in trigger points of patients with TTH compared with healthy control subjects.[309] The appearance of active trigger points is thought to be related to muscle trauma, particularly eccentric muscle lengthening during contraction.[54] However, experiments directed at inducing such damage have been largely inconclusive.

Some researchers have suggested that muscle hypoperfusion (diminished blood flow) may be the primary factor in initiating muscle pain, possibly because of changes in sympathetic control.[310] Moreover, the unchecked motor end plates previously described develop sensitivity to sympathetic nervous system activity.[54] Similarly, sensitized nociceptors may be activated by sympathetic activity. Thus, the sympathetic nervous system is capable of independently initiating all the features of MFP.[310,311] However, there is still insufficient data at present to entirely endorse or refute this hypothesis.

Lifestyle

Very little research has been performed on the relationship between various lifestyle habits, such as nutrition, exercise, and smoking, and the presence and treatment of MFP. In one patient population study, current tobacco use was associated with unfavorable demographic variables and more pain interference in subjects with TMDs, but these effects were less pronounced in the case of myofascial pain.[312] Cigarette smoking and its extent have been positively correlated with pain intensity in patients with TMDs, though there were no differences between articular pain and MFP.[141,313,314] In a recent, population-based questionnaire study, current tobacco use was significantly greater in patients with MFP relative to those with painful TMJs or to control subjects.[315] Maintenance

of an organized nutritional schedule was found significantly less frequently in patients with MFP.[315] The potential future applications of established lifestyle risk factors in MFP are particularly interesting as they may be relatively easy avenues for initial and conservative treatment.

Genetics

No heritability has been found in humans for any TMD. In a study on monozygotic and dizygotic twins, no concordance in TMD signs and symptoms was found.[316] A study on female patients with MFP and their first-degree relatives also revealed no evidence of familial aggregation.[317] However, genetic influences on TMD development have been found.[115,318] A significant association between polymorphisms in the serotonin transporter gene and TMD has been shown in a Japanese population.[318] A relationship between clinical phenotypes of TMDs (joint versus muscle) and *COMT* polymorphisms has also been reported,[319] but neither the clinical criteria used nor the terminology (*myofacial* versus *myofascial*) are in line with current thinking. Further work on COMT has identified three genetic variants (haplotypes) of the *COMT*-encoding gene, which were designated as low pain sensitivity, average pain sensitivity, and high pain sensitivity. These haplotypes encompass 96% of the human population, and five combinations of these haplotypes were shown to be strongly associated with sensitivity to experimental pain. The presence of even a single low pain sensitivity haplotype diminished the risk of developing MFP by as much as 2.3 times. The low pain sensitivity haplotype produces much higher levels of COMT enzymatic activity compared with the average pain sensitivity or high pain sensitivity haplotypes. Inhibition of COMT in rats results in a profound increase in pain sensitivity. Thus, COMT activity substantially influences pain sensitivity, and the three major haplotypes determine COMT activity in humans, which inversely correlates with pain sensitivity and the risk of developing MFP.[115] In a further study examining beta-adrenergic receptor haplotypes, positive or negative imbalances in receptor function increased the vulnerability to persistent pain conditions such as TMDs.[320] The same group later showed the first direct evidence that low

COMT activity leads to increased pain sensitivity via a beta-adrenergic mechanism.[178] This study was a major breakthrough, but it must be stressed that the genetic variation in *COMT* seems to be specific not to MFP but rather to pain sensitivity and the development of persistent pain in general,[321] and it acts via the opioid system.[322] Several new genetic risk factors for TMDs, including glucocorticoid receptors (NR3C1), protein kinase (CAMK4), muscarinic receptors (CHRM2), transcription coregulators (IFRD1), and phosphorylators of G proteins (GRK5) have been recently identified.[323] Moreover, the OPPERA study demonstrated that nonspecific orofacial symptoms, but not TMD pain itself, were associated with voltage-gated sodium channel, type I, alpha subunit, and angiotensin I-converting enzyme 2 and that global psychologic symptoms, stress, and negative affectivity were associated with prostaglandin-endoperoxide synthase 1 (PTGS1) and amyloid-β (A4) precursor protein (APP), indicating new genetic pathways influencing the risk of TMDs.[25]

Although these findings need to be replicated in independent cohorts, the genes potentially represent important markers of risk for TMDs, and they identify potential targets for therapeutic intervention. For example, pain conditions resulting from low COMT activity and/or elevated catecholamine levels can be treated with pharmacologic agents that block both beta (2)- and beta (3)-adrenergic receptors. Adrenergic dysregulation has been seen in patients with TMDs or fibromyalgia,[177] and acute treatment with low-dose propranolol has led to short-term improvement. However, the clinical effectiveness of propranolol is dependent on the *COMT* haplotype.[116] These studies lead the way in establishing pharmacogenomics in the management of MFP.

Sleep disturbance

Associations between pain and sleep disturbance have been documented in several samples of patients with persistent pain, usually in association with depression.[324] Recent research suggests bidirectional interactions between the experience of pain and the process of sleep. Pain interferes with the ability to obtain sleep, and disrupted sleep contributes to enhanced pain perception. Moreover, it was recently suggested that poor sleep may interfere with endogenous pain modulation.[325,326] Some pain conditions, such as cluster headache and fibromyalgia, present with disturbed sleep as an expression of a common pathophysiology.

In general, pain severity seems to be a major parameter in the occurrence of disturbed sleep.[327] Indeed, pain disturbances and pain-related awakenings are common in persistent orofacial pain and are related to pain intensity.[328–330] Patients with MFP often report poor sleep and have been objectively shown to have poorer sleep quality than patients with painful TMJs or CDH.[145,151,239,331,332] These data suggest that in some patients with MFP, sleep disruption may not just be a result of the pain but, as in fibromyalgia, may form part of the disease process itself. Pain-related awakenings occur in about a quarter of patients with MFP and are related to pain intensity and the degree of muscle pain.[328] Primary insomnia has been associated with reduced mechanical and thermal pain thresholds in the orofacial muscles even after controlling for multiple potential confounders.[333] Chapter 5 specifically deals with the relationship between sleep and facial pain.

Comorbidities

MFP has been significantly associated with a number of comorbidities, such as irritable bowel syndrome,[334] fibromyalgia,[335,336] migraine,[337–339] vulvodynia,[145] and TTH.[340,341] Some patients with MFP present with widespread pain and some do not, and they seem to respond to therapy differently.[104] Some indications suggest that these comorbidities and MFP share a basic disorder in pain modulation and psychosocial factors. The study of these associations will no doubt shed new light on the pathophysiology of MFP. MFP is possibly a graded phenomenon from regional to widespread with other comorbidities; or alternatively there may be two subsets of MFP—people with and people without widespread pain and comorbidity.

Pathophysiology: Summary

Clearly, many factors may be active in the etiology of TMDs in general and MFP in particular (see Fig 8-6). Host susceptibility plays a role in MFP at a number of levels. Some patients may be more prone than others to develop trigger points secondary to muscle injury; that is, they may have a genetically influenced injury response. Other genetically influenced physical traits, such as pain modulation and pharmacogenomics, may then interact with psychologic traits to determine disease onset and progression and indeed whether pain develops. Additionally, environmental parameters such as ethnicity, culture, and stress are essential variables in the patient's coping abilities and demand for treatment. The effects of sex are paramount and may be expressed via interactions between hormones and nociceptive pathways as well as environmental and cultural issues.

Any of the etiologic agents discussed may contribute to MFP in one patient but not in another; some require a single etiologic factor and some a combination of etiologic factors to develop MFP in accordance with the suggestion of heterogenous multisystem dysregulations in TMD pain.[76] Clinicians, however, are still unable to accurately identify these factors in individual patients so as to tailor a focused, mechanism-based treatment plan.

Tension-Type Headaches

TTHs are extremely common, and most people will experience at least one in their lifetime. The IHS subclassifies TTH into episodic (infrequent and frequent), chronic, and probable TTH (see Tables 8-4 and 8-5). The individual attacks in these subentities have similar clinical features with some subtle differences; severity and the occurrence of mild nausea tend to increase with frequency. Pericranial muscle tenderness is an extremely common feature in patients with TTH, but because some patients do not demonstrate this feature, the IHS subclassifies TTH as with or without pericranial tenderness. Note that there is a perhaps somewhat overlapping diagnosis of headache attributed to TMD in accordance with the DC/TMD criteria[7] and the IHS criteria.

Epidemiology and genetics of TTH

Evidence indicates that TTH varies across continents and is most common in European countries.[342] In Europe, TTH has a 1-year prevalence in adults of more than 80%, an incidence that is higher than migraine, and a lifetime prevalence of more than 80%.[6] In North America, the prevalence is around 38%; taking world statistics together, the global prevalence of TTH is much lower at around 30%.[342]

European population studies indicate that infrequent episodic TTH that occurs on average once per month is most common (48% to 59%) but does not usually require medical attention.[343,344] One-year prevalence of frequent episodic TTH is 18% to 43%, and 10% to 25% report weekly headaches.[344,345]

The frequency and severity of TTH attacks are fundamental in estimating socioeconomic and personal impact. By definition, patients with frequent episodic TTH suffer more than one attack monthly but less than a headache every other day, which can have a significant effect on quality of life. Indeed, patients with frequent episodic TTH report missing, on average, 3 days of work per month.[346] In one study, 12% of patients with TTH reported absence from work during the previous year because of headache.[347] Considering the high prevalence of TTH, this is a significant problem. TTH, in particular chronic TTH, is thought to account for more than 10% of disease-related absenteeism in Denmark.[348] Chronic TTH has a profound negative effect on the well-being of patients and significantly reduces quality of life.[349]

The average onset age of TTH is 20 to 30 years, and peak prevalence is in the 30s to 50s.[343] However, up to 25% of schoolchildren report having TTH,[347] and in the older population (> 60 years), the prevalence is 20% to 30%. Postadolescent women are only slightly more affected than men (ratio of 5:4).[343,345]

Genetic studies reveal that first-degree relatives of sufferers of chronic TTH are three times as likely to also suffer headaches relative to the population.[350] This suggests that chronic TTH has important genetic factors. Frequent episodic TTH is significantly affected by environmental factors, and there is evidence for only a minor genetic contribution.[351] For example, it has been shown that variants of the COMT gene (see previous sections) do not contribute specifically to the predisposition to suffer from chronic TTH in children.

Episodic tension-type headache

Clinical features

Location. Episodic TTH is almost exclusively bilateral (> 90%) and is usually described as bandlike or caplike. It affects, in order of frequency, the occipital, parietal, temporal, and frontal areas (see Fig 8-2). Pain site may vary with intensity and among patients.[352]

Quality and severity. The vast majority of patients describe the quality of pain as pressure-like, dull, or a sensation of tightness. A throbbing character is rare in TTH, but it has been reported in 14% to 20% of patients, particularly during more severe attacks.[353]

Pain of TTH is considered milder than migraine pain, but the differences may not always be as striking as expected. Usually TTH is mild to moderate in intensity and graded at around 5 to 7 on a VAS,[354,355] but it may become moderate to severe with an increase in headache frequency. This is in contrast to the pattern observed in migraine, an all or none phenomena where pain severity is largely unaffected by headache frequency (see chapter 10). Many patients with TTH suffer from pain in the neck and shoulder muscles, and this increases in chronic TTH.[356]

Temporal pattern. The temporal features of individual episodic TTHs are extremely variable both within and among patients. TTH duration may range from 30 minutes to 7 days, and the reported median duration ranges from 4 to 13 hours.[346,357] The median frequency in the population ranges from one headache every 2 months to two headache days per month, whereas in a clinic population it is expectedly higher at 6 days per month.[346,354] The IHS classification lists five diagnostic criteria for episodic TTH (listed A through E), with the first criterion (A) distinguishing, by temporal features, between infrequent and frequent episodic TTH (Table 8-4).

Long-term follow-up indicates that most patients (75%) with episodic TTH continue to suffer episodic attacks, but 25% report evolving into chronic TTH.[345,358] However, in another study, 45% of patients with frequent episodic TTH or chronic TTH experienced remission over a follow-up period of 12 years, which suggests that some patients with TTH have a good long-term prognosis.[359] Negative prognostic factors for TTH included not being married, no physical activity, and poor sleep.[359] Episodic TTH is a chronic condition with an average duration before treatment of 9 to 12 years.[354,359]

Precipitating or aggravating factors. Episodic TTH is commonly precipitated by a number of factors; stress, fatigue, disturbed meals, menstruation, alcohol, and lack of sleep.[360,361] These are similar to those reported by migraineurs (see chapter 10).

TTH is usually not aggravated by physical activity.[352] This has been considered a major differentiating factor from migraine, with more than 95% of migraineurs reporting aggravation by exercise.[362] However, there are reports that exercise may aggravate pain in 16% to 28% of patients with TTH.[363,364]

Associated signs. A proportion of sufferers from episodic TTH experience significant disability related to pain severity, frequency, and accompanying features, such as poor sleep.[365] Sleep disturbances are common in persons with TTH,[366] and fatigue is reported very often. Lack of sleep is a common precipitant of TTH.

Accompanying symptoms are rare in the less frequent forms of TTH, but mild to moderate anorexia is reported by 18% of patients.[367] Occasional and mild photophobia (10%) or phonophobia (7%) has been observed.[352,367]

Many patients will suffer from both migraines and TTHs that may further affect quality of life. Interestingly, episodic TTH in migraine sufferers responds to sumatriptan, a migraine-specific drug, whereas in nonmigraine patients it does not.[368] This may suggest that mild migraines may be phenotypically very similar to episodic TTH (see chapter 10).

Chronic tension-type headache

Chronic TTH is one of the subtypes of a more recent diagnostic family simply termed *chronic daily headaches*. The umbrella diagnosis of CDH is based on the daily or near-daily occurrence of headaches.

see p. 226

225

Table 8-4	Diagnostic criteria for episodic TTH*	
Infrequent episodic TTH		**Notes**
A. At least 10 episodes of headache occurring on < 1 day per month on average (< 12 days per year) and fulfilling criteria B through D		Patients with TTH often present with clinical pericranial muscle tenderness. However, some patients do not, and the role of muscle tenderness and hyperactivity is unclear. Infrequent episodic TTH and frequent episodic TTH have therefore been subclassified as with or without pericranial tenderness.
Frequent episodic TTH		
A. At least 10 episodes occurring 1 to 14 days per month on average for > 3 months (≥ 12 and < 180 days per year) and fulfilling criteria B through D		
Both infrequent and frequent episodic TTH		
B. Headache lasting from 30 minutes to 7 days		
C. At least two of the following four characteristics: 1. Bilateral location 2. Pressing or tightening (nonpulsating) quality 3. Mild or moderate intensity 4. Not aggravated by routine physical activity, such as walking or climbing stairs		Accumulating evidence suggests that some TTHs may be aggravated by exercise (see text). The diagnostic difficulty most often encountered is to discriminate episodic TTH from mild migraine without aura. This is especially so because patients with frequent headaches often suffer from both disorders. Criteria D are very common in migraines.
D. Both of the following: 1. No nausea or vomiting 2. No more than one of photophobia or phonophobia		
E. Not better accounted for by another *International Classification of Headache Disorders,* third edition diagnosis		Secondary headache has been excluded by history, examination, and imaging if appropriate.

*Reproduced with permission from the International Headache Society.

Chronic daily headache   CDH

The diagnosis of CDH is based on specific criteria that have been shown to accurately classify most cases.[369] Most importantly, CDH is defined as headaches occurring on at least 15 days per month and may be subdivided into two forms: primary or secondary (attributable to specific pathology). The most common secondary type of CDH is medication-overuse headache (see chapter 14). Primary CDH may be short or long lasting (> 4 hours per attack) and include chronic migraine (see chapter 10); chronic trigeminal autonomic cephalalgias, including hemicrania continua (see chapter 11); chronic TTH; and new daily persistent headache (NDPH). The latter two entities are phenotypically similar and are described in this section. The diagnosis of NDPH is reserved for patients with daily headache and strictly no history of episodic migraine or episodic TTH. As most patients with daily headache have a tendency to abuse analgesics[370] that themselves potentially induce headache, the primary CDH must occur without drug abuse. The concept of CDH is clinically and epidemiologically useful, but because it represents a family of entities with different therapeutic responses, a specific diagnosis is essential for successful management.

The prevalence of CDH in the population, from children to the elderly, is about 2.5% to 5% and remains consistent across global studies.[347,371,372] Chronic TTH has a global prevalence of 2% to 3%,[344,345] and chronic migraine has been estimated to occur in 1.3% to 2.5% of the population (see chapter 10). Therefore, the vast majority of CDH patients in the population suffer from chronic TTH or chronic migraine. CDH is very common in headache clinics. In one study, 45% of 171 patients with a primary complaint of headache were diagnosed as suffering from CDH; 62% of them had chronic migraine, 34% had chronic TTH, 2.6% had NDPH, and 1.3% were diagnosed with hemicrania continua.[373] In pediatric headache clinics, CDH may be rare and account for about 5% of primary

CDH definition

Table 8-5	Diagnostic criteria for chronic TTH*
Diagnostic criteria	**Notes**
A. Headache occurring on ≥ 15 days per month on average for > 3 months (≥ 180 days per year), fulfilling criteria B through D	Chronic TTH evolves from episodic TTH. Chronic headache starting de novo should be classified as NDPH (see Table 8-7).
B. Headache lasting hours to days or unremitting	
C. At least two of the following four characteristics: 1. Bilateral location 2. Pressing/tightening (nonpulsating) quality 3. Mild or moderate intensity 4. Not aggravated by routine physical activity such as walking or climbing stairs	Chronic TTH is subdivided into with or without pericranial tenderness.
D. Both of the following: 1. No more than one of photophobia or phonophobia or mild nausea 2. Neither moderate/severe nausea nor vomiting	These criteria may complicate differentiation with chronic migraine (see chapter 10), and patients may need careful follow-up (pain diaries) to accurately diagnose their headaches. Chronic TTH is bilateral.
E. Not better accounted for by another *International Classification of Headache Disorders,* third edition diagnosis	Secondary headaches have been ruled out. Medication overuse is common in chronic headache and may lead to medication-overuse headache (see text and chapter 14).

*Reproduced with permission from the International Headache Society.

headaches.[374] Most studies demonstrate that 25% to 38% of patients with CDH are abusing analgesics.[375–377] This would require persistence of symptoms after cessation of drug abuse and before final diagnosis. Treatment of CDH depends on the specific diagnosis and is based on prophylactic regimens involving many classes of drugs (see chapters 10, 11, and 14 on the relevant disorders and chapters 16 and 17 on the drugs commonly used).

Clinical features of chronic TTH

Classically, the typical patient with chronic TTH is a middle-aged woman with a long headache history who originally had episodic headaches 10 to 20 years previously that slowly increased in frequency.[370,378,379] The clinical features of chronic TTH are largely similar to those in frequent episodic TTH, but there are differences in accompanying features, treatment response, and impact on quality of life (Table 8-5).

Location and quality. In 80% to 98% of patients, chronic TTH is bilateral and usually located in the frontal, temporal, or frontotemporal regions.[367,379,380] Headaches limited to the occipital region have also been reported.[381]

Pain quality is similar to that reported in episodic TTH and is mostly pressure-like and bilateral.[367] Severity of chronic TTH in population and clinic studies reveal that most patients (78%) suffer moderate pain, some (14.8% to 16%) mild, and very few (4% to 7.4%) severe.[367,382]

Temporal pattern. Chronic TTH is characterized by a continuous or daily headache. Mean frequency obtained from patient diaries is 23 to 30 headache days per month.[380,383]

Associated signs. Many patients with chronic TTH demonstrate increased pericranial tenderness in regional muscles. This is more severe in trapezius, neck, and sternocleidomastoid muscles but is also detectable in masseter and temporalis muscles.[384] Extracranial tenderness may also be present.[385] Headaches are often accompanied (32% of patients) by photophobia or phonophobia.[381] As reported for episodic TTH, physical activity may worsen pain in a subgroup of patients with chronic TTH.[367,382]

Persons who suffer from TTH report a lack of sufficient and restorative sleep, but this is a common finding in patients with chronic pain and may also be related to depression.[386] Indeed, as observed in other chronic pain conditions, depression and anxiety are common in patients with chronic TTH.[387]

Photophobia or phonophobia was reported by 17% of a population and 32% of subjects in a clinic-based study on patients with chronic TTH.[367,381] Nausea was reported by 25% of patients with chronic TTH in the population. Chronic TTH may be diagnosed in patients with only one of the conditions of photophobia, phonophobia, or mild nausea (see Table 8-5).[388]

Treatment of TTH

Patient education is essential, and there are websites that explain headaches and their treatment (eg, www.achenet.org/). The dangers of analgesic drug abuse must be made clear to the patient and every effort made to control it. Many patients with frequent episodic TTH or chronic TTH suffer from impaired function and quality of life, often accompanied by emotional distress and drug abuse that needs careful and professional attention.

Pharmacologic

The pharmacologic management of TTH may be subdivided into abortive (individually treat the acute attack) or prophylactic approaches; the choice depends on headache frequency, patient preference, and other factors. Abortive approaches are largely pharmacologic, whereas psychologic, physiotherapeutic, and TMD-aimed treatments have all been used in the prophylactic treatment of TTH with varying degrees of success. Abortive pharmacotherapy should not be used in chronic TTH because the high headache frequency may lead to analgesic abuse and medication-overuse headache (see chapter 14).

As abortive therapy, mild analgesics or NSAIDs have been consistently proven efficacious and are considered the first choice (Table 8-6). Mild headaches may respond favorably to 1 g of acetaminophen or aspirin.[389] Ibuprofen (200 to 400 mg) is superior to ac-

etaminophen and aspirin and provides better and faster pain relief.[390] Low-dose diclofenac is comparable with 400 mg of ibuprofen.[391] The more rapidly absorbed naproxen formulation, naproxen sodium (375 to 550 mg), is effective in TTH, and the higher dose was superior to 1 g of acetaminophen.[392] Overall, however, onset of pain relief is delayed in most of these drugs.[393] Based on efficacy and safety profiles, expert recommendations suggest ibuprofen or naproxen sodium as drugs of choice[393,394] (see Table 8-6). The exact dosages should be titrated individually according to response and adverse effects. Combination analgesics are often used but may offer small advantage over single drugs and may increase the risk of medication-overuse headache. However, caffeine at doses up to 200 mg has been proven to increase the efficacy of ibuprofen and other mild analgesics in the treatment of TTH, but caffeine carries a high addiction profile and should be carefully monitored.[395] In patients with chronic TTH, or coexisting migraine and episodic TTH, triptans have induced significant pain relief.[396,397]

Tricyclic antidepressants have been extensively studied as prophylactic agents and are superior to serotonin-selective agents in TTH.[398] Amitriptyline is consistently efficacious in prophylactically reducing frequency, duration, and severity of chronic TTH.[399] Interpreting these results and applying them to clinical practice and patient expectations require extreme care; often, statistically significant reductions in headache duration (eg, from 11 to 8 hours) may be of doubtful value to the patient.[12] Nevertheless, amitriptyline and other tricyclic antidepressants are widely used for chronic TTH. Indeed, amitriptyline is effective in chronic TTH but not in episodic TTH, which suggests different pathophysiologic mechanisms. Amitriptyline should be initiated at 10 mg daily taken just before bedtime (see chapter 17) and then titrated according to response and side effects. Studies on patients with chronic TTH show that a higher dose is often needed (75 mg).[12] Venlafaxine (150 mg/day), a serotonin noradrenaline reuptake inhibitor, may be a good second choice.[394] Based on the high frequency of pericranial muscle tenderness in TTH, investigators have tried muscle relaxants such as tizanidine with mixed results.[400]

Table 8-6   **Evidence-based recommendations for the abortive therapy of TTH***

Drug	Dose (mg)	Notes
Ibuprofen	200–800	Gastrointestinal irritation, bleeding risk
Aspirin	500–1,000	Gastrointestinal irritation, bleeding risk
Naproxen	275–825	Gastrointestinal irritation, bleeding risk
Acetaminophen	1,000	Hepatic considerations
Caffeine in analgesic combinations	65–200	Increased efficacy of ibuprofen and acetaminophen but addictive and increases risk of medication-overuse headache

*Reproduced with permission from the International Headache Society.

Nonpharmacologic interventions

Commonly used behavioral interventions for TTH include relaxation training, biofeedback training, and cognitive-behavioral (stress-management) therapy.[394,401] These treatments attempt to influence the frequency and severity of headaches and emphasize the prevention of headache episodes. Relaxation and EMG biofeedback therapies are effective mainly in episodic TTH and provide on average a 50% reduction in headache activity.[402] However, in patients with chronic TTH, the combination of stress management with a tricyclic antidepressant (amitriptyline ≤ 100 mg/day or nortriptyline ≤ 75 mg/day) was more likely to produce clinically significant reductions in headache index scores than each therapy alone or placebo.[403]

Physical or manual therapies are often integrated into the treatment plan of those suffering from TTH. Physiotherapy is more effective than massage therapy or acupuncture for the treatment of TTH and appears to be most beneficial for patients with a high frequency of headache episodes. Chiropractic manipulation may be beneficial for TTH, but the evidence is weak. Data are lacking regarding the efficacy of these treatments in reducing headache frequency, intensity, duration, and disability in many commonly encountered clinical situations. Many of the published case series and controlled studies are of low quality, and there is very little rigorous evidence clearly supporting the use of these modalities.[404]

Botulinum toxin injection has not been of any significant benefit to those suffering from TTH.[405] Repeated local lidocaine injections into the trigger points located in the pericrani-al muscles are reasonably effective in frequent episodic TTH and may be an alternative or adjunctive treatment.[355] Additionally, acupuncture has emerged as a valuable nonpharmacologic tool in patients with frequent episodic TTH or chronic TTH.[406]

Temporomandibular disorder therapies in the treatment of TTH. Interpretation of the relevant literature is hampered by the overwhelming majority of studies (> 95%) that are not randomized, controlled, or blinded. Uncontrolled studies show a reduction in severity and frequency of headaches after use of occlusal splints, occlusal adjustments, or physiotherapy.[407] With no placebo control and poor definition of headache types, these studies are of limited applicability. The newest version of the IHS and DC/TMD should help clinicians and researchers to better characterize and phenotype their patients with overlapping signs and symptoms of headache and TMDs. The use of stabilization splints in headache patients with concurrent TMDs resulted in a significant reduction in headache frequency and analgesic use relative to a group treated by a neurologist.[408] This would seem to make sense in that comprehensive treatment planning to include all pain-related problems is more likely to produce beneficial results. Moreover, the splint group was examined more often by the treating physician, which may have subconscious beneficial effects on treatment outcome. No significant effect of occlusal adjustment was observed on headache frequency.[409] The use of a new type of bite plate, the nociceptive trigeminal inhibition tension suppression system, for the treatment of migraines and TTH has recently been proposed.[89] The original studies were all open and have not been duplicated. Moreover, the nociceptive trigeminal inhibition tension suppression system provides occlusal contacts in the anterior region only and may, with overuse, cause permanent occlusal changes.

In summary, standard TMD therapies may help some patients with TTH, particularly those with concomitant MFP. However, as previously stated, irreversible destruction of tooth structure, as in occlusal adjustment, does not have enough evidence in the authors' view. In selected cases, a trial with a flat occlusal splint may be justified.

A later section has a brief discussion of NDPH as it represents a differential diagnosis to CDH and chronic TTH.

→p. 226

Pathophysiology of TTH. Interrelationships among peripheral and central mechanisms probably underlie the initiation of TTH, but the exact etiology is uncertain. Note that the same etiologic factors are considered in TTH and in MFP, which further suggests a common pathophysiology.

Pericranial muscles as a source of pain. Whether the presence of pericranial muscle tenderness is the cause or the result of the headache is unclear. Moreover, many patients with TTH present without pericranial myofascial tenderness. Notwithstanding, many patients with TTH display increased myofascial sensitivity, and this is considered important in the pathophysiology of this group of patients.[3,410]

Human experiments with intramuscular injection of algesic substances (usually hypertonic saline) induce pain and referral patterns characteristic of craniofacial myofascial conditions. Injections into the sternocleidomastoid and trapezius muscles produce localized pain with referral to regions associated with TTH location.[53,411–413] In contrast, injection into the masseter, medial, or lateral pterygoids refers pain to the teeth, angle of the mandible, and TMJ and resembles the pain pattern observed in MFP.[53,412] Quality and intensity of resultant pain do not differ significantly among injection sites. This would suggest a prominent role for muscle nociceptors in the location and referral patterns of reported pain in TTH and MFP. Pain-referral patterns also involve central convergence of peripheral afferents onto second-order neurons in the subnucleus caudalis, central sensitization with expansion of receptive fields,[414] and activation of convergent thalamic neurons.[415]

Muscle hyperactivity. Excessive contraction of pericranial muscles has been thought to play a major role in the pathophysiology of many myofascial disorders, including TTH. Pericranial muscle activity in patients with TTH has been shown to be variably normal or increased. Later studies have similarly been inconclusive, but in summary, there is no substantial evidence to support a causal relationship between pericranial muscle hyperactivity and TTH. Some patients with TTH do have increased muscle activity, but this may be in line with the protective mechanisms proposed by the pain adaptation model.[301] Moreover, contamination of EMG recordings by the muscles of facial expression is an important confounding variable.

p. 2

Experimental chewing (concentric exercises) with or without temporal artery ischemia induces a bilateral dull head pain.[416] TTH was induced by prolonged tooth clenching with muscle tenderness that preceded the onset of headache by several hours.[417] Prolonged experimental frontalis muscle contraction, however, failed to produce headaches in a group with relatively frequent TTHs.[418] Moreover, a further study on patients with TTH showed no significant differences in the induction of headache between active clenching and holding a toothpick between their lips as a control procedure.[419] Both groups, however, developed more headaches than did patients without TTH under the same experimental conditions. This would suggest that abnormalities in central pain transmission or modulation alter the susceptibility of patients to develop headache and are more important than muscle strain induced, for example, by jaw clenching. Similar conclusions may be derived from an experiment testing headache onset after static contraction of the trapezius muscle; although more patients with TTH developed headache than did control subjects, there was no significant difference in headache development between the active and the placebo procedure (tibial muscle contraction) in patients or control subjects.[420] Eccentric exercises are proposed to induce ultrastructural muscle damage and thus lead to inflammatory pain. This has been postulated to involve abnormalities in muscle blood flow, but experiments show this is normal in patients with chronic TTH.[421] During static contraction, diminished flow was noted but was unassociated with ischemia or inflammation.[421] Headache has been produced after various experimental muscle exercises but is usually short lasting, even after prolonged exercises.[422] Thus, the role of pericranial muscle tenderness in TTH remains unclear; in patients with TTH and muscle tenderness, it has been suggested that the mechanisms involve persistent nociceptive input leading to central sensitization that is negatively affected by faulty central modulation. This hypothesis is very similar to that proposed for MFP but leaves the origin of the peripheral nociceptive activity unanswered. Most likely, a combination of and interaction among several factors will be needed in accordance with the conceptual model presented in Fig 8-6. (p. 213)

Biopsychosocial parameters. The complex relationships between chronic pain and psychosocial pathology have been increasingly investigated, including in the field of headache. Significant psychopathology is observed in a minority of headache patients in the population, although those with significant problems are more likely to seek treatment for their headaches.[423] For example, patients with recurrent headaches (eg, TTH or migraines) exhibit significantly more psychiatric comorbidity.[424] Significant psychopathology complicates headache management and is associated with a reduced prognosis. People with recurrent TTH report more stressful events and judge them to have more impact on their lives.[425] Those suffering from TTH also seem to use different coping strategies for stress and pain.[425] However, there is little evidence of differences in physiologic responses to stressful events.[425] Recent findings suggest that stress contributes to headache, in part, by aggravating existing hyperalgesia.[426] Coping abilities have not been extensively studied in TTH, but catastrophizing may be more common in persons suffering from TTH. In summary, the cause-and-effect relationship between TTH and psychosocial problems is unclear but may affect treatment outcome.

Peripheral and central neural mechanisms. In both episodic TTH and chronic TTH,

there is a high proportion of patients with tenderness of the myofascial tissues (including tendons) that is present during and between attacks, which suggests peripheral sensitization.[419,427] Interestingly, muscle tenderness correlates with frequency and intensity of TTH, and often the relief of TTH is accompanied by reduced muscle tenderness.[428] Once again, the peripheral mechanism associated with these findings remains unclear.

However, it has been suggested that sensitivity in the pericranial muscles may be secondary to changes in the central nervous system. In a trial on the initiation of TTH by tooth clenching, it was found that patients with frequent episodic TTH who did not develop headache developed increased pressure-pain thresholds, which suggests that clenching activated their antinociceptive system.[417] Interestingly, the patients who did develop headache had no change in pressure-pain thresholds, which suggests that patients unable to recruit endogenous antinociceptive pathways are more likely to develop headache.[417] This lends support to the hypothesis that muscle tenderness may be secondary to central sensitization and/or faulty supraspinal inhibitory or facilitatory mechanisms.[429] The presence of central sensitization in chronic TTH is supported by findings of increased sensitivity to pressure, electrical stimuli, and thermal stimuli at craniofacial and general body sites.[384,430] In most studies, pain detection and tolerance thresholds are also reduced in patients with chronic TTH.[384,430] In contrast, patients with episodic TTH, other than those with frequent episodic TTH, demonstrate normal pain-detection thresholds.[357,431] In chronic TTH, there is a significant correlation between generalized sensitivity and pericranial tenderness.[384,432] Because chronic TTH is most often a progression from frequent episodic TTH, it is likely that central sensitization in patients with chronic TTH is induced by prolonged nociceptive inputs from myofascial tissues.[433] Increased pain sensitivity seems to accompany the transformation of episodic TTH to chronic TTH, but it is most likely a result rather than the cause of increased headaches.[434,435] Impairment of endogenous supraspinal pain-modulation systems after experimental pain has been shown in patients with chronic TTH,[436,437] and there is significant gray-matter decrease in regions known to be

CS
∅.
P. ☐
237

CATASTROPHIZING P. 106

Table 8-7 **Diagnostic criteria for NDPH***

Diagnostic criteria	Notes
A. Persistent headache fulfilling criteria B and C	Headache is daily from onset and very soon unremitting. Prior headache is not contraindicated, but onset of NDPH is not preceded by increasing frequency of migraine or TTH.
B. Distinct and clearly remembered onset, with pain becoming continuous and unremitting within 24 hours	Essential for accurate diagnosis. If headache evolves from TTH, the diagnosis should be chronic TTH.
C. Headache present for > 3 months	There are two subforms: a self-limiting subform that typically resolves within several months without therapy, and a refractory form that is resistant to aggressive treatment regimens.
D. Not better accounted for by another *International Classification of Headache Disorders,* third edition diagnosis	Secondary headaches have been ruled out. Medication overuse is common in chronic headache and may lead to medication-overuse headache (see text).

*Reproduced with permission from the International Headache Society.

involved in pain processing.[438] The evidence thus suggests that peripheral mechanisms play a major role in episodic TTH, whereas central mechanisms such as faulty inhibitory mechanisms and central sensitization are prominent in chronic TTH.

New daily persistent headache. The NDPH type of chronic headache was previously termed *chronic headache with acute onset.* Presentation may be heterogenous, as exemplified by case studies.[439] The headache, as defined by the IHS, must become chronic within 3 days of onset (Table 8-7), and this is the major differentiating feature in relation to chronic TTH[388] (compare with Tables 8-4 and 8-5). In the current definition, patients with a history of migraine or TTH are not excluded from the diagnosis of NDPH, but the NDPH headache should take on a sudden daily frequency without any gradual increase in frequency of the underlying headache.[3,440]

Clinical features

Location

Pain is bilateral in most patients.[441–443] Location involves the temporal region alone (20% of patients) or in combination with other sites (46% of patients). In one series, retro-orbital pain was reported by 40% of patients.[441] Occipital areas are involved in 40% to 60% of cases, and a minority will describe pain throughout the head.[441]

Quality and severity

Pressure (54%) and throbbing (10% to 55%) qualities are the individual descriptors most commonly reported.[441,442] Pain quality is varied, and many patients describe their pain with combinations of descriptors such as pressure and tightening (73%).[442] Stabbing (45%), aching (43%), dull (37%), and tightness (36%) are also frequently used. More rarely, burning (23%) or searing (4%) pain is reported.

Most patients (66%) report headache severity as usually moderate (4 to 6 on a 10-cm VAS); some (21%), however, report persistently severe pain (> 6 VAS).[441] In a series of 30 Japanese patients with NDPH, all reported severe unbearable pain.[442] These cases excluded post-viral cases (discussed later), so the differences in pain severity may reflect a diagnostic subgroup or cultural differences.[442]

Temporal features

Many patients can accurately recall the exact date of headache onset with a subsequently rapid progression to chronic pain (< 3 days).[441]

Vertigo (handwritten)

TopAMAX – Broad Spectrum Anti-convulsant (handwritten)

Tension-Type Headaches

The vast majority will report headache that is present continuously, but about one-fifth suffer from a daily headache lasting a number of hours.[441,442] More recent characterization of these patients suggests they may be subdivided based on temporal pattern and prognosis: *(1)* persistent type with a continuous headache from onset, *(2)* remitting type with complete resolution of headaches that occur fewer than 5 days per month for 3 months, and *(3)* relapsing-remitting type with pain-free breaks between bouts of continuous headache.[444]

Headache onset

Flu (handwritten)

A recent infection or flulike illness is reported in 30% of patients.[441] Extracranial surgery (12%) or a stressful life event (12% to 20%) are also common precipitators, but 46% to 80% of patients had no identifiable precipitating factors.[441,442] One series excluded patients with post-viral NDPH, so the contribution of viral infections to NDPH onset and phenotype remains unclear.[442]

Accompanying signs/symptoms

Associated migrainous symptoms may be present in more than 50% of patients.[445,446] These include nausea or vomiting, phonophobia, and photophobia.[441,442,447] Other more general symptoms include lightheadedness, stiff neck, blurred vision, and vertigo. Aura-type symptoms have been observed in a small fraction of patients.[441] Patients with NDPH commonly report a history of anxiety/panic disorder and/or depression.[444,448]

Vertigo P. 189 (handwritten)

Aggravating/relieving factors

Stress, physical exertion, and bright light were reported as aggravating factors in a third to 40% of patients.[441] Headache relief was obtained by lying down in two-thirds of patients or by being in a dark room by almost half of patients.[441] Massage relieved pain in about a quarter and sleep only in a minority of patients (9%).[441]

Epidemiology

Based on available studies, a female preponderance is apparent.[441,442] Age of onset in women (20s to 30s) occurs earlier than in men (50s).[441]

As discussed previously, CDH has a prevalence of about 2.5% to 5% in the general population. In a Spanish population, NDPH was found in 0.1% of patients and formed only 2% to 6.7% of all the cases of CDH identified.[375,449] In specialist clinics, the proportion of CDH cases diagnosed as NDPH increases to 11% to 14%.[370,450]

Treatment

NDPH seems to have two subgroups: those refractory to treatment[442] and those who have a benign progression and will improve, with or without therapy, within a few months.[3,440] Complete resolution was reported in 86% of male patients and 73% of female patients over a period of 2 years.

Specifically for patients with post-viral NDPH, early treatment with methylprednisone may be effective.[451] Based on case reports, botulinum toxin may provide relief for some patients.[440,452]   *229* (handwritten)

Elevated levels of tumor necrosis factor alpha in the cerebrospinal fluid (CSF) of patients with NDPH led to a successful trial of doxycycline and subsequently nimodipine (anti–tumor necrosis factor alpha properties).[440,453]

Anecdotal evidence suggests that the novel antiepileptic drugs, such as gabapentin and topiramate, may be useful in the prophylactic treatment of NDPH.[440] Using a stepped approach that began with muscle relaxants and progressed through tricyclic antidepressants, selective serotonin reuptake inhibitors, and antiepileptic drugs, it was found that 30% of patients graded the result as moderate or very improved, but only two patients were cured.[442] The drugs that were moderately to very successful were tricyclic antidepressants in 33% of patients and antiepileptic drugs or muscle relaxants in 22% of patients each.[442] However, gabapentin and topiramate were not tested.

Positive findings for the use of naratriptan for the treatment of CDH, including some patients that may have had NDPH, suggest its utility in the treatment of NDPH.[454–456] Naratriptan was used for 3 months to 1 year in these patients.

Differential diagnosis

NDPH is phenotypically similar to chronic TTH, but onset of NDPH is independent of episod-

Blurred Vision (handwritten)

HSV   CMV

ic TTH or migraine that increases in frequency, and NDPH may be very refractory to treatment.[457] Both NDPH and hemicrania continua are continuous from onset. Hemicrania continua is usually accompanied by ipsilateral autonomic signs and responds to treatment with indomethacin.

A number of disorders may also give rise to NDPH-like headaches.[458,459] Low CSF-volume headache is commonly encountered after lumbar puncture and is characteristically relieved by bed rest. Patients with chronic CSF leaks may report a history of lumbar puncture or epidural injection or vigorous exercises that involve strong Valsalva maneuvers (eg, lifting heavy objects). Headache is absent on waking and worsens during the day; lying down rapidly improves pain. Magnetic resonance imaging with gadolinium enhancement will usually identify the leak. Raised CSF pressure may occur secondary to tumors and induce headache. Subarachnoid hemorrhage may be present with a normal or near normal neurologic examination and cause headache of moderate to severe intensity. Onset of subarachnoid hemorrhage headache may be instantaneous in about half of patients or develop over about 5 minutes.[458] Benign thunderclap headache is also of sudden onset, reaching maximum intensity within 30 seconds. The headache may last several hours, but a less severe headache may persist for weeks. Some consider benign thunderclap headache to be symptomatic of subarachnoid hemorrhage, cervical artery dissection (see chapter 14), or cerebral venous thrombosis.[388] These entities should therefore be excluded in patients suspected of secondary NDPH.

Pathophysiology

Because about one-third of patients describe a viral illness before headache onset, it has been hypothesized that NDPH has an infectious etiology. In support, more than 80% of patients with NDPH had evidence of active Epstein-Barr virus infection, a percentage significantly higher than in control subjects.[460] More than 60% of patients with NDPH were actively excreting Epstein-Barr virus in the oropharynx. Past but not active Epstein-Barr virus infection was found in five of seven patients tested in a later study.[441] Other viral infections, such as recent herpes simplex virus infection and cytomegalovirus, have also been identified in patients with NDPH.[461] Moreover, bacterial agents have been associated with NDPH, but the highly frequent reports of fever (34.2%) and painful cervical lymphadenopathy (56.5%) reported in other studies suggests that this may be a distinct subgroup.[462] In a pediatric population with NDPH, 43% reported onset of their symptoms during an infection, and positive Epstein-Barr virus serology was detected in half of these. However, how a viral infection leads to NDPH is unclear. Some suggest that subclinical meningitis may be involved,[458] and in support, new onset headache after meningitis is quite common.[463]

Minor head injuries (23%) and surgery were also common precipitators of headaches, which suggests that posttraumatic mechanisms may also be involved (see chapter 12). Stressful life events are also frequently reported in patients with NDPH, but it is unclear how these cause onset of headache.

In view of the heterogenous presentation of NDPH, the unreliable response to treatment, and the relationship between onset and a variable list of triggers, it has been suggested that NDPH be viewed as a syndrome rather than a discrete disorder.[464]

Headache, Myofascial Pains, and Fibromyalgia

Masticatory muscle pain has been suggested to be a localized expression of a spectrum of myofascial disorders with many similarities among MFP, TTH, and fibromyalgia; it is not unusual that these entities coexist in patients.[465] Indeed, the segregation of MFP from other myofascial pain disorders of a more generalized type, such as fibromyalgia, has been questioned.[466] The new DC/TMD[7] has suggested a distinction among local myalgia, myofascial pain, and myofascial pain with referral based on the response to standardized palpation of the masseter and temporalis muscle: In local myalgia there is only pain specifically located to the site of palpation, in myofascial pain there is a spread of pain on palpation but within the boundaries of the muscle being palpated, and myofascial pain with referral is linked to a spread of pain outside the boundaries of the muscle during palpation. One simple view could be that there is a progression from myalgia to myofascial pain to myofascial pain with referral and therefore that the suggested subdivision of MFP may represent different stages and pathophysiologic mechanisms, perhaps with clinical implications. However, another view is that pain spreading/referral could represent epiphenomena of deep nociceptive activity. Further studies are needed to address these issues.

TMDs, fibromyalgia, and some headaches are characterized by central sensitization and have been termed *central sensitivity syndromes*. These central sensitivity syndromes also include irritable bowel syndrome, restless legs syndrome, chronic fatigue syndrome, and other similar chronic painful conditions that are based on central sensitization.[467]

Headache and masticatory myofascial pain

Headache has been reported to be more common in adult patients with TMDs than in those without,[235,468] but often these results are not replicated in other studies or age groups.[469] Patients suffering from headache and those suffering from MFP show great similarities and possible overlap. Age distribution, female preponderance, and contributing psychophysiologic mechanisms are shared. Muscle tenderness is a frequent finding in patients with migraine and TTH, the distribution of which may be distinctly similar to that in patients with MFP. Thus, two of the fundamental symptoms of MFP—daily occurrence of pain and tenderness of muscles to palpation—fail to properly differentiate between patients with headache and those with MFP.

Migraineurs suffer no more TMDs than control subjects, and this association does not change with increasing frequency of migraine.[470] The rate of migraine in patients with MFP does not differ from that in the general population, so patients with MFP and those with migraine seem to be separate groups.[471] Children with migraine and migraine-type headaches were recently shown to have the highest incidence of more severe TMD signs.[469,472] Mi-

graine sufferers have been found to report significantly more clenching habits that may relate to some forms of muscle pain.[473] An association between migraine and MFP is not clearly apparent; pathophysiology and clinical presentation are distinctly different. The role that neurovascular mechanisms, such as neurogenic inflammation, play in MFP is not entirely clear. Vascular headache is rapid eye movement locked, and some data point to a rapid eye movement–locked destructive form of bruxism that may link certain forms of muscle pain with vascular mechanisms.[474,475] Moreover, recent associations between migraine and fibromyalgia suggest that a relationship with MFP may yet become apparent.[476]

In spite of stated similarities, most patients with MFP have pain and muscle tenderness on palpation unilaterally, whereas TTH and fibromyalgia are predominantly bilateral pain conditions. Patients with TMDs report headaches significantly more frequently and of higher severity,[468] and patients with MFP report a significantly higher incidence of TTH than control subjects.[144] Limited evidence supports a finding of masticatory muscle tenderness (possibly equivalent to MFP) in patients with TTH. However, there is considerable overlap in the tender muscles needed for the diagnosis of MFP and TTH, and this may suggest that MFP and TTH share pathophysiologic mechanisms and often coexist. Therefore, there is no convincing evidence for the role of TMDs in the initiation of TTH. However, both the DC/TMD and IHS criteria include a diagnostic subgroup termed *headache attributed to TMD* (see Table 8-1).

Fibromyalgia

Diagnosis

Fibromyalgia is a common condition characterized by widespread pain.[477] In the past, diagnosis was made based on the physical finding of at least 11 points of tenderness out of the 18 anatomical sites defined by the American College of Rheumatology.[478] More recently, these criteria have been revised, and the need for tender points as a central element in diagnosis has been removed.[479] Additionally, the new criteria introduce a quantitative measure of the number of sites with pain, termed the *widespread pain index* (WPI), and a measure of the severity of symptoms associated with fibromyalgia, the symptom severity scale (SSS). The WPI is the number of painful areas reported by the patient from a list of 19 sites, so the score may vary from 0 to 19. Notably, physical examination is no longer required for diagnosis but is strongly recommended.[480] The SSS is derived from the sum of a 0 to 3 scoring on the severity of associated fatigue, waking unrefreshed, cognitive symptoms, and the overall extent of somatic symptoms (scores thus range from 0 to 12). Importantly, these criteria recognize fibromyalgia as a disease spectrum with altering and fluctuating symptoms.[481] A diagnosis is justified when the WPI ≥ 7 and the SSS ≥ 5, or the WPI = 2–3 and the SSS ≥ 9. In addition, symptoms have been present for 3 months or more and no better diagnosis explains the patient's symptoms. These new criteria have not met with universal acceptance but have been widely applied.[482] The Research Criteria, a self-report version of the 2010 criteria, was developed for research purposes,[483] and there is strong evidence that it accurately identifies fibromyalgia as diagnosed by clinicians. These criteria have comfortably combined the WPI and the SSS into one scale, the polysymptomatic distress scale (PSD). This removes the need to calculate the ranges of the WPI and SSS; the case definition is then a PSD score ≥ 12.[483]

Without a clear diagnostic biomarker, fibromyalgia remains controversial.[56,484] Moreover, the boundaries between fibromyalgia and regional myofascial pains, such as MFP, are at times poorly demarcated in spite of established criteria. A major differentiating feature between fibromyalgia and regional myofascial pain is the presence of trigger points and a palpable band of tight muscle in regional myofascial pain as opposed to multiple tender points in fibromyalgia. For MFP, trigger points are not an integral part of the RDC/TMD or DC/TMD criteria. By definition, trigger points, on palpation, refer pain to a distant site, but this condition for trigger points has been suggested as unnecessary, and trigger points may be considered active or latent, which further clouds the boundaries between regional myofascial pain and fibromyalgia. Moreover, only regional pain and tenderness have been validated in fibromyalgia and regional myofascial pain; the presence of

trigger points may be unnecessary.[485] The other basic difference is the chronic, widespread, systemic character of fibromyalgia as opposed to the acute, localized nature of myofascial pains. However, fibromyalgia often begins as a localized pain disorder and later becomes widespread, whereas persistent myofascial pains may involve multiple sites and cause systemic symptoms.[486] Many of the perpetuating factors in myofascial pains are the modulating factors of fibromyalgia: physical activity, cold, stress, and weather changes. Indeed, it has been suggested that fibromyalgia and regional myofascial pains represent an overlapping spectrum.[465]

Clinical features

Fibromyalgia symptomatology is complex and affects multiple modalities; widespread pain is universal, but other common complaints include fatigue (75% to 90%), a feeling of swelling or paresthesia (50% each), vertigo (60%), nonrestorative sleep (70%), and psychologic symptoms (60%).

Pain in fibromyalgia is usually located in the lower back, neck, shoulder, arms, hands, hips, thighs, knees, legs, and feet. Complaints of joint pains may accompany fibromyalgia and may be the prominent feature in some patients. In the vast majority (85%) of patients with fibromyalgia, pain is accompanied by stiffness, particularly in the morning. Both pain and stiffness are aggravated by cold or humid weather, anxiety or stress, inactivity, and poor sleep. Fatigue, usually expressed by patients as feeling drained, is correlated to pain and poor sleep.[487,488]

Paresthesias and swelling usually affect the extremities and need careful neurologic examination. Vertigo or dizziness is considered to be central in origin and may be accompanied by phonophobia or tinnitus. Sleep disturbances include difficulties in falling asleep (increased sleep latency), waking up during the night (decreased sleep efficiency), and feeling tired in the morning (nonrefreshing sleep). Poor sleep correlates with pain, psychologic distress, and fatigue.[489,490] Anxiety, depression, and stress are prevalent in patients with fibromyalgia, and psychologic distress correlates with disease severity.[491] Rarer signs include Raynaud phenomenon, symptoms similar to those in Sjögren syndrome, and cognitive dysfunction. In established fibromyalgia cases, long-term follow-up shows that there is usually no further deterioration in symptomatology.[492]

Studies indicate that the vast majority (84%) of patients with fibromyalgia suffer a significant medical comorbidity.[493] Most commonly, they have other musculoskeletal conditions (67%), psychologic disorders (35%), gastrointestinal disorders (27%), cardiovascular disorders (23.5%), and endocrinologic disorders (19%). Patients with fibromyalgia are two to seven times more likely to have one or more of the following comorbid conditions: depression, anxiety, headache, irritable bowel syndrome, chronic fatigue syndrome, systemic lupus erythematosus, and rheumatoid arthritis.[494]

Epidemiology

The point prevalence of fibromyalgia is about 2.7%; women (4.1%) are affected more than men (1.4%),[487,495] and its prevalence increases with age.[481,493] Most commonly, fibromyalgia occurs in women aged 40 to 60 years.[496]

Risk factors and pathophysiology

The pathophysiology of fibromyalgia remains unclear.[497] However, the risk of developing symptoms is significantly affected by a number of factors, including physical trauma, sleep disturbance, psychologic distress, socioeconomic status, lifestyle, genetics, and dysfunctional pain modulation.[497] Fibromyalgia onset is often linked to a preceding viral infection or mental stress.[498]

Fibromyalgia may begin as a regional pain. In a prospective trial, back pain predicted fibromyalgia, whereas tender points and pain in the neck did not. Self-assessed depression, long-lasting pain, and the presence of three or more associated symptoms were significant predictors for progression.[499]

Lack of consistent peripheral tissue abnormalities has shifted the focus to the central nervous system as a source of pain and other features in fibromyalgia. Many patients display paresthesias, allodynia, augmented central nervous system processing of pain (central sensitization), and a deficit of endogenous pain

inhibition, all of which are characteristic of neuropathic pain.[336,500] In support, imaging studies suggest that there is less functional connectivity in areas of the descending pain modulatory system.[501,502] Studies provide moderate evidence for increased activation of the pain matrix and lowered pain thresholds.[501] Specific decreases in gray matter volume with unchanged global gray matter are difficult to establish as a cause-and-effect relationship.[501,502] However, clinical pain is correlated to the level of gray matter loss in the medial frontal gyrus.[502] Other consequences of these changes are unclear, but patients with fibromyalgia experience more gray matter loss per year than control subjects with possible deterioration in cognitive function and pain processing.[502] However, a peripheral nociceptive input from sensitized nociceptors in deep tissues and muscle may produce all the observed central effects.[503] In view of the evidence, a peripheral input in the pathophysiology of fibromyalgia cannot be ruled out.

Patients with fibromyalgia have increased neural sympathetic activation and lack an adequate sympathetic response to stressor or cardiovascular challenges.[167,171] The data suggest that fibromyalgia may be a generalized form of sympathetically maintained neuropathic pain. As suggested, an alternative description for fibromyalgia could be neuroplastic pain in order to differentiate it from the recently proposed definition of neuropathic pain with emphasis on a lesion or disease of the somatosensory system and avoidance of the term *dysfunction*.[504] Dysfunction of the hypothalamic-pituitary-adrenal axis is thought to partly underlie sleep disorders, some pain symptoms, and autonomic nervous system imbalance.[171]

HPA

Management

Many pharmacologic and nonpharmacologic approaches have been used to treat fibromyalgia. Treatment aims at controlling pain and associated signs and improving functional and psychologic disability. Nonpharmacologic management involves the initiation of an aerobic exercise program, relaxation, CBT, and pacing (matching activity to pain levels).[505] Tricyclic or other antidepressants and antiepileptic drugs are probably the most effective pharmacologic agents.[505–507] Combining these with aerobic

p. 32

Cognitive-Behavioral Therapy — p. 107

exercise and CBT may increase efficacy.[508] Acupuncture, hypnosis/guided imagery, and tai chi may offer relief for some patients and are recommended modalities.[509] Novel therapies that may find a place in the management of fibromyalgia include cannabinoids and sodium oxybate.[510]

Pot !

GHB

Temporomandibular disorders and fibromyalgia

Early reports on MFP/fibromyalgia comorbidity suggested that a connection might exist between these entities. Fibromyalgia, by definition, is characterized by widespread pain, so it is not surprising that many patients with fibromyalgia have signs of MFP. Additionally, pain outside the craniofacial region is common among patients with TMDs. Some patients with MFP (18%) have signs suggestive of fibromyalgia, and up to 75% of patients with fibromyalgia demonstrate comorbid MFP.[43,335,467,511–513] Female patients with widespread pain are at significantly increased risk of developing TMDs, which suggests that TMDs may be related, and in continuum, to generalized muscle disorders.[144,514] Indeed, patients with fibromyalgia, regional myofascial pain such as MFP, and chronic fatigue syndrome share many clinical features, including myalgia, fatigue, and disturbed sleep, which suggests a common etiology.[515] Additionally, patients with fibromyalgia and TMDs have significantly elevated prevalence rates of irritable bowel syndrome, sleep disturbances, and concentration difficulties.[516] Fatigued patients are four times more likely to suffer from TMDs than nonfatigued twin control subjects. Thus, fatigue and fatigue-related symptoms are common in TMDs but are also frequently reported by all patients with chronic pain and are probably related to somatization and depression.[517]

In many cases of MFP, muscle tenderness affects many sites in the head and neck, but trigger points may be hard to find. These patients often have tender points and characteristics associating them with fibromyalgia (eg, disturbed sleep, anxiety, and general fatigue). When the symptoms of patients with fibromyalgia are compared with those of patients with MFP, no symptoms are specific to MFP, which suggests that such local conditions of myofascial pain should be compiled to form one entity. Focusing on the one region in which pain is greatest may account for a restricted diagnosis, such as MFP, when in effect this disorder can be a local symptom of a more generalized condition. Findings of faulty pain processing in patients with MFP would seem to support this contention.[148,150] However, not surprisingly, patients with TMDs are distinguishable from patients with fibromyalgia by a high prevalence of masticatory muscle tenderness and a reduced prevalence of fatigue, muscle weakness, migratory arthralgias, and burning or shooting muscle pains.[516] Patients with fibromyalgia may also demonstrate lower pain thresholds and lower tolerance levels to experimental facial pain than patients with TMDs, which suggests differential processing of external stimuli.[158] The vast majority of patients with fibromyalgia (94%) reported local pain from the temporomandibular region, most frequently the temple, the TMJ, and the neck.[518] About 50% of the patients complained about difficulties in jaw movements, and about three-quarters reported tiredness of the jaws. Generalized body pain had a significantly longer duration than the onset of TMD symptoms, suggesting that fibromyalgia starts in other parts of the body and later extends to the masticatory system. In a large study, jaw pain was found in 35.4% of patients with fibromyalgia and in about 19% each of patients with osteoarthritis and rheumatoid arthritis.[519] Jaw pain is associated with disease severity and the presence of jaw pain in patients with fibromyalgia, correlated with a significantly reduced quality of life relative to fibromyalgia without jaw pain.[519]

Female patients (n = 162) with a previous diagnosis of MFP were reexamined 7 years later to elicit a history of comorbid fibromyalgia.[520] Thirty-eight patients (23.5%) had a positive history of fibromyalgia but showed no difference in presenting signs and symptoms relating to MFP. However, patients with a positive history of fibromyalgia reported more MFP symptoms accompanied by more severe pain and increased emotional distress. In conclusion, increased chronicity was observed for patients with MFP and comorbid fibromyalgia, which also seemed to be more resistant to occlusal splint treatment.[104]

The data suggest similarities between MFP and generalized muscle disorders.[76,145] Although it is clear that in many cases MFP is a local pain condition with minimal complaints in other areas of the body, many patients present with complaints suggestive of a generalized widespread disorder. Possibly, there are two distinct MFP subgroups (with and without fibromyalgia/widespread pain), or the MFP phenotype may be part of a spectrum of a possible progression to fibromyalgia. However, which patients with MFP progress to fibromyalgia remains unclear.

Headache and fibromyalgia

The prevalence of fibromyalgia in patients attending a headache clinic with a diagnosis of primary headache was between 6.9% and 59%.[493] Data indicate that TTH is most commonly associated with fibromyalgia.[521] Similarities have been observed in the distribution of muscle tender points between patients with recurrent headache and those with fibromyalgia. A bidirectional association between fibromyalgia and TTH is suggested by the finding that twins with chronic TTH have 6.6 times more fibromyalgia and patients with fibromyalgia have 5.0 times more chronic TTH.[522] In patients with concomitant CDH and fibromyalgia, there was significantly more insomnia and more incapacitating headaches than in headache patients without fibromyalgia.[523] Within CDH, both migrainous and nonmigrainous headaches have been similarly associated with generalized muscle pains.[524] The most significant headache parameter associated with muscle pain was headache frequency and not headache diagnosis. These findings may indicate that musculoskeletal pains and chronic headaches (irrespective of diagnosis) may share central sensitization as a common etiologic factor.[521,524] In this and further studies, a highly significant correlation was found between headaches and muscle pain in the upper body area, which may suggest segmental effects.

Data on central nervous system dysregulation and widespread allodynia in migraine (see chapter 10) suggest that in some patients migraine may form part of more widespread pain disorders, such as fibromyalgia. Migraines occur frequently in patients with fibromyalgia.[525] Conversely, fibromyalgia was found in 36% of patients with transformed migraine, and the comorbidity was predicted by concomitant depression and insomnia.[526] A recent study on 100 patients with fibromyalgia found that 76% had headaches, most of which began before onset of fibromyalgia,[476] and the most common headache diagnosis was migraine alone or in combination with TTH. Characteristics of fibromyalgia patients with headache were not different from those without headache, so that they are not a distinct subgroup. The data suggest that migraine may form part of the fibromyalgia phenotype. Based on the data showing considerable overlap among migraine, MFP, fibromyalgia, and TTH, comorbidity in any given patient is highly likely.

Future of MFP

In this chapter, the current knowledge of MFP pathophysiology and treatment implications have been reviewed; however, it is evident that although the field has progressed substantially over the past decades, there are still significant gaps in the understanding of the neurobiologic mechanisms involved in the efficacy of treatment. The ultimate goal is to provide mechanism-specific diagnosis of MFP and its overlapping phenotypic representations followed by individualized management. A major challenge is the integration of all the detailed research-based information on the multiple dimensions of pain into a sufficiently simple clinical context. A better understanding of the interactions and relative timing and significance of multiple risk factors is needed in order to build treatment algorithms based on underlying mechanisms. Important steps have been taken to allow this progression. First, the taxonomic classifications of TMDs and headaches have improved, and second, longitudinal studies have been undertaken that may pave the road for further insights into MFP.

References

1. Peck CC, Goulet JP, Lobbezoo F, et al. Expanding the taxonomy of the diagnostic criteria for temporomandibular disorders. J Oral Rehabil 2014;41:2–23.
2. Schiffman EL, Velly AM, Look JO, et al. Effects of four treatment strategies for temporomandibular joint closed lock. Int J Oral Maxillofac Surg 2014;43:217–226.

3. Headache Classification Subcommittee of the International Headache Society. The International Classification of Headache Disorders, 3rd Edition (beta version). Cephalalgia 2013;33:629–808.

4. Dworkin SF, LeResche L. Research diagnostic criteria for temporomandibular disorders: Review, criteria, examinations and specifications, critique. J Craniomandib Disord 1992;6:301–355.

5. Ohrbach R, Turner JA, Sherman JJ, et al. The Research Diagnostic Criteria for Temporomandibular Disorders. IV: Evaluation of psychometric properties of the Axis II measures. J Orofac Pain 2010;24:48–62.

6. Lyngberg AC, Rasmussen BK, Jørgensen T, Jensen R. Incidence of primary headache: A Danish epidemiologic follow-up study. Am J Epidemiol 2005;161:1066–1073.

7. Schiffman E, Ohrbach R, Truelove E, et al. Diagnostic Criteria for Temporomandibular Disorders (DC/TMD) for clinical and research applications: Recommendations of the International RDC/TMD Consortium Network and Orofacial Pain Special Interest Group. J Oral Facial Pain Headache 2014;28:6–27.

8. John MT, Dworkin SF, Mancl LA. Reliability of clinical temporomandibular disorder diagnoses. Pain 2005;118:61–69.

9. Leher A, Graf K, PhoDuc JM, Rammelsberg P. Is there a difference in the reliable measurement of temporomandibular disorder signs between experienced and inexperienced examiners? J Orofac Pain 2005;19:58–64.

10. Futarmal S, Kothari M, Ayesh E, Baad-Hansen L, Svensson P. New palpometer with implications for assessment of deep pain sensitivity. J Dent Res 2011;90:918–922.

11. Benoliel R, Birman N, Eliav E, Sharav Y. The International Classification of Headache Disorders: Accurate diagnosis of orofacial pain? Cephalalgia 2008;28:752–762.

12. Fumal A, Schoenen J. Chronic tension-type headache. In: Goadsby PJ, Silberstein SD, Dodick D, (eds). Chronic Daily Headache. Hamilton: BC Decker, 2005:57–64.

13. Benoliel R, Sharav Y. Tender muscles and masticatory myofascial pain diagnosis: How many or how much? J Orofac Pain 2009;23:300–301.

14. LeResche L. Epidemiology of temporomandibular disorders: Implications for the investigation of etiologic factors. Crit Rev Oral Biol Med 1997;8:291–305.

15. Yap AU, Dworkin SF, Chua EK, List T, Tan KB, Tan HH. Prevalence of temporomandibular disorder subtypes, psychologic distress, and psychosocial dysfunction in Asian patients. J Orofac Pain 2003;17:21–28.

16. Slade GD, Bair E, Greenspan JD, et al. Signs and symptoms of first-onset TMD and sociodemographic predictors of its development: The OPPERA Prospective Cohort Study. J Pain 2013;14(12, suppl):T20–T32;e21–e23.

17. Magnusson T, Egermark I, Carlsson GE. A longitudinal epidemiologic study of signs and symptoms of temporomandibular disorders from 15 to 35 years of age. J Orofac Pain 2000;14:310–319.

18. Macfarlane TV, Blinkhorn AS, Davies RM, Kincey J, Worthington HV. Oro-facial pain in the community: Prevalence and associated impact. Community Dent Oral Epidemiol 2002;30:52–60.

19. Nilsson IM, List T, Drangsholt M. Prevalence of temporomandibular pain and subsequent dental treatment in Swedish adolescents. J Orofac Pain 2005;19:144–150.

20. Goulet JP, Lavigne GJ, Lund JP. Jaw pain prevalence among French-speaking Canadians in Québec and related symptoms of temporomandibular disorders. J Dent Res 1995;74:1738–1744.

21. Gesch D, Bernhardt O, Alte D, et al. Prevalence of signs and symptoms of temporomandibular disorders in an urban and rural German population: Results of a population-based Study of Health in Pomerania. Quintessence 2004;35:143–150.

22. Katz J, Heft M. The epidemiology of self-reported TMJ sounds and pain in young adults in Israel. J Public Health Dent 2002;62:177–179.

23. Kamisaka M, Yatani H, Kuboki T, Matsuka Y, Minakuchi H. Four-year longitudinal course of TMD symptoms in an adult population and the estimation of risk factors in relation to symptoms. J Orofac Pain 2000;14:224–232.

24. Rammelsberg P, LeResche L, Dworkin S, Mancl L. Longitudinal outcome of temporomandibular disorders: A 5-year epidemiologic study of muscle disorders defined by research diagnostic criteria for temporomandibular disorders. J Orofac Pain 2003;17:9–20.

25. Smith SB, Mir E, Bair E, et al. Genetic variants associated with development of TMD and its intermediate phenotypes: The genetic architecture of TMD in the OPPERA Prospective Cohort Study. J Pain 2013;14(12, suppl):T91–T101;e101–e103.

26. Slade GD, Sanders AE, Bair E, et al. Preclinical episodes of orofacial pain symptoms and their association with health care behaviors in the OPPERA Prospective Cohort Study. Pain 2013;154:750–760.

27. Thilander B, Rubio G, Pena L, de Mayorga C. Prevalence of temporomandibular dysfunction and its association with malocclusion in children and adolescents: An epidemiologic study related to specified stages of dental development. Angle Orthod 2002;72:146–154.

28. Wahlund K. Temporomandibular disorders in adolescents. Epidemiological and methodological studies and a randomized controlled trial. Swed Dent J Suppl 2003;(164):2–64.

29. Dervis E. Changes in temporomandibular disorders after treatment with new complete dentures. J Oral Rehabil 2004;31:320–326.

30. Schmitter M, Rammelsberg P, Hassel A. The prevalence of signs and symptoms of temporomandibular disorders in very old subjects. J Oral Rehabil 2005;32:467–473.

31. Osterberg T, Carlsson GE, Wedel A, Johansson U. A cross-sectional and longitudinal study of craniomandibular dysfunction in an elderly population. J Craniomandib Disord 1992;6:237–245.

32. Anastassaki A, Magnusson T. Patients referred to a specialist clinic because of suspected temporomandibular disorders: A survey of 3194 patients in respect of diagnoses, treatments, and treatment outcome. Acta Odontol Scand 2004;62:183–192.

33. White BA, Williams LA, Leben JR. Health care utilization and cost among health maintenance organization members with temporomandibular disorders. J Orofac Pain 2001;15:158–169.

34. LeResche L, Mancl LA, Drangsholt MT, Saunders K, Von Korff M. Relationship of pain and symptoms to pubertal development in adolescents. Pain 2005;118:201–209.

35. Schmid-Schwap M, Bristela M, Kundi M, Piehslinger E. Sex-specific differences in patients with temporomandibular disorders. J Orofac Pain 2013;27:42–50.

36. LeResche L, Sherman JJ, Huggins K, et al. Musculoskeletal orofacial pain and other signs and symptoms of temporomandibular disorders during pregnancy: A prospective study. J Orofac Pain 2005;19:193–201.

37. LeResche L, Mancl L, Sherman JJ, Gandara B, Dworkin SF. Changes in temporomandibular pain and other symptoms across the menstrual cycle. Pain 2003;106:253–261.

38. Dworkin SF, LeResche L. Temporomandibular disorder pain: Epidemiologic data. APS Bulletin 1993;12–13.

39. Pierce CJ, Weyant RJ, Block HM, Nemir DC. Dental splint prescription patterns: A survey. J Am Dent Assoc 1995;126:248–254.

40. Wright EF. Referred craniofacial pain patterns in patients with temporomandibular disorder. J Am Dent Assoc 2000;131:1307–1315.

41. Svensson P, Graven-Nielsen T. Craniofacial muscle pain: Review of mechanisms and clinical manifestations. J Orofac Pain 2001;15:117–145.

42. Fernández-de-Las-Peñas C, Galán-Del-Río F, Alonso-Blanco C, Jiménez-García R, Arendt-Nielsen L, Svensson P. Referred pain from muscle trigger points in the masticatory and neck-shoulder musculature in women with temporomandibular disorders. J Pain 2010;11:1295–1304.

43. Rhodus NL, Fricton J, Carlson P, Messner R. Oral symptoms associated with fibromyalgia syndrome. J Rheumatol 2003;30:1841–1845.

44. Kino K, Sugisaki M, Haketa T, et al. The comparison between pains, difficulties in function, and associating factors of patients in subtypes of temporomandibular disorders. J Oral Rehabil 2005;32:315–325.

45. van Grootel RJ, van der Glas HW, Buchner R, de Leeuw JR, Passchier J. Patterns of pain variation related to myogenous temporomandibular disorders. Clin J Pain 2005;21:154–165.

46. Benoliel R, Eliav E, Sharav Y. Self-reports of pain-related awakenings in persistent orofacial pain patients. J Orofac Pain 2009;23:330–338.

47. Camparis CM, Formigoni G, Teixeira MJ, Siqueira JT. Clinical evaluation of tinnitus in patients with sleep bruxism: Prevalence and characteristics. J Oral Rehabil 2005;32:808–814.

48. Saldanha AD, Hilgenberg PB, Pinto LM, Conti PC. Are temporomandibular disorders and tinnitus associated? Cranio 2012;30:166–171.

49. Hilgenberg PB, Saldanha AD, Cunha CO, Rubo JH, Conti PC. Temporomandibular disorders, otologic symptoms and depression levels in tinnitus patients. J Oral Rehabil 2012;39:239–244.

50. Schmitter M, Kress B, Rammelsberg P. Temporomandibular joint pathosis in patients with myofascial pain: A comparative analysis of magnetic resonance imaging and a clinical examination based on a specific set of criteria. Oral Surg Oral Med Oral Pathol Oral Radiol Endod 2004;97:318–324.

51. Alonso-Blanco C, Fernández-de-Las-Peñas C, de-la-Llave-Rincón AI, Zarco-Moreno P, Galán-Del-Río F, Svensson P. Characteristics of referred muscle pain to the head from active trigger points in women with myofascial temporomandibular pain and fibromyalgia syndrome. J Headache Pain 2012;13:625–637.

52. Stohler CS, Kowalski CJ, Lund JP. Muscle pain inhibits cutaneous touch perception. Pain 2001;92:327–333.

53. Svensson P, Bak J, Troest T. Spread and referral of experimental pain in different jaw muscles. J Orofac Pain 2003;17:214–223.

54. Gerwin RD, Dommerholt J, Shah JP. An expansion of Simons' integrated hypothesis of trigger point formation. Curr Pain Headache Rep 2004;8:468–475.

55. Simons DG. Review of enigmatic MTrPs as a common cause of enigmatic musculoskeletal pain and dysfunction. J Electromyogr Kinesiol 2004;14:95–107.

56. Wolfe F. Stop using the American College of Rheumatology Criteria in the clinic. J Rheumatol 2003;30:1671–1672.

57. Chen H, Slade G, Lim PF, Miller V, Maixner W, Diatchenko L. Relationship between temporomandibular disorders, widespread palpation tenderness, and multiple pain conditions: A case-control study. J Pain 2012;13:1016–1027.

58. Pfau DB, Rolke R, Nickel R, Treede RD, Daublaender M. Somatosensory profiles in subgroups of patients with myogenic temporomandibular disorders and fibromyalgia syndrome. Pain 2009;147:72–83.

59. Koutris M, Lobbezoo F, Sümer NC, Atis ES, Türker KS, Naeije M. Is myofascial pain in temporomandibular disorder patients a manifestation of delayed-onset muscle soreness? Clin J Pain 2013;29:712–716.

60. Mostafapour SP, Futran ND. Tumors and tumorous masses presenting as temporomandibular joint syndrome. Otolaryngol Head Neck Surg 2000;123:459–464.

61. Treasure T. External auditory canal carcinoma involving the temporomandibular joint: Two cases presenting as temporomandibular disorders. J Oral Maxillofac Surg 2002;60:465–469.

62. Baba K, Tsukiyama Y, Yamazaki M, Clark GT. A review of temporomandibular disorder diagnostic techniques. J Prosthet Dent 2001;86:184–194.

63. Lund JP, Murray G, Svensson P. Pain and motor reflexes. In: Sessle BJ, Lavigne GJ, Lund JP, Dubner R (eds). Orofacial Pain: From Basic Science to Clinical Management, ed 2. Chicago: Quintessence, 2009:109–116.

64. Svensson P, Baad-Hansen L, Pigg M, et al. Guidelines and recommendations for assessment of somatosensory function in oro-facial pain conditions—A taskforce report. J Oral Rehabil 2011;38:366–394.

65. Eliav E, Teich S, Nitzan D, et al. Facial arthralgia and myalgia: Can they be differentiated by trigeminal sensory assessment? Pain 2003;104:481–490.

66. Quek SY, Grunwerg BS. Masseteric nerve block for masseter muscle pain—A clinical note. Quintessence 2009;40:87–91.

67. De Laat A, Stappaerts K, Papy S. Counseling and physical therapy as treatment for myofascial pain of the masticatory system. J Orofac Pain 2003;17:42–49.

68. Dworkin SF, Huggins KH, Wilson L, et al. A randomized clinical trial using research diagnostic criteria for temporomandibular disorders-axis II to target clinic cases for a tailored self-care TMD treatment program. J Orofac Pain 2002;16:48–63.

69. Michelotti A, Steenks MH, Farella M, Parisini F, Cimino R, Martina R. The additional value of a home physical therapy regimen versus patient education only for the treatment of myofascial pain of the jaw muscles: Short-term results of a randomized clinical trial. J Orofac Pain 2004;18:114–125.

70. Ekberg E, Nilner M. Treatment outcome of appliance therapy in temporomandibular disorder patients with myofascial pain after 6 and 12 months. Acta Odontol Scand 2004;62:343–349.

71. List T, Axelsson S. Management of TMD: Evidence from systematic reviews and meta-analyses. J Oral Rehabil 2010;37:430–451.

72. Benoliel R, Sharav Y, Tal M, Eliav E. Management of chronic orofacial pain: today and tomorrow. Compend Contin Educ Dent 2003;24:909–920;922–904;926–908.

73. Sherman JJ, Turk DC. Nonpharmacologic approaches to the management of myofascial temporomandibular disorders. Curr Pain Headache Rep 2001;5:421–431.

74. Dworkin RH, Turk DC, Wyrwich KW, et al. Interpreting the clinical importance of treatment outcomes in chronic pain clinical trials: IMMPACT recommendations. J Pain 2008;9:105–121.

75. Grossi ML, Goldberg MB, Locker D, Tenenbaum HC. Reduced neuropsychologic measures as predictors of treatment outcome in patients with temporomandibular disorders. J Orofac Pain 2001;15:329–339.

76. Chen H, Nackley A, Miller V, Diatchenko L, Maixner W. Multisystem dysregulation in painful temporomandibular disorders. J Pain 2013;14:983–996.

77. Gavish A, Winocur E, Menashe S, Halachmi M, Eli I, Gazit E. Experimental chewing in myofascial pain patients. J Orofac Pain 2002;16:22–28.

78. Craane B, Dijkstra PU, Stappaerts K, De Laat A. One-year evaluation of the effect of physical therapy for masticatory muscle pain: A randomized controlled trial. Eur J Pain 2012;16:737–747.

79. Cetiner S, Kahraman SA, Yücetaş S. Evaluation of low-level laser therapy in the treatment of temporomandibular disorders. Photomed Laser Surg 2006;24:637–641.

80. Kulekcioglu S, Sivrioglu K, Ozcan O, Parlak M. Effectiveness of low-level laser therapy in temporomandibular disorder. Scand J Rheumatol 2003;32:114–118.

81. Petrucci A, Sgolastra F, Gatto R, Mattei A, Monaco A. Effectiveness of low-level laser therapy in temporomandibular disorders: A systematic review and meta-analysis. J Orofac Pain 2011;25:298–307.

82. Carlson CR, Bertrand PM, Ehrlich AD, Maxwell AW, Burton RG. Physical self-regulation training for the management of temporomandibular disorders. J Orofac Pain 2001;15:47–55.

83. Michelotti A, Iodice G. The role of orthodontics in temporomandibular disorders. J Oral Rehabil 2010;37:411–429.

84. Pullinger A. Establishing better biological models to understand occlusion. I: TM joint anatomic relationships. J Oral Rehabil 2013;40:296–318.

85. Türp JC, Schindler H. The dental occlusion as a suspected cause for TMDs: Epidemiological and etiological considerations. J Oral Rehabil 2012;39:502–512.

86. Hellsing G. Occlusal adjustment and occlusal stability. J Prosthet Dent 1988;59:696–702.

87. De Boever JA, Carlsson GE, Klineberg IJ. Need for occlusal therapy and prosthodontic treatment in the management of temporomandibular disorders. Part I. Occlusal interferences and occlusal adjustment. J Oral Rehabil 2000;27:367–379.

88. McNamara JA Jr. Orthodontic treatment and temporomandibular disorders. Oral Surg Oral Med Oral Pathol Oral Radiol Endod 1997;83:107–117.

89. Shankland WE. Nociceptive trigeminal inhibition—Tension suppression system: A method of preventing migraine and tension headaches. Compend Contin Educ Dent 2002;23:105–108;110;112–103.

90. Türp JC, Komine F, Hugger A. Efficacy of stabilization splints for the management of patients with masticatory muscle pain: A qualitative systematic review. Clin Oral Investig 2004;8:179–195.

91. Eberhard D, Bantleon HP, Steger W. The efficacy of anterior repositioning splint therapy studied by magnetic resonance imaging. Eur J Orthod 2002;24:343–352.

92. Lundh H, Westesson PL. Long-term follow-up after occlusal treatment to correct abnormal temporomandibular joint disk position. Oral Surg Oral Med Oral Pathol 1989;67:2–10.

93. Tallents RH, Katzberg RW, Macher DJ, Roberts CA. Use of protrusive splint therapy in anterior disk displacement of the temporomandibular joint: A 1- to 3-year follow-up. J Prosthet Dent 1990;63:336–341.

94. Tecco S, Festa F, Salini V, Epifania E, D'Attilio M. Treatment of joint pain and joint noises associated with a recent TMJ internal derangement: A comparison of an anterior repositioning splint, a full-arch maxillary stabilization splint, and an untreated control group. Cranio 2004;22:209–219.

95. Nitzan DW. Intraarticular pressure in the functioning human temporomandibular joint and its alteration by uniform elevation of the occlusal plane. J Oral Maxillofac Surg 1994;52:671–679.

96. Ekberg E. Treatment of temporomandibular disorders of arthrogeneous origin. Controlled double-blind studies of a non-steroidal anti-inflammatory drug and a stabilisation appliance. Swed Dent J Suppl 1998;131:1–57.

97. Conti PC, dos Santos CN, Kogawa EM, de Castro Ferreira Conti AC, de Araujo Cdos R. The treatment of painful temporomandibular joint clicking with oral splints: A randomized clinical trial. J Am Dent Assoc 2006;137:1108–1114.

98. Magnusson T, Adiels AM, Nilsson HL, Helkimo M. Treatment effect on signs and symptoms of temporomandibular disorders—Comparison between stabilisation splint and a new type of splint (NTI). A pilot study. Swed Dent J 2004;28:11–20.

99. Al Quran FA, Kamal MS. Anterior midline point stop device (AMPS) in the treatment of myogenous TMDs: Comparison with the stabilization splint and control group. Oral Surg Oral Med Oral Pathol Oral Radiol Endod 2006;101:741–747.

100. Forssell H, Kalso E. Application of principles of evidence-based medicine to occlusal treatment for temporomandibular disorders: Are there lessons to be learned? J Orofac Pain 2004;18:9–22.

101. Al-Ani Z, Gray RJ, Davies SJ, Sloan P, Glenny AM. Stabilization splint therapy for the treatment of temporomandibular myofascial pain: A systematic review. J Dent Educ 2005;69:1242–1250.

102. Kuttila M, Le Bell Y, Savolainen-Niemi E, Kuttila S, Alanen P. Efficiency of occlusal appliance therapy in secondary otalgia and temporomandibular disorders. Acta Odontol Scand 2002;60:248–254.

103. Wassell RW, Adams N, Kelly PJ. The treatment of temporomandibular disorders with stabilizing splints in general dental practice: One-year follow-up. J Am Dent Assoc 2006;137:1089–1098.

104. Raphael KG, Marbach JJ. Widespread pain and the effectiveness of oral splints in myofascial face pain. J Am Dent Assoc 2001;132:305–316.

105. Truelove E, Huggins KH, Mancl L, Dworkin SF. The efficacy of traditional, low-cost and nonsplint therapies for temporomandibular disorder: A randomized controlled trial. J Am Dent Assoc 2006;137:1099–1107.

106. Dubé C, Rompré PH, Manzini C, Guitard F, de Grandmont P, Lavigne GJ. Quantitative polygraphic controlled study on efficacy and safety of oral splint devices in tooth-grinding subjects. J Dent Res 2004;83:398–403.

107. Harada T, Ichiki R, Tsukiyama Y, Koyano K. The effect of oral splint devices on sleep bruxism: A 6-week observation with an ambulatory electromyographic recording device. J Oral Rehabil 2006;33:482–488.

108. Chung SC, Kim YK, Kim HS. Prevalence and patterns of nocturnal bruxofacets on stabilization splints in temporomandibular disorder patients. Cranio 2000;18:92–97.

109. Sharav Y, Singer E, Schmidt E, Dionne RA, Dubner R. The analgesic effect of amitriptyline on chronic facial pain. Pain 1987;31:199–209.

110. Plesh O, Curtis D, Levine J, McCall WD Jr. Amitriptyline treatment of chronic pain in patients with temporomandibular disorders. J Oral Rehabil 2000;27:834–841.

111. Benoliel R, Eliav E, Elishoov H, Sharav Y. Diagnosis and treatment of persistent pain after trauma to the head and neck. J Oral Maxillofac Surg 1994;52:1138–1147.

112. Harkins S, Linford J, Cohen J, Kramer T, Cueva L. Administration of clonazepam in the treatment of TMD and associated myofascial pain: A double-blind pilot study. J Craniomandib Disord 1991;5:179–186.

113. Herman CR, Schiffman EL, Look JO, Rindal DB. The effectiveness of adding pharmacologic treatment with clonazepam or cyclobenzaprine to patient education and self-care for the treatment of jaw pain upon awakening: A randomized clinical trial. J Orofac Pain 2002;16:64–70.

114. Kimos P, Biggs C, Mah J, et al. Analgesic action of gabapentin on chronic pain in the masticatory muscles: A randomized controlled trial. Pain 2006;127:151–160.

115. Diatchenko L, Slade GD, Nackley AG, et al. Genetic basis for individual variations in pain perception and the development of a chronic pain condition. Hum Mol Genet 2005;14:135–143.

116. Tchivileva IE, Lim PF, Smith SB, et al. Effect of catechol-O-methyltransferase polymorphism on response to propranolol therapy in chronic musculoskeletal pain: A randomized, double-blind, placebo-controlled, crossover pilot study. Pharmacogenet Genomics 2010;20:239–248.

117. Dworkin RH, Turk DC, Farrar JT, et al. Core outcome measures for chronic pain clinical trials: IMMPACT recommendations. Pain 2005;113:9–19.

118. Brousseau M, Manzini C, Thie N, Lavigne G. Understanding and managing the interaction between sleep and pain: An update for the dentist. J Can Dent Assoc 2003;69:437–442.

119. Turner JA, Dworkin SF. Screening for psychosocial risk factors in patients with chronic orofacial pain: Recent advances. J Am Dent Assoc 2004;135:1119–1125.

120. Turner JA, Holtzman S, Mancl L. Mediators, moderators, and predictors of therapeutic change in cognitive-behavioral therapy for chronic pain. Pain 2007;127:276–286.

121. Crider AB, Glaros AG. A meta-analysis of EMG biofeedback treatment of temporomandibular disorders. J Orofac Pain 1999;13:29–37.

122. Borgeat F, Elie R, Larouche LM. Pain response to voluntary muscle tension increases and biofeedback efficacy in tension headache. Headache 1985;25:387–391.

123. Flor H, Birbaumer N. Comparison of the efficacy of electromyographic biofeedback, cognitive-behavioral therapy, and conservative medical interventions in the treatment of chronic musculoskeletal pain. J Consult Clin Psychol 1993;61:653–658.

124. Gardea MA, Gatchel RJ, Mishra KD. Long-term efficacy of biobehavioral treatment of temporomandibular disorders. J Behav Med 2001;24:341–359.

125. Mishra KD, Gatchel RJ, Gardea MA. The relative efficacy of three cognitive-behavioral treatment approaches to temporomandibular disorders. J Behav Med 2000;23:293–309.

126. Graboski CL, Gray DS, Burnham RS. Botulinum toxin A versus bupivacaine trigger point injections for the treatment of myofascial pain syndrome: A randomised double blind crossover study. Pain 2005;118:170–175.

127. Ernberg M, Hedenberg-Magnusson B, List T, Svensson P. Efficacy of botulinum toxin type A for treatment of persistent myofascial TMD pain: A randomized, controlled, double-blind multicenter study. Pain 2011;152:1988–1996.

P. 을지
2 / 0

128. Nixdorf DR, Heo G, Major PW. Randomized controlled trial of botulinum toxin A for chronic myogenous orofacial pain. Pain 2002;99:465–473.

129. Cummings TM, White AR. Needling therapies in the management of myofascial trigger point pain: A systematic review. Arch Phys Med Rehabil 2001;82:986–992.

130. Wexler GB, McKinney MW. Temporomandibular treatment outcomes within five diagnostic categories. Cranio 1999;17:30–37.

131. Mense S. The pathogenesis of muscle pain. Curr Pain Headache Rep 2003;7:419–425.

132. Diatchenko L, Nackley AG, Slade GD, Fillingim RB, Maixner W. Idiopathic pain disorders—Pathways of vulnerability. Pain 2006;123:226–230.

133. Tracey I, Mantyh PW. The cerebral signature for pain perception and its modulation. Neuron 2007;55:377–391.

134. Galdón MJ, Durá E, Andreu Y, Ferrando M, Poveda R, Bagán JV. Multidimensional approach to the differences between muscular and articular temporomandibular patients: Coping, distress, and pain characteristics. Oral Surg Oral Med Oral Pathol Oral Radiol Endod 2006;102:40–46.

135. Ferrando M, Andreu Y, Galdón MJ, Durá E, Poveda R, Bagán JV. Psychological variables and temporomandibular disorders: Distress, coping, and personality. Oral Surg Oral Med Oral Pathol Oral Radiol Endod 2004;98:153–160.

136. Suvinen TI, Reade PC, Hanes KR, Könönen M, Kemppainen P. Temporomandibular disorder subtypes according to self-reported physical and psychosocial variables in female patients: A re-evaluation. J Oral Rehabil 2005;32:166–173.

137. Woda A, Pionchon P. A unified concept of idiopathic orofacial pain: Clinical features. J Orofac Pain 1999;13:172–184.

138. Dworkin SF, Burgess JA. Orofacial pain of psychogenic origin: Current concepts and classification. J Am Dent Assoc 1987;115:565–571.

139. Suvinen TI, Reade PC, Kemppainen P, Könönen M, Dworkin SF. Review of aetiological concepts of temporomandibular pain disorders: Towards a biopsychosocial model for integration of physical disorder factors with psychological and psychosocial illness impact factors. Eur J Pain 2005;9:613–633.

140. Maixner W, Diatchenko L, Dubner R, et al. Orofacial Pain Prospective Evaluation and Risk Assessment study—the OPPERA study. J Pain 2011;12(11, suppl):T4–T11.

141. Ohrbach R, Fillingim RB, Mulkey F, et al. Clinical findings and pain symptoms as potential risk factors for chronic TMD: Descriptive data and empirically identified domains from the OPPERA case-control study. J Pain 2011;12(11, suppl):T27–T45.

142. Slade GD, Bair E, By K, et al. Study methods, recruitment, sociodemographic findings, and demographic representativeness in the OPPERA study. J Pain 2011;12(11, suppl):T12–T26.

143. Lorduy KM, Liegey-Dougall A, Haggard R, Sanders CN, Gatchel RJ. The prevalence of comorbid symptoms of central sensitization syndrome among three different groups of temporomandibular disorder patients. Pain Pract 2013;13:604–613.

144. John MT, Miglioretti DL, LeResche L, Von Korff M, Critchlow CW. Widespread pain as a risk factor for dysfunctional temporomandibular disorder pain. Pain 2003;102:257–263.

145. Sanders AE, Slade GD, Bair E, et al. General health status and incidence of first-onset temporomandibular disorder: The OPPERA prospective cohort study. J Pain 2013;14(12, suppl):T51–T62.

146. Türp JC, Kowalski CJ, O'Leary N, Stohler CS. Pain maps from facial pain patients indicate a broad pain geography. J Dent Res 1998;77:1465–1472.

147. Plesh O, Adams SH, Gansky SA. Temporomandibular joint and muscle disorder-type pain and comorbid pains in a national US sample. J Orofac Pain 2011;25:190–198.

148. Fillingim RB, Fillingim LA, Hollins M, Sigurdsson A, Maixner W. Generalized vibrotactile allodynia in a patient with temporomandibular disorder. Pain 1998;78:75–78.

149. Maixner W, Fillingim R, Booker D, Sigurdsson A. Sensitivity of patients with painful temporomandibular disorders to experimentally evoked pain. Pain 1995;63:341–351.

150. Maixner W, Fillingim R, Sigurdsson A, Kincaid S, Silva S. Sensitivity of patients with painful temporomandibular disorders to experimentally evoked pain: Evidence for altered temporal summation of pain. Pain 1998;76:71–81.

151. Carlson CR, Reid KI, Curran SL, et al. Psychological and physiological parameters of masticatory muscle pain. Pain 1998;76:297–307.

152. Svensson P, Graven-Nielsen T, Arendt-Nielsen L. Mechanical hyperesthesia of human facial skin induced by tonic painful stimulation of jaw muscles. Pain 1998;74:93–100.

153. Sipilä K, Suominen AL, Alanen P, Heliövaara M, Tiittanen P, Könönen M. Association of clinical findings of temporomandibular disorders (TMD) with self-reported musculoskeletal pains. Eur J Pain 2011;15:1061–1067.

154. King CD, Wong F, Currie T, Mauderli AP, Fillingim RB, Riley JL 3rd. Deficiency in endogenous modulation of prolonged heat pain in patients with irritable bowel syndrome and temporomandibular disorder. Pain 2009;143:172–178.

155. Raphael KG, Janal MN, Anathan S, Cook DB, Staud R. Temporal summation of heat pain in temporomandibular disorder patients. J Orofac Pain 2009;23:54–64.

156. Sarlani E, Grace EG, Reynolds MA, Greenspan JD. Evidence for up-regulated central nociceptive processing in patients with masticatory myofascial pain. J Orofac Pain 2004;18:41–55.

157. Svensson P, List T, Hector G. Analysis of stimulus-evoked pain in patients with myofascial temporomandibular pain disorders. Pain 2001;92:399–409.

158. Hedenberg-Magnusson B, Ernberg M, Kopp S. Symptoms and signs of temporomandibular disorders in patients with fibromyalgia and local myalgia of the temporomandibular system. A comparative study. Acta Odontol Scand 1997;55:344–349.

159. Fernández-de-las-Peñas C, Galán-del-Río F, Fernández-Carnero J, Pesquera J, Arendt-Nielsen L, Svensson P. Bilateral widespread mechanical pain sensitivity in women with myofascial temporomandibular disorder: Evidence of impairment in central nociceptive processing. J Pain 2009;10:1170–1178.

160. Fernández-de-las-Peñas C, Galán-del-Río F, Ortega-Santiago R, Jiménez-García R, Arendt-Nielsen L, Svensson P. Bilateral thermal hyperalgesia in trigeminal and extra-trigeminal regions in patients with myofascial temporomandibular disorders. Exp Brain Res 2010;202:171–179.

161. Greenspan JD, Slade GD, Bair E, et al. Pain sensitivity risk factors for chronic TMD: Descriptive data and empirically identified domains from the OPPERA case control study. J Pain 2011;12(11, suppl):T61–T74.

162. Sherman JJ, LeResche L, Huggins KH, Mancl LA, Sage JC, Dworkin SF. The relationship of somatization and depression to experimental pain response in women with temporomandibular disorders. Psychosom Med 2004;66:852–860.

163. Horjales-Araujo E, Demontis D, Lund EK, et al. Emotional modulation of muscle pain is associated with polymorphisms in the serotonin transporter gene. Pain 2013;154:1469–1476.

164. Gustin SM, Peck CC, Wilcox SL, Nash PG, Murray GM, Henderson LA. Different pain, different brain: Thalamic anatomy in neuropathic and non-neuropathic chronic pain syndromes. J Neurosci 2011;31:5956–5964.

165. Moayedi M, Weissman-Fogel I, Salomons TV, et al. White matter brain and trigeminal nerve abnormalities in temporomandibular disorder. Pain 2012;153:1467–1477.

166. Younger JW, Shen YF, Goddard G, Mackey SC. Chronic myofascial temporomandibular pain is associated with neural abnormalities in the trigeminal and limbic systems. Pain 2010;149:222–228.

167. Martinez-Lavin M. Fibromyalgia as a sympathetically maintained pain syndrome. Curr Pain Headache Rep 2004;8:385–389.

168. Galli U, Gaab J, Ettlin DA, Ruggia F, Ehlert U, Palla S. Enhanced negative feedback sensitivity of the hypothalamus-pituitary-adrenal axis in chronic myogenous facial pain. Eur J Pain 2009;13:600–605.

169. Demitrack MA, Crofford LJ. Evidence for and pathophysiologic implications of hypothalamic-pituitary-adrenal axis dysregulation in fibromyalgia and chronic fatigue syndrome. Ann N Y Acad Sci 1998;840:684–697.

170. Drewes AM. Pain and sleep disturbances with special reference to fibromyalgia and rheumatoid arthritis. Rheumatology (Oxford) 1999;38:1035–1038.

171. Sarzi-Puttini P, Atzeni F, Diana A, Doria A, Furlan R. Increased neural sympathetic activation in fibromyalgia syndrome. Ann N Y Acad Sci 2006;1069:109–117.

172. Vgontzas AN, Chrousos GP. Sleep, the hypothalamic-pituitary-adrenal axis, and cytokines: Multiple interactions and disturbances in sleep disorders. Endocrinol Metab Clin North Am 2002;31:15–36.

173. Maixner W, Greenspan JD, Dubner R, et al. Potential autonomic risk factors for chronic TMD: Descriptive data and empirically identified domains from the OPPERA case-control study. J Pain 2011;12(11, suppl):T75–T91.

174. Evaskus DS, Laskin DM. A biochemical measure of stress in patients with myofascial pain-dysfunction syndrome. J Dent Res 1972;51:1464–1466.

175. Marbach JJ, Levitt M. Erythrocyte catechol-O-methyltransferase activity in facial pain patients. J Dent Res 1976;55:711.

176. Reid KI, Carlson CR, Sherman JJ, Curran SL, Gracely RH. Influence of a sympathomimetic amine on masticatory and trapezius pain/pressure thresholds and electromyographic levels. Oral Surg Oral Med Oral Pathol Oral Radiol Endod 1996;82:525–531.

177. Light KC, Bragdon EE, Grewen KM, Brownley KA, Girdler SS, Maixner W. Adrenergic dysregulation and pain with and without acute beta-blockade in women with fibromyalgia and temporomandibular disorder. J Pain 2009;10:542–552.

178. Nackley AG, Tan KS, Fecho K, Flood P, Diatchenko L, Maixner W. Catechol-O-methyltransferase inhibition increases pain sensitivity through activation of both beta2- and beta3-adrenergic receptors. Pain 2007;128:199–208.

179. Greenspan JD, Slade GD, Bair E, et al. Pain sensitivity and autonomic factors associated with development of TMD: The OPPERA prospective cohort study. J Pain 2013;14(12, suppl):T63–T74.

180. Kopp S. Neuroendocrine, immune, and local responses related to temporomandibular disorders. J Orofac Pain 2001;15:9–28.

181. Cairns BE, Gambarota G, Svensson P, Arendt-Nielsen L, Berde CB. Glutamate-induced sensitization of rat masseter muscle fibers. Neuroscience 2002;109:389–399.

182. Cairns BE, Svensson P, Wang K, et al. Activation of peripheral NMDA receptors contributes to human pain and rat afferent discharges evoked by injection of glutamate into the masseter muscle. J Neurophysiol 2003;90:2098–2105.

183. Cairns BE, Wang K, Hu JW, Sessle BJ, Arendt-Nielsen L, Svensson P. The effect of glutamate-evoked masseter muscle pain on the human jaw-stretch reflex differs in men and women. J Orofac Pain 2003;17:317–325.

184. Castrillon EE, Cairns BE, Wang K, Arendt-Nielsen L, Svensson P. Comparison of glutamate-evoked pain between the temporalis and masseter muscles in men and women. Pain 2012;153:823–829.

185. Ro JY, Capra NF, Masri R. Contribution of peripheral N-methyl-D-aspartate receptors to c-fos expression in the trigeminal spinal nucleus following acute masseteric inflammation. Neuroscience 2004;123:213–219.

186. Lee JS, Ro JY. Peripheral metabotropic glutamate receptor 5 mediates mechanical hypersensitivity in craniofacial muscle via protein kinase C dependent mechanisms. Neuroscience 2007;146:375–383.

187. Cairns BE, Hu JW, Arendt-Nielsen L, Sessle BJ, Svensson P. Sex-related differences in human pain and rat afferent discharge evoked by injection of glutamate into the masseter muscle. J Neurophysiol 2001;86:782–791.

188. Mann MK, Dong XD, Svensson P, Cairns BE. Influence of intramuscular nerve growth factor injection on the response properties of rat masseter muscle afferent fibers. J Orofac Pain 2006;20:325–336.

189. Svensson P, Cairns BE, Wang K, Arendt-Nielsen L. Injection of nerve growth factor into human masseter muscle evokes long-lasting mechanical allodynia and hyperalgesia. Pain 2003;104:241–247.

190. Svensson P, Castrillon E, Cairns BE. Nerve growth factor-evoked masseter muscle sensitization and perturbation of jaw motor function in healthy women. J Orofac Pain 2008;22:340–348.

191. Svensson P, Wang K, Arendt-Nielsen L, Cairns BE. Effects of NGF-induced muscle sensitization on proprioception and nociception. Exp Brain Res 2008;189:1–10.

192. Svensson P, Wang MW, Dong XD, Kumar U, Cairns BE. Human nerve growth factor sensitizes masseter muscle nociceptors in female rats. Pain 2010;148:473–480.

193. Castrillon EE, Cairns BE, Ernberg M, et al. Effect of peripheral NMDA receptor blockade with ketamine on chronic myofascial pain in temporomandibular disorder patients: A randomized, double-blinded, placebo-controlled trial. J Orofac Pain 2008;22:122–130.

194. Castrillon EE, Cairns BE, Ernberg M, et al. Effect of a peripheral NMDA receptor antagonist on glutamate-evoked masseter muscle pain and mechanical sensitization in women. J Orofac Pain 2007;21:216–224.

195. Ernberg M, Hedenberg-Magnusson B, Alstergren P, Kopp S. The level of serotonin in the superficial masseter muscle in relation to local pain and allodynia. Life Sci 1999;65:313–325.

196. Wang K, Svensson P, Sessle BJ, Cairns BE, Arendt-Nielsen L. Interactions of glutamate and capsaicin-evoked muscle pain on jaw motor functions of men. Clin Neurophysiol 2010;121:950–956.

197. Mørk H, Ashina M, Bendtsen L, Olesen J, Jensen R. Experimental muscle pain and tenderness following infusion of endogenous substances in humans. Eur J Pain 2003;7:145–153.

198. Mørk H, Ashina M, Bendtsen L, Olesen J, Jensen R. Possible mechanisms of pain perception in patients with episodic tension-type headache. A new experimental model of myofascial pain. Cephalalgia 2004;24:466–475.

199. Fischer DJ, Mueller BA, Critchlow CW, LeResche L. The association of temporomandibular disorder pain with history of head and neck injury in adolescents. J Orofac Pain 2006;20:191–198.

200. Inglese M, Makani S, Johnson G, et al. Diffuse axonal injury in mild traumatic brain injury: A diffusion tensor imaging study. J Neurosurg 2005;103:298–303.

201. Povlishock JT, Katz DI. Update of neuropathology and neurological recovery after traumatic brain injury. J Head Trauma Rehabil 2005;20:76–94.

202. Huang GJ, LeResche L, Critchlow CW, Martin MD, Drangsholt MT. Risk factors for diagnostic subgroups of painful temporomandibular disorders (TMD). J Dent Res 2002;81:284–288.

203. Macfarlane TV, Blinkhorn AS, Davies RM, Kincey J, Worthington HV. Factors associated with health care seeking behaviour for orofacial pain in the general population. Community Dent Health 2003;20:20–26.

204. Macfarlane TV, Gray RJM, Kincey J, Worthington HV. Factors associated with the temporomandibular disorder, pain dysfunction syndrome (PDS): Manchester case-control study. Oral Dis 2001;7:321–330.

205. Velly AM, Gornitsky M, Philippe P. Contributing factors to chronic myofascial pain: A case-control study. Pain 2003;104:491–499.

206. Plesh O, Gansky SA, Curtis DA, Pogrel MA. The relationship between chronic facial pain and a history of trauma and surgery. Oral Surg Oral Med Oral Pathol Oral Radiol Endod 1999;88:16–21.

207. Huang GJ, Rue TC. Third-molar extraction as a risk factor for temporomandibular disorder. J Am Dent Assoc 2006;137:1547–1554.

208. De Boever JA, Keersmaekers K. Trauma in patients with temporomandibular disorders: Frequency and treatment outcome. J Oral Rehabil 1996;23:91–96.

209. Kolbinson DA, Epstein JB, Senthilselvan A, Burgess JA. A comparison of TMD patients with or without prior motor vehicle accident involvement: Initial signs, symptoms, and diagnostic characteristics. J Orofac Pain 1997;11:206–214.

210. Steed PA, Wexler GB. Temporomandibular disorders—Traumatic etiology vs. nontraumatic etiology: A clinical and methodological inquiry into symptomatology and treatment outcomes. Cranio 2001;19:188–194.

211. Klobas L, Tegelberg A, Axelsson S. Symptoms and signs of temporomandibular disorders in individuals with chronic whiplash-associated disorders. Swed Dent J 2004;28:29–36.

212. Pérez del Palomar A, Doblaré M. Dynamic 3D FE modelling of the human temporomandibular joint during whiplash. Med Eng Phys 2008;30:700–709.

213. Salé H, Isberg A. Delayed temporomandibular joint pain and dysfunction induced by whiplash trauma: A controlled prospective study. J Am Dent Assoc 2007;138:1084–1091.

214. Häggman-Henrikson B, Lampa E, Nordh E. Altered thermal sensitivity in facial skin in chronic whiplash-associated disorders. Int J Oral Sci 2013;5:150–154.

215. Häggman-Henrikson B, Grönqvist J, Eriksson PO. Frequent jaw-face pain in chronic whiplash-associated disorders. Swed Dent J 2011;35:123–131.

216. Ciancaglini R, Testa M, Radaelli G. Association of neck pain with symptoms of temporomandibular dysfunction in the general adult population. Scand J Rehabil Med 1999;31:17–22.

217. Bartsch T, Goadsby PJ. The trigeminocervical complex and migraine: Current concepts and synthesis. Curr Pain Headache Rep 2003;7:371–376.

218. Ge HY, Wang K, Madeleine P, Svensson P, Sessle BJ, Arendt-Nielsen L. Simultaneous modulation of the exteroceptive suppression periods in the trapezius and temporalis muscles by experimental muscle pain. Clin Neurophysiol 2004;115:1399–1408.

219. Wiesinger B, Häggman-Henrikson B, Hellström F, Wänman A. Experimental masseter muscle pain alters jaw-neck motor strategy. Eur J Pain 2013;17:995–1004.

220. Eriksson PO, Zafar H, Häggman-Henrikson B. Deranged jaw-neck motor control in whiplash-associated disorders. Eur J Oral Sci 2004;112:25–32.

221. Grönqvist J, Häggman-Henrikson B, Eriksson PO. Impaired jaw function and eating difficulties in whiplash-associated disorders. Swed Dent J 2008;32:171–177.

222. Häggman-Henrikson B, Osterlund C, Eriksson PO. Endurance during chewing in whiplash-associated disorders and TMD. J Dent Res 2004;83:946–950.

223. Häggman-Henrikson B, Zafar H, Eriksson PO. Disturbed jaw behavior in whiplash-associated disorders during rhythmic jaw movements. J Dent Res 2002;81:747–751.

224. Barnsley L, Lord S, Bogduk N. Whiplash injury. Pain 1994;58:283–307.

225. Ferrari R, Schrader H, Obelieniene D. Prevalence of temporomandibular disorders associated with whiplash injury in Lithuania. Oral Surg Oral Med Oral Pathol Oral Radiol Endod 1999;87:653–657.

226. Kasch H, Hjorth T, Svensson P, Nyhuus L, Jensen TS. Temporomandibular disorders after whiplash injury: A controlled, prospective study. J Orofac Pain 2002;16:118–128.

227. Carroll LJ, Ferrari R, Cassidy JD. Reduced or painful jaw movement after collision-related injuries: A population-based study. J Am Dent Assoc 2007;138:86–93.

228. Visscher C, Hofman N, Mes C, Lousberg R, Naeije M. Is temporomandibular pain in chronic whiplash-associated disorders part of a more widespread pain syndrome? Clin J Pain 2005;21:353–357.

229. Häggman-Henrikson B, Rezvani M, List T. Prevalence of whiplash trauma in TMD patients: A systematic review. J Oral Rehabil 2014;41:59–68.

230. Häggman-Henrikson B, List T, Westergren HT, Axelsson SH. Temporomandibular disorder pain after whiplash trauma: A systematic review. J Orofac Pain 2013;27:217–226.

231. Epker J, Gatchel RJ. Coping profile differences in the biopsychosocial functioning of patients with temporomandibular disorder. Psychosom Med 2000;62:69–75.

232. Raphael KG, Marbach JJ, Gallagher RM. Somatosensory amplification and affective inhibition are elevated in myofascial face pain. Pain Med 2000;1:247–253.

233. Fillingim RB, Ohrbach R, Greenspan JD, et al. Potential psychosocial risk factors for chronic TMD: Descriptive data and empirically identified domains from the OPPERA case-control study. J Pain 2011;12(11, suppl):T46–T60.

234. Schnurr RF, Rollman GB, Brooke RI. Are there psychologic predictors of treatment outcome in temporomandibular joint pain and dysfunction? Oral Surg Oral Med Oral Pathol 1991;72:550–558.

235. Aaron LA, Buchwald D. Chronic diffuse musculoskeletal pain, fibromyalgia and co-morbid unexplained clinical conditions. Best Pract Res Clin Rheumatol 2003;17:563–574.

236. Türp JC, Kowalski CJ, Stohler CS. Temporomandibular disorders—Pain outside the head and face is rarely acknowledged in the chief complaint. J Prosthet Dent 1997;78:592–595.

237. Epker J, Gatchel RJ, Ellis E 3rd. A model for predicting chronic TMD: Practical application in clinical settings. J Am Dent Assoc 1999;130:1470–1475.

238. Selaimen CM, Jeronymo JC, Brilhante DP, Grossi ML. Sleep and depression as risk indicators for temporomandibular disorders in a cross-cultural perspective: A case-control study. Int J Prosthodont 2006;19:154–161.

239. Vazquez-Delgado E, Schmidt JE, Carlson C, De Leeuw R, Okeson J. Psychological and sleep quality differences between chronic daily headache and temporomandibular disorders patients. Cephalalgia 2004;24:446–454.

240. Velly AM, Look JO, Schiffman E, et al. The effect of fibromyalgia and widespread pain on the clinically significant temporomandibular muscle and joint pain disorders—A prospective 18-month cohort study. J Pain 2010;11:1155–1164.

241. Garofalo JP, Gatchel RJ, Wesley AL, Ellis E 3rd. Predicting chronicity in acute temporomandibular joint disorders using the research diagnostic criteria. J Am Dent Assoc 1998;129:438–447.

242. Fillingim RB, Ohrbach R, Greenspan JD, et al. Psychological factors associated with development of TMD: the OPPERA prospective cohort study. J Pain 2013;14(12, suppl):T75–T90.

243. Brister H, Turner JA, Aaron LA, Mancl L. Self-efficacy is associated with pain, functioning, and coping in patients with chronic temporomandibular disorder pain. J Orofac Pain 2006;20:115–124.

244. Michelotti A, Cioffi I, Landino D, Galeone C, Farella M. Effects of experimental occlusal interferences in individuals reporting different levels of wake-time parafunctions. J Orofac Pain 2012;26:168–175.

245. Michelotti A, Farella M, Gallo LM, Veltri A, Palla S, Martina R. Effect of occlusal interference on habitual activity of human masseter. J Dent Res 2005;84:644–648.

246. van der Meulen MJ, Lobbezoo F, Aartman IH, Naeije M. Self-reported oral parafunctions and pain intensity in temporomandibular disorder patients. J Orofac Pain 2006;20:31–35.

247. Svensson P, Jadidi F, Arima T, Baad-Hansen L, Sessle BJ. Relationships between craniofacial pain and bruxism. J Oral Rehabil 2008;35:524–547.

248. Pergamalian A, Rudy TE, Zaki HS, Greco CM. The association between wear facets, bruxism, and severity of facial pain in patients with temporomandibular disorders. J Prosthet Dent 2003;90:194–200.

249. Carlsson GE, Egermark I, Magnusson T. Predictors of signs and symptoms of temporomandibular disorders: A 20-year follow-up study from childhood to adulthood. Acta Odontol Scand 2002;60:180–185.

250. Clark GT, Tsukiyama Y, Baba K, Watanabe T. Sixty-eight years of experimental occlusal interference studies: What have we learned? J Prosthet Dent 1999;82:704–713.

251. Magnusson T, Egermarki I, Carlsson GE. A prospective investigation over two decades on signs and symptoms of temporomandibular disorders and associated variables. A final summary. Acta Odontol Scand 2005;63:99–109.

252. Pereira LJ, Pereira-Cenci T, Del Bel Cury AA, et al. Risk indicators of temporomandibular disorder incidences in early adolescence. Pediatr Dent 2010;32:324–328.

253. Marklund S, Wänman A. Risk factors associated with incidence and persistence of signs and symptoms of temporomandibular disorders. Acta Odontol Scand 2010;68:289–299.

254. Manfredini D, Peretta R, Guarda-Nardini L, Ferronato G. Predictive value of combined clinically diagnosed bruxism and occlusal features for TMJ pain. Cranio 2010;28:105–113.

255. Gesch D, Bernhardt O, Alte D, Kocher T, John U, Hensel E. Malocclusions and clinical signs or subjective symptoms of temporomandibular disorders (TMD) in adults. Results of the population-based Study of Health in Pomerania (SHIP) [in German]. J Orofac Orthop 2004;65:88–103.

256. Henrikson T, Nilner M. Temporomandibular disorders, occlusion and orthodontic treatment. J Orthod 2003;30:129–137.

257. Sonnesen L, Svensson P. Temporomandibular disorders and psychological status in adult patients with a deep bite. Eur J Orthod 2008;30:621–629.

258. Le Bell Y, Niemi PM, Jämsä T, Kylmälä M, Alanen P. Subjective reactions to intervention with artificial interferences in subjects with and without a history of temporomandibular disorders. Acta Odontol Scand 2006;64:59–63.

259. Gesch D, Bernhardt O, Kirbschus A. Association of malocclusion and functional occlusion with temporomandibular disorders (TMD) in adults: A systematic review of population-based studies. Quintessence 2004;35:211–221.

260. Pahkala R, Qvarnström M. Can temporomandibular dysfunction signs be predicted by early morphological or functional variables? Eur J Orthod 2004;26:367–373.

261. Gesch D, Bernhardt O, Mack F, John U, Kocher T, Alte D. Association of malocclusion and functional occlusion with subjective symptoms of TMD in adults: Results of the Study of Health in Pomerania (SHIP). Angle Orthod 2005;75:183–190.

262. Farella M, Bakke M, Michelotti A, Rapuano A, Martina R. Masseter thickness, endurance and exercise-induced pain in subjects with different vertical craniofacial morphology. Eur J Oral Sci 2003;111:183–188.

263. Egermark I, Carlsson GE, Magnusson T. A 20-year longitudinal study of subjective symptoms of temporomandibular disorders from childhood to adulthood. Acta Odontol Scand 2001;59:40–48.

264. Mohlin BO, Derweduwen K, Pilley R, Kingdon A, Shaw WC, Kenealy P. Malocclusion and temporomandibular disorder: A comparison of adolescents with moderate to severe dysfunction with those without signs and symptoms of temporomandibular disorder and their further development to 30 years of age. Angle Orthod 2004;74:319–327.

265. Egermark I, Carlsson GE, Magnusson T. A prospective long-term study of signs and symptoms of temporomandibular disorders in patients who received orthodontic treatment in childhood. Angle Orthod 2005;75:645–650.

266. Macfarlane TV, Kenealy P, Kingdon HA, et al. Twenty-year cohort study of health gain from orthodontic treatment: Temporomandibular disorders. Am J Orthod Dentofacial Orthop 2009;135:692;e691–e698.

267. Hirsch C. No increased risk of temporomandibular disorders and bruxism in children and adolescents during orthodontic therapy. J Orofac Orthop 2009;70:39–50.

268. Kim MR, Graber TM, Viana MA. Orthodontics and temporomandibular disorder: A meta-analysis. Am J Orthod Dentofacial Orthop 2002;121:438–446.

269. Luther F, Layton S, McDonald F. Orthodontics for treating temporomandibular joint (TMJ) disorders. Cochrane Database Syst Rev 2010;(7).

270. McNamara JA Jr, Seligman DA, Okeson JP. Occlusion, orthodontic treatment, and temporomandibular disorders: A review. J Orofac Pain 1995;9:73–90.

271. How CK. Orthodontic treatment has little to do with temporomandibular disorders. Evid Based Dent 2004;5:75.

272. Slade GD, Diatchenko L, Ohrbach R, Maixner W. Orthodontic treatment, genetic factors and risk of temporomandibular disorder. Semin Orthod 2008;14:146–156.

273. Al-Riyami S, Cunningham SJ, Moles DR. Orthognathic treatment and temporomandibular disorders: A systematic review. Part 2. Signs and symptoms and meta-analyses. Am J Orthod Dentofacial Orthop 2009;136:626;e621–e616.

274. Sessle BJ, Hu JW. Mechanisms of pain arising from articular tissues. Can J Physiol Pharmacol 1991;69:617–626.

275. Schiffman EL, Anderson GC, Fricton JR, Lindgren BR. The relationship between level of mandibular pain and dysfunction and stage of temporomandibular joint internal derangement. J Dent Res 1992;71:1812–1815.

276. Sessle BJ. The neural basis of temporomandibular joint and masticatory muscle pain. J Orofac Pain 1999;13:238–245.

277. Sessle BJ. Acute and chronic craniofacial pain: Brainstem mechanisms of nociceptive transmission and neuroplasticity, and their clinical correlates. Crit Rev Oral Biol Med 2000;11:57–91.

278. Broton JG, Sessle BJ. Reflex excitation of masticatory muscles induced by algesic chemicals applied to the temporomandibular joint of the cat. Arch Oral Biol 1988;33:741–747.

279. Kato T, Thie NM, Huynh N, Miyawaki S, Lavigne GJ. Topical review: Sleep bruxism and the role of peripheral sensory influences. J Orofac Pain 2003;17:191–213.

280. Winocur E, Gavish A, Voikovitch M, Emodi-Perlman A, Eli I. Drugs and bruxism: A critical review. J Orofac Pain 2003;17:99–111.

281. Ahlberg J, Savolainen A, Rantala M, Lindholm H, Könönen M. Reported bruxism and biopsychosocial symptoms: A longitudinal study. Community Dent Oral Epidemiol 2004;32:307–311.

282. Bader G, Lavigne G. Sleep bruxism; An overview of an oromandibular sleep movement disorder. Review article. Sleep Med Rev 2000;4:27–43.

283. Lavigne GJ, Rompré PH, Poirier G, Huard H, Kato T, Montplaisir JY. Rhythmic masticatory muscle activity during sleep in humans. J Dent Res 2001;80:443–448.

284. Ariji Y, Sakuma S, Izumi M, et al. Ultrasonographic features of the masseter muscle in female patients with temporomandibular disorder associated with myofascial pain. Oral Surg Oral Med Oral Pathol Oral Radiol Endod 2004;98:337–341.

285. Clark GT, Adler RC, Lee JJ. Jaw pain and tenderness levels during and after repeated sustained maximum voluntary protrusion. Pain 1991;45:17–22.

286. Gay T, Maton B, Rendell J, Majourau A. Characteristics of muscle fatigue in patients with myofascial pain-dysfunction syndrome. Arch Oral Biol 1994;39:847–852.

287. Türp JC, Schindler HJ, Pritsch M, Rong Q. Anteroposterior activity changes in the superficial masseter muscle after exposure to experimental pain. Eur J Oral Sci 2002;110:83–91.

288. Lund JP, Stohler CS. Effects of pain on muscular activity in temporomandibular disorders and related conditions. In: Stohler CS, Carlson DS (eds). Biological and Psychological Aspects of Orofacial Pain. Ann Arbor: University of Michigan, 1994:74–91.

289. Shiau YY, Peng CC, Wen SC, Lin LD, Wang JS, Lou KL. The effects of masseter muscle pain on biting performance. J Oral Rehabil 2003;30:978–984.

290. Buchner R, Van der Glas HW, Brouwers JE, Bosman F. Electromyographic parameters related to clenching level and jaw-jerk reflex in patients with a simple type of myogenous cranio-mandibular disorder. J Oral Rehabil 1992;19:495–511.

291. Glaros AG, Burton E. Parafunctional clenching, pain, and effort in temporomandibular disorders. J Behav Med 2004;27:91–100.

292. Glaros AG, Tabacchi KN, Glass EG. Effect of parafunctional clenching on TMD pain. J Orofac Pain 1998;12:145–152.

293. Zennaro D, Läubli T, Krebs D, Klipstein A, Krueger H. Continuous, intermitted and sporadic motor unit activity in the trapezius muscle during prolonged computer work. J Electromyogr Kinesiol 2003;13:113–124.

294. Sjøgaard G, Søgaard K. Muscle injury in repetitive motion disorders. Clin Orthop Relat Res 1998;(351):21–31.

295. Farella M, De Oliveira ME, Gallo LM, et al. Firing duration of masseter motor units during prolonged low-level contractions. Clin Neurophysiol 2011;122:2433–2440.

296. Lobbezoo F, van Selms MK, Naeije M. Masticatory muscle pain and disordered jaw motor behaviour: Literature review over the past decade. Arch Oral Biol 2006;51:713–720.

297. Macfarlane TV, Blinkhorn AS, Davies RM, Worthington HV. Association between local mechanical factors and orofacial pain: Survey in the community. J Dent 2003;31:535–542.

298. Manfredini D, Lobbezoo F. Relationship between bruxism and temporomandibular disorders: A systematic review of literature from 1998 to 2008. Oral Surg Oral Med Oral Pathol Oral Radiol Endod 2010;109:e26–e50.

299. Marbach JJ, Raphael KG, Janal MN, Hirschkorn-Roth R. Reliability of clinician judgements of bruxism. J Oral Rehabil 2003;30:113–118.

300. Johansson A, Unell L, Carlsson GE, Söderfeldt B, Halling A. Risk factors associated with symptoms of temporomandibular disorders in a population of 50- and 60-year-old subjects. J Oral Rehabil 2006;33:473–481.

301. Lund JP, Donga R, Widmer CG, Stohler CS. The pain-adaptation model: A discussion of the relationship between chronic musculoskeletal pain and motor activity. Can J Physiol Pharmacol 1991;69:683–694.

302. Graven-Nielsen T, Svensson P, Arendt-Nielsen L. Effects of experimental muscle pain on muscle activity and co-ordination during static and dynamic motor function. Electroencephalogr Clin Neurophysiol 1997;105:156–164.

303. Svensson P, Arendt-Nielsen L, Houe L. Muscle pain modulates mastication: An experimental study in humans. J Orofac Pain 1998;12:7–16.

304. Murray GM, Peck CC. Orofacial pain and jaw muscle activity: A new model. J Orofac Pain 2007;21:263–278.

305. Lavigne GJ, Rompré PH, Montplaisir JY. Sleep bruxism: Validity of clinical research diagnostic criteria in a controlled polysomnographic study. J Dent Res 1996;75:546–552.

306. Raphael KG, Sirois DA, Janal MN, et al. Sleep bruxism and myofascial temporomandibular disorders: A laboratory-based polysomnographic investigation. J Am Dent Assoc 2012;143:1223–1231.

307. Raphael KG, Janal MN, Sirois DA, et al. Masticatory muscle sleep background electromyographic activity is elevated in myofascial temporomandibular disorder patients. J Oral Rehabil 2013;40:883–891.

308. Shah JP, Phillips TM, Danoff JV, Gerber LH. An in vivo microanalytical technique for measuring the local biochemical milieu of human skeletal muscle. J Appl Physiol 2005;99:1977–1984.

309. Couppé C, Torelli P, Fuglsang-Frederiksen A, Andersen KV, Jensen R. Myofascial trigger points are very prevalent in patients with chronic tension-type headache: A double-blinded controlled study. Clin J Pain 2007;23:23–27.

310. Maekawa K, Clark GT, Kuboki T. Intramuscular hypoperfusion, adrenergic receptors, and chronic muscle pain. J Pain 2002;3:251–260.

311. Mense S. Do we know enough to put forward a unifying hypothesis? J Pain 2002;3:264–267.

312. Weingarten TN, Iverson BC, Shi Y, Schroeder DR, Warner DO, Reid KI. Impact of tobacco use on the symptoms of painful temporomandibular joint disorders. Pain 2009;147:67–71.

313. Melis M, Lobo SL, Ceneviz C, et al. Effect of cigarette smoking on pain intensity of TMD patients: A pilot study. Cranio 2010;28:187–192.

314. Sanders AE, Maixner W, Nackley AG, et al. Excess risk of temporomandibular disorder associated with cigarette smoking in young adults. J Pain 2012;13:21–31.

315. Benoliel R, Sela G, Teich S, Sharav Y. Painful temporomandibular disorders and headaches in 359 dental and medical students. Quintessence 2011;42:73–78.

316. Michalowicz BS, Pihlstrom BL, Hodges JS, Bouchard TJ Jr. No heritability of temporomandibular joint signs and symptoms. J Dent Res 2000;79:1573–1578.

317. Raphael KG, Marbach JJ, Gallagher RM, Dohrenwend BP. Myofascial TMD does not run in families. Pain 1999;80:15–22.

318. Ojima K, Watanabe N, Narita N, Narita M. Temporomandibular disorder is associated with a serotonin transporter gene polymorphism in the Japanese population. Biopsychosoc Med 2007;1:3.

319. Erdal ME, Herken H, Mutlu MN, Bayazit YA. Significance of catechol-O-methyltransferase gene polymorphism in myofacial pain syndrome. Pain Clin 2003;15:309–313.

320. Diatchenko L, Anderson AD, Slade GD, et al. Three major haplotypes of the beta2 adrenergic receptor define psychological profile, blood pressure, and the risk for development of a common musculoskeletal pain disorder. Am J Med Genet B Neuropsychiatr Genet 2006;141B:449–462.

321. Diatchenko L, Nackley AG, Slade GD, et al. Catechol-O-methyltransferase gene polymorphisms are associated with multiple pain-evoking stimuli. Pain 2006;125:216–224.

322. Zubieta JK, Heitzeg MM, Smith YR, et al. COMT val158met genotype affects mu-opioid neurotransmitter responses to a pain stressor. Science 2003;299:1240–1243.

323. Smith SB, Maixner DW, Greenspan JD, et al. Potential genetic risk factors for chronic TMD: Genetic associations from the OPPERA case control study. J Pain 2011;12(11, suppl):T92–T101.

324. Ohayon MM. Relationship between chronic painful physical condition and insomnia. J Psychiatr Res 2005;39:151–159.

325. Edwards RR, Grace E, Peterson S, Klick B, Haythornthwaite JA, Smith MT. Sleep continuity and architecture: Associations with pain-inhibitory processes in patients with temporomandibular joint disorder. Eur J Pain 2009;13:1043–1047.

326. Smith MT, Edwards RR, McCann UD, Haythornthwaite JA. The effects of sleep deprivation on pain inhibition and spontaneous pain in women. Sleep 2007;30:494–505.

327. Smith MT, Haythornthwaite JA. How do sleep disturbance and chronic pain inter-relate? Insights from the longitudinal and cognitive-behavioral clinical trials literature. Sleep Med Rev 2004;8:119–132.

328. Benoliel R, Eliav E, Sharav Y. Self-reports of pain-related awakenings in persistent orofacial pain patients. J Orofac Pain 2009;23:330–338.

329. Riley JL 3rd, Benson MB, Gremillion HA, et al. Sleep disturbance in orofacial pain patients: Pain-related or emotional distress? Cranio 2001;19:106–113.

330. Wong MC, McMillan AS, Zheng J, Lam CL. The consequences of orofacial pain symptoms: A population-based study in Hong Kong. Community Dent Oral Epidemiol 2008;36:417–424.

331. Yatani H, Studts J, Cordova M, Carlson CR, Okeson JP. Comparison of sleep quality and clinical and psychologic characteristics in patients with temporomandibular disorders. J Orofac Pain 2002;16:221–228.

332. Lindroth JE, Schmidt JE, Carlson CR. A comparison between masticatory muscle pain patients and intracapsular pain patients on behavioral and psychosocial domains. J Orofac Pain 2002;16:277–283.

333. Smith MT, Wickwire EM, Grace EG, et al. Sleep disorders and their association with laboratory pain sensitivity in temporomandibular joint disorder. Sleep 2009;32:779–790.

334. Grossi ML, Goldberg MB, Locker D, Tenenbaum HC. Irritable bowel syndrome patients versus responding and nonresponding temporomandibular disorder patients: A neuropsychologic profile comparative study. Int J Prosthodont 2008;21:201–209.

335. Balasubramaniam R, de Leeuw R, Zhu H, Nickerson RB, Okeson JP, Carlson CR. Prevalence of temporomandibular disorders in fibromyalgia and failed back syndrome patients: A blinded prospective comparison study. Oral Surg Oral Med Oral Pathol Oral Radiol Endod 2007;104:204–216.

336. Clauw DJ. Fibromyalgia: An overview. Am J Med 2009;122(12, suppl):S3–S13.

337. Di Paolo C, Di Nunno A, Vanacore N, Bruti G. ID migraine questionnaire in temporomandibular disorders with craniofacial pain: A study by using a multidisciplinary approach. Neurol Sci 2009;30:295–299.

338. Franco AL, Gonçalves DA, Castanharo SM, Speciali JG, Bigal ME, Camparis CM. Migraine is the most prevalent primary headache in individuals with temporomandibular disorders. J Orofac Pain 2010;24:287–292.

339. Stuginski-Barbosa J, Macedo HR, Bigal ME, Speciali JG. Signs of temporomandibular disorders in migraine patients: A prospective, controlled study. Clin J Pain 2010;26:418–421.

340. Gonçalves DA, Bigal ME, Jales LC, Camparis CM, Speciali JG. Headache and symptoms of temporomandibular disorder: An epidemiological study. Headache 2010;50:231–241.

341. Ballegaard V, Thede-Schmidt-Hansen P, Svensson P, Jensen R. Are headache and temporomandibular disorders related? A blinded study. Cephalalgia 2008;28:832–841.

342. Sahler K. Epidemiology and cultural differences in tension-type headache. Curr Pain Headache Rep 2012;16:525–532.

343. Lyngberg AC, Rasmussen BK, Jørgensen T, Jensen R. Has the prevalence of migraine and tension-type headache changed over a 12-year period? A Danish population survey. Eur J Epidemiol 2005;20:243–249.

344. Russell MB. Tension-type headache in 40-year-olds: A Danish population-based sample of 4000. J Headache Pain 2005;6:441–447.

345. Jensen R, Symon D. Epidemiology of tension-type headache. In: Olesen J, Goadsby PJ, Ramadan NM, Tfelt-Hansen P, Welch KMA (eds). The Headaches, ed 3. Philadelphia: Lippincott Williams & Wilkins, 2006:621–624.

346. Pryse-Phillips W, Findlay H, Tugwell P, Edmeads J, Murray TJ, Nelson RF. A Canadian population survey on the clinical, epidemiologic and societal impact of migraine and tension-type headache. Can J Neurol Sci 1992;19:333–339.

347. Stovner LJ, Zwart JA, Hagen K, Terwindt GM, Pascual J. Epidemiology of headache in Europe. Eur J Neurol 2006;13:333–345.

348. Rasmussen BK, Jensen R, Olesen J. Impact of headache on sickness absence and utilisation of medical services: A Danish population study. J Epidemiol Community Health 1992;46:443–446.

349. Holroyd KA, Stensland M, Lipchik GL, Hill KR, O'Donnell FS, Cordingley G. Psychosocial correlates and impact of chronic tension-type headaches. Headache 2000;40:3–16.

350. Ostergaard S, Russell MB, Bendtsen L, Olesen J. Comparison of first degree relatives and spouses of people with chronic tension headache. BMJ 1997;314:1092–1093.

351. Ulrich V, Gervil M, Olesen J. The relative influence of environment and genes in episodic tension-type headache. Neurology 2004;62:2065–2069.

352. Iversen HK, Langemark M, Andersson PG, Hansen PE, Olesen J. Clinical characteristics of migraine and episodic tension-type headache in relation to old and new diagnostic criteria. Headache 1990;30:514–519.

353. Inan LE, Tulunay FC, Guvener A, Tokgoz G, Inan N. Characteristics of headache in migraine without aura and episodic tension-type headache in the Turkish population according to the IHS classification. Cephalalgia 1994;14:171–173.

354. Göbel H, Petersen-Braun M, Soyka D. The epidemiology of headache in Germany: A nationwide survey of a representative sample on the basis of the headache classification of the International Headache Society. Cephalalgia 1994;14:97–106.

355. Karadas Ö, Gül HL, Inan LE. Lidocaine injection of pericranial myofascial trigger points in the treatment of frequent episodic tension-type headache. J Headache Pain 2013;14:44.

356. Blaschek A, Milde-Busch A, Straube A, et al. Self-reported muscle pain in adolescents with migraine and tension-type headache. Cephalalgia 2012;32:241–249.

357. Jensen R. Mechanisms of spontaneous tension-type headaches: An analysis of tenderness, pain thresholds and EMG. Pain 1996;64:251–256.

358. Couch JR. The long-term prognosis of tension-type headache. Curr Pain Headache Rep 2005;9:436–441.

359. Lyngberg AC, Rasmussen BK, Jørgensen T, Jensen R. Prognosis of migraine and tension-type headache: A population-based follow-up study. Neurology 2005;65:580–585.

360. Karli N, Zarifoglu M, Calisir N, Akgoz S. Comparison of pre-headache phases and trigger factors of migraine and episodic tension-type headache: Do they share similar clinical pathophysiology? Cephalalgia 2005;25:444–451.

361. Spierings EL, Ranke AH, Honkoop PC. Precipitating and aggravating factors of migraine versus tension-type headache. Headache 2001;41:554–558.

362. Rasmussen BK, Jensen R, Schroll M, Olesen J. Interrelations between migraine and tension-type headache in the general population. Arch Neurol 1992;49:914–918.

363. Ulrich V, Russell MB, Jensen R, Olesen J. A comparison of tension-type headache in migraineurs and in non-migraineurs: A population-based study. Pain 1996;67:501–506.

364. Köseoglu E, Naçar M, Talaslioglu A, Cetinkaya F. Epidemiological and clinical characteristics of migraine and tension type headache in 1146 females in Kayseri, Turkey. Cephalalgia 2003;23:381–388.

365. Lipton RB, Cady RK, Stewart WF, Wilks K, Hall C. Diagnostic lessons from the spectrum study. Neurology 2002;58(9, suppl):S27–S31.

366. Engstrøm M, Hagen K, Bjørk M, Stovner L, Stjern M, Sand T. Sleep quality, arousal and pain thresholds in tension-type headache: A blinded controlled polysomnographic study. Cephalalgia 2014;34:455–463.

367. Rasmussen BK, Jensen R, Olesen J. A population-based analysis of the diagnostic criteria of the International Headache Society. Cephalalgia 1991;11:129–134.

368. Lipton RB, Stewart WF, Cady R, et al. 2000 Wolfe Award. Sumatriptan for the range of headaches in migraine sufferers: Results of the Spectrum Study. Headache 2000;40:783–791.

369. Silberstein SD, Lipton RB, Sliwinski M. Classification of daily and near-daily headaches: Field trial of revised IHS criteria. Neurology 1996;47:871–875.

370. Bigal ME, Sheftell FD, Rapoport AM, Lipton RB, Tepper SJ. Chronic daily headache in a tertiary care population: Correlation between the International Headache Society Diagnostic Criteria and proposed revisions of criteria for chronic daily headache. Cephalalgia 2002;22:432–438.

371. Lantéri-Minet M, Auray JP, El Hasnaoui A, et al. Prevalence and description of chronic daily headache in the general population in France. Pain 2003;102:143–149.

372. Hagen K, Zwart JA, Vatten L, Stovner LJ, Bovim G. Prevalence of migraine and non-migrainous headache—Head-HUNT, a large population-based study. Cephalalgia 2000;20:900–906.

373. Deleu D, Hanssens Y. Primary chronic daily headache: Clinical and pharmacological aspects. A clinic-based study in Oman. Headache 1999;39:432–436.

374. Raieli V, Eliseo M, Pandolfi E, et al. Recurrent and chronic headaches in children below 6 years of age. J Headache Pain 2005;6:135–142.

375. Castillo J, Munoz P, Guitera V, Pascual J. Epidemiology of chronic daily headache in the general population. Headache 1999;39:190–196.

376. Prencipe M, Casini AR, Ferretti C, et al. Prevalence of headache in an elderly population: Attack frequency, disability, and use of medication. J Neurol Neurosurg Psychiatry 2001;70:377–381.

377. Wang SJ, Fuh JL, Lu SR, et al. Chronic daily headache in Chinese elderly: Prevalence, risk factors, and biannual follow-up. Neurology 2000;54:314–319.

378. Scher AI, Stewart WF, Ricci JA, Lipton RB. Factors associated with the onset and remission of chronic daily headache in a population-based study. Pain 2003;106:81-89.

379. Solomon S, Lipton RB, Newman LC. Clinical features of chronic daily headache. Headache 1992;32:325–329.

380. Bendtsen L, Jensen R. Mirtazapine is effective in the prophylactic treatment of chronic tension-type headache. Neurology 2004;62:1706–1711.

381. Langemark M, Olesen J, Poulsen DL, Bech P. Clinical characterization of patients with chronic tension headache. Headache 1988;28:590–596.

382. Manzoni GC, Granella F, Sandrini G, Cavallini A, Zanferrari C, Nappi G. Classification of chronic daily headache by International Headache Society criteria: Limits and new proposals. Cephalalgia 1995;15:37–43.

383. Jensen R, Rasmussen BK. Muscular disorders in tension-type headache. Cephalalgia 1996;16:97–103.

384. Bendtsen L, Jensen R, Olesen J. Decreased pain detection and tolerance thresholds in chronic tension-type headache. Arch Neurol 1996;53:373–376.

385. Prakash S, Kumar M, Belani P, Susvirkar A, Ahuja S. Interrelationships between chronic tension-type headache, musculoskeletal pain, and vitamin D deficiency: Is osteomalacia responsible for both headache and musculoskeletal pain? Ann Indian Acad Neurol 2013;16:650–658.

386. Palermo TM, Kiska R. Subjective sleep disturbances in adolescents with chronic pain: Relationship to daily functioning and quality of life. J Pain 2005;6:201–207.

387. de Filippis S, Salvatori E, Coloprisco G, Martelletti P. Headache and mood disorders. J Headache Pain 2005;6:250–253.

388. Olesen J, Bousser M-G, Diener HC, et al. The International Classification of Headache Disorders, 2nd Edition. Cephalalgia 2004;24(1, suppl):24–150.

389. Steiner TJ, Lange R, Voelker M. Aspirin in episodic tension-type headache: Placebo-controlled dose-ranging comparison with paracetamol. Cephalalgia 2003;23:59–66.

390. Schachtel BP, Furey SA, Thoden WR. Nonprescription ibuprofen and acetaminophen in the treatment of tension-type headache. J Clin Pharmacol 1996;36:1120–1125.

391. Kubitzek F, Ziegler G, Gold MS, Liu JM, Ionescu E. Low-dose diclofenac potassium in the treatment of episodic tension-type headache. Eur J Pain 2003;7:155–162.

392. Prior MJ, Cooper KM, May LG, Bowen DL. Efficacy and safety of acetaminophen and naproxen in the treatment of tension-type headache. A randomized, double-blind, placebo-controlled trial. Cephalalgia 2002;22:740–748.

393. Mathew NT, Ashina M. Acute pharmacotherapy of tension-type headaches. In: Olesen J, Goadsby PJ, Ramadan NM, Tfelt-Hansen P, Welch KMA (eds). The Headaches, ed 3. Philadelphia: Lippincott Williams & Wilkins, 2006:727–733.

394. Bendtsen L, Evers S, Linde M, et al. EFNS guideline on the treatment of tension-type headache—Report of an EFNS task force. Eur J Neurol 2010;17:1318–1325.

395. Diamond S, Freitag FG. The use of ibuprofen plus caffeine to treat tension-type headache. Curr Pain Headache Rep 2001;5:472–478.

396. Brennum J, Kjeldsen M, Olesen J. The 5-HT1-like agonist sumatriptan has a significant effect in chronic tension-type headache. Cephalalgia 1992;12:375–379.

397. Cady RK, Gutterman D, Saiers JA, Beach ME. Responsiveness of non-IHS migraine and tension-type headache to sumatriptan. Cephalalgia 1997;17:588–590.

398. Bendtsen L, Jensen R, Olesen J. A non-selective (amitriptyline), but not a selective (citalopram), serotonin reuptake inhibitor is effective in the prophylactic treatment of chronic tension-type headache. J Neurol Neurosurg Psychiatry 1996;61:285–290.

399. Tomkins GE, Jackson JL, O'Malley PG, Balden E, Santoro JE. Treatment of chronic headache with antidepressants: A meta-analysis. Am J Med 2001;111:54–63.

400. Stillman MJ. Pharmacotherapy of tension-type headaches. Curr Pain Headache Rep 2002;6:408–413.

401. Holroyd KA. Behavioral and psychologic aspects of the pathophysiology and management of tension-type headache. Curr Pain Headache Rep 2002;6:401–407.

402. Bogaards MC, ter Kuile MM. Treatment of recurrent tension headache: A meta-analytic review. Clin J Pain 1994;10:174–190.

403. Holroyd KA, O'Donnell FJ, Stensland M, Lipchik GL, Cordingley GE, Carlson BW. Management of chronic tension-type headache with tricyclic antidepressant medication, stress management therapy, and their combination: A randomized controlled trial. JAMA 2001;285:2208–2215.

404. Fernandez-de-Las-Penas C, Alonso-Blanco C, Cuadrado ML, Miangolarra JC, Barriga FJ, Pareja JA. Are manual therapies effective in reducing pain from tension-type headache?: A systematic review. Clin J Pain 2006;22:278–285.

405. Ashkenazi A, Blumenfeld A. OnabotulinumtoxinA for the treatment of headache. Headache 2013;53(suppl 2):54–61.

406. Linde K, Allais G, Brinkhaus B, Manheimer E, Vickers A, White AR. Acupuncture for tension-type headache. Cochrane Database Syst Rev 2009:CD007587.

407. Magnusson T, Carlsson GE. A 2½-year follow-up of changes in headache and mandibular dysfunction after stomatognathic treatment. J Prosthet Dent 1983;49:398–402.

408. Schokker RP, Hansson TL, Ansink BJ. The result of treatment of the masticatory system of chronic headache patients. J Craniomandib Disord 1990;4:126–130.

409. Vallon D, Ekberg E, Nilner M, Kopp S. Occlusal adjustment in patients with craniomandibular disorders including headaches. A 3- and 6-month follow-up. Acta Odontol Scand 1995;53:55–59.

410. Bendtsen L, Fernandez-de-la-Penas C. The role of muscles in tension-type headache. Curr Pain Headache Rep 2011;15:451–458.

411. Jensen K, Norup M. Experimental pain in human temporal muscle induced by hypertonic saline, potassium and acidity. Cephalalgia 1992;12:101–106.

412. Schmidt-Hansen P, Svensson P, Jensen T, Graven-Nielsen T, Bach F. Patterns of experimentally induced pain in pericranial muscles. Cephalalgia 2006;26:568–577.

413. Simons DG, Travell JG, Simons LS. Head and neck pain. In: Travell JG, Simons DG (eds). Myofascial Pain and Dysfunction: The Trigger Point Manual, ed 2. Baltimore: Williams and Wilkins, 1999:237–483.

414. Svensson P, Cairns BE, Wang K, et al. Glutamate-evoked pain and mechanical allodynia in the human masseter muscle. Pain 2003;101:221–227.

415. Kawakita K, Dostrovsky JO, Tang JS, Chiang CY. Responses of neurons in the rat thalamic nucleus submedius to cutaneous, muscle and visceral nociceptive stimuli. Pain 1993;55:327–338.

416. Gobel H, Cordes P. Circadian variation of pain sensitivity in pericranial musculature. Headache 1990;30:418–422.

417. Jensen R, Olesen J. Initiating mechanisms of experimentally induced tension-type headache. Cephalalgia 1996;16:175–182.

418. Lacroix JM, Corbett L. An experimental test of the muscle tension hypothesis of tension-type headache. Int J Psychophysiol 1990;10:47–51.

419. Neufeld JD, Holroyd KA, Lipchik GL. Dynamic assessment of abnormalities in central pain transmission and modulation in tension-type headache sufferers. Headache 2000;40:142–151.

420. Christensen MB, Bendtsen L, Ashina M, Jensen R. Experimental induction of muscle tenderness and headache in tension-type headache patients. Cephalalgia 2005;25:1061–1067.

421. Ashina M. Neurobiology of chronic tension-type headache. Cephalalgia 2004;24:161–172.

422. Arima T, Svensson P, Arendt-Nielsen L. Experimental grinding in healthy subjects: A model for postexercise jaw muscle soreness? J Orofac Pain 1999;13:104–114.

423. Lake AE 3rd, Rains JC, Penzien DB, Lipchik GL. Headache and psychiatric comorbidity: Historical context, clinical implications, and research relevance. Headache 2005;45:493–506.

424. Breslau N, Lipton RB, Stewart WF, Schultz LR, Welch KM. Comorbidity of migraine and depression: Investigating potential etiology and prognosis. Neurology 2003;60:1308–1312.

425. Wittrock DA, Myers TC. The comparison of individuals with recurrent tension-type headache and headache-free controls in physiological response, appraisal, and coping with stressors: a review of the literature. Ann Behav Med 1998;20:118–134.

426. Cathcart S, Bhullar N, Immink M, Della Vedova C, Hayball J. Pain sensitivity mediates the relationship between stress and headache intensity in chronic tension-type headache. Pain Res Manag 2012;17:377–380.

427. Lipchik GL, Holroyd KA, O'Donnell FJ, et al. Exteroceptive suppression periods and pericranial muscle tenderness in chronic tension-type headache: Effects of psychopathology, chronicity and disability. Cephalalgia 2000;20:638–646.

428. Bendtsen L, Jensen R. Amitriptyline reduces myofascial tenderness in patients with chronic tension-type headache. Cephalalgia 2000;20:603–610.

429. Pielsticker A, Haag G, Zaudig M, Lautenbacher S. Impairment of pain inhibition in chronic tension-type headache. Pain 2005;118:215–223.

430. Langemark M, Bach FW, Jensen TS, Olesen J. Decreased nociceptive flexion reflex threshold in chronic tension-type headache. Arch Neurol 1993;50:1061–1064.

431. Jensen R, Rasmussen BK, Pedersen B, Olesen J. Muscle tenderness and pressure pain thresholds in headache. A population study. Pain 1993;52:193–199.

432. Jensen R, Bendtsen L, Olesen J. Muscular factors are of importance in tension-type headache. Headache 1998;38:10–17.

433. Bendtsen L. Central sensitization in tension-type headache—Possible pathophysiological mechanisms. Cephalalgia 2000;20:486–508.

434. Buchgreitz L, Lyngberg AC, Bendtsen L, Jensen R. Increased pain sensitivity is not a risk factor but a consequence of frequent headache: A population-based follow-up study. Pain 2008;137:623–630.

435. Buchgreitz L, Lyngberg AC, Bendtsen L, Jensen R. Increased prevalence of tension-type headache over a 12-year period is related to increased pain sensitivity. A population study. Cephalalgia 2007;27:145–152.

436. Sandrini G, Rossi P, Milanov I, Serrao M, Cecchini A, Nappi G. Abnormal modulatory influence of diffuse noxious inhibitory controls in migraine and chronic tension-type headache patients. Cephalalgia 2006;26:782–789.

437. Buchgreitz L, Egsgaard LL, Jensen R, Arendt-Nielsen L, Bendtsen L. Abnormal pain processing in chronic tension-type headache: A high-density EEG brain mapping study. Brain 2008;131(Pt 12):3232–3238.

438. Schmidt-Wilcke T, Leinisch E, Straube A, et al. Gray matter decrease in patients with chronic tension type headache. Neurology 2005;65:1483–1486.

439. Robbins MS, Evans RW. The heterogeneity of new daily persistent headache. Headache 2012;52:1579–1589.

440. Joshi SG, Mathew PG, Markley HG. New daily persistent headache and potential new therapeutic agents. Curr Neurol Neurosci Rep 2014;14:425.

441. Li D, Rozen TD. The clinical characteristics of new daily persistent headache. Cephalalgia 2002;22:66–69.

442. Takase Y, Nakano M, Tatsumi C, Matsuyama T. Clinical features, effectiveness of drug-based treatment, and prognosis of new daily persistent headache (NDPH): 30 cases in Japan. Cephalalgia 2004;24:955–959.

443. Li N, Wang J, Huang Q, Tan G, Chen L, Zhou J. Clinical features of new daily persistent headache in a tertiary outpatient population. Headache 2012;52:1546–1552.

444. Robbins MS, Grosberg BM, Napchan U, Crystal SC, Lipton RB. Clinical and prognostic subforms of new daily-persistent headache. Neurology 2010;74:1358–1364.

445. Evans RW. New daily persistent headache. Headache 2012;52(suppl 1):40–44.

446. Peng KP, Fuh JL, Yuan HK, Shia BC, Wang SJ. New daily persistent headache: Should migrainous features be incorporated? Cephalalgia 2011;31:1561–1569.

447. Prakash S, Saini S, Rana KR, Mahato P. Refining clinical features and therapeutic options of new daily persistent headache: A retrospective study of 63 patients in India. J Headache Pain 2012;13:477–485.

448. Peres MF, Lucchetti G, Mercante JP, Young WB. New daily persistent headache and panic disorder. Cephalalgia 2011;31:250–253.

449. Colás R, Muñoz P, Temprano R, Gómez C, Pascual J. Chronic daily headache with analgesic overuse: Epidemiology and impact on quality of life. Neurology 2004;62:1338–1342.

450. Koenig MA, Gladstein J, McCarter RJ, Hershey AD, Wasiewski W. Chronic daily headache in children and adolescents presenting to tertiary headache clinics. Headache 2002;42:491–500.

451. Prakash S, Shah ND. Post-infectious new daily persistent headache may respond to intravenous methylprednisolone. J Headache Pain 2010;11:59–66.

452. Spears RC. Efficacy of botulinum toxin type A in new daily persistent headache. J Headache Pain 2008;9:405–406.

453. Rozen TD, Beams JL. New daily persistent headache with a thunderclap headache onset and complete response to nimodipine (a new distinct subtype of NDPH). J Headache Pain 2013;14:100.

454. Gallagher RM, Mueller L. Managing intractable migraine with naratriptan. Headache 2003;43:991–993.

455. Rapoport AM, Bigal ME, Volcy M, Sheftell FD, Feleppa M, Tepper SJ. Naratriptan in the preventive treatment of refractory chronic migraine: A review of 27 cases. Headache 2003;43:482–489.

456. Sheftell FD, Rapoport AM, Tepper SJ, Bigal ME. Naratriptan in the preventive treatment of refractory transformed migraine: A prospective pilot study. Headache 2005;45:1400–1406.

457. Robbins MS, Crystal SC. New daily-persistent headache versus tension-type headache. Curr Pain Headache Rep 2010;14:431–435.

458. Evans RW. New daily persistent headache. Curr Pain Headache Rep 2003;7:303–307.

459. Goadsby PJ, Boes C. New daily persistent headache. J Neurol Neurosurg Psychiatry 2002;72(2, suppl):6–9.

460. Diaz-Mitoma F, Vanast WJ, Tyrrell DL. Increased frequency of Epstein-Barr virus excretion in patients with new daily persistent headaches. Lancet 1987;1(8530):411–415.

461. Meineri P, Torre E, Rota E, Grasso E. New daily persistent headache: Clinical and serological characteristics in a retrospective study. Neurol Sci 2004;25(suppl 3):S281–S282.

462. Santoni JR, Santoni-Williams CJ. Headache and painful lymphadenopathy in extracranial or systemic infection: Etiology of new daily persistent headaches. Intern Med 1993;32:530–532.

463. Neufeld MY, Treves TA, Chistik V, Korczyn AD. Post-meningitis headache. Headache 1999;39:132–134.

464. Goadsby PJ. New daily persistent headache: A syndrome, not a discrete disorder. Headache 2011;51:650–653.

465. Meyer HP. Myofascial pain syndrome and its suggested role in the pathogenesis and treatment of fibromyalgia syndrome. Curr Pain Headache Rep 2002;6:274–283.

466. Widmer CG. Chronic muscle pain syndromes: An overview. Can J Physiol Pharmacol 1991;69:659–661.

467. Yunus MB. The prevalence of fibromyalgia in other chronic pain conditions. Pain Res Treat 2012;(2012).

468. Ciancaglini R, Radaelli G. The relationship between headache and symptoms of temporomandibular disorder in the general population. J Dent 2001;29:93–98.

469. Liljeström MR, Jämsä A, Le Bell Y, et al. Signs and symptoms of temporomandibular disorders in children with different types of headache. Acta Odontol Scand 2001;59:413–417.

470. Jensen R, Rasmussen BK, Lous I. Oromandibular dysfunctions and provocation of headache. In: Olesen J, Schoenen J (eds). Tension-Type Headache: Classification, Mechanisms and Treatment. New York: Raven, 1993:210–223.

471. Watts PG, Peet KM, Juniper RP. Migraine and the temporomandibular joint: The final answer? Br Dent J 1986;161:170–173.

472. Liljeström MR, Le Bell Y, Anttila P, et al. Headache children with temporomandibular disorders have several types of pain and other symptoms. Cephalalgia 2005;25:1054–1060.

473. Steele JG, Lamey PJ, Sharkey SW, Smith GM. Occlusal abnormalities, pericranial muscle and joint tenderness and tooth wear in a group of migraine patients. J Oral Rehabil 1991;18:453–458.

474. Dodick DW, Eross EJ, Parish JM, Silber M. Clinical, anatomical, and physiologic relationship between sleep and headache. Headache 2003;43:282–292.

475. Ware JC, Rugh JD. Destructive bruxism: Sleep stage relationship. Sleep 1988;11:172–181.

476. Marcus DA, Bernstein C, Rudy TE. Fibromyalgia and headache: An epidemiological study supporting migraine as part of the fibromyalgia syndrome. Clin Rheumatol 2005;24:595–601.

477. Yunus MB, Inanici F, Aldag JC, Mangold RF. Fibromyalgia in men: Comparison of clinical features with women. J Rheumatol 2000;27:485–490.

478. Wolfe F, Smythe HA, Yunus MB, et al. The American College of Rheumatology 1990 criteria for the classification of fibromyalgia. Report of the Multicenter Criteria Committee. Arthritis Rheum 1990;33:160–172.

479. Wolfe F, Clauw DJ, Fitzcharles MA, et al. The American College of Rheumatology preliminary diagnostic criteria for fibromyalgia and measurement of symptom severity. Arthritis Care Res (Hoboken) 2010;62:600–610.

480. Wolfe F. New American College of Rheumatology criteria for fibromyalgia: A twenty-year journey. Arthritis Care Res (Hoboken) 2010;62:583–584.

481. Wolfe F, Brähler E, Hinz A, Häuser W. Fibromyalgia prevalence, somatic symptom reporting, and the dimensionality of polysymptomatic distress: Results from a survey of the general population. Arthritis Care Res (Hoboken) 2013;65:777–785.

482. Wolfe F. Fibromyalgia research criteria. J Rheumatol 2014;41:187.

483. Wolfe F, Clauw DJ, Fitzcharles MA, et al. Fibromyalgia criteria and severity scales for clinical and epidemiological studies: A modification of the ACR preliminary diagnostic criteria for fibromyalgia. J Rheumatol 2011;38:1113–1122.

484. Crofford LJ, Clauw DJ. Fibromyalgia: Where are we a decade after the American College of Rheumatology classification criteria were developed? Arthritis Rheum 2002;46:1136–1138.

485. Wolfe F, Simons DG, Fricton J, et al. The fibromyalgia and myofascial pain syndromes: A preliminary study of tender points and trigger points in persons with fibromyalgia, myofascial pain syndrome and no disease. J Rheumatol 1992;19:944–951.

486. Inanici F, Yunus MB, Aldag JC. Clinical features and psychological factors in regional soft tissue pain: Comparison with fibromyalgia syndrome. J Musculoskelet Pain 1999;7:293–301.

487. White KP, Speechley M, Harth M, Ostbye T. The London Fibromyalgia Epidemiology Study: The prevalence of fibromyalgia syndrome in London, Ontario. J Rheumatol 1999;26:1570–1576.

488. Yunus M, Masi AT, Calabro JJ, Miller KA, Feigenbaum SL. Primary fibromyalgia (fibrositis): Clinical study of 50 patients with matched normal controls. Semin Arthritis Rheum 1981;11:151–171.

489. Moldofsky H. Management of sleep disorders in fibromyalgia. Rheum Dis Clin North Am 2002;28:353–365.

490. Moldofsky H. Sleep and pain. Sleep Med Rev 2001;5:385–396.

491. Yunus MB, Ahles TA, Aldag JC, Masi AT. Relationship of clinical features with psychological status in primary fibromyalgia. Arthritis Rheum 1991;34:15–21.

492. Wolfe F, Anderson J, Harkness D, et al. Health status and disease severity in fibromyalgia: Results of a six-center longitudinal study. Arthritis Rheum 1997;40:1571–1579.

493. Queiroz LP. Worldwide epidemiology of fibromyalgia. Curr Pain Headache Rep 2013;17:356.

494. Weir PT, Harlan GA, Nkoy FL, et al. The incidence of fibromyalgia and its associated comorbidities: A population-based retrospective cohort study based on International Classification of Diseases, 9th revision codes. J Clin Rheumatol 2006;12:124–128.

495. Wolfe F, Ross K, Anderson J, Russell IJ, Hebert L. The prevalence and characteristics of fibromyalgia in the general population. Arthritis Rheum 1995;38:19–28.

496. Neumann L, Buskila D. Epidemiology of fibromyalgia. Curr Pain Headache Rep 2003;7:362–368.

497. McBeth J, Mulvey MR. Fibromyalgia: Mechanisms and potential impact of the ACR 2010 classification criteria. Nat Rev Rheumatol 2012;8:108–116.

498. Buskila D. Fibromyalgia, chronic fatigue syndrome, and myofascial pain syndrome. Curr Opin Rheumatol 2001;13:117–127.

499. Forseth KO, Husby G, Gran JT, Førre O. Prognostic factors for the development of fibromyalgia in women with self-reported musculoskeletal pain. A prospective study. J Rheumatol 1999;26:2458–2467.

500. Staud R. Abnormal endogenous pain modulation is a shared characteristic of many chronic pain conditions. Expert Rev Neurother 2012;12:577–585.

501. Cagnie B, Coppieters I, Denecker S, Six J, Danneels L, Meeus M. Central sensitization in fibromyalgia? A systematic review on structural and functional brain MRI. Semin Arthritis Rheum 2014;44:68–75.

502. Staud R. Brain imaging in fibromyalgia syndrome. Clin Exp Rheumatol 2011;29(6, suppl):S109–S117.

503. Vierck CJ Jr. Mechanisms underlying development of spatially distributed chronic pain (fibromyalgia). Pain 2006;124:242–263.

504. Jensen TS, Baron R, Haanpää M, et al. A new definition of neuropathic pain. Pain 2011;152:2204–2205.

505. Carville SF, Arendt-Nielsen S, Bliddal H, et al. EULAR evidence-based recommendations for the management of fibromyalgia syndrome. Ann Rheum Dis 2008;67:536–541.

506. Wiffen PJ, Derry S, Moore RA, et al. Antiepileptic drugs for neuropathic pain and fibromyalgia—An overview of Cochrane reviews. Cochrane Database Syst Rev 2013;(11).

507. Häuser W, Thieme K, Türk DC. Guidelines on the management of fibromyalgia syndrome—A systematic review. Eur J Pain 2010;14:5–10.

508. Rao SG, Clauw DJ. The management of fibromyalgia. Drugs Today (Barc) 2004;40:539–554.

509. Ablin J, Fitzcharles MA, Buskila D, Shir Y, Sommer C, Haäuser W. Treatment of fibromyalgia syndrome: Recommendations of recent evidence-based interdisciplinary guidelines with special emphasis on complementary and alternative therapies. Evid Based Complement Alternat Med 2013;2013.

510. Ablin JN, Buskila D. Fibromyalgia syndrome—Novel therapeutic targets. Maturitas 2013;75:335–340.

511. Pimentel MJ, Gui MS, Martins de Aquino LM, Rizzatti-Barbosa CM. Features of temporomandibular disorders in fibromyalgia syndrome. Cranio 2013;31:40–45.

512. Smythe HA. Temporomandibular joint disorder and other medically unexplained symptoms in rheumatoid arthritis, osteoarthritis, and fibromyalgia. J Rheumatol 2005;32:2288–2290.

513. Fraga BP, Santos EB, Farias Neto JP, et al. Signs and symptoms of temporomandibular dysfunction in fibromyalgic patients. J Craniofac Surg 2012;23:615–618.

514. Velly AM, Look JO, Schiffman E, et al. The effect of fibromyalgia and widespread pain on the clinically significant temporomandibular muscle and joint pain disorders—A prospective 18-month cohort study. J Pain 2010;11:1155–1164.

515. Cimino R, Michelotti A, Stradi R, Farinaro C. Comparison of clinical and psychologic features of fibromyalgia and masticatory myofascial pain. J Orofac Pain 1998;12:35–41.

516. Aaron LA, Burke MM, Buchwald D. Overlapping conditions among patients with chronic fatigue syndrome, fibromyalgia, and temporomandibular disorder. Arch Intern Med 2000;160:221–227.

517. de Leeuw R, Studts JL, Carlson CR. Fatigue and fatigue-related symptoms in an orofacial pain population. Oral Surg Oral Med Oral Pathol Oral Radiol Endod 2005;99:168–174.

518. Hedenberg-Magnusson B, Ernberg M, Kopp S. Presence of orofacial pain and temporomandibular disorder in fibromyalgia. A study by questionnaire. Swed Dent J 1999;23:185–192.

519. Wolfe F, Katz RS, Michaud K. Jaw pain: Its prevalence and meaning in patients with rheumatoid arthritis, osteoarthritis, and fibromyalgia. J Rheumatol 2005;32:2421–2428.

520. Raphael KG, Marbach JJ, Klausner J. Myofascial face pain. Clinical characteristics of those with regional vs. widespread pain. J Am Dent Assoc 2000;131:161–171.
521. de Tommaso M. Prevalence, clinical features and potential therapies for fibromyalgia in primary headaches. Expert Rev Neurother 2012;12:287–295.
522. Schur EA, Afari N, Furberg H, et al. Feeling bad in more ways than one: Comorbidity patterns of medically unexplained and psychiatric conditions. J Gen Intern Med 2007;22:818–821.
523. Peres MF, Kaup AO, Zukerman OE, Feldman D. Fibromyalgia and chronic daily headache. Cephalalgia 2000;20:302–303.
524. Hagen K, Einarsen C, Zwart JA, Svebak S, Bovim G. The co-occurrence of headache and musculoskeletal symptoms amongst 51 050 adults in Norway. Eur J Neurol 2002;9:527–533.
525. Hudson JI, Goldenberg DL, Pope HG Jr, Keck PE Jr, Schlesinger L. Comorbidity of fibromyalgia with medical and psychiatric disorders. Am J Med 1992;92:363–367.
526. Peres MF, Young WB, Kaup AO, Zukerman E, Silberstein SD. Fibromyalgia is common in patients with transformed migraine. Neurology 2001;57:1326–1328.

Pain and Dysfunction of the Temporomandibular Joint

Dorrit W. Nitzan, DMD
Gary M. Heir, DMD
M. Franklin Dolwick, DMD, PhD
Rafael Benoliel, BDS, LDS

9

p. 257 - 318

Temporomandibular disorders (TMDs) refer to various painful and nonpainful conditions affecting the temporomandibular joint (TMJ), masticatory muscles, and contiguous tissue components. Two common types of painful TMDs are encountered: *(1)* myogenous, or muscle-generated pain, and *(2)* arthrogenous, or joint-generated pain. As discussed in chapter 8 and in this chapter, the use of the term *TMD* is problematic because it attempts to integrate these two distinct biologic entities into one. The pooling of data from epidemiologic, clinical, and therapeutic studies of "TMD" is therefore misleading. An overview of the overall epidemiology and general characteristics of TMDs is presented in chapter 8.

The Diagnostic Criteria for Temporomandibular Disorders (DC/TMD)[1] further subdivides myalgic and arthralgic TMDs into subgroups, including local myalgia, myofascial pain with and without referral, disc displacement disorders, degenerative joint disease, and subluxation. The DC/TMD also includes headache attributed to TMDs, which is covered elsewhere in this text.

This chapter focuses on pain and dysfunction originating from within the TMJ proper, particularly as a result of disc derangements or osteoarthritis. Other relatively rare joint-related entities that may present with TMJ pain are extremely important in the differential diagnosis but are beyond the scope of this chapter. Some have been partially covered in other chapters (Table 9-1).

The term *internal derangement* is often used as a diagnosis for TMJ disorders. However, internal derangement is a classification or descriptive term, not a diagnosis, and includes disc displacements (joint derangements) and degeneration of the TMJ.[2] *Joint derangement* refers to a biomechanical disturbance in joint function. For an accurate diagnosis, the structures and the mechanical problem must be clearly defined—for example, painful disc displacement with reduction (DDwR), limited mouth opening associated with disc displacement without reduction (DDwoR), intermittent locking, and anchored disc phenomenon. When there is damage to the condyle and/or eminence, it is referred to as *joint degeneration, degenerative joint disease,* or *TMJ osteoarthritis*. This process is

Table 9-1	Differential diagnosis: Entities not covered in this chapter that may be associated with TMJ pain		
Mechanism	**Structure/entity**	**Notes**	**Chapter**
Referred			
Regional	Dental	Referral related to pain intensity	6
	Ear	Very common	7
	Muscular	Very common; pterygoids, masseter	8
	Neurovascular	Hemicrania continua	11
	Neuropathic	Glossopharyngeal, nervus intermedius neuralgias	12
Distant	Cardiac	Usually left-sided, associated with exertion	14
Systemic			
Autoimmune	Rheumatoid arthritis, psoriasis, systemic lupus erythematosus, mixed connective tissue disease, ankylosing spondylitis, systemic sclerosis	Patient's primary disorder has usually been diagnosed and requires specific TMJ-related management	14
Infectious			
Primary	Bacterial	Usually staphylococcal	14
Reactive	Reiter syndrome *p. 492*		14
Tumor			
Benign	Usually bone or cartilage	Uncommon; new-onset malocclusion, painless swelling	14
Malignant	Primary	Uncommon; usually chondrosarcoma, painful mass	14
	Metastatic	More common than primary; breast, lung, prostate	14
	Referred pain	Nasopharyngeal carcinoma	14
	After therapy	Surgery, radiotherapy	14

associated with clear tissue damage and disintegration leading to pathologic changes of the joint components that are not necessarily associated with signs and symptoms.

Many patients report the onset of TMJ pain or dysfunction secondary to trauma; others describe an insidious onset with no apparent cause. However, accumulating data suggest that many TMJ disorders may be primarily due to overuse or overloading of the system. Included in this chapter is a review of current thinking on pathogenesis, diagnosis, and treatment as well as a discussion of pain, dysfunction, and degenerative changes of the TMJ based on the biomechanical and biochemical events underlying these conditions. Although knowledge of the etiology of TMJ disorders is limited, the prognosis of most of these is favorable, and many patients improve spontaneously in terms of signs and symptoms. Treatment should therefore be in line with the natural process

of healing. Adopting a conservative treatment approach with an aim toward reducing inflammation, encouraging healing and repair by reducing joint load, and restoring function consistently results in a successful outcome for most patients.

Classification

The DC/TMD,[1] a validated tool recommended for clinical and research purposes, states that it is "intended for use within any clinical setting and supports the full range of diagnostic activities from screening to definitive evaluation and diagnosis." However, the DC/TMD criteria does not include other syndromes of orofacial pain, which limits its wider application. The American Academy of Orofacial Pain[3] offers guidelines (rather than classifications) and coordinates and integrates with the International Headache

Society Classification of Headache Disorders.[4] The authors' recommendation for diagnostic purposes is to combine these systems, which allows for extensive diagnostic options.

Patient Assessment

Interview and clinical examination

A detailed and thorough patient interview and evaluation are essential for an accurate diagnosis. This is the key to appropriate treatment. Bear in mind that information taken or given out of context may be misleading. Therefore, it is crucial to evaluate each patient as if assembling a new puzzle. A conclusion can be drawn only when all pieces are collected and properly assessed; missing pieces should be looked for, and misleading pieces should be recognized and discarded (see chapter 1).

Examination of the TMJ is rarely performed without a thorough head and neck examination, including masticatory, neck, and pericranial muscles. A complete examination of the head and neck musculature is essential to diagnose comorbid muscle problems (see chapter 8). The basic examination techniques and anamnestic approach to patients with orofacial pain were reviewed in chapters 1 and 8. Therefore, presented here are only those aspects of the diagnostic process relevant to patients with TMJ problems.

A useful diagnostic aid is a self-completed questionnaire detailing demographic information and a comprehensive history of the primary complaints in the patient's own words. Some very good questionnaires are available,[5] and although there is some debate as to their true utility, they can be timesaving and extremely useful. Information includes initial symptoms and their characteristics, onset and duration, triggering, modifying or aggravating factors, and oral habits (eg, clenching). TMJ and masticatory muscle pain (but not referred pain) is usually accompanied by complaints of dysfunction, such as a reduced chewing ability. Location and referral patterns should be described in words and illustrated by the patient on a diagram of the head and neck region. Patients with intra-articular pain usually locate complaints around the joint and ear that may radiate to adjacent structures. Pain is increased on forced opening, biting and/or chewing, and joint loading. Pain is typically induced on the contralateral side, and indeed, patients are often puzzled when reporting that eating on the affected side is therefore easier. The severity of pain at rest and during function, as well as the extent of any dysfunction, should be assessed by using a visual analog scales (VAS) (see chapter 3). In addition to quantifying the patient's subjective experience, VAS records enable the clinician to assess changes over time and treatment response in a more objective manner (see also use of pain diaries in chapter 1).

A dental history and examination (see chapter 6) are essential to exclude primary dental pathology or secondary occlusal problems, such as deviation of the dental midline, missing teeth, and collapsed or open bites. The patient's previous treatments, such as medications and their dosages and duration as well as physical exercises and the result obtained, should be recorded. The patient's compliance with prior treatment protocols is important; prescribed treatment, if not carefully followed, often leads to a misperceived treatment failure. General health problems and current or past medications are highly relevant to diagnosis and treatment planning (see drug interactions and contraindications in chapters 15 and 16). Psychosocial factors are important modifiers of disease onset, progression, and treatment response, and a basic psychosocial history, with or without the aid of pre-prepared forms, may be useful (see chapters 4 and 8). The DC/TMD clinical examination protocols and techniques are highly recommended. They include careful observation, determination, and recording of clinical signs and symptoms. Additionally, the Axis II tools offer a rapid assessment of psychosocial issues.

Clinical examination of the TMJ should begin with the clinician becoming familiar with the patient's behavior, relative sensitivity, and primary complaint (eg, limited function, pain with function, and/or joint sounds). The examination and interview should be performed with the clinician facing the patient so that responses can be adequately assessed and any asymmetry of form or movement may be observed. After the initial interview, the lateral pole of the joint is palpated in the preauricular and intra-auricular areas,

*HARD END-feel

Box 9-1   **Defining joint sounds**

Click
- A brief and distinct sound of limited duration occurring during mandibular movement.
- The sound is usually of a sharp or popping nature.
- Clicking noises may occur during opening or closing jaw movements; when they occur on both, the click is termed *reciprocal*.
- Reproducible clicks refer to sounds consistently present on clinical examination and not only as a patient complaint.

Crepitus
- A sound that is present continuously during jaw movement and is therefore not brief, like a click.
- Crepitus reflects the noise of bone grinding against bone or cartilage on cartilage, and it sounds or feels like the grinding of stones or walking on snow or sand.
- DC/TMD considers crepitus, either coarse or fine, as a sign of degenerative joint disease. Because coarse and fine are clinically difficult to distinguish, there is no need to do so; the presence of crepitus is sufficient.

---

and the patient is instructed to perform basic jaw movements; this also familiarizes the patient with the examination procedures to follow. The joint should be carefully palpated with uniform pressure (the DC/TMD suggests palpation of 0.5 kg to 1 kg for muscles and joints). Palpation should be performed from the lateral aspect, around the joint area, and intra-auricularly in both the open and closed positions. The degree of resultant tenderness and pain may be recorded on a simple ordinal scale (0 = no pain, 1 = mild pain, 2 = moderate pain, and 3 = severe pain) or using a 10-cm VAS.

The presence and characteristics of joint sounds should be recorded. This may be performed manually via light palpation over the TMJs where joint sounds may be perceived or via stethoscopic auscultation. Joint sounds may be present continuously throughout movement or at a particular position; the point at which sounds occur should be recorded. Definitions of joint sounds are noted in Box 9-1. Maximal unassisted and assisted interincisal mouth opening should be accurately measured with a millimeter ruler; the presence and pattern of deviation or deflections, if either exists, should be recorded. For example, persistent deviation to one side is characteristic of ipsilateral osteoarthritis disc derangement without reduction, anchored disc phenomenon, osteoarthritis, or even muscular pain. Deviation during opening with the classic S-shape and associated with a joint sound is characteristic of ipsilateral DDwR. Pain produced on assisted opening, its severi-

ty, and, very importantly, its location should be carefully noted (Fig 9-1).

Other characteristics associated with limitation in jaw movement should be recorded when present. Anchored disc phenomenon is associated with a strictly limited mouth opening (hard end feel), whereas other disorders may allow increased opening with manual assistance (soft end feel). Other jaw movements, such as protrusion and lateral excursions, should be accurately assessed and measured on a millimeter scale, and the exact location of resultant pain should be recorded. Be aware that the distance between the joint and the posterior border of the masseter is 5 to 10 mm. These measurements are reliable in differentiating patients with TMJ from control subjects.[6–8] A useful approach is the joint-loading test, which is performed by instructing the patient to bite on a wooden stick on the canines and molars on both sides and then point to the pain location and define its intensity (Fig 9-2a). Intra-articular inflammatory processes are characterized by pain or sensitivity when the patient bites contralaterally to the affected TMJ, whereas muscle disorders usually result in pain ipsilateral to the loading (Fig 9-2b). Care should be taken that any complaints reported by patients are those for which they seek treatment, that is, familiar pain.

Imaging

Imaging of the TMJ is an adjunctive diagnostic modality to the clinical examination and may be

ORDINAL Scale

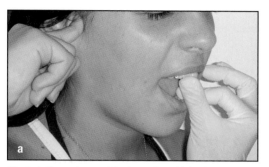 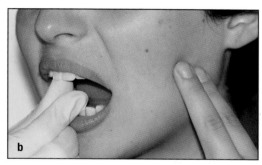

Fig 9-1 Forced or assisted opening. *(a)* Assisted opening will often induce strong pain in the affected TMJ. *(b)* In masticatory myofascial pain, this is often localized over the masseter muscle. Additionally, this examination demonstrates the amount of additional opening that may be gained by mild force; in muscle this may be substantial (≥ 5 mm), in DDwoR this may be moderate (< 4 mm), and in anchored disc phenomenon the limitation is hard and has no possibility of increase.

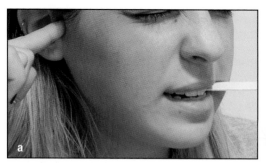 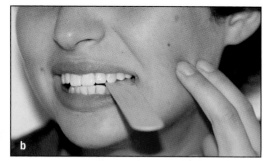

Fig 9-2 Loading test. *(a)* In patients with painful intra-articular disorders or degeneration of the TMJs, loading by clenching the teeth on a wooden stick or spatula induces pain located to the contralateral joint. *(b)* In muscle disorders, clenching usually induces ipsilateral pain over the masseter muscle.

Q # 7, 6

used to confirm a diagnosis, aid in treatment planning, and assess disease progress. Imaging techniques, such as arthrography (radiography with contrast medium), have greatly contributed to our understanding of TMJ disorders and the high correlation between specific clinical signs and anatomical disc derangements. The correlation is such that arthrography is no longer necessary[9] and has been replaced by magnetic resonance imaging (MRI). Indeed, clinical examination and the co-occurrence of certain signs may accurately predict the presence of abnormalities often demonstrated on MRI, such as effusion.[10] However, in some cases, clinical findings do not always accurately predict the precise intra-articular disorder. Although dependent on the clinician, the predictability of the clinical examination in disc displacement and TMJ osteoarthritis is generally low compared with MRI or arthroscopy.[11–14]

Findings suggest that computed tomography (CT) is needed to accurately assess osteoarthritis and that MRI is needed to assess disc position and effusion.[15] Therefore, after a clinical assessment, imaging studies may be required to complete the diagnostic process, but careful patient selection is important.[16]

Gross changes in the TMJ may be detected with panoramic radiographs. However, the panoramic images are typically distorted, and often there is superimposition from the zygomatic process.[17] Panoramic radiographs have poor reliability and low sensitivity for detecting TMJ osseous changes and are of limited use for evaluating the TMJ.[15] Two-dimensional radiographs, such as transpharyngeal and transcranial views in the closed- and open-mouth positions, provide limited information on the hard tissue structures and range of movement and thus should be used sparingly.[18] These

P. 305

ANAMNESTIC - Recollection

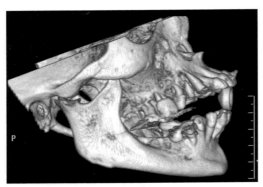

Fig 9-3 Reconstruction of CT images provides a three-dimensional image that is especially useful for assessing TMJ anatomy. In this case, the right TMJ shows degenerative changes consistent with osteoarthritis and the presence of ankylosis.

1p. 289

views also suffer from significant superimposition of the overlying structures, which compromises the clinician's ability to detect pathologic TMJ changes. The decision to obtain more advanced imaging modalities of the TMJ, such as CT, MRI, cone beam CT (CBCT), or bone scan should be considered when findings indicate their need.[19,20] In choosing the modality, consider whether the clinical question can be answered using the specific technique. CT and CBCT scanning provide the most complete three-dimensional reproduction of TMJ bony anatomy but are not essential for a diagnosis (Fig 9-3). CT and CBCT are valuable in assessing the degree of joint degeneration or the possible presence of ankylosis and can be essential before open surgical intervention (see Fig 9-3). CBCT has the advantage of providing a lower radiation dose, producing multiplanar images with excellent resolution relative to standard CT, and detecting most osseous abnormalities in adults and children.[21,22] Although CT has been recommended for the TMJ,[15] CBCT is rapidly superseding it as the modality of choice to image the osseous components of the TMJ.[23]

However, accurate information of all the soft tissue elements of the TMJ can only be obtained using MRI. Indeed, MRI may depict joint abnormalities not seen with any other imaging technique and, thus, is the best method for obtaining a thorough imaging assessment of the TMJ when indicated.[24] When MRI is used, some disc displacements may be detected in

asymptomatic persons. Consecutive MRI images may be performed to create a dynamic representation of joint movement, and this clearly shows the causes for limitation, such as anchored disc or disc displacements without reduction. Additionally, MRI is able to detect joint effusion and mandibular condyle marrow abnormalities.[25,26] It is important to realize, however, that MRI as a sole modality is not sufficient for the diagnosis of TMJ pathologies and must be integrated with clinical and anamnestic findings.[27,28] Indeed, clinical examination remains central to the diagnosis. Notwithstanding, MRI has dramatically improved clinicians' diagnostic abilities, and it is therefore important to use it selectively. Figure 9-4 presents a case where the use of MRI was critical to the diagnosis and subsequent management of the patient.

Bone scanning (scintigraphy or radionuclide studies) offers information on the metabolic activity of bone and can show increased activity in osteoarthritic joints,[29] even in the absence of radiographic changes.[29–31] Severe osteoarthritic joint degeneration associated with a negative bone scan indicates inactive disease, making scintigraphy an invaluable tool. Conversely, a positive bone scan indicates active disease and should be an integral consideration before any invasive or other definitive therapies in conditions such as idiopathic condylar resorption (discussed later).

Other special tests

Joint sounds

Diagnosis of many intra-articular disorders relies on the clinical detection and characterization of joint sounds, but different examiners may not agree on the presence and characteristics of these sounds. Patient confirmation of digitally detected sounds improves the agreement between two independent examiners to approximately 90%.[32] Techniques using vibration or sound sensors to characterize specific TMJ dysfunction conditions have been tested, but these studies suffer from research design flaws that make the conclusions questionable.[33] Poor reproducibility of joint sounds can be best explained by the fact that joint sounds vary over time.[34] A systematic review of the literature and meta-analysis of diagnostic mea-

p. 306

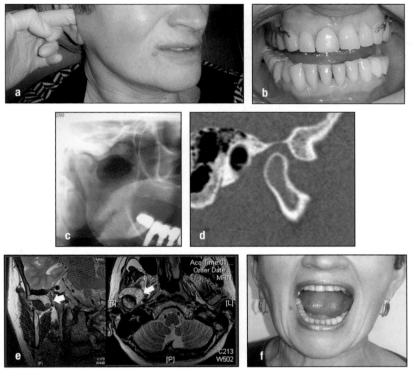

Fig 9-4 *(a and b)* A patient presenting with severe joint pain and limited mouth opening. *(c and d)* The panoramic radiograph and CT scan were clinically normal. Conventional treatment, including arthrocentesis, was unsuccessful. *(e)* An MRI finally revealed the cause of pain in the relevant axial and coronal sections. The *white arrows* point to widespread synovial chondromatosis. *(f)* Removal of the affected tissue was associated with pain relief and normal opening.

sures used to detect TMDs[35] evaluated seven diagnostic techniques, including the evaluation of joint sounds, and found that only three studies included in the literature review met the standards of a high-quality study. This included reviews of research on joint sounds. The DC/TMD has removed the distinction between fine and coarse crepitation as noncontributory to diagnostic accuracy. The DC/TMD does refer to clicking as a criteria for disc displacement but notes that the presence of clicking has a low sensitivity for this diagnosis as patients with disc displacement may not necessarily have a discernible click.[36]

Laboratory findings

Clear biomarkers for TMJ disorders remain elusive, and isolated TMJ disorders are rarely accompanied by changes in hematologic, biochemical, or autoimmune profiles. Salivary markers of TMJ pain are also being investigated but are not ready for clinical use.[37] TMJ involvement in polyarthritides, however, is accompanied by a number of diagnostic and prognostic markers.

Direct markers of disease provide a measure of cellular responses or changes in the affected tissues and are largely metabolic markers. One example is antigenic keratin sulfate, which is found almost exclusively in cartilage aggrecan. Destruction of cartilage releases high levels of antigenic keratin sulfate into body fluids, allowing its detection in most patients with polyarticular osteoarthritis.[38] Aggrecanase, a proteolytic enzyme that acts on aggrecan, is increased in the synovial fluid of patients with TMJ osteoarthritis.[39] Indirect markers have the ability to influence the metabolism of cells in the affected tissues and include proteolytic enzymes, growth factors, and proinflammatory agents. Proteoglycan biomarkers can be detected as soon as 8 hours after an intra-articular inflammatory event, resulting in matrix metalloproteinase (MMP) activation. This can lead to a sustained increase in collagen II biomarkers.[40] Erythrocyte sedimentation rate and C-reactive protein are indirect systemic markers of inflammation, but unless there is severe disease, these will not be altered. In patients with hip or TMJ disease that warranted surgery, significantly higher levels of bone morphogenetic proteins 2 (BMP-2) and 4 (BMP-4) and lower levels of alpha-2 HS-glycoprotein in serum were found compared with healthy control subjects.[41] Inflammatory markers may also be assessed from synovial fluid, as described in the section on pathophysiology. Synovial fluid analysis is probably the most promising test in intra-articular disorders but is relatively more invasive than venipuncture. Ultimately, the final diagnosis is based on the skillful integration and interpretation of the patient's complaint (pain, dysfunction), the history, the clinical examination, and the radiographic and laboratory findings.

Diagnosis of TMJ Disorders

Historical perspective

As late as the 1980s, disorders of the TMJ and the muscles of mastication were pooled together under a variety of diagnostic terms, such as *temporomandibular dysfunction syndrome*. However, it became apparent that temporomandibular dysfunction syndrome included both muscle- and joint-based problems, which required separate categorization.[42] Concomitantly, disc displacement was the postulated cause of joint pain, limited mandibular movement, and joint sounds.[43-45] Naturally, at this point a variety of surgical interventions were developed to restore normal TMJ anatomy (disc displacements) and function that led to apparently successful outcomes. However, these procedures were based on limited awareness of the differential diagnosis and pathogenesis of TMJ pain and dysfunction. For example, patients with painless clicking joints but severe muscle pain underwent unwarranted surgical intervention.

The result was severe joint and muscle pain accompanied by an inability to exercise the jaw, leading to further complications. Subsequently, many patients complained of recurring and severe signs and symptoms after surgery, leading to further, multiple surgical interventions. These repeated interventions often resulted in severe complications that created a need and demand for prosthetic joint replacements.[46-48] Thus, although TMJ pain and dysfunction as a clinical entity has been given much attention, efforts to explain the factor(s) underlying this phenomenon appeared only at a later stage.[49,50]

Current thinking

The reported results of therapeutic interventions aimed at disc displacements and data from recent research stimulated a rethinking of the role played by disc displacement in TMJ complaints.[51] Disc displacement may be a physiologic change,[52] often observed in healthy persons and not associated with joint pain.[53] More than one-third of joints in asymptomatic volunteers were found to have moderately or severely displaced discs.[16,54,55] Contralateral discs in asymptomatic joints of patients with unilateral TMJ problems were found to be displaced as often as the disc on the symptomatic side.[56] Conversely, normal disc position is observed on imaging in about a quarter of clicking joints.[56] Clearly, disc displacement is not always the underlying cause of clicking joints.

In addition, lavage of the upper joint compartment using arthroscopy[57,58] or arthrocentesis,[59] neither of which change the disc position,[60,61] were found to markedly improve function and alleviate pain. Disc displacement is a common finding in persons who are not seeking or in need of care.[36] When disc displacement was evaluated in patients with mild symptoms, 90% were found to have TMJ disc displacement, a rate similar to that of patients seeking treatment.[36] However, nearly 30% of subjects in the same study who did not have jaw pain or dysfunction also showed evidence of similar disc displacement. Therefore, there is a high prevalence of disc displacement in healthy populations, and care must be taken to distinguish whether discal displacement is a symptomatic finding or the cause of the patient's complaint.[36] Clearly, disc position does not dictate the presence of such symptoms as pain and dysfunction.

Thus, accurate diagnosis of the origin of pain and/or dysfunction is crucial before any treatment recommendations are given. Gradually, studies on the position of the disc have shifted to the search for the intra-articular, biomechanical, and biochemical events underlying joint pain and dysfunction.[59,62] A greater understanding of the role of peripheral and central sensitization secondary to intracapsular inflammation, as well as pain-referral patterns that mimic TMJ pain, has led to more specific therapeutic targets for extracapsular sources of pain with the potential to mimic TMJ pathology previously assumed to be related to disc displacement.

Taken together, these studies indicate that disc displacement is not an indication for surgery, especially in an asymptomatic patient or for those with a normal mandibular range of motion.

The Temporomandibular Joint

Understanding the functional anatomy of the TMJ is essential for a thorough clinical examination, interpretation of findings, and understanding the intricacies of the disorders that afflict this joint. The maintenance of a healthy and functional joint involves the interactions among its constituent tissues: bone cartilage, synovium, capsule, disc, blood vessels, and innervation. Because much of the articular cartilage is avascular, it is dependent on the synovial fluid for its nutrients, lubricating agents, and metabolic homeostasis.

Anatomy and function

The TMJ is a ginglymoarthrodial synovial joint, that is, a joint capable of hingelike (rotational) and sliding (translational) movements. The TMJ is encapsulated, bathed in synovial fluid, stress-bearing, and capable of allowing opening, lateral, and protrusive movement of the mandibular body. Condylar movements are protected from direct contact with the bony architecture of the fossa through an intricate system of fibrocartilage and synovial structures. Compared with other load-bearing joints, the TMJ is unique in anatomical functional and genetic regulation.[63]

The TMJ is a complex joint with two joint compartments separated by an articular disc and, thus, four articular surfaces within the joint capsule. The articular disc is made of dense fibrous connective tissue and divides the joint cavity into upper and lower joint spaces. The disc is shaped to match the condyle and fossa: concave inferiorly and convex superiorly. If sectioned anteroposteriorly, the anterior portion (or anterior band) is thicker than its central portion (or intermediate zone). Posteriorly, the articular disc (or posterior band) is thickest. Both the posterior band and the intermediate zone become thinner laterally. Laterally and medially, collateral ligaments attach the disc to the condylar head. Some have suggested that the disc imparts the TMJ with abilities to withstand impressive and prolonged compression, relative to joints without a disc.[64] Significantly, however, patients present with excellent function 30 years after meniscectomy.[65–68]

Joint rotation (hinge movement) occurs largely in the lower joint space, and sliding (translation) occurs within the upper joint space. The articular surfaces, including the disc, are all fibrocartilage rather than the chondrocartilage found in other joints. Fibrocartilage is more resistant to tensile or shear forces associated with full-range mandibular movements. Articular cartilage is made up of collagen, proteoglycan, and chondrocytes. A dense network of aggrecan (aggregating chondroitin sulfate proteoglycan) and collagen fibers provides the cartilage with the necessary biomechanical properties (see loading, discussed later). The TMJ is the only joint in the body with vascularized tissue within the capsular ligament. Jaw movements require bilateral participation and coordination between TMJs.

During function, the lateral and medial discal collateral ligaments, which attach the disc to the condyle, allow for rotational movement of the condyle on the inferior surface of the disc. The superior surface of the disc translates or slides along the posterior aspect of the articular eminence during full mouth opening. Limited lateral movements are also possible. During all movements of a normal TMJ, the interarticular disc is always positioned between the fossa/eminence

hinge

and condyle by the action of the superior lateral pterygoid muscle and the uppermost elastic properties of the posterior attachment known as the *posterior, superior retrodiscal lamina of the retrodiscal tissue*. Translation of the condyle occurs as a result of the action of the inferior lateral pterygoid muscle, which protrudes the mandible, acting in concert with other mandibular depressors and the infrahyoid and suprahyoid musculature. Movement of the disc is controlled during opening by the superior retrodiscal lamina, which passively pulls the disc posteriorly as the condyle translates anteriorly. During closing, the superior lateral pterygoid muscle contracts eccentrically, stabilizing the disc against the distal slope of the articular eminence.

Load distribution and lubrication

The arrangement of the teeth, muscles, and TMJ functions as a class 3 lever system, predicting that during clenching the TMJ is loaded proportionally to the relative lengths of both lever arms. Experimental evidence demonstrates that forces acting on the TMJ are both compressive and tensile.[69,70] The bone architecture of the condyle includes fine, vertically oriented bony trabeculae ideally suited for compressive loading. The articular eminence has a thick cortex with the trabeculae oriented approximately transversely and suited for tensile and shearing forces.[70] The articular disc is also subjected to both compression and shearing forces.[69]

The articular surfaces are smooth and possess a high surface energy, thus requiring an efficient lubrication system.[71–73] Note that there is ongoing debate as to just how smooth the normal articular surfaces are.[74] The smooth movements of the TMJ are possible as a result of sophisticated lubricating and shock-absorbing mechanisms. The synovial membrane, which lines the two compartments within the joint capsule, including the disc (except for the articulating surface), produces synovial fluid when subjected to pressure (hydrostatic lubrication) and supplies the nutritional needs of the joint.[75] The lubricating abilities depend on the synovial membrane and fluid, the disc, and the articular cartilage. The latter are microporous, allowing permeability of the synovial fluid. The permeability and mechanical response of the joint are mutually dependent.[76] *Boundary lubrication* refers to lubricants that bind to articular surfaces separating the frictional elements. These lubricants include hyaluronic acid, lubricin, and surface-active phospholipids.[77] An important point to understand is that TMJ movements are responsible for the efficient generation of lubrication, blood supply, load absorption, and normal mandibular growth.

In situ, the joint space is filled by the highly viscous synovial fluid, which contains hyaluronic acid and the glycoprotein lubricin.[78,79] Hyaluronic acid is a polymer of d-glucuronic acid and N-acetylglucosamine, which are highly unstable and degrade under inflammatory conditions.[80] Lubricin is composed of about 44% protein, about 45% carbohydrates, and about 11% surface-active phospholipids[78] and is suggested to facilitate joint lubrication.[81,82] The surface-active phospholipids protect the articular surfaces and are highly effective as major boundary lubricants.[81,83] Lubricin and proteolipid, which have been isolated from synovial fluid, seem to facilitate surface-active phospholipid deposition at articular surfaces.[81]

An electron-dense layer has been identified in the TMJ that maintains proper joint function and prevents adherence of the articular surfaces.[84] Osmiophilic layers with embedded vesicular structures have been demonstrated in the TMJ.[85] The dominant presence of phosphatidylcholine, a surface-active phospholipid, in rat TMJs was demonstrated in connection with hyaluronic acid and fibronectin.[86] Upon exposure to phospholipase A2 (PLA2), the osmiophilic droplet cluster in centrifuged synovial fluid degraded, and the immunolabeling for phosphatidylcholine was clearly decreased.[86] PLA2, which is part of the inflammatory process, is naturally secreted into the synovial fluid by the synoviocytes, chondrocytes, and osteoblasts and probably acts specifically on phospholipids. Adding PLA2 to the synovial fluid in vitro significantly increases the measured friction.[87]

Hyaluronic acid, although not itself a lubricant, forms a full-fluid film that separates the articular surfaces and acts as a cushion, preventing the generation of friction.[80] An in vitro study revealed that hyaluronic acid protects phospholipid membranes (liposomes) from lysis by PLA2 by their mutual adherence, thus having an indirect role in synovial joint lubrication.[80,86] The lubricating mechanism is therefore intricate and may be disturbed by disruption of any one of its elements.

Lubricin and hyaluronic acid are theoretically protective of joint wear.[88] Although lubricin has been shown to function as a boundary lubricant, conflicting evidence exists as to hyaluronic acid's ability as a boundary lubricant. The articular cartilage surface contains hydrophilic and hydrophobic elements.[88] Adding lubricin significantly reduced friction between hydrophobic surfaces and slightly increased friction between hydrophilic surfaces. Adding hyaluronic acid did not alter the frictional behavior between the model surfaces, and a physiologic mixture of lubricin and hyaluronic acid had no synergistic effect on friction behavior.[88] Thus, lubricin can mediate the frictional response between hydrophilic and hydrophobic surfaces and likely prevents direct surface-to-surface contact. These experiments suggest that hyaluronic acid provides considerably less boundary lubrication, so therapy by the specific injection of hyaluronic acid is of questionable value.[88] In clinical studies on patients with TMJ osteoarthritis, the effect of hyaluronic acid injections was compared with that of arthrocentesis only.[89,90] The reported efficacy of treatment was similar, and hyaluronic acid showed no significant benefit over arthrocentesis, thus raising questions about the value of hyaluronic acid injection.[89,90]

Normal subchondral bone contains (fatty) bone marrow and trabecular bone with many arterial terminal branches. Subchondral bone marrow accounts for more than 50% of the glucose, oxygen, and water requirements of cartilage and is therefore important for cartilage metabolism.[91] Additionally, shock absorption in synovial joints is shared by the articular cartilage and the subchondral bone; 1% to 3% of load forces are attenuated by cartilage, whereas normal subchondral bone is able to attenuate about 30% of the loads.[91] Thus, the subchondral bone has a role protecting articular cartilage from damage caused by excessive loading.

Various methods have been used to assess the amount of load generated in the TMJ. Forces of up to 17.7 kg have been recorded in macaques, and contact stress in human TMJs is similar to that in the hip and knee joints.[92,93] Intra-articular pressure indirectly measures load; it is negative under most conditions and reaches high positive values in synovial joints only at the extremes of movement.[94] In weanling pigs, intra-articular pressure in the superior TMJ compartment was as high as 20 mmHg during masticatory movement.[94] In awake humans, intra-articular pressure in the open-mouth position is negative and becomes positive in the clenched-mouth position.[95] These fluctuating intra-articular pressures play a major role in governing joint nutrition, waste removal, and condylar growth.[95]

Innervation

The TMJ is innervated by small-diameter afferents (nociceptors), proprioceptors (including Ruffini, Pacinian), and sympathetic and parasympathetic efferents.[96–101] Surprisingly, the articular proprioceptors become active only at extremes of jaw movement, and it is postulated that muscle proprioceptors control routine jaw movements. Animal experiments indicate the presence of TMJ neurons encoding at least joint position and displacement in the physiologic range of mandibular displacement.[102] Sensory innervation is derived primarily from the mandibular division of the trigeminal nerve via the auriculotemporal branch, although the masseteric and deep temporal nerves also participate.[101,103] Additionally, fibers originating from the upper cervical dorsal root ganglia may be important in patterns of pain referral.[101] The intra-articular distribution pattern of these fibers is anatomically peripheral (ie, present in the capsule and synovium), and the central parts of the articular disc, condylar head, and fossa are largely noninnervated. The periphery of the human articular disc is, however, sparsely innervated.[97]

The sensation of pain requires the presence and activity of nociceptors, but in normal circumstances most of the articular disc is avascular and largely noninnervated. Additionally, the articular surfaces of the fossa, eminence, and condyle are not innervated. Thus, pain from within the joint is usually due to inflammation or injury of the capsule, the highly vascularized and innervated retrodiscal tissues, or inflammation of the synovial tissues. The autonomic nervous system, particularly the sympathetic nervous system, is involved in pain modulation. Autonomic fibers probably originate in the su-

OLD-World Monkey   ATTenuATed

[handwritten: ,8.38,46]

[handwritten: OTIC Ganglion - glossopharyngeal Nerve And parotid glan]

perior cervical, stellate, and otic ganglia[104] (see chapters 2 and 12).

[handwritten: I Just Below The Foramen ovale]

Effects of inflammation

After inflammation, clinical and experimental evidence suggests significant changes in the innervation pattern and neuronal characteristics of the TMJ. Nerve sprouting into the central portion of the articular disc has been shown after TMJ arthritis was produced experimentally in rats.[105] This was associated with behavioral changes, such as reduced food and water intake, suggestive of pain. TMJ inflammation significantly increased the numbers of heat-sensitive units and induced a lowered heat threshold.[106] Mechanical thresholds also tended to be lower, suggesting that inflammation may sensitize nociceptors in the TMJ and cause hyperalgesia and allodynia.[106] This phenomenon remains controversial in humans. Evidence also exists for the establishment of central sensitization after TMJ inflammation. Expanded receptive fields, reduced thresholds to mechanostimulation, and prolonged neuronal discharges have been documented after TMJ inflammation.[107–111] The sympathetic nervous system has a significant pain-modulating capacity that has been demonstrated in experimental arthritis of the TMJ.[112]

Clinical correlates of these inflammatory and central changes are difficult but have been documented. Inflammation of the TMJ is clinically characterized by synovitis with increased vascularity and synovial hyperplasia, which is usually accompanied by neuronal structures.[113–115] Sensory thresholds of the skin overlying inflamed TMJs were significantly lower than in noninflamed TMJs, indicating peripheral sensitization.[116] These changes, and patients' pain ratings, were reversed by arthrocentesis, suggesting that inflammatory cytokines may have been responsible. Immunohistochemical analysis of articular discs from humans with disc displacements revealed more intense substance P–like reactivity than in control subjects.[117]

Taken together, the evidence points to a dynamic response of the TMJ's constituent tissues to inflammation and includes neuronal plasticity and neuroanatomical changes. Clinically, this should be interpreted as indications for early, effective (but conservative) interventions in painful TMJ conditions.

Pathophysiology of TMJ Disorders: General Factors

In the following section, the pathophysiologic events associated with TMJ disorders are discussed under two major headings: intra-articular and extra-articular factors. These may be involved to various degrees in different pathologies; factors known to be specifically associated with particular diagnoses are further elaborated in individual sections.

Intra-articular

Joint derangements are generally accepted to involve a complex interaction among its constituent tissues; these components may individually initiate disease but also interact to modify disease progression.[2,118] Debate continues regarding the initiating factor or event in joint derangements. Overloading, immobilization, and trauma are the major factors associated with joint derangement and disruption of its integrity.[119,120] Parafunction, such as clenching, is a good example of repetitive jaw motion associated with possibly high and unevenly distributed impact loading that may elicit marked damage to the TMJ.[95,121] The involvement of such parafunctions and overload may suggest that certain types of malocclusion that overload the joint may lead to or worsen existing TMJ osteoarthritis.[122,123]

Overloading is capable of inducing direct and indirect cellular events, neuronal activation, and the triggering of a cascade of molecular events that lead to the degradation of the joint constituents by a number of mechanisms. These events include the release of free radicals, neuropeptides, cytokines, proinflammatory agents, enzymes, and growth factors (reviewed later). This leads to the establishment of conditions for joint derangement, degeneration, and chronic pain. Excessive force, as in macrotrauma, leads to direct cellular and tissue damage with an additional massive release of intracellular contents. This type of injury with microbleeding may also be the source of re-

[handwritten: Parafunction Repetitive]

Redox Active iron

Substance P

dox active iron,[124] which acts much in the same way as free radicals (discussed later). Even in the presence of these events, joint function remains normal as long as its adaptive capacity is not compromised.[43,93,95,120]

Production of free radicals

Free radicals are highly unstable and reactive and will rapidly interact with surrounding molecules to initiate chemical reactions and/or induce tissue injury. Cells such as synoviocytes generate free radicals in response to excessive loading and inflammatory cytokines.[125–127] Free radicals may also be generated as a result of hypoxic-reperfusion cycles associated with overloading.[128,129] Temporary hypoxia is a natural outcome of TMJ capillary bed compression occurring during loading (eg, tooth clenching), a time when the intra-articular pressure may exceed end-capillary perfusion pressure.[95] Reoxygenation upon cessation of overloading may initiate a hypoxic-reperfusion cycle evoking nonenzymatic release of reactive oxygen species (ROS), that is, superoxide and hydroxyl anions.[128,129] The highly reactive ROS may enter into rapid chemical reactions in various tissues or with important molecules in the synovial joint.[130] ROS have a number of detrimental effects that may lead to joint disease[131]:

- Induction of neuropeptide release by sensory afferents (discussed later).
- Initiation of the formation of adhesions.[130,132]
- Induction of inflammatory cytokines and activation of transcription of genes involved in the pathogenesis of joint disease.[125]
- Inhibition of hyaluronic acid biosynthesis and initiation of its degradation,[50] thus decreasing the viscosity of synovial fluid.[129] ROS degradation of hyaluronic acid removes an essential protection mechanism. An in vitro study has shown that in the degraded form, hyaluronic acid fails to protect continuity of the surface-active phospholipid layer.[80,133] Thus, PLA2 secreted into the synovial fluid after any inflammatory event is able to extensively lyse surface-active phospholipids.[80,133] This will reduce or eliminate the continuity of the boundary surfactant layer essential to the integrity of articular surfaces. In the TMJ, un-

covering of the articular surface is speculated to be an initiating factor in joint derangement such as disc displacement. PLA2 is also a key element in the production of fatty acid derivatives such as prostaglandins and leukotrienes.

- Inhibition of the activity of proteolytic enzyme inhibitors by oxidation, for example, tissue inhibitor of metalloproteinases,[50,134,135] thus removing an important homeostatic mechanism.

Neuropeptides

Proinflammatory and nociceptive neuropeptides are released in the TMJ by nociceptive trigeminal nerve terminals found in the retrodiscal tissue and capsular ligaments. These include substance P, calcitonin gene-related peptide (CGRP), neuropeptide Y (NPY), and vasoactive intestinal peptide (VIP).[136–139] Substance P and CGRP are released by sensory fibers, NPY by sympathetic fibers, and VIP by parasympathetic fibers. Analysis of the synovial fluid of patients with TMJ disorders has shown elevated levels of CGRP,[140] substance P,[141] NPY. and VIP,[142] providing further evidence that the human TMJ is innervated as described in rodent experiments.[97] Neuropeptide release can be initiated by intra-articular mechanical and nociceptive stimuli, as in overload; this effect is reversible by opioids. The primary effects (nociceptor activity, neurogenic inflammation) are followed by the appearance of various enzymes and cytokines that were linked by in vitro and in vivo studies to the biologic activities leading to the typical degenerative alterations.[143,144] It is important to appreciate that neuropeptides released by nerve terminals and the resultant neurogenic inflammation are normally essential elements of healing and repair, and a disruption in this balance occurs in arthritis.[145]

Vascular endothelial growth factor (VEGF) is a signal protein produced by cells that stimulates vasculogenesis and angiogenesis. VEGF forms part of a system that maintains the oxygen supply to tissues when blood circulation is compromised. VEGF expression in normal cartilage vanishes in adults, but it is expressed in chondrocytes of osteoarthritic cartilage.[146] Overload and hypoxia will induce the secre-

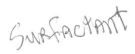

Surfactant

tion of hypoxia-inducible factor-1 (HIF-1)[147] and subsequently VEGF.[146–149] Both induce osteo-clastogenesis, and VEGF induces subchondral bone sclerosis, so they may have a role in initiating joint degradation.[146–149] Correspondingly, osteoarthritis was induced when VEGF was injected intra-articularly in an animal model.[150] In humans, VEGF levels in synovial fluid of the TMJ correlates with levels of arthroscopically observed synovitis.[151]

Cytokines

Cytokines are small proteins released by cells that have specific effects on cell-cell communication, or interaction, and cell behavior. The cytokines includes the interleukins (ILs), lymphokines, cell signal molecules (eg, tumor necrosis factor [TNF]), and the interferons, which trigger inflammation. Proinflammatory cytokines are barely detectable in the synovial fluid of healthy TMJs.[152] Among the cytokines reported in osteoarthritic joints are IL-1, IL-6, and TNF-α, all of which are associated with cartilage degradation.[149,153–158] Some of these molecules are correlated with disease severity and may be used to predict therapeutic outcomes.[158–160] Cytokines exert their effects via a number of mechanisms:

- Potent proinflammatory effects, such as accumulation of prostaglandins and other molecules (discussed later)
- IL-1 and TNF-α, which are known inducers of the synthesis and activation of metalloproteinases by chondrocytes, possibly leading to increased tissue destruction
- Stimulation of sensory nerve endings, inducing pain and the release of proinflammatory neuropeptides
- Generation of free radicals (discussed earlier)

Proinflammatory agents

A number of molecules active in the inflammatory process (see chapter 15) have been identified in disorders of the TMJ; some are closely related to clinical symptoms and therapeutic response.[160–162] Significant correlations include the levels of prostaglandin E_2 with pain on movement.[161] Prostaglandin E_2 is involved in the pathogenesis of osteoarthritis and induces the production of cytokines, proteases, and ROS.

Enzymes

Enzymes are released within the osteoarthritic joint by chondrocytes of the articular cartilage, by the cells lining the synovial membrane, and by the osteoblasts in subchondral bone. They are mainly metalloproteinases, serine proteases, thiolproteases, and aggrecanases; all are known for their collagen and proteoglycan lysis activity and have been detected in human TMJ disorders.[134,158,163]

Bone morphogenetic proteins and growth factors

Development of chondrocytes in articular cartilage is arrested before final maturation by growth factors that circumvent mineralization and apoptosis. The exact role these factors play in joint disease is unclear; they may be involved in attempts at repair (decompensation). On the other hand, some growth factors have been shown to induce catabolic processes and activate proteases.[118] In osteoarthritic joints, cartilage and osteophytes express growth factor genes, such as BMP-2 and BMP-4, which are probably involved in allowing the cells to complete the maturation cycle.[118] Insulinlike growth factor, BMP-2, and transforming growth factor-β, which are related to matrix synthesis, have been identified in the synovial fluid of TMJ disorders.[164,165] Once the exact mechanisms underlying the effect of the various factors in osteoarthritis are elucidated, some of these may be beneficial in the treatment of TMJ disorders.[166,167]

Interactions and progressive damage

The continued presence of proinflammatory agents and neuropeptides will themselves activate trigeminal fibers and further drive the production of neuropeptides; these interactions are schematically represented in Fig 9-5. As a result of the accumulation of free radicals, neuropeptides, cytokines, and proteases, there is damage to the lubrication system and the collagen structure of the cartilage as well as an increased volume of proteoglycans. Damage to

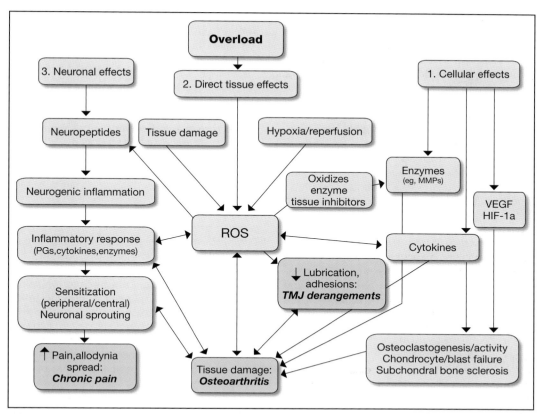

Fig 9-5 Schematic summary of events leading to pain and TMJ disorders. Overload is considered to be a major factor in the initiation of articular tissue damage. Note that extra-articular factors, such as nutrition, atheromatous disease (hypoxia), or obesity, may predispose a person to joint disease; the overload may therefore be relative. Female sex is also a significant predisposing factor. Overload exerts its damaging effects via a number of mechanisms, including direct tissue, cellular, and neuronal effects. 1. Cellular effects include the induction of cytokine and enzyme release from resident tissue cells. Released cytokines are proinflammatory and algesic molecules that are also known to induce the release of ROS. The cellular enzymes released are largely proteases that induce tissue damage. Mechanical overload induces the production of VEGF within the cartilage disc. This is mediated by HIF. VEGF induces subchondral bone sclerosis and initiates joint degradation. Mechanical overload also leads to increased activity of osteoclasts and chondrocyte/chondroblast failure, thereby disturbing the TMJ's repair capabilities and increasing tissue destruction. 2. Direct tissue effects are the result of damage (macrotrauma with massive tissue injury) and hypoxia-reperfusion injury induced by repetitive capillary bed compression and release (eg, clenching). Hypoxia-reperfusion cycles result in the production of ROS that have multiple deleterious efects on joint function. ROS are able to induce direct tissue damage. They also induce the release of neuropeptides from afferent fibers and cytokines and enzymes from cells as well as the oxidation of tissue inhibitors of enzymatic proteases, thus increasing tissue destruction. The lubrication system is severely affected by ROS, including the inhibition of hyaluronic acid biosynthesis and its increased degradation, which leads to increased friction and the formation of adhesions. This may underlie the initiation of some TMJ derangements. 3. Neuronal effects are caused by mechanical activation of trigeminal afferents inducing peripheral release of neuropeptides and subsequent neurogenic inflammation. If unchecked, neurogenic inflammation induces an inflammatory response with classic proinflammatory agents (eg, prostaglandins [PGs]) and induces the release of cytokines and tissue-damaging enzymes. Prolonged inflammation will result in neuronal changes (plasticity), including peripheral and central sensitization and neuronal sprouting into the central portion of the articular disc. These events are clinically represented as ongoing (spontaneous) pain, allodynia (pain on movement, touch), and spread of pain to adjacent structures (ear, temple, mandible).

the lubrication system may lead to stickiness of the disc and derangements.

More rarely, severe damage to the joint ensues. Cartilage swelling and softening occurs (chondromalacia) followed by the breakdown of cartilage by proteases[76] and release of proteoglycans into the synovial fluid.[168,169] This results in weakened cartilage that is unable to withstand loads and, thus, deforms. Signs of fibrocartilage disintegration include the appearance of vertical and horizontal cracks or fractures and thinning of the cartilage.[76,170] Moreover, tissue loading results in chondroblast and chondrocyte failure and osteoclastic bone destruction, which leads to impaired repair capacities and structural damage.[2]

TMJ pain usually impairs mandibular movement. The maintenance of joint movement (with normal loading) is stressed because it is essential for eliminating damaging by-products and promoting healing. Therefore, limitation of joint function secondary to pain is also a contributing factor to progressive damage.

Extra-articular

Recent evidence suggests that a number of extra-articular factors may significantly affect the initiation and progression of joint disease. These include nutrition, bone physiology, genetics, and sex.

Nutrition

In general, suppressed or abnormal synthesis related to insufficient or disturbed nutrition may manifest as degenerative disease. A direct connection between deficient nutrition and joint disorders in general (TMJ disorders included) is rare and has not been clearly established.[171] However, recent research demonstrates that certain foods or nutritional supplements may offer protection from or alleviate joint disorders.[172,173] The anti-inflammatory effects of omega-3 fatty acids (see chapter 17) are well established, and these supplements have been successfully applied in patients with rheumatoid arthritis.[174] Preliminary evidence also supports the beneficial effects of vitamins C and D in arthritic conditions.[175] Glucosamine, with or without chondroitin sulfate, is beneficial in arthritic conditions but its effect is of slow on-

set.[176] Evidence suggests that these may be useful in TMJ disorders, but the clinical significance is unclear.[177–181] However, a recent placebo-controlled study found no evidence for the efficacy of glucosamine sulfate.[182] Therefore, it is unclear whether these agents will provide clinically significant improvement in TMJ disorders. As data accumulate, a decision may be made as to whether these supplements may be gradually incorporated into the management of TMJ disorders.

Genetics

Genetic variations in the initiation and maintenance of chronic pain syndromes, including TMDs,[183] have been extensively studied (see chapters 8 and 10 through 12). Genetic risk factors are believed to combine with environmental exposures and contribute to the risk of developing TMDs.[184] Certain single-nucleotide polymorphisms have been associated with intermediate phenotypes shown to be predictive of TMD onset, including psychologic symptoms and pain sensitivity.[183] The onset of TMDs and masticatory muscle pain has been linked to variants (haplotype) of the gene encoding catecholamine-O-methyltransferase (COMT).[185] Candidate gene studies for TMD susceptibility have identified several other genes, including beta-2 adrenergic receptor (ADRB2)[186] and 5-hydroxytryptamine (serotonin) receptor 2A (HTR2A).[187] Note, however, that these cases are categorized under the umbrella term of TMDs.

Mutations in genes encoding collagen have been associated with degenerative joint disease.[171] Specifically, the ankylosis, progressive homolog (ANKH) gene has been associated with TMJ closed lock[188] and the estrogen receptor 1 (ESR1) with pain in female patients with TMJ osteoarthritis.[189] A haplotype of ESR1 was subsequently associated with the risk of TMJ bone changes.[190] An MMP 1 gene polymorphism has also been associated with degenerative changes of the TMJ.[191]

In a genome-wide association study, researchers examined 146 patients with TMJ degeneration and 374 control subjects from an East Asian population.[192] TMJ osteoarthritis was diagnosed by examining panoramic radiographs, MRI, or CT images. The researchers

haplotype

identified 22 independent loci showing suggestive association signals with degenerative bony changes of the TMJ. However, none of these replicated polymorphisms were located on genes that were reported to be associated with TMDs or TMJ osteoarthritis in previous studies.

Sex

Pain, dysfunction, and clinical signs of TMJ osteoarthritis are slightly more common in females than males.[193–195] Additionally, TMD symptoms were reported to be more severe in females than males.[196] Although the reasons for this are unclear, they are probably linked to the following findings:

- Evidence indicates that female hormones modulate the release of neuropeptides from trigeminal ganglion cells.[197]
- TMJ afferent activity after intra-articular glutamate injection (excitatory neurotransmitter) is greater in female than male rats.[198] Estrogen increases the excitability of rat TMJ afferents and amplifies sensitization secondary to inflammation.[199,200] Experimental data suggest that testosterone may reduce TMJ damage by modifying the inflammatory response.[199]   *p. 398*
- The central integration of pain signals originating from the TMJ region differs between male and female rats[201] and varies over the estrus cycle.[202] Proestrus female rats showed a higher level of central neuronal activation after TMJ inflammation than male rats.[201] Additionally, morphine caused a greater dose-related reduction in nociceptive markers in males than in females.
- Various cell types within TMJs, including synoviocytes and neurons, express estrogen receptors, and their activation is thought to contribute to joint hypermobility, increased MMP activity, and decreased content of collagen and protein in the articular disc.[203,204]
- The combined data suggest that females are more prone to tissue damage in the TMJ and that this damage expresses itself more severely. Females may also be more resistant to pharmacologic treatment. Experiential and sociocultural differences in pain experience between men and women that are related to

hormonally and genetically driven sex differences in brain neurochemistry probably underlie these differences.[205]

The Painful TMJ

Arthralgia, a term used in the DC/TMD classification, is defined as "pain of joint origin that is affected by jaw movement, function, or parafunction, and replication of this pain occurs with provocation testing of the TMJ" (Table 9-2). These signs usually indicate capsulitis or synovitis.

Many disorders and degenerative diseases of the TMJ are painless. When pain is present, it usually indicates an active inflammatory and/or a neuropathic process (see the earlier section on innervation). The following sections deal with individual clinical conditions: joint inflammation, derangements, and joint degeneration. Within each section, the clinical features are described, specific pathophysiologic events are highlighted, and general treatment options are outlined. These entities may present with or without joint pain (arthralgia), and the diagnosis should clearly state this. Full descriptions of the individual treatment options can be found at the end of the chapter.

Arthralgia: Capsulitis and synovitis

The DC/TMD classifies capsulitis and synovitis together under *arthralgia*. In the following section, these conditions are discussed separately in an attempt to differentiate between them.

Capsulitis

Although little data exist concerning the clinical presentation of capsulitis, patients typically complain of pain around the affected TMJ, particularly during jaw movements that stretch the capsule, and the joint is tender to pressure. Usually, there is no pain on loading. In pure capsulitis, there are no joint sounds and no findings on plain radiography. However, capsulitis may accompany disc derangements.

Treatment should initially include analgesics or nonsteroidal anti-inflammatory drugs (NSAIDs; see chapter 15) and physiotherapy to

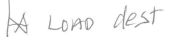

Table 9-2	Diagnostic criteria and symptomatology of capsulitis/synovitis and arthralgia[1,206]	
	Capsulitis	**Arthralgia (DC/TMD)**
Description	Painful disorder of the TMJ induced by inflammation of the articular tissues. Considered the equivalent of *arthritis*, as defined by DC/TMD	Pain of joint origin that is affected by jaw movement, function, or parafunction; replication of this pain occurs with provocation testing of the TMJ.
History	Localized TMJ pain; pain is exacerbated by function and palpation	Positive for both of the following: 1. Pain* in the jaw, temple, ear, or in front of the ear AND 2. Pain modified with jaw movement, function, or parafunction
Examination	Pain may be present at rest; pain may cause limited range of movement; fluctuant swelling may be found over the affected TMJ; ear pain; pain may be exacerbated by contralateral joint loading[†]	Positive for both of the following: 1. Confirmation[‡] of pain location in the area of the TMJ(s) AND 2. Report of familiar pain[§] in the TMJ with at least one of the following provocation tests: a. Palpation of the lateral pole or around the lateral pole b. Maximum unassisted or assisted opening, right or left lateral, or protrusive movement(s)[‖]
Imaging	A bright MRI (T2 weighted) signal may be detected if an effusion is present; no extensive osteoarthritic changes	Not included

*Refers to a history of pain in the previous 30 days.
[†]In the authors' opinion, synovitis is usually distinguishable from capsulitis by the presence of pain on joint loading with contralaterally applied occlusal force (load test).
[‡]The clinician must review with patient.
[§]Pain is induced by provocation that mimics the patient's complaint (sensitivity = 0.89; specificity = 0.98). In the authors' view, arthralgia is a nonspecific term with specific criteria reminiscent of capsulitis; it has proven invaluable for research purposes. The authors recommend that clinicians attempt to reach a clinical diagnosis that may have features of capsulitis, synovitis, and so on.
[‖]Pain not better accounted for by another diagnosis.

maintain joint mobility. Alternatively, periarticular steroids have proven beneficial.

Synovitis

Characteristically, TMJ synovitis results in local pain and tenderness to palpation and evoked pain on mandibular movement. Pain on joint loading is a particular feature of synovitis that is not present in capsulitis. Rarely, fullness over the joint is detectable due to joint effusion and may induce a sense of acute ipsilateral open bite (mild). In this case, joint effusion may be detectable with a T2-weighted MRI. Synovitis may occur after external trauma to the joint (falls, blows, traffic accidents) or from joint overload, such as repetitive and prolonged clenching. Treatment includes analgesics or NSAIDs, physiotherapy (with no loading) to maintain joint mobility, and reduction of joint loading with an intraoral appliance (discussed later). In resistant cases, arthrocentesis and/or intra-articular steroids have proven beneficial. Autoimmune etiologies for joint effusions may be considered in the absence of trauma or if there is a consistent medical history.

Derangements of the TMJ

In its broadest sense, the term *internal derangements of the TMJ* includes all of the intra-articular disorders characterized by dysfunction based on localized anatomical faults.[2] Derangements that are accompanied by significant dysfunction, including clicking joints, intermittent locking, limited mouth opening, and open lock are discussed. The DC/TMD has classified internal derangements of the TMJ as disc displacement with reduction, with reduction and with intermittent locking, without reduction and with limited opening, without reduction and without limited opening, and degenerative joint disease.

The clicking joint

Clicking sounds from TMJs are very common and are reported in patients not seeking treatment; the incidence has been reported as 8.9% in children[207] and 6% to 48% in larger population studies.[194,208] Most often clicking joints are detected by clinicians in patients previously unaware they had joint sounds,[209] which suggests that patients do not view clicking as a significant treatment-seeking symptom.

Although clicking is commonly considered the first sign of a TMJ derangement, the clinical value of a clicking joint as a diagnosis is doubtful. Clicking sounds per se are of no prognostic value and are not an absolute indication for treatment; only 7% of patients with clicking joints progressed over 1 to 7.5 years to a bothersome problem.[210] In a large study that followed up patients over a 20-year period, joint sounds rarely progressed to clinically significant problems.[211] ~p. 311)

Clicking may not be a permanent feature of jaw movements and is typically referred to as *intermittent clicking*, a condition that is largely asymptomatic. Persistent clicking is a condition characterized by joint sounds consistently occurring during function, usually at variable points during mandibular movement.

Persistent click

The patient may present with clicking sounds upon mouth opening, closing, or both. Mouth opening is not limited, but when the clicking is unilateral the mandible may deviate to the affected side on mouth opening. Clicking may be associated with mild to severe pain and sensitivity to palpation or on loading. However, this is rare, and regional muscles should be eliminated as a source of pain. These symptoms may cause limitation in function. Some patients may experience intermittent locking, where they are unable to open the jaw to the normal range, but

this may be eliminated by active manipulation of the jaw. Joint noise may often be associated with, but is not caused by, muscular pain.

Most often, persistent clicking is produced when an anteriorly displaced disc is reduced to its proper relationship with the condyle during mouth opening (Fig 9-6). After reduction, the disc-condyle complex slides down the posterior slope of the articular eminence, resulting in normal mouth opening in most cases. Upon closure of the mouth, the disc slips to its anteriorly displaced position, and this is associated with a clicking sound during closure (see Fig 9-6). This pattern of joint clicking on opening and closing is referred to as a *reciprocal click* and is pathognomonic of DDwR.

Disc displacements

Disc displacement is defined as an abnormal anatomical relationship between the condylar head and the articular disc; in most cases, the disc is anteriorly displaced. Disc displacements may be divided into two major categories: disc displacement with reduction (DDwR) and disc displacement without reduction (DDwoR) (see Fig 9-6). Patients with DDwR or DDwoR account for about 9% of clinic patients and may also be seen in conjunction with muscular disorders (8%) or together with osteoarthritis, joint pain, and muscle disorders (12%).[212] Disc displacements as diagnosed with the previous Research Diagnostic Criteria for Temporomandibular Disorders (RDC/TMD) are relatively rare in the community—about 3%—and are more commonly seen with muscle disorders (8%).[212]

Disc displacement with reduction

Displacement of the articular disc is usually anteriorly or anteromedially,[213] but other rare displacements have been described[214,215] (see Fig 9-6). DDwR is characterized by a reproducible joint noise occurring during opening and closing mandibular movements[1] (Table 9-3). The click during opening occurs at about a 20- to 25-mm interincisal opening; the click on closing invariably occurs at a smaller interincisal opening (15 to 20 mm).[216] Jaw movements on opening have a classic S shape with initial deviation to the affected side; after the click, it returns to undeviated and unrestricted maximal opening.

Classic "S" shape

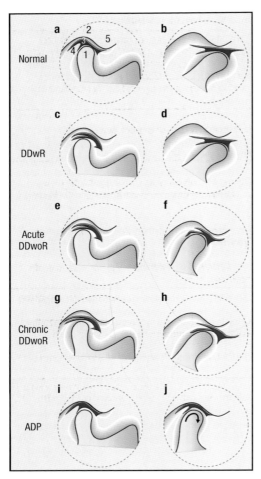

Fig 9-6 Schematic representation of condyle and articular disc movements in various disorders. *(a)* Under normal circumstances, the condyle (1) is located in the fossa (2) with the articular disc (3) located superiorly and slightly anteriorly. The highly vascular and innervated retrodiscal tissues (4) do not articulate (5 = articular eminence). *(b)* During opening and closing, the disc and condyle are coordinated and move smoothly together. *(c)* In DDwR, the disc is anteriorly displaced. During opening, the condyle meets the displaced disc, which causes a temporary obstacle to movement and thus deviation to the affected side. *(d)* The condyle is able to reduce under the disc (opening click), and subsequently opening is undeviated and unlimited. On closing, the condyle-disc relation is again disturbed (closing click), leaving the disc displaced anteriorly. *(e to h)* DDwoR may be acute *(e)* or chronic *(g)*. *(f)* In acute DDwoR, the disc remains anteriorly displaced during opening movements (with limited mouth opening ≤ 35 mm). The repetitive forces during mouth opening eventually deform the disc structure and stretch the posterior attachment, leading to chronic DDwoR *(g and h)*. In this situation, the disc has been pushed anteriorly by stretching the posterior attachment that has undergone adaptive changes to act as an articulating disc. Consequently, mouth opening is far less limited (> 35 mm) and may even approach normal values *(h)*. In anchored disc phenomenon (ADP), the disc adheres to the fossa *(i)* and allows for rotatory movements only *(j)*; thus, mouth opening is severely limited (< 30 mm).

Patients with DDwR are usually asymptomatic and may not even be aware of their joint sounds. TMJ sensitivity and pain may occur spontaneously or secondary to joint loading or other function. When present, pain is usually moderate but may occasionally be more severe (VAS scores up to 7).[217] When a patient is asked to protrude the jaw and then open it, the click is usually eliminated.[216]

Pathogenesis of disc displacement. Many etiologic factors have been proposed to explain the occurrence of disc displacement. The suggestion that spasm of the superior head of the lateral pterygoid muscle is responsible for the displacement of the disc was rejected.[218,219]

Joint laxity might be a contributing factor but is not prevalent enough relative to the prevalence of disc displacement.[220] Trauma was thought to cause disc displacement; however, several studies have failed to confirm significant relationships between indirect trauma and disc displacement.[54,221] For example, the prevalence of disc displacement is similar in patients with and without history of whiplash.[222]

Displacement of the disc seems to be caused by impairment of free articular movements as a result of disruption of the lubrication system.[120,223-226] Some researchers have suggested that even with prolonged compression, the lubrication system in the TMJ is relatively stable compared with other joints without disc

Table 9-3	Diagnostic criteria for disc displacement with reduction[1,206]
Description*	An intracapsular biomechanical disorder involving the condyle-disc complex. In the closed-mouth position, the disc is in an anterior position relative to the condylar head, and the disc reduces upon opening of the mouth. Medial and lateral displacement of the disc may also be present. Clicking, popping, or snapping noises may occur with disc reduction. A history of prior locking in the closed position, coupled with interference in mastication, precludes this diagnosis.
History	Positive for at least one of the following: 1. In the previous 30 days, any TMJ noise(s) present with jaw movement or function OR 2. Patient report of any noise present during the examination
Examination	Positive for at least one of the following: 1. Clicking, popping, and/or snapping noise during both opening and closing movements detected with palpation during at least one of three repetitions of jaw opening and closing movements OR 2a. Clicking, popping, and/or snapping noise detected with palpation during at least one of three repetitions of opening or closing movement(s) AND 2b. Clicking, popping, and/or snapping noise detected with palpation during at least one of three repetitions of right or left lateral or protrusive movement(s)
Imaging	When this diagnosis needs to be confirmed, TMJ MRI criteria should be positive for both of the following: 1. In the maximal intercuspal position, the posterior band of the disc is located anterior to the 11:30 position, and the intermediate zone of the disc is anterior to the condylar head AND 2. On full opening, the intermediate zone of the disc is located between the condylar head and the articular eminence

*DDwR may also occur with intermittent locking and is separately defined by the DC/TMD. The patient reports that the jaw locks with limited mouth opening, even for a moment, then unlocks. Otherwise, the diagnostic criteria are the same as in DDwR (sensitivity = 0.34; specificity = 0.92); imaging is the reference standard.

displacement.[227] Still, the adaptive capacity of the joint structures is often exceeded by prolonged overloading, and the viscoelastic properties are affected. This leads to increased shear stress in the disc, which in turn leads to fatigue and damage. This is associated with generation of free radicals[228] that are detrimental to the lubrication system[229,230] (see Fig 9-5). As a result of repetitive disc hesitation, the ligaments seem to gradually stretch.[223] The disc adheres to the fossa, decreasing disc mobility and finally inducing its displacement[2,120,225] (Fig 9-7). In support, TMJ arthrography in DDwR demonstrates disfiguration of the lower compartment caused by the condyle sliding under the hesitating disc and stretching the anterior wall of the capsule.

Accumulating data are driving research in the direction of the biologic mechanisms of joint lubrication; thus, disc mobility may be much more important than disc position.[231–233] Additional mechanisms potentially involved in disruption of disc mobility were discussed earlier (see general factors).

Diagnostic criteria and symptomatology of intermittent clicking

Not all clicking joints have verifiable disc displacement, and the question that arises is what causes clicking in these cases. Intermittent clicking may also be caused by disc hesitation or lagging as a result of stickiness in the upper compartment after transient overloading

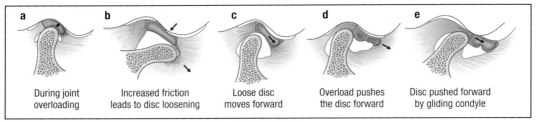

a	b	c	d	e
During joint overloading	Increased friction leads to disc loosening	Loose disc moves forward	Overload pushes the disc forward	Disc pushed forward by gliding condyle

Fig 9-7 Pathophysiology of disc displacements.[225] Displacement of the disc is thought to begin by the disruption of the lubrication system, leading to increased friction during articular movements and subsequent tissue disruption. *(a)* In prolonged overloading, the viscoelastic properties of the disc are damaged. Concomitant generation of free radicals disrupts the lubrication system, resulting in repetitive disc hesitation and gradual stretching of the ligaments. The disc adheres to the fossa, increasing disc mobility *(b)* and finally inducing its displacement *(c)*. *(d and e)* The displaced disc is now repetitively pushed forward, causing further displacement on clenching and on opening as well as overloading of the posterior attachment.

or clenching.[234] The clicking noise is assumed to occur upon release of the disc or while the condyle moves against the lagging disc. Other possible mechanisms that may induce intermittent or persistent clicking include joint hypermobility,[235] enlargement of the lateral pole of the condyle,[236] irregularities of the articular eminence,[237] and adhesions or intra-articular bodies.[60,238]

Clicking joint: Treatment guidelines

The treatment of a clicking joint, including DDwR, is dictated primarily by the presence of pain or dysfunction. Reciprocal or intermittent click with no significant symptoms should not be treated. Most patients with DDwR do not progress to DDwoR.[239,240] Unfortunately, there are currently no means by which to predict which patients will deteriorate (see also the discussion on prognosis of disc displacements). In the presence of pain or dysfunction, therapy should begin with conservative options, such as joint unloading (appliances, behavioral modification), physiotherapy, and medication. This will improve pain but leaves clicking largely unaffected. When clicking is associated with severe joint pain with no response to nonsurgical treatment, arthrocentesis may improve symptoms, but clicking usually remains or recurs. Surgical arthroscopy, disc repositioning, condylotomy, discectomy, or disc anchorage may be considered when an intolerable loud sound and/or pain resistant to conservative therapy

persists. Each procedure should be enhanced by reducing joint loading and by physical therapy. Recurrence of clicking often occurs but is usually less annoying to the patient.

In cases where clicking is secondary to adhesions, lavage of the upper compartment releases the disc and enables the condyle and disc to move simultaneously, thereby preventing the clicking noise. Alternatively, if clicking is caused by irregularities, anatomical changes, or loose bodies, an alternative approach such as arthroscopy or surgery is recommended.[241–245] Alleviation of symptoms is obtained regardless of the posttreatment disc position, which usually remains anteriorly displaced.[232,233] Therefore, it has become evident that disc position may be relatively unimportant in TMJ disorders.[246]

Limited mouth opening

In general, the TMJ itself accounts for only a small proportion of disorders causing limitation. Most TMJ disorders are muscular in origin,[212] and these account for most cases of limitation of mouth opening. TMJ disorders underlying limited mouth opening include closed lock[159,247–249] (the term includes DDwoR[25,250,251] and anchored disc phenomenon[226]), fibrous ankylosis,[252] and osteoarthritis.[253] Arthrocentesis seems efficient for these entities, other than for fibrous ankylosis.[25,60,254,255] However, it is important to realize that each of these is an independent disorder that requires an individually tailored approach based on clear diagnostic criteria.

Table 9-4	Diagnostic criteria for disc displacement without reduction with limited opening[1,206]
Description*	An intracapsular biomechanical disorder involving the condyle-disc complex. In the closed-mouth position, the disc is in an anterior position relative to the condylar head, and the disc does not reduce with opening of the mouth. Medial and lateral displacement of the disc may also be present. This disorder is associated with persistent limited mandibular opening that does not resolve when the clinician or patient performs a specific manipulative maneuver. This is also referred to as *closed lock*.
History	Positive for both of the following: 1. Jaw locked so that the mouth will not open all the way AND 2. Limitation in jaw opening is severe enough to limit jaw opening and interfere with the ability to eat
Examination	Positive for maximum assisted opening (passive stretch) movement, including vertical incisal overlap < 40 mm.[†]
Imaging	When this diagnosis needs to be confirmed, TMJ MRI criteria should be positive for both of the following: 1. In the maximal intercuspal position, the posterior band of the disc is located anterior to the 11:30 position, and the intermediate zone of the disc is anterior to the condylar head AND 2. On full opening, the intermediate zone of the disc is located anterior to the condylar head[‡]

*The current definition of acute DDwoR includes a subgroup of limited mouth opening caused by anchored disc phenomenon. The major factor that may finally differentiate is clinical response (mouth opening, pain) to arthrocentesis, which is dramatic in anchored disc phenomenon and not so significant in DDwoR (sensitivity = 0.80; specificity = 0.97).
[†]Presence of TMJ noise (eg, click during opening) does not exclude this diagnosis.
[‡]Maximum assisted opening < 40 mm is determined clinically.

Table 9-5	Diagnostic criteria for disc displacement without reduction without limited opening[1,206]
Description*	An intracapsular biomechanical disorder involving the condyle-disc complex. In the closed-mouth position, the disc is in an anterior position relative to the condylar head, and the disc does not reduce with opening of the mouth. Medial and lateral displacement of the disc may also be present. This disorder is not associated with limited mandibular opening.
History	Positive for history of both of the following: 1. Jaw locked so that the mouth will not open all the way AND 2. Limitation in jaw opening is severe enough to limit jaw opening and interfere with the ability to eat
Examination	Positive for maximum assisted opening (passive stretch) movement, including vertical incisal overlap ≥ 40 mm.[†]
Imaging	When this diagnosis needs to be confirmed, TMJ MRI criteria are the same as for disc displacement without reduction with limited opening.[‡]

*The definition of limited mouth opening in the authors' view includes an opening that is significantly less than the patient's original normal value (sensitivity = 0.54; specificity = 0.79).
[†]Presence of TMJ noise (eg, click during opening) does not exclude this diagnosis.
[‡]Maximum assisted opening ≥ 40 mm is determined clinically.

Disc displacement without reduction

The basic alteration of disc position in DDwoR is the same as in DDwR, but in DDwoR the condyle is unable to reduce onto the disc during opening (Tables 9-4 and 9-5; see also Fig 9-5). Accumulating data have shown that DDwoR may occur with or without clinically significant limited mouth opening.[216] Clinically significant limited mouth opening is defined as less than

40 mm interincisally or when the patient subjectively reports discomfort/dysfunction associated with an opening that is less than their usual maximal opening.

DDwoR is characterized by limited mouth opening (usually 25 to 35 mm) that usually develops gradually. A history of clicking must be present to make this diagnosis.[256] Mouth opening is associated with deviation to the affected side, and lateral excursion to the contralateral side is markedly limited. Assisted mouth opening may be painful but usually results in an increase of about 4 mm or less. The clinician must determine if the elicited pain is articular or muscular. The affected joint may be symptomatic, and localized pain may occur spontaneously or on jaw movements. Pain over the affected TMJ is usually moderate (with VAS scores of about 6) but may be more severe, particularly in patients seeking treatment. Patients often complain of chewing problems and reduced masticatory efficiency.[257] Pain is usually present on palpation of the affected joint and on loading (see Fig 9-1). Pain is due to stretching and overloading of the yet unadapted and highly innervated retrodiscal tissue. In the absence of problematic limitation of opening or pain, this disorder might remain unnoticed by an affected person. Plain open-mouth or CT radiographs of the TMJ invariably demonstrate some condylar sliding, however limited. In arthrography and MRI, the disc is located anterior to the condyle in closed-mouth and open-mouth positions.

Over time, pain may be markedly reduced (VAS scores 1 to 2), and maximal opening may approach normal values.[258–260] This stage is termed *chronic DDwoR* by the American Academy of Orofacial Pain[256] and *DDwoR without limited opening* by the RDC/TMD.[216]

Pathogenesis of DDwoR. The pathogenesis of DDwoR is thought to involve similar processes discussed earlier (see general pathophysiologic processes and Fig 9-5) and particular processes associated with DDwR (see Fig 9-7).

Prognosis of disc displacements

Some studies have suggested that disc displacements will naturally progress to osteoarthritis.[261,262] However, osteoarthritis can afflict TMJs with or without discs[65,66,68] and may ap-

pear before signs of disc displacement,[170,263] which suggests that these disorders may be independent. Degenerative changes in the condyle are related more to female sex, joint immobilization, increased load, atheromatous disease, increased age, and a reduced dental arch length and less to disc position.[119,264,265] Most prospective studies have shown that the vast majority of patients with symptomatic DDwoR either remain static or improve spontaneously.[259,266,267] The reduction in symptoms and restoration of function in patients with DDwoR probably reflect adaptive intracapsular changes that include an increase in dense connective tissue, decreased vascularity, and decreased innervation.[268,269] These changes are also present in elderly people, irrespective of disc position, so they may be both adaptive and age-related events.[265,270,271] The end result is that the retrodiscal tissues are modified and able to act as a functional disc.

More recently, disc mobility and not disc position has emerged as highly important in the prognosis of TMJ disorders.[231] This is interesting in that it links the lack of adequate joint lubrication to the development of advanced TMJ disorders.

Treatment of disc displacement without reduction

In patients with early (acute) DDwoR and pain, conservative management may improve symptoms, but mouth opening usually remains limited. Arthrocentesis will improve symptoms and marginally increase mouth opening; this is to be expected because arthrocentesis does not alter disc position. Arthrocentesis should be accompanied by conservative options, such as joint unloading, appliances, behavioral modification, physiotherapy, and analgesic or anti-inflammatory medication. This supportive mode of treatment encourages adaptation of the posterior attachment to act as a disc.[271]

The decision to treat chronic DDwoR (or disc displacement with no limited mouth opening) depends largely on the assessment of functional capabilities as described by the patient and the presence of localized joint pain. If treatment is offered, it should include conservative options with or without arthrocentesis. Surgical options are considered for patients who still have localized joint pain and significant dysfunction despite conservative management.

Anchored disc phenomenon *ADP*

Anchored disc phenomenon is characterized by sudden, severe, and persistent limited mouth opening, ranging from 10 to 30 mm (considerably lower than in DDwoR), with deviation toward the affected side of the mandibular midline on opening (see Figs 9-6i and 9-6j). The movement toward the contralateral side is limited and often painful. On protrusion, the mandible deviates toward the ipsilateral side. History of clicking is *not* obligatory (see DDwoR) but may be present in up to 70% of patients. Usually, there is no pain in the TMJ upon loading. Forced mouth opening evokes pain in the affected joint and is characterized by an inability to increase maximal opening; the limitation in anchored disc phenomenon feels hard relative to that of DDwoR. In long-lasting anchored disc phenomenon, the clinical characteristics are less pronounced. In plain open-mouth radiographs and CT scans, the TMJ shows evidence of a nonsliding but normally structured condyle; however, rotatory movements are present.[59,226,272] In MRI, the disc appears stuck to the articular eminence, and the condyle slides underneath it.[272,273]

Pathogenesis of anchored disc phenomenon

The cause of limitation has been suggested to originate from a suction-cup effect, whereby the disc that clings to the articular eminence is responsible for the limitation of movement.[58,274] However, introducing one needle into the upper joint space to abolish the vacuum does not cure this limitation, so other adhesive forces between the disc and fossa have been suggested.[226,272,275] Overloading of the joint is assumed to damage the normal lubrication of the joint (see Figs 9-5 and 9-7). Apparently, in the presence of suboptimal lubrication, adhesive forces can be generated between the pressed, denuded, smooth, elastic disc and the eminence.[226,272,275] The disc might be in a normal or displaced position. Even a limited area of adhesion between the two opposing surfaces is capable of suddenly holding the disc from

sliding down the slope of the eminence. Forced opening is not recommended, as the condyle is pulled away from the adhered disc. Such stretching of the joint's ligaments may traumatically disrupt the anatomical relationship between the condyle and the disc.

Treatment of anchored disc phenomenon

Case 9-1 describes a young woman with anchored disc phenomenon who responded very well to arthrocentesis and joint unloading and showed good long-term stability (Fig 9-8). Arthrocentesis neutralizes the adhesive forces, separates the flexible disc from the rigid surface of the eminence, and enables smooth, normal opening.[59,272] Arthrocentesis should be enhanced by reducing joint loading and by physical therapy. The latter, which is not indicated as long as the disc is stuck, should be intensively used after disc release. Under these circumstances, recurrence is rare, probably because of patient awareness and the low likelihood that the two opposing articular surfaces will again become uncovered and adhere.[59]

TMJ disorders characterized by inability to close the mouth

Open lock versus TMJ condylar dislocation

Open lock is characterized by a sudden inability to close the mouth and is usually released by the patient's manipulation. Mouth opening during open lock is usually less extreme than in condylar dislocation (Table 9-6) and may range from 25 to 30 mm.[276] In plain radiographs and CT scans, the condyle in open lock is located inferior to and not in front of the eminence, as would be expected in condylar dislocation. MRIs show the condyle to be located anterior to the lagging disc.[276] The cause for open lock probably involves diminished lubrication with increased friction between the disc and the eminence. The disc, which normally moves together with the condyle, lags behind it, and consequently the condyle slides under and in front of the disc and cannot return to its former position in the fossa; hence, the mouth remains open.

A 30-year-old woman with anchored disc phenomenon.

CASE 9-1

Present complaint: Limited mouth opening. The patient reports that she cannot even bite a sandwich and has to cut food into small pieces. She also cannot chew on the left side due to pain.

History of present complaint: Three months before her referral, she woke up in the morning and could not open her mouth. Her dentist referred her to physiotherapy, but there was no improvement. The patient claimed she had no joint clicking in the past.

General health: Healthy.

Patient evaluation: On a 10-cm VAS, her pain level was 7.8 when opening was forced. Pain was specifically located at her right TMJ. Dysfunction was graded 8 of 10.

Clinical examination: Maximal mouth opening was about 24 mm with deviation to the right (see Fig 9-8a). Upon forced passive opening, pain was located in the right TMJ, but mouth opening remained unchanged. Lateral movements to the right were unrestricted, but the patient felt she was unable to freely move her jaw to the left (see Fig 9-8b). Protrusion was also restricted, with deviation to the right. Upon palpation, there was no TMJ pain and no masticatory muscles tenderness, except for slight tenderness in her right external pterygoid. No clicking was observed, and pain was not generated upon right and left loading.

Imaging: Plain radiographs revealed normal anatomy. The condyle, however, demonstrated no sliding down the slope of the eminence. MRI demonstrated that at maximal opening, the disc was stuck to the temporal bone, and the condyle was only able to rotate under the stuck disc.

Diagnosis: The absence of a history of clicking, the sudden onset, the extremely limited mouth opening, and the absolute resistance of the mandible to increase interincisal opening during active assistance suggested anchored disc phenomenon.

Treatment: Joint unloading by an interocclusal appliance followed by arthrocentesis with immediate rehabilitation of all joint movements. At the 4-year follow-up, there was no recurrence.

Discussion: Clinicians should begin with conservative therapy, such as unloading with an intraoral appliance, which may release the disc in 10% of patients. This is followed by arthrocentesis.

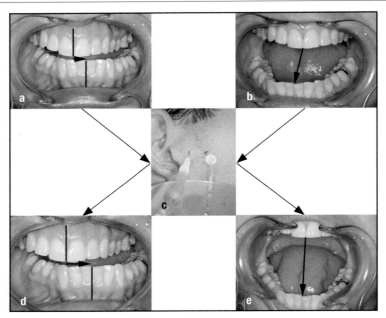

Fig 9-8 Patient from Case 9-1 with anchored disc phenomenon of the right TMJ. Before arthrocentesis, mouth opening was limited and deviated to the affected side *(a)*, and lateral excursion to the contralateral side was limited *(b)*. After superior joint space lavage *(c)*, mouth opening improved markedly without deviation *(d)*, and normal lateral excursion was regained *(e)*.

Table 9-6	Comparison between the characteristics of open lock and condylar dislocation	
Characteristic	**Open lock**	**Condylar dislocation**
Age	Younger	Older
Occurrence	Spontaneous in joints with internal derangement	Maximal opening (yawning, shouting, neurogenic, neuroleptic drugs, joint laxity)
Maximal mouth opening during the event	Maximal opening with protrusion	Increased maximal opening
Reduction	Difficult but self-corrected	Usually professional
Condyle location on radiographs and CT	Anterior and inferior to eminence	Anterior and superior to eminence
MRI (open-mouth position)	Trapped condyle; located anterior to the lagging disc	Condyle located anterior to the eminence
Treatment	Arthrocentesis and unloading	Surgery if recurrent

Dislocation of the TMJ occurs when the mandibular condyle is displaced anteriorly beyond the articular eminence, and the patient is unable to self-reduce the condyle. This is in contrast to *subluxation*, which is generally defined as a displacement of the condyle out of the glenoid fossa and anterosuperior to the articular eminence, which can be self-reduced by the patient.[277] Dislocation has multiple causes, which may be related to endogenous factors, such as a lack of integrity of the joint ligaments or problems with the bony architecture of the joint surfaces.[277] Exogenous factors that may induce dislocation include trauma and imbalanced activity of the musculature acting on the joint, sometimes habitual or secondary to medications. Final diagnosis of open lock or dislocation must be supported by imaging at the time of occurrence (see Table 9-6).

Treatment of open lock/dislocation

For open lock, nonsurgical means are usually effective, and if not, lavage of the upper compartment can restore sliding of the disc, allowing it and the condyle to move simultaneously. Preventing the condyle from moving anterior to the disc provides relief, and long-term recurrence is rare.

For chronic dislocation, injection of sclerosing solution (sodium morrhuate or sodium tetradecyl sulfate) has been suggested, which induces scarring of the capsule and may pre-

vent recurrence in some patients.[277] Similarly, injection of botulinum toxin to the lateral pterygoid muscle is claimed to be effective, but the treatment is temporary. Surgical treatments for recurrent condylar dislocation include eminectomy,[278] capsule tightening, introducing an obstacle (eg, bone) to prevent dislocation, and surgical stripping of the lateral pterygoid muscle.[277]

p. 202

Degenerative Joint Disease of the TMJ: Osteoarthritis

As in other synovial load-bearing joints, the TMJ is subject to pathologic overload or systemic disease that may lead to tissue breakdown, pain, and dysfunction. The DC/TMD classifies osteoarthritis and osteoarthrosis as subclasses of degenerative joint disease (Table 9-7). Under the DC/TMD, osteoarthritis is symptomatic, whereas osteoarthrosis shares all the same signs and symptoms of joint damage and dysfunction but there is no pain. The presence of ongoing pain is suggested to reflect inflammation, hence the terminology. Indeed, degenerative joint disease or osteoarthritis has historically been considered a noninflammatory disorder. However, accumulating evidence indicated the presence of inflammation involving the synovium.[279] Sustained intra-articular inflammation induces degeneration of TMJ structures.[280] Clear evidence now exists that synovitis is associated

Table 9-7	Diagnostic criteria for degenerative joint disease (osteoarthritis or osteoarthrosis)[1,206]
Description*	A degenerative disorder involving the joint characterized by deterioration of articular tissue with concomitant osseous changes in the condyle and/or articular eminence. Degenerative joint disease (DJD) can be subclassified: DJD without arthralgia is osteoarthrosis, and DJD with arthralgia is osteoarthritis. Flattening and/or cortical sclerosis are considered indeterminant findings for DJD and may represent normal variation, aging, remodeling, or a precursor to frank DJD. DJD can result in malocclusions, including an anterior open bite (especially when present bilaterally) or a contralateral posterior open bite (when present unilaterally).
History 1	Positive for at least one of the following: 1. In the previous 30 days, any TMJ noise(s) present with jaw movement or function OR 2. Patient report of any noise present during the examination
History 2	3. Arthralgia*
Examination	Positive for crepitus detected with palpation during at least one of the following: opening, closing, right or left lateral or protrusive movement(s) Rheumatologic consultation when needed: 1. Negative for rheumatologic disease
Imaging	When this diagnosis needs to be confirmed, then TMJ CT criteria are positive for at least one of the following: subchondral cyst(s), erosion(s), generalized sclerosis, or osteophyte(s).†

*When arthralgia (pain) is present, the diagnosis is osteoarthritis. With no pain, the diagnosis is osteoarthrosis. The DC/TMD also allows for the diagnosis of DJD with or without arthralgia and simplifies the ongoing taxonomic discussion on osteoarthritis or osteoarthrosis (sensitivity = 0.55; specificity = 0.61).

†Osteoarthritis has an extremely variable clinical expression. It may present with no pain, minimal or no dysfunction, and extensive radiographic degeneration only. Conversely, there may be extreme pain and dysfunction in patients with minimal radiographic findings. These are difficult to classify with the current criteria.

P. 313

with pain and dysfunction and that it promotes cartilage destruction in osteoarthritic joints.[281,282]

In view of the fact that secondary synovitis develops rapidly in most patients,[2,11] the authors support the use of the term *osteoarthritis*. Some patients with clinical and radiographic signs of degenerative joint disease have minimal if any symptoms or signs; they probably represent a subacute or chronic form of osteoarthritis. The appearance of symptoms is associated with the identification of intra-articular inflammatory molecules.[138,283] Accordingly, the authors adopt the thinking that osteoarthritis is the most appropriate terminology[2] and suggest that this simply be further characterized as with or without pain and/or dysfunction. Alternatively, the terminology of degenerative joint disease with or without arthralgia is a good alternative.[1,206]

Epidemiology and clinical features

Osteoarthritis increases with age and may be related to mechanical factors, such as loss of molar support with shortening of the dental arch.[264] The condition is more common in women than in men, particularly after the age of 40 to 50 years. In one study, about 10% of women and 5% of men aged 65 years were found to have TMJ crepitation, compared with about 5% and 4%, respectively, in 35-year-olds.[284] Radiographic evidence of osteoarthritis is very common (14% to 50%) in asymptomatic people, mostly unilaterally, but only 8% to 16% will have clinically detectable disease.[285–288] Both clinical and radiographic findings are found in about 5% of patients.[212,285,286] These figures are comparable with those found in other joints of the body.[289] Patients with osteoarthritis or pain of the TMJ make up about 6% of clinic samples; most often these entities are seen together with muscle pain with (18%) or without (35%) disc displacements.[212]

In the acute painful phase of TMJ osteoarthritis, patients typically complain of early-morning joint stiffness that lasts more than 30 minutes. This may be accompanied by severe joint pain at rest and during jaw movement as well as difficulty in yawning, biting, and chewing. Sometimes the symptoms are accompanied by a sensation of swelling in the TMJ area.[290,291] The most frequent complaints include a variable combination of pain and tenderness of the joint, stiffness and roughness, difficulty during mouth opening, and diminished range of jaw movements (with or without pain). Crepitation in the arthritic joint may occur during jaw movement, and the history of clicking is variable.

On physical examination, findings include painful limited mouth opening; furthermore, lateral excursions in both directions induce pain in the affected joint (even if only one joint is affected), and attempts to protrude the jaw beyond the limits imposed by the disorder elicit considerable pain in the affected joint (Case 9-2). Crepitation in the arthritic joint, with or without clicking, may occur during jaw movement. Palpation of the affected joint can evoke mild to severe pain. In general, these patients do not present any distinctive description, complaining of all or some of the symptoms with severity varying considerably from mild to severe.[290] Occlusal changes/interference might be found sequential to joint effusion or condylar resorption (open bite in the affected joint or in the contralateral joint, respectively) or contributing to the degenerative changes, such as posterior bite collapse or premature tooth contact.

Imaging of an osteoarthritic joint may show only mild changes; however, advanced stages typically show erosion of the cortical outline, loss of intra-articular space, osteophytes, marginal spurs, subcortical cysts, subchondral bone sclerosis, reduced joint space, and a perforated disc, among other features[91,168,292] (see Fig 9-9). Within a symptomatic group of patients with TMJ osteoarthritis, there may be some correlation between bone changes and clinical measures of dysfunction,[293] but the issue remains debatable. Moreover, inconsistency may exist between the clinical symptoms and imaging: Mild clinical disease might be associated with severe imaging appearance and vice versa. Indeed, early osteoarthritis may not be detectable by radiographic imaging,[18,290,294,295] and conversely, radiographic changes are present in many asymptomatic persons.[295,296] MRI may show the presence of a joint effusion, particularly in painful joints.[26] Scintigraphy is useful to assess the degree of disease activity.

Table 9-8 summarizes the differences between the clinical signs and symptoms and imaging data of anchored disc phenomenon, DDwoR, and osteoarthritis.

Specific comments on the pathogenesis of osteoarthritis

Synovial joints constantly adapt to their functional needs. Symptomatic osteoarthritis results when joint loading (intrinsic or extrinsic) exceeds the joint's adaptive capacity. Osteoarthritis involves the concomitant actions of inflammation, degeneration, and attempts at repair. Degeneration is, in essence, a maladaptive response, a failure of the tissues to respond to the demands made of it. In osteoarthritis, the usually well-kept balance between tissue synthesis (repair mechanisms) and breakdown (damage) is disturbed.[297] The authors believe that the TMJ has a higher adaptation potential because of the highly potent proliferative layer that is not found in other adult synovial joints.

Recent research has shown that osteoarthritis is much more complicated than previously thought, and the variable presentation is probably a result of the variety of factors linked with the disease. Awareness of these factors is essential for improving insight into the origin of the signs and symptoms and thereby the treatment approach.

As discussed earlier in the section on general pathophysiology, a number of processes may result from joint overloading (see Fig 9-5). When overloading exceeds the joint's repair capacity, a cascade of deterioration may be initiated. This may lead to disruption of the lubrication system and wear of the articular cartilage that gradually penetrates the underlying bone.[290,298,299] Concomitantly, overloading is associated with a variety of mutilations to the subchondral bone, which leads to microfractures that induce subchondral bone sclerosis. When sclerosed, the subchondral bone does not provide enough nutrition to the cartilage and does not function as an efficient shock absorber, both of which are crucial for the integrity of the articular cartilage. Some researchers have suggested that, subsequent to these bony changes, the cartilage is degraded and separates from the underlying bone.[150,300] Other factors such as obesity and cardiovascular diseases may induce hypoxia and subchondral bone sclerosis and predis-

CASE 9-2

A 45-year-old man with TMJ osteoarthritis.

Present complaint: Sudden severe pain in his right joint associated with severely limited mouth opening. He was unable to talk without suffering pain, and eating had progressively become nearly impossible.

History of present complaint: The patient, a lawyer experiencing an especially demanding period, had a normal but very intensive life until a month ago when sharp pain on the right side of the face woke him up at night. Since then he has not been able to bite or chew on the left side. Various medications, such as analgesic NSAIDs have been tried with no improvement. He has no history of clicking or trauma. The patient reports no generalized joint pain and feels well. Recent routine laboratory tests revealed a normal differential blood count, liver function, and electrolytes.

Medical history: Hypercholesterolemia controlled with 20 mg simvastatin daily.

Clinical evaluation: The patient evaluated his pain and dysfunction as 9 and 7.8, respectively, on a 10-cm VAS.

Clinical examination: Maximal mouth opening was 22 mm with slight deviation to the right. Upon slight forced opening, excruciating pain was generated in the right TMJ. Lateral movements to the right were unrestricted but were painful and limited to the left; both were associated with severe pain in the right TMJ. Protrusion was limited with deviation to the right and severe pain on the right side. The patient had a deep overbite and a deviated dental midline (to the left) but a well-maintained dentition. Upon contralateral loading, severe pain was generated in the right joint.

Imaging: A CT scan demonstrated typical degenerative changes on the right TMJ, limited movement, and no widening of the intra-articular space (Fig 9-9).

Diagnosis: The signs and symptoms are typical of osteoarthritis.

Treatment: Joint unloading and right TMJ arthrocentesis were followed by immediate improvement in mandibular movements (Fig 9-10). Intensive physiotherapy was supported by analgesic medication.

Discussion: The purpose of the treatment is to aid the patient and provide optimal conditions for healing and restored function. This is performed by providing an intraoral appliance and anti-inflammatory medication to reduce internal and external load. These controlled the pain but only marginally improved maximal mouth opening. Arthrocentesis eliminated the use of inflammatory products and was followed by immediate rehabilitation of movement. Interestingly, local anesthesia applied before arthrocentesis eliminated pain but did not improve mouth opening. Physiotherapy is an essential component and maintains adequate function.

The severe degenerative changes demonstrated by the CT are not to be misinterpreted as contraindicating arthrocentesis. In the authors' experience, there is no correlation between the severity of the degeneration (as shown by CT scan) and the results of arthrocentesis.

pose the joint to damage. Indeed, a primary role for the subchondral bone in inducing damage to the articular cartilage and the development of TMJ osteoarthritis is suggested from experimental findings in mice.[150,300,301] More recently, the metabolic syndrome, which involves the combination of obesity, dyslipidemia, cardiovascular disease, hyperglycemia, and hypertension, has been implicated in osteoarthritis.

Imbalance in bone physiology

The main radiologic features of osteoarthritis are joint-space narrowing and extensive remodeling of subchondral bone that is generally sclerotic. Bone changes may precede cartilage destruction, and prominent alterations in subchondral bone suggest that this tissue plays a key role in the initiation of TMJ disease. Cartilage loss in knee osteoarthritis can often be predicted by the enhanced uptake of radioactive markers (scintigraphy), specifically by subchondral bone.[302] Moreover, scintigraphic activity precedes episodes of radiographic degeneration. Bone cells, contrary to cartilage cells, are well supported by a capillary plexus. This, however, also exposes them to secondary effects of local or systemic disease that may affect local blood flow (see the cardiovascular disease section later in the chapter).

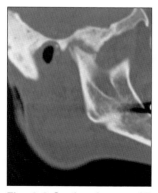

Fig 9-9 Section from a CT showing osteoarthritis in the patient from Case 9-2. The sagittal view shows the right TMJ. The head of the condyle is severely degenerated with flattening and osteophyte formation.

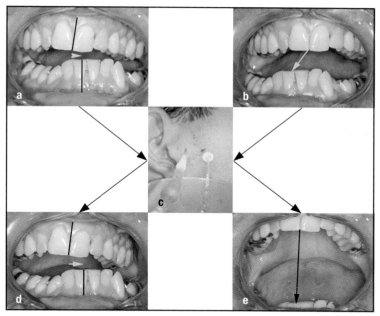

Fig 9-10 Patient from Case 9-2 with osteoarthritis of the right TMJ. Before arthrocentesis, mouth opening was limited and deviated to the affected side *(a)*, lateral excursion to the contralateral side was limited *(b)*, and both caused severe pain. After superior joint space lavage *(c)*, mouth opening improved markedly without deviation *(d)*, and normal range of lateral excursion was regained *(e)*.

Table 9-8	Comparison of the common characteristics of anchored disc phenomenon, DDwoR, and osteoarthritis		
Characteristic	**Anchored disc phenomenon**	**DDwoR**	**Osteoarthritis**
Occurrence	Sudden	Gradual	Sudden/gradual
Past clicks	No (30%)	Yes	No/yes
Maximal mouth opening	15 to 25 mm	30 to 45 mm	10 to 30 mm
Contralateral	Limited	Limited	Limited
Ipsilateral movement	Normal	Normal	Limited
Pain (self-assessment)	−	+	Severe to none
Dysfunction (self-assessment)	+	−	− to +++
MRI (open-mouth position)	Disc stuck, located superior to and behind the condyle	Disc displaced/ deformed, located anterior to the condyle	Effusion +/− Adhesion +/− Disc displaced +/− Deformed disc +/− Perforated disc +/−
Effect of arthrocentesis	Excellent	Moderate	Very good (70%)

Bone mass. Sinigaglia et al[303] found that patients with osteoarthritis have a significantly increased bone mass and less osteoporosis. A high bone mass has been shown to play a role in the development of erosive changes in the TMJ.[304] Osteoarthritis is characterized by an in-

Leptin

Adipocytes

crease in material density in subchondral bone, constituting increased collagen matrix and abnormal mineralization.[118] Osteoarthritic bone of the femoral neck is significantly stiffer than that of control subjects.[305] On the one hand, this results in relative protection from fractures, but on the other hand it results in uncompliant subchondral bone structure that is inadequate support for the articular cartilage; shear forces are generated, and cartilage damage with cleft formation and separation from bone occurs.[150]

Although the debate is ongoing,[171,306] osteoarthritis seems less common in patients with osteoporosis, possibly because osteoporosis renders the bone more flexible.[303] Cartilage separation allows the cytokines, growth factors, and prostaglandins produced by the subchondral bone tissue to cross through the bone-cartilage interface and damage the cartilage.[91,307] In support, osteoarthritic subchondral bone has significantly increased levels of cytokines, inflammatory mediators, and MMP activity.[308,309] Recent data have shown that bone resorption pits in subchondral bone may release MMPs derived from bone marrow cells into the articular cartilage.[118]

Metabolic syndrome and osteoarthritis

Metabolic syndrome is the name for a group of risk factors that raises the risk for heart disease and other health problems, such as diabetes. More recently, metabolic syndrome has been linked to osteoarthritis.[310] The syndrome consists of obesity, dyslipidemia, increased blood pressure, and hyperglycemia. Some of these factors have individually been identified as osteoarthritis risk factors.

Cardiovascular diseases. Osteoarthritis is associated with an increased prevalence of hypertension, particularly in younger people. The association remained even when obesity was controlled for.[311] The proposed mechanism begins with narrowing of blood vessels and reduced blood flow, resulting in ischemia of the subchondral bone.[312] In rat models of hypertension, osteocyte apoptosis and bone necrosis develop even without osteoarthritis.[313,314] Additionally, atheromatous diseases are highly correlated with osteoarthritis,[315] and compromised blood supply to the subchondral bone is a pos-

sible inducer of osteoarthritis. This provides an explanation for the occurrence of osteoarthritis in older patients with atheromatous diseases even in unloaded joints.[144]

Obesity. Obesity is a well-known risk factor for osteoarthritis and is thought to act via increased joint loading. However, increased osteoarthritis of the hand in patients who are obese suggests that other, probably metabolic, factors are at play.[171,316,317] The hormone leptin, derived from adipocytes, may be key to this relationship. Leptin plays a major role in preventing obesity by effects at the hypothalamic level, and leptin resistance is associated with obesity. Levels of leptin are increased in osteoblasts within osteoarthritic subchondral bone and in the synovial fluid of patients who are obese.[118,316] Leptin exhibits, in synergy with other proinflammatory cytokines, a detrimental effect on articular cartilage cells by inducing the production of MMPs—proinflammatory mediators—and promoting nitric oxide synthesis in chondrocytes.[316,318] Adiponectin is a hormone that increases the oxidation of fatty acids and reduces the synthesis of glucose in the liver. Some evidence suggests that adiponectin may act as an intra-articular proinflammatory and could be involved in matrix degradation.[319,320]

A connection between obesity and the TMJ has not been shown; this may be due to differential metabolic control of the TMJ relative to other joints.[63] This difference is supported by experimental findings where diet-induced obesity caused osteoarthritis in the knee joint but not the TMJ of mice.[321]

Jaw movement

Immobilization is presently considered among the principal causes for joint deterioration, mainly because of the absence of natural elimination of the virulent inflammatory core. Movements of the joint are necessary to induce fluctuating intra-articular pressures that function like a pump and are crucial for joint homeostasis.[95] ~ *p. 308*

Although most damage is associated with movement, immobilization of the joint is a dominant factor in joint deterioration. Interestingly, prolonged opening has led to osteoarthritis in mice,[322] and immobilizing the joint in primates leads to marked thinning of the articular cartilage.[323]

Early and correct diagnosis associated with the appropriate treatment aimed at bringing the joint back to normal movements is crucial. Adequate mobilization also avoids further complications, such as ankylosis (see Fig 9-3).

P. 262

Treatment of osteoarthritis

The physician's role is supportive, establishing ideal conditions for healing by unloading and enabling movement. As the synovial joint is believed to be an adaptable organ, the goal is to bring the symptomatic joint from an unadaptable state to an adaptable one, bearing in mind that clinicians treat the patient and not the radiographic image. A paucity of high-level evidence exists for the effectiveness of interventions for the management of TMJ osteoarthritis.[324,325] Especially in this disorder, surgery should not be recommended unless nonsurgical means have failed.[43,146,226,291,326–329] The prognosis of osteoarthritis after conservative management has been shown to be good and stable; although radiographic bone changes may show deterioration, clinical signs and symptoms tend to improve.[261,330–332] Treatment should focus on joint unloading, joint mobilization, and pain control. Joint unloading is crucial for restoring lubrication and allowing healing of the cartilage. External loads may be reduced by such modalities as intraoral appliances (IOAs), soft diet, and behavioral treatments. Reduction of internal factors, such as the inflammatory exudate, may be attained by medication provided orally, intramuscularly, or intra-articularly. Arthrocentesis is also able to mechanically rinse the joint and remove proinflammatory agents; this unloads the joint, provides analgesia, and releases adhesions, thus promoting joint mobility. Results are often dramatic (see Case 9-2 and Figs 9-9 and 9-10). ~ P. 287   P. 261

To attain joint mobilization, maximal pain control must be attained. Pain relief is rapidly achieved by pharmacologic means (NSAIDs, analgesics; see chapter 15) or by joint unloading with an IOA or arthrocentesis. Reports indicate a similar degree of effectiveness with intra-articular injections consisting of sodium hyaluronate or corticosteroid preparations and equivalent analgesia with diclofenac sodium compared with IOA.[325] Glucosamine appears to be just as effective as ibuprofen for the management of TMJ osteoarthritis.[324] Physiotherapy is a critical component essential for overcoming the acute stage of the disorder. Better functional performance allows for nutrition, efficient removal of waste, and increased joint lubrication, thus establishing conditions that will allow healing of the TMJ constituents.

If pain and dysfunction are not eliminated, surgical intervention should be planned. In the authors' experience,[333] arthrocentesis obviates the need for corrective surgery in 68.4% of patients who did not respond to other non-surgical treatment and were candidates for surgery. The authors investigated 79 patients with osteoarthritis of the TMJ (67 women, 12 men) and found a relatively young mean age of 36.9 ± 1.66 years (unpublished data), which is in contrast to the findings for symptomatic osteoarthritis in other joints.[334,335] These patients presented with 83 osteoarthritic joints that had not responded to conservative treatment and subsequently underwent arthrocentesis. Long-term success was examined (mean, 54.33 ± 6.95 months) and was determined by self-assessment questionnaires, clinical examination, and radiologic examination. Arthrocentesis resulted in significant improvement in 81% of the patients; after the arthrocentesis, maximal mouth opening increased from about 24 to 43 mm. Over a mean follow-up period of about 20 months (range, 6 to 62 months), pain levels decreased substantially from VAS scores of 6.92 to 2.36, and dysfunction scores were reduced from 7.37 to 2.24 on a VAS. The patients' overall satisfaction with the treatment was high (8.78 on a scale of 0 to 10). These outcomes are not perfect but certainly suffice to obviate corrective surgery. However, in the remaining 31.6% of patients, similar symptoms were caused by joint pathologies, such as bone spicules or fibrous ankylosis, which are not amenable to lavage (see Fig 9-3). A similar rationale explains the effect of arthrocentesis in the treatment of TMJ rheumatoid arthritis and other polyarthritides.

No correlation was found between the severity of the clinical signs and symptoms and the severity of the degenerative changes seen in imaging. Similarly, response to arthrocentesis did not correlate with disease severity on imaging. Thus, imaging has no definite role in deciding whether arthrocentesis should be performed. Clearly, arthrocentesis, and not imaging, acts as a diagnostic tool that determines whether there is a need for further surgical intervention.

When arthrocentesis fails, surgical intervention is recommended: surgical arthroscopy, disc repair and repositioning, and discectomy. In very severe cases with marked loss of vertical dimension and malocclusion, joint replacement is required and is accomplished by autogenic bone or an artificial joint (discussed later).

Secondary osteoarthritis

A number of systemic disorders may induce a degenerative process within the TMJ that is often clinically and radiologically indistinguishable from primary osteoarthritis[336] (Table 9-9). However, these entities are usually accompanied by symptoms associated with the systemic disease, such as fatigue, pyrexia, anemia, and serology. Table 9-10 summarizes salient features of systemic conditions that may induce TMJ pain and degeneration.[337–343]

Idiopathic condylar resorption (condylysis)

Degenerative conditions of the condyle are usually primary and associated with articular loading. Secondary osteoarthritis is related to a number of factors, such as trauma or infection, or is due to systemic conditions that may involve the TMJ. Some cases have been reported after orthognathic surgery,[344,345] and prolonged steroid use has been associated with destructive joint disease.

However, there are patients, usually females aged 15 to 35 years, who present with condylar resorption with no apparent cause.[346,347] These conditions have been termed *idiopathic condylar resorption (ICR)* or *condylysis*[256]; the authors adopt the former term. The patients complain of an anterior open bite and a variable degree of dysfunction. The presence of pain and sensitivity to pressure over the joints is inconsistent. Clinical findings also include a number of skeletal and occlusal features suggested to be involved in its pathogenesis.[348] Radiography

usually reveals bilateral condylar damage similar to that observed in osteoarthritis, and scintigraphy is useful in assessing the current activity of bone destruction. By definition, ICR must be seronegative and display no biochemical or hematologic abnormalities.

ICR is often a dramatic condition characterized by aggressive loss of the condyle associated with severe signs and symptoms in young healthy females. The underlying etiology of ICR appears to be joint loading (intrinsic or extrinsic) that exceeds the joint's adaptive capacity.[349] Internal derangement parafunction, macrotrauma, and unstable occlusion are also considered possible contributing factors.[350] Researchers speculate that the balance between tissue breakdown and synthesis may be interrupted because the joint tissues fail to adapt to functional or parafunctional demands, resulting in destructive changes in the articular cartilage and destruction of the underlying bone.[351,352] ICR may be a severe form of osteoarthritis or may be related to disturbed blood supply to subchondral bone, as observed in hip joints. The high predilection for females suggests that hormonal influences are important.

Nonsurgical management of ICR

The treatment of ICR is divided into two phases: the first aims to arrest resorption (assessed by bone scan) and the second to correct the occlusion and malformation. Assuming that joint overloading plays a major role in this resorption process, Mercuri[353] summarized the noninvasive modalities aimed at arresting the process: anti-inflammatories, muscle relaxant medications, IOAs, soft diet, and physiotherapy. Avoiding heavy-loading exercises that compress the joint and reconstructing the occlusion when required are recommended. Minimally invasive modalities, such as intra-articular injections of hyaluronic acid and corticosteroids, arthrocentesis, and arthroscopy, may help arrest the active resorption process. Gunson et al[349] suggest medical therapy aimed at the underlying pathophysiologic processes. They include the use of antioxidants, tetracyclines, omega-3 fatty acids, NSAIDs, and inflammatory cytokine inhibitors to help prevent and control articular bone loss, including osseous mandibular condylar resorption.[349] More aggressive medical

Table 9-9	Involvement of the TMJ in systemic arthritides: Secondary osteoarthritis[1,206]
History	Positive for both of the following: 1. Rheumatologic diagnosis of a systemic inflammatory joint disease AND 2a. In the past month, any TMJ pain present OR 2b. TMJ pain that worsens with episodes/exacerbations of the systemic inflammatory joint disease
Examination	Positive for both of the following: 1. Rheumatologic diagnosis of a systemic joint disease AND 2a. Arthritis* signs and symptoms as defined in I.1.B OR 2b. Crepitus detected with palpation during maximum unassisted opening, maximum assisted opening, right or left lateral movements, or protrusive movements
Imaging	If osseous changes are present, TMJ CT/CBCT or MRI is positive for at least one of the following: 1. Subchondral cyst(s) OR 2. Erosion(s) OR 3. Generalized sclerosis OR 4. Osteophyte(s)

*Arthritis as used by the DC/TMD is equivalent to capsulitis or synovitis. Often the TMJ symptoms occur as part of disease progression. Secondary osteoarthritis may also occur after trauma, which is not discussed in this chapter.

Table 9-10	Laboratory findings of osteoarthritis that may involve the TMJ			
Diagnosis	**Prevalence**	**Peak onset**	**Laboratory findings**	**Clinical findings**
Rheumatoid	2% to 2.5%	40 to 60 years	Rheumatoid factors (70% to 80%), antinuclear antibody (15%), elevated erythrocyte sedimentation rate (90%), mild anemia (25%), HLA-Dw5 HLA-DrW (50%)	Bilateral arthralgia with crepitation, open bite, radiographic evidence of osteoarthritis; TMJ involvement occurs in 50% to 75% of patients and signifies severe disease and usually is not a presenting symptom
Psoriatic	0.07%	35 to 45 years	Seronegative, HLA-B27	Fatigue, weight loss, pyrexia, myalgia; often unilateral pain of the TMJ; psoriasis itself affects 1% to 2% of the population, but arthritis is a rare complication, and TMJ involvement is even rarer
Ankylosing spondylitis	0.4% to 1.6%	20 to 30 years	Seronegative, elevated erythroctye sedimentation rate (70%), HLA-B27	Arthralgia, stiffness of the TMJ that may result in ankylosis; TMJ involvement occurs in patients late in the disease
Reiter syndrome	Reactive to infection	20 to 30 years	Seronegative	Fatigue, weight loss, pyrexia, lymphadenopathy, acute unilateral arthralgia

HLA, human leukocyte antigen.

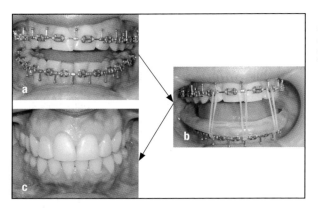

Fig 9-11 Patient with an anterior open bite induced by ICR. *(a)* Anterior open bite. *(b)* Treatment according to the principles of closed reduction. *(c)* The open bite was closed within 1 month, and follow-up for 2 years showed no relapse.

intervention, including anti-TNF-α biologics, is warranted in view of the rapid bone loss some patients experience.[350] Surgical interventions include correcting disc location by arthroscopy[354] or arthroplasty, including removal of hyperplastic synovial and bilaminar tissue if well documented by MRI.[355]

The authors have found that in cases of progressing anterior or posterior open bite caused by ICR, the open bite can be corrected by the principles of closed reduction. The authors add an appliance to increase the effect of the maxillomandibular fixation (unpublished data). Figure 9-11 shows the closure of a severe anterior open bite with orthodontic elastics. The adaptability of the facial musculoskeletal system to the normal occlusion and excellent function in the presence of deficient condylar height is a fascinating phenomenon. Therefore, anterior open bite can be eliminated with this approach and should be considered before any surgical intervention. Treatment may be provided in close collaboration with orthodontists and orofacial pain practitioners.

Surgical management of ICR

To correct occlusion and malformation, orthognathic surgery is commonly used.[355] However, orthognathic surgery may be associated with a complication rate (relapse or TMJ dysfunction) of approximately 45% (8 of 18 patients).[356] In contrast, condylectomy and costochondral grafting appeared to produce stable and functional results. Because orthognathic surgery is

associated with a high risk of relapse, special care is necessary to prevent joint loading during the process. Removal of the affected condyle and reconstruction with a costochondral (rib) or alloplast (total joint replacement) has been suggested.[357]

Clinicians commonly claim, however, that patients with ICR experience minor pain and a normal range of motion, and this approach of eliminating the joint seems radical to most. In any event, all of these methods include complications, and failure, overgrowth, infection, and limited range of motion, among others, have been reported. Distraction osteogenesis and transport distraction osteogenesis are other methods attempted to overcome bone deficiency, especially loss of condylar height. Considering the impact of failure, the most conservative approach should be considered before joint reconstruction.

Pain in the TMJ: Differential Diagnosis

Common pathologies within the joint that presents with pain and/or dysfunction have been reviewed. However, the location of the TMJ in the midst of the skull, with resultant referral of pain, often makes patient evaluation complex (see chapter 1). Importantly, the differential diagnosis of pain felt in the TMJ, but not originating from the joint, includes a number of causes. Masticatory myofascial pain, a far more common condition that affects the lateral and/or medial pterygoids and/or the masseter will often refer pain specifically to the TMJ (see chapter 8). Many other adjacent structures may refer pain to the TMJ area, including intraoral pathology (see chapter 6), the ear (see chapter 7), neurovascular syndromes (see chapters 10 and 11), or neuropathic syndromes (see chapter 12). In addition, a variety of extra-articular systemic disorders may directly affect joint growth, anatomy, and function (see Tables 9-1 and 9-10). Although rare, primary tumors (benign/malignant) may originate from TMJ structures, and distant tumors may metastasize to the TMJ, presenting with joint pain or sensitivity[358,359] (see also chapter 14). Most tumors arising in the TMJ will be of bone or cartilage origin.[360,361] In any clinical evaluation, careful data collection and examination are crucial for avoiding misdiagnosis, and imaging is a complementary tool. Figure 9-12 is a simplified algorithm to aid clinicians in the diagnosis of painful TMJ disorders that may be accompanied by limited mouth opening and/or joint sounds.

Treatment of TMJ Disorders

Because the etiology of TMJ disorders is considered multifactorial, numerous forms of ostensibly targeted therapies have been designed. Modalities include mechanistic approaches, such as orthotic or occlusal therapies, and biopsychosocial approaches that integrate behavioral therapies into the standard medical model of disease. Interestingly, many of these interventions, alone or in combination, have an equally positive effect in reducing or eliminating a patient's symptoms. Studies clearly show no superiority of any one treatment for patients with TMJ disorders; successful treatment outcomes typically follow a multimodal and often multidisciplinary approach.

Treatment of TMJ problems may be compared with the treatment of any other skeletal disorder. The ultimate goals are to decrease pain and increase function. Indeed, TMJ pain and/or dysfunction are the clearest indicators that treatment should be offered. Dysfunction includes limited mandibular range of motion and reduced functionality. However, it is im-

portant to clearly state the treatment objectives to the patient, because elimination or alleviation of pain and dysfunction may not always be accompanied by eradication of joint sounds. The clinician should stress to the patient that long-term follow-up of clicking joints shows no significant deterioration in the vast majority of patients[210] and no advantage of surgical over nonsurgical techniques in controlling deterioration.[362] The American Association for Dental Research strongly recommended that, unless there are specific and justifiable indications to the contrary, treatment of patients with TMDs should initially be based on the use of conservative, reversible, and evidence-based therapeutic modalities.[363]

A conservative approach is successful for most patients, but on the rare occasion when a patient complains of a disturbing joint sound, even in the absence of pain or dysfunction, surgical treatment may be offered (discussed later).

Nonsurgical treatment options

Nonsurgical treatment of painful, dysfunctional TMJs commonly relies on the use of patient education and awareness techniques, joint unloading by functional modification or appliances, physical therapy or manipulation,[364,365] bite appliances,[366–368] medications,[366] or cognitive-behavioral therapy. Other less common modalities include warming,[369] soft laser,[370] and complementary or alternative medicine[371,372] (see chapter 17), but their efficacy is unclear. Because most patients with painful TMJs have a good prognosis, the aim of treatment is palliative and supportive. Even in patients with DDwoR, the use of a conservative approach is effective[373] and is in no way inferior to surgical intervention in controlling signs and symptoms.[374] However, patients with a history of persistently limited mouth opening (< 30 mm) have been shown to be relatively resistant to nonsurgical intervention.[375]

Joint unloading: Functional behavioral modification

In some patients, clenching or other parafunctional habits (protrusion) may be associated with TMJ pain; behavioral modification to stop these may alleviate symptoms. However, in

Mechanistic

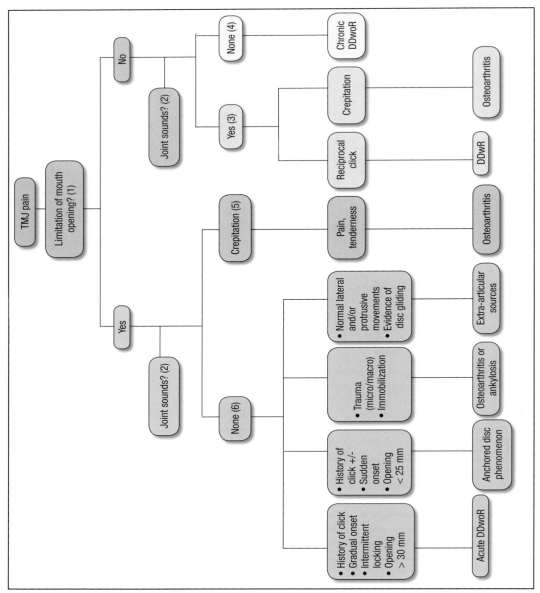

Fig 9-12 Algorithm to aid in the diagnosis of painful TMDs. A possible approach (1) is to initially separate patients with and without limitation of mouth opening. The presence of joint sounds (2) further subdivides these groups. In patients with no limitation in mouth opening and joint sounds (3), the quality of the sound may rapidly aid in diagnosis; crepitation is a classic sign of osteoarthritis and reciprocal clicking of DDwR. No limitation of mouth opening in the absence of joint sounds (4) may be due to long-standing or chronic DDwoR. Limited mouth opening with crepitation is often present in active osteoarthritis (5) (see also Case 9-2). The absence of joint sounds accompanied by limited mouth opening and a symptomatic TMJ is often difficult to diagnose (6). A history of clicking joints with a gradual onset of locking or limitation of opening that is around 30 mm suggest acute DDwoR. In contrast, an acute onset of limited mouth opening of less than 25 mm in a young patient with no history of clicks suggests anchored disc phenomenon. A history of clicks in the past does not exclude anchored disc phenomenon. Macrotrauma, TMJ surgery, or long-standing osteoarthritis that has been inadequately managed suggests that ankylosis is present (see Fig 9-3). Muscle disorders are a common extra-articular cause of limitation of mouth opening. Rare causes, such as coronoid hyperplasia and tumors, should be kept in mind (not shown).

some patients, further evaluation of parafunctional disorders may lead to a diagnosis of a movement disorder, such as a focal dystonia. A review of the patient medication profile and possible neurologic consultations, including referral for a sleep study (polysomnography), may be indicated.[376] In most cases of pain, an initial period of rest and a soft diet are also useful. Rest, which is beneficial for any symptomatic synovial joint, is not totally relevant for the TMJ because it is involved in essentially daily functions, such as eating, swallowing, and speech. Moreover, sleep parafunction is a major source of TMJ overloading and is not controllable by the patient, so appliances are indicated. The use of appliances is described later in this chapter and more extensively in chapter 8.

Encouraging the patient to actively participate in the treatment with the aim to identify and reduce potentially damaging parafunction is essential. This approach may be enhanced with the use of biofeedback and stress management (see chapters 4 and 8).

Physical therapy

Joint mobilization is essential in maintaining long-term function and joint integrity.[95] This functionality acts as a pump that stimulates local cellular activity[377] and encourages blood flow and the effective removal of intra-articular metabolites.[95] Exercises can be taught by the treating physician, but in difficult cases or when cooperation is not achieved, it is essential to refer the patient to a professional physiotherapist. Exercises that the authors prescribe include passive and active symmetric movements in all directions[365]; upon maximal movement, further stretching exercises are recommended to increase range of motion. Exercises combined with anti-inflammatory drugs are an effective strategy.[378] Careful follow-up and meticulous recording of the extent of motion are essential. In addition, the patient should be actively involved in goal setting and follow-up.

Intraoral appliances

The etiology of parafunction is unclear, whether it is an acquired habit, medication induced, or a neurologically based movement disorder. However, the effects of parafunction may be palliated by the short-term use of IOAs (see also chapter 8). Numerous studies on the therapeutic effect and efficacy of IOAs have been published with limited results. Of the various proposed therapeutic mechanisms suggested, none have adequate support in the literature.[379] With few exceptions, most studies were of limited quality; lacked a standardized diagnosis and outcome measures; and had small sample sizes, a short evaluation period, inadequate selection of controls, and limited follow-up. Regardless of these factors, in the short term, parafunctional habits may temporarily diminish with appliances or medications and thus may reduce joint loading, but habits tend to recur when appliances are removed or after long-term use.[380–382] Although the therapeutic mechanism is unclear, oral orthotics may be useful in providing relief of masticatory muscle pain and TMJ dysfunction.[379,383]

Some studies in the literature suggest that appliances are beneficial for reducing pain severity in patients with painful joint disorders, at rest and on palpation, compared with no treatment.[366,384,385] Repositioning appliances have been advocated to treat internal derangements and to recapture the disc. However, in the long term, clicks or abnormal disc positions tend to recur,[386,387] and these appliances fail to recapture the disc in internal derangement without reduction.[388]

In long-standing DDwoR, return to a normal disc-condyle relationship is unlikely, even with the use of protrusion appliances.[388] Indeed, repositioning appliances have no significant benefit over stabilization appliances in the treatment of TMJ sounds[389] and may induce irreversible occlusal changes. Recent data suggest that flat centric splints will relieve clinical symptoms more efficiently than repositioning splints in patients with DDwoR.[390] In a randomized clinical trial, a group of patients with painful DDwR were treated with three types of bite plates: flat occlusal, canine guided, and nonoccluding.[217] After 6 months, all patients with occluding splints had significant improvement in pain with no difference between the type of guidance.[217] Interestingly, the frequency of joint noises decreased over time, and there were no significant differences among the three groups. This effect has also been observed in nontreatment groups in a similar study, which suggests a natural fluctuation in the expression of clicks.[391] In contrast, a Cochrane review concluded that there is weak evidence that stabilization splints reduce pain at rest and on palpation compared with no treatment.[392] However, the review examined the effect on patients with "pain dysfunction syndrome," an unclear diagnosis that is not clinically applicable.

Reduction of TMJ loading may be obtained by constructing an appliance with occlusal contacts in the posterior region only.[95] This type of interocclusal appliance reduces the pressure generated in the joint during active clenching by 81.2%.[95] The use of techniques to offload the TMJ is not unlike the effect of different bandaging techniques as an adjunct to orthopedic management. Informing patients that IOAs are a temporary means of management is imperative, as long-term use is associated with uncontrolled changes in occlusion.

Medications

Most patients with TMJ pain will improve with the use of mild analgesics and NSAIDs. NSAIDs, both topically and systemically, have been shown to be effective in TMJ disorders.[181,366,393] Some data suggest that the nonspecific NSAIDs, such as naproxen, may be more effective than specific cyclooxygenase-2 (COX-2) inhibitors in the management of TMJ pain.[394] Because naproxen has a better cardiovascular safety profile than COX-2 inhibitors, this would suggest their preferential use (see chapter 15). In severe cases, the combination of initial steroid therapy followed by an NSAID was as effective as surgical or other management of DDwoR.[374]

In the absence of extensive and specific research on drug use in inflammatory TMJ disorders,[395] results of experimental models or clinical trials of other joints affected by osteoarthritis may be extrapolated. For example, both acetaminophen and COX-2 inhibitors were able to reverse the behavioral effects of experimental TMJ inflammation in rats.[396] Celecoxib (200 to 400 mg/day) was compared with acetaminophen (slow-release formulation 3,990 mg/day) in patients with osteoarthritis in various sites.[397] Most patients found acetaminophen to be as effective as celecoxib.[397] A systematic review on the treatment of osteoarthritis of the knee

or hip concluded that acetaminophen in doses of about 4 g daily is clinically effective and superior to placebo.[398] However, NSAIDs (eg, ibuprofen 1,200 mg/day, diclofenac 75 to 150 mg/day, celecoxib 200 mg/day) improve pain, function, and stiffness more than acetaminophen, especially in moderate to severe cases. Patients taking traditional NSAIDs were more likely to have adverse gastrointestinal effects, but otherwise there was no major difference in side effects relative to acetaminophen. This would suggest that NSAIDs should also be used in TMJ osteoarthritis; however, most of the studies lasted only about 6 weeks.[398] For long-term management, the efficacy of NSAIDs must be countered with severe side effects on the gastrointestinal, renal, and cardiovascular systems, factors that may favor the use of acetaminophen. Renal and cardiovascular risks are particularly relevant for the specific COX-2 inhibitors that also involve increased cost. Systemic side effects may be minimized by the use of topical application of diclofenac (see chapter 16). Topical diclofenac may have an additional analgesic effect via peripheral N-methyl-D-aspartate–type glutamate receptors.[399]

Taken together, the data suggest that for short-term management of TMJ pain and osteoarthritis, NSAIDs (naproxen, ibuprofen) are most likely to be effective and have minimal side effects. Emphasizing that renal and cardiovascular risks are increased within 1 month of NSAID use is important (see chapter 15), so the authors suggest titrating clinical response and transferring patients at the earliest opportunity to other analgesics. Particularly in patients with medical comorbidity (cardiovascular, renal), acetaminophen is the drug of choice, although in patients with gastrointestinal problems, NSAIDs may be used in conjunction with a proton pump inhibitor (consult the managing physician). For long-term management, the use of mild analgesics, such as acetaminophen, is effective for patients with TMJ pain and certainly safer. The advantages of mild analgesics over NSAIDs are discussed in chapter 15. Rarely, stronger analgesics, such as mild opioids, may be needed for short-term therapy in severe cases or postoperatively. All of the aforementioned medications, drug dosages, schedules, and side-effect profiles are extensively reviewed in chapter 15. More recent data suggest that drugs specifically acting on cytokines may be clinically useful.[400] Infliximab, an anti–TNF-α agent, was given systemically to patients with TMJ pain, who reported significantly reduced pain levels.[400]

When comorbid muscle pain is present, the use of adjuvant analgesics is beneficial. These drugs include muscle relaxants (cyclobenzaprine), antidepressants (amitriptyline), and anticonvulsants (gabapentin, clonazepam), which are reviewed in chapter 16. The analgesic effects of antidepressants may account for their use in patients with articular disorders.[401–403] Based on two pilot studies, chondroitin sulfate or glucosamine hydrochloride is effective in TMJ pain[178,181] (see the earlier nutrition section).

TMJ surgery

Surgery of the TMJ plays a small but important role in the management of patients with TMJ disorders.[326,404] The literature has shown that approximately 5% of patients with TMJ disorders require surgical intervention, and a spectrum of invasive procedures, from simple arthrocentesis to more complex open-joint surgical procedures, is available. Consideration of each surgical procedure should conform to strict criteria. However, each procedure has its enthusiastic supporters, and specific criteria are lacking for the most appropriate intervention in each diagnosis. Thus, the literature is based more on observation than scientifically controlled studies. Recognizing that scientifically proven criteria are lacking, the authors discuss the criteria for each procedure, including indications, brief descriptions of techniques, outcomes, and complications.

Indications

Indications for surgery of the TMJ may be divided into relative and absolute.[326,404] Absolute indications are reserved for those conditions where surgery has an undisputed role, such as tumors, growth anomalies, and ankylosis of the TMJ.

Surgical intervention of a dysfunctional or painful joint must be based on clearly defined criteria, such as:

1. Pain and/or dysfunction of such a magnitude as to constitute a disability to the patient

2. Failure of nonsurgical therapy to resolve the problem
3. Documentation of TMJ intracapsular pathologic condition or anatomical derangement that is a major source of the patient's pain and/or dysfunction
4. The condition is amenable to surgical intervention

Although the indications for surgery may appear clear, they are, in fact, nonspecific. The first criterion—significant TMJ pain and dysfunction—may be the most important. What distinguishes a surgical candidate from nonsurgical patients is localization of the pain and dysfunction to the TMJ. The more localized the pain and dysfunction are to the TMJ, the better the prognosis for a successful surgical outcome. Conversely, the more diffuse the pain and dysfunction, the less likely surgical intervention will succeed. The decision for surgical intervention should be made based on the clinical findings in conjunction with assessment of how the pain and dysfunction affect the patient's well-being, balanced against the prognosis if surgery is not performed. Surgical candidates should have localized, continuous TMJ pain that is moderate to severe and becomes worse during mandibular function (ie, talking or chewing). The patient may present with limited movements with or without pain or other signs of dysfunction, such as painful clicking, crepitation, or locking of the TMJ.

The second criterion—failure of nonsurgical treatment—is also nonspecific. TMDs encompass a wide variety of etiologies and complaints, and therefore no clear consensus exists on protocols for conservative or nonsurgical treatment. Nonetheless, most clinicians understand what nonsurgical or conservative therapy involves: typically, a combination of patient education, medication, physical therapy, an occlusal appliance, and possibly counseling or behavioral therapy. Most patients will respond successfully to this treatment, though others may see a reduction in symptoms over time, even in the absence of treatment. Therefore, surgical consideration should be reserved for patients who fail to respond successfully over a reasonable period of time. However, it must also be stressed that not all patients who fail nonsurgical treatment are surgical candidates.

Surgical treatment must be limited to those who respond to the first criterion of pain and dysfunction arising from within the TMJ. Patients who have pain and dysfunction arising from the masticatory muscles or other non-TMJ sources are not surgical candidates and may be made worse by surgical intervention. Myofascial pain referral and referral from numerous other extracapsular sources of pain must be considered before a surgical intervention.

The third criterion—imaging evidence of disease—appears to be the most objective; however, imaging should not be interpreted in isolation. The correlation of disc derangement, dysfunction, and osteoarthrosis found on imaging with pain is poor.[53,405] Therefore, imaging should be used only to confirm and support the clinical findings. Surgery cannot be performed on the basis of imaging alone.

The mere presence of a disc displacement is clearly not an indication for surgery. Results of a recent study found that approximately 90% of persons with mild TMD symptoms displayed TMJ disc displacement of a magnitude similar to that of patients seeking treatment. Moreover, nearly a third of persons without any jaw pain or dysfunction (asymptomatic volunteers) also showed evidence of disc displacement. The prevalence of disc displacement is common in the general population, and care needs to be taken to distinguish symptomatic and asymptomatic persons.[36]

Surgical interventions include arthrocentesis, arthroscopy, condylotomy, and open joint procedures, such as disc repositioning and discectomy. Randomized clinical trials comparing these procedures do not exist, so the surgical procedure selected is based mostly on the surgeon's experience. Each procedure has specific benefits and risks. Therefore, the procedure that has the highest potential for success with the lowest risks and most cost-effectiveness should be chosen for the patient's specific problem.

Based on the authors' experience, arthrocentesis and arthroscopic lavage and lysis should be used for TMJ pain during function, intermittent clicking, or limited opening.[406] Condylotomy for TMJ pain with little or no restriction of opening and open TMJ surgery should be reserved for advanced cases of internal derangement and osteoarthrosis.

TMJ arthrocentesis

In the authors' view, arthrocentesis is probably the first surgical procedure that should be used in patients with TMJ pain and dysfunction that have not responded to conservative therapy. Studies on the effect of arthrocentesis on DDwoR have shown consistently improved mouth opening and decreased pain.[250,251,253,407] The authors' clinical experience suggests that range of jaw movements in DDwoR only improve marginally after arthrocentesis: Interincisal opening may increase from about 32 to 36 mm, and lateral excursions from 8 to 8.5 mm. These findings are expected, as arthrocentesis and arthroscopic lavage are incapable of changing the disc's shape or position.[60,61] The marked improvement described in the literature was probably in a group of patients that were not strictly defined and may have included other disorders. After arthrocentesis, pain and dysfunction levels are improved more rapidly than with conservative care.[408,409]

In a group of patients with disc displacements resistant to conservative therapy, arthrocentesis was not significantly different from arthroscopy for decreasing patient reports of pain and increasing functional mobility of the mandible.[410] Because arthrocentesis is a simple outpatient procedure performed under local anesthetic and is relatively safer than arthroscopy, it should be tried first.

Technique. Murakami et al[411] were the first to offer a systematic description of TMJ arthrocentesis, which they described as "manipulation technique followed by pumping and hydraulic pressure." Arthrocentesis of the TMJ, as presented here, is a modification of the traditional method in which two needles instead of one are introduced into the upper joint space. This adaptation permits massive lavage of the joint, in addition to aspiration and injection.[412]

The patient is seated inclined at a 45-degree angle, with the head turned to the unaffected side to provide an easy approach to the affected joint. After proper preparation of the target site, the external auditory meatus is blocked with cotton soaked in mineral oil. The points of needle insertion are marked on the skin as follows. A line is drawn from the middle of the tragus to the outer canthus. The posterior en-

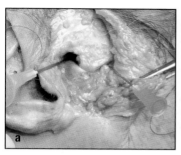 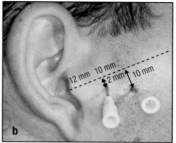 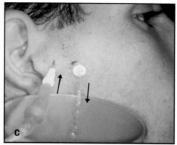

Fig 9-13 Arthrocentesis. *(a)* The positioning of the arthrocentesis needles is shown on a cadaver. With the jaw in an open position, two needles are placed: one in the posterior (left needle) and one in the anterior (right needle) recesses of the upper joint space. *(b)* To locate these points in patients, a line is drawn from the middle of the tragus to the outer canthus. The posterior entrance point is located along the canthotragal line, 10 to 12 mm from the middle of the tragus and 2 mm below the line. The anterior point of entry is placed 10 mm farther along the line and 8 to 10 mm below it. *(c)* Irrigation is then performed as described in the text.

trance point is located along the canthotragal line, 10 to 12 mm from the middle of the tragus and 2 mm below the line (Fig 9-13). The anterior point of entry is placed 10 mm farther along the line and 8 to 10 mm below it. These markings over the skin indicate the location of the articular fossa and the eminence of the TMJ but should always be verified clinically. Using these points as guides is important because the precise location needs to be confirmed by careful examination of the patient's anatomy.

Stages in arthrocentesis. Following are the stages involved in arthrocentesis:

1. A local anesthetic is injected at the planned entrance points, taking care to avoid penetration into the joint and injection into the synovial fluid.
2. If samples of synovial fluid are needed for research or diagnostic assessment, the procedure is continued by injecting 1 mL of lactated Ringer's solution into the superior compartment at the posterior point and immediately aspirated. This procedure is repeated three times to obtain a sufficient amount of fluid for diagnostic and research purposes.
3. If the procedure is purely for therapeutic purposes, stage 2 is omitted. Surface anesthesia from stage 1 is then followed by injection of 2 to 3 mL bupivacaine 0.5% through the posterior point, using a syringe with a 19-gauge needle, to distend the up-

per joint space and anesthetize the adjacent tissues. A second 19-gauge needle is then inserted into the distended compartment in the area of the articular eminence (anterior point of entry) to enable free flow of Ringer's solution through the superior compartment (see Fig 9-13). Slight adjustment of the needle position may be necessary. In cases of sluggish outflow, additional needles may be inserted into the distended compartment to enhance the transport of the solution. A free flow of 100 mL of Ringer's solution is recommended[413] because denatured hemoglobin and various proteinases have been recovered in this fraction. Later studies suggested that 300 to 400 mL should be used for the washout of bradykinin, IL-6, and proteins.[414] A simplified procedure is one in which the second needle is inserted next to the first one, into the posterior rather than the anterior recess, and saline is then flushed through the upper compartment. During the lavage, the mandible is moved through opening, excursive, and protrusive movements to facilitate lysis of adhesions.[415]

Mode of action. By forcing apart the flexible disc from the fossa and by washing away degraded particles and inflammatory components, arthrocentesis reduces load and pain and reestablishes joint movements, which is the hallmark of joint health. Upon termination of the procedure and after the removal of one needle, medication can be injected into the joint space. Hyaluronic acid is an example of such a supplement of arthrocentesis,[62,416] though its effectiveness is still debated.[417] The potency of hyaluronic acid will be minimal if inflammatory products in the affected joint are allowed to degrade it, but with the removal of the inflammatory products by arthrocentesis, the hyaluronic acid remains intact and is probably more effective.

Reports on the elimination of products from the diseased TMJ by arthrocentesis suggest that this may be a major mode of action (see the earlier section on pathophysiology). Arthrocentesis is also an important diagnostic tool. Adhesions or osteophytes are not always unambiguously diagnosed as the causes of limitation or pain by available imaging techniques. Failure of lavage suggests that surgical means may be required and are legitimate ways to release the joint and restore movement. Indeed, arthrocentesis is a prerequisite for most TMJ surgical intervention.

Complications. Temporary facial weakness or paralysis, as a result of the use of a local anesthetic, and/or swelling of the neighboring tissues caused by perfusion of Ringer's solution might occur during arthrocentesis. Both signs are transient and disappear within hours. Numerous other complications have been described as a result of arthrocentesis, including extradural hematoma. Correct diagnosis, appropriate treatment approach, and careful surgical technique should prevent complications.

TMJ arthroscopy

TMJ arthroscopy is a minimally invasive procedure but is usually performed under general anesthesia in the operating room. The procedure is very much equipment dependent and requires considerable manual dexterity on the part of the surgeon. TMJ arthroscopy now plays a major role in the surgical management of TMJ internal derangement and osteoarthrosis.

Technique. TMJ arthroscopy involves the placement of an arthroscopic telescope (1.8 to 2.6 mm in diameter) into the upper joint space of the TMJ. A camera is attached to the arthroscope to project the image onto a television

monitor. The surgeon must conceptualize a three-dimensional space on a two-dimensional image. A second access instrument is placed approximately 10 to 15 mm in front of the arthroscope. This access point provides an outflow portal for irrigation and access for instrumentation of the joint space. The examination is started posteriorly by identifying the posterior attachment tissue. The synovial lining is inspected for the presence of inflammation, such as increased capillary hyperemia. The junction of the posterior band of the disc and posterior attachment tissues can be identified. Movement of the joint allows for the identification of clicking or restriction in movement of the disc. As the arthroscope is moved through the upper joint space, the articular cartilage is inspected for the presence of degenerative changes, such as softness, fibrillation, or tears. The joint space is also inspected for the presence of adhesions, loose bodies, or other pathology. The integrity of the disc, or perforations of the disc or posterior attachment tissues, can be identified. Although the lower joint space is not usually examined, the presence of a perforation in the disc or posterior attachment may allow limited examination of the lower joint space and condyle. Although sophisticated operative techniques ranging from ablation of adhesions with lasers to plication of the disc have been developed, most surgeons limit the use of arthroscopy to lysis of adhesions and lavage of the upper joint space. Lysis of adhesions is accomplished most often by sweeping the arthroscope or the irrigation cannula through the adhesions and tearing them. After completion of the examination, the joint space is thoroughly irrigated to remove debris and small blood clots. The patient is usually discharged the same day after recovering from the anesthesia. Postoperative care includes a nonchew soft diet for a few days, range-of-motion exercises for several days, an IOA, and analgesics as necessary for pain control.

Multiple studies report an 80% to 90% success rate with arthroscopic lysis and lavage for the management of patients with painful limited mouth opening.[243,244,249,374,418,419] Most patients have decreased pain and improved mouth opening. Studies with 5- and 10-year follow-up have shown that the arthroscopic lysis and lavage technique is successful for all stages of internal derangement, and results are comparable with those obtained using open surgery procedures.[418,419] Data from surgical arthroscopic techniques, such as disc repositioning, are difficult to interpret, and it is unclear whether the outcomes are better than those obtained with simple lysis and lavage.

Mode of action. Basically, arthroscopy is a sophisticated method for lavage and lysis of adhesions in the TMJ (see the earlier arthrocentesis section). The technique offers the additional benefits of allowing the use of rotatory instruments, lasers, and other microsurgical implements to modify anatomy, cauterize tissues, repair the disc, and remove loose bodies.

Complications. The advantages of TMJ arthroscopy are that it is minimally invasive and causes less surgical trauma to the joint. Surgical complications are rare and mostly limited to reversible effects, some similar to those observed in arthrocentesis.[242] Patient recovery is rapid, and healing time is shorter than with open surgical procedures. The disadvantages include the surgical limitations, the necessity for sophisticated equipment, and the high level of training needed.

Modified condylotomy

Modified TMJ condylotomy, the only TMJ surgical procedure that does not invade the joint structures, is a modification of the transoral vertical ramus osteotomy used in orthognathic surgery. Although some authors recommend modified condylotomy as the surgical treatment of choice for all stages of TMJ internal derangement, it seems to be most successful when used to treat painful TMJ internal derangement without reduced mouth opening.[420]

Mode of action. The objective of the procedure is to surgically increase the joint space between the condyle and the fossa, thus allowing repositioning of the condyle anteriorly and inferiorly beneath the displaced disc. Good pain relief was reported in about 90% of 400 patients treated over a 9-year period with modified condylotomies.[420] In follow-up studies, a 94% success rate has been reported in patients with DDwR. Interestingly, 72% of these

patients had a normal disc position when evaluated with follow-up MRIs.[421] This would suggest that the procedure is able to provide optimal conditions for the restoration of a clinically normal disc-condyle relationship. However, in a group of patients with DDwoR, the success rate for modified condylotomy was slightly lower at 88%.[421]

Technique. The modified condylotomy is performed under general anesthesia, usually as an outpatient procedure, but it may require an overnight stay in the hospital. An incision is made intraorally along the anterior border of the mandibular ramus. After exposure of the lateral aspect of the mandibular ramus, a vertical cut is made posteriorly to the lingula from the coronoid notch to the mandibular angle. After mobilization of the condylar segment, the medial pterygoid muscle is stripped from the segment. The mandible is then immobilized using maxillomandibular fixation. Although the surgery is simple, there is a period of postoperative rehabilitation involving 2 or 3 weeks of maxillomandibular fixation followed by training elastics so that the occlusion is maintained.

Complications. The most significant potential complication of the modified condylotomy is excessive condylar sag resulting in malocclusion. In one series of cases, the complication rate was only 4% and consisted primarily of minor occlusal discrepancies.[422] In spite of the simplicity of the procedure and its high success rate, the procedure has not become widely used. The reasons for this are unclear but are most likely related to the necessity for maxillomandibular fixation and the fear of excessive condylar sag that could result in an unstable condylar position with malocclusion.

Open joint surgery (arthrotomy)

Open joint surgery is indicated for those patients with TMJ internal derangement and osteoarthritis who have failed to respond to simpler surgical procedures or have failed previous open surgery. In cases where previous surgery failed, the surgeon must be very hesitant to operate again because the success rate for repeat surgery is very low; in fact, after two surgeries, it may approach zero. The surgeon must be certain that the source of the pain and/or dysfunction arises from within the joint. Severe mechanical interference, such as loud, hard clicking or intermittent locking associated with loud, hard clicking, is an indication to perform open surgery without first performing simpler procedures because experience indicates that simpler procedures are rarely successful in these cases.

Although the use of open joint surgery has decreased significantly, it still has a small but important role in the surgical management of TMJ disorders. Although other surgical procedures provide a limited range of options, open TMJ surgery provides the surgeon with an unlimited scope of procedures ranging from simple debridement of the joint to the removal of the disc. Disc repositioning procedures are less commonly performed today than in the 1980s and 1990s because most patients with discs that can be preserved are successfully treated with simpler procedures. Advanced cases of internal derangement with degenerative discs and severe arthritic changes may require partial discectomy. Arthroplasty in the form of bone contouring of the articular eminence or condyle is sometimes necessary, particularly with disc repositioning procedures.

Open joint surgery is performed under general anesthesia in the hospital and usually requires a 1- or 2-day stay. The most common surgical approach is via a preauricular incision. Incorporating the tragus of the ear into the incision line is often used for cosmetic purposes. Exposure of the capsule is carefully performed to protect the temporal branches of the facial nerve. After exposure of the capsule, the upper joint space is entered and inspected for the presence of adhesions. The contour and integrity of the fossa and eminence are evaluated, and lastly the disc is visualized. Evaluation of the disc includes its color, position, mobility, shape, and integrity.

Disc repositioning. If the disc is intact, not deformed, and can be repositioned without tension, then repositioning can be performed by removing excess tissue from the posterior attachment tissues, repositioning the disc, and stabilizing it with sutures. Some surgeons advise release of the anterior attachment.[354] Bone recontouring of the glenoid fossa and/or articular eminence is generally performed, especially in cases of gross mechanical interference or advanced degenerative joint disease. The goal of disc repositioning surgery is to eliminate mechanical interferences to smooth joint function. After completion of the intra-articular procedures, the superior joint space is irrigated and the soft tissues closed. Exercises to improve range of motion are begun immediately after the surgery. Continuation of postoperative conservative treatment is essential to ensure a successful outcome. A soft, nontextured diet is recommended for 6 weeks after surgery.

The literature indicates that disc repositioning surgery is successful in 80% to 95% of patients; however, experience indicates that this may be an overestimation.[423–427] Although disc repositioning surgery significantly reduced pain and dysfunction in 51 subjects evaluated up to 6 years postoperatively, improvement in disc position was not maintained for most patients over the follow-up period.[428] In spite of these findings, the preservation of a healthy, freely mobile disc is justified. Moreover, the primary treatment for persons with disc displacements should consist of medical management or rehabilitation.[374] The use of this approach will avoid unnecessary surgical procedures.

Discectomy. A diseased or deformed disc that interferes with smooth function of the joint and cannot be repositioned should be removed. Only the diseased or deformed portion of the disc needs to be removed. The synovial tissues should be preserved as much as possible. After removal of the disc, only minimal bone recontouring should be performed because exposure of bone marrow may result in heterotopic bone formation. Limitation caused by the heterotopic bone can be prevented by intensive physiotherapy. To minimize the risk of heterotopic bone formation, placement of an interpositional fat graft into the joint space is recommended. After completion of the intra-articular procedures, the joint space is irrigated and the soft tissues closed.

The postoperative findings are the same after discectomy as described for disc repositioning. The postoperative recommendations are also the same except that a soft nonchew diet is recommended for 6 months.

Discectomy of the TMJ has the longest follow-up studies of any procedure for management of TMJ internal derangement. Four studies with at least 30 years' follow-up report excellent reduction in pain and improvement in function in most patients.[65–68] Postoperative imaging studies of patients after discectomy generally show significant changes in condylar morphology.[68] These changes are thought to be adaptive and not degenerative. Despite the excellent long-term success associated with TMJ discectomy, surgeons seem reluctant to perform this procedure.

Immediately after the surgery, the patient may experience swelling in front of the ear and a slight change in occlusion and limited mouth opening, which usually resolves in about 2 weeks. All patients experience some numbness in front of the ear, which resolves in about 6 weeks. Patients normally have moderate discomfort lasting 1 or 2 weeks. The most significant complication associated with open surgery is facial nerve injury. Although total facial nerve paralysis is possible, it is rare. Inability to raise the eyebrow is the most commonly observed finding and occurs in about 5% of cases. The problem usually resolves within 3 months and is permanent in less than 1% of patients. Other complications are limited opening and minor occlusal changes. The complications associated with discectomy are similar to those associated with disc repositioning. The growth of heterotopic bone is more common after discectomy than other TMJ surgical procedures. This can be a significant complication that can result in complete ankylosis of the joint. The frequency of occurrence of heterotopic bone formation is unclear.

TMJ replacement. A complete discussion of total TMJ replacement is beyond the scope of this chapter. The discussion here is limited to alloplastic total joint replacement in adult patients who have advanced degenerative joint disease, ankylosis, or complications of previously performed open surgery. The use of alloplastic materials to reconstruct or replace the diseased tissues of the TMJ caused disastrous results in the 1980s and 1990s. The use of Proplast/Teflon and silastic implants caused significant foreign body reactions with severe destruction of the TMJ structures.[292,429–431] This experience has led some surgeons to reject the use of alloplastic TMJ prostheses in favor

of autogenous tissues, such as costochondral grafts, for TMJ reconstruction.[432] Though there are advantages to using autogenous tissues, recently developed alloplastic TMJ prostheses provide safe and predictably successful reconstruction of the TMJ.[433,434]

Two basic prosthetic joints are discussed in this section: a patient-fitted prosthesis and a stock prosthesis. A patient-fitted prosthesis is a type of custom-made implant that has been available for more than 10 years.[433] The prosthesis consists of a glenoid fossa implant that has an articular surface made of high–molecular weight polyethylene attached to a pure titanium mesh. The body of the condylar prosthesis is made of medical-grade titanium alloy with a cobalt-chromium-molybdenum condylar head. The process for making the prosthesis requires a head CT, from which an acrylic model of the patient's skull is made. The planned surgery is performed on the model. The prosthesis is designed on the model and sent to the surgeon for approval. After approval, the patient's prosthesis is made using computer-aided design/computer-assisted manufacturing (CAD/CAM) technology.

In contrast, a stock prosthesis is a prefabricated implant available in various sizes (small, medium, and large) for the fossa and three lengths (45, 50, and 55 mm) for the condyle. The prosthesis includes a glenoid fossa component made of high–molecular weight polyethylene and a condylar component made of cobalt-chromium-molybdenum alloy. The articular surface is the same on all three implants; only the flange varies in size.

The surgical placement is essentially the same for both types of implants. The surgery requires preauricular and retromandibular incisions for access to the TMJ and mandibular ramus. A gap arthroplasty is performed by removing the diseased condyle or ankylosed bone. Generally, a coronoidectomy is also performed. After the teeth are placed into maxillomandibular fixation, the implants are fitted and secured using titanium screws. Stock implants are more difficult to place than patient-fitted implants because the bony structures must be reshaped to fit the implants. The maxillomandibular fixation is released, the occlusion is verified, and the range of motion is determined. If these are acceptable, the wounds are irrigated, a fat graft is placed around the condyle, and the soft tissues are closed.

The criteria used to determine success in patients with complex, chronic TMJ pain are somewhat relative, so precise success rates are difficult to determine. A successful outcome generally means that the patient has reduced pain levels, increased range of motion, improved function, and an absence of surgical complications. Using these criteria, the success rates are high for both types of prostheses.

Patients who have had multiple TMJ surgical procedures and who suffer from chronic pain generally experience about 50% pain reduction and gain 10 to 15 mm of mandibular opening. However, total TMJ replacement is not necessarily a solution to the management of chronic TMJ pain. The TMJ prosthesis can be used to predictably restore occlusion and increase range of motion, but pain relief is variable. On the other hand, both types of TMJ prostheses predictably provide pain-free restoration of occlusion and range of motion for patients who have TMJ reconstruction for ankylosis, tumors, or other conditions where pain is not an original component of the condition. This may suggest that the presence of preexisting pain is a negative prognostic factor and may be related to plastic changes of the nervous system in persistent pain states (see chapters 2 and 12).

The most significant complication after TMJ reconstruction with alloplastic implants is facial nerve injury. Although uncommon, it does occur more frequently than after routine open joint surgery, especially in patients who have had multiple TMJ surgeries previously. Formation of heterotopic bone is a common complication that occurs in as many as 20% of patients. Other complications, such as infection, foreign body and allergic reactions, malocclusion, and implant failure can occur but are rare. Complications requiring implant removal are unusual.

Unquestionably, the patient-fitted prosthesis provides the best TMJ reconstruction. The surgery is easier to perform, and the implants fit more accurately than a stock prosthesis. However, there is a need for both types of implants. Patient-fitted implants require 1 to 3 months to manufacture, so immediate TMJ reconstruction is not possible. They are also more expensive than stock prostheses. In addition, in several situations two surgeries are necessary to use a patient-fitted prosthesis: (1) patients who require significant mandibular repositioning to correct large malocclusions; (2) patients with extensive bony ankylosis requiring large amounts of bone removal; (3) patients with foreign bodies, such as previously placed alloplastic TMJ prostheses that must be removed before an accurate CT can be obtained; and (4) combinations of 1 and 2. When two surgeries are required, it can be problematic to maintain occlusion and function after the first surgery as well as during the time the prosthesis is being constructed. Additionally, two surgeries are inconvenient for the patient, prolong healing time, expose the patient to greater risks of complications, and are more expensive. Stock joint prostheses can provide adequate reconstruction with a single operation in these situations. Conversely, in some situations a stock prosthesis cannot be used, for example, in patients who have extensive bone loss at the lateral aspect of the fossa and articular eminence or the mandibular ramus, which results in inadequate bone for placement of a stock prosthesis. The design of patient-fitted prostheses offers great flexibility and allows them to be adapted to a variety of complex clinical situations. Surgeons must be familiar with both types of prostheses so they can successfully meet the needs of the variety of patient conditions requiring TMJ replacement.

Summary

Complex referral patterns in the head and neck make an accurate diagnosis of TMJ-related pain difficult. The roles of inflammation, peripheral sensitization, and central sensitization add to the diagnostic complexity. Additionally, diagnostic criteria are often not adhered to, which can lead to misdiagnosis of muscle-related pain as a TMJ disorder.

Most painful disorders of the TMJ may be successfully treated by conservative means. Frequently, recovery occurs with minimal palliative or conservative management. Surgical techniques include minimally invasive options, such as arthrocentesis and arthroscopy, which have been shown to be highly effective in many patients resistant to conservative management. Relative indications for open surgical intervention include failed conservative therapy and structural abnormalities that cause pain and dysfunction. Open surgery allows for the most flexible treatment options but carries the greatest morbidity. However, open surgery is absolutely indicated for some limited TMJ disorders, mainly tumors and ankylosis. In a minority of cases, prosthetic replacement of the TMJ may be required, and custom or stock options are available. Ensuring that practitioners are familiar with all surgical techniques is essential so that they will be able to discuss options with the oral and maxillofacial surgeon. This will result in more optimal management of patients with orofacial pain.

References

1. Schiffman E, Ohrbach R, Truelove E, et al. Diagnostic Criteria for Temporomandibular Disorders (DC/TMD) for clinical and research applications: Recommendations of the International RDC/TMD Consortium Network and Orofacial Pain Special Interest Group. J Oral Facial Pain Headache 2014;28:6–27.
2. Stegenga B. Osteoarthritis of the temporomandibular joint organ and its relationship to disc displacement. J Orofac Pain 2001;15:193–205.
3. de Leeuw JR, Klasser G (eds). Orofacial Pain: Guidelines for Assessment, Diagnosis and Management. Chicago: Quintessence, 2013.
4. Headache Classification Subcommittee of the International Headache Society. The International Classification of Headache Disorders, 3rd edition (beta version). Cephalalgia 2013;33:629–808.
5. Gonzalez YM, Schiffman E, Gordon SM, et al. Development of a brief and effective temporomandibular disorder pain screening questionnaire: Reliability and validity. J Am Dent Assoc 2011;142:1183–1191.
6. Celić R, Jerolimov V, Knezović Zlatarić D, Klaić B. Measurement of mandibular movements in patients with temporomandibular disorders and in asymptomatic subjects. Coll Antropol 2003;27(2, suppl):43–49.
7. Dworkin SF, Sherman J, Mancl L, Ohrbach R, LeResche L, Truelove E. Reliability, validity, and clinical utility of the Research Diagnostic Criteria for Temporomandibular Disorders Axis II Scales: Depression, nonspecific physical symptoms, and graded chronic pain. J Orofac Pain 2002;16:207–220.
8. Look JO, Schiffman EL, Truelove EL, Ahmad M. Reliability and validity of Axis I of the Research Diagnostic Criteria for Temporomandibular Disorders (RDC/TMD) with proposed revisions. J Oral Rehabil 2010;37:744–759.
9. Nitzan DW, Dolwick FM, Marmary Y. The value of arthrography in the decision-making process regarding surgery for internal derangement of the temporomandibular joint. J Oral Maxillofac Surg 1991;49:375–379.
10. Manfredini D, Tognini F, Zampa V, Bosco M. Predictive value of clinical findings for temporomandibular joint effusion. Oral Surg Oral Med Oral Pathol Oral Radiol Endod 2003;96:521–526.
11. Israel HA, Diamond B, Saed-Nejad F, Ratcliffe A. Osteoarthritis and synovitis as major pathoses of the temporomandibular joint: Comparison of clinical diagnosis with arthroscopic morphology. J Oral Maxillofac Surg 1998;56:1023–1027.
12. Paesani D, Westesson PL, Hatala MP, Tallents RH, Brooks SL. Accuracy of clinical diagnosis for TMJ internal derangement and arthrosis. Oral Surg Oral Med Oral Pathol 1992;73:360–363.
13. Roberts C, Katzberg RW, Tallents RH, Espeland MA, Handelman SL. The clinical predictability of internal derangements of the temporomandibular joint. Oral Surg Oral Med Oral Pathol 1991;71:412–414.
14. Schiffman EL, Ohrbach R, Truelove EL, et al. The Research Diagnostic Criteria for Temporomandibular Disorders. V: Methods used to establish and validate revised axis I diagnostic algorithms. J Orofac Pain 2010;24:63–78.
15. Ahmad M, Hollender L, Anderson Q, et al. Research diagnostic criteria for temporomandibular disorders (RDC/TMD): Development of image analysis criteria and examiner reliability for image analysis. Oral Surg Oral Med Oral Pathol Oral Radiol Endod 2009;107:844–860.
16. Maizlin ZV, Nutiu N, Dent PB, et al. Displacement of the temporomandibular joint disk: Correlation between clinical findings and MRI characteristics. J Can Dent Assoc 2010;76:a3.
17. Crow HC, Parks E, Campbell JH, Stucki DS, Daggy J. The utility of panoramic radiography in temporomandibular joint assessment. Dentomaxillofac Radiol 2005;34:91–95.
18. Brooks SL, Brand JW, Gibbs SJ, et al. Imaging of the temporomandibular joint: A position paper of the American Academy of Oral and Maxillofacial Radiology. Oral Surg Oral Med Oral Pathol Oral Radiol Endod 1997;83:609–618.
19. Boeddinghaus R, Whyte A. Computed tomography of the temporomandibular joint. J Med Imaging Radiat Oncol 2013;57:448–454.
20. Hunter A, Kalathingal S. Diagnostic imaging for temporomandibular disorders and orofacial pain. Dent Clin North Am 2013;57:405–418.
21. Honda K, Larheim TA, Maruhashi K, Matsumoto K, Iwai K. Osseous abnormalities of the mandibular condyle: Diagnostic reliability of cone beam computed tomography compared with helical computed tomography based on an autopsy material. Dentomaxillofac Radiol 2006;35:152–157.
22. Sakabe R, Sakabe J, Kuroki Y, Nakajima I, Kijima N, Honda K. Evaluation of temporomandibular disorders in children using limited cone-beam computed tomography: A case report. J Clin Pediatr Dent 2006;31:14–16.
23. Barghan S, Tetradis S, Mallya S. Application of cone beam computed tomography for assessment of the temporomandibular joints. Aust Dent J 2012;57(suppl 1):109–118.

24. Larheim TA. Role of magnetic resonance imaging in the clinical diagnosis of the temporomandibular joint. Cells Tissues Organs 2005;180:6–21.

25. Guler N, Uckan S, Imirzalioglu P, Acikgozoglu S. Temporomandibular joint internal derangement: Relationship between joint pain and MR grading of effusion and total protein concentration in the joint fluid. Dentomaxillofac Radiol 2005;34:175–181.

26. Takahashi T, Nagai H, Seki H, Fukuda M. Relationship between joint effusion, joint pain, and protein levels in joint lavage fluid of patients with internal derangement and osteoarthritis of the temporomandibular joint. J Oral Maxillofac Surg 1999;57:1187–1193.

27. Emshoff R, Brandlmaier I, Bertram S, Rudisch A. Relative odds of temporomandibular joint pain as a function of magnetic resonance imaging findings of internal derangement, osteoarthrosis, effusion, and bone marrow edema. Oral Surg Oral Med Oral Pathol Oral Radiol Endod 2003;95:437–445.

28. Widmalm SE, Brooks SL, Sano T, Upton LG, McKay DC. Limitation of the diagnostic value of MR images for diagnosing temporomandibular joint disorders. Dentomaxillofac Radiol 2006;35:334–338.

29. Kim JH, Kim YK, Kim SG, Yun PY, Kim JD, Min JH. Effectiveness of bone scans in the diagnosis of osteoarthritis of the temporomandibular joint. Dentomaxillofac Radiol 2012;41:224–229.

30. Epstein JB, Rea A, Chahal O. The use of bone scintigraphy in temporomandibular joint disorders. Oral Dis 2002;8:47–53.

31. Lee JW, Lee SM, Kim SJ, Choi JW, Baek KW. Clinical utility of fluoride-18 positron emission tomography/CT in temporomandibular disorder with osteoarthritis: Comparisons with 99mTc-MDP bone scan. Dentomaxillofac Radiol 2013;42:29292350.

32. Goulet JP, Clark GT. Clinical TMJ examination methods. J Calif Dent Assoc 1990;18:25–33.

33. Baba K, Tsukiyama Y, Yamazaki M, Clark GT. A review of temporomandibular disorder diagnostic techniques. J Prosthet Dent 2001;86:184–194.

34. Kalaykova S, Lobbezoo F, Naeije M. Two-year natural course of anterior disc displacement with reduction. J Orofac Pain 2010;24:373–378.

35. Reneker J, Paz J, Petrosino C, Cook C. Diagnostic accuracy of clinical tests and signs of temporomandibular joint disorders: A systematic review of the literature. J Orthop Sports Phys Ther 2011;41:408–416.

36. Sale H, Bryndahl F, Isberg A. Temporomandibular joints in asymptomatic and symptomatic nonpatient volunteers: A prospective 15-year follow-up clinical and MR imaging study. Radiology 2013;267:183–194.

37. Rodríguez de Sotillo D, Velly AM, Hadley M, Fricton JR. Evidence of oxidative stress in temporomandibular disorders: A pilot study. J Oral Rehabil 2011;38:722–728.

38. Thonar EJ, Lenz ME, Klintworth GK, et al. Quantification of keratan sulfate in blood as a marker of cartilage catabolism. Arthritis Rheum 1985;28:1367–1376.

39. Yoshida K, Takatsuka S, Tanaka A, et al. Aggrecanase analysis of synovial fluid of temporomandibular joint disorders. Oral Dis 2005;11:299–302.

40. de Grauw JC, van de Lest CH, Brama PA, Rambags BP, van Weeren PR. In vivo effects of meloxicam on inflammatory mediators, MMP activity and cartilage biomarkers in equine joints with acute synovitis. Equine Vet J 2009;41:693–699.

41. Albilia JB, Tenenbaum HC, Clokie CM, et al. Serum levels of BMP-2, 4, 7 and AHSG in patients with degenerative joint disease requiring total arthroplasty of the hip and temporomandibular joints. J Orthop Res 2013;31:44–52.

42. Eversole LR, Machado L. Temporomandibular joint internal derangements and associated neuromuscular disorders. J Am Dent Assoc 1985;110:69–79.

43. Milam SB, Schmitz JP. Molecular biology of temporomandibular joint disorders: Proposed mechanisms of disease. J Oral Maxillofac Surg 1995;53:1448–1454.

44. Westesson PL, Rohlin M. Internal derangement related to osteoarthrosis in temporomandibular joint autopsy specimens. Oral Surg Oral Med Oral Pathol 1984;57:17–22.

45. Wilkes C. Internal derangement of the TMJ. Arch Otolaryngol Head Neck Surg 1989;115:469–477.

46. Dolwick MF, Dimitroulis G. Is there a role for temporomandibular joint surgery? Br J Oral Maxillofac Surg 1994;32:307–313.

47. Mercuri LG. Are we getting out of TMJ surgery? J Oral Maxillofac Surg 2006;64:996.

48. Mercuri LG, Wolford LM, Sanders B, White RD, Hurder A, Henderson W. Custom CAD/CAM total temporomandibular joint reconstruction system: Preliminary multicenter report. J Oral Maxillofac Surg 1995;53:106–115.

49. Haskin CL, Milam SB, Cameron IL. Pathogenesis of degenerative joint disease in the human temporomandibular joint. Crit Rev Oral Biol Med 1995;6:248–277.

50. Zardeneta G, Milam SB, Lee T, Schmitz JP. Detection and preliminary characterization of matrix metalloproteinase activity in temporomandibular joint lavage fluid. Int J Oral Maxillofac Surg 1998;27:397–403.

51. Hall HD. Intra-articular disc displacement. Part II: Its significant role in TMJ pathology. J Oral Maxillofac Surg 1995;53:1073–1079.

52. Scapino RP. Histopathology associated with malposition of the human temporomandibular joint disc. Oral Surg Oral Med Oral Pathol 1983;55:382–397.

53. Kircos LT, Ortendahl DA, Mark AS, Arakawa M. Magnetic resonance imaging of the TMJ disc in asymptomatic volunteers. J Oral Maxillofac Surg 1987;45:852–854.

54. Katzberg RW, Westesson PL, Tallents RH, Drake CM. Anatomic disorders of the temporomandibular joint disc in asymptomatic subjects. J Oral Maxillofac Surg 1996;54:147–153.

55. Tallents RH, Katzberg RW, Murphy W, Proskin H. Magnetic resonance imaging findings in asymptomatic volunteers and symptomatic patients with temporomandibular disorders. J Prosthet Dent 1996;75:529–533.

56. Davant TS 6th, Greene CS, Perry HT, Lautenschlager EP. A quantitative computer-assisted analysis of disc displacement in patients with internal derangement using sagittal view magnetic resonance imaging. J Oral Maxillofac Surg 1993;51:974–979.

57. Nitzan DW, Dolwick MF, Heft MW. Arthroscopic lavage and lysis of the temporomandibular joint: A change in perspective. J Oral Maxillofac Surg 1990;48:798–801.

58. Sanders B. Arthroscopic surgery of the temporomandibular joint: Treatment of internal derangement with persistent closed lock. Oral Surg Oral Med Oral Pathol 1986;62:361–372.

59. Nitzan DW, Samson B, Better H. Long-term outcome of arthrocentesis for sudden-onset, persistent, severe closed lock of the temporomandibular joint. J Oral Maxillofac Surg 1997;55:151–157.

60. Montgomery MT, Van Sickels JE, Harms SE, Thrash WJ. Arthroscopic TMJ surgery: Effects on signs, symptoms, and disc position. J Oral Maxillofac Surg 1989;47:1263–1271.

61. Moses JJ, Poker ID. TMJ arthroscopic surgery: An analysis of 237 patients. J Oral Maxillofac Surg 1989;47:790–794.

62. Xinmin Y, Jian H. Treatment of temporomandibular joint osteoarthritis with viscosupplementation and arthrocentesis on rabbit model. Oral Surg Oral Med Oral Pathol Oral Radiol Endod 2005;100:e35–e38.

63. Luyten FP. A scientific basis for the biologic regeneration of synovial joints. Oral Surg Oral Med Oral Pathol Oral Radiol Endod 1997;83:167–169.

64. Tanaka E, Kawai N, Hanaoka K, et al. Shear properties of the temporomandibular joint disc in relation to compressive and shear strain. J Dent Res 2004;83:476–479.

65. Tolvanen M, Oikarinen VJ, Wolf J. A 30-year follow-up study of temporomandibular joint meniscectomies: A report on five patients. Br J Oral Maxillofac Surg 1988;26:311–316.

66. Takaku S, Toyoda T. Long-term evaluation of discectomy of the temporomandibular joint. J Oral Maxillofac Surg 1994;52:722–726.

67. Silver CM. Long-term results of meniscectomy of the temporomandibular joint. Cranio 1984;3:46–57.

68. Eriksson L, Westesson PL. Long-term evaluation of meniscectomy of the temporomandibular joint. J Oral Maxillofac Surg 1985;43:263–269.

69. Sindelar BJ, Herring SW. Soft tissue mechanics of the temporomandibular joint. Cells Tissues Organs 2005;180:36–43.

70. Herring SW, Liu ZJ. Loading of the temporomandibular joint: Anatomical and in vivo evidence from the bones. Cells Tissues Organs 2001;169:193–200.

71. Hills BA. Synovial surfactant and the hydrophobic articular surface. J Rheumatol 1996;23:1323–1325.

72. Ghadially FN, Yong NK, Lalonde JM. A transmission electron microscopic comparison of the articular surface of cartilage processed attached to bone and detached from bone. J Anat 1982;135:685–706.

73. Bloebaum RD, Radley KM. Three-dimensional surface analysis of young adult human articular cartilage. J Anat 1995;187:293–301.

74. Tanaka E, Detamore MS, Tanimoto K, Kawai N. Lubrication of the temporomandibular joint. Ann Biomed Eng 2008;36:14–29.

75. Dijkgraaf LC, de Bont LG, Boering G, Liem RS. Structure of the normal synovial membrane of the temporomandibular joint: A review of the literature. J Oral Maxillofac Surg 1996;54:332–338.

76. de Bont LG, Liem RS, Boering G. Ultrastructure of the articular cartilage of the mandibular condyle: Aging and degeneration. Oral Surg Oral Med Oral Pathol 1985;60:631–641.

77. Moskalewski S, Jankowska-Steifer E. Hydrostatic and boundary lubrication of joints—Nature of boundary lubricant. Ortop Traumatol Rehabil 2012;14:13–21.

78. Swann DA, Slayter HS, Silver FH. The molecular structure of lubricating glycoprotein-I, the boundary lubricant for articular cartilage. J Biol Chem 1981;256:5921–5925.

79. Kawai N, Tanaka E, Takata T, et al. Influence of additive hyaluronic acid on the lubricating ability in the temporomandibular joint. J Biomed Mater Res A 2004;70:149–153.

80. Nitzan DW, Nitzan U, Dan P, Yedgar S. The role of hyaluronic acid in protecting surface-active phospholipids from lysis by exogenous phospholipase A(2). Rheumatology (Oxford) 2001;40:336–340.

81. Schwarz IM, Hills BA. Surface-active phospholipid as the lubricating component of lubricin. Br J Rheumatol 1998;37:21–26.

82. Hills BA, Butler BD. Surfactants identified in synovial fluid and their ability to act as boundary lubricants. Ann Rheum Dis 1984;43:641–648.

83. Hills BA. Boundary lubrication in vivo. Proc Inst Mech Eng H 2000;214:83–94.

84. Marchetti C, Bernasconi G, Reguzzoni M, Farina A. The articular disc surface in different functional conditions of the human temporo-mandibular joint. J Oral Pathol Med 1997;26:278–282.

85. Clark JM, Norman AG, Kääb MJ, Nötzli HP. The surface contour of articular cartilage in an intact, loaded joint. J Anat 1999;195:45–56.

86. Zea-Aragon Z, Terada N, Ohtsuki K, Ohnishi M, Ohno S. Immunohistochemical localization of phosphatidylcholine in rat mandibular condylar surface and lower joint cavity by cryotechniques. Histol Histopathol 2005;20:531–536.

87. Hills BA, Monds MK. Enzymatic identification of the load-bearing boundary lubricant in the joint. Br J Rheumatol 1998;37:137–142.

88. Chang DP, Abu-Lail NI, Coles JM, Guilak F, Jay GD, Zauscher S. Friction force microscopy of lubricin and hyaluronic acid between hydrophobic and hydrophilic surfaces. Soft Matter 2009;5:3438–3445.

89. Guarda-Nardini L, Rossi A, Ramonda R, Punzi L, Ferronato G, Manfredini D. Effectiveness of treatment with viscosupplementation in temporomandibular joints with or without effusion. Int J Oral Maxillofac Surg 2014;43:1218–1223.

90. Manfredini D, Arveda N, Guarda-Nardini L, Segù M, Collesano V. Distribution of diagnoses in a population of patients with temporomandibular disorders. Oral Surg Oral Med Oral Pathol Oral Radiol 2012;114:e35–e41.

91. Imhof H, Sulzbacher I, Grampp S, Czerny C, Youssefzadeh S, Kainberger F. Subchondral bone and cartilage disease: A rediscovered functional unit. Invest Radiol 2000;35:581–588.

92. Chen J, Xu L. A finite element analysis of the human temporomandibular joint. J Biomech Eng 1994;116:401–407.

93. Boyd RL, Gibbs CH, Mahan PE, Richmond AF, Laskin JL. Temporomandibular joint forces measured at the condyle of *Macaca arctoides*. Am J Orthod Dentofacial Orthop 1990;97:472–479.

94. Ward DM, Behrents RG, Goldberg JS. Temporomandibular synovial fluid pressure response to altered mandibular positions. Am J Orthod Dentofacial Orthop 1990;98:22–28.

95. Nitzan DW. Intraarticular pressure in the functioning human temporomandibular joint and its alteration by uniform elevation of the occlusal plane. J Oral Maxillofac Surg 1994;52:671–679.

96. Dreessen D, Halata Z, Strasmann T. Sensory innervation of the temporomandibular joint in the mouse. Acta Anat (Basel) 1990;139:154–160.

97. Haeuchi Y, Matsumoto K, Ichikawa H, Maeda S. Immunohistochemical demonstration of neuropeptides in the articular disk of the human temporomandibular joint. Cells Tissues Organs 1999;164:205–211.

98. Kido MA, Kiyoshima T, Ibuki T, et al. A topographical and ultrastructural study of sensory trigeminal nerve endings in the rat temporomandibular joint as demonstrated by anterograde transport of wheat germ agglutinin-horseradish peroxidase (WGA-HRP). J Dent Res 1995;74:1353–1359.

99. Kido MA, Kiyoshima T, Kondo T, et al. Distribution of substance P and calcitonin gene-related peptide-like immunoreactive nerve fibers in the rat temporomandibular joint. J Dent Res 1993;72:592–598.

100. Kido MA, Zhang JQ, Muroya H, Yamaza T, Terada Y, Tanaka T. Topography and distribution of sympathetic nerve fibers in the rat temporomandibular joint: Immunocytochemistry and ultrastructure. Anat Embryol (Berl) 2001;203:357–366.

101. Uddman R, Grunditz T, Kato J, Sundler F. Distribution and origin of nerve fibers in the rat temporomandibular joint capsule. Anat Embryol (Berl) 1998;197:273–282.

102. Suzuki O, Tsuboi A, Tabata T, Takafuji Y, Sakurai T, Watanabe M. Response properties of temporomandibular joint mechanosensitive neurons in the trigeminal sensory complex of the rabbit. Exp Brain Res 2012;222:113–123.

103. Davidson JA, Metzinger SE, Tufaro AP, Dellon AL. Clinical implications of the innervation of the temporomandibular joint. J Craniofac Surg 2003;14:235–239.

104. Damico JP, Ervolino E, Torres KR, et al. Phenotypic alterations of neuropeptide Y and calcitonin gene-related peptide-containing neurons innervating the rat temporomandibular joint during carrageenan-induced arthritis. Eur J Histochem 2012;56:e31.

105. Shinoda M, Honda T, Ozaki N, et al. Nerve terminals extend into the temporomandibular joint of adjuvant arthritic rats. Eur J Pain 2003;7:493–505.

106. Takeuchi Y, Zeredo JL, Fujiyama R, Amagasa T, Toda K. Effects of experimentally induced inflammation on temporomandibular joint nociceptors in rats. Neurosci Lett 2004;354:172–174.

107. Takeda M, Tanimoto T, Ikeda M, et al. Temporomandibular joint inflammation potentiates the excitability of trigeminal root ganglion neurons innervating the facial skin in rats. J Neurophysiol 2005;93:2723–2738.

108. Sessle BJ, Hu JW. Mechanisms of pain arising from articular tissues. Can J Physiol Pharmacol 1991;69:617–626.

109. Lam DK, Sessle BJ, Cairns BE, Hu JW. Neural mechanisms of temporomandibular joint and masticatory muscle pain: A possible role for peripheral glutamate receptor mechanisms. Pain Res Manag 2005;10:145–152.

110. Iwata K, Tashiro A, Tsuboi Y, et al. Medullary dorsal horn neuronal activity in rats with persistent temporomandibular joint and perioral inflammation. J Neurophysiol 1999;82:1244–1253.

111. Broton JG, Hu JW, Sessle BJ. Effects of temporomandibular joint stimulation on nociceptive and nonnociceptive neurons of the cat's trigeminal subnucleus caudalis (medullary dorsal horn). J Neurophysiol 1988;59:1575–1589.

112. Rodrigues LL, Oliveira MC, Pelegrini-da-Silva A, de Arruda Veiga MC, Parada CA, Tambeli CH. Peripheral sympathetic component of the temporomandibular joint inflammatory pain in rats. J Pain 2006;7:929–936.

113. Gynther GW, Dijkgraaf LC, Reinholt FP, Holmlund AB, Liem RS, de Bont LG. Synovial inflammation in arthroscopically obtained biopsy specimens from the temporomandibular joint: A review of the literature and a proposed histologic grading system. J Oral Maxillofac Surg 1998;56:1281–1286.

114. Gynther GW, Holmlund AB, Reinholt FP. Synovitis in internal derangement of the temporomandibular joint: Correlation between arthroscopic and histologic findings. J Oral Maxillofac Surg 1994;52:913–917.

115. Murakami K, Segami N, Fujimura K, Iizuka T. Correlation between pain and synovitis in patients with internal derangement of the temporomandibular joint. J Oral Maxillofac Surg 1991;49:1159–1161.

116. Eliav E, Teich S, Nitzan D, et al. Facial arthralgia and myalgia: Can they be differentiated by trigeminal sensory assessment? Pain 2003;104:481–490.

117. Yoshida H, Fujita S, Nishida M, Iizuka T. The expression of substance P in human temporomandibular joint samples: An immunohistochemical study. J Oral Rehabil 1999;26:338–344.

118. Martel-Pelletier J, Lajeunesse D, Fahmi H, Tardif G, Pelletier JP. New thoughts on the pathophysiology of osteoarthritis: One more step toward new therapeutic targets. Curr Rheumatol Rep 2006;8:30–36.

119. Alexander CJ. Idiopathic osteoarthritis: Time to change paradigms? Skeletal Radiol 2004;33:321–324.

120. Stegenga B, de Bont LG, Boering G, van Willigen JD. Tissue responses to degenerative changes in the temporomandibular joint: A review. J Oral Maxillofac Surg 1991;49:1079–1088.

121. Commisso MS, Martínez-Reina J, Mayo J. A study of the temporomandibular joint during bruxism. Int J Oral Sci 2014;6:116–123.

122. Wang YL, Zhang J, Zhang M, et al. Cartilage degradation in temporomandibular joint induced by unilateral anterior crossbite prosthesis. Oral Dis 2014;20:301–306.

123. Ishizuka Y, Shibukawa Y, Nagayama M, et al. TMJ degeneration in SAMP8 mice is accompanied by deranged Ihh signaling. J Dent Res 2014;93:281–287.

124. Zardeneta G, Milam SB, Schmitz JP. Iron-dependent generation of free radicals: Plausible mechanisms in the progressive deterioration of the temporomandibular joint. J Oral Maxillofac Surg 2000;58:302–308.

125. Fukuoka Y, Hagihara M, Nagatsu T, Kaneda T. The relationship between collagen metabolism and temporomandibular joint osteoarthrosis in mice. J Oral Maxillofac Surg 1993;51:288–291.

126. Green DM, Noble PC, Ahuero JS, Birdsall HH. Cellular events leading to chondrocyte death after cartilage impact injury. Arthritis Rheum 2006;54:1509–1517.

127. Kawai Y, Kubota E, Okabe E. Reactive oxygen species participation in experimentally induced arthritis of the temporomandibular joint in rats. J Dent Res 2000;79:1489–1495.

128. Blake DR, Merry P, Unsworth J, et al. Hypoxic-reperfusion injury in the inflamed human joint. Lancet 1989;1(8633):289–293.

129. Merry P, Williams R, Cox N, King JB, Blake DR. Comparative study of intra-articular pressure dynamics in joints with acute traumatic and chronic inflammatory effusions: Potential implications for hypoxic-reperfusion injury. Ann Rheum Dis 1991;50:917–920.

130. Sheets DW Jr, Okamoto T, Dijkgraaf LC, Milam SB, Schmitz JP, Zardeneta G. Free radical damage in facsimile synovium: Correlation with adhesion formation in osteoarthritic TMJs. J Prosthodont 2006;15:9–19.

131. Milam SB, Zardeneta G, Schmitz JP. Oxidative stress and degenerative temporomandibular joint disease: A proposed hypothesis. J Oral Maxillofac Surg 1998;56:214–223.

132. Dijkgraaf LC, Zardeneta G, Cordewener FW, et al. Crosslinking of fibrinogen and fibronectin by free radicals: A possible initial step in adhesion formation in osteoarthritis of the temporomandibular joint. J Oral Maxillofac Surg 2003;61:101–111.

133. Dan P, Nitzan DW, Dagan A, Ginsburg I, Yedgar S. H2O2 renders cells accessible to lysis by exogenous phospholipase A2: A novel mechanism for cell damage in inflammatory processes. FEBS Lett 1996;383:75–78.

134. Kanyama M, Kuboki T, Kojima S, et al. Matrix metalloproteinases and tissue inhibitors of metalloproteinases in synovial fluids of patients with temporomandibular joint osteoarthritis. J Orofac Pain 2000;14:20–30.

135. Shinoda C, Takaku S. Interleukin-1 beta, interleukin-6, and tissue inhibitor of metalloproteinase-1 in the synovial fluid of the temporomandibular joint with respect to cartilage destruction. Oral Dis 2000;6:383–390.

136. Appelgren A, Appelgren B, Kopp S, Lundeberg T, Theodorsson E. Neuropeptides in the arthritic TMJ and symptoms and signs from the stomatognathic system with special consideration to rheumatoid arthritis. J Orofac Pain 1995;9:215–225.

137. Appelgren A, Appelgren B, Kopp S, Lundeberg T, Theodorsson E. Substance P-associated increase of intra-articular temperature and pain threshold in the arthritic TMJ. J Orofac Pain 1998;12:101–107.

138. Holmlund A, Ekblom A, Hansson P, Lind J, Lundeberg T, Theodorsson E. Concentrations of neuropeptides substance P, neurokinin A, calcitonin gene-related peptide, neuropeptide Y and vasoactive intestinal polypeptide in synovial fluid of the human temporomandibular joint. A correlation with symptoms, signs and arthroscopic findings. Int J Oral Maxillofac Surg 1991;20:228–231.

139. Kopp S. Neuroendocrine, immune, and local responses related to temporomandibular disorders. J Orofac Pain 2001;15:9–28.

140. Sato J, Segami N, Kaneyama K, Yoshimura H, Fujimura K, Yoshitake Y. Relationship of calcitonin gene-related peptide in synovial tissues and temporomandibular joint pain in humans. Oral Surg Oral Med Oral Pathol Oral Radiol Endod 2004;98:533–540.

141. Henry CH, Wolford LM. Substance P and mast cells: Preliminary histologic analysis of the human temporomandibular joint. Oral Surg Oral Med Oral Pathol Oral Radiol Endod 2001;92:384–389.

142. Alstergren P, Appelgren A, Appelgren B, Kopp S, Lundeberg T, Theodorsson E. Co-variation of neuropeptide Y, calcitonin gene-related peptide, substance P and neurokinin A in joint fluid from patients with temporomandibular joint arthritis. Arch Oral Biol 1995;40:127–135.

143. van der Kraan PM, van den Berg WB. Anabolic and destructive mediators in osteoarthritis. Curr Opin Clin Nutr Metab Care 2000;3:205–211.

144. Pufe T, Harde V, Petersen W, Goldring MB, Tillmann B, Mentlein R. Vascular endothelial growth factor (VEGF) induces matrix metalloproteinase expression in immortalized chondrocytes. J Pathol 2004;202:367–374.

145. Levine JD, Khasar SG, Green PG. Neurogenic inflammation and arthritis. Ann NY Acad Sci 2006;1069:155–167.

146. Tanaka E, Aoyama J, Miyauchi M, et al. Vascular endothelial growth factor plays an important autocrine/paracrine role in the progression of osteoarthritis. Histochem Cell Biol 2005;123:275–281.

147. Shirakura M, Tanimoto K, Eguchi H, et al. Activation of the hypoxia-inducible factor-1 in overloaded temporomandibular joint, and induction of osteoclastogenesis. Biochem Biophys Res Commun 2010;393:800–805.

148. Murata M, Yudoh K, Nakamura H, et al. Distinct signaling pathways are involved in hypoxia- and IL-1-induced VEGF expression in human articular chondrocytes. J Orthop Res 2006;24:1544–1554.

149. Pufe T, Lemke A, Kurz B, et al. Mechanical overload induces VEGF in cartilage discs via hypoxia-inducible factor. Am J Pathol 2004;164:185–192.

150. Ludin A, Sela JJ, Schroeder A, Samuni Y, Nitzan DW, Amir G. Injection of vascular endothelial growth factor into knee joints induces osteoarthritis in mice. Osteoarthritis Cartilage 2013;21:491–497.

151. Kumagai K, Hamada Y, Holmlund AB, et al. The levels of vascular endothelial growth factor in the synovial fluid correlated with the severity of arthroscopically observed synovitis and clinical outcome after temporomandibular joint irrigation in patients with chronic closed lock. Oral Surg Oral Med Oral Pathol Oral Radiol Endod 2010;109:185–190.

152. Kristensen KD, Alstergren P, Stoustrup P, Küseler A, Herlin T, Pedersen TK. Cytokines in healthy temporomandibular joint synovial fluid. J Oral Rehabil 2014;41:250–256.

153. Kaneyama K, Segami N, Yoshimura H, Honjo M, Demura N. Increased levels of soluble cytokine receptors in the synovial fluid of temporomandibular joint disorders in relation to joint effusion on magnetic resonance images. J Oral Maxillofac Surg 2010;68:1088–1093.

154. Lee JK, Cho YS, Song SI. Relationship of synovial tumor necrosis factor alpha and interleukin 6 to temporomandibular disorder. J Oral Maxillofac Surg 2010;68:1064–1068.

155. Ogura N, Satoh K, Akutsu M, et al. MCP-1 production in temporomandibular joint inflammation. J Dent Res 2010;89:1117–1122.

156. Ogura N, Tobe M, Sakamaki H, et al. Interleukin-1 beta induces interleukin-6 mRNA expression and protein production in synovial cells from human temporomandibular joint. J Oral Pathol Med 2002;31:353–360.

157. Ogura N, Tobe M, Sakamaki H, Nagura H, Abiko Y, Kondoh T. Tumor necrosis factor-alpha increases chemokine gene expression and production in synovial fibroblasts from human temporomandibular joint. J Oral Pathol Med 2005;34:357–363.

158. Kubota E, Kubota T, Matsumoto J, Shibata T, Murakami KI. Synovial fluid cytokines and proteinases as markers of temporomandibular joint disease. J Oral Maxillofac Surg 1998;56:192–198.

159. Hamada Y, Kondoh T, Holmlund AB, et al. Inflammatory cytokines correlated with clinical outcome of temporomandibular joint irrigation in patients with chronic closed lock. Oral Surg Oral Med Oral Pathol Oral Radiol Endod 2006;102:596–601.

160. Kaneyama K, Segami N, Sato J, Fujimura K, Nagao T, Yoshimura H. Prognostic factors in arthrocentesis of the temporomandibular joint: Comparison of bradykinin, leukotriene B4, prostaglandin E2, and substance P level in synovial fluid between successful and unsuccessful cases. J Oral Maxillofac Surg 2007;65:242–247.

161. Alstergren P, Kopp S. Prostaglandin E2 in temporomandibular joint synovial fluid and its relation to pain and inflammatory disorders. J Oral Maxillofac Surg 2000;58:180–186.

162. Murakami KI, Shibata T, Kubota E, Maeda H. Intraarticular levels of prostaglandin E2, hyaluronic acid, and chondroitin-4 and -6 sulfates in the temporomandibular joint synovial fluid of patients with internal derangement. J Oral Maxillofac Surg 1998;56:199–203.

163. Yoshida K, Takatsuka S, Hatada E, et al. Expression of matrix metalloproteinases and aggrecanase in the synovial fluids of patients with symptomatic temporomandibular disorders. Oral Surg Oral Med Oral Pathol Oral Radiol Endod 2006;102:22–27.

164. Götz W, Dührˍ S, Jäger A. Distribution of components of the insulin-like growth factor system in the temporomandibular joint of the aging mouse. Growth Dev Aging 2005;69:67–79.

165. Matsumoto K, Honda K, Ohshima M, et al. Cytokine profile in synovial fluid from patients with internal derangement of the temporomandibular joint: A preliminary study. Dentomaxillofac Radiol 2006;35:432–441.

166. Almarza AJ, Athanasiou KA. Evaluation of three growth factors in combinations of two for temporomandibular joint disc tissue engineering. Arch Oral Biol 2006;51:215–221.

167. Detamore MS, Athanasiou KA. Evaluation of three growth factors for TMJ disc tissue engineering. Ann Biomed Eng 2005;33:383–390.

168. Israel HA, Diamond BE, Saed-Nejad F, Ratcliffe A. Correlation between arthroscopic diagnosis of osteoarthritis and synovitis of the human temporomandibular joint and keratan sulfate levels in the synovial fluid. J Oral Maxillofac Surg 1997;55:210–217.

169. Ratcliffe A, Israel HA, Saed-Nejad F, Diamond B. Proteoglycans in the synovial fluid of the temporomandibular joint as an indicator of changes in cartilage metabolism during primary and secondary osteoarthritis. J Oral Maxillofac Surg 1998;56:204–208.

170. de Bont LG, Boering G, Liem RS, Eulderink F, Westesson PL. Osteoarthritis and internal derangement of the temporomandibular joint: A light microscopic study. J Oral Maxillofac Surg 1986;44:634–643.

171. Cimmino MA, Parodi M. Risk factors for osteoarthritis. Semin Arthritis Rheum 2005;34(6, suppl):29–34.

172. Lopez HL. Nutritional interventions to prevent and treat osteoarthritis. Part II: Focus on micronutrients and supportive nutraceuticals. PM R 2012;4(5, suppl):S155–S168.

173. Lopez HL. Nutritional interventions to prevent and treat osteoarthritis. Part I: Focus on fatty acids and macronutrients. PM R 2012;4(5, suppl):S145–S154.

174. Goldberg RJ, Katz J. A meta-analysis of the analgesic effects of omega-3 polyunsaturated fatty acid supplementation for inflammatory joint pain. Pain 2007;129:210–223.

175. McAlindon TE. Nutraceuticals: Do they work and when should we use them? Best Pract Res Clin Rheumatol 2006;20:99–115.

176. Reginster JY, Neuprez A, Lecart MP, Sarlet N, Bruyere O. Role of glucosamine in the treatment for osteoarthritis. Rheumatol Int 2012;32:2959–2967.

177. Haghighat A, Behnia A, Kaviani N, Khorami B. Evaluation of glucosamine sulfate and Ibuprofen effects in patients with temporomandibular joint osteoarthritis symptom. J Res Pharm Pract 2013;2:34–39.

178. Nguyen P, Mohamed SE, Gardiner D, Salinas T. A randomized double-blind clinical trial of the effect of chondroitin sulfate and glucosamine hydrochloride on temporomandibular joint disorders: A pilot study. Cranio 2001;19:130–139.

179. Shankland WE 2nd. The effects of glucosamine and chondroitin sulfate on osteoarthritis of the TMJ: A preliminary report of 50 patients. Cranio 1998;16:230–235.

180. Su N, Yang X, Liu Y, Huang Y, Shi Z. Evaluation of arthrocentesis with hyaluronic acid injection plus oral glucosamine hydrochloride for temporomandibular joint osteoarthritis in oral-health-related quality of life. J Craniomaxillofac Surg 2014;42:846–851.

181. Thie NM, Prasad NG, Major PW. Evaluation of glucosamine sulfate compared to ibuprofen for the treatment of temporomandibular joint osteoarthritis: A randomized double blind controlled 3 month clinical trial. J Rheumatol 2001;28:1347–1355.

182. Cahlin BJ, Dahlström L. No effect of glucosamine sulfate on osteoarthritis in the temporomandibular joints—A randomized, controlled, short-term study. Oral Surg Oral Med Oral Pathol Oral Radiol Endod 2011;112:760–766.

183. Smith SB, Mir E, Bair E, et al. Genetic variants associated with development of TMD and its intermediate phenotypes: The genetic architecture of TMD in the OPPERA prospective cohort study. J Pain 2013;14(suppl 12):T91–T101.

184. Maixner W, Diatchenko L, Dubner R, et al. Orofacial pain prospective evaluation and risk assessment study—The OPPERA study. J Pain 2011;12(suppl 11):T4–T11.

185. Diatchenko L, Slade GD, Nackley AG, et al. Genetic basis for individual variations in pain perception and the development of a chronic pain condition. Hum Mol Genet 2005;14:135–143.

186. Diatchenko L, Anderson AD, Slade GD, et al. Three major haplotypes of the beta2 adrenergic receptor define psychological profile, blood pressure, and the risk for development of a common musculoskeletal pain disorder. Am J Med Genet B Neuropsychiatr Genet 2006;141B:449–462.

187. Mutlu N, Erdal ME, Herken H, Oz G, Bayazit YA. T102C polymorphism of the 5-HT2A receptor gene may be associated with temporomandibular dysfunction. Oral Dis 2004;10:349–352.

188. Huang B, Takahashi K, Sakata T, et al. Increased risk of temporomandibular joint closed lock: A case-control study of ANKH polymorphisms. PLoS One 2011;6:e25503.

189. Kang SC, Lee DG, Choi JH, Kim ST, Kim YK, Ahn HJ. Association between estrogen receptor polymorphism and pain susceptibility in female temporomandibular joint osteoarthritis patients. Int J Oral Maxillofac Surg 2007;36:391–394.

190. Kim BS, Kim YK, Yun PY, Lee E, Bae J. The effects of estrogen receptor alpha polymorphism on the prevalence of symptomatic temporomandibular disorders. J Oral Maxillofac Surg 2010;68:2975–2979.

191. Planello AC, Campos MI, Meloto CB, et al. Association of matrix metalloproteinase gene polymorphism with temporomandibular joint degeneration. Eur J Oral Sci 2011;119:1–6.

192. Yamaguchi T, Nakaoka H, Yamamoto K, et al. Genome-wide association study of degenerative bony changes of the temporomandibular joint. Oral Dis 2014;20:409–415.

193. Yap AU, Dworkin SF, Chua EK, List T, Tan KB, Tan HH. Prevalence of temporomandibular disorder subtypes, psychologic distress, and psychosocial dysfunction in Asian patients. J Orofac Pain 2003;17:21–28.

194. De Kanter RJ, Truin GJ, Burgersdijk RC, et al. Prevalence in the Dutch adult population and a meta-analysis of signs and symptoms of temporomandibular disorder. J Dent Res 1993;72:1509–1518.

195. Agerberg G, Inkapööl I. Craniomandibular disorders in an urban Swedish population. J Craniomandib Disord 1990;4:154–164.

196. Schmid-Schwap M, Bristela M, Kundi M, Piehslinger E. Sex-specific differences in patients with temporomandibular disorders. J Orofac Pain 2013;27:42–50.

197. Puri V, Cui L, Liverman CS, et al. Ovarian steroids regulate neuropeptides in the trigeminal ganglion. Neuropeptides 2005;39:409–417.

198. Cairns BE, Sessle BJ, Hu JW. Characteristics of glutamate-evoked temporomandibular joint afferent activity in the rat. J Neurophysiol 2001;85:2446–2454.

199. Flake NM, Hermanstyne TO, Gold MS. Testosterone and estrogen have opposing actions on inflammation-induced plasma extravasation in the rat temporomandibular joint. Am J Physiol Regul Integr Comp Physiol 2006;291:R343–R348.

200. Flake NM, Bonebreak DB, Gold MS. Estrogen and inflammation increase the excitability of rat temporomandibular joint afferent neurons. J Neurophysiol 2005;93:1585–1597.

201. Bereiter DA, Shen S, Benetti AP. Sex differences in amino acid release from rostral trigeminal subnucleus caudalis after acute injury to the TMJ region. Pain 2002;98:89–99.

202. Okamoto K, Hirata H, Takeshita S, Bereiter DA. Response properties of TMJ units in superficial laminae at the spinomedullary junction of female rats vary over the estrous cycle. J Neurophysiol 2003;89:1467–1477.

203. Abubaker AO, Hebda PC, Gunsolley JN. Effects of sex hormones on protein and collagen content of the temporomandibular joint disc of the rat. J Oral Maxillofac Surg 1996;54:721–727.

204. Abubaker AO, Raslan WF, Sotereanos GC. Estrogen and progesterone receptors in temporomandibular joint discs of symptomatic and asymptomatic persons: A preliminary study. J Oral Maxillofac Surg 1993;51:1096–1100.

205. Mogil JS. Sex differences in pain and pain inhibition: Multiple explanations of a controversial phenomenon. Nat Rev Neurosci 2012;13:859–866.

206. Peck CC, Goulet JP, Lobbezoo F, et al. Expanding the taxonomy of the Diagnostic Criteria for Temporomandibular Disorders. J Oral Rehabil 2014;41:2–23.

207. Keeling SD, McGorray S, Wheeler TT, King GJ. Risk factors associated with temporomandibular joint sounds in children 6 to 12 years of age. Am J Orthod Dentofacial Orthop 1994;105:279–287.

208. Locker D, Slade G. Prevalence of symptoms associated with temporomandibular disorders in a Canadian population. Community Dent Oral Epidemiol 1988;16:310–313.

209. Hardison JD, Okeson JP. Comparison of three clinical techniques for evaluating joint sounds. Cranio 1990;8:307–311.

210. Randolph CS, Greene CS, Moretti R, Forbes D, Perry HT. Conservative management of temporomandibular disorders: A posttreatment comparison between patients from a university clinic and from private practice. Am J Orthod Dentofacial Orthop 1990;98:77–82.

211. Magnusson T, Egermark I, Carlsson GE. A longitudinal epidemiologic study of signs and symptoms of temporomandibular disorders from 15 to 35 years of age. J Orofac Pain 2000;14:310–319.

212. Lobbezoo F, Drangsholt M, Peck C, Sato H, Kopp S, Svensson P. Topical review: New insights into the pathology and diagnosis of disorders of the temporomandibular joint. J Orofac Pain 2004;18:181–191.

213. Prinz JF. Correlation of the characteristics of temporomandibular joint and tooth contact sounds. J Oral Rehabil 1998;25:194–198.

214. Huddleston Slater JJ, Lobbezoo F, Hofman N, Naeije M. Case report of a posterior disc displacement without and with reduction. J Orofac Pain 2005;19:337–342.

215. Westesson PL, Kurita K, Eriksson L, Katzberg RW. Cryosectional observations of functional anatomy of the temporomandibular joint. Oral Surg Oral Med Oral Pathol 1989;68:247–251.

216. Dworkin SF, LeResche L. Research diagnostic criteria for temporomandibular disorders: Review, criteria, examinations and specifications, critique. J Craniomandib Disord 1992;6:301–355.

217. Conti PC, dos Santos CN, Kogawa EM, de Castro Ferreira Conti AC, de Araujo Cdos R. The treatment of painful temporomandibular joint clicking with oral splints: A randomized clinical trial. J Am Dent Assoc 2006;137:1108–1114.

218. Eriksson PO, Eriksson A, Ringqvist M, Thornell LE. Special histochemical muscle-fibre characteristics of the human lateral pterygoid muscle. Arch Oral Biol 1981;26:495–507.

219. Mao J, Stein RB, Osborn JW. The size and distribution of fiber types in jaw muscles: A review. J Craniomandib Disord 1992;6:192–201.

220. Westling L. Temporomandibular joint dysfunction and systemic joint laxity. Swed Dent J Suppl 1992;81:1–79.

221. Isacsson G, Linde C, Isberg A. Subjective symptoms in patients with temporomandibular joint disk displacement versus patients with myogenic craniomandibular disorders. J Prosthet Dent 1989;61:70–77.

222. Tasaki MM, Westesson PL, Isberg AM, Ren YF, Tallents RH. Classification and prevalence of temporomandibular joint disk displacement in patients and symptom-free volunteers. Am J Orthod Dentofacial Orthop 1996;109:249–262.

223. Ogus H. Common Disorders of the Temporomandibular Joint. Bristol: Wright, 1981.

224. Ogus H. The mandibular joint: Internal rearrangement. Br J Oral Maxillofac Surg 1987;25:218–226.

225. Nitzan DW. The process of lubrication impairment and its involvement in temporomandibular joint disc displacement: A theoretical concept. J Oral Maxillofac Surg 2001;59:36–45.

226. Nitzan DW. 'Friction and adhesive forces'—Possible underlying causes for temporomandibular joint internal derangement. Cells Tissues Organs 2003;174:6–16.

227. Tanaka E, Kawai N, Tanaka M, et al. The frictional coefficient of the temporomandibular joint and its dependency on the magnitude and duration of joint loading. J Dent Res 2004;83:404–407.

228. Cai HX, Luo JM, Long X, Li XD, Cheng Y. Free-radical oxidation and superoxide dismutase activity in synovial fluid of patients with temporomandibular disorders. J Orofac Pain 2006;20:53–58.

229. Takahashi T, Kondoh T, Kamei K, et al. Elevated levels of nitric oxide in synovial fluid from patients with temporomandibular disorders. Oral Surg Oral Med Oral Pathol Oral Radiol Endod 1996;82:505–509.

230. Nitzan DW, Goldfarb A, Gati I, Kohen R. Changes in the reducing power of synovial fluid from temporomandibular joints with "anchored disc phenomenon". J Oral Maxillofac Surg 2002;60:735–740.

231. Benito C, Casares G, Benito C. TMJ static disk: Correlation between clinical findings and pseudodynamic magnetic resonance images. Cranio 1998;16:242–251.

232. Ohnuki T, Fukuda M, Nakata A, et al. Evaluation of the position, mobility, and morphology of the disc by MRI before and after four different treatments for temporomandibular joint disorders. Dentomaxillofac Radiol 2006;35:103–109.

233. Takatsuka S, Yoshida K, Ueki K, Marukawa K, Nakagawa K, Yamamoto E. Disc and condyle translation in patients with temporomandibular disorder. Oral Surg Oral Med Oral Pathol Oral Radiol Endod 2005;99:614–621.

234. Prinz JF. Resonant characteristics of the human head in relation to temporomandibular joint sounds. J Oral Rehabil 1998;25:954–960.

235. Johansson AS, Isberg A. The anterosuperior insertion of the temporomandibular joint capsule and condylar mobility in joints with and without internal derangement: A double-contrast arthrotomographic investigation. J Oral Maxillofac Surg 1991;49:1142–1148.

236. Griffin CJ. The prevalence of the lateral subcondylar tubercle of the mandible in fossil and recent man with particular reference to Anglo-Saxons. Arch Oral Biol 1977;22:633–639.

237. Pereira FJ Jr, Lundh H, Westesson PL, Carlsson LE. Clinical findings related to morphologic changes in TMJ autopsy specimens. Oral Surg Oral Med Oral Pathol 1994;78:288–295.

238. Bewyer DC. Biomechanical and physiologic processes leading to internal derangement with adhesion. J Craniomandib Disord 1989;3:44–49.

239. Sato S, Goto S, Nasu F, Motegi K. Natural course of disc displacement with reduction of the temporomandibular joint: Changes in clinical signs and symptoms. J Oral Maxillofac Surg 2003;61:32–34.

240. Manfredini D, Favero L, Gregorini G, Cocilovo F, Guarda-Nardini L. Natural course of temporomandibular disorders with low pain-related impairment: A 2-to-3-year follow-up study. J Oral Rehabil 2013;40:436–442.

241. Dolwick MF. Temporomandibular joint surgery for internal derangement. Dent Clin North Am 2007;51:195–208.

242. González-García R, Rodríguez-Campo FJ, Escorial-Hernández V, et al. Complications of temporomandibular joint arthroscopy: A retrospective analytic study of 670 arthroscopic procedures. J Oral Maxillofac Surg 2006;64:1587–1591.

243. Hall HD, Indresano AT, Kirk WS, Dietrich MS. Prospective multicenter comparison of 4 temporomandibular joint operations. J Oral Maxillofac Surg 2005;63:1174–1179.

244. Smolka W, Iizuka T. Arthroscopic lysis and lavage in different stages of internal derangement of the temporomandibular joint: Correlation of preoperative staging to arthroscopic findings and treatment outcome. J Oral Maxillofac Surg 2005;63:471–478.

245. Undt G, Murakami K, Rasse M, Ewers R. Open versus arthroscopic surgery for internal derangement of the temporomandibular joint: A retrospective study comparing two centres' results using the Jaw Pain and Function Questionnaire. J Craniomaxillofac Surg 2006;34:234–241.

246. Dolwick MF. Intra-articular disc displacement. Part I: Its questionable role in temporomandibular joint pathology. J Oral Maxillofac Surg 1995;53:1069–1072.

247. Emshoff R, Puffer P, Strobl H, Gassner R. Effect of temporomandibular joint arthrocentesis on synovial fluid mediator level of tumor necrosis factor-alpha: Implications for treatment outcome. Int J Oral Maxillofac Surg 2000;29:176–182.

248. Emshoff R, Rudisch A, Bösch R, Gassner R. Effect of arthrocentesis and hydraulic distension on the temporomandibular joint disk position. Oral Surg Oral Med Oral Pathol Oral Radiol Endod 2000;89:271–277.

249. Reston JT, Turkelson CM. Meta-analysis of surgical treatments for temporomandibular articular disorders. J Oral Maxillofac Surg 2003;61:3–10.

250. Carvajal WA, Laskin DM. Long-term evaluation of arthrocentesis for the treatment of internal derangements of the temporomandibular joint. J Oral Maxillofac Surg 2000;58:852–855.

251. Han Z, Ha Q, Yang C. Arthrocentesis and lavage of TMJ for the treatment of anterior disc displacement without reduction [in Chinese]. Zhonghua Kou Qiang Yi Xue Za Zhi 1999;34:269–271.

252. McCain JP, Sanders B, Koslin MG, Quinn JH, Peters PB, Indresano AT. Temporomandibular joint arthroscopy: A 6-year multicenter retrospective study of 4,831 joints. J Oral Maxillofac Surg 1992;50:926–930.

253. Emshoff R, Rudisch A, Bösch R, Strobl H. Prognostic indicators of the outcome of arthrocentesis: A short-term follow-up study. Oral Surg Oral Med Oral Pathol Oral Radiol Endod 2003;96:1218.

254. Alpaslan GH, Alpaslan C. Efficacy of temporomandibular joint arthrocentesis with and without injection of sodium hyaluronate in treatment of internal derangements. J Oral Maxillofac Surg 2001;59:613–618.

255. Goudot P, Jaquinet AR, Hugonnet S, Haefliger W, Richter M. Improvement of pain and function after arthroscopy and arthrocentesis of the temporomandibular joint: A comparative study. J Craniomaxillofac Surg 2000;28:39–43.

256. Okeson JP. Orofacial Pain: Guidelines for Assessment, Classification, and Management. Chicago: Quintessence, 1996.

257. Peroz I, Tai S. Masticatory performance in patients with anterior disk displacement without reduction in comparison with symptom-free volunteers. Eur J Oral Sci 2002;110:341–344.

258. Choi BH, Yoo JH, Lee WY. Comparison of magnetic resonance imaging before and after nonsurgical treatment of closed lock. Oral Surg Oral Med Oral Pathol 1994;78:301–305.

259. Sato S, Goto S, Kawamura H, Motegi K. The natural course of nonreducing disc displacement of the TMJ: Relationship of clinical findings at initial visit to outcome after 12 months without treatment. J Orofac Pain 1997;11:315–320.

260. Sato S, Sakamoto M, Kawamura H, Motegi K. Long-term changes in clinical signs and symptoms and disc position and morphology in patients with nonreducing disc displacement in the temporomandibular joint. J Oral Maxillofac Surg 1999;57:23–29.

261. de Leeuw R, Boering G, Stegenga B, de Bont LG. Clinical signs of TMJ osteoarthrosis and internal derangement 30 years after nonsurgical treatment. J Orofac Pain 1994;8:18–24.

262. Rasmussen OC. Description of population and progress of symptoms in a longitudinal study of temporomandibular arthropathy. J Dent Res 1981;89:196–203.

263. Pereira FJ Jr, Lundh H, Westesson PL. Morphologic changes in the temporomandibular joint in different age groups. An autopsy investigation. Oral Surg Oral Med Oral Pathol 1994;78:279–287.

264. Luder HU. Factors affecting degeneration in human temporomandibular joints as assessed histologically. Eur J Oral Sci 2002;110:106–113.

265. Luder HU, Bobst P, Schroeder HE. Histometric study of synovial cavity dimensions of human temporomandibular joints with normal and anterior disc position. J Orofac Pain 1993;7:263–274.

266. Kurita K, Westesson PL, Yuasa H, Toyama M, Machida J, Ogi N. Natural course of untreated symptomatic temporomandibular joint disc displacement without reduction. J Dent Res 1998;77:361–365.

267. Lundh H, Westesson PL, Eriksson L, Brooks SL. Temporomandibular joint disk displacement without reduction. Treatment with flat occlusal splint versus no treatment. Oral Surg Oral Med Oral Pathol 1992;73:655–658.

268. Isberg A, Isacsson G. Tissue reactions associated with internal derangement of the temporomandibular joint. A radiographic, cryomorphologic, and histologic study. Acta Odontol Scand 1986;44:160–164.

269. Kurita K, Westesson PL, Sternby NH, et al. Histologic features of the temporomandibular joint disk and posterior disk attachment: Comparison of symptom-free persons with normally positioned disks and patients with internal derangement. Oral Surg Oral Med Oral Pathol 1989;67:635–643.

270. Pereira FJ, Lundh H, Eriksson L, Westesson PL. Microscopic changes in the retrodiscal tissues of painful temporomandibular joints. J Oral Maxillofac Surg 1996;54:461–468.

271. Scapino RP. The posterior attachment: Its structure, function, and appearance in TMJ imaging studies. Part 1. J Craniomandib Disord 1991;5:83–95.

272. Sanromán JF. Closed lock (MRI fixed disc): A comparison of arthrocentesis and arthroscopy. Int J Oral Maxillofac Surg 2004;33:344–348.

273. Rao VM, Farole A, Karasick D. Temporomandibular joint dysfunction: Correlation of MR imaging, arthrography, and arthroscopy. Radiology 1990;174:663–667.

274. Xu Y, Zhang ZG, Zheng YH. Measurement and analysis of the intra-articular pressure in temporomandibular joint with sudden-onset, severe closed lock [in Chinese]. Hua Xi Kou Qiang Yi Xue Za Zhi 2005;23:41–42.

275. Nitzan DW, Etsion I. Adhesive force: The underlying cause of the disc anchorage to the fossa and/or eminence in the temporomandibular joint—A new concept. Int J Oral Maxillofac Surg 2002;31:94–99.

276. Nitzan DW. Temporomandibular joint "open lock" versus condylar dislocation: Signs and symptoms, imaging, treatment, and pathogenesis. J Oral Maxillofac Surg 2002;60:506–511.

277. Shorey CW, Campbell JH. Dislocation of the temporomandibular joint. Oral Surg Oral Med Oral Pathol Oral Radiol Endod 2000;89:662–668.

278. Güven O. Inappropriate treatments in temporomandibular joint chronic recurrent dislocation: A literature review presenting three particular cases. J Craniofac Surg 2005;16:449–452.

P. 284

279. Oehler S, Neureiter D, Meyer-Scholten C, Aigner T. Subtyping of osteoarthritic synoviopathy. Clin Exp Rheumatol 2002;20:633–640.

280. Wang XD, Kou XX, Mao JJ, Gan YH, Zhou YH. Sustained inflammation induces degeneration of the temporomandibular joint. J Dent Res 2012;91:499–505.

281. Scanzello CR, McKeon B, Swaim BH, et al. Synovial inflammation in patients undergoing arthroscopic meniscectomy: Molecular characterization and relationship to symptoms. Arthritis Rheum 2011;63:391–400.

282. Walsh DA, Bonnet CS, Turner EL, Wilson D, Situ M, McWilliams DF. Angiogenesis in the synovium and at the osteochondral junction in osteoarthritis. Osteoarthritis Cartilage 2007;15:743–751.

283. Israel HA, Saed-Nejad F, Ratcliffe A. Early diagnosis of osteoarthrosis of the temporomandibular joint: Correlation between arthroscopic diagnosis and keratan sulfate levels in the synovial fluid. J Oral Maxillofac Surg 1991;49:708–711.

284. Agerberg G, Bergenholtz A. Craniomandibular disorders in adult populations of West Bothnia, Sweden. Acta Odontol Scand 1989;47:129–140.

285. Sato H, Osterberg T, Ahlqwist M, Carlsson GE, Gröndahl HG, Rubinstein B. Association between radiographic findings in the mandibular condyle and temporomandibular dysfunction in an elderly population. Acta Odontol Scand 1996;54:384–390.

286. Touré G, Duboucher C, Vacher C. Anatomical modifications of the temporomandibular joint during ageing. Surg Radiol Anat 2005;27:51–55.

287. dos Anjos Pontual ML, Freire JS, Barbosa JM, Frazão MA, dos Anjos Pontual A. Evaluation of bone changes in the temporomandibular joint using cone beam CT. Dentomaxillofac Radiol 2012;41:24–29.

288. Koyama J, Nishiyama H, Hayashi T. Follow-up study of condylar bony changes using helical computed tomography in patients with temporomandibular disorder. Dentomaxillofac Radiol 2007;36:472–477.

289. Cimmino MA, Sarzi-Puttini P, Scarpa R, et al. Clinical presentation of osteoarthritis in general practice: Determinants of pain in Italian patients in the AMICA study. Semin Arthritis Rheum 2005;35(suppl 1):17–23.

290. Zarb GA, Carlsson GE. Temporomandibular disorders: Osteoarthritis. J Orofac Pain 1999;13:295–306.

291. Kopp S. Degenerative and inflammatory diseases of the temporomandibular joint [in German]. Schweiz Monatsschr Zahnmed 1985;95:950–962.

292. Dolwick MF, Aufdemorte TB. Silicone-induced foreign body reaction and lymphadenopathy after temporomandibular joint arthroplasty. Oral Surg Oral Med Oral Pathol 1985;59:449–452.

293. Su N, Liu Y, Yang X, Luo Z, Shi Z. Correlation between bony changes measured with cone beam computed tomography and clinical dysfunction index in patients with temporomandibular joint osteoarthritis. J Craniomaxillofac Surg 2014;42:1402–1407.

294. Brooks SL, Westesson PL, Eriksson L, Hansson LG, Barsotti JB. Prevalence of osseous changes in the temporomandibular joint of asymptomatic persons without internal derangement. Oral Surg Oral Med Oral Pathol 1992;73:118–122.

295. Holmlund A, Hellsing G. Arthroscopy of the temporomandibular joint. A comparative study of arthroscopic and tomographic findings. Int J Oral Maxillofac Surg 1988;17:128–133.

296. Ericson S, Lundberg M. Structural changes in the finger, wrist and temporomandiblar joints. A comparative radiologic study. Acta Odontol Scand 1968;26:111–126.

297. Lee AS, Ellman MB, Yan D, et al. A current review of molecular mechanisms regarding osteoarthritis and pain. Gene 2013;527:440–447.

298. Malemud CJ, Islam N, Haqqi TM. Pathophysiological mechanisms in osteoarthritis lead to novel therapeutic strategies. Cells Tissues Organs 2003;174:34–48.

299. Mow VC, Ateshian GA. Lubrication and wear of diarthrodial joints. In: Mow VC, Hayes WC (eds). Basic Orthopaedic Biomechanics, ed 2. Philadelphia: Lippincott-Raven, 1997:275–315.

300. Amir G, Goldfarb AW, Nyska M, Redlich M, Nyska A, Nitzan DW. 2-Butoxyethanol model of haemolysis and disseminated thrombosis in female rats: A preliminary study of the vascular mechanism of osteoarthritis in the temporomandibular joint. Br J Oral Maxillofac Surg 2011;49:21–25.

301. Jiao K, Zhang M, Niu L, et al. Overexpressed TGF-beta in subchondral bone leads to mandibular condyle degradation. J Dent Res 2014;93:140–147.

302. Dieppe P, Cushnaghan J, Young P, Kirwan J. Prediction of the progression of joint space narrowing in osteoarthritis of the knee by bone scintigraphy. Ann Rheum Dis 1993;52:557–563.

303. Sinigaglia L, Varenna M, Casari S. Bone involvement in osteoarthritis. Semin Arthritis Rheum 2005;34:44–46.

304. Flygare L, Hosoki H, Petersson A, Rohlin M, Akerman S. Bone volume in human temporomandibular autopsy joints with and without erosive changes. Acta Odontol Scand 1997;55:167–172.

305. Li B, Aspden RM. Material properties of bone from the femoral neck and calcar femorale of patients with osteoporosis or osteoarthritis. Osteoporos Int 1997;7:450–456.

306. McDonald Blumer MH. Bone mineral content versus bone density in a population with osteoarthritis: A new twist to the controversy? J Rheumatol 2005;32:1868–1869.

307. Lajeunesse D, Reboul P. Subchondral bone in osteoarthritis: A biologic link with articular cartilage leading to abnormal remodeling. Curr Opin Rheumatol 2003;15:628–633.

308. Mansell JP, Bailey AJ. Abnormal cancellous bone collagen metabolism in osteoarthritis. J Clin Invest 1998;101:1596–1603.

309. Martel-Pelletier J, Pelletier JP. New insights into the major pathophysiological processes responsible for the development of osteoarthritis. Semin Arthritis Rheum 2005;34(6, suppl):6–8.

310. Zhuo Q, Yang W, Chen J, Wang Y. Metabolic syndrome meets osteoarthritis. Nat Rev Rheumatol 2012;8:729–737.

311. Puenpatom RA, Victor TW. Increased prevalence of metabolic syndrome in individuals with osteoarthritis: An analysis of NHANES III data. Postgrad Med 2009;121(6):9–20.

312. Findlay DM. Vascular pathology and osteoarthritis. Rheumatology (Oxford) 2007;46:1763–1768.

313. Kerachian MA, Harvey EJ, Cournoyer D, Chow TY, Nahal A, Séguin C. A rat model of early stage osteonecrosis induced by glucocorticoids. J Orthop Surg Res 2011;6:62.

314. Shibahara M, Nishida K, Asahara H, et al. Increased osteocyte apoptosis during the development of femoral head osteonecrosis in spontaneously hypertensive rats. Acta Med Okayama 2000;54:67–74.

315. Conaghan PG, Vanharanta H, Dieppe PA. Is progressive osteoarthritis an atheromatous vascular disease? Ann Rheum Dis 2005;64:1539–1541.

316. Vuolteenaho K, Koskinen A, Moilanen E. Leptin—A link between obesity and osteoarthritis. Applications for prevention and treatment. Basic Clin Pharmacol Toxicol 2014;114:103–108.

317. Bay-Jensen AC, Slagboom E, Chen-An P, et al. Role of hormones in cartilage and joint metabolism: Understanding an unhealthy metabolic phenotype in osteoarthritis. Menopause 2013;20:578–586.

318. Otero M, Lago R, Gomez R, et al. Towards a proinflammatory and immunomodulatory emerging role of leptin. Rheumatology (Oxford) 2006;45:944–950.

319. Poonpet T, Honsawek S. Adipokines: Biomarkers for osteoarthritis? World J Orthop 2014;5:319–327.

320. Scotece M, Conde J, Lopez V, et al. Leptin in joint and bone diseases: New insights. Curr Med Chem 2013;20:3416–3425.

321. Griffin TM, Fermor B, Huebner JL, et al. Diet-induced obesity differentially regulates behavioral, biomechanical, and molecular risk factors for osteoarthritis in mice. Arthritis Res Ther 2010;12:R130.

322. Fujisawa T, Kuboki T, Kasai T, et al. A repetitive, steady mouth opening induced an osteoarthritis-like lesion in the rabbit temporomandibular joint. J Dent Res 2003;82:731–735.

323. Glineburg RW, Laskin DM, Blaustein DI. The effects of immobilization on the primate temporomandibular joint: A histologic and histochemical study. J Oral Maxillofac Surg 1982;40:3–8.

324. de Souza RF, Lovato da Silva CH, Nasser M, Fedorowicz Z, Al-Muharraqi MA. Interventions for the management of temporomandibular joint osteoarthritis. Cochrane Database Syst Rev 2012;4.

325. Patel DN, Manfredini D. Two commentaries on interventions for the management of temporomandibular joint osteoarthritis. Evid Based Dent 2013;14:5–7.

326. Dimitroulis G. The role of surgery in the management of disorders of the temporomandibular joint: A critical review of the literature. Part 2. Int J Oral Maxillofac Surg 2005;34:231–237.

327. Kurita H, Uehara S, Yokochi M, Nakatsuka A, Kobayashi H, Kurashina K. A long-term follow-up study of radiographically evident degenerative changes in the temporomandibular joint with different conditions of disk displacement. Int J Oral Maxillofac Surg 2006;35:49–54.

328. Kurita H, Kojima Y, Nakatsuka A, Koike T, Kobayashi H, Kurashina K. Relationship between temporomandibular joint (TMJ)-related pain and morphological changes of the TMJ condyle in patients with temporomandibular disorders. Dentomaxillofac Radiol 2004;33:329–333.

329. Martinez Blanco M, Bagán JV, Fons A, Poveda Roda R. Osteoarthrosis of the temporomandibular joint. A clinical and radiological study of 16 patients. Med Oral 2004;9:106–110;110–115.

330. de Leeuw R, Boering G, Stegenga B, de Bont LG. Symptoms of temporomandibular joint osteoarthrosis and internal derangement 30 years after nonsurgical treatment. Cranio 1995;13:81–88.

331. de Leeuw R, Boering G, Stegenga B, de Bont LG. Radiographic signs of temporomandibular joint osteoarthrosis and internal derangement 30 years after nonsurgical treatment. Oral Surg Oral Med Oral Pathol Oral Radiol Endod 1995;79:382–392.

332. de Leeuw R, Boering G, van der Kuijl B, Stegenga B. Hard and soft tissue imaging of the temporomandibular joint 30 years after diagnosis of osteoarthrosis and internal derangement. J Oral Maxillofac Surg 1996;54:1270–1280.

333. Nitzan DW, Price A. The use of arthrocentesis for the treatment of osteoarthritic temporomandibular joints. J Oral Maxillofac Surg 2001;59:1154–1159.

334. Manfredini D, Piccotti F, Ferronato G, Guarda-Nardini L. Age peaks of different RDC/TMD diagnoses in a patient population. J Dent 2010;38:392–399.

335. Pereira D, Peleteiro B, Araújo J, Branco J, Santos RA, Ramos E. The effect of osteoarthritis definition on prevalence and incidence estimates: A systematic review. Osteoarthritis Cartilage 2011;19:1270–1285.

336. Uchiyama Y, Murakami S, Furukawa S. Temporomandibular joints in patients with rheumatoid arthritis using magnetic resonance imaging. Clin Rheumatol 2013;32:1613–1618.

337. Celiker R, Gökçe-Kutsal Y, Eryilmaz M. Temporomandibular joint involvement in rheumatoid arthritis. Relationship with disease activity. Scand J Rheumatol 1995;24:22–25.

338. Tegelberg A, Kopp S. Subjective symptoms from the stomatognathic system in individuals with rheumatoid arthritis and osteoarthrosis. Swed Dent J 1987;11:11–22.

339. Tegelberg A, Kopp S. A 3-year follow-up of temporomandibular disorders in rheumatoid arthritis and ankylosing spondylitis. Acta Odontol Scand 1996;54:14–18.

340. Yoshida A, Higuchi Y, Kondo M, Tabata O, Ohishi M. Range of motion of the temporomandibular joint in rheumatoid arthritis: Relationship to the severity of disease. Cranio 1998;16:162–167.

341. Helenius LM, Hallikainen D, Helenius I, et al. Clinical and radiographic findings of the temporomandibular joint in patients with various rheumatic diseases. A case-control study. Oral Surg Oral Med Oral Pathol Oral Radiol Endod 2005;99:455–463.

342. Helenius LM, Tervahartiala P, Helenius I, et al. Clinical, radiographic and MRI findings of the temporomandibular joint in patients with different rheumatic diseases. Int J Oral Maxillofac Surg 2006;35:983–989.

343. Voog U, Alstergren P, Eliasson S, Leibur E, Kallikorm R, Kopp S. Inflammatory mediators and radiographic changes in temporomandibular joints of patients with rheumatoid arthritis. Acta Odontol Scand 2003;61:57–64.

344. Bouwman JP, Kerstens HC, Tuinzing DB. Condylar resorption in orthognathic surgery. The role of inter-maxillary fixation. Oral Surg Oral Med Oral Pathol 1994;78:138–141.

345. Kerstens HC, Tuinzing DB, Golding RP, van der Kwast WA. Condylar atrophy and osteoarthrosis after bimaxillary surgery. Oral Surg Oral Med Oral Pathol 1990;69:274–280.

346. Arnett GW, Milam SB, Gottesman L. Progressive mandibular retrusion-idiopathic condylar resorption. Part II. Am J Orthod Dentofacial Orthop 1996;110:117–127.

347. Arnett GW, Milam SB, Gottesman L. Progressive mandibular retrusion—Idiopathic condylar resorption. Part I. Am J Orthod Dentofacial Orthop 1996;110:8–15.

348. Wolford LM, Cardenas L. Idiopathic condylar resorption: Diagnosis, treatment protocol, and outcomes. Am J Orthod Dentofacial Orthop 1999;116:667–677.

349. Gunson MJ, Arnett GW, Milam SB. Pathophysiology and pharmacologic control of osseous mandibular condylar resorption. J Oral Maxillofac Surg 2012;70:1918–1934.

350. Arnett GW, Gunson MJ. Risk factors in the initiation of condylar resorption. Semin Orthod 2013;19:81–88.

351. Tanaka E, Detamore MS, Mercuri LG. Degenerative disorders of the temporomandibular joint: Etiology, diagnosis, and treatment. J Dent Res 2008;87:296–307.

352. Milam SB. Pathogenesis of degenerative temporomandibular joint arthritides. Odontology 2005;93:7–15.

353. Mercuri LG. Osteoarthritis, osteoarthrosis, and idiopathic condylar resorption. Oral Maxillofac Surg Clin North Am 2008;20:169–183.

354. Yang C, Cai XY, Chen MJ, Zhang SY. New arthroscopic disc repositioning and suturing technique for treating an anteriorly displaced disc of the temporomandibular joint: Part I—Technique introduction. Int J Oral Maxillofac Surg 2012;41:1058–1063.

355. Wolford LM. Idiopathic condylar resorption of the temporomandibular joint in teenage girls (cheerleaders syndrome). Proc (Bayl Univ Med Cent) 2001;14:246–252.

356. Huang YL, Pogrel MA, Kaban LB. Diagnosis and management of condylar resorption. J Oral Maxillofac Surg 1997;55:114–119.

357. Mercuri LG. A rationale for total alloplastic temporomandibular joint reconstruction in the management of idiopathic/progressive condylar resorption. J Oral Maxillofac Surg 2007;65:1600–1609.

358. Allias-Montmayeur F, Durroux R, Dodart L, Combelles R. Tumours and pseudotumorous lesions of the temporomandibular joint: A diagnostic challenge. J Laryngol Otol 1997;111:776–781.

359. Nwoku AL, Koch H. The temporomandibular joint: A rare localisation for bone tumours. J Maxillofac Surg 1974;2:113–119.

360. Bavitz JB, Chewning LC. Malignant disease as temporomandibular joint dysfunction: Review of the literature and report of case. J Am Dent Assoc 1990;120:163–166.

361. Warner BF, Luna MA, Robert Newland T. Temporomandibular joint neoplasms and pseudotumors. Adv Anat Pathol 2000;7:365–381.

362. Greene CS, Laskin DM. Long-term status of TMJ clicking in patients with myofascial pain and dysfunction. J Am Dent Assoc 1988;117:461–465.

363. Temporomandibular Disorders (TMD). Alexandria: American Association for Dental Research, 2010.

364. Jagger RG. Mandibular manipulation of anterior disc displacement without reduction. J Oral Rehabil 1991;18:497–500.

365. Nicolakis P, Erdogmus B, Kopf A, et al. Effectiveness of exercise therapy in patients with internal derangement of the temporomandibular joint. J Oral Rehabil 2001;28:1158–1164.

366. Ekberg E. Treatment of temporomandibular disorders of arthrogeneous origin. Controlled double-blind studies of a nonsteroidal anti-inflammatory drug and a stabilisation appliance. Swed Dent J Suppl 1998;131:1–57.

367. Ekberg E, Nilner M. A 6- and 12-month follow-up of appliance therapy in TMD patients: A follow-up of a controlled trial. Int J Prosthodont 2002;15:564–570.

368. Ekberg EC, Vallon D, Nilner M. Occlusal appliance therapy in patients with temporomandibular disorders. A double-blind controlled study in a short-term perspective. Acta Odontol Scand 1998;56:122–128.

369. Dahlström L. Conservative treatment methods in craniomandibular disorder. Swed Dent J 1992;16:217–230.

370. Fikácková H, Dostálová T, Vosická R, Peterová V, Navrátil L, Lesák J. Arthralgia of the temporomandibular joint and low-level laser therapy. Photomed Laser Surg 2006;24:522–527.

371. DeBar LL, Vuckovic N, Schneider J, Ritenbaugh C. Use of complementary and alternative medicine for temporomandibular disorders. J Orofac Pain 2003;17:224–236.

372. Ernst E, White AR. Acupuncture as a treatment for temporomandibular joint dysfunction: A systematic review of randomized trials. Arch Otolaryngol Head Neck Surg 1999;125:269–272.

373. Murakami K, Kaneshita S, Kanoh C, Yamamura I. Ten-year outcome of nonsurgical treatment for the internal derangement of the temporomandibular joint with closed lock. Oral Surg Oral Med Oral Pathol Oral Radiol Endod 2002;94:572–575.

374. Schiffman EL, Look JO, Hodges JS, et al. Randomized effectiveness study of four therapeutic strategies for TMJ closed lock. J Dent Res 2007;86:58–63.

375. Iwase H, Sasaki T, Asakura S, et al. Characterization of patients with disc displacement without reduction unresponsive to nonsurgical treatment: A preliminary study. J Oral Maxillofac Surg 2005;63:1115–1122.

376. Silber MH. Sleep-related movement disorders. Continuum (Minneap Minn) 2013;19:170–184.

377. Xu T, Wu MJ, Feng JY, Lin XP, Gu ZY. Combination of intermittent hydrostatic pressure linking TGF-beta1, TNF-alpha on modulation of proteoglycan 4 metabolism in rat temporomandibular synovial fibroblasts. Oral Surg Oral Med Oral Pathol Oral Radiol 2012;114:183–192.

378. Yuasa H, Kurita K. Randomized clinical trial of primary treatment for temporomandibular joint disk displacement without reduction and without osseous changes: A combination of NSAIDs and mouth-opening exercise versus no treatment. Oral Surg Oral Med Oral Pathol Oral Radiol Endod 2001;91:671–675.

379. Dao TT, Lavigne GJ. Oral splints: The crutches for temporomandibular disorders and bruxism? Crit Rev Oral Biol Med 1998;9:345–361.

380. Rugh JD, Harlan J. Nocturnal bruxism and temporomandibular disorders. Adv Neurol 1988;49:329–341.

381. Sheikholeslam A, Holmgren K, Riise C. A clinical and electromyographic study of the long-term effects of an occlusal splint on the temporal and masseter muscles in patients with functional disorders and nocturnal bruxism. J Oral Rehabil 1986;13:137–145.

382. Solberg WK, Clark GT, Rugh JD. Nocturnal electromyographic evaluation of bruxism patients undergoing short term splint therapy. J Oral Rehabil 1975;2:215–223.

383. Dao TT, Lavigne GJ, Charbonneau A, Feine JS, Lund JP. The efficacy of oral splints in the treatment of myofascial pain of the jaw muscles: A controlled clinical trial. Pain 1994;56:85–94.

384. Ekberg E, Vallon D, Nilner M. Treatment outcome of headache after occlusal appliance therapy in a randomised controlled trial among patients with temporomandibular disorders of mainly arthrogenous origin. Swed Dent J 2002;26:115–124.

385. Forssell H, Kalso E. Application of principles of evidence-based medicine to occlusal treatment for temporomandibular disorders: Are there lessons to be learned? J Orofac Pain 2004;18:9–22.

386. Lundh H, Westesson PL, Kopp S, Tillström B. Anterior repositioning splint in the treatment of temporomandibular joints with reciprocal clicking: Comparison with a flat occlusal splint and an untreated control group. Oral Surg Oral Med Oral Pathol 1985;60:131–136.

387. Tallents RH, Katzberg RW, Macher DJ, Roberts CA. Use of protrusive splint therapy in anterior disk displacement of the temporomandibular joint: A 1- to 3-year follow-up. J Prosthet Dent 1990;63:336–341.

388. Eberhard D, Bantleon HP, Steger W. The efficacy of anterior repositioning splint therapy studied by magnetic resonance imaging. Eur J Orthod 2002;24:343–352.

389. Tecco S, Festa F, Salini V, Epifania E, D'Attilio M. Treatment of joint pain and joint noises associated with a recent TMJ internal derangement: A comparison of an anterior repositioning splint, a full-arch maxillary stabilization splint, and an untreated control group. Cranio 2004;22:209–219.

390. Schmitter M, Zahran M, Duc JM, Henschel V, Rammelsberg P. Conservative therapy in patients with anterior disc displacement without reduction using 2 common splints: A randomized clinical trial. J Oral Maxillofac Surg 2005;63:1295–1303.

391. Conti PC, Miranda JE, Conti AC, Pegoraro LF, Araújo CR. Partial time use of anterior repositioning splints in the management of TMJ pain and dysfunction: A one-year controlled study. J Appl Oral Sci 2005;13:345–350.

392. Al-Ani MZ, Davies SJ, Gray RJ, Sloan P, Glenny AM. Stabilisation splint therapy for temporomandibular pain dysfunction syndrome. Cochrane Database Syst Rev 2004;(1).

393. Di Rienzo Businco L, Di Rienzo Businco A, D'Emilia M, Lauriello M, Coen Tirelli G. Topical versus systemic diclofenac in the treatment of temporo-mandibular joint dysfunction symptoms. Acta Otorhinolaryngol Ital 2004;24:279–283.

394. Ta LE, Dionne RA. Treatment of painful temporomandibular joints with a cyclooxygenase-2 inhibitor: A randomized placebo-controlled comparison of celecoxib to naproxen. Pain 2004;111:13–21.

395. List T, Axelsson S, Leijon G. Pharmacologic interventions in the treatment of temporomandibular disorders, atypical facial pain, and burning mouth syndrome. A qualitative systematic review. J Orofac Pain 2003;17:301–310.

396. Ahn DK, Chae JM, Choi HS, et al. Central cyclooxygenase inhibitors reduced IL-1beta-induced hyperalgesia in temporomandibular joint of freely moving rats. Pain 2005;117:204–213.

397. Yelland MJ, Nikles CJ, McNairn N, Del Mar CB, Schluter PJ, Brown RM. Celecoxib compared with sustained-release paracetamol for osteoarthritis: A series of n-of-1 trials. Rheumatology (Oxford) 2007;46:135–140.

398. Towheed TE, Maxwell L, Judd MG, Catton M, Hochberg MC, Wells G. Acetaminophen for osteoarthritis. Cochrane Database Syst Rev 2006;(1).

399. Dong XD, Svensson P, Cairns BE. The analgesic action of topical diclofenac may be mediated through peripheral NMDA receptor antagonism. Pain 2009;147:36–45.

400. Kopp S, Alstergren P, Ernestam S, Nordahl S, Morin P, Bratt J. Reduction of temporomandibular joint pain after treatment with a combination of methotrexate and infliximab is associated with changes in synovial fluid and plasma cytokines in rheumatoid arthritis. Cells Tissues Organs 2005;180:22–30.

401. Johansson Cahlin B, Samuelsson N, Dahlström L. Utilization of pharmaceuticals among patients with temporomandibular disorders: A controlled study. Acta Odontol Scand 2006;64:187–192.

402. Plesh O, Curtis D, Levine J, McCall WD Jr. Amitriptyline treatment of chronic pain in patients with temporomandibular disorders. J Oral Rehabil 2000;27:834–841.

403. Rizzatti-Barbosa CM, Nogueira MT, de Andrade ED, Ambrosano GM, de Barbosa JR. Clinical evaluation of amitriptyline for the control of chronic pain caused by temporomandibular joint disorders. Cranio 2003;21:221–225.

404. Dimitroulis G. The role of surgery in the management of disorders of the temporomandibular joint: A critical review of the literature. Part 1. Int J Oral Maxillofac Surg 2005;34:107–113.

405. Kozeniauskas JJ, Ralph WJ. Bilateral arthrographic evaluation of unilateral temporomandibular joint pain and dysfunction. J Prosthet Dent 1988;60:98–105.

406. Kendell BD, Frost DE. Arthrocentesis. Atlas Oral Maxillofac Surg Clin North Am 1996;4(2):1–14.

407. Yura S, Totsuka Y. Relationship between effectiveness of arthrocentesis under sufficient pressure and conditions of the temporomandibular joint. J Oral Maxillofac Surg 2005;63:225–228.

408. Vos LM, Huddleston Slater JJ, Stegenga B. Lavage therapy versus nonsurgical therapy for the treatment of arthralgia of the temporomandibular joint: A systematic review of randomized controlled trials. J Orofac Pain 2013;27:171–179.

409. Vos LM, Huddleston Slater JJ, Stegenga B. Arthrocentesis as initial treatment for temporomandibular joint arthropathy: A randomized controlled trial. J Craniomaxillofac Surg 2014;42:e134–e139.

410. Fridrich KL, Wise JM, Zeitler DL. Prospective comparison of arthroscopy and arthrocentesis for temporomandibular joint disorders. J Oral Maxillofac Surg 1996;54:816–820.

411. Murakami KI, Iizuka T, Matsuki M, Ono T. Recapturing the persistent anteriorly displaced disk by mandibular manipulation after pumping and hydraulic pressure to the upper joint cavity of the temporomandibular joint. Cranio 1987;5:17–24.

412. Nitzan DW, Dolwick MF, Martínez GA. Temporomandibular joint arthrocentesis: A simplified treatment for severe, limited mouth opening. J Oral Maxillofac Surg 1991;49:1163–1167.

413. Zardeneta G, Milam SB, Schmitz JP. Elution of proteins by continuous temporomandibular joint arthrocentesis. J Oral Maxillofac Surg 1997;55:709–716.

414. Kaneyama K, Segami N, Nishimura M, Sato J, Fujimura K, Yoshimura H. The ideal lavage volume for removing bradykinin, interleukin-6, and protein from the temporomandibular joint by arthrocentesis. J Oral Maxillofac Surg 2004;62:657–661.

415. Segami N, Murakami K, Iizuka T. Arthrographic evaluation of disk position following mandibular manipulation technique for internal derangement with closed lock of the temporomandibular joint. J Craniomandib Disord 1990;4:99–108.

416. Alpaslan C, Bilgihan A, Alpaslan GH, Güner B, Ozgür Yis M, Erbaş D. Effect of arthrocentesis and sodium hyaluronate injection on nitrite, nitrate, and thiobarbituric acid-reactive substance levels in the synovial fluid. Oral Surg Oral Med Oral Pathol Oral Radiol Endod 2000;89:686–690.

417. Shi Z, Guo C, Awad M. Hyaluronate for temporomandibular joint disorders. Cochrane Database Syst Rev 2003;(1).

418. Murakami K, Segami N, Okamoto M, Yamamura I, Takahashi K, Tsuboi Y. Outcome of arthroscopic surgery for internal derangement of the temporomandibular joint: Long-term results covering 10 years. J Craniomaxillofac Surg 2000;28:264–271.

419. Murakami KI, Tsuboi Y, Bessho K, Yokoe Y, Nishida M, Iizuka T. Outcome of arthroscopic surgery to the temporomandibular joint correlates with stage of internal derangement: Five-year follow-up study. Br J Oral Maxillofac Surg 1998;36:30–34.

420. Hall HD, Nickerson JW Jr, McKenna SJ. Modified condylotomy for treatment of the painful temporomandibular joint with a reducing disc. J Oral Maxillofac Surg 1993;51:133–142.

421. Hall HD, Navarro EZ, Gibbs SJ. Prospective study of modified condylotomy for treatment of nonreducing disk displacement. Oral Surg Oral Med Oral Pathol Oral Radiol Endod 2000;89:147–158.

422. Hall HD, Navarro EZ, Gibbs SJ. One- and three-year prospective outcome study of modified condylotomy for treatment of reducing disc displacement. J Oral Maxillofac Surg 2000;58:7–17.

423. Marciani RD, Ziegler RC. Temporomandibular joint surgery: A review of fifty-one operations. Oral Surg Oral Med Oral Pathol 1983;56:472–476.

424. Hall MB. Meniscoplasty of the displaced temporomandibular joint meniscus without violating the inferior joint space. J Oral Maxillofac Surg 1984;42:788–792.

425. Piper MA. Microscopic disc preservation surgery of the temporomandibular joint. Oral Maxillofac Clinic North Am 1989;1:279–302.

426. Dolwick MF, Nitzan DW. TMJ disk surgery: 8-year follow-up evaluation [in German]. Fortschr Kiefer Gesichtschir 1990;35:162–163.

427. Dolwick MF, Nitzan DW. The role of disc repositioning surgery for internal derangement of the temporomandibular joint. Oral Maxillofac Clin North Am 1994;6:271–275.

428. Montgomery MT, Gordon SM, Van Sickels JE, Harms SE. Changes in signs and symptoms following temporomandibular joint disc repositioning surgery. J Oral Maxillofac Surg 1992;50:320–328.

429. Heffez L, Mafee MF, Rosenberg H, Langer B. CT evaluation of TMJ disc replacement with a Proplast-Teflon laminate. J Oral Maxillofac Surg 1987;45:657–665.

430. Westesson PL, Eriksson L, Lindström C. Destructive lesions of the mandibular condyle following diskectomy with temporary silicone implant. Oral Surg Oral Med Oral Pathol 1987;63:143–150.

431. Kaplan PA, Ruskin JD, Tu HK, Knibbe MA. Erosive arthritis of the temporomandibular joint caused by Teflon-Proplast implants: Plain film features. AJR Am J Roentgenol 1988;151:337–339.

432. MacIntosh RB. The use of autogenous tissues for temporomandibular joint reconstruction. J Oral Maxillofac Surg 2000;58:63–69.

433. Mercuri LG. The use of alloplastic prostheses for temporomandibular joint reconstruction. J Oral Maxillofac Surg 2000;58:70–75.

434. Quinn PD. Alloplastic reconstruction of the temporomandibular joint. Sel Read Oral Maxillofac Surg 2000;7:1.

Migraine and Possible Facial Variants: Neurovascular Orofacial Pain

10

Yair Sharav, DMD, MS

Zaza Katsarava, MD, PhD, MSc

Rafael Benoliel, BDS

Chapters 10 and 11 deal with primary neurovascular craniofacial pain (NVCP) and emphasize the orofacial clinical equivalents. NVCP includes migraines and trigeminal autonomic cephalalgias (TACs), which include cluster headache, paroxysmal hemicrania, short-lasting unilateral neuralgiform headache attacks with conjunctival injection and tearing (SUNCT), and hemicrania continua[1] (see chapter 11). The term *neurovascular* better reflects the suspected etiology of the pain, which is considered to result, at least partly, from an interaction between the nervous and vascular systems.[2] Although sharing common pathophysiologic pathways of activation of the trigeminal vascular system as well as many signs and symptoms, NVCPs are clearly classified based on well-defined criteria of location, attack frequency, duration, accompanying signs or symptoms, and treatment response.

Referral of pain to oral structures is common in NVCPs, and pain quality often resembles dental pathologies so that patients with NVCP are often encountered by dental practitioners and later in orofacial pain clinics.[3,4] The authors collected cases describing patients with NVCP and, applying International Headache Society (IHS) criteria, found that 52% were unclassifiable; these were later grouped into an entity termed _neurovascular orofacial pain_ (NVOP).[5,6] Migraines and TACs are classically located around the ocular and frontal regions. Yet primary neurovascular type pain in the lower two-thirds of the face has been reported in the literature.[5,7,8] These patients are not easily classified with IHS criteria and have been assigned diagnoses of facial migraine, lower-half facial migraine, or NVOP.[3–5,7–12]

In 1997, the authors hypothesized that a primary neurovascular pain may exist that is separate from migraines or TACs.[5] They called the pain *NVOP* because it is more descriptive than the term *facial migraine* and because it is important to differentiate NVOP from dental pulpal pathology, with which it is often confused due to the presence of dental sensitivity during attacks. In addition to the location outside the conventional calvarial boundaries of the head, NVOP clinical features contain a distinctive combination of signs and symptoms common to both migraine and TACs. Thus, the rationale for introducing NVOP is based on its specific features that separate it from other primary NVCP

* NAUSEA

Table 10-1   IHS classification of migraine subtypes*

Category	Classification	Notes
1.1	Migraine without aura	Detailed in text
1.2	Migraine with aura	Detailed in text
1.2.1	Typical aura with migraine headache	Detailed in text
1.2.2	Typical aura with nonmigraine headache	Aura may accompany headaches other than migraine
1.2.3	Typical aura without headache	Aura that occurs with no headache
1.2.4	Familial hemiplegic migraine	Familial migraine with unilateral motor symptoms
1.2.5	Sporadic hemiplegic migraine	Nonfamilial appearance of 1.2.4
1.2.6	Basilar-type migraine	Migraine with aura symptoms clearly of brainstem origin or from both hemispheres
1.3	Childhood periodic syndromes that are common precursors of migraine	
1.3.1	Cyclical vomiting	Vomiting/nausea accompanied by pallor; self-limiting condition
1.3.2	Abdominal migraine	Episodic midline abdominal pain, moderate to severe and lasting 1 to 72 hours; associated with vasomotor symptoms, ✻ nausea/vomiting
1.3.3	Benign paroxysmal vertigo of childhood	Recurrent and brief vertigo, with spontaneous resolution
1.4	Retinal migraine	Repeated monocular visual disturbances (may include blindness) preceding migraine without aura
1.5	Complications of migraine	
1.5.1	Chronic migraine	Detailed in text
1.5.2	Status migrainosus	Migraine attacks lasting > 72 hours
1.5.3	Persistent aura without infarction	Long-lasting (> 1 week) aura symptoms without evidence of brain infarct (neuroimaging)
1.5.4	Migrainous infarction	One or more migraine aura symptoms accompanying an ischemic brain lesion (neuroimaging)
1.5.5	Migraine-triggered seizure	Epileptic seizure triggered by migraine
1.6	Probable migraine	Headaches or related symptomatology missing a feature that otherwise would classify it as a disorder from 1.1 to 1.5
1.6.1	Probable migraine without aura	
1.6.2	Probable migraine with aura	
1.6.3	Probable chronic migraine	

*Criteria adapted from the International Headache Society[1] with permission.

and its intraoral and perioral location, which has great diagnostic and therapeutic importance for differentiating NVOP from dental pathology.[3–6] A clear classification and terminology, discussed later in this chapter, will help clinicians avoid misdiagnosis and dental mutilation.

Migraine

Migraine is a common primary headache with an additional number of rarer related syndromes[1] (Table 10-1). The combination of high prevalence, severe pain, and debilitating neurologic symptoms increases the social impact of migraine to beyond that of other primary headaches. The two most common types of migraine headaches are migraine without aura (MWoA) and migraine with aura (MWA), which are often confused in clinics and in the literature.[13] This section describes MWoA, MWA, and chronic migraine.

The clinical features of the headache phase in MWoA or MWA are very similar and are described under the section for MWoA. Features specific to MWA are discussed under that section.

Migraine without aura

Clinical features

MWoA is the most common form of migraine.[1] MWoA is a disease affecting the young, and onset occurs before the age of 20 years in about half of patients.[14] Case 10-1 describes MWoA that is typical in presentation and clinical behavior (Figs 10-1 and 10-2).

Location. Headache is typically unilateral with no side preference, but it is reported bilaterally in some patients.[15–17] Migraine that occurs persistently in the same side (side-locked migraine) has been observed in up to half of migraineurs.[17]

A single location is rarely encountered, and migraines commonly occur in the ocular, temporal, and frontal regions. Other areas often involved are the occipital and neck regions, while the vertex and diffuse locations are rarer[17] (Fig 10-3). A migraine-like headache reported to occur in the lower half of the face[8,10] is discussed in detail in the section on NVOP pain.

Quality. Typically, pain is throbbing or pulsating (47% to 82% of patients) but may occasionally be pressing[16,18,19] (Table 10-2). Pain intensity is moderate to severe, and on average, a visual analog scale (VAS) rating of 7.5 is reported.[14] However, pain intensity is not uniform; mild to moderate (VAS 3 to 6) and moderate to severe (VAS 7 to 8) pain are each reported by about 40% of migraineurs, and 15% report very severe pain (VAS 9 to 10).[19] Some patients (24%) describe exacerbations of pain within an attack.[19] Others report interictal, short, sharp, periorbital pain, often described as ice pick pains.[20]

A feature of MWoA is that it is almost invariably (95% of patients) aggravated by routine physical activity such as walking or climbing stairs.[16,18] Many patients report that even moving the head, coughing, or holding their breath will accentuate headaches.

Temporal pattern. Headache development is often insidious, and it may take a half hour to 2 hours for a mild nonspecific ache to progress to a typical migraine.[21] Migraine is a periodic headache lasting 4 to 72 hours, and longer-lasting attacks are considered status migrainosus.[1] In about half of migraineurs, pain duration was 5 to 24 hours, in a third more than 25 hours, and in a small number (16.4%) less than 5 hours.[19]

For most migraineurs, headache frequency is less than one per month[14,22] but may vary considerably from 6 to 12 per year (46% of patients) to 1 or 2 per month (20% of patients) and up to 2 to 4 per month (16% of patients).[19] Clinic populations report more frequent headaches, and a third of these patients suffer more than four attacks per month.[23] MWoA has a higher average attack frequency and is usually more debilitating than MWA. Seasonal or cyclic patterns have been associated with migraine attacks, often correlating with light hours.[24]

Time delay from onset to diagnosis of MWoA in a tertiary center for headache was less than 1 year in 16.5% of patients, from 1 to 5 years in 30%, and more than 5 years in 53.5%. Younger age at migraine onset and a lower level of education were significantly associated with a longer time to diagnosis.[25] A minority (15.6%) of migraineurs describe daily or near-daily headaches,[19] or *chronic migraine*, which is described later.

Associated signs. On average, 50% of migraineurs vomit during an attack, 80% report nausea, and more than 80% report photophobia or phonophobia.[15,16] Associated signs are more prominent and common in severe headaches.[16] However, not all headaches are accompanied by the same signs, even in the same patient.[19]

Migraine may present with ipsilateral autonomic signs, most usually lacrimation (≈ 50% of patients), demonstrating significant correlation with unilateral and severe attacks.[26] The prevalence of one or more autonomic symptoms in 786 migraine patients was 56% and did not differ among migraine subtypes,[27] whereas the population-based prevalence was 26.9% of patients. Migraine patients with facial pain suffer significantly more trigemino-autonomic symptoms (conjunctival injection, tearing, miosis, ptosis, eyelid edema, nasal congestion, facial flush) than patients without facial pain (47.8% versus 7.9%).[28] Remarkably, most pediatric migraineurs (62%) had one or more cranial autonomic symptoms, and symptoms tended to be bilateral. Age, sex, laterality of headache, presence of aura, and whether the migraine was ep-

Migraine without aura in a 41-year-old woman.

Present complaint: Strong pain (visual analog scale [VAS] 8) around the eye, forehead, and maxillary teeth. Usually the pain is unilateral (left) side, but side shift does occur (see Fig 10-1). Pain is throbbing, often with superimposed sharp pain, and lasts from 9 to 48 hours depending on rest and response to treatment. Rarely, she suffers a milder bilateral headache that is pressing in quality and located frontally and occipitally.

History of present complaint: Similar though milder unilateral pain attacks began at the age of 15 years (frequency, one every 2 or 3 months). Over the years, the pain became stronger and more frequent, particularly during stressful periods. At the time of examination, frequency had increased dramatically. Pain is menstrually related. During some attacks, she feels a throbbing pain in the ipsilateral molars. Premonitory signs include repeated yawning and tiredness. Pain is accompanied by photophobia, phonophobia, nausea, and, when intense pain is present, ipsilateral ptosis and nasal congestion. During attacks, she is unable to brush her hair as this is very painful. On resolution of symptoms, she feels very tired. Interictal jabs of severe pain (ice pick) around the left eye occur with no warning signs and independent of migraine. These are very severe (VAS 9), last seconds, and occur in clusters or individually (see Fig 10-2).

Physical examination: Pericranial muscle tenderness (bilateral) was present with no limitation of jaw movement. The cranial nerve examination was normal. Intraoral examination (including bitewing radiographs) revealed no dental or other pathology.

Relevant medical history: The patient has had hypothyroidism since age 35 years, for which she takes 50 µg levothyroxine. She has been taking oral contraceptive pills for 5 years with no change in headache parameters. Her mother suffered from severe migraines until menopause.

Diagnosis: Migraine without aura; infrequent tension-type headache (TTH) with pericranial muscle tenderness.

Diagnostic and treatment considerations: The early onset and associated family history are typical of migraine. Because of the change in headache frequency, the patient underwent a brain computed tomography scan, which was normal. The long duration, premonitory signs, accompanying features, and headache resolution phase make migraine without aura the most likely diagnosis. The intraoral pain is secondary to migraine, as a dental source was excluded. The patient's pain diary confirmed that the headaches were menstrually related, and there were few attacks between cycles (see Fig 10-2). The patient also reported infrequent (2 or 3 per month) attacks of very sharp, short-lasting pain around the eye but not within a migraine. The bilateral headaches were rarer and matched a diagnosis of TTH; these responded to mild analgesics.

Abortive therapy was initiated with sumatriptan, which caused intolerable side effects. Similar results were obtained with rizatriptan. The patient also reported only mild resolution of symptoms with the triptans used. Soluble aspirin (1 g immediately) produced significant reduction in pain intensity and duration in about 70% of attacks. Similar results were obtained with naproxen sodium (775 mg immediately). The patient has thus far opted to remain on abortive therapy and refuses prophylactic therapy.

---

isodic or chronic did not influence the likelihood of having cranial autonomic symptoms.[29]

Premonitory symptoms and headache resolution phase. Premonitory symptoms may begin hours or a day or two before the other symptoms of a migraine attack (with or without aura). They include various combinations of fatigue, difficulty in concentrating, neck stiffness, sensitivity to light and/or sound, nausea, blurred vision, yawning, and pallor. The terms *prodrome* and *warning symptoms* are best avoided, how-ever, because they are often mistakenly used to include aura.[1] Additionally, hyper- or hypo-activity, depression, and food craving are often reported. Some of these signs have been found to be predictive of headache, such as speech difficulty, reading/writing difficulty, yawning, emotional changes, blurred vision, and phono-phobia.[30] Most premonitory signs are actually part of the migraine complex and not a trigger. The headache resolution phase is gradual in most patients, and the signs are similar to those observed in the premonitory phase.[30]

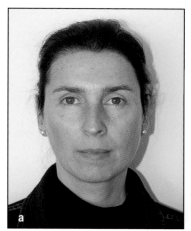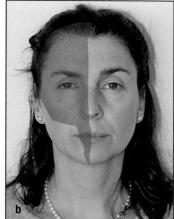

Fig 10-1 *(a and b)* Pain location for the patient described in Case 10-1 was commonly unilateral affecting the orbital, frontal, temporal, maxillary, and intraoral regions *(shaded area)*. Note the difference in expression and mild ipsilateral ptosis when the patient has a migraine *(b)*.

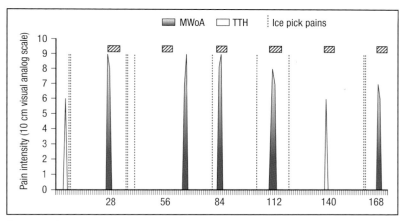

Fig 10-2 The pain diary kept by the patient described in Case 10-1 over a period of six menstrual cycles. Note that the migraines without aura (MWoA) are menstrually related but not exclusively so; MWoA occurs at other points of the menstrual cycle and not at every menstruation (marked by *rectangles*) and generally lasts for 1 or 2 days. On rare occasions, the patient suffers from a bilateral dull headache that is shorter and less severe and has no accompanying signs (see day 140); these are infrequent episodic tension-type headaches (TTHs). Additionally, she experiences sharp, severe jabs of momentary pain around the eye (ice pick pain), which is marked by *vertical dotted lines*.

Migraine triggers

Several factors reported as initiators of migraine attack have been termed *triggers* or *precipitating factors*[31] (Table 10-3). One or more such factors are reported by up to 90% of migraineurs.[32,33] However, only a subgroup of migraineurs react to specific triggers and do not always develop a headache with the same precipitant. Common triggers include foods (eg, chocolate, cheese), alcoholic beverages (eg, wine), menstruation, sensory stimuli, fatigue, and changes in weather. Often patients report more than one factor that may act together or individually.[32,33] Although precipitants are accepted as clinically relevant, there is a

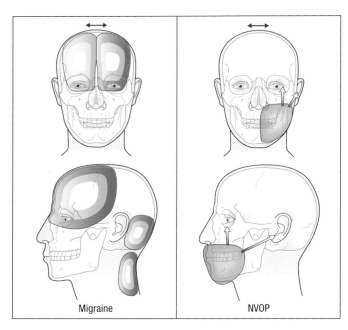

Fig 10-3 Pain location in migraine and NVOP. Migraine pain is typically periorbital and frontotemporal with referral to the suboccipital and neck regions; it is usually unilateral but may be bilateral in up to 30% of patients (marked by a *lighter shaded area* contralaterally). NVOP is characterized by its location in the lower two-thirds of the face, with intraoral and perioral areas frequently involved as primary sites. The *double-headed arrows* above the diagrams indicate side shifts of headache.

Migraine

NVOP

Table 10-2	**Diagnostic criteria for migraine without aura***
Diagnostic criteria	**Notes**
A. At least 5 attacks fulfilling criteria B through D	People who otherwise meet criteria for migraine without aura but have had fewer than five attacks should be coded as probable migraine without aura.
B. Headache attacks lasting 4 to 72 hours (untreated or unsuccessfully treated)	When the patient falls asleep during migraine and wakes up without it, duration of the attack is calculated until the time of awakening.
C. Headache has at least two of the following characteristics: 1. Unilateral location 2. Pulsating quality 3. Moderate or severe pain intensity 4. Aggravation by or causing avoidance of routine physical activity	Migraine headache is commonly bilateral in young children. Occipital headache in children is rare and calls for diagnostic caution; many cases are attributable to structural lesions. *Pulsating* means throbbing or varying with the heartbeat.
D. During headache, at least one of the following: 1. Nausea and/or vomiting 2. Photophobia or phonophobia	In young children, photophobia and phonophobia may be inferred from the child's behavior.
E. Not attributed to another disorder	History and physical examination do not suggest any structural lesion or other disorders, or such disorder is ruled out by appropriate investigation, or the attacks do not occur for the first time in close temporal relation to the disorder.

*Criteria adapted from the International Headache Society[1] with permission.

paucity of research that conclusively and consistently links most of these to migraine.[34] Interestingly, precipitants were identical between tension-type headache (TTH) and migraine and largely induced more severe headaches in migraineurs.[32]

Table 10-3 Common migraine triggers*

Group	Example
Endogenous factors	
Hormonal changes	Menstruation (4), contraceptive pill, hormone replacement therapy
Fatigue (1)	
Mental	Stress (2), cessation of stress (weekend headache)
Exogenous factors	
Alcoholic beverages (3)	Red wine, beer
Foodstuffs	Chocolate, cheese, hot dogs
Drugs	
Chemical additives	Nitrites, monosodium glutamate, aspartame, caffeine (or withdrawal), amines (eg, histamine, phenylethylamine, tyramine)
Strong or flickering lights	
Weather changes (5)	
Head trauma	"Footballer's headache"
Behavioral factors	
Missed meals	
Oversleeping	
Physical exertion	

*Numbers in parentheses rate the most common precipitants according to frequency reported: 1 = most frequent, 5 = least. Some of the factors have overlapping mechanisms (eg, wine contains alcohol and nitrites, and some cheeses contain tyramine).

Dietary. Foods and drinks are significantly and consistently related to headache onset in migraineurs.[32] The most consistent are chocolate, cheese, fruit, and alcoholic beverages. However, double-blind studies of chocolate as a migraine trigger have been inconclusive.[35] The significance of dietary factors as triggers is limited by the lack of prospective studies with clear experimental designs. Nevertheless, the high frequency of possible specific dietary triggers validates efforts to reveal the involvement of food-related factors in precipitating migraines.[36] Although foods trigger TTHs and migraines, chocolate and cheese seem highly related to migraine.[37] Alcoholic drinks precipitate headache in many migraineurs, and many principally identify red wine.[33]

Migraine and sleep. The relationship between sleep and headaches is well established.[38] Many migraineurs report that sleeping, even for a couple of hours, will abolish headache, so migraineurs frequently go to sleep to relieve headaches.[39] Moreover, a lack of sleep and disturbed or excessive sleep can trigger a headache. The sleep association and inherent periodicity of migraine headaches suggests involvement of central sites linked to biologic rhythm. In humans, these are located in the posterior hypothalamic gray, an area termed the *suprachiasmatic nucleus*.[40] Nearly two-thirds of migraineurs report symptoms suggestive of hypothalamic dysfunction, and disturbed sleep patterns are present during nights preceding headache.[41] Additionally, many (71%) patients reported at least occasionally being woken from sleep by a migraine.[39] Migraines are more likely to occur during periods of rapid eye movement sleep and with morning arousals.[38] The relationship between sleep and pain is further discussed in chapter 5.

Migraine and the menstrual cycle. Estrogen has long been considered to play a role in headache. In addition to its better-known functions, estrogen is a central neuromodulator,[42] and its withdrawal can induce estrogen withdrawal headache. Furthermore, many women report improvement or resolution of migraine headaches during late pregnancy.[18] Because sex differences persist past menopause, other major influences on migraine headaches are clearly involved.

Variations in hormone levels during puberty, menstruation, or menopause, or use of exogenous hormones (contraceptives, hormone

Table 10-4 Diagnostic criteria for typical aura with migraine headache*	
Diagnostic criteria	**Notes**
A. At least two attacks fulfilling criteria B through D	
B. Aura consisting of at least one of the following but no motor weakness: 1. Fully reversible visual symptoms, including positive features (ie, flickering lights, spots, or lines) and/or negative features (ie, loss of vision) 2. Fully reversible sensory symptoms, including positive features (ie, pins and needles) and/or negative features (ie, numbness) 3. Fully reversible dysphasic speech disturbances	If the headache includes motor weakness, code the patient as familial or sporadic hemiplegic migraine. Do not mistake sensory loss for weakness. Symptoms usually follow one another in succession, beginning with visual and then sensory symptoms and dysphagia, but the reverse and other orders have been noted.
C. At least two of the following: 1. Homonymous visual symptoms and/or unilateral sensory symptoms 2. At least one aura symptom develops gradually over 5 minutes and/or different aura symptoms occur in succession over 5 minutes Each symptom lasts more than 5 and less than 60 minutes	Additional loss or blurring of central vision may occur.
D. Headache fulfilling criteria B through D for migraine without aura begins during the aura or follows aura within 60 minutes	
E. Not attributed to another disorder	History and physical examination do not suggest any structural lesion or other disorders, or such disorder is ruled out by appropriate investigation, or the attacks do not occur for the first time in close temporal relation to the disorder.

*Criteria adapted from the International Headache Society[1] with permission.

replacement), are associated with migraine onset and changes in headache pattern (more in MWoA than in MWA). Headaches in general are very common around menstruation, and up to a quarter of women report menstrual-related migraine.[43] In the clinic, however, more than half of the female patients report menstruation as a common migraine precipitant, though it occurs more often in MWoA.[32] Indeed, MWoA often has a prominent menstrual relation, and in the IHS classification it has been subclassified in the appendix as *pure menstrual migraine* and *menstrually related migraine.*[1] Pure menstrual migraine is classified as MWoA with attacks occurring exclusively from 2 days before to 2 days after onset of endometrial bleeding; it is proposed that it may respond better to hormone replacement.[1] Menstrually related migraine headaches are significantly longer, more severe, and resistant to abortive treatment than attacks at any other time of the menstrual cycle.[44]

Estrogen receptors have been localized to the brain in regions involved in migraine patho-

genesis, and migraine-linked variation has been demonstrated in the estrogen SR1 gene, suggesting a role in migraine susceptibility.[45] The neuropeptides galanin and neuropeptide Y are modulated during the natural estrous cycle in trigeminal ganglia, suggesting a contribution to estrogen-related changes in trigeminal excitability and headache.[46]

Migraine with aura

Typical aura with migraine headache is the most common migraine syndrome associated with aura[1] (Table 10-4). MWA is a recurrent disorder manifesting in attacks of reversible focal neurologic symptoms that usually develop gradually over 5 to 20 minutes and last for less than 60 minutes. These neurologic symptoms (the aura) are reported by about 40% of migraineurs and are followed in about 10 minutes by a headache fulfilling the criteria for MWoA.[47] In most cases, headache follows the aura (93%), and in a few cases, headache and aura occur simultaneously (4%) or the aura follows headache (3%).[48] Less commonly, the headache lacks migrainous features or is completely absent. The discussion in this section is limited to typical aura with migraine headache.

The typical aura consists of visual and/or sensory and/or speech symptoms, develops gradually, and lasts no longer than an hour. The focal neurologic symptoms that usually precede or sometimes accompany the headache consist of one or more of the following: visual disturbances, unilateral paresthesia and/or numbness, unilateral weakness, and aphasia or unclassifiable speech difficulty.[1] In a large population-based study[48] visual symptoms were most frequent (99%), followed by sensory (31%), aphasic (18%), and motor (6%) symptoms. Visual aura was invariably present when several types of aura symptoms were reported.[47,48] The typical visual aura starts as a flickering, uncolored, zigzag line in the center of the visual field and affects the central vision—a fortification spectrum. Areas of lost vision (scotoma) may also be observed at this stage. The area progresses toward the periphery of one hemifield and often leaves a residual scotoma.

Next in frequency are sensory disturbances (pins and needles), which affect a variable part of one side of the body and face. The typical sensory aura is unilateral, starts in the hand, progresses toward the arm, and then affects the face and tongue. Less frequent are speech disturbances, usually dysphasic but often hard to categorize. The typical motor aura is half-sided and affects the hand and arm. Complete reversibility characterizes a headache-associated aura; the visual, sensory, and aphasic auras rarely last more than 1 hour, though in many cases the motor aura may persist.[48] Diagnostic criteria for typical aura with migraine headache are presented in Table 10-4.

Migraine Epidemiology

Globally, the percentages of the adult population with an active headache disorder are 46% for headache in general, 42% for TTH, 11% for migraine, and 3% for chronic daily headache.[49] New cases of migraine are uncommon among men but relatively common among women in their late 20s; the highest rates are found in 25-

to 34-year-olds (men, 6.5 per 1,000; women 22.8 per 1,000).[50] Among males and females younger than 30 years, the incidence rate for migraine with visual aura appears to peak earlier than MWoA.[50] Both MWA and MWoA peak earlier in boys, which explains why in childhood boys have a higher prevalence of migraine than girls.[51] At age 11 years, a female preponderance appears, possibly linked to female hormones. Although migraine itself tends to decline with age, the transformation of migraine to a higher-frequency disorder progresses steadily such that by age 70 years the occurrence of migraine 10 or more days per month is nearly double that in the 40s. The characteristic unilateral nature of migraine occurs in only 38% of older patients compared with 57% of those in the prime adult years, and there is a decline in throbbing, unilaterality, severity, and exertion exacerbation. Similarly, nausea, photophobia, and phonophobia also tended to decline with advancing age, though the occurrence of aura increased.[52,53]

In most studies, MWoA is more prevalent than MWA.[15] The 1-year prevalence of MWA is 2% to 5.8% (females, 6% to 9%; males, 1.3% to 4%). Race differences have been demonstrated in epidemiologic studies of migraine, suggesting altered genetic susceptibility.[34] In a recent study, the sex differences in the prevalence, symptoms, and associated features of migraine and probable migraine were investigated. "Severe headache" was reported in 17.4% (females, 23.5%; males, 6%), 11.8% met *International Classification of Headache Disorders,* second edition (ICHD-2) criteria for migraine (females, 17.3%; males, 5.7%), and 4.6% met criteria for probable migraine (females, 5.3%; males, 3.9%).[54] Females with migraine and probable migraine had higher rates of most migraine symptoms—aura, greater associated impairment, and higher health care resource utilization—than males.

Migraines and Disability

Due to its high prevalence and high socioeconomic and personal impacts, the *Global Burden of Disease Survey 2010* ranked migraine as the third most prevalent disorder and the seventh-highest specific cause of disability worldwide.[1] Eighty percent of migraineurs will report disability secondary to headaches, and more than half of the attacks result in significant interference with daily activities.[14] The most relevant psychosocial difficulties related to migraine were reduced vitality and fatigue, emotional problems, pain, difficulties at work, general physical and mental health problems, social functioning issues, and global disability.[55] Migraineurs were found to have elevated odds ratios (ORs) for depression (women, OR = 1.89; men, OR = 2.02) and suicidal ideation (women, OR = 1.72; men, OR = 1.70), even when adjusting for sociodemographic variables and disability status.[56] A significant increase in psychosocial impairment related to the number of headache days per month was found at lower headache frequencies but leveled off at higher headache frequencies (around 13.3 headache days/month).[57] The high prevalence during the most productive years of life imposes a substantial cost in lost work days.[14,51] An estimated 5.7 working days/year are lost for every working or student migraineur, although most of this effect is produced by the most disabled 10%.[14] However, it is important to notice that personal and societal costs of headache disorders are likely to be reduced when headache patients receive appropriate treatments and when continuity of care is offered.[58]

Pain diaries may be used to assess headache disability, but these give data only on headache frequency and intensity. A recommended approach is to apply the migraine disability assessment (MIDAS) questionnaire, which is simple to use and has been shown to capture unique information relating to the disabling consequences of headache beyond frequency and intensity.[19]

Migraine Comorbidity

Migraine is frequently associated with fibromyalgia syndrome, which may have a common pathophysiologic basis.[59] An association was found among painful temporomandibular disorders, migraine, and TTH ($P < .01$). The magnitude of association was higher for chronic migraine (OR = 95.9), followed by episodic migraine (OR = 7.0) and episodic TTH (OR = 3.7).[60] However, no significant correlation was found between headache diagnosis (episodic

TTHs or migraines) and the presence of painful temporomandibular disorders in another study.[61] The difference in findings could stem from different sampling; the study by Fernandes et al[60] was on patients seeking help for temporomandibular disorders, while that by Benoliel et al[61] was on healthy students. Indeed, another patient population with episodic or chronic migraine was more likely to have tenderness at the temporomandibular joint and on the masticatory muscles relative to control subjects without headaches.[62] Strong evidence suggests a relationship between migraine and depression or anxiety, stroke (particularly in smokers with MWA), other pain syndromes, and allergies. Among persons with episodic MWoA, depression was associated with an increased risk of chronic migraine, after adjusting for sociodemographic variables and headache characteristics,[63] and an increased risk of suicide attempt.[64]

Genetics

An up to twofold increase of MWoA is found among first-degree relatives of probands suffering from MWoA and a fourfold increase in MWA.[65] Twin studies of MWoA and MWA reveal a maximum proband concordance rate of 50% in monozygotic and dizygotic twins (higher in females).[66] These and other studies of inheritance factors emphasize that MWoA and MWA are caused by the combined effects of environment and genetics and suggest a multifactorial inheritance pattern.[67]

A severe form of MWoA is linked to an autosomal dominant disease termed *familial hemiplegic migraine*. A recent review summarizes the three genes that have been identified in families with familial hemiplegic migraine. The first was identified as *CACNA1A*. A second gene, *FHM2*, has been mapped to chromosome 1q21-23. The defect is a new mutation in the $\alpha2$ subunit of the Na/K pump (*ATP1A2*). A third gene (*FHM3*) has been linked to chromosome 2q24 and is due to a missense mutation in gene *SCN1A* (*Gln1489Lys*), which encodes an $\alpha1$ subunit of a neuronal voltage-gated Na^+ channel. A role has been suggested for the two-pore domain potassium channel, that is, the TWIK-related spinal cord potassium channel. The TWIK-related spinal cord potassium channel is in-

Table 10-5	Differentiating signs and symptoms for migraine without aura and episodic TTH	
Parameter	**Migraine without aura**	**Episodic TTH**
Location	Unilateral	Bilateral
Quality	Throbbing	Aching/pressing
Severity	Moderate to severe	Mild to moderate
Duration	4 to 72 hours	30 minutes to 7 days
Physical activity aggravates pain	Yes	Occasionally
Photophobia and phonophobia	May have both	Only one
Anorexia	Yes	Yes
Nausea/vomiting	May have both	None
Associated autonomic signs	In severe attacks	None
Wakes from sleep	Yes	No
Menstrual trigger	High association	Low association

volved in migraine by screening the *KCNK18* gene in subjects diagnosed with migraine.[68]

Differential Diagnosis

Tension-type headache

Although clinical overlap between MWoA and episodic TTH is prominent, the overall profile of signs and symptoms differs (Table 10-5). The similarities may at times be very marked, such as mild nausea, photophobia, and phonophobia, and some believe them to be clinical phenotypes of a common pathophysiology—the convergence hypothesis.[69] However, these signs are usually more severe and frequent in MWoA; therefore, routinely grading them in the clinic (mild, moderate, severe) is recommended.[16,70] TTH is mostly bilateral, while MWoA is largely unilateral, although bilateral migraine and unilateral TTH may be observed in significant proportions.[17,70] Pain is consistently more intense in migraine relative to TTH and may be a sensitive marker.[16,71] Similarly, attack duration in MWoA is usually longer than in episodic TTH but may overlap, particularly as migraine attacks longer than 5 hours have been observed.[19] Autonomic signs may occur in migraine to a higher degree than previously considered, and this has not been reported in TTH. Classically, TTH is not exacerbated by physical activity, whereas MWoA is. However, TTH aggravated by exercise has been reported.[22,70] A careful history and assessment of individual pain characteristics will usually facilitate the correct diagnosis.[71] Routine use of pain diaries and careful reassessment will identify misdiagnosed patients. Response to triptans can further help in diagnosis.

Sinusitis

Large population studies suggest that migraine is often misdiagnosed as a sinus headache.[72] This is confirmed in studies of patients with purported sinus headache in primary care.[73] From both studies, the reported pain location emerged as the most confounding sign. It seems therefore that migraine pain occurs commonly over the maxillary sinuses and, if accompanied by rhinorrhea (nasal discharge), for example, could be a confusing presentation.

A later study specifically examined the diagnostic relationship between migraine, allergies, and sinus pain.[74] In patients with self-diagnosed sinus headache, migraine was the most common correct diagnosis, and the features most commonly found in these patients included nasal congestion or rhinorrhea (81%) and eyelid edema (37%). Once again, the pain location was one of the most common reasons for misdiagnosis (see discussion of migraine and sinus headache in chapter 7).

Secondary migraine

Headaches with migraine characteristics may occur for the first time in close approximation to a primary organic cause. Vascular disorders such as transient ischemic attacks, thromboembolic stroke, intracranial hematoma, and subarachnoid hemorrhage may cause migraine-like headaches. Intracranial tumors and infections may also cause migraine-like headaches. Many of these are sudden-onset headaches or are accompanied by atypical neurologic signs and symptoms and need referral for imaging and neurologic management.[1] Neurovascular type headaches have been described after head and neck trauma.[75] Very often cervicogenic headache is similar in its clinical presentation to that seen in migraine and other neurovascular headaches. This entity is described in detail in chapter 14 and is also discussed with TACs in chapter 11. Indications for neuroimaging in headaches are discussed at the end of this chapter.

Treatment

Migraine currently has no cure, but adequate control can be achieved for most patients. Patient education, symptomatic treatments, and prophylactic treatments are the essential foundation of successful treatment in all headaches. Because patients with migraine have severe and disabling attacks, usually of headache with other symptoms of sensory disturbance (eg, light and sound sensitivity), medical treatment is often required. Medication overuse is an important concern in migraine therapeutics and needs to be identified and managed. In most patients, migraine can be improved with careful attention to the details of therapy.[76]

Patient education includes providing accurate and comprehensible information about the disorder and explaining the importance of contributing factors, such as sleep, diet, and other lifestyle practices that may precipitate attacks.[77] Some patients may, for health or personal reasons or because of intolerable side effects, prefer nonpharmacologic therapies

such as stress-management training, acupuncture, and physical therapy.[78] Often, combining modalities with each other or with pharmacologic agents may improve outcomes.[78] Pharmacologic treatment can be abortive (acute, symptomatic) or preventive (chronic, prophylactic). Abortive treatment is taken during, or preferably just before, attack onset with the aim of stopping the pain attack, whereas prophylactic medication is taken on a daily basis to reduce the severity, duration, and frequency of migraine attacks. In spite of the severe disability associated with migraine, up to half of migraineurs will not seek medical advice and will self-medicate, mostly (22% to 54%) with simple over-the-counter analgesics.[79] Although the symptoms are often well characterized and have been present for many years, for most patients (53.5%), the time elapsed between the first clinical manifestations and the diagnosis of migraine was more than 5 years, and the diagnosis was significantly associated with patients consulting a large number of specialists and nonspecialist physicians, who often prescribed expensive and unnecessary diagnostic investigations.[28] Nonspecific medication may be rated as satisfactory, but a trial of triptans resulted in improved quality of life.[80] In a study of triptan use in a headache center, 72% of patients intended to continue to use triptans, above all for their efficacy, and most of those who discontinued their use reported adverse effects.[81]

Alternative management strategies used by patients include avoidance of trigger factors, stress management, relaxation therapy, regular exercise, and herbal/homeopathic remedies[79,82] (see chapter 17). In particular, bed rest is commonly used (62%) to supplement care,[79] which suggests that patients are not optimally managed.

Patients may often need to manage a pain diary and return for reassessment before definitive therapy is initiated. The following section reviews drug therapies for migraine; whenever relevant, figures for the number needed to treat (NNT) and number needed to harm (NNH) are provided (see also chapters 15 and 16).

Abortive treatment

Abortive therapy is typically used when a patient has fewer than four attacks per month, but it may be augmented with prophylactic medications in special circumstances. Additionally, abortive drugs are often used to supplement prophylactic regimens that do not totally eradicate headaches; in these situations, the drugs are often referred to as escape medications. The major goals of abortive therapy are to rapidly (< 2 hours) relieve headache with no recurrence, cause minimal side effects, restore function, and reduce additional medication use.[83,84] An attempt should also be made to identify persons at risk and prevent disease progression into chronic migraine.[83] Many therapies not only relieve headache but also alleviate nausea and other associated symptoms.[76] Acute migraine therapy can be strategically approached in three ways: *(1)* step care within an attack, *(2)* step care between attacks, and *(3)* stratified care.[83] In step care, the first-line medication will often be a relatively inexpensive analgesic with a good safety profile. Nonresponders are *stepped up* to a more specific drug (eg, a triptan) until a satisfactory outcome is obtained. This strategy can be applied within a single attack or between a number of attacks. In stratified care, the initial treatment is selected based on assessment of the severity of attacks and associated disability. Stratified care provides a significantly better and faster clinical outcome and is more cost-effective than the two other strategies.[85]

Nonspecific medication

The patient's preference, including cost and past experience, as well as any contraindications must be taken into consideration.[76] Efficacy of abortive therapy is maximized when an appropriate dose is initiated as early in the course of the attack as possible. Analgesics and anti-inflammatory drugs are to be considered first, and if these are not effective, triptans should be used. Analgesics such as 1,000 mg of aspirin, preferably as an effervescent tablet, are good first-line drugs in the acute treatment of migraine.[84,86] For ibuprofen 400 mg, NNTs for 2-hour headache relief and 24-hour sustained headache relief were 3.2 and 4.0, respectively. Soluble formulations of ibuprofen 400 mg were better than standard tablets for 1-hour but not 2-hour headache relief.[87] For patients unable to take nonsteroidal anti-inflammatory drugs

(NSAIDs), 1,000 mg of acetaminophen may be effective (NNT = 5.2).[88] For mild to moderate headaches, a fixed-dose combination, such as aspirin with acetaminophen and caffeine (NNT = 3.9), may provide excellent response rates, superior to that of sumatriptan 50 mg.[84,86] Aspirin with the antiemetic metoclopramide (NNT = 3.5) or acetaminophen with codeine also have proven clinical efficacy.[84,89] If these fail, 550 to 825 mg of naproxen sodium can be tried.[84,89] However, because most of these analgesics and NSAIDs can be obtained over the counter, they are associated with abuse and the risk of serious side effects, such as gastric complications, liver failure, or withdrawal/abuse headaches.

Several calcitonin gene-related peptide (CGRP) receptor antagonists (discussed later) are being evaluated for acute treatment of episodic migraine. Likely it is just a matter of time until CGRP antagonists are approved for the acute treatment of migraine, given that proof of efficacy has already been established.[90] A summary of the more commonly used abortive medications for migraine is presented in Table 10-6.

Triptans

Triptans (selective **5-hydroxytryptamine 1B/D** [5-HT$_{1B/1D}$] receptor agonists) have become the drug of choice for abortive treatment of migraine as they relieve pain and associated signs.[84] A study of the pharmacoepidemiology of triptans in a headache center indicated that 72% of patients continued to use triptans, above all for their efficacy.[81] Response to triptans is not, however, considered pathognomonic of migraine; patients with cluster headache also respond. Triptans are thought to act peripherally and centrally at a number of sites (see chapter 16).

The introduction of sumatriptan represented a remarkable advancement in the treatment and research of migraine headache and stimulated the development of several second-generation agents, such as zolmitriptan, naratriptan, rizatriptan, almotriptan, eletriptan, and frovatriptan.[89] Eletriptan, naratriptan, rizatriptan, and zolmitriptan display increased stability to first-pass metabolic inactivation by monoamine oxidase and decreased hydrophilicity, resulting in a 2.5-fold increase in oral bioavailability relative

Table 10-6	Some common abortive treatments for migraine	
Class	Drugs	Initial oral dose (mg)
Analgesics	Aspirin	500 to 1,000
Combinations	Aspirin / acetaminophen / caffeine	500 to 600 / 200 to 400 / 50 to 200
	Acetaminophen and codeine	400 / 25
Ergot alkaloids	Dihydroergotamine NS	2
NSAIDs:		
Nonspecific	Naproxen sodium	550 to 825
	Ibuprofen	400 to 800
	Diclofenac	50 to 100
Selective cyclooxygenase 2 inhibitors	Celecoxib	200 to 400
Triptans (5HT agonist)	Sumatriptan	50 to 100
	Sumatriptan NS	20 (1 NS metered dose)
	Sumatriptan SC	6
	Naratriptan	2.5
	Eletriptan	40
	Rizatriptan	10
	Zolmitriptan	2.5
	Zolmitriptan NS	2.5 (1 NS metered dose)

NS, nasal spray; SC, subcutaneous injection.

Table 10-7	The triptans (5HT agonists): Summary of efficacy and side-effect profile*		
Drug/route	Dose (mg)	NNT (95% CI)	NNH (95% CI)
Sumatriptan	50	3.87 (3.21 to 4.89)	23.38 (8.26 to −28.13)
Sumatriptan SC	6	2.64 (1.82 to 4.80)	3.25 (2.81 to 3.85)
Naratriptan	2.5	6.49 (5.25 to 8.50)	−98.50 (22.09 to −15.25)
Rizatriptan	10	3.15 (2.89 to 3.46)	7.10 (5.37 to 10.45)
Zolmitriptan	2.5	5.92 (4.47 to 8.73)	26.82 (10.32 to −44.70)

*Efficacy = pain free at 2 hours; side-effect profiles = all adverse effects.
CI, confidence interval; SC, subcutaneous injection.

to sumatriptan.[91] Rizatriptan and zolmitriptan are also available in a rapidly dissolving wafer formulation, which can be taken without water, a particular advantage for patients with nausea.[92] Unfortunately, these new drugs are not superior in such parameters as speed of onset and recurrence rates.[93] Sumatriptan nasal spray (20 mg) is significantly better than placebo, but the difference is modest (NNT = 6.7) and inconsistent, and the drug has an unpleasant taste.[94] Zolmitriptan 5 mg intranasal spray (NNT = 2.85) has a rapid onset (15 minutes), has good tolerability, and is the drug of choice for this route of administration.[95] A summary of triptan efficacy and adverse effects, as measured by NNTs and NNHs, is shown in Table 10-7.

In a series of recent Cochrane reviews, the effectiveness of sumatriptan for acute migraine attacks in adults was evaluated for oral, rectal, intranasal, and subcutaneous routes; the drug was found to be effective in all routes for relieving pain, nausea, photophobia, phonophobia, and functional disability.[96–99] However, recent expert opinions concluded that sumatriptan has failed to show superiority over more standard and cheaper treatments, such as aspirin or aspirin plus metoclopramide. Additionally, oral sumatriptan at 100 mg kept patients pain free for 24 hours in only 20% of patients, so the authors concluded that there is a need to develop new, non-triptan antimigraine drugs.[100] Unfortunately, attempts to develop new drugs based on CGRP receptor antagonists and inducible nitric oxide synthase inhibitors have failed.[101]

Combining a triptan with an NSAID makes sense because they have different modes of action and adverse-effect profiles. The US Food and Drug Administration (FDA) cleared a fixed-dose combination of 85 mg sumatriptan and 500 mg naproxen sodium. This combination provides superior results than either drug alone.[102,103] More recently, frovatriptan (2.5 mg) was tested in combination with dexketoprofen (25 mg or 37.5 mg), and the combinations were found to be superior to frovatriptan alone at 2-hour and 24-hour follow-ups.[104]

Efficiency and side effects may not be similar across patients, however. Differences among the triptans may be clinically significant, and experts suggest that rizatriptan 10 mg will consistently provide rapid relief.[105,106] Almotriptan (12.5 mg) has good efficacy and tolerability, while eletriptan provides high efficacy with low recurrence but low tolerability.[106] A good starting point is low doses of rizatriptan (5 mg) or eletriptan (40 mg) with titration as necessary. Sumatriptan remains the most versatile drug with oral, intranasal, subcutaneous, and rectal formulations. Indeed, the subcutaneous format provides the most consistent and efficacious relief from migraine but with a high frequency of side effects and the need to self-inject (see Table 10-7).

Eletriptan is an orally administered, lipophilic, and highly selective serotonin $5\text{-HT}_{1B/1D}$ receptor agonist with a rapid onset of action, as early as 30 minutes after the administration of a single 40- or 80-mg oral dose, which is used in the acute treatment of moderate to severe migraine attacks in adults.[107] In a comparative study of efficacy for the 2-hour end points, eletriptan was significantly superior to sumatriptan, almotriptan, naratriptan, and frovatriptan. Rizatriptan yielded the second-highest treatment effects, followed by zolmitriptan. For the 24-hour end points, eletriptan was significantly superior to sumatriptan, rizatriptan, almotriptan, and naratriptan. Frovatriptan data were not available at that end point.[108]

Frovatriptan is one of the newest triptans. The drug's high affinity for $5\text{-HT}_{1B/1D}$ receptors and long half-life of about 26 hours in blood contribute to its sustained and prolonged effect compared with other triptans. A study in patients with coronary artery disease or at high risk of coronary artery disease found that frovatriptan was no different to placebo in bringing about clinically significant electrocardiogram (ECG) changes or cardiac rhythm disturbances.[109] Thus, frovatriptan is one of the safest triptans and has the lowest risk of treatment-emergent adverse events, and it has now gained a grade A recommendation from the guidelines for short-term prophylaxis of menstrual migraine[110] and for the management of oral contraceptive–induced menstrual migraine.[111]

Recently, the 5-HT_{1F} receptor agonist lasmiditan has shown efficacy in the treatment of migraines and is considered safe in patients with cardiovascular disorders. However, its central nervous system–related adverse events may considerably limit its clinical use.[112]

Side effects and safety. The most frequent adverse events of triptans are dizziness, somnolence, nausea, fatigue, chest symptoms, and paresthesia.[113,114] Adverse events occur less frequently with naratriptan and almotriptan than with rizatriptan, sumatriptan, zolmitriptan, and eletriptan, and the tolerability profile of almotriptan 12.5 mg resembles that of placebo.[93] Almotriptan and naratriptan appear to have fewer chest symptoms than sumatriptan or zolmitriptan but do not confer superior cardiovascular safety.[93,114] A sensation of chest tightness is a well-documented adverse effect with sumatriptan that occurs in 3% to 5% of patients,[115] but it is not associated with ECG changes, coronary vasoconstriction, or cardiac ischemia.[116] Also, in a positron emission tomography study, subcutaneous sumatriptan (6 mg) did not affect myocardial perfusion in a group of subjects without cardiovascular disease.[117] The risk of severe cardiovascular adverse events after the use of a sumatriptan is estimated at 1:100,000 treated attacks, which makes it unsuitable in patients with a history, symptoms, or signs of ischemic vascular disease.[118] Another study comparing triptan users with and without cardiovascular risks found no relationship between the overuse of triptans and cardiac outcomes.[119] As mentioned previously, in patients with coronary artery disease or at high risk of coronary artery disease, frovatriptan did not increase the occurrence of clinically significant ECG changes or cardiac rhythm disturbances compared with placebo; thus, it is considered one of the safest triptans.[109]

Some triptans have the potential for significant drug interactions, such as sumatriptan, rizatriptan, and zolmitriptan with monoamine oxidase inhibitors; zolmitriptan with cimetidine; and eletriptan with P-glycoprotein pump inhibitors. Other interactions should be considered with medications such as propranolol, serotonin selective reuptake inhibitors (SSRIs), and ergot derivatives.[120] The serotonin syndrome is a potential complication when co-prescribing triptans with SSRIs; however, it seems to be very rare.[121]

Triptan therapy during pregnancy was not associated with an overall increased risk of congenital malformations.[122] A slight increase in the risk of atonic uterus and hemorrhage was associated with triptan use during the second and/or third trimester.[123]

Prophylactic treatment

Migraine is a chronic disorder with episodic manifestations that is progressive in some people and that has profound social and economic costs. Cognitive-behavioral therapy plus amitriptyline resulted in greater reductions in days with headache and migraine-related disability compared with use of headache education plus amitriptyline.[124] Exercise may be an option in patients who do not benefit from or do not want to take daily medication, in particular because no difference in mean reduction of attacks was found among the exercise, relaxation, and topiramate groups.[125] Nonetheless, most studies did not find a significant reduction of headache attacks or headache duration with aerobic exercise.[126] Consequently, instituting lifestyle changes such as diet, physical activity, rest, and sleep and using a cognitive-behavioral minimal contact program focused on pain acceptance, reducing pain catastrophizing, and improving functional pain coping could be used instead of or in addition to pharmacologic intervention. Also, prevention of medication overuse in patients with migraine was achieved effec-tively with a cognitive-behavioral minimal contact program and an educational brochure.[127] A recent Cochrane review points to the efficacy of acupuncture for migraine prophylaxis, which is as effective as, or possibly more effective than, prophylactic drug treatment and has fewer adverse effects[128] (see also chapter 17).

Epidemiologic studies suggest that approximately 38% of migraineurs need preventive therapy but only 3% to 13% currently use it.[129] Moreover, patients on prophylactic treatment have poor adherence; specifically, patients on propranolol, amitriptyline, and topiramate showed adherence rates of 77%, 55%, and 57%, respectively, at 16 to 26 weeks.[130] Among patients with episodic migraine and chronic migraine, antidepressants were used most frequently (episodic migraine, 60.9%; chronic migraine, 54.7%), followed by beta-blockers (episodic migraine, 35.4%; chronic migraine, 36.8%) and antiepileptics (episodic migraine, 28.6%; chronic migraine, 36.3%). Odds of continuation of preventive medication use were higher among patients with chronic migraine than those with episodic migraine (OR = 2.72).[131]

The goals of migraine preventive therapy are to reduce attack frequency, severity, and duration; to enhance responsiveness to treatment of acute attacks (synergy); and to improve or restore function and reduce disability.[132] Indications for prophylactic treatment include four or more attacks per month, more than two attacks per month that induce disability for 3 or more days, contraindication or ineffectiveness of abortive therapies, and use of abortive medications more than twice weekly.[132] Chronic migraine typically evolves from repetitive episodic migraine in susceptible persons due to central sensitization. Prevention of chronic migraine is therefore an important goal in the management of episodic migraine.[133] Best remission was obtained when migraine prophylaxis was maintained for 24 months after patients became pain free. Patients were using a combination of atenolol (25 to 50 mg/day), nortriptyline (10 to 20 mg/day), and flunarizine (2.5 to 4 mg/day).[134] Of the patients in the group that maintained prophylaxis for another 2 years, 76.0% (19/25) remained pain free at a 5-year follow-up versus 44.0% (11/25) for the group that maintained prophylaxis for just another 1 year (P = .001). Prolonged use of a combination of drugs seems to act on more than one neurotransmitter, which may be needed to achieve prolonged remission.[134]

In 2012, a Quality Standards Subcommittee of the American Academy of Neurology and the American Headache Society provided an updated evidence-based recommendation for the preventive treatment of migraine headache, which revised the 2000 guidelines of the American Academy of Neurology. Based on new data, some drugs were downgraded or listed as not effective. Following is a partial list of recommendations[135]:

1. Level A: Medications with established efficacy
   - Antiepileptic: divalproex sodium, sodium valproate, topiramate
   - Beta-blockers: metoprolol, propranolol
   - Triptans: frovatriptan (for short-term use in menstrual migraine)
2. Level B: Medications that are probably effective
   - Antidepressants: amitriptyline, venlafaxine
   - Beta-blockers: atenolol, nadolol
   - Triptans: naratriptan, zolmitriptan (for short-term use in menstrual migraine)
3. Level C: Medications that are possibly effective
   - Angiotensin-receptor blockers: candesartan
   - Antiepileptic: carbamazepine (no new data, based on original guidelines)
4. Level U: Inadequate or conflicting data to support or refute medication use
   - Antiepileptic drug: gabapentin
5. Established as not effective
   - Lamotrigine

On March 11, 2014, the FDA cleared the first transcutaneous electrical nerve stimulation (TENS) device for use in the prophylaxis of MWA. The user attaches it just above the eyes (supraorbital TENS). The FDA evaluated the safety and effectiveness of the device based on data from a clinical study. After 3 months of treatment, the mean number of migraine days decreased significantly in the verum group (6.94 versus 4.88) but not in the sham group (6.54 versus 6.22). The therapeutic gain (26%) is within the range of other preventive drug and nondrug treatments.[136]

The choice of prophylactic medicine is influenced by medical contraindications, possible side effects, and the need to treat comorbidities, such as insomnia, TTH, depression, and hypertension. Cost is an additional consideration in a long-term prophylactic schedule. Inexpensive prophylactic medications (eg, generic beta-blockers or tricyclic antidepressants) and behavioral interventions using limited delivery formats, such as minimal-contact cognitive-behavioral therapy, are the least costly of the empirically validated interventions.[137]

Principles of preventive therapy

In clinical practice, a patient may have to test a number of migraine preventive drugs for a complete therapeutic trial (2 to 6 months) before the drug of choice is found. The patient should understand the process, and the patient's preferences should be taken into account to obtain full cooperation. Comorbidity should also be considered when choosing the most appropriate drug (Table 10-8 and Fig 10-4). The drug should be started at a low dose and titrated up until a therapeutic effect is reached or side effects become intolerable. Pharmacokinetics have interindividual variations; therefore, fixed dosing may lead to poor compliance and is not recommended.[138] In light of recent evidence, it seems prudent to continue prophylactic treatment for long periods, possibly for years; after all, prophylactic drugs are used indefinitely in such conditions as hypertension, epilepsy, and diabetes.[134] The possibility of using a combination of different classes of drugs, in order to act on more than one neurotransmitter, is also worth considering.[134] Breakthrough headache is not an indication to alter therapy.[139] Women of childbearing potential must be informed of potential risks of relevant drugs to conception or the fetus with consideration to the risk-benefit value of prophylaxis.

Three main drug groups are presently considered most effective and have relatively few and minor side effects and low cost: anticonvulsants, beta-adrenoreceptor blocking drugs, and tricyclic antidepressants (see Table 10-8); a possible short-term prophylaxis of menstrual migraine with triptans may also be considered.[135] On average, two-thirds of patients will experience a 50% reduction in headache fre-

Table 10-8	Choice of migraine preventive treatment*			
Drug	Dose (mg)	Adverse events	Contraindications	Relative indications
Divalproex sodium	500 to 1,000	Nausea/vomiting, alopecia, tremor, weight gain/loss	Liver disease, bleeding disorder	Mania, epilepsy, anxiety
Propranolol (sustained release)	80 to 240	Bradycardia, hypotension, fatigue, sleep disturbances, dyspepsia, depression	Asthma, depression, cardiac failure, Raynaud phenomenon, diabetes	Hypertension, angina
Amitriptyline	10 to 50	Sedation, weight gain, dry mouth, blurred vision, constipation, urinary retention, postural hypotension	Mania, urinary retention, heart block	Insomnia, anxiety, depression, TTH, other chronic pains

*The three most effective and commonly used drugs are presented. Choice is influenced by adverse events, comorbidity, and relative indications.

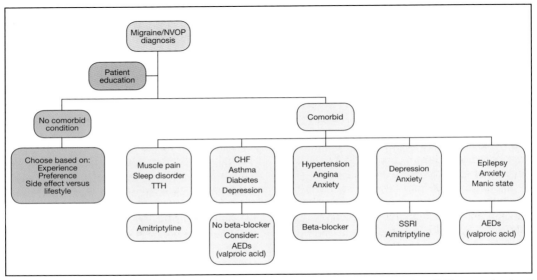

Fig 10-4 Algorithm for preventive treatment of migraine and NVOP affected by comorbidity. CHF, congestive heart failure; AED, antiepileptic drugs.

quency on most preventive therapies,[140] with a somewhat better rate for valproate sodium.[138]

Anticonvulsants

Placebo-controlled studies clearly point to anticonvulsant medication as increasingly recommended for migraine prevention.[135] Meta-analysis of published studies suggests that anticonvulsants significantly reduce migraine frequency by about 1 or 2 attacks per month, with an overall NNT of 3.8.[141] Of the anticonvulsants, the related compounds divalproex (a

stable complex comprising valproate sodium and valproic acid in a 1:1 molar ratio) and valproic acid have been the most extensively studied.[141] Sodium valproate has an NNT of 3.1 and divalproex sodium an NNT of 4.8.[141] Divalproex sodium is effective at an initial dose of 500 mg, which may be raised to 1,000 mg; the extended-release form has adverse-effect rates comparable with those of placebo.[142] For valproate sodium and divalproex sodium, the most common side effect is nausea (NNH = 6.6), though vomiting and gastrointestinal distress are also frequent and are dose related. Fatigue, tremor, weight gain, and dizziness are rare (< 8%) and are also dose related; at 1,500 mg of valproic acid per day, dizziness and tremor were particularly pronounced.[141] Safety and efficacy of divalproex sodium during 6 years of use revealed no hepatotoxicity and negligible weight gain.[143] Overall evidence from multiple well-designed clinical trials is sufficient to establish divalproex sodium and valproate sodium as a first-line prophylactic therapy for migraine.[135] A recent Cochrane review points to very similar results.[144] No significant difference was found in the proportion of responders between valproate sodium versus flunarizine or between divalproex sodium versus propranolol. For placebo-controlled trials of valproate sodium and divalproex sodium, NNHs for clinically important adverse events ranged from 7 to 14.[144]

The effect of another anticonvulsant—gabapentin—on the prevention of migraine was less favorable than valproic acid, placing gabapentin at level U[135] (see the earlier list). Trials of gabapentin suggest that it is not efficacious for the prophylaxis of episodic migraine in adults and should not be used in routine clinical practice.[145] No published evidence has been found from controlled trials of pregabalin for the prophylaxis of episodic migraine in adults.[145]

Topiramate (100 mg/day) was found to significantly reduce the frequency of migraine attacks and the quantity of escape drugs (NNT = 3.5).[141] Topiramate was classified as an A-level medication for the prevention of acute migraine.[135] This provides good evidence to support its use in routine clinical management.[146] Efficacy of topiramate versus placebo was comparable for dosages of 50, 100, and 200 mg, but it seems that 200 mg is no more effective than 100 mg and has more side effects.[146] With regard to mean headache frequency and/or responder rate, trials found no significant difference between topiramate and amitriptyline, topiramate and flunarizine, topiramate and propranolol, and topiramate and relaxation, but topiramate had a slight significant advantage over valproate sodium. As for migraine-specific quality of life, it improved significantly more by relaxation than by topiramate.[146] Adverse events reported for topiramate were usually mild; for topiramate 50 mg, except for taste disturbance and weight loss, adverse events were comparable to those of placebo. Adverse events were significantly more common with topiramate 100 mg (NNH = 3 to 25) and even higher for topiramate 200 mg (NNH = 2 to 17).[146] At a dose of 100 mg daily, the most common unwanted effect of topiramate is paresthesia (NNH = 2.4); less frequent (< 9%) adverse events include taste disturbance, weight loss, language problems, and anorexia.[141] Paresthesias are transient and, if bothersome to the patient, respond to potassium supplementation. The mechanisms by which anticonvulsants exert their actions in pain and headache are discussed in chapter 16.

Beta-adrenergic blockers

Beta-adrenergic blockers are the most widely used class of drugs in the prophylaxis of migraine.[147,148] Metoprolol, a selective β1-blocker, and propranolol, a nonselective β-blocker, were classified as A-level medications for the preventive treatment of acute migraine.[135] Metoprolol (200 mg/day) was more effective than aspirin (300 mg/day) in achieving 50% migraine frequency reduction (metoprolol, 45.2%; aspirin, 29.6%). From start to week 20, attack frequencies decreased from 3.36 to 2.37 for aspirin and from 3.55 to 1.82 for metoprolol. No significant adverse events were reported.[149] Evidence for the efficacy of propranolol (120 to 240 mg daily) is consistent, and there is no significant correlation between dose and clinical outcome.[148] Based on a meta-analysis, propranolol prophylaxis has an NNT of 3.3 for a significant reduction in migraine activity.[150] Whether these effects are stable after stopping propranolol is not clear.[148] Propranolol and amitriptyline are equally effective in migraine prophylaxis,[151] but propranolol is more efficacious in patients with migraine alone while amitriptyline is superior for patients with migraine and TTH.[152] Initial dose of 80 mg of the slow-release preparation is titrated according to side effects versus treatment response and may reach 240 mg daily (see chapter 16). If no response is achieved within 4 to 6 weeks at the maximum dosage, therapy should be gradually discontinued over a 2-week period. However, the efficacy of propranolol may increase progressively between 3 and 12 months of therapy. A longer trial period is therefore indicated, particularly in patients with a partial response.[153]

Adverse events most commonly reported with beta-blockers were fatigue, depression, nausea, dizziness, and insomnia, but the drugs are usually fairly well tolerated. Congestive heart failure, asthma, and type 1 diabetes are contraindications to the use of nonselective beta-blockers.[142] Metoprolol, a selective β1-blocker, can be considered as an alternative. Atenolol is another selective β1-blocker that has fewer side effects than propranolol, but its effectiveness in migraine prophylaxis achieved a B-level rating.[135] In patients on escape medication with zolmitriptan, an interaction with a metabolite of propranolol mandates a zolmitriptan dosage reduction to 5 mg.[91]

P. 91

Antidepressants

Sedative effects of antidepressant drugs make them an attractive option in patients with sleep problems, and comorbidity with depression or TTH often indicates their use. By pooling treatment outcomes for chronic headaches, a meta-analysis found an NNT of 3.2 for all antidepressant drugs.[154] In an updated evidence-based recommendation, amitriptyline was downgraded to B level (ie, probably effective), making it probably as effective as topiramate and possibly as effective as venlafaxine for migraine prevention.[135] Amitriptyline, a tricyclic antidepressant, is a serotonin and norepinephrine reuptake inhibitor (SNRI), and its efficacy in migraine treatment has been shown to be independent of its antidepressant action.[155] Thus, the optimum dosage for two-thirds of subjects was less than 50 mg per day.[156] In the authors' experience, a dose of 25 to 35 mg at bedtime is often effective; therapy is usually initiated with 10 mg at bedtime and titrated according to response and side effects. Response is normally seen within 10 days but may take longer.[139] Divalproex sodium extended release is more effective at 3 months than amitriptyline; however, at 6 months both are equally effective in migraine prophylaxis. The composite side effects were also similar, but hair loss, menstrual irregularity, polycystic ovary, and weight gain were more common in the divalproex sodium group.[157] The mechanisms involved in the effect of amitriptyline on headaches are discussed in chapter 16.

Venlafaxine, a structurally novel SNRI antidepressant, was compared with amitriptyline in the prophylactic treatment of migraine.[158] Amitriptyline (75 mg/day) and venlafaxine (150 mg/day) reduced significantly and equally the frequency, duration, and severity of migraine attacks. Venlafaxine has mechanisms of action similar to those of amitriptyline but with fewer side effects; sedation, dry mouth, and difficulty in concentration were higher in the amitriptyline group, but the dose of amitriptyline used in the study (75 mg) was considerably higher than that used in common practice. Venlafaxine is graded B level for migraine prevention.[135]

Duloxetine is also a structurally novel SNRI antidepressant. A prospective study on duloxetine treatment was carried out on episodic migraine headache.[159] Patients who did not have depression were titrated to a goal dose of 120 mg (mean, 110 mg). Subjects went from 9.2 ± 2.7 headache days per month to 4.5 ± 3.4 ($P < .001$), but there were no differences in headache duration, severity, maximum attack severity, and level of functioning.[159] Duloxetine has not been graded in the updated evidence-based recommendations for preventing migraine.[135] Unlike SNRIs, SSRIs are no more efficacious than placebo in patients with migraine. In patients with chronic TTH, SSRIs are less efficacious than SNRIs.[160]

Transcranial magnetic stimulation. In recent years, noninvasive brain-stimulation techniques based on magnetic fields have been shown to be safe and effective tools to explore the issue of cortical excitability, activation, and plasticity in migraine. Transcranial magnetic stimulation (TMS) and repetitive TMS have been explored as potential therapeutics.

On December 13, 2013, the FDA cleared the first TMS device in abortive treatment of MWA. In patients with episodic migraine, headache frequency, VAS score, and functional disability improved significantly at 1 month in the repetitive TMS group compared with the sham stimulation group.[161] Active high-frequency repetitive TMS was not effective, however, for the prophylaxis of chronic migraine.[162] Nevertheless, a position paper of the European Headache Federation calls for further controlled studies to validate and strengthen the use of neurostimulation.[163] Furthermore, until these data are available, the European Headache Federation recommends that neurostimulation devices "only

SNRI

be used in patients with medically intractable syndromes in tertiary headache centers, either as part of a valid study or have [sic] shown to be effective in such controlled studies with an acceptable side effect profile."[163]

Migraine therapy in pregnancy

Women in their reproductive years are the most predominant migraineurs. Migraine attacks may subside during pregnancy, particularly toward the third trimester. However, migraines commonly occur during the first trimester at the time of fetal organogenesis and require careful management.[164] For example, ergot alkaloids are contraindicated, whereas opioids and codeine have no teratogenic hazard. The use of aspirin during the first two trimesters seems safe, but all NSAIDs should be avoided in the third trimester because of the danger of premature closure of the ductus arteriosus and pulmonary hypertension in the neonate.[164] Acetaminophen, if efficient, is a safe alternative (see chapter 15 for a full discussion of acetaminophen and NSAIDs during pregnancy).

The risk of all major birth defects after first-trimester exposure to sumatriptan was 4.6% (2.9% to 7.2%). This, coupled with a consistent failure of additional epidemiologic studies to observe teratogenicity, gives a level of reassurance concerning the safety of sumatriptan in pregnancy. Acetaminophen, NSAIDs, and sumatriptan should therefore be the preferred drugs for the treatment of acute migraine attacks in pregnant women.[122] Research, however, does not exclude the risk of individual or rare congenital malformations with the use of triptans. A slight increase in the risk of atonic uterus and hemorrhage was associated with triptan use during the second and/or third trimester.[123]

Prophylaxis is not advised but, if unavoidable, should begin only in the second trimester and only when patients experience at least three prolonged severe attacks a month that are particularly incapacitating or unresponsive to symptomatic therapy; propranolol is the recommended drug.[164] Nonpharmacologic approaches are preferred, but if ineffective, preventive treatment should include low doses of beta-blockers or amitriptyline.[165] Amitriptyline and propranolol are classified for pregnancy risk at category C (ie, use with caution if benefits outweigh risks). Lactation is not recommended with amitriptyline and is controversial with propranolol.

On May 6, 2013, the FDA advised that valproate sodium, valproic acid, and divalproex sodium should not be taken by pregnant women for the prevention of migraine headaches. Pregnancy category for migraine use was changed from D to X (ie, the risk of use in pregnant women clearly outweighs any possible benefit of the drug). Indeed, an increase in risk of neurodevelopmental disorders was observed in children exposed in utero to monotherapy with valproate sodium (OR = 6.05 to 24.53) or to polytherapy (OR = 9.97 to 49.40) compared with control children. Autistic spectrum disorder was the most frequent diagnosis.[166] This should be considered whenever prescribing valproates for migraine prophylaxis in women of childbearing age.

Migraine in Children and Adolescents

Migraines are very common in children and adolescents, but diagnosis may be more difficult because of problems in obtaining an accurate history and the somewhat different symptomatology (eg, there is often a bilateral location). Researchers have suggested that the diagnosis of migraine in children should include severe headache associated with nausea, even if the criteria of location, quality, and aggravation by physical activity are not fulfilled.[167] Moreover, migraine criteria lack sensitivity in children; of 64 patients with confirmed diagnoses of migraine, only 45% had headaches that fulfilled the ICHD-2 migraine criteria.[168] Also, brief migraine episodes (5 to 45 minutes), defined as *atypical migraine* by ICHD-2, are common in children and adolescents. The researchers concluded that if duration of head pain is less than 1 hour, two additional features should be included to diagnose definitive migraine: one parent or sibling with migraine and one of the migraine trigger precipitants.[169] The estimated overall mean prevalence of headache in children and adolescents was 54.4%, and the overall mean prevalence of migraine was 9.1%.[170] Unpredictably, in one study, most children with migraine showed little or no disability regarding daily life activities.[171] Cranial autonomic symptoms are common in children and tend to be bilateral. Age, sex, laterality of headache, presence of aura, and whether migraine was episodic versus chronic did not influence the likelihood of having cranial autonomic symptoms.[29]

On the whole, evidence for the pharmacologic treatment of acute migraine in children is very poor.[172] High placebo response rates represent the principal challenge in pediatric trials of drugs for abortive treatment of migraine, and triptans show a very low therapeutic gain because of a high placebo rate.[173,174] Recommendations for the acute treatment of migraine in children younger than 6 years include ibuprofen (effective) and acetaminophen (probably effective).[175] Prophylactic magnesium pretreatment induced a significant decrease in pain intensity and pain frequency in acetaminophen-treated and ibuprofen-treated children.[176] For adolescents older than 12 years, acute treatment of migraine with sumatriptan nasal spray is recommended. Topiramate is an effective and well-tolerated prophylactic therapy for use in pediatric patients with migraine. Doses of 100 and 200 mg/day (1.47 to 2.0 mg/kg/day) effectively decreased the frequency of migraine headaches, with 100 mg/day providing the optimal benefit-to-risk ratio.[177] Recently, it was shown that frequency, severity, and duration of headache decreased on 3 mg/kg/day of topiramate or 1 mg/kg/day of propranolol at the end of 3 months. Topiramate was more effective than propranolol, and transient mild side effects were seen in 18% of subjects in the topiramate group and 10% in the propranolol group ($P = .249$).[178] Data concerning divalproex sodium is insufficient to recommend its use in children.[179]

Prognosis

Migraine is a chronic illness, and although some may suffer increased attacks as they reach middle age, many will report long-term remissions.[180] Favorable prognostic factors were short duration of migraine (from onset in years), male sex, and a solely visual aura.[181] In people over 50 years old, the prevalence of migraine rapidly declines such that by age 70 years

the prevalence of migraine approximates that of the middle teen years.[182] The characteristic unilateral nature of migraine was found to occur in only 38% of older patients with migraine compared with 57% of those in the prime adult years. A decline in the pain characteristics of migraine with increasing age was observed, such as reduced severity and reduced exacerbation on throbbing and on exertion. Similarly, nausea, photophobia, and phonophobia also tended to decline. On the other hand, the occurrence of aura increased with increasing age.[183] Although the prevalence of migraine tends to decline with age, the transformation of migraine to a higher-frequency disorder progresses steadily through the adult years such that by age 70 years, the occurrence of migraine 10 or more days per month can be nearly double that seen in a person's 40s.[184] Thus, a small group of patients will develop increased frequency of migraine headache with reduced intensity, ultimately transforming into chronic migraine.[185]

Chronic Migraine

Definition and characteristics

Chronic migraine is defined as headache that occurs on 15 or more days per month for more than 3 months, has the features of migraine headache on at least 8 days per month, and/or responds to migraine-specific treatment in a patient with a lifetime history of at least five prior migraine attacks and no medication overuse.[1] Results of electrophysiologic and functional imaging studies indicate that chronic migraine is associated with abnormalities in the brainstem that may be progressive. Additionally, chronic migraine is associated with a greater degree of impairment in cortical processing of sensory stimuli than in episodic migraine, perhaps because there is more pervasive or persistent cortical hyperexcitability.[133] Because of these distinctions, it is critical to focus on chronic migraine as a unique condition, even though its relationship to episodic migraine, primarily as a predisposing condition, is acknowledged.[133] Interictal CGRP levels were significantly increased in peripheral blood in women with chronic migraine (74.90 pg/mL) compared with healthy control women (33.74 pg/mL) or women with episodic migraine (46.37 pg/mL); peripheral CGRP levels may be a biomarker for chronic migraine.[186]

Typically, the headache location is bilateral in the frontotemporal region but may be strictly unilateral in up to half of patients. Headache is mostly mild to moderate with a dull and pressing quality. Truly continuous headache is observed in less than half of patients, and although most patients do not awaken with a headache, many will develop it during the early morning. Nighttime arousals due to headache were reported, particularly by women.[187]

Epidemiology and predictors for chronicity

About 3% of episodic migraine cases progress to chronic migraine. The clinical evolution appears to occur gradually over months or years, and some people progress from infrequent attacks (2 to 104 headache days/year) or frequent episodic attacks (105 to 179/year) to chronic migraine.[188] A recent global prevalence study reported that the 1-year sex-stratified prevalence for chronic migraine was 1.3% for women and 0.5% for men. Chronic migraine prevalence rates also varied by age and were highest for women (1.9%) and men (0.8%) in the age range of 40 to 49 years. The authors also reported that chronic migraine represents 7.7% of the total migraine population.[189]

Factors associated with the progression of episodic to chronic migraine include female sex, lower socioeconomic status, and marital status (unmarried). Other factors include obesity, snoring, other pain syndromes, previous neck or head injury, stressful life events, caffeine intake, and use of acute headache medication. Sleep disorders, psychopathology (especially anxiety and depression), and gastrointestinal disorders also occur more frequently in those with chronic migraine than in those with episodic migraine.[190] Sociodemographic profiles differed also; persons with chronic migraine reported significantly lower household income levels, were less likely to be employed full-time, and were more likely to be occupationally disabled than persons with episodic migraine.[191] Depression was a significant predictor of the transformation from episodic to chronic migraine (OR = 1.65). A depression dose effect was found; relative to participants with no or mild depression, those with moderate (OR = 1.77) and severe depression (OR = 2.53) were at increased risk for the onset of chronic migraine.[63]

Additionally MWoA is most prone to accelerate to chronic migraine with frequent use of symptomatic medication, resulting in a new type of headache termed *medication-overuse headache*.[1] About 50% of patients who supposedly have chronic migraine revert to an episodic migraine subtype after drug withdrawal; such patients are in a sense wrongly diagnosed as having chronic migraine. After drug withdrawal, migraine will either revert to the episodic subtype or remain chronic and be rediagnosed accordingly.[1] In an interdisciplinary pain clinic, chronic headache was more prevalent among patients with analgesic overuse (39.8%) than without analgesic overuse (18%), with an OR of 13.1 to have chronic headache with history of primary headache compared with patients without a primary headache syndrome. Consequently, primary headaches have a high risk for progressing to chronic in patients who are overusing analgesics for other pain disorders.[192] Medication overuse is defined as intake of simple analgesics (eg, aspirin, acetaminophen, ibuprofen) on more than 15 days per month or the intake of combination analgesics, opioids, ergots, or triptans on more than 10 days per month.[193] Overuse of acute pain medication or specific migraine medication is reported in about 66% to 75% of adults with chronic migraine.[192] Recent experiments in animals after exposure to opioids and triptans resulted in enhanced sensitivity to nitric oxide, which has been demonstrated to trigger migraine in humans, and may offer insights into the possible pathology of chronic migraine.[194]

Disability and comorbidity

Chronic migraine and episodic migraine are part of the spectrum of migraine disorders, but they are distinct clinical entities in terms of clinical, sociodemographic, and comorbidity profiles. Population-based studies have shown that those with chronic migraine demonstrate higher individual and societal burden because they are significantly more disabled than those with episodic migraine and have greater impairment in quality of life.[195] Patients with chronic migraine were significantly less likely to be employed full-time and almost twice as likely to be occupationally disabled. In addition, patients with chronic migraine were nearly twice as likely to have anxiety, chronic pain, or depression. Furthermore, patients with chronic migraine had higher cardiovascular and respiratory risk; 40% were more likely to have heart disease and angina, and 70% were more likely to have a history of stroke.[196]

Treatment

The management of chronic migraine requires identifying and managing risk factors (eg, sleep apnea, caffeine consumption), establishing limits on acute pain medications to less than 10 days per month, initiating nonpharmacologic treatment if appropriate, initiating preventive treatment, and assessing and treating neuropsychiatric disorders and other comorbid conditions that could contribute to increased attack frequency (eg, obesity).[193]

Pharmacotherapy. Preventive treatment, even in the presence of overuse of acute pain medication, has been shown to effectively reduce migraine frequency and disability. Drug selection should be individualized based on comorbid or coexistent illness/disorders, specifically avoiding drugs that may exacerbate another underlying condition.[193] Only two pharmacologic treatments have been shown to be effective in patients with chronic migraine with and without medication overuse: topiramate and local injection of botulinum toxin.

Two large clinical trials were performed with topiramate in patients with chronic migraine, one in the United States and the other in Europe.[193] These trials were similar in design. They included patients with chronic migraine with and without medication overuse, had a 16-week double-blind phase, and used topiramate 100 mg as a target dose. In the US trial, monthly migraine reduction was 5.6 ± 6.0 days compared with placebo (4.1 ± 6.1 days; P = .032). In the European trial, monthly migraine reduction was 3.5 ± 6.3 days compared with placebo (0.2 ± 4.7 days; P = .02). Based on these two

studies, it was concluded[197] that topiramate at a dose of 100 mg daily is effective and generally well tolerated by patients with chronic migraine. A lower dosage of topiramate, 50 mg per day, may be effective as well. General treatment effects were independent from medication overuse. This would indicate a change in strategy; it may not be necessary to withdraw patients with chronic migraine from medication overuse before treatment with topiramate. Only patients who fail this treatment or cannot tolerate topiramate need to undergo a formal withdrawal program.

Several other drugs were tried for prophylactic treatment of chronic daily headache, but data are still rare and studies statistically underpowered. One group studied gabapentin, 2,400 mg daily, in patients with chronic daily headache. After 12 weeks of treatment, the median 4-week migraine rate was 2.7 (baseline = 4.2) in the treatment group and 3.5 (baseline = 4.1) in the placebo group (P = .006). Adverse events were observed in 13 of 98 gabapentin-treated patients (13.3%) and included mainly somnolence and dizziness.[198] An open-label trial investigated the efficacy of pregabalin in the treatment of chronic migraine on an initial dosage of 75 mg, which was subsequently adjusted. Results showed a significant decrease in headache frequency, headache severity, and rescue medication intake. Frequent adverse events included dizziness (40%), somnolence (29%), abnormal thinking (17%), and constipation and fatigue (13%).[199]

Botulinum toxin – see also p. 229

Botulinum toxin A is FDA cleared (as of 2013) for prophylactic treatment of chronic migraine. Pooled analyses demonstrated a decrease from baseline in frequency of headache days, favoring botulinum toxin A over placebo at week 24 (–8.4 versus –6.6; P < .001),[200] and the treatment is considered cost-effective in the United Kingdom.[201] Although botulinum toxin A had a modest benefit for chronic daily headache and chronic migraine, it was not associated with a reduction in episodic migraine or chronic TTH.[202] The injection paradigm consists of delivering a total of 155 units administered as 5-unit injections per site (31 sites) using a sterile 30-gauge, short (0.5-in) needle.[203] The sites

p. 233

Chronic migraine in a 41-year-old woman.

Present complaint: Continuous headache over the eye and frontotemporal region (see Fig 10-5). The headache is unilateral (usually on right side) but may also be bilateral in the same areas. The character is pressing and dull, often with a pulsating quality, and it may wake the patient in the early morning. Pain intensity is mostly constant (VAS 5 or 6), with frequent exacerbations of VAS 7 or 8. When pain is exacerbated, it is accompanied by photophobia, phonophobia, and often nasal congestion. Pain refers to the ipsilateral maxilla and feels like a toothache.

History of present complaint: The patient has a 26-year history of episodic MWoA successfully treated with nonspecific abortive medications (largely NSAIDs). Mean attack frequency for MWoA had been 2 or 3 per month. About 2 or 3 years ago, the frequency increased, but the attacks were successfully treated with propranolol. However, the patient stopped taking medication about 2 years ago. A short time after this, over a period of some months, frequency gradually increased to a point where she was rarely free from headaches and suffered constant pain of variable intensity. In addition to daily pain, the patient reported significant social and work disability; she is currently unemployed because of the headaches.

Physical examination: Pericranial and masticatory muscle tenderness were present bilaterally. Relevant medical history: Eight months earlier, the patient had an epidermoid cyst removed via craniotomy. The patient was treated with carbamazepine postoperatively, and there was no change in the chronic headache pattern.

Diagnosis: Chronic daily headache; chronic migraine (transformed migraine).

Diagnostic and treatment considerations: Primary chronic daily headaches include chronic migraine, chronic TTH, hemicrania continua, and new daily persistent headache. Often the subentities are difficult to distinguish, and a definitive diagnosis is based on the history and treatment response. A trial of indomethacin up to 100 mg daily had not provided relief, suggesting that the patient's condition was not hemicrania continua. A common secondary cause would be analgesic-abuse headache, but the patient had no history of such drug abuse. Posttraumatic headache is not relevant because the craniotomy had been performed more than 1 year after the onset of chronic migraine, and surgery had not altered the headache pattern. Therapy was initiated with valproic acid starting at 200 mg daily and escalating by 200 mg every 3 days to a maintenance dose of 600 mg daily in three doses. The effect was remarkable, and pain relief occurred very rapidly (see Fig 10-6). The patient returned to part-time employment within 2 months of therapy. The patient was followed up for 4 years (2.5 years are shown Fig 10-6) and, with occasional dose titrations (400 to 800 mg daily) of valproic acid, has maintained long-term relief of pain and disability. Note that occasional exacerbations in pain occur, but overall a VAS less than 2.5 was obtained. This follow-up suggests that 800 mg was superior to 600 mg valproic acid in providing pain relief but was accompanied by increased side effects, so the patient preferred a 600-mg maintenance dose.

---

injected are the corrugator, procerus, frontalis, temporalis, occipital, cervical paraspinal group, and trapezius muscles bilaterally (see chapter 16).

Clinical example

The patient described in Case 10-2 had a typical history of episodic migraine that evolved into chronic migraine over a period of 2 to 3 years (Figs 10-5 and 10-6). Compare this case to Case 10-4.

Neurovascular Orofacial Pain or Facial Migraine

Cases of isolated orofacial pain with neurovascular features have been reported, and most reports suggest that these are *facial migraines*.[8,11,12] Or, in cases in which the patient has a history of migraines, the term *relocated migraines* may be used.[204,205] However, although facial pain was not unusual in migraine (8.9%), isolated facial migraine was exceptionally rare

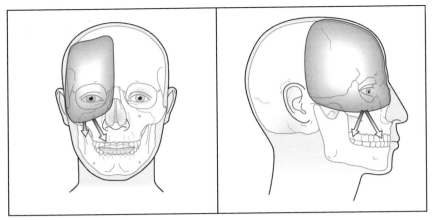

Fig 10-5 Pain location for the patient described in Case 10-2.

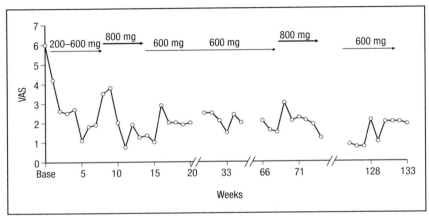

Fig 10-6 Mean weekly VAS rating for the patient described in Case 10-2. Since initiation of therapy with valproic acid, a marked and relatively rapid improvement was observed. Note that exacerbations do occur, even on prophylactic regimens, and some dose response is apparent (ie, 800 mg is more efficient than 600 mg). The *arrows* and amounts in milligrams denote the duration and dosage of valproic acid administration.

(0.2%).[28] In 1997, the authors hypothesized that a primary, isolated neurovascular pain, separate from migraines or TACs, may exist.[5] As noted earlier, the authors consider the term *neurovascular orofacial pain* to be more descriptive than *facial migraine*. However, in addition to the location outside the conventional calvarial boundaries of the head, the clinical features of NVOP contain a distinctive combination of signs and symptoms common to both migraine and TACs.[3–5] Furthermore, primary orofacial pain of neurovascular origin is of great diagnostic and therapeutic importance for differentiat-

ing NVOP from dental pulpal pathology, which are often confused because of the presence of dental sensitivity during attacks.[4–6] A clear classification and terminology will prevent misdiagnosis and dental mutilation.

Clinical features

Location

The vast majority of patients (93%) report unilateral pain.[5,8] Pain occurs primarily intraorally, and teeth are often affected (see Case 10-3)

Table 10-9 | **Suggested criteria for neurovascular orofacial pain (NVOP)**

Diagnostic criteria	Notes
A. At least five attacks of facial pain fulfilling criteria B through E	
B. Severe, unilateral oral and/or perioral pain	May refer to orbital and/or temporal regions. Side shift may occur, but bilateral cases are rarely reported.

C. At least one of the following characteristics:
  1. Toothache with no local pathology
  2. Throbbing
  3. Wakes patient from sleep
	Frequently, painful vital teeth will be hypersensitive to cold stimuli. Some of the teeth in the painful region may have undergone root canal therapy with no long-standing pain relief.

D. Episodic attacks lasting minutes to more than 24 hours	Chronic unremitting cases have been observed that may result in subclassification into episodic and chronic forms.

E. Accompanied by at least one of the following:
  1. Ipsilateral lacrimation and/or conjunctival injection
  2. Ipsilateral rhinorrhea and/or nasal congestion
  3. Ipsilateral cheek swelling
  4. Photophobia and/or phonophobia
  5. Nausea and/or vomiting	

F. Not attributed to another disorder	Dental pathology may be very difficult to differentiate and needs careful assessment.

around the alveolar process (62%) and mucosal sites (32%).[5,7] Pain referral was to perioral structures (eg, lips, chin) in 35% of patients, to the periorbital region (usually infraorbital) in 35%, and to the preauricular region in 30%[5] (see Fig 10-3).

Quality and temporal pattern

NVOP is characterized by moderate to strong, pulsating, episodic, and unilateral pain.[3,5-8] In 48% of patients, the pain throbs, and in 35% of patients, the pain wakes them from sleep.[3,5] Pain may last from minutes to hours (45% to 72% of patients) or, more rarely, continues for more than 24 hours (28% to 55% of patients).[5,7,8] Many cases are characterized by a chronic high-frequency pattern.

Accompanying phenomena

Pain can be accompanied by various local autonomic signs, and these were found in 36% of patients.[7] Specifically, tearing (10%), nasal congestion (7%), a complaint of excessive sweating (7%), and a feeling of swelling or fullness (7%),

particularly in the cheek, were reported.[5] Other phenomena, such as photophobia or phonophobia (14%) and nausea (24%) are observed.[5,7,8] Often, patients report dental hypersensitivity to cold, which may lead to diagnostic confusion.[4,6] Pain may be aggravated by physical activity.[8] Based on these conditions, the diagnostic criteria outlined in Table 10-9 are suggested.

Clinical examples

The clinical experiences of the authors suggest that two temporal patterns are common: an episodic form and a chronic form. Case 10-3 describes an episodic type of NVOP in which pain attacks were spaced apart and no background pain was experienced (Fig 10-7). However, the patient suffered high-frequency pain (six to seven attacks per 24 hours) lasting up to 1 hour and similar in some ways to an atypical paroxysmal hemicrania. Treatment with indomethacin was unsuccessful, but propranolol provided long-term relief. Because of the high frequency, preventive therapy was used.

The patient described in Case 10-4, on the other hand, is representative of a chronic

CASE 10-3

NVOP (episodic type) in a 21-year-old woman.

Present complaint: Strong paroxysmal pain in the right mandibular area. The pain is spontaneous and wakes the patient from sleep. Six or seven attacks typically occur within 24 hours, each lasting from 20 to 60 minutes. Pain is typically evoked by ingestion of cold or hot drinks.

History of present complaint: Pain started about 5 months ago, and its frequency, intensity, and duration increased with time. Pain responded minimally to analgesics. The referring physician suspected paroxysmal hemicrania and prescribed indomethacin with no response.

Physical examination: Oral structures and the masticatory system were clinically normal. No caries lesions were detected on physical and radiographic examinations (see Fig 10-7). Cold application evoked strong pain, lasting about 30 seconds after application (overshoot) in most of the right mandibular teeth (from central incisor to first molar) and the adjacent vestibular area.

Relevant medical history: The patients is healthy and has no history of migraine.

Diagnosis: NVOP.

Diagnostic and treatment considerations: The type, duration, and frequency of the pain are highly suggestive of paroxysmal hemicrania. However, lack of response to indomethacin and the very high sensitivity to cold application in the teeth led to the diagnosis of NVOP. The patient was started on 80 mg of slow-release propranolol that was increased to 160 mg/day within 3 days. Pain improved markedly within 1 week; the spontaneous pain almost completely disappeared and no longer woke the patient.

Upon examination a week after drug initiation, only the teeth were sensitive to cold, but there was no overshoot. The dosage was adjusted to 80 mg/day, and the patient was symptom free 4 weeks after initiation of treatment. The patient was monitored for another 6 months. Certain points typical of this condition should be emphasized: the quick response to propranolol (1 week), the cold allodynia not only of the teeth but also the adjacent vestibular area, and the high daily frequency (six or seven a day) and short duration (20 to 60 minutes) of attacks, which is not typical of migraine.

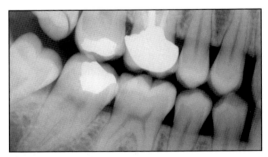

Fig 10-7 Bitewing radiograph of the patient described in Case 10-3. Very high sensitivity with overshoot to cold application was found for all right mandibular teeth and the adjacent vestibular area. No local pathology was identified.

type of NVOP in which a constant, throbbing, low-grade pain is present in the mandibular area with severe exacerbations accompanied by migrainous features (Figs 10-8 and 10-9). Etodolac (a cyclooxygenase 2 inhibitor; see chapter 15) and analgesic combination drugs were unsuccessful. Rizatriptan provided rapid relief of attacks, and prophylactic therapy was indicated because of the high frequency observed in pain diaries and the background pain. Note the similarities to chronic daily headache, particularly hemicrania continua and chronic migraine.

Epidemiology

The onset of NVOP is around 40 to 50 years of age (mean, 43 years), and there is a female-male ratio of 3.25:1.[5,7] Time to diagnosis was around 34 to 101 months (range, 1 to 528 months), which attests to the diagnostic difficulties presented by these patients.[5,7] In 38% to 45% of patients, the pain was diagnosed as secondary to dental pathology, and patients underwent dental treatment with no success.[4,5,7] Some patients (36%) underwent repeated extractions in the same quadrant.[7]

Treatment

Low-dose amitriptyline, propranolol, and NSAIDs have been successful in the treatment of NVOP,[4–7] and response to triptan was reported in all patients in one study.[8] The drugs

CASE 10-4

NVOP (chronic type) in a 24-year-old woman.

Present complaint: Strong (VAS 5 to 9.5), pulsating pain in the posterior mandibular area, sometimes on the right side and sometimes on the left but never bilateral. When pain is very strong, it radiates to the temporal area (see Fig 10-8). Pain wakes the patient from sleep and may be associated with nausea, dizziness, and sometimes vomiting.

History of present complaint: Pain started about 2 years ago with a variable frequency of once a week to once a month. Each pain attack lasts from half a day to 4 days and is not related to menstrual period. During an attack, chewing and physical activity increase pain. Since the pain started, she has been wearing a bite guard, and arthrocentesis was performed on both temporomandibular joints. None of these treatments eased her pain.

Physical examination: Both right and left masseters and sternomastoid muscles were very tender to palpation. Mouth opening was normal (46 mm), and the temporomandibular joints were not tender to palpation and moved freely. No tenderness was detected from other masticatory or pericranial muscles, including the temporalis.

Relevant medical history: For the past couple of years, the patient has been taking 100 mg fluvoxamine per day for anxiety and depressive episodes as well as 3.75 mg zopiclone at bedtime to aid sleep onset. The patient has multiple allergies, and asthma is suspected.

Diagnosis: NVOP.

Diagnostic and treatment considerations: Although the symptomatology of this patient is similar to MWoA, the strict confinement of the pain to the mandibular area justifies a distinct diagnosis of NVOP. Unfortunately, because of the pain location, the patient was mistreated with a bite guard and arthrocentesis of the temporomandibular joint. The continuous nature suggests similarity to chronic migraine.

Initially, the patient had reported that the pain was episodic in nature, so treatment with an abortive strategy was begun. Nonspecific abortives were unsuccessful, including etodolac 600 mg and an analgesic-antiemetic combination (Migraleve: buclizine 6.25 mg, acetaminophen 500 mg, codeine 8 mg, dioctyl sodium sulphosuccinate 10 mg). The next resort was rizatriptan 10 mg, which proved very effective in shortening attacks but caused dizziness and tiredness; hence, the dose was reduced to 5 mg. The pain diary revealed interictal, low-grade background pain and a high frequency of attacks (see Fig 10-9), so the patient was started on a prophylactic regimen of slow-release divalproex. This was preferred over amitriptyline because the patient already was on an SSRI, and propranolol was contraindicated because of the possibility of asthma.

and guidelines outlined in the migraine treatment section are relevant for NVOP, as is the treatment algorithm (see Fig 10-4). Abortive or prophylactic treatments should be considered, but it has been the authors' experience that prophylactic treatment is usually indicated because of the daily or almost daily pain and the high sensitivity to cold food ingestion.

Differential diagnosis

Because of the dental thermal hypersensitivity observed in NVOP, the differential diagnosis includes irreversible pulpitis and cold-stimulus (or ice-cream) headache. Cold-stimulus headache occurs particularly in persons with a history of migraine and is not associated with dental pathology[206] (Table 10-10). Pain follows the passage of cold material over the palate and posterior pharyngeal wall and does not originate in the teeth; facial pain is produced in the midfrontal region or around the ears, probably referred by the trigeminal and glossopharyngeal nerves, respectively. No treatment other than sensible caution is needed. Prolonged gingival cold allodynia should be considered in patients with atypical odontalgia, but these cases are relatively rare, and their background pain pattern is very different from that of NVOP.[207] Although initially pulpal pain may resemble NVCPs, careful history and examination should easily differentiate the two conditions (see Table 10-10). Additionally, trial triptan treatment should be considered in more complicated cases. Successful treatment with triptans might subsequently lead to implementation of migraine prophylaxis.[8]

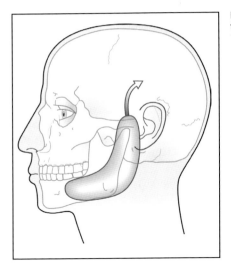

Fig 10-8 Pain location for the patient described in Case 10-4.

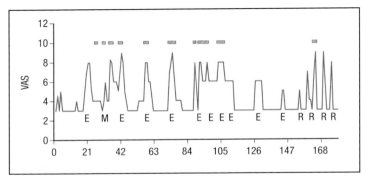

Fig 10-9 Mean daily VAS for the patient described in Case 10-4. The patient suffered constant low-grade background pain (VAS 3). Superimposed on these, there were exacerbations of moderate to severe pain (VAS 6 to 8). The *gray rectangles* above the plot show when the patient was woken by nocturnal pain. The patient tried abortive therapies with etodolac (E), Migraleve (M; Pfizer), and rizatriptan (R). Only rizatriptan significantly shortened the attack duration. Because of the high frequency of attacks, the patient was started on sustained-release divalproex.

Nosologic issues

Descriptions of perioral pain with distinct neurovascular-type features have been reported that may be a manifestation of migraine at atypical locations or a discrete diagnostic entity.[5,7,8] Continued use of the term *lower-half migraine* may be tempting,[7] yet although facial pain was not unusual in migraine (8.9%), isolated facial migraine was exceptionally rare (0.2%).[28] The authors believe lower-half migraines may form a distinct subdiagnosis and deserve classification.[3–5] Indeed, until recently no attempt had been made to characterize or categorize these patients.[3-5,7,8] NVOP has enough differentiating factors to distinctly classify it, the most prominent being oral and perioral or midface[9] location, late age of onset, neurovascular pain secondary to trauma, and neurovascular pulpitis.[5–8,12] As a migraine variant, one would expect to see most patients with longer pain attacks, a younger onset, and more photophobia, phonophobia, and nausea.[5,8] The similarities to the cluster headache

Table 10-10 Craniofacial pain in response to cold ingestion: Comparative features

Parameter	NVOP	Irreversible pulpitis	Cold-stimulus headache
History of			
Migraine	+	−	+
Past endodontics	+	−	−
Autonomic/systemic signs	+	−	−
Treatment/effectiveness			
Endodontics	−	++	−
NSAIDs	+	+/−	−
Amitriptyline	++	−	−
Beta-adrenergic blocker	++	−	−
Clinical signs			
Teeth:			
Hypersensitive to cold	+	++	−*
Tender to percussion	−	++ (80%)	−
Pain changes location/side shift	+	−	−
Carious (clinical/radiologic)	−	++	−
Soft tissues:			
Swelling	+	−	−
Redness	+	−	−

*Pain is induced by cold application to palatal and pharyngeal mucosa.

Table 10-11 Differential diagnosis: Migraine and NVOP

Parameter	Migraine	NVOP
Age of onset (years)	20 to 40	40 to 50
Male-female ratio	1:2	1:2.5
Location (mostly unilateral)	Forehead, temple	Intraoral/lower face
Duration	Hours to days	Minutes to hours
Character of pain	Throbbing, deep, continuous	Throbbing, paroxysmal
Pain intensity	Moderate to severe	Moderate to severe
Precipitating factors	Stress, hunger, menstrual period, and others	Sometimes cold foods
Associated signs	Nausea, photophobia, visual aura	Cheek swelling and redness, tearing
Treatment: abortive	NSAIDs, triptans	NSAIDs, triptans
Treatment: prophylactic	Amitriptyline, beta-blockers, valproate	Amitriptyline, beta-blockers, valproate

group are limited by the fact that there is an overwhelming female preponderance and that treatment response is not similar. Although some patients with NVOP had features similar to those observed in hemicrania continua, they did not respond to indomethacin. Treatment of NVOP with classic antimigraine drugs has been successful and firmly establishes an association with migraine.[5–8] In chronic cases, good results have been achieved with prophylactic propranolol, divalproex sodium, or, when muscle tenderness is prominent, amitriptyline. Some cases of episodic NVOP respond quite well to NSAIDs, particularly naproxen sodium. Similarly, some patients respond excellently to triptans, but the response rate seems to be lower than that in typical migraine.[3] A summary of migraine and NVOP features is presented in

Table 10-11. NVOP is characterized by a chronic pain pattern, and some patients describe a history of episodic migraine, which suggests similarities to chronic migraine.[5,7] However, unlike chronic migraine, pain in NVOP is largely unilateral and throbbing, and exacerbations of pain are not characterized by more prominent or typical migrainous features as in chronic migraine. They also differ in treatment response.

To conclude, although the head and face are intimately related, diagnostic classifications of headache and orofacial pain are not sufficiently integrated. The IHS classification system for headaches[1] does not adequately cover currently accepted orofacial pain entities.[3] As a result, it states that "a subset, of otherwise typical patients, has facial location of pain, which is called 'facial migraine' in the literature; there is no evidence that these patients form a separate subgroup of migraine patients."[1] Regrettably, in the *International Classification of Headache Disorders,* third edition,[1] the bibliography for the "Headache or facial pain attributed to other disorder of cranium, neck, eyes, ears, nose, sinuses, teeth, mouth or other facial or cervical structure" section is limited to references no later than 2001. Newer data are required to make a prudent decision on the classification of NVOP.

Pathophysiology of Migraine

Historically, migraine was considered to be a vascular phenomenon. The aura was due to transient ischemia secondary to vasoconstriction, and the headache was secondary to rebound vasodilation and mechanical activation of perivascular nociceptors.[114] Current evidence, however, does not support this hypothesis. Magnetic resonance angiography has clearly shown that changes in flow or vessel diameter in migraine are a result of pain in the trigeminal ophthalmic division.[208] Vasodilation of meningeal and/or extracranial arteries is neither necessary nor sufficient to cause migraine pain.[209] Researchers believe migraine headache is a manifestation of a brain state of altered excitability capable of activating the trigeminovascular system in genetically suscep-

tible people.[210] Advances in in vivo and in vitro technologies indicate that cortical spreading depression and activation of the trigeminovascular system and its constituent neuropeptides, as well as neuronal and glial ion channels and transporters, contribute to the putative cortical excitatory/inhibitory imbalance that renders migraineurs susceptible to an attack.[209]

The trigeminovascular system

The trigeminovascular system consists of trigeminal neurons (mainly ophthalmic) and the blood vessels (usually cerebral) they innervate (Fig 10-10). The peripheral axons synapse with cranial structures and craniofacial blood vessels (predominantly pain-producing large cranial vessels), and the centrally projecting fibers synapse in the trigeminal nucleus caudalis and the upper two cervical divisions, that is, the trigeminocervical complex.[211] A plexus of mainly unmyelinated fibers from the ophthalmic division and the upper cervical dorsal roots surrounds the cerebral and pial vessels, the large venous sinuses, and the dura mater. These fibers contain substance P and CGRP, which are released when the trigeminal ganglion is stimulated.[212] Nerve fibers vary in their neuropeptide content. Sensory fibers are rich in substance P, CGRP, nitric oxide, and neurokinin A; parasympathetic fibers contain vasoactive intestinal polypeptide (VIP) and nitric oxide; and sympathetic fibers express neuropeptide Y.[213,214] These peptides (nitric oxide, substance P, CGRP, VIP) induce vasodilation and plasma extravasation and are released into the bloodstream; therefore, they are assayed as indicators of trigeminal and autonomic nerve fiber activation. Recently, a novel retinothalamocortical pathway that carries photic signals from the retina to the thalamic trigeminovascular neurons was discovered, and photic signals that converge on the nociceptive pathway provide data on the mechanism by which light intensifies migraine headache.[215]

Neurogenic inflammation

Neurogenic inflammation occurs when trigeminal afferents are stimulated antidromically and release vasoactive neuropeptides that induce mast-cell degranulation and plasma extravasation, which play a central role in the initiation

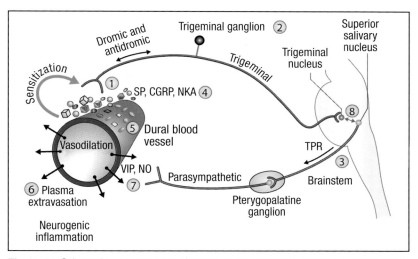

Fig 10-10 Schematic representation of events at the trigeminal-cerebrovascular junction (1). Cell bodies of cerebrovascular and other orofacial nociceptors reside in the trigeminal ganglion (2) with their second-order neurons in the trigeminal nucleus caudalis (3). Neurogenic inflammation: Vasoactive peptides such as CGRP, substance P (SP), and neurokinin A (NKA) are released from trigeminal C fibers (4) after antidromic activation, possibly secondary to brainstem dysfunction. These peptides bind to receptors (5) and induce vasodilation (6), plasma extravasation, and further nociceptor activation. Although rare, local autonomic signs such as lacrimation have been reported in migraine. This is thought to be secondary to reflex parasympathetic activation (the trigeminal-parasympathetic reflex, with the parasympathetic fibers containing vasoactive intestinal polypeptide [VIP] and nitric oxide [NO]) (7) mediated by connections between the trigeminal system and the superior salivary nucleus (8) at brainstem level (see also chapter 11). Similar processes may also occur within oral and dental tissues leading to a primary NVOP syndrome.

of neurovascular-type headaches. Although the main function of trigeminal sensory neurons is the transduction of orthodromic information, additional roles have become apparent, such as an antidromic neuropeptide release at the periphery. These neuropeptides include substance P, neurokinin A, and CGRP—the most potent vasodilator. The fibers releasing these neuropeptides are characteristic of thin, unmyelinated C fibers. When released, the neuropeptides initiate a cascade of events, including mast-cell degranulation, platelet aggregation, vasodilation, and plasma extravasation,[216] that is, neurogenic inflammation (see Fig 10-10). CGRP receptors are localized in the trigeminal nucleus in a fiber network partially colocalized with granular CGRP-immunoreactive structures but not on second-order neurons, which suggests the possibility of CGRP-mediated signaling between central terminals of primary afferents.[217]

The headache phase of migraine depends on the activation and sensitization of trigeminal nociceptors that innervate the large blood vessels in the meninges. These processes then lead to sequential activation (and, in most patients, sensitization) of second- and third-order central trigeminovascular neurons, which in turn activate different areas of the brainstem and forebrain, resulting in pain and other migrainous symptoms.[209] Also consistent with the neurogenic inflammation hypothesis is the evidence that the headache-triggering substance ethanol activates peptidergic meningeal trigeminal afferents (via different receptors: TRPV1 and TRPA1), causing CGRP release and neurogenic dura inflammatory responses in animals used experimentally.[218] However, the mechanisms of action of CGRP during a migraine attack and the mechanisms underlying the hypersensitivity of migraineurs to CGRP-mediated modulation of nociceptive pathways remain unclear.[209]

Additionally, the vasodilatory effect is thought to be partly mediated by reflex activation of the parasympathetic system and the release of VIP[219] (see Fig 10-10). Noxious stimulation of the superior sagittal sinus induces activity in neurons of the superior salivary nucleus,[220] an important relay in the cranial parasympathetic outflow to the lacrimal and nasal glands, as well as autonomic signs.

However, vasodilation of meningeal and/or extracranial arteries is neither necessary nor sufficient to cause migraine pain. Neurogenic inflammation is one key mechanism that may underlie the activation and sensitization of perivascular meningeal nociceptors, but the endogenous processes promoting the inflammation during migraine attacks remain unclear.[209] Furthermore, functional analysis of familial hemiplegic migraine in mouse models supports the view of migraine as a disorder of brain excitability characterized by deficient regulation of the cortical excitatory/inhibitory balance as well as the view of cortical spreading depression as a key migraine trigger. In fact, the familial hemiplegic migraine mouse models show enhanced cortical excitatory synaptic transmission with unaltered inhibitory synaptic transmission and facilitation of induction and propagation of cortical spreading depression due to enhanced glutamatergic neurotransmission.[209]

The trigeminocervical complex

After meningeal irritation, neuronal activation is detected in the spinal trigeminal nucleus caudalis (SpVC), thus accounting for the referral of pain to the neck that is commonly observed in the clinic. Activation of trigeminal neurons in the subnucleus caudalis was detected, accompanied by vasodilation and plasma extravasation; all were attenuated by trigeminal nerve section.[221] Available data describe projections of functionally identified trigeminovascular neurons from SpVC to the parabrachial area; anterior hypothalamic, lateral hypothalamic, and perifornical hypothalamic areas; and lateral preoptic, zona incerta, ventral posteromedial, and parafascicular thalamic nuclei. In addition, the ventrolateral area of the upper cervical and medullary dorsal horn, an area containing most of the second-order trigeminovascular neurons, projects to the ventrolateral periaqueductal gray (PAG) matter, rostral trigeminal spinal nuclei, nucleus of the solitary tract, brainstem reticular areas, superior salivary nuclei, and cuneiform nuclei.[210]

Stimulation of a lateralized structure, the middle meningeal artery, activated neurons bilaterally in the cat and monkey brain,[222] a finding that is consistent with the fact that up to one-third of patients complain of bilateral pain.

Central pain activation and modulation

Increasing evidence from animal studies supports the idea that cortical spreading depression can cause sustained activation of meningeal nociceptors and central trigeminovascular neurons and can thus initiate headache mechanisms. Also, in the period between attacks, migraineurs show abnormal processing of sensory information due to dysfunctional regulation of cortical excitability.[209] A central noxious event has been shown to activate trigeminal afferents (ie, pain) with reflex parasympathetic activation. Parasympathetic nerve section attenuated vasodilation but not plasma extravasation.[221] Plasma extravasation was thus clearly shown to be under trigeminal nerve control, though vasodilation seemed to be dependent on intact trigeminal and parasympathetic systems, which suggests involvement of a trigeminal-parasympathetic reflex. A wide variety of symptoms that are associated with migraine headache, such as irritability, fatigue, sleepiness, exaggerated emotional responses, nausea, and loss of appetite, may appear before or after the onset of the headache. Most likely, the symptoms that appear before the onset of migraine (ie, prodrome) are related to abnormal neuronal activity in cortical, diencephalic, and/or brainstem structures. In contrast, the most likely explanation for symptoms that appear after the onset of migraine is the bombardment of supramedullary brain structures involved in sensory, affective, endocrine, and autonomic functions by intracranial pain signals originating in the meninges.[210]

During MWoA, human positron emission tomography studies demonstrate activation of the PAG matter in the region of the dorsal raphe nucleus, the dorsal pons, and near the locus coeruleus.[223] Neuronal inhibition via 5-hydroxytryptamine (5-HT) receptors can occur at two levels: *(1)* prejunctional, which will inhibit neuropeptide release from primary afferents and neurotransmission,[224] and *(2)* postjunctional, which inhibits neurons in SpVC.[225]

This activity may reflect 5-HT$_{1B}$, 5-HT$_{1D}$, or 5-HT$_{1F}$ receptor agonist action, or a combination of these.[226] Solid evidence exists for the synthesis of 5-HT$_{1D}$ and 5-HT$_{1F}$ receptors in human trigeminal ganglion,[227] and these locate to small and medium-sized neurons, often co-localizing with glutamate and CGRP.[228] Thus, 5-HT$_{1D}$ and 5-HT$_{1F}$ receptors are in a prime location to inhibit release of the neuropeptides that are intimately involved in the pathogenesis of migraine. Migraine-like headaches are induced when PAG areas are electrically stimulated[229] or triggered by structural pathologies affecting the PAG matter.[230] Iron homeostasis in the PAG matter has been demonstrated to be progressively impaired in MWA, MWoA, and chronic headache.[231] These results support the hypothesis that PAG is a major element in the pathophysiology of migraine attacks, possibly acting as a central generator or as a permissive dysfunctional control of trigeminovascular nociception.

Observed widespread allodynia is consistent with third-order neuronal sensitization, such as in thalamic neurons clearly supporting a central nervous system component to the pathophysiology of migraine.[232] The establishment of sensitization is a crucial negative factor in determining the outcome of triptan treatment, so early and aggressive intervention is advised; migraine attacks in humans treated with triptans before onset of allodynia respond significantly better than those accompanied by allodynia.[232]

Figure 10-10 summarizes the brainstem regions, the neurovascular interaction, and higher brain centers thought to underlie pain in migraine and NVOP.

Pathophysiology of Neurovascular Orofacial Pain

Primary NVOP in the lower two-thirds of the face accompanied by systemic and autonomic signs raises various issues relating to mechanisms. The pathophysiology of NVOP may be based on migraine. If so, researchers need to analyze the possibility that neurogenic inflammation occurs in the oral and perioral tissues and therefore must consider its possible role in the phenotype of NVOP.

Neurogenic inflammation in oral tissues and dental pulp

Nerve fibers entering the dental pulp have been identified as unmyelinated C fibers and autonomic nerves and myelinated Aδ and Aβ fibers (see chapters 2 and 6). Nerve fibers exhibiting substance P– and CGRP-positive immunoreactivity are present in the dental pulp and oral mucosa in several species, including humans.[214] The levels of these two sensory neuropeptides as well as two endogenous opioids, methionine-enkephalin and β-endorphin, were studied in human dental pulp. After 24 hours of an intrusive stimulus associated with discomfort, only substance P significantly increased, clarifying the role of neurogenic inflammation in early injury response.[233] Analysis of human dental pulp revealed significantly greater expression of CGRP, substance P, and VIP in permanent teeth relative to primary counterparts.[234] This may explain the lack of children in reports of NVOP.[5,7] After antidromic electrical nerve stimulation, neurogenic inflammation has been demonstrated in the dental pulp of dogs and in the dental pulp, lower lip, and oral mucosa of rats.[235,236] This effect was not attenuated after sympathectomy.[237] Involvement of adjacent teeth suggests that collateral C-fiber innervation exists within the pulps of molar teeth in the same dental quadrant[237] and may partly explain referral patterns in primary NVOP. The anatomical substrate for neurovascular tooth pain is therefore present.

Because neurogenic inflammation in the trigeminovascular system seems to play a central role in the genesis of NVCP, the same mechanism could function in the oral mucosa and teeth. Researchers have postulated that the trigeminovascular system causes some of its effects by neurovascular activation within the space limited by the skull, a closed system that may rapidly lead to pressure buildup and increased nociceptor activation. This system is replicated in the dental pulp, which is similarly confined by the surrounding dental hard tissues; it is feasible that pressure buildup plays a role in intrapulpal nociceptor activation. For example, Aδ fibers have been shown to be sensitive to the increased intrapulpal pressure after plasma extravasation.[238] However, homeostatic mechanisms limit pressure buildup in the pulp after antidromic stimulation,[239] probably by reabsorption into the circulation. This may explain clinical observations that in spite of pulpitis-like symptoms in teeth of patients with NVOP, spontaneous pulp necrosis is rare.

Additionally, activation of 5-HT$_{1B/1D}$ receptors, by local injection of naratriptan into ventrolateral PAG matter, produces selective inhibition of trigeminovascular nociceptive afferent input but not facial afferents.[240] This finding may have important consequences for the treatment of other neurovascular pains located in the orofacial region, such as cluster headache and NVOP.

The trigeminal-parasympathetic reflex in the orofacial region

The trigeminal-parasympathetic reflex is thought to be important in the clinical phenotype of migraine and TACs. Trigeminal pain, particularly in the ophthalmic branch, initiates reflex activation of the parasympathetic afferents and induces autonomic signs. In NVOP isolated to the lower face, the question is whether the trigeminal-parasympathetic reflex is also activated.

The trigeminal-parasympathetic reflex has been shown in animals after stimulation of the lingual nerve.[241] Stimulation of the infraorbital nerve and the maxillary buccal gingiva in cats[216] or painful stimulation of tooth pulp in humans induces an increase in ipsilateral blood flow to the lip.[242] Reflex salivation secondary to experimental lingual nerve stimulation has been reported and has also been observed in patients with craniofacial pain.

An oral trigeminal-parasympathetic reflex that is activated by intradermatomal stimuli is therefore apparent. However, some patients with NVOP present with tearing and mandibular pain, that is, cross-dermatomal activation of the trigeminal-parasympathetic reflex. Cross-dermatomal activation has been experimentally demonstrated; electrical stimuli to the infraorbital nerve induce vasodilation in the ipsilateral lower lip of cats.[216] Such cross-dermatomal reflexes could therefore explain clinical reports of lacrimation in mandibular and maxillary pain syndromes (eg, in NVOP of mandibular teeth). However, there is no experimental evidence of ocular autonomic signs after peripheral stimuli to the mandibular region. Capsaicin injected into the forehead induces a rapid ipsilateral autonomic response, but injection of capsaicin into the mandibular region (third trigeminal division) does not.[243] In mild to moderate experimental pain in the mandibular branches of the trigeminal nerve, the authors found no reflex lacrimation (unpublished observations). Experimental ophthalmic pain will induce vasodilation in the internal carotid artery, whereas mandibular pain will not.[244] From these data, the authors conclude that patients with pain in the distribution of the mandibular divisions accompanied by such ocular autonomic signs as lacrimation are not driven via peripheral activation of the trigeminal-parasympathetic reflex; therefore, central mechanisms are likely candidates. This may also explain the relative paucity of autonomic signs in NVOP.

Conclusion

Migraine is a common and debilitating condition with clear but complex genetic components. Clinical presentation is heterogenous with features that include neurologic disturbances, alterations in sensory sensitivity, mood changes, and autonomic dysfunction. The introduction of triptans represented a remarkable advancement in the treatment of and research on migraine headache. However, recent expert opinions concluded that triptans have failed to show superiority over more standard and cheaper drugs such as aspirin or aspirin plus metoclopramide; thus, there is a need to develop new non-triptan antimigraine drugs. Unfortunately, attempts to develop new drugs based on CGRP receptor antagonists and inducible nitric oxide synthase inhibitors have so far failed. Research suggests that episodic dysfunction of brainstem regions may play a key role in migraine pain, either as central generators or as faulty modulation, particularly the PAG matter, a pain-inhibiting structure. These studies have relied on advanced neuroimaging that may evolve into a diagnostic test. Much importance has been given to mechanisms underlying the cortical excitability that has been suggested to be dysfunctional in migraine. TMS and TENS have opened an interesting perspective for noninvasive neurostimulation for symptomatic and preventive treatment of migraine. The management of migraine is in the midst of far-reaching changes because of advancements in neuroimaging, pharmacogenomics, and molecular biology techniques. The discovery of the genes underlying familial hemiplegic migraine suggests that migraine may involve at least one or more channelopathies and will lead to new therapeutic targets for headache.

The nosologic status of primary NVCP in the lower face is at present unclear. Although the head and face are intimately related, diagnostic classifications of headache and orofacial pain are not sufficiently integrated. The authors suggest that this entity be referred to as *NVOP*, a descriptive term that stresses the anatomical location and suspected unique mechanisms of this type of pain. The relationship between NVOP and migraine needs more research to clarify common and specific mechanisms and responses to therapy.

Choosing wisely

In an effort to draw attention to tests and procedures associated with low-value care in headache medicine, the American Headache Society joined the Choosing Wisely initiative of the American Board of Internal Medicine Foundation. Following are the five recommendations approved by the American Headache Society's board of directors[245]:

1. Do not perform neuroimaging studies in patients with stable headaches that meet criteria for migraine.
2. Do not perform computed tomography imaging for headache when magnetic resonance imaging is available, except in emergency settings.
3. Do not recommend surgical deactivation of migraine trigger points outside of a clinical trial.
4. Do not prescribe opioid- or butalbital-containing medications as a first-line treatment for recurrent headache disorders.

5. Do not recommend prolonged or frequent use of over-the-counter pain medications for headache.

References

1. Headache Classification Committee of the International Headache Society. The International Classification of Headache Disorders, ed 3 (beta version). Cephalalgia 2013;33:629–808.
2. Goadsby PJ. Neuroimaging in headache. Microsc Res Tech 2001;53:179–187.
3. Benoliel R, Birman N, Eliav E, Sharav Y. The International Classification of Headache Disorders: Accurate diagnosis of orofacial pain? Cephalalgia 2008;28:752–762.
4. Benoliel R, Sharav Y, Eliav E. Neurovascular orofacial pain. J Am Dent Assoc 2010;141:1094–1096.
5. Benoliel R, Elishoov H, Sharav Y. Orofacial pain with vascular-type features. Oral Surg Oral Med Oral Pathol Oral Radiol Endod 1997;84:506–512.
6. Czerninsky R, Benoliel R, Sharav Y. Odontalgia in vascular orofacial pain. J Orofac Pain 1999;13:196–200.
7. Peñarrocha M, Bandrés A, Peñarrocha M, Bagán JV. Lower-half facial migraine: A report of 11 cases. J Oral Maxillofac Surg 2004;62:1453–1456.
8. Obermann M, Mueller D, Yoon MS, Pageler L, Diener H, Katsarava Z. Migraine with isolated facial pain: A diagnostic challenge. Cephalalgia 2007;27:1278–1282.
9. Daudia AT, Jones NS. Facial migraine in a rhinological setting. Clin Otolaryngol Allied Sci 2002;27:521–525.
10. Lance JW, Goadsby PJ. Mechanism and Management of Headache. Philadelphia: Elsevier, 2005.
11. Gaul C, Sándor PS, Galli U, Palla S, Ettlin DA. Orofacial migraine. Cephalalgia 2007;27:950–952.
12. Dodick DW. Migraine with isolated facial pain: A diagnostic challenge. Cephalalgia 2007;27:1199–1200.
13. Olesen J. The migraines: Introduction. In: Olesen J, Tfelt-Hansen P, Welch KMA (eds). The Headaches, ed 2. Philadelphia: Lippincott Williams & Wilkins, 2000:223–225.
14. Steiner TJ, Scher AI, Stewart WF, Kolodner K, Liberman J, Lipton RB. The prevalence and disability burden of adult migraine in England and their relationships to age, gender and ethnicity. Cephalalgia 2003;23:519–527.
15. Rasmussen BK, Olesen J. Migraine with aura and migraine without aura: An epidemiological study. Cephalalgia 1992;12:221–228.
16. Rasmussen BK, Jensen R, Olesen J. A population-based analysis of the diagnostic criteria of the International Headache Society. Cephalalgia 1991;11:129–134.
17. Kelman L. Migraine pain location: A tertiary care study of 1283 migraineurs. Headache 2005;45:1038–1047.
18. Russell MB, Rasmussen BK, Fenger K, Olesen J. Migraine without aura and migraine with aura are distinct clinical entities: A study of four hundred and eighty-four male and female migraineurs from the general population. Cephalalgia 1996;16:239–245.

19. Stewart WF, Lipton RB, Kolodner K. Migraine disability assessment (MIDAS) score: Relation to headache frequency, pain intensity, and headache symptoms. Headache 2003;43:258–265.

20. Rasmussen BK, Olesen J. Symptomatic and non-symptomatic headaches in a general population. Neurology 1992;42:1225–1231.

21. Zagami AS, Rasmussen BK. Symptomatology of migraine. In: Olesen J, Tfelt-Hansen P, Welch KMA (eds). The Headaches, ed 2. Philadelphia: Lippincott Williams & Wilkins, 2000:337–343.

22. Pryse-Phillips W, Findlay H, Tugwell P, Edmeads J, Murray TJ, Nelson RF. A Canadian population survey on the clinical, epidemiologic and societal impact of migraine and tension-type headache. Can J Neurol Sci 1992;19:333–339.

23. Magnusson JE, Becker WJ. Migraine frequency and intensity: Relationship with disability and psychological factors. Headache 2003;43:1049–1059.

24. Alstadhaug KB, Salvesen R, Bekkelund SI. Seasonal variation in migraine. Cephalalgia 2005;25:811–816.

25. Viticchi G, Silvestrini M, Falsetti L, et al. Time delay from onset to diagnosis of migraine. Headache 2011;51:232–236.

26. Kaup AO, Mathew NT, Levyman C, Kailasam J, Meadors LA, Villarreal SS. 'Side locked' migraine and trigeminal autonomic cephalgias: Evidence for clinical overlap. Cephalalgia 2003;23:43–49.

27. Lai TH, Fuh JL, Wang SJ. Cranial autonomic symptoms in migraine: Characteristics and comparison with cluster headache. J Neurol Neurosurg Psychiatry 2009;80:1116–1119.

28. Yoon MS, Mueller D, Hansen N, et al. Prevalence of facial pain in migraine: A population-based study. Cephalalgia 2010;30:92–96.

29. Gelfand AA, Reider AC, Goadsby PJ. Cranial autonomic symptoms in pediatric migraine are the rule, not the exception. Neurology 2013;81:431–436.

30. Giffin NJ, Ruggiero L, Lipton RB, et al. Premonitory symptoms in migraine: An electronic diary study. Neurology 2003;60:935–940.

31. Martin VT, Behbehani MM. Toward a rational understanding of migraine trigger factors. Med Clin North Am 2001;85:911–941.

32. Chabriat H, Danchot J, Michel P, Joire JE, Henry P. Precipitating factors of headache. A prospective study in a national control-matched survey in migraineurs and nonmigraineurs. Headache 1999;39:335–338.

33. Rasmussen BK. Migraine and tension-type headache in a general population: Precipitating factors, female hormones, sleep pattern and relation to lifestyle. Pain 1993;53:65–72.

34. Breslau N, Rasmussen BK. The impact of migraine: Epidemiology, risk factors, and co-morbidities. Neurology 2001;56(6, suppl):S4–S12.

35. Marcus DA, Scharff L, Turk D, Gourley LM. A double-blind provocative study of chocolate as a trigger of headache. Cephalalgia 1997;17:855–862.

36. Rockett FC, de Oliveira VR, Castro K, Chaves ML, Perla Ada S, Perry ID. Dietary aspects of migraine trigger factors. Nutr Rev 2012;70:337–356.

37. Smetana GW. The diagnostic value of historical features in primary headache syndromes: A comprehensive review. Arch Intern Med 2000;160:2729–2737.

38. Dodick DW, Eross EJ, Parish JM, Silber M. Clinical, anatomical, and physiologic relationship between sleep and headache. Headache 2003;43:282–292.

39. Kelman L, Rains JC. Headache and sleep: Examination of sleep patterns and complaints in a large clinical sample of migraineurs. Headache 2005;45:904–910.

40. Leone M, Bussone G. A review of hormonal findings in cluster headache. Evidence for hypothalamic involvement. Cephalalgia 1993;13:309–317.

41. Göder R, Fritzer G, Kapsokalyvas A, et al. Polysomnographic findings in nights preceding a migraine attack. Cephalalgia 2001;21:31–37.

42. Ceccarelli I, Fiorenzani P, Grasso G, et al. Estrogen and mu-opioid receptor antagonists counteract the 17 beta-estradiol-induced licking increase and interferon-gamma reduction occurring during the formalin test in male rats. Pain 2004;111:181–190.

43. Martin VT, Wernke S, Mandell K, et al. Defining the relationship between ovarian hormones and migraine headache. Headache 2005;45:1190–1201.

44. Granella F, Sances G, Allais G, et al. Characteristics of menstrual and nonmenstrual attacks in women with menstrually related migraine referred to headache centres. Cephalalgia 2004;24:707–716.

45. Colson NJ, Lea RA, Quinlan S, MacMillan J, Griffiths LR. The estrogen receptor 1 G594A polymorphism is associated with migraine susceptibility in two independent case/control groups. Neurogenetics 2004;5:129–133.

46. Puri V, Cui L, Liverman CS, et al. Ovarian steroids regulate neuropeptides in the trigeminal ganglion. Neuropeptides 2005;39:409–417.

47. Kelman L. The aura: A tertiary care study of 952 migraine patients. Cephalalgia 2004;24:728–734.

48. Russell MB, Olesen J. A nosographic analysis of the migraine aura in a general population. Brain 1996;119(Pt 2):355–361.

49. Stovner L, Hagen K, Jensen R, et al. The global burden of headache: A documentation of headache prevalence and disability worldwide. Cephalalgia 2007;27:193–210.

50. Stewart WF, Linet MS, Celentano DD, Van Natta M, Ziegler D. Age- and sex-specific incidence rates of migraine with and without visual aura. Am J Epidemiol 1991;134:1111–1120.

51. Lipton RB, Bigal ME. Migraine: epidemiology, impact, and risk factors for progression. Headache 2005;45(1, suppl):S3–S13.

52. Bigal ME, Liberman JN, Lipton RB. Age-dependent prevalence and clinical features of migraine. Neurology 2006;67:246–251.

53. Martins KM, Bordini CA, Bigal ME, Speciali JG. Migraine in the elderly: A comparison with migraine in young adults. Headache 2006;46:312–316.

54. Buse DC, Loder EW, Gorman JA, et al. Sex differences in the prevalence, symptoms, and associated features of migraine, probable migraine and other severe headache: results of the American Migraine Prevalence and Prevention (AMPP) Study. Headache 2013;53:1278–1299.

55. Raggi A, Giovannetti AM, Quintas R, et al. A systematic review of the psychosocial difficulties relevant to patients with migraine. J Headache Pain 2012;13:595–606.

56. Fuller-Thomson E, Schrumm M, Brennenstuhl S. Migraine and despair: Factors associated with depression and suicidal ideation among Canadian migraineurs in a population-based study. Depress Res Treat 2013;2013.

57. Ruscheweyh R, Müller M, Blum B, Straube A. Correlation of headache frequency and psychosocial impairment in migraine: A cross-sectional study. Headache 2013;54:861–871.

58. D'Amico D, Grazzi L, Usai S, Leonardi M, Raggi A. Disability and quality of life in headache: Where we are now and where we are heading. Neurol Sci 2013;34(suppl 1):S1–S5.

59. Evans RW, de Tommaso M. Migraine and fibromyalgia. Headache 2011;51:295–299.

60. Fernandes G, Franco AL, Gonçalves DA, Speciali JG, Bigal ME, Camparis CM. Temporomandibular disorders, sleep bruxism, and primary headaches are mutually associated. J Orofac Pain 2013;27:14–20.

61. Benoliel R, Sela G, Teich S, Sharav Y. Painful temporomandibular disorders and headaches in 359 dental and medical students. Quintessence 2011;42:73–78.

62. Stuginski-Barbosa J, Macedo HR, Bigal ME, Speciali JG. Signs of temporomandibular disorders in migraine patients: A prospective, controlled study. Clin J Pain 2010;26:418–421.

63. Ashina S, Serrano D, Lipton RB, et al. Depression and risk of transformation of episodic to chronic migraine. J Headache Pain 2012;13:615–624.

64. Breslau N, Schultz L, Lipton R, Peterson E, Welch KM. Migraine headaches and suicide attempt. Headache 2012;52:723–731.

65. Russell MB, Olesen J. Increased familial risk and evidence of genetic factor in migraine. BMJ 1995;311:541–544.

66. Gervil M, Ulrich V, Kaprio J, Olesen J, Russell MB. The relative role of genetic and environmental factors in migraine without aura. Neurology 1999;53:995–999.

67. Ferrari MD, Russell MB. Genetics of migraine. In: Olesen J, Tfelt-Hansen P, Welch KMA (eds). The Headaches, ed 2. Philadelphia: Lippincott Williams & Wilkins, 2000:241–254.

68. Silberstein SD, Dodick DW. Migraine genetics: Part II. Headache 2013;53:1218–1229.

69. Cady R, Schreiber C, Farmer K, Sheftell F. Primary headaches: A convergence hypothesis. Headache 2002;42:204–216.

70. Köseoglu E, Naçar M, Talaslioglu A, Cetinkaya F. Epidemiological and clinical characteristics of migraine and tension type headache in 1146 females in Kayseri, Turkey. Cephalalgia 2003;23:381–388.

71. Zebenholzer K, Wöber C, Kienbacher C, Wöber-Bingöl C. Migrainous disorder and headache of the tension-type not fulfilling the criteria: A follow-up study in children and adolescents. Cephalalgia 2000;20:611–616.

72. Lipton RB, Stewart WF, Diamond S, Diamond ML, Reed M. Prevalence and burden of migraine in the United States: Data from the American Migraine Study II. Headache 2001;41:646–657.

73. Schreiber CP, Hutchinson S, Webster CJ, Ames M, Richardson MS, Powers C. Prevalence of migraine in patients with a history of self-reported or physician-diagnosed "sinus" headache. Arch Intern Med 2004;164:1769–1772.

74. Eross E, Dodick D, Eross M. The Sinus, Allergy and Migraine Study (SAMS). Headache 2007;47:213–224.

75. Baandrup L, Jensen R. Chronic post-traumatic headache—A clinical analysis in relation to the International Headache Classification 2nd edition. Cephalalgia 2005;25:132–138.

76. Goadsby PJ, Sprenger T. Current practice and future directions in the prevention and acute management of migraine. Lancet Neurol 2010;9:285–298.

77. Pryse-Phillips WE, Dodick DW, Edmeads JG, et al. Guidelines for the nonpharmacologic management of migraine in clinical practice. Canadian Headache Society. CMAJ 1998;159:47–54.

78. Campbell JK, Penzien DB, Wall EM. US Headache Consortium: Evidence-Based Guidelines for Migraine Headache: Behavioral and Physical Treatments, 2000.

79. MacGregor EA, Brandes J, Eikermann A. Migraine prevalence and treatment patterns: The Global Migraine and Zolmitriptan Evaluation Survey. Headache 2003;43:19–26.

80. Robbins L. Triptans versus analgesics. Headache 2002;42:903–907.

81. Ferrari A, Spaccapelo L, Sternieri E. Pharmacoepidemiology of triptans in a headache centre. Cephalalgia 2010;30:847–854.

82. Adams J, Barbery G, Lui CW. Complementary and alternative medicine use for headache and migraine: A critical review of the literature. Headache 2013;53:459–473.

83. Diamond M, Cady R. Initiating and optimizing acute therapy for migraine: The role of patient-centered stratified care. Am J Med 2005;118(1, suppl):18S–27S.

84. Matchar DB, Young WB, Rosenberg JH, et al. US Headache Consortium: Evidence-Based Guidelines for Migraine Headache in the Primary Care Setting: Pharmacological Management of Acute Attacks: American Academy of Neurology, 2000.

85. Lipton RB, Stewart WF, Stone AM, Láinez MJ, Sawyer JP. Stratified care vs step care strategies for migraine: The Disability in Strategies of Care (DISC) Study: A randomized trial. JAMA 2000;284:2599–2605.

86. Diener HC, Pfaffenrath V, Pageler L, Peil H, Aicher B. The fixed combination of acetylsalicylic acid, paracetamol and caffeine is more effective than single substances and dual combination for the treatment of headache: A multicentre, randomized, double-blind, single-dose, placebo-controlled parallel group study. Cephalalgia 2005;25:776–787.

87. Rabbie R, Derry S, Moore RA. Ibuprofen with or without an antiemetic for acute migraine headaches in adults. Cochrane Database Syst Rev 2013;4.

88. Moore A, Edwards J, Barden J, McQuay H. Bandolier's Little Book of Pain. Oxford: Oxford University, 2003.

89. Tfelt-Hansen P, McEwen J. Nonsteroidal antiinflammatory drugs in the acute treatment of migraine. In: Olesen J, Tfelt-Hansen P, Welch KMA (eds). The Headaches, ed 2. Philadelphia: Lippincott Williams & Wilkins, 2000:391–397.

90. Bigal ME, Walter S, Rapoport AM. Calcitonin generelated peptide (CGRP) and migraine current understanding and state of development. Headache 2013;53:1230–1244.

91. Millson DS, Tepper SJ, Rapoport AM. Migraine pharmacotherapy with oral triptans: A rational approach to clinical management. Expert Opin Pharmacother 2000;1:391–404.

92. Dahlöf CG, Rapoport AM, Sheftell FD, Lines CR. Rizatriptan in the treatment of migraine. Clin Ther 1999;21:1823–1836.

93. Dahlöf CG, Dodick D, Dowson AJ, Pascual J. How does almotriptan compare with other triptans? A review of data from placebo-controlled clinical trials. Headache 2002;42:99–113.

94. Dahlöf C. Clinical applications of new therapeutic deliveries in migraine. Neurology 2003;61(8, suppl):S31–S34.

95. Dodick D, Brandes J, Elkind A, Mathew N, Rodichok L. Speed of onset, efficacy and tolerability of zolmitriptan nasal spray in the acute treatment of migraine: A randomised, double-blind, placebo-controlled study. CNS Drugs 2005;19:125–136.

96. Derry CJ, Derry S, Moore RA. Sumatriptan (oral route of administration) for acute migraine attacks in adults. Cochrane Database Syst Rev 2012;2.

97. Derry CJ, Derry S, Moore RA. Sumatriptan (rectal route of administration) for acute migraine attacks in adults. Cochrane Database Syst Rev 2012;2.

98. Derry CJ, Derry S, Moore RA. Sumatriptan (intranasal route of administration) for acute migraine attacks in adults. Cochrane Database Syst Rev 2012;2.

99. Derry CJ, Derry S, Moore RA. Sumatriptan (subcutaneous route of administration) for acute migraine attacks in adults. Cochrane Database Syst Rev 2012;2.

100. Tfelt-Hansen P, Hougaard A. Sumatriptan: A review of its pharmacokinetics, pharmacodynamics and efficacy in the acute treatment of migraine. Expert Opin Drug Metab Toxicol 2013;9:91–103.

101. Hoffmann J, Goadsby PJ. New agents for acute treatment of migraine: CGRP receptor antagonists, iNOS inhibitors. Curr Treat Options Neurol 2012;14:50–59.

102. Smith TR, Sunshine A, Stark SR, Littlefield DE, Spruill SE, Alexander WJ. Sumatriptan and naproxen sodium for the acute treatment of migraine. Headache 2005;45:983–991.

103. Mathew NT, Landy S, Stark S, et al. Fixed-dose sumatriptan and naproxen in poor responders to triptans with a short half-life. Headache 2009;49:971–982.

104. Tullo V, Valguarnera F, Barbanti P, et al. Comparison of frovatriptan plus dexketoprofen (25 mg or 37.5 mg) with frovatriptan alone in the treatment of migraine attacks with or without aura: A randomized study. Cephalalgia 2014;34:434–445.

105. Dodick DW, Lipton RB, Ferrari MD, et al. Prioritizing treatment attributes and their impact on selecting an oral triptan: Results from the TRIPSTAR Project. Curr Pain Headache Rep 2004;8:435–442.

106. Ferrari MD, Goadsby PJ, Roon KI, Lipton RB. Triptans (serotonin, 5-HT1B/1D agonists) in migraine: Detailed results and methods of a meta-analysis of 53 trials. Cephalalgia 2002;22:633–658.

107. McCormack PL, Keating GM. Eletriptan: A review of its use in the acute treatment of migraine. Drugs 2006;66:1129–1149.

108. Thorlund K, Mills EJ, Wu P, et al. Comparative efficacy of triptans for the abortive treatment of migraine: A multiple treatment comparison meta-analysis. Cephalalgia 2013;34:258–267.

109. Sanford M. Frovatriptan: A review of its use in the acute treatment of migraine. CNS Drugs 2012;26:791–811.

110. Allais G, Benedetto C. A review of the use of frovatriptan in the treatment of menstrually related migraine. Ther Adv Neurol Disord 2013;6:55–67.

111. Allais G, Tullo V, Omboni S, et al. Frovatriptan vs. other triptans for the acute treatment of oral contraceptive-induced menstrual migraine: pooled analysis of three double-blind, randomized, crossover, multicenter studies. Neurol Sci 2013;34(suppl 1):S83–S86.

112. Tfelt-Hansen PC, Pihl T, Hougaard A, Mitsikostas DD. Drugs targeting 5-hydroxytryptamine receptors in acute treatments of migraine attacks. A review of new drugs and new administration forms of established drugs. Expert Opin Investig Drugs 2014;23:375–385.

113. Ferrari MD, Roon KI, Lipton RB, Goadsby PJ. Oral triptans (serotonin 5-HT(1B/1D) agonists) in acute migraine treatment: A meta-analysis of 53 trials. Lancet 2001;358:1668–1675.

114. Goadsby PJ, Lipton RB, Ferrari MD. Migraine—Current understanding and treatment. N Engl J Med 2002;346:257–270.

115. Dahlöf CG, Ekbom K, Persson L. Clinical experiences from Sweden on the use of subcutaneously administered sumatriptan in migraine and cluster headache. Arch Neurol 1994;51:1256–1261.

116. Dahlöf CG, Mathew N. Cardiovascular safety of 5HT-1B/1D agonists—is there a cause for concern? Cephalalgia 1998;18:539–545.

117. Lewis PJ, Barrington SF, Marsden PK, Maisey MN, Lewis LD. A study of the effects of sumatriptan on myocardial perfusion in healthy female migraineurs using 13NH3 positron emission tomography. Neurology 1997;48:1542–1550.

118. Barra S, Lanero S, Madrid A, et al. Sumatriptan therapy for headache and acute myocardial infarction. Expert Opin Pharmacother 2010;11:2727–2737.

119. Lugardon S, Roussel H, Sciortino V, Montastruc JL, Lapeyre-Mestre M. Triptan use and risk of cardiovascular events: A nested-case-control study from the French health system database. Eur J Clin Pharmacol 2007;63:801–807.

120. Ferrari MD. Current perspectives on effective migraine treatments: Are small clinical differences important for patients? Drugs Today (Barc) 2003;39(suppl D):37–41.

121. Putnam GP, O'Quinn S, Bolden-Watson CP, Davis RL, Gutterman DL, Fox AW. Migraine polypharmacy and the tolerability of sumatriptan: A large-scale, prospective study. Cephalalgia 1999;19:668–675.

122. Cunnington M, Ephross S, Churchill P. The safety of sumatriptan and naratriptan in pregnancy: What have we learned? Headache 2009;49:1414–1422.

123. Nezvalová-Henriksen K, Spigset O, Nordeng H. Triptan exposure during pregnancy and the risk of major congenital malformations and adverse pregnancy outcomes: Results from the Norwegian Mother and Child Cohort Study. Headache 2010;50:563–575.

124. Powers SW, Kashikar-Zuck SM, Allen JR, et al. Cognitive behavioral therapy plus amitriptyline for chronic migraine in children and adolescents: A randomized clinical trial. JAMA 2013;310:2622–2630.

125. Varkey E, Cider A, Carlsson J, Linde M. Exercise as migraine prophylaxis: A randomized study using relaxation and topiramate as controls. Cephalalgia 2011;31:1428–1438.

126. Busch V, Gaul C. Exercise in migraine therapy—Is there any evidence for efficacy? A critical review. Headache 2008;48:890–899.

127. Fritsche G, Frettlöh J, Hüppe M, et al. Prevention of medication overuse in patients with migraine. Pain 2010;151:404–413.

128. Linde K, Allais G, Brinkhaus B, Manheimer E, Vickers A, White AR. Acupuncture for migraine prophylaxis. Cochrane Database Syst Rev 2009;(1).

129. Lipton RB, Bigal ME, Diamond M, et al. Migraine prevalence, disease burden, and the need for preventive therapy. Neurology 2007;68:343–349.

130. Hepp Z, Bloudek LM, Varon SF. Systematic review of migraine prophylaxis adherence and persistence. J Manag Care Pharm 2014;20:22–33.

131. Blumenfeld AM, Bloudek LM, Becker WJ, et al. Patterns of use and reasons for discontinuation of prophylactic medications for episodic migraine and chronic migraine: Results from the second international burden of migraine study (IBMS-II). Headache 2013;53:644–655.

132. Ramadan NM, Silberstein SD, Freitag FG, Gilbert TT, Frishberg BM. US Headache Consortium: Evidence-based guidelines for migraine headache in the primary care setting: Pharmacological management for prevention of migraine: American Academy of Neurology, 2000.

133. Aurora SK, Kulthia A, Barrodale PM. Mechanism of chronic migraine. Curr Pain Headache Rep 2011;15:57–63.

134. Silva-Néto RP, Almeida KJ, Bernardino SN. Analysis of the duration of migraine prophylaxis. J Neurol Sci 2014;337:38–41.

135. Silberstein SD, Holland S, Freitag F, et al. Evidence-based guideline update: Pharmacologic treatment for episodic migraine prevention in adults: Report of the Quality Standards Subcommittee of the American Academy of Neurology and the American Headache Society. Neurology 2012;78:1337–1345.

136. Schoenen J, Vandersmissen B, Jeangette S, et al. Migraine prevention with a supraorbital transcutaneous stimulator: A randomized controlled trial. Neurology 2013;80:697–704.

137. Schafer AM, Rains JC, Penzien DB, Groban L, Smitherman TA, Houle TT. Direct costs of preventive headache treatments: Comparison of behavioral and pharmacologic approaches. Headache 2011;51:985–991.

138. Dahlof CGH. Management of primary headaches: Current and future aspects. In: Giamberardino MA (ed). Pain 2002—An Updated Review: Refresher Course. Seattle: IASP, 2002:85–112.

139. Silberstein SD, Saper JR, Freitag FG. Migraine: Diagnosis and treatment. In: Silberstein SD, Lipton RB, Dalessio DJ (eds). Wolff's Headache and Other Head Pains, ed 7. Oxford: Oxford University, 2001:121–237.

140. Goadsby PJ. Advances in the understanding of headache. Br Med Bull 2005;73–74:83–92.

141. Chronicle E, Mulleners W. Anticonvulsant drugs for migraine prophylaxis. Cochrane Database Syst Rev 2004;(3).

142. Silberstein SD, Goadsby PJ. Migraine: Preventive treatment. Cephalalgia 2002;22:491–512.

143. Freitag FG, Diamond S, Diamond ML, Urban GJ. Divalproex in the long-term treatment of chronic daily headache. Headache 2001;41:271–278.

144. Linde M, Mulleners WM, Chronicle EP, McCrory DC. Valproate (valproic acid or sodium valproate or a combination of the two) for the prophylaxis of episodic migraine in adults. Cochrane Database Syst Rev 2013;6.

145. Linde M, Mulleners WM, Chronicle EP, McCrory DC. Gabapentin or pregabalin for the prophylaxis of episodic migraine in adults. Cochrane Database Syst Rev 2013;6.

146. Linde M, Mulleners WM, Chronicle EP, McCrory DC. Topiramate for the prophylaxis of episodic migraine in adults. Cochrane Database Syst Rev 2013;6.

147. Loder E, Biondi D. General principles of migraine management: The changing role of prevention. Headache 2005;45(suppl 1):S33–S47.

148. Linde K, Rossnagel K. Propranolol for migraine prophylaxis. Cochrane Database Syst Rev 2004;(2).

149. Diener HC, Hartung E, Chrubasik J, et al. A comparative study of oral acetylsalicyclic acid and metoprolol for the prophylactic treatment of migraine. A randomized, controlled, double-blind, parallel group phase III study. Cephalalgia 2001;21:120–128.

150. Holroyd KA, Penzien DB, Cordingley GE. Propranolol in the management of recurrent migraine: A meta-analytic review. Headache 1991;31:333–340.

151. Ziegler DK, Hurwitz A, Hassanein RS, Kodanaz HA, Preskorn SH, Mason J. Migraine prophylaxis. A comparison of propranolol and amitriptyline. Arch Neurol 1987;44:486–489.

152. Mathew NT. Prophylaxis of migraine and mixed headache. A randomized controlled study. Headache 1981;21:105–109.

153. Diamond S, Kudrow L, Stevens J, Shapiro DB. Long-term study of propranolol in the treatment of migraine. Headache 1982;22:268–271.

154. Tomkins GE, Jackson JL, O'Malley PG, Balden E, Santoro JE. Treatment of chronic headache with antidepressants: A meta-analysis. Am J Med 2001;111:54–63.

155. Couch JR, Hassanein RS. Amitriptyline in migraine prophylaxis. Arch Neurol 1979;36:695–699.

156. Gomersall JD, Stuart A. Amitriptyline in migraine prophylaxis. Changes in pattern of attacks during a controlled clinical trial. J Neurol Neurosurg Psychiatry 1973;36:684–690.

157. Kalita J, Bhoi SK, Misra UK. Amitriptyline vs divalproate in migraine prophylaxis: A randomized controlled trial. Acta Neurol Scand 2013;128:65–72.

158. Bulut S, Berilgen MS, Baran A, Tekatas A, Atmaca M, Mungen B. Venlafaxine versus amitriptyline in the prophylactic treatment of migraine: Randomized, double-blind, crossover study. Clin Neurol Neurosurg 2004;107:44–48.

159. Young WB, Bradley KC, Anjum MW, Gebeline-Myers C. Duloxetine prophylaxis for episodic migraine in persons without depression: A prospective study. Headache 2013;53:1430–1437.

160. Moja PL, Cusi C, Sterzi RR, Canepari C. Selective serotonin re-uptake inhibitors (SSRIs) for preventing migraine and tension-type headaches. Cochrane Database Syst Rev 2005;(3).

161. Misra UK, Kalita J, Bhoi SK. High-rate repetitive transcranial magnetic stimulation in migraine prophylaxis: A randomized, placebo-controlled study. J Neurol 2013;260:2793–2801.

162. Conforto AB, Amaro E Jr, Gonçalves AL, et al. Randomized, proof-of-principle clinical trial of active transcranial magnetic stimulation in chronic migraine. Cephalalgia 2013;34:464–472.

163. Martelletti P, Jensen RH, Antal A, et al. Neuromodulation of chronic headaches: Position statement from the European Headache Federation. J Headache Pain 2013;14:86.

164. Fox AW, Diamond ML, Spierings EL. Migraine during pregnancy: Options for therapy. CNS Drugs 2005;19:465–481.

165. Cassina M, Di Gianantonio E, Toldo I, Battistella PA, Clementi M. Migraine therapy during pregnancy and lactation. Expert Opin Drug Saf 2010;9:937–948.

166. Bromley RL, Mawer GE, Briggs M, et al. The prevalence of neurodevelopmental disorders in children prenatally exposed to antiepileptic drugs. J Neurol Neurosurg Psychiatry 2013;84:637–643.

167. Wöber-Bingöl C, Wöber C, Wagner-Ennsgraber C, et al. IHS criteria and gender: A study on migraine and tension-type headache in children and adolescents. Cephalalgia 1996;16:107–112.

168. Trottier ED, Bailey B, Lucas N, Lortie A. Diagnosis of migraine in the pediatric emergency department. Pediatr Neurol 2013;49:40–45.

169. Francis MV. Brief migraine episodes in children and adolescents—A modification to International Headache Society Pediatric Migraine (without aura) Diagnostic Criteria. Springerplus 2013;2:77.

170. Wöber-Bingöl C. Epidemiology of migraine and headache in children and adolescents. Curr Pain Headache Rep 2013;17:341.

171. Ferracini GN, Dach F, Speciali JG. Quality of life and health-related disability in children with migraine. Headache 2014;54:325–334.

172. Wöber-Bingöl C. Pharmacological treatment of acute migraine in adolescents and children. Paediatr Drugs 2013;15:235–246.

173. Evers S. The efficacy of triptans in childhood and adolescence migraine. Curr Pain Headache Rep 2013;17:342.

174. Sun H, Bastings E, Temeck J, et al. Migraine therapeutics in adolescents: A systematic analysis and historic perspectives of triptan trials in adolescents. JAMA Pediatr 2013;167:243–249.

175. Lewis D, Ashwal S, Hershey A, Hirtz D, Yonker M, Silberstein S. Practice parameter: Pharmacological treatment of migraine headache in children and adolescents: Report of the American Academy of Neurology Quality Standards Subcommittee and the Practice Committee of the Child Neurology Society. Neurology 2004;63:2215–2224.

176. Gallelli L, Avenoso T, Falcone D, et al. Effects of acetaminophen and ibuprofen in children with migraine receiving preventive treatment with magnesium. Headache 2014;54:313–324.

177. Deaton TL, Mauro LS. Topiramate for migraine prophylaxis in pediatric patients. Ann Pharmacother 2014;48:638–643.

178. Fallah R, Divanizadeh MS, Karimi M, Mirouliaei M, Shamsazadeh A. Topiramate and propranolol for prophylaxis of migraine. Indian J Pediatr 2013;80:920–924.

179. Bakola E, Skapinakis P, Tzoufi M, Damigos D, Mavreas V. Anticonvulsant drugs for pediatric migraine prevention: An evidence-based review. Eur J Pain 2009;13:893–901.

180. Lipton RB, Stewart WF, Scher AI. Epidemiology of migraine. In: Diener HC (ed). Drug Treatment of Migraine and Other Headaches, vol 17. Basel: Karger, 2000:2–15.

181. Eriksen MK, Thomsen LL, Russell MB. Prognosis of migraine with aura. Cephalalgia 2004;24:18–22.

182. Victor TW, Hu X, Campbell JC, Buse DC, Lipton RB. Migraine prevalence by age and sex in the United States: A life-span study. Cephalalgia 2010;30:1065–1072.

183. Freitag FG. Why do migraines often decrease as we age? Curr Pain Headache Rep 2013;17:366.

184. Bigal ME, Lipton RB. Migraine at all ages. Curr Pain Headache Rep 2006;10:207–213.

185. Mathew NT, Reuveni U, Perez F. Transformed or evolutive migraine. Headache 1987;27:102–106.

186. Cernuda-Morollón E, Larrosa D, Ramón C, Vega J, Martínez-Camblor P, Pascual J. Interictal increase of CGRP levels in peripheral blood as a biomarker for chronic migraine. Neurology 2013;81:1191–1196.

187. Krymchantowski AV, Moreira PF. Clinical presentation of transformed migraine: Possible differences among male and female patients. Cephalalgia 2001;21:558–566.

188. Bigal ME, Lipton RB. Concepts and mechanisms of migraine chronification. Headache 2008;48:7–15.

189. Natoli JL, Manack A, Dean B, et al. Global prevalence of chronic migraine: A systematic review. Cephalalgia 2010;30:599–609.

190. Scher AI, Midgette LA, Lipton RB. Risk factors for headache chronification. Headache 2008;48:16–25.

191. Buse DC, Manack A, Serrano D, Turkel C, Lipton RB. Sociodemographic and comorbidity profiles of chronic migraine and episodic migraine sufferers. J Neurol Neurosurg Psychiatry 2010;81:428–432.

192. Schmid CW, Maurer K, Schmid DM, et al. Prevalence of medication overuse headache in an interdisciplinary pain clinic. J Headache Pain 2013;14:4.

193. Diener HC, Holle D, Dodick D. Treatment of chronic migraine. Curr Pain Headache Rep 2011;15:64–69.

194. De Felice M, Ossipov MH, Wang R, et al. Triptan-induced latent sensitization: A possible basis for medication overuse headache. Ann Neurol 2010;67:325–337.

195. Katsarava Z, Buse DC, Manack AN, Lipton RB. Defining the differences between episodic migraine and chronic migraine. Curr Pain Headache Rep 2012;16:86–92.

196. Lipton RB. Chronic migraine, classification, differential diagnosis, and epidemiology. Headache 2011;51(suppl 2):77–83.

197. Silberstein S, Diener HC, Lipton R, et al. Epidemiology, risk factors, and treatment of chronic migraine: A focus on topiramate. Headache 2008;48:1087–1095.

198. Mathew NT, Rapoport A, Saper J, et al. Efficacy of gabapentin in migraine prophylaxis. Headache 2001;41:119–128.

199. Calandre EP, García-Leiva JM, Rico-Villademoros F, Vilchez JS, Rodríguez-López CM. Pregabalin in the treatment of chronic migraine: An open-label study. Clin Neuropharmacol 2010;33:35–39.

200. Dodick DW, Turkel CC, Degryse RE, et al. OnabotulinumtoxinA for treatment of chronic migraine: A response. Headache 2011;51:1005–1008.

201. Batty AJ, Hansen RN, Bloudek LM, et al. The cost-effectiveness of onabotulinumtoxinA for the prophylaxis of headache in adults with chronic migraine in the UK. J Med Econ 2013;16:877–887.

202. Jackson JL, Kuriyama A, Hayashino Y. Botulinum toxin A for prophylactic treatment of migraine and tension headaches in adults: A meta-analysis. JAMA 2012;307:1736–1745.

203. Blumenfeld A, Silberstein SD, Dodick DW, Aurora SK, Turkel CC, Binder WJ. Method of injection of botulinumtoxinA for chronic migraine: A safe, well-tolerated, and effective treatment paradigm based on the PREEMPT clinical program. Headache 2010;50:1406–1418.

204. Benoliel R, Sharav Y. Pain remapping in migraine to the orofacial region. Headache 2009;49:1353–1354.

205. Hussain A, Stiles MA, Oshinsky ML. Pain remapping in migraine: A novel characteristic following trigeminal nerve injury. Headache 2010;50:669–671.

206. Fuh JL, Wang SJ, Lu SR, Juang KD. Ice-cream headache—A large survey of 8359 adolescents. Cephalalgia 2003;23:977–981.

207. Zagury JG, Eliav E, Heir GM, et al. Prolonged gingival cold allodynia: A novel finding in patients with atypical odontalgia. Oral Surg Oral Med Oral Pathol Oral Radiol Endod 2011;111:312–319.

208. Bahra A, Matharu MS, Buchel C, Frackowiak RS, Goadsby PJ. Brainstem activation specific to migraine headache. Lancet 2001;357:1016–1017.

209. Pietrobon D, Moskowitz MA. Pathophysiology of migraine. Annu Rev Physiol 2013;75:365–391.

210. Noseda R, Burstein R. Migraine pathophysiology: Anatomy of the trigeminovascular pathway and associated neurological symptoms, CSD, sensitization and modulation of pain. Pain 2013;154(suppl 1):S44–S53.

211. Goadsby PJ, Hoskin KL. The distribution of trigeminovascular afferents in the nonhuman primate brain Macaca nemestrina: A c-fos immunocytochemical study. J Anat 1997;190(Pt 3):367–375.

212. Goadsby PJ, Edvinsson L, Ekman R. Release of vasoactive peptides in the extracerebral circulation of humans and the cat during activation of the trigeminovascular system. Ann Neurol 1988;23:193–196.

213. Tajti J, Möller S, Uddman R, Bodi I, Edvinsson L. The human superior cervical ganglion: Neuropeptides and peptide receptors. Neurosci Lett 1999;263:121–124.

214. Tajti J, Uddman R, Möller S, Sundler F, Edvinsson L. Messenger molecules and receptor mRNA in the human trigeminal ganglion. J Auton Nerv Syst 1999;76:176–183.

215. Noseda R, Burstein R. Advances in understanding the mechanisms of migraine-type photophobia. Curr Opin Neurol 2011;24:197–202.

216. Izumi H. Nervous control of blood flow in the orofacial region. Pharmacol Ther 1999;81:141–161.

217. Lennerz JK, Rühle V, Ceppa EP, et al. Calcitonin receptor-like receptor (CLR), receptor activity-modifying protein 1 (RAMP1), and calcitonin gene-related peptide (CGRP) immunoreactivity in the rat trigeminovascular system: Differences between peripheral and central CGRP receptor distribution. J Comp Neurol 2008;507:1277–1299.

218. Nicoletti P, Trevisani M, Manconi M, et al. Ethanol causes neurogenic vasodilation by TRPV1 activation and CGRP release in the trigeminovascular system of the guinea pig. Cephalalgia 2008;28:9–17.

219. Goadsby PJ, Edvinsson L. Human in vivo evidence for trigeminovascular activation in cluster headache. Neuropeptide changes and effects of acute attacks therapies. Brain 1994;117(Pt 3):427–434.

220. Knight YE, Classey JD, Lasalandra MP, et al. Patterns of fos expression in the rostral medulla and caudal pons evoked by noxious craniovascular stimulation and periaqueductal gray stimulation in the cat. Brain Res 2005;1045:1–11.

221. Bolay H, Reuter U, Dunn AK, Huang Z, Boas DA, Moskowitz MA. Intrinsic brain activity triggers trigeminal meningeal afferents in a migraine model. Nat Med 2002;8:136–142.

222. Hoskin KL, Zagami AS, Goadsby PJ. Stimulation of the middle meningeal artery leads to Fos expression in the trigeminocervical nucleus: A comparative study of monkey and cat. J Anat 1999;194(Pt 4):579–588.

223. Afridi SK, Giffin NJ, Kaube H, et al. A positron emission tomographic study in spontaneous migraine. Arch Neurol 2005;62:1270–1275.

224. Buzzi MG, Moskowitz MA. Evidence for 5-HT$_{1B/1D}$ receptors mediating the antimigraine effect of sumatriptan and dihydroergotamine. Cephalalgia 1991;11:165–168.

225. Kaube H, Hoskin KL, Goadsby PJ. Inhibition by sumatriptan of central trigeminal neurones only after blood-brain barrier disruption. Br J Pharmacol 1993;109:788–792.

226. Goadsby PJ, Classey JD. Evidence for serotonin (5-HT)1B, 5-HT1D and 5-HT1F receptor inhibitory effects on trigeminal neurons with craniovascular input. Neuroscience 2003;122:491–498.

227. Bouchelet I, Cohen Z, Case B, Séguéla P, Hamel E. Differential expression of sumatriptan-sensitive 5-hydroxytryptamine receptors in human trigeminal ganglia and cerebral blood vessels. Mol Pharmacol 1996;50:219–223.

228. Ma QP, Hill R, Sirinathsinghji D. Colocalization of CGRP with 5-HT1B/1D receptors and substance P in trigeminal ganglion neurons in rats. Eur J Neurosci 2001;13:2099–2104.

229. Veloso F, Kumar K, Toth C. Headache secondary to deep brain implantation. Headache 1998;38:507–515.

230. Goadsby PJ. Neurovascular headache and a midbrain vascular malformation: Evidence for a role of the brainstem in chronic migraine. Cephalalgia 2002;22:107–111.

231. Welch KM, Nagesh V, Aurora SK, Gelman N. Periaqueductal gray matter dysfunction in migraine: Cause or the burden of illness? Headache 2001;41:629–637.

232. Burstein R, Collins B, Jakubowski M. Defeating migraine pain with triptans: A race against the development of cutaneous allodynia. Ann Neurol 2004;55:19–26.

233. Chavarría-Bolaños D, Martinez-Zumaran A, Lombana N, Flores-Reyes H, Pozos-Guillen A. Expression of substance P, calcitonin gene-related peptide, ß-endorphin and methionine-enkephalin in human dental pulp tissue after orthodontic intrusion: A pilot study. Angle Orthod 2013;84:521–526.

234. Rodd HD, Boissonade FM. Comparative immunohistochemical analysis of the peptidergic innervation of human primary and permanent tooth pulp. Arch Oral Biol 2002;47:375–385.

235. Izumi H, Karita K. Vasodilator responses following intracranial stimulation of the trigeminal, facial and glossopharyngeal nerves in the cat gingiva. Brain Res 1991;560:71–75.

236. Ohkubo T, Shibata M, Yamada Y, Kaya H, Takahashi H. Role of substance P in neurogenic inflammation in the rat incisor pulp and the lower lip. Arch Oral Biol 1993;38:151–158.

237. Komorowski RC, Torneck CD, Hu JW. Neurogenic inflammation and tooth pulp innervation pattern in sympathectomized rats. J Endod 1996;22:414–417.

238. Byers MR, Närhi MV. Dental injury models: Experimental tools for understanding neuroinflammatory interactions and polymodal nociceptor functions. Crit Rev Oral Biol Med 1999;10:4–39.

239. Heyeraas KJ, Kvinnsland I. Tissue pressure and blood flow in pulpal inflammation. Proc Finn Dent Soc 1992;88(suppl 1):393–401.

240. Bartsch T, Knight YE, Goadsby PJ. Activation of 5-HT(1B/1D) receptor in the periaqueductal gray inhibits nociception. Ann Neurol 2004;56:371–381.

241. Mizuta K, Izumi H. Bulbar pathway for contralateral lingual nerve-evoked reflex vasodilatation in cat palate. Brain Res 2004;1020:86–94.

242. Kemppainen P, Leppänen H, Jyväsjärvi E, Pertovaara A. Blood flow increase in the orofacial area of humans induced by painful stimulation. Brain Res Bull 1994;33:655–662.

243. Frese A, Evers S, May A. Autonomic activation in experimental trigeminal pain. Cephalalgia 2003;23:67–68.

244. May A, Büchel C, Turner R, Goadsby PJ. Magnetic resonance angiography in facial and other pain: Neurovascular mechanisms of trigeminal sensation. J Cereb Blood Flow Metab 2001;21:1171–1176.

245. Loder E, Weizenbaum E, Frishberg B, Silberstein S. Choosing wisely in headache medicine: The American Headache Society's list of five things physicians and patients should question. Headache 2013;53:1651–1659.

The Trigeminal Autonomic Cephalalgias

Rafael Benoliel, BDS
Yair Sharav, DMD, MS

The most recent International Headache Society (IHS) classification modifies the trigeminal auto-nomic cephalalgias (TACs) to a group that now includes hemicrania continua together with cluster headache, paroxysmal hemicrania, and short-lasting neuralgiform headache attacks[1] (Box 11-1). This is based on accumulating data that hemicrania continua is phenotypically and pathophysio-logically similar to the TACs.[2,3] In relation to short-lasting unilateral neuralgiform headache attacks with conjunctival injection and tearing (SUNCT) and short-lasting unilateral neuralgiform headache attacks with cranial autonomic symptoms (SUNA), there has been a conceptual change. The clas-sification now describes short-lasting unilateral neuralgiform headache attacks (SUNHA), which are then subdivided into SUNCT and SUNA (see Box 11-1). Additionally, there have been a number of changes throughout the diagnostic criteria of TACs.

TACs are characterized by a shared clinical phenotype of trigeminal pain accompanied by prom-inent autonomic signs, which suggests a common pathophysiology.[1] Common diagnostic features of TACs include episodic pain that is unilateral, pulsatile, or sharp; is of severe intensity; is accom-panied by autonomic phenomena, such as tearing and rhinorrhea; and often causes waking from sleep.[1] However, TACs have been individually classified based on well-defined criteria of location, attack frequency, duration, and accompanying signs and symptoms with a specific and distinctive response to therapy. Pain quality in TACs and dental pulpitis is similar, and dentists are often the first health care providers consulted.[4–6]

<table>
<tr><td>Box 11-1</td><td>The IHS classification of trigeminal autonomic cephalalgias (TACs)</td></tr>
</table>

3.1 Cluster headache
    3.1.1 Episodic
    3.1.2 Chronic
3.2 Paroxysmal hemicrania
    3.2.1 Episodic
    3.2.2 Chronic
3.3 Short-lasting unilateral neuralgiform headache attacks
    3.3.1 With conjunctival injection and tearing (SUNCT)
        3.3.1.1 Episodic
        3.3.1.2 Chronic
    3.3.2 With cranial autonomic symptoms (SUNA)
        3.3.2.1 Episodic
        3.3.2.2 Chronic
3.4 Hemicrania continua
3.5 Probable TAC

Cluster Headache

Cluster headache is essentially the archetypal TAC with severe pain and major autonomic activation[1] (Table 11-1). Pain in cluster headache is probably the most severe of the primary headaches and approaches that for trigeminal neuralgia; some patients even consider suicide because of the pain.[7,8]

In spite of dramatic symptomatology, cluster headache often remains misdiagnosed, sometimes for more than 10 years.[9] The median interval between the first episode and final diagnosis is about 3 years: 34% to 45% of patients had consulted a dentist and 27% to 33% an otolaryngologist before the diagnosis was accurately established.[5,6] In some cases, it still takes around 3 to 6 years and three or four physicians to diagnose cluster headache.[5,10,11] Common misdiagnoses include migraine, sinusitis, and dental problems.[9] Factors that increase the diagnostic delay are a young age of onset and female sex, both of which are suggestive of migraines.[9] Additionally, diagnosis is delayed with the presence of photophobia or phonophobia, nausea, and an episodic attack pattern; again, these signs are more typical of migraine. Many patients with cluster headache describe toothache-like pain,[12] and incorrect diagnosis may lead to dental treatment that is misguided and unjustified; 15% of patients with cluster headache reported having dental extractions in an attempt to treat their pain.[9]

Clinical features

Cluster headache attacks tend to occur in clusters that last for a variable period of time (weeks to years).[7] Based on the distinct temporal patterns of these cluster periods, two clinical presentations of cluster headache are described. Most patients (80% to 85%) suffer from the episodic type, which is characterized by considerable pain-free periods between clusters. The IHS defines *episodic* as at least two cluster periods lasting 7 to 365 days and separated by pain-free periods of at least 1 month. In chronic cluster headache, repeated attacks recur over more than a year without remission or with remission periods lasting less than 1 month. Interictal pain may also be present between attacks or between clusters.[6]

Only 15% of patients with cluster headache suffer from the chronic form. In two-thirds of these patients, the cluster headache begins as chronic, while in the remaining one-third it evolves from the episodic form. Up to half of patients with chronic cluster headache report transition to an episodic pattern. Over the course of the disease, attack duration tends to lengthen in both episodic and chronic cluster headache, whereas concomitantly frequency tends to increase in episodic and decrease in chronic cluster headache.[13]

Clinical example

Examine Case 11-1. Note the prominent autonomic signs that are particularly pronounced in this patient (Fig 11-1); in other TACs, they may be subtler. Relative to other TACs, the pattern is low-frequency, long-lasting headaches with a nocturnal occurrence (Fig 11-2).

Location

Cluster headache is strictly unilateral, but attacks may change sides in about 20% of patients.[7,12,13] A recent population survey indicated that bilateral cluster headache may occur in about 3% of patients.[9] Attacks that alternate

Table 11-1   Diagnostic criteria for cluster headache*

Diagnostic criteria	Notes
A. At least five attacks fulfilling criteria B through D	Attacks usually occur in clusters lasting weeks/months separated by months/years. Of patients, 10% to 15% will suffer continuous attacks with no remission (chronic type). Age at onset is 20 to 40 years. The male-female ratio is 3:1.
B. Severe to very severe unilateral orbital, supraorbital, and/or temporal region pain lasting 15 to 180 minutes if untreated	During less than half of the time course, attacks may be less severe and/or shorter/longer. Interictal pain or discomfort may occur. During active periods, attacks may be provoked by alcohol, histamine, or nitroglycerin.

C. Headache is accompanied by either or both of the following:
  1. At least one of the following symptoms or signs, ipsilateral to the headache:
    a. Conjunctival injection and/or lacrimation
    b. Nasal congestion and/or rhinorrhea
    c. Eyelid edema
    d. Forehead and facial sweating
    e. Forehead and facial flushing
    f. Sensation of fullness in the ear
    g. Miosis and/or ptosis
 	
  2. A sense of restlessness or agitation
	Cases have been reported where autonomic signs appear with no headache and vice versa.
	
	During the worst attacks, patients are usually unable to lie down and become characteristically agitated (eg, pace the floor).

D. Attack frequency ranges from one every other day to eight per day for more than half of the time when the disorder is active *Episodic:* At least two cluster periods lasting 7 to 365 days (when untreated) and separated by pain-free remissions lasting at least 1 month *Chronic:* Occurring without remission periods or with remission periods lasting less than 1 month for at least 1 year.	During part (but less than half) of the time course, attacks may be less severe and/or of shorter or longer duration.
E. Not better accounted for by another *International Classification of Headache Disorders,* third edition diagnosis	Of patients with pituitary tumor, 4% suffer from cluster headache

*Reproduced with permission from the International Headache Society.

sides are more common between clusters than between attacks in the same cluster.[7] Peak pain intensity in cluster headache is classically felt periorbitally or in the eye.[7,14]

Lower and upper subtypes of cluster headache have been reported. Pain in lower cluster headache is ocular, temporal, and suboccipital with radiation to the teeth, jaws, and neck.[7,15] Intraoral/perioral radiation of pain includes the jaws (37%), teeth (maxillary, 50%; mandibular, 32%), and the cheeks (45%).[6,14] In upper clus-ter headache, pain is periorbital but radiates to the forehead, temporal, and parietal regions.[7] Note that radiation to the teeth (44%), the jaws (37%), and the ear (28%) is extremely common, irrespective of subtype.[9]

Quality

Cluster headache is severe and rated as 8 to 10 on a 10-point visual analog scale (VAS).[7,8] Nearly all patients describe their pain as sharp[9] and,

CASE 11-1

Cluster headache in a 29-year-old man.

Present complaint: Attacks of extremely severe pain (visual analog scale 9) periorbitally radiating to the ipsilateral temple, cheek, and maxillary molars. Pain is stabbing and sometimes throbbing. Most attacks last 30 to 60 minutes, but the patient has suffered more prolonged attacks of up to 4 hours.

History of present complaint: For the past 11 years, he has suffered repeated pain attacks that often wake him from sleep in the early hours of the morning. The attacks occur during specific periods (cluster periods), sometimes lasting 2 to 14 weeks; however, at other times, he does not suffer from any pain, and these remission periods may last up to 6 months. Once an attack begins, he is unable to continue working and becomes irritated and extremely agitated. Attacks are accompanied by ipsilateral tearing, rhinorrhea, and ptosis (see Fig 11-1). The longer attacks are very often accompanied by nausea and photophobia. The patient reported onset of pain in the waiting room; the pain was preceded by a strange sensation around the right cheek and eye (twinges) and rapidly (< 5 minutes) reached peak intensity with clear local signs.

Physical examination: Head and neck examination between attacks was unremarkable. During attacks, the findings described in Fig 11-1 were present.

Relevant medical history: None.

Diagnosis: A tentative diagnosis of episodic cluster headache was made, and the patient was instructed to use oxygen (5 L/min) as abortive therapy.

Diagnostic and treatment considerations: At follow-up, the patient reported that oxygen was very effective in either eradicating or significantly reducing pain attacks (see Fig 11-2a). However, in spite of relatively easy access to oxygen, the patient often found that it took too long to obtain and requested alternative therapy. Preventive treatment with verapamil was offered, but the patient was unwilling to be on permanent medication; therefore, sumatriptan 6 mg SC was prescribed with excellent response.

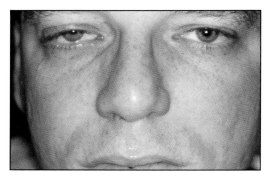

Fig 11-1 Photograph of the patient described in Case 11-1 taken during a right-sided painful attack. Note the ipsilateral ptosis and miosis. Additionally, there is obvious ipsilateral lacrimation and rhinorrhea (see upper lip).

less frequently, throbbing or pressure-like.[8,13] A small number describe combined characteristics of sharp and throbbing pain. Descriptions of a "hot poker" or a "stabbing" feeling in the eye are common.[7,14] The extensive array of descriptors used by patients attests to the wide variety of presentation.[8] In addition, sudden jabs of intense pain are often felt and may be an integral part of some cluster headache variants.[13] In one recent series, about 40% of patients with cluster headache described their pain as "toothache-like," which may partly explain the extensive misdiagnosis with dental pain.[12]

Temporal pattern of individual attacks

Nearly half of patients report that the most common time for a cluster headache is around 2 am, and a further one-third report the most common time as 1 am or 3 am.[9] Peak intensity is usually reached within 9 or 10 minutes of onset but may develop rapidly, within 3 minutes.[8] Most attacks last 30 minutes to 1 hour (average, 45 to 90 minutes; range, 15 to 180 minutes), but attacks rarely may last from 3 to 48 hours.[6,7,12] The most common attack frequency is two per day but may reach eight per day.[9] Most patients report daily attacks during active clusters.[9] See Fig 11-2 to compare the duration of attacks with those of other TACs (paroxysmal hemicrania and SUNCT).

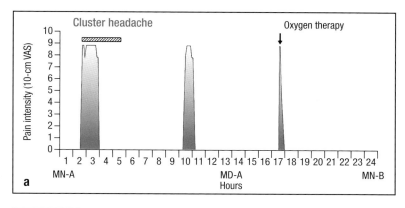

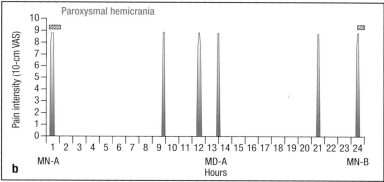

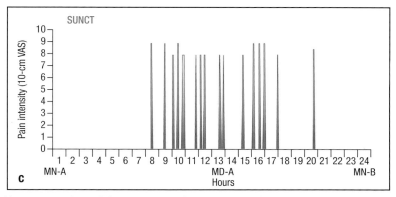

Fig 11-2 Graphic representations of the pain diaries of the patients in Case 11-1, Case 11-2, and Case 11-3 over a 24-hour period (from midnight [MN] on day A to midnight on day B). *(a)* Cluster headache (Case 11-1). Pain duration varied from 45 to 90 minutes, and frequency over this period was three per 24 hours; one attack woke him about 2 hours after sleep onset *(shaded rectangle)*. Pain intensity was severe (visual analog scale 8 to 9). The third attack (at 5:00 pm) occurred when access to oxygen was available, and inhalation rapidly aborted the attack. *(b)* Paroxysmal hemicrania (Case 11-2). Pain duration varied from 10 to 15 minutes, and frequency over this period was six per 24 hours; two attacks woke the patient from sleep *(shaded rectangles)*. Pain intensity was moderate to severe (VAS 7 to 9). *(c)* Shortlasting unilateral neuralgiform headache attacks (Case 11-3). Pain duration varied from 3 to 5 minutes to a rare duration of 10 minutes. Frequency over this period was 16 per 24 hours; no attacks woke the patient from sleep. Pain intensity was moderate to severe (VAS 9 to 10).

After a first cluster headache attack, a quarter of patients were found to have no further recurrence over a mean follow-up of 8 years,[16] but because only the one attack occurred it would not be classified as cluster headache. Most patients (65%) had subsequent episodic attacks, most within 3 to 5 years.[16]

Nocturnal attacks

Frequency of nocturnal cluster headache is high (51% to 73%), and pain often awakens patients 90 minutes after sleep initiation, at about the onset of rapid eye movement (REM) sleep[14] (see Case 11-1 and Fig 11-2a). An association between episodic cluster headache and REM sleep has been shown, less so with chronic cluster headache (see chapter 5). Sleep deprivation, resulting from high-frequency attacks, leads to early-onset REM, which often triggers further attacks. Severity of nocturnal pain is either stronger than[9] or no different from that occurring during the day.[7]

Interictal pain

Lower-level pain persisting between attacks seems to be common in cluster headache and is associated with parameters of disease severity, such as prolonged disease duration, poor response to sumatriptan, allodynia during and between attacks, and a diagnosis of chronic cluster headache.[17]

Cluster periods

Episodic cluster headache commonly occurs at least once daily for a period of weeks. At low frequencies, cluster headache attacks tend to occur at the same time of day or night with surprising clockwork regularity.[7] Active periods (average 6 to 12 weeks) are followed by a temporary remission or an inactive period that may last from weeks to years (average, 12 months). Attacks tend to be shorter and less severe at the beginning and toward the end of each cluster period.[13] Particularly at the initial onset of cluster headache, active periods are seasonal, occurring around spring or autumn.[7,9,18] Correlation between daylight hours and cluster headache occurrence and frequency has also been noted. However, as cluster headache de-

velops, the active periods become less predictable, and variations in the length of active and inactive periods are apparent.[7]

Triggers

Alcohol, even in small amounts, may precipitate cluster headache attacks during active cluster periods.[9,19] Patients with cluster headache, particularly those whose condition evolves into chronic cluster headache, are high consumers of alcohol and tobacco.[20] Dietary factors are unimportant in cluster headache.

Nitroglycerin provocative test

Nitroglycerin administration provokes headaches during active clusters and has been considered diagnostic. However, nitroglycerin will induce headaches in patients with cluster headache, in migraineurs, and in sufferers from chronic tension-type headache and is therefore not specific.[21]

Autonomic signs

Ipsilateral autonomic signs are very common in cluster headache; lacrimation, the most frequent, occurs in up to 90% of patients.[9,12,14] Autonomic signs overwhelmingly occur with the headache rather than before or after.[22] About 50% to 75% of patients may have multiple autonomic signs, such as conjunctival injection, nasal congestion, ptosis, and/or miosis and rhinorrhea[12,14] (see Case 11-1 and Fig 11-1). Autonomic signs are transient and resolve with the headache, but rarely, ptosis and miosis (partial Horner syndrome) may persist. Forehead sweating may be observed and is usually bilateral.[9,22] Patients with lower cluster headache reported not only a higher overall rate of autonomic signs but also a higher predominance of nasal congestion, ptosis, and forehead and facial sweating.[15]

A small number of patients with cluster headache (3% to 7%) may not have autonomic signs during attacks, and this may make diagnosis difficult.[23,24] Cluster headache with autonomic signs is significantly more painful than cluster headache without autonomic signs.[23,25] Additionally, autonomic signs are significantly more frequent in males than females and in

Same as Rhythmicity?

episodic rather than chronic cluster headache but are probably related to differences in attack intensity.[23]

Migrainous features

Migrainous features are common in cluster headache attacks and affect around a quarter of patients with the condition.[26] The most frequently reported features vary but include photophobia, phonophobia, nausea, vomiting, and, more rarely, gustatory, olfactory, ocular, and behavioral phenomena.[9,14,26] Rarely, patients may complain of concomitant ipsilateral limb pain that may alternate sides. Cluster headache associated with transient hemiparesis has been reported to be also accompanied by visual symptoms, photophobia, phonophobia, and nausea.[27] This clinical phenotype is strikingly similar to side-locked migraine. Up to 8% of patients with cluster headache may suffer comorbid migraine; however, the presence of migrainous features is not dependent on the presence of comorbid migraine.[12]

Laterality of features

Clearly, the ipsilaterality of features—particularly lacrimation and photophobia, but also conjunctival injection, phonophobia, and others—are of diagnostic importance.[22,28] This is particularly useful in the differential diagnosis of cluster headache and hemicrania continua versus migraine. In migraine, photophobia and phonophobia are bilateral in about 90% of patients, whereas in TACs they occur unilaterally in more than half of patients.[29] The only consistently bilateral feature in both cluster headache and migraine is forehead/facial sweating.[22]

Systemic features

Changes in cardiovascular parameters include increases and decreases in heart rate at onset and during attacks, respectively, and arrhythmias. Increases in systolic and diastolic blood pressure have been reported. These changes are probably mediated by connections between the trigeminal and the parabrachial nuclei involved in autonomic control of cardiovascular function.

Prodromata and premonitory symptoms

In cluster headache, specific symptoms may occur minutes to days before pain onset.[8,14,30,31] Prodromes precede headache onset by minutes and are reported by almost all patients.[8] Local prodromes include autonomic signs and mild pain or nonpainful sensations in the area that subsequently become painful, for example, twinges, pressure, tingling, and a pulsating feeling.[8] Additionally, blurred vision, sensitivity to smells, nausea, dyspepsia, hunger, irritability, tiredness, and tenseness are described. Symptoms specific to the oral cavity include dry mouth, metallic taste, and a tight feeling in the teeth. General psychic symptoms are also common.[8] Premonitory symptoms may predict cluster headache days before onset and are reported in 40% of patients with cluster headache.[8] These may be similar to those experienced by migraineurs and include body numbness, neck pain, irritability, lethargy, and sleepiness. Aura-like symptoms are found in 14% to 21% of patients.[9,14,32]

Patient behavior

Restlessness during attacks is so frequent (> 80%) that it has been included as a cluster headache diagnostic criterion.[8,12,17] Patients are agitated[9]; they continually move around and change body position, particularly during severe attacks. This is in sharp contrast to the quiet-seeking behavior observed in migraine.

Prognosis

Remission periods may increase in many patients with time, and active cluster headache beyond the age of 65 to 75 years is rare so that long-term prognosis may be good.[13,33]

Patient burden is a significant concern, and many patients lose a number of workdays or even become unemployed because of cluster headache.[9] Furthermore, 2% of patients with cluster headache report attempting suicide.[9]

Symptomatic cluster headache

The clinical presentation may be quite typical,[34] and no specific pattern is associated with symptomatic cluster headache.[35] Atypical attack duration and/or frequency, an abnormal neurologic examination, and resistance to standard therapy should raise suspicion.[34,36] Furthermore, some patients may present with typical cluster headache and only subsequently develop atypical signs leading to the diagnosis of symptomatic cluster headache.[34] For these reasons, it seems wise to refer all patients with cluster headache for brain imaging, and magnetic resonance imaging (MRI) is the preferred modality.[34,35]

Pituitary adenomas seem to be a common cause of symptomatic TACs in general and cluster headache in particular.[34–36] The size of the pituitary tumor seems unrelated to headache, suggesting that functional tumor activity may be important.[37] In patients with pituitary tumor, associated headaches were usually unilateral, located orbitally, severe, and associated with photophobia and nausea.[38] During exacerbations, some patients reported lacrimation and conjunctival injection. This clinical phenotype is reminiscent of cluster headache or other TACs, and when the authors applied IHS criteria, 4% fitted a diagnosis of cluster headache and a further 6% fit a diagnosis of SUNCT or hemicrania continua.[38] In view of this, MRI imaging with pituitary views and tests of pituitary function are indicated for all TACs.[39]

Symptomatic cluster headache has been described as a result of inflammatory orbital myositis, inflammatory myeloblastic pseudotumor of the posterior fossa, sphenoidal aspergillosis, and multiple sclerosis.[34,40,41] Vascular lesions with cluster headache symptomatology may occur in carotid artery dissection, arteriovenous malformation of the middle cerebellar artery, and vertebral artery injury.[34] Cluster headache secondary to posttraumatic head injury is commonly observed.[9] Case studies of cluster headache with onset after tooth extraction have been published, but the importance of such peripheral nerve lesions in the etiology of cluster headache is unclear.[42,43] Nonmetastatic and brain-metastasized lung cancer have presented with cluster headache.[44] Careful review of such cases reveals that telltale signs were often present in the neurologic examination and in the behavior, presentation, and symptomatology of the headaches.[45]

Epidemiology

Several studies of the general population show that cluster headache is a relatively rare syndrome that affects men about five times more than women.[46,47] Based on epidemiologic data, the closest approximation to actual 1-year prevalence of cluster headache is proposed to be 0.53%.[48,49] A higher proportion of male sufferers is reported with a male-female ratio of 4.3:1.[49] The possible increase in women has been postulated to be associated with the proliferation of alcohol and tobacco use among women but may also be due to increased recognition of cluster headache in women.[48,50] This is in line with findings that women with cluster headache suffer from a longer delay to diagnosis.[51] Further subtle differences are found between male and female patients with cluster headache: age of onset in men is around the third decade, whereas peak onset in women is bimodal in the second (major) and the fifth to sixth (minor) decades.[51,52] Mean attack duration in women is shorter, miosis and ptosis are less common, and nausea and vomiting are more frequent than in men.[52] Additionally, in women pain around the jaws and teeth is more common, and response to sumatriptan is not as good.[51] Cluster headache has also been described in children aged 5 to 16 years and in the elderly.[53,54]

Genetics

A genetic basis is inferred by family and twin studies, but the mode of transmission seems to vary, and the degree of heritability is unclear.[55] First-degree relatives of patients with cluster headache are up to 39 times and second-degree relatives eight times more likely to have cluster headache than the general population.[56,57] A family history is present in 0.8% to 18% of patients with cluster headache (in women more frequently than in men), and accumulated evidence indicates that cluster headache is inherited.[9,58] High concordance is also found in monozygotic and dizygotic twins.[59] Cluster headache is likely to have an autosomal dominant gene with low penetrance and to be present in 3% to 4% of men and 7% to 10% of women, but autosomal recessive or multifactorial inheritance may also occur.

Co-occurrence of cluster headache and migraine suggests a common inheritance; however, the incidence of migraine in patients with cluster headache is not significantly different from that observed in the general population.[14,60] Moreover, no mutations of the calcium channel gene (CACNA1A) implicated in migraine were found in cluster headache.[61,62] Actions of the nitric oxide synthase enzyme induce nitric oxide release, a molecule important in the etiology of cluster headache, but no significant nitric oxide synthase polymorphism associations have been found.[63]

The circadian rhythm of cluster headache suggests that the genes involved (clock genes) may display polymorphisms, but again no significant associations were observed between genotype and phenotype.[64] The neuropeptide hypocretin is found exclusively in the posterolateral hypothalamus, an area highly associated with cluster headache. Moreover, functions of hypocretin include pain modulation[65] and regulation of the sleep-wake cycle. A significant association has been found between a polymorphism in the hypocretin receptor 2 gene and cluster headache[66] but accounts for only a part of the genetic susceptibility. Pharmacogenetic studies have suggested a possible polymorphism involved in the treatment response to triptans.[55]

Treatment

The three treatment approaches for cluster headache are abortive, transitional (intermediate), and prophylactic[67–70] (see Tables 11-2 to 11-4). The choice depends on a host of factors, including attack frequency and patient preference. Patients should be instructed to avoid daytime naps, alcoholic beverages, and other triggers, such as volatile substances (eg, paints). Although smoking cessation is advised, smoking may not have a significant effect on headaches.[71,72] Altitude hypoxemia may trigger an attack during active periods but may be pharmacologically prevented.[7,72] A clear explanation of mechanisms, treatment options, and prognosis is essential.

Abortive

Table 11-2 outlines abortive treatment options for cluster headache. Oxygen at 12 to 15 L per minute for 15 to 20 minutes will provide relief in about 70% of patients; higher flow rates may be successful in previously resistant patients.[73] The response rates in young men are higher (87%) than in older patients with chronic cluster headache (57%) and in women (59%).[74] Hyperbaric oxygen is also effective but is difficult to access.[67] Oxygen seems to act specifically on the parasympathetic innervation of the cranial vasculature and inhibits evoked trigeminovascular activation and activation of the autonomic pathway during cluster headache attacks.[75] Interestingly, oxygen has no direct effect on trigeminal afferents, which explains why it has no effect in migraine.

Subcutaneous (SC) and, more recently, intranasal spray sumatriptan is effective in the acute treatment of cluster headache, resulting in few side effects even with prolonged usage and high dosing.[76,77] SC sumatriptan (6 mg) is effective in 50% to 80% of patients within 15 minutes of administration but is slightly less effective in chronic cluster headache.[68] Based on placebo-controlled studies, SC sumatriptan (6 mg) has a number needed to treat (NNT) of about 2.2 and is currently the most efficient abortive therapy (see Table 11-2). When multiple doses are required on a daily basis, sumatriptan 3 mg SC remains an effective and safe option.[72] However, there have been reports that continued use of sumatriptan may lead to increased frequency of cluster headache attacks or even medication overuse headache, which was not thought to be an issue in cluster headache.[78,79] Intranasal sumatriptan (20 mg) provides some relief within 30 minutes but is inferior to the SC formulation (NNT of 3.5) and has an unpleasant taste.[77] Oral zolmitriptan 5 to 10 mg is efficient in episodic but not in chronic cluster headache, and although the drug is more tolerable, it takes more than 30 minutes to be effective and is inferior to sumatriptan (NNTs of 6.7 and 5.6, respectively).[80] When intranasal zolmitriptan 5 to 10 mg was used, improved NNTs were obtained depending on whether episodic or chronic cluster headache was being treated[67,68,81] (see Table 11-2). Intravenous dihydroergotamine has been successfully used in cluster headache but is impractical. Oral ergot formulations have also been used, but absorption may not be rapid enough to be effective, and nasal inha-

| | | **Table 11-2** | **Selected abortive pharmacologic treatment options for cluster headache** | | |

Agent	NNT	Dose	Notes	Side effects
Oxygen (inhaled via face mask)	2.04	5 to 10 L/min for 15 min; 10 to 15 L/min may be tried	First line but cumbersome; hyperbaric oxygen also efficacious but impractical	Mild dizziness
Sumatriptan	2.2	6 to 12 mg SC	First line, fast, and efficacious; 12 mg as effective as 6 mg but has more side effects; marginally less effective in chronic cluster headache; contraindicated in cardiovascular disease	Fatigue, nausea/vomiting, chest symptoms, skin reactions over puncture wound
	3.45	20 mg intranasal	Less effective but easier to use; contraindicated in cardiovascular disease	As above with added nose irritation
Zolmitriptan	6.7 to 5.6	5 to 10 mg oral	Limited efficacy; alternative to intranasal sumatriptan; contraindicated in cardiovascular disease; only for episodic cluster headache	Chest pain or pressure in the chest or neck; sensation of burning, warmth, heat, numbness, tightness or tingling; abdominal pain
	6.2 to 2.6	Episodic cluster headache, 5 to 10 mg intranasal	Limited efficacy; alternative to intranasal sumatriptan; contraindicated in cardiovascular disease; more effective in episodic than chronic cluster headache	Unusual taste, dry mouth, nasal discomfort, tingling/numbness, nausea, weakness, drowsiness, or dizziness; chest/jaw/neck tightness
	4.2 to 4.0	Chronic cluster headache, 5 to 10 mg intranasal	Limited efficacy; alternative to intranasal sumatriptan; contraindicated in cardiovascular disease; more effective in episodic than chronic cluster headache	
Dihydroergotamine	–	0.5 to 1.0 mg intranasal (bilateral)	Reduces severity but not frequency; risk of rebound; contraindicated in cardiovascular disease; do not use with triptan	Irritation in the nose/throat and/or disturbances in taste; blood pressure increase; vasospastic phenomena such as muscle pains, numbness, coldness, pallor, and cyanosis of the digits
Lignocaine	–	1 mL of 4% to 10% solution applied intranasally on cotton pledget bilaterally	Pain is decreased, but not enough studies have been conducted to confirm; needs to be inserted deep near the pterygopalatine foramen	Bitter taste

NNT, number needed to treat; SC, subcutaneous.

lation seems only to reduce attack intensity. Intranasal lidocaine may be partially effective in up to one-third of patients and is therefore considered adjunctive therapy.[72]

Transitional

Table 11-3 outlines transitional treatment options for episodic cluster headache. Cortico-

Table 11-3 Transitional treatment options for episodic cluster headache

Agent	Dose	Notes	Side effects
Steroid/local analgesic	–	Occipital nerve blocks	Local hematoma, irritation
Prednisolone	60 to 100 mg/day orally for at least 5 days	Transitional therapy until, for example, verapamil takes effect; prolonged use is not recommended because of side effects; taper over 10 to 21 days	Increased appetite, nervousness, hyperglycemia, insomnia, headaches

Table 11-4 Prophylactic treatment options for episodic and chronic cluster headache

Agent	Dose	Notes	Side effects
Episodic			
Verapamil	480 to 720 mg/day orally	First-line treatment; perform baseline electrocardiogram and after reaching 480 mg/day; renew after every 80 mg; increase thereafter	Hypotension, bradycardia, heart block, dizziness, fatigue
Valproic acid	600 to 2,000 mg/day orally	Efficacious in patients with pronounced migrainous features; monitor liver function	Nausea, dizziness, dyspepsia, thrombocytopenia
Topiramate	25 to 200 mg/day orally	Increase by 25 mg/day every 5 days	Cognitive effects, paresthesias, dizziness
Gabapentin	900 mg/day orally	Few studies but promising results	Drowsiness
Melatonin	9 to 10 mg/day orally at night	Few studies	Short-term feelings of depression, daytime sleepiness, dizziness and irritability
Chronic			
Verapamil	480 to 720 mg/day orally	First-line treatment; perform baseline electrocardiogram and after reaching 480 mg/day; renew after every 80 mg; increase thereafter	Hypotension, bradycardia, heart block, dizziness, fatigue
Lithium carbonate	300 to 900 mg/day orally	Requires monitoring of renal and thyroid function and serum concentrations (best at 0.4 to 0.8 mEq/L); more side effects than verapamil	Weakness, nausea, tremor, slurred speech, blurred vision

steroids are effective in about 70% to 80% of patients and may induce remission of a cluster period in about one quarter of patients.[70,82] Currently, their main use is in attaining rapid transitional prophylaxis.[83,84] This period allows the patient to comfortably initiate prophylactic therapy, which takes time to fully control headaches. Oral prednisone at 60 to 100 mg daily in the morning should be continued for 5 to 7 days then tapered by 10 mg every 2 or 3 days[70,72] (see Table 11-3). Intravenous methylprednisolone (250 to 500 mg daily) for 3 to 5 days is very effective.[85]

Blockade of the greater occipital nerve with steroids and local analgesics may also provide transitional relief and, if repeated monthly, may be a useful prophylactic addition.[86–89] Occipital nerve blocks have provided pain relief and certainly seem to be a logical option before any invasive modalities.[90–92]

Prophylactic

Table 11-4 outlines prophylactic treatment options for episodic and chronic cluster headache. During prolonged periods of active episodic and chronic cluster headache, continuous abortive therapy is impractical and may be associated with unacceptable side effects. Prevention is often initiated with verapamil,[7] which is efficacious for long-term management of episodic and chronic cluster headache but

---

Box 11-2   **Assessment of intractable cluster headache before surgery**

1. Rule out or reassess organic pathology.
2. Reassess diagnosis versus other entities, such as:
   a. Side-locked migraine
   b. Paroxysmal hemicrania
   c. SUNCT
3. Review pharmacotherapy.
   a. Adequate monotherapy?
      i. Have the frontline drugs all been tested?
      ii. At adequate dosing/duration?
   b. Adequate polytherapy as above?
4. Consider referral:
   a. For reassessment and diagnosis
   b. For inpatient treatment with intravenous medication
5. Is the patient fit for neurosurgery?
   a. Medically
   b. Psychologically
6. Patients with strictly unilateral pain are the best candidates.
   a. Pain that has alternated sides is a poor prognostic factor.
7. Patients must understand that surgical failure is a possibility and attacks or autonomic signs (or both) may continue.

---

requires doses of 480 to 720 mg daily.[67] Reports document the use of verapamil at a 1,200 mg dose. Verapamil should be initiated at 240 mg daily and increased by 80 mg at 2-week intervals[39]; dosages in chronic cluster headache are usually higher. The doses used in cluster headache are very high, and patients' electrocardiograms should be monitored at each dose escalation and routinely once established.[39,93] For chronic cluster headache, lithium carbonate is an established prophylactic therapy that may induce remission (see Table 11-4). Lithium has been shown to be as efficient as verapamil, albeit with more side effects. In addition, it requires monitoring of serum concentrations because of its narrow therapeutic window. Anticonvulsant drugs have also been tested in cluster headache with mixed success; topiramate (100 to 200 mg/day) is associated with clinical improvement in some patients, and valproic acid is inconsistent but may be efficacious in cluster headache with migrainous features.[94,95]

Cluster headache refractory to pharmacotherapy

Medically resistant cluster headache is a distressing condition; up to 10% to 20% patients experience excruciating pain that is unresponsive to a number of therapies.[50] Some patients may respond to medical therapy but suffer intolerable side effects that severely compromise their quality of life. In these situations, surgical intervention or deep brain stimulation may be considered.

Invasive procedures. Who should undergo these? Strict selection criteria for invasive interventions should be met and include accurate diagnosis of long-lasting (more than 2 years) unilateral chronic cluster headache, pharmacotherapy that has been exhausted, a patient medical, neurologic, and psychologic profile that does not contraindicate surgery or electrode stimulation, clinically normal neuroimaging studies, and a patient who does not smoke or consume alcohol.[96]

Procedures may be aimed at the trigeminal ganglion or nerve, the sphenopalatine ganglion, and the superior petrosal nerve. Microvascular decompression and trigeminal nerve root resection, as in the management of trigeminal neuralgia, have also been used. However, some patients will remain symptomatic after these procedures.[97] Thus, patient selection for surgery needs to include careful assessment and considerations (Box 11-2).

Neurostimulation and surgery. Relevant neurosurgical treatments are discussed in chapter

13; see also Hong and Roberts.[98] The options range from application of glycerol or local anesthetics onto the trigeminal ganglion to radiofrequency rhizotomy of the trigeminal ganglion, microvascular decompression, and resection or blockade of the superior petrosal nerve or the sphenopalatine ganglion. However, the efficacy of these surgical interventions is questionable, and when neurostimulation offers a safe and efficacious alternative, there is no indication for destructive procedures.[39]

Recent technical advances offer the opportunity to apply neurostimulation to virtually any target. The exact mechanism by which neurostimulation exerts its effects is unclear, although a neuronal functional block seems likely. Targets for cluster headache include the hypothalamus, the occipital nerve, and the sphenopalatine ganglion.[99,100]

The hypothalamus is considered important in the pathogenesis of cluster headache (see pathophysiology), and stimulation of specific hypothalamic areas has resulted in excellent pain control.[101] Patient follow-up of about 9 years has shown that significant pain relief may be attained in around 50% to 60% of patients.[99,101] The major application of hypothalamic stimulation has been in the prophylactic treatment of cluster headache,[101] and usually there is a latency for this effect to develop, which suggests a complex mechanism that possibly involves brain plasticity.[99] Hypothalamic stimulation induces activity in areas associated with the pain matrix, which suggests that some of its effects are mediated by restoring function in some of these hypofunctional regions and reestablishing efficient top-down pain modulation.[102] Interestingly, after years of stimulation, a persistently pain-free state can be achieved even if the stimulator is turned off, which suggests a disease-altering potential for hypothalamic stimulation.[101] Hypothalamic stimulation has also been tested for the abortion of acute cluster headache attacks but has not been successful. Associated morbidity and mortality are a real concern, but recent technical advances have reduced these. Bilateral chronic cluster headache is a negative prognostic factor in hypothalamic stimulation.[101]

Occipital nerve stimulation for the prophylaxis of cluster headache has gained popularity and seems to offer significant relief.[103,104] Pares-thesia in the dermatome of the greater occipital nerve may accompany clinical improvement in patients with chronic cluster headache.[105]

Pain and autonomic signs in cluster headache result from the activation of the trigeminal parasympathetic reflex, mediated through the sphenopalatine ganglion. Low-frequency activation of the sphenopalatine ganglion induces cluster headache attacks.[106] Targeting facial parasympathetic output by modulating, blocking, treating, or lesioning the sphenopalatine ganglion makes scientific sense. High-frequency stimulation of the sphenopalatine ganglion has shown efficacy in the acute treatment and prevention of cluster headache, but these were small studies.[105–107] Blocking the sphenopalatine ganglion with local analgesics[108] or treating the sphenopalatine ganglion directly with steroids relieves pain in episodic cluster headache.[109]

Paroxysmal Hemicrania

Paroxysmal hemicrania was initially thought to be a rare variant of cluster headache. However, a separate category for paroxysmal hemicrania was created based on a number of features that distinguish it from cluster headache (Table 11-5).

Clinical features

Clinical example

Examine Case 11-2 (Fig 11-3). Notice the similar pain location in cluster headache and paroxysmal hemicrania. In this case, duration and frequency were typical. Referral of pain to dental structures is very common and often leads to misguided dental treatment. Indomethacin very often causes gastric side effects, and in these instances, combination with an antacid is indicated.

Location

Pain occurs typically in the temporal, periorbital, periauricular, and maxillary areas[110–113] but is probably more widespread in its location than previously recognized.[113] Extratrigeminal distribution of pain in paroxysmal hemicrania is in-

Table 11-5 Diagnostic criteria for paroxysmal hemicrania*

Diagnostic criteria	Notes
A. At least 20 attacks fulfilling criteria B through E	Onset is usually in adulthood, although childhood cases are reported. Unlike cluster headache, there is no male predominance.
B. Several unilateral orbital, supraorbital, or temporal pain attacks lasting 2 to 30 minutes	Attacks are similar to cluster headache but are shorter lasting and more frequent.
C. At least one of the following signs or symptoms ipsilateral to the pain: 1. Conjunctival injection and/or lacrimation 2. Nasal congestion and/or rhinorrhea 3. Eyelid edema 4. Forehead and facial sweating 5. Forehead and facial flushing 6. Sensation of fullness in the ear 7. Miosis and/or ptosis	
D. Attacks have frequency of more than five per day for more than half of the time • *Episodic:* At least two bouts lasting from 7 days to 1 year (when untreated) and separated by pain-free remission periods of ≥ 1 month. • *Chronic:* Occurring without a remission period or with remissions lasting < 1 month for at least 1 year.	During less than half of the time, attacks may be less frequent.
E. Attacks are prevented absolutely by therapeutic doses of indomethacin	In adults, oral indomethacin should be used initially in a dose of at least 150 mg daily and increased if necessary up to 225 mg daily. The dose by injection is 100 to 200 mg. Smaller maintenance doses are often used.
F. Not better accounted for by another *International Classification of Headache Disorders,* third edition diagnosis	It has been suggested that chronic paroxysmal hemicrania secondary to organic disease may be the rule rather than the exception and requires careful workup in these cases.

*Reproduced with permission from the International Headache Society.

creasingly reported.[110,113] Pain felt in the shoulder, neck, and arm is quite common.[110,111]

Pain is unilateral, rarely changes sides, and extremely rarely becomes bilateral.[110,111,113–115] However, strong pain may cross the midline.[110]

Quality

A number of descriptors may be used, often by the same patient, but sharp and stabbing, throbbing, or boring are used most commonly.[110–113,116] Pain is severe and rated as 7 to 10 on a VAS.[113]

Temporal pattern

Pain onset is rapid and mostly peaks in less than 5 minutes.[110] The attacks in paroxysmal hemicrania are short; the average duration is seconds to 30 minutes, but attacks may last over an hour and are usually sharp and excruciating.[110,112,113]

Most attacks are spontaneous, but common triggers include stress; exercise; alcohol; pressure on the C2 root, the C4 to C5 transverse processes, or the occipital nerve; and neck movement.[113] Interictal pain is milder than that in hemicrania continua and is more common in long-standing paroxysmal hemicrania with comorbid migraine.[112,113]

Frequency is high, about eight attacks per 24 hours, but it can reach as many as 30 to 50.[111,113] Lower frequencies of one to five attacks per 24 hours have also been reported.[110,113] The temporal similarity to cluster headache behavior has led to the term *modified cluster pattern*, which describes the frequent attacks of paroxysmal hemicrania.[111]

CASE 11-2

Paroxysmal hemicrania in a 56-year-old man.

Present complaint: Left facial pain, excruciating (VAS 9) and sharp, located periorbitally, peri-auricularly, and radiating to the neck (see Fig 11-3). Onset may be preceded by pain over the ipsilateral premolar and molar teeth and adjoining alveolar bone. The pain can awaken the patient from sleep but has also occurred equally frequently throughout the day. Attacks last up to 15 minutes (see Fig 11-2b).

History of present complaint: The problem began 12 months previously and occurred frequently. The patient experienced an approximate maximum of up to six attacks daily and a minimum of three per day, with increasing frequency over the previous few months. The pain was invariably accompanied by conjunctival injection, nasal congestion, and occasional ptosis. Dental treatment has included extraction of a left mandibular molar, but this resulted in no change in pain character or quality. Computed tomography of the temporomandibular joints was clinically normal, as were two full sets of full-mouth intraoral periapical radiographs.

Physical examination: No relevant findings.

Relevant medical history: None.

Diagnosis: Trigeminal autonomic cephalalgia: paroxysmal hemicrania.

Diagnostic and treatment considerations: This case was difficult to diagnose because the pain often began intraorally. Because of the extensive reports on organic pathology underlying paroxysmal hemicrania, the patient was referred for a computed tomography scan of the head, which was clinically normal. Indomethacin (75 mg daily) provided significant relief. Per-schedule antacids were added for dyspepsia; however, any attempt at reducing the indomethacin caused pain relapse. The patient continues to take indomethacin for pain relief.

The first reported cases of paroxysmal hemicrania were of a continuous nature and were categorized as chronic paroxysmal hemicrania. Only a scant number of paroxysmal hemicranias behaved episodically,[110] and many of these eventually developed into a chronic form.

Paroxysmal hemicrania does not characteristically occur at night.[39] However, some patients report nocturnal attacks that wake them from sleep, and researchers have found that these are REM-sleep related.[112,113]

Autonomic phenomena

Autonomic signs may occur bilaterally but are more pronounced on the symptomatic side.[113] The most commonly seen are ipsilateral lacrimation, nasal congestion, conjunctival injection, and rhinnorrhea.[112,113,116] More rarely, eyelid swelling and fullness in the ear are described.[113] Heart rate changes (bradycardia, tachycardia, extrasystole), increased local sweating, and salivation are not common.[111,113] Pain in paroxysmal hemicrania is not considered secondary to autonomic activation as pain continues in spite of these phenomena being blocked.

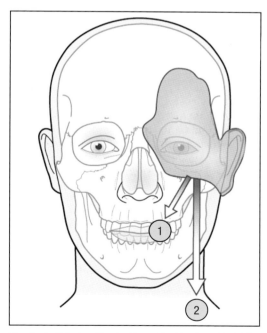

Fig 11-3 Pain location for the patient in Case 11-2. The patient indicated pain primarily in the periorbital and periauricular area and radiating to the teeth and neck (1 and 2, respectively).

Cluster headache–like features

A significant number of patients with paroxysmal hemicrania report agitation, restlessness, and verbal aggression during attacks.[112,113] A seasonal pattern of attacks has been described in patients with paroxysmal hemicrania.[29,113,117,118]

Migrainous features

Phonophobia or photophobia is present in up to 65% of patients with paroxysmal hemicrania and is mostly unilateral, thus differentiating these patients from migraine patients.[29,110,113] Motion sensitivity, osmophobia, nausea, and vomiting have also been reported to affect 40% to 50% of patients with paroxysmal hemicrania.[113]

Epidemiology

Paroxysmal hemicrania is rare, and large population-based studies are needed to accurately assess its prevalence. Based on cluster headache figures and patient populations, the prevalence of paroxysmal hemicrania has been estimated to be between 0.02% and 0.07%.[111,119] Some believe paroxysmal hemicrania is more common than previously thought, and as it shares many clinical characteristics with dental pain, it will frequently be seen in orofacial pain clinics.

A family history of paroxysmal hemicrania in patient samples is rare.[113] Family history of any of the neurovascular-type headaches was examined in patients with paroxysmal hemicrania, but no significantly increased prevalence was found.[111] Initial reported cases were largely female, but in recent reviews the female-male ratio approaches 1:1.[111,113]

Mean age of onset is usually 34 to 41 years, but children aged 6 and adults aged 81 years have been reported, and the average illness duration is 13 years.[110,112,113,120] The episodic form is considered to have an earlier mean age of onset (27 years) than the chronic form (37 years).

Symptomatic paroxysmal hemicrania

Many patients with chronic paroxysmal hemicrania (22%) report head and neck trauma.

However, this prevalence is no different from that found in cluster headache or migraine.[111]

Malignancy, central nervous system disease, and benign tumors have been implicated in symptomatic paroxysmal hemicrania.[41] A case of parotid gland epidermoid carcinoma with cerebral metastasis causing paroxysmal hemicrania has been reported.[121]

Literature reviews suggest that systemic diseases are common in paroxysmal hemicrania, including connective tissue disease and thrombocytopenia.[41] Thus, it has been suggested that chronic paroxysmal hemicrania secondary to organic disease may be the rule rather than the exception and thus requires careful workup, including imaging.

Treatment

Attacks of paroxysmal hemicrania are generally so short that an abortive approach is impractical. Paroxysmal hemicrania is supposed to have an absolute response to indomethacin,[122] but the mechanism is poorly understood. Moreover, some patients with paroxysmal hemicrania do not respond to indomethacin fully or even at all.[112] The inclusion of an absolute indomethacin response as part of the criteria for paroxysmal hemicrania has been questioned, but its usefulness outweighs any disadvantage. Most patients respond within 24 hours, many within 8 hours.[72] If response is partial, trial therapy should be continued for 4 days at 75 mg daily followed, if needed, by 150 mg daily for a further 3 days. Some patients may require 200 to 300 mg daily for full prophylaxis,[113] but persistently high dosage requirements may be an indication of underlying pathology.[72] Prognosis in paroxysmal hemicrania is good, and long-term remission has been reported.

Long-term treatment with indomethacin may be complicated by gastrointestinal and other complications. The use of antacids may reduce the gastrointestinal morbidity. A time-dependent decrease of up to 60% in indomethacin dosage requirements has been documented.[123] The underlying mechanisms are unknown but may be related to disease-modifying capabilities of indomethacin.[124]

Indomethacin-resistant paroxysmal hemicrania has been treated with calcium channel blockers, steroids, naproxen, topiramate, and

Table 11-6	Pharmacotherapy for paroxysmal hemicrania, SUNCT, and hemicrania continua			
Condition	**Drug of choice**	**Dose (route)**	**Second line**	
Paroxysmal hemicrania	Indomethacin	75 to 225 mg/day orally	Other NSAIDs, verapamil, acetazolamide	
SUNCT	Lamotrigine	100 to 300 mg/day orally	Gabapentin 900 to 2,700 mg/day, topiramate 50 to 200 mg/day	
Hemicrania continua	Indomethacin	25 to 300 mg/day orally	Other NSAIDs, piroxicam-beta-cyclodextrin	

NSAID, nonsteroidal anti-inflammatory drug.

carbamazepine.[72] Topiramate has been recommended as second-line therapy.[125] The gastrointestinal effects of indomethacin can be severe, so selective cyclooxygenase-2 (COX-2) inhibitors, such as celecoxib, have also been tried, at times quite successfully, but again long-term morbidity is a problem.[117,126,127] Acetazolamide, a diuretic with anticonvulsant properties, is partially effective in paroxysmal hemicrania. Sumatriptan, which is beneficial in cluster headache and migraine, may be effective in a minority of patients with paroxysmal hemicrania.[113] Table 11-6 summarizes the pharmacotherapeutic options for treatment of paroxysmal hemicrania, SUNCT, and hemicrania continua.

The indomethacin effect

The striking response of paroxysmal hemicrania and hemicrania continua to indomethacin but not other nonsteroidal anti-inflammatory drugs is an interesting and still unclear phenomenon. Another indomethacin-responsive headache is the less known long-lasting autonomic symptoms with hemicrania (LASH) syndrome.[128] Paroxysmal hemicrania, hemicrania continua, and LASH are clinically quite distinct, but their shared treatment response has led to the term *indomethacin-responsive headache*[129] or *indomethacin-responsive TACs*.[130]

Indomethacin crosses the blood-brain barrier better than naproxen and ibuprofen, making a central action in headache treatment plausible.[131] Indeed indomethacin is able to block central sensitization at the level of the trigeminocervical complex.[132]

Inhibiting the production of prostaglandins and inflammatory processes via COX enzyme inhibition is not exclusive to indomethacin.

However, in vitro experiments indicate that indomethacin has a better binding profile to COX than naproxen and ibuprofen.[132] Indomethacin inhibits neurogenic inflammation in rat dura mater induced by electrical stimulation of the trigeminal ganglion and at higher concentrations was able to inhibit substance P–induced extravasation.[133]

Low concentrations of indomethacin enhance the vasoconstriction induced by endothelin-1 in human artery.[134] A COX-2 dependent pathway of cytokine-induced calcitonin gene-related peptide (CGRP) release in trigeminal ganglia neurons that is not affected by 5-hydroxytryptamine 1B/D (5-HT$_{1B/D}$) receptor activation has been described.[135] As a consequence of the blockage of prostaglandin-E release, the release of CGRP was inhibited.[135] These actions may explain indomethacin-induced reductions in regional cerebral blood flow found in experiments with animals and humans.

Nitric oxide (NO)–induced effects in headache pathophysiology are of great interest because it is known that application of NO donors induces an acute headache, followed by a later-onset headache.[21] Glyceryltrinitrate-induced paroxysmal hemicrania starts immediately after NO administration, but this is both unpredictable and irregular.[113] This indicates that the NO mechanism is not a major component in the pathophysiology of paroxysmal hemicrania pathophysiology and suggests other mechanisms for indomethacin's actions. However, findings from an experimental pain model suggest that an interaction between indomethacin and local NO synthesis is involved in the antinociceptive effects of indomethacin.[136] Indomethacin inhibits NO production by

Table 11-7	Diagnostic criteria for SUNHA*
Diagnostic criteria	**Notes**
A. At least 20 attacks fulfilling criteria B through D	May coexist with trigeminal neuralgia; in such patients, there is overlap of signs and symptoms, and the differentiation is clinically difficult.
B. Moderate or severe unilateral head pain, with orbital, supraorbital, temporal, and/or other trigeminal distribution, lasting for 1 to 600 seconds and occurring as single stabs, as a series of stabs, or in a sawtooth pattern	This is the shortest of the TACs. Longer-duration attacks are characterized by multiple stabs or a sawtooth pain pattern.
C. At least one of the following cranial autonomic symptoms or signs, ipsilateral to the pain: 1. Conjunctival injection and/or lacrimation 2. Nasal congestion and/or rhinorrhea 3. Eyelid edema 4. Forehead and facial sweating 5. Forehead and facial flushing 6. Sensation of fullness in the ear 7. Miosis and/or ptosis	Patients may be seen with only one of these cranial autonomic symptoms or signs
D. Attacks have a frequency of at least one a day for more than half of the time when the disorder is active	SUNCT and SUNA are usually triggerable without a refractory period. This is in contrast to trigeminal neuralgia, which usually has a refractory period after each attack.
E. Not better accounted for by another *International Classification of Headache Disorders,* third edition diagnosis	The most common mimics of SUNCT are lesions in the posterior fossa or involving the pituitary gland.

*Reproduced with permission from the International Headache Society.

endothelial and inducible NO synthase[137] and is effective in inhibiting NO-induced dural vasodilation.[138] This seems specific because indomethacin, but not naproxen or ibuprofen, had an effect on NO-induced vasodilation.[131]

An inhibitory effect of indomethacin was shown on trigeminal nociceptive firing that was elicited by stimulation of the superior salivary nucleus and recorded in the trigeminocervical complex itself.[139] Indomethacin also inhibited trigeminoautonomic activation. Indomethacin, oxygen, and sumatriptan were effective, and naproxen was not, which reflects the pharmacotherapeutic profile of TACs. Only indomethacin was able to inhibit blood-flow changes in the rat lacrimal gland after stimulation of the superior salivary nucleus as a model for activation of autonomic symptoms, which demonstrates a direct effect on the craniovascular outflow.[139] All of these mechanisms are likely involved in indomethacin's ability to relieve paroxysmal hemicrania, hemicrania continua, and LASH syndrome.

Short-Lasting Unilateral Neuralgiform Headache Attacks

Short-lasting unilateral neuralgiform headache attacks (SUNHA) are characterized by attacks of moderate or severe, strictly unilateral head pain lasting seconds to minutes. They occur at least once a day and are usually associated with prominent lacrimation and conjunctival injection of the ipsilateral eye.

The most recent IHS classification specifically classifies two subtypes of SUNHA: short-lasting unilateral neuralgiform headache attacks with conjunctival injection and tearing (SUNCT) and short-lasting unilateral neuralgiform headache attacks with cranial autonomic symptoms (SUNA) (Table 11-7 and Box 11-3). SUNCT is likely a subform of SUNA, but until data accumulate, the classification retains this separation.

Box 11-3	Criteria for SUNCT and SUNA*

3.3.1 SUNCT

A. Attacks fulfilling criteria for SUNHA and criterion B below

B. Both conjunctival injection and lacrimation (tearing)
- *Episodic:* Meets criteria A and B with at least two bouts lasting from 7 days to 1 year and separated by pain-free remission periods ≥ 1 month.
- *Chronic:* Meets criteria A and B and occurs without a remission period or with remissions lasting < 1 month for at least 1 year.

3.3.2 SUNA

A. Attacks fulfilling criteria for SUNHA and criterion B below

B. Only one or neither of conjunctival injection and lacrimation (tearing)
- *Episodic:* Meets criteria A and B with at least two bouts lasting from 7 days to 1 year and separated by pain-free remission periods ≥ 1 month.
- *Chronic:* Meets criteria A and B and occurs without a remission period or with remissions lasting < 1 month for at least 1 year.

*Reproduced with permission from the International Headache Society.

SUNCT and SUNA are differentiated on the basis of accompanying autonomic signs—both conjunctival injection and tearing in SUNCT but only one or neither of these in SUNA. Otherwise they are identical in clinical presentation as described later.

Clinical presentation

The similarities of this syndrome to trigeminal neuralgia are marked, particularly the triggering mechanism, and many believe SUNCT to be a trigeminal neuralgia variant.

Clinical example

Case 11-3 (Fig 11-4) clearly shows the difficulty in differentiating between SUNCT and trigeminal neuralgia of the ophthalmic branch. Trigeminal neuralgia with lacrimation is a particularly difficult differential diagnosis (see chapter 12).

Location

Pain is unilateral with no obvious side predilection and located in the temporal, auricular, and occipital regions.[140] Side-variable attacks may be seen in a minority of patients and rarely bilateral pain.[141] Although usually located in the ocular and periocular regions, it may involve any of the areas of the head/face.[141] Pain spreading across the midline or changing sides is rare.[140]

Quality

SUNCT is considered a moderate to severe pain syndrome,[140–142] and SUNA may be slightly less severe.[141] The pain is rarely pulsatile and is usually burning, stabbing, and sometimes electric.[141,143,144]

Temporal pattern

Multiple attacks occur, usually during the daytime; fewer than 2% occur at night.[144] A bimodal distribution of attacks occurring in the morning and late afternoon has been observed.[144] Remissions have been observed and may last for several months.[145]

Attacks begin rapidly and end abruptly.[144] Each attack lasts from 1 to 600 seconds with a mean duration of about 1 minute,[141] but longer attacks of 250 seconds, 600 seconds, and even 2 or 3 hours have been reported.[141,146]

Frequency ranges from 2 to 600 daily, with an average of 59 per day; many patients have such frequent attacks that they may be unable to quantify them[141] (see Fig 11-2c). A clusterlike pattern has been reported with active and inactive episodes but is variably present. Rarely, SUNCT status occurs, which consists of pain lasting for the better part of the day for 1 to 3 days. Low-grade background (interictal) pain or local discomfort may also be part of SUNCT, even in the absence of medication overuse[140,141] (Fig 11-5).

CASE 11-3

A 57 year-old-man with SUNCT.

Present complaint: Severe periorbital pain (see Fig 11-4) with an electric, spasmlike quality that severely interferes with normal activity. He experiences at least 10 attacks per day (usually more) with duration of up to 3 to 5 minutes (very rarely more) (see Fig 11-2c). The pain is referred to the left temporal area and intraorally. Pain can be induced by mechanical stimulation around the lips (such as shaving and eating) and by intraoral stimuli (such as tooth brushing). However, the vast majority of attacks are spontaneous, have no clear trigger preceding onset, and are always accompanied by ipsilateral lacrimation and conjunctival injection.

History of present complaint: Attacks began 1.5 years previously. Pain did not wake the patient from sleep. Neurologic examination and brain computed tomography scan were clinically normal. In the past, the patient has received carbamazepine, baclofen, and amitriptyline in adequate doses with no pain relief. The pain has recently been worsening.

Physical examination: Clinically normal. Blood chemistry and hematology were within normal limits.

Relevant medical history: None.

Diagnosis: Trigeminal autonomic cephalalgia; SUNCT.

Diagnostic and treatment considerations: The occasionally longer attacks are not typical of SUNCT, and therefore, trial treatment with indomethacin 75 mg daily was initiated. Four weeks later, the patient returned complaining of strong pain and lacrimation, although there was improvement. The dose was increased to 150 mg indomethacin daily with no change in symptoms. Clonazepam 0.5 mg to aid in sleep helped him during the night, but the diurnal pain was unaffected. An MRI of the brain was clinically normal. A period of spontaneous remission followed for some weeks, but the pain returned. The patient was then prescribed lamotrigine 100 to 200 mg daily, and although this was only partially successful, the difference was considered clinically significant by the patient.

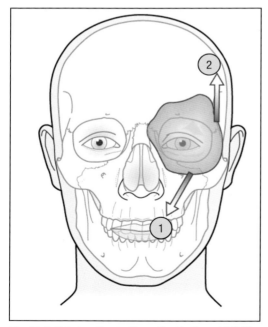

Fig 11-4 Pain location for the patient in Case 11-3. The patient indicated pain primarily in the periorbital area and radiating to the teeth and temporal areas (1 and 2, respectively).

An irregular pattern of attacks is characteristic. However, a number of patterns of typical attacks have been described; single attacks may last a bit longer and have a plateau-like pattern.[147] Shorter attacks in rapid succession or repetitive attacks are also recognized. Sawtooth-like attacks may also occur, in which consecutive spike-like paroxysms occur without reaching the pain-free baseline. A mixture of short attacks on top of the typical plateau pattern, termed *plateau-like plus exacerbations*, has also been described[141,142,144] (see Fig 11-5).

Triggering

Pain in SUNCT/SUNA may be triggered by light mechanical stimuli in the areas innervated by the trigeminal nerve, chewing, tooth brushing, or wind.[141,142] SUNA seems to have a lower incidence of triggers than SUNCT.[141,142] Extratrigeminal triggers, including neck movements, have also been shown to precipitate attacks.[144] Alcohol is not usually reported to worsen pain.

In contrast to trigeminal neuralgia, refractory periods in SUNCT/SUNA are either absent

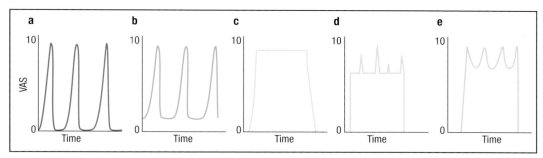

Fig 11-5 Temporal patterns of SUNHA attacks. Shorter-lasting attacks in rapid succession, or repetitive attacks, are recognized (a). Sawtooth-like attacks are also possible, in which consecutive spikelike paroxysms occur without reaching the pain-free baseline (b). Single attacks may last a bit longer and have a plateau-like pattern (c). There can also be a mixture of short attacks on top of the typical plateau pattern, termed *plateau-like plus exacerbations* (d). When attacks are very frequent, the pattern may take on a "sawtooth" appearance (e). (Adapted from Pareja and Sjaastad[147] with permission.)

or extremely rare, and this is a major differentiating sign.[141,142,148] Additionally, local analgesic blockade is ineffective in SUNCT/SUNA.[144]

Autonomic signs

By definition, SUNHAs are accompanied by autonomic signs. In SUNCT, marked ipsilateral conjunctival injection and lacrimation appear rapidly with onset of pain.[140] Nasal stuffiness and rhinorrhea are common, whereas sweating may accompany attacks but is rare and often subclinical. Autonomic signs appear irrespective of the site of pain, which may occur in the maxillary or mandibular dermatomes.[141]

Migrainous symptoms

A minority of patients with SUNCT/SUNA may report migrainous features.[141] These include photophobia, phonophobia, and nausea. All of these patients, however, had coexisting migraine headaches. Auralike symptoms, including tingling of facial skin, have been reported.[142,149]

Patient behavior

Reports suggest that some patients with SUNCT/SUNA become agitated during attacks, much like patients with cluster headache.[141]

Associated phenomena

Respiratory studies have indicated that patients with SUNCT hyperventilate during attacks. Heart rate may also decrease during attacks in patients

with SUNCT. Increased intraocular pressure with increased facial temperature periocularly has been reported.[144] Orbital phlebography studies show abnormalities on the painful side and may indicate venous vasculitis. Imaging studies during attacks are essentially normal, but cerebral blood flow may be abnormal in SUNCT.

Epidemiology

SUNHA seems to be a very rare syndrome, but it is possible that the clinical similarities with trigeminal neuralgia and cluster headache lead to the misdiagnosis of many patients.[140] SUNHA may therefore be more common than estimates based on the sparse case reports. A study in Australia estimated the prevalence of SUNCT/SUNA at 0.0066%.[142] Cases have been reported from childhood to old age, with a mean onset of about 50 years.[140,150]

The exact male-female ratio is unclear.[140,142,143] Initially, the male preponderance was 7:1, but with more female cases appearing, SUNCT is presently considered only slightly more common in males, about 1.5:1.[140,141,143]

SUNCT occurring in siblings, or familial SUNCT, has been reported[151] and raises the possibility that SUNCT, together with migraine, cluster headache, and possibly other TACs, will eventually be considered to have a genetic predisposition.

Symptomatic SUNHA

Symptomatic SUNCT/SUNA presents similarly to primary cases.[141] Diagnoses in symptomatic

SUNCT include brainstem infarction, cerebellopontine arteriovenous malformations, cerebellopontine astrocytoma or other tumors, cavernous hemangioma of the brainstem, cavernous sinus tumor, extraorbital cystic mass, and neurofibromatosis.[41,140] Post-traumatic SUNCT, including eye trauma, has been reported.[140,152] Rare reports include SUNCT related to HIV and osteogenesis imperfecta.[41]

TACs and SUNCT/SUNA have been associated with underlying pathology of the pituitary gland.[141,153] In a series of patients with pituitary tumor, 5% were found to suffer from pain that could be diagnosed as SUNCT.[38] Symptomatic causes are diagnosable with MRI, and all patients with SUNCT should therefore be referred for appropriate imaging.[140]

A number of cases of SUNCT/SUNA with neurovascular compression have been described, similar to that in classical trigeminal neuralgia.[154] These findings add to the ongoing discussion of SUNCT/SUNA's relation to trigeminal neuralgia. However, the question arises as to whether this is an incidental finding or indeed the underlying pathophysiology in these cases.

Treatment

Pharmacotherapy

A distinct factor in SUNCT/SUNA is resistance to a large number of drugs. Lamotrigine is the treatment of choice and is recommended as initial therapy[70,142] (see Table 11-6). The standard dose is 100 to 300 mg/day, but dosages ranging from 25 to 600 mg/day may be needed.[144] Lamotrigine seems to be more effective in episodic than in chronic SUNCT/SUNA.[142]

Other anticonvulsant drugs may produce some improvement; carbamazepine may induce relief in about one-third of patients with SUNCT but is usually ineffective in SUNA.[40,72] SUNCT, and less so SUNA, responds to treatment with relatively new anticonvulsants, such as topiramate.[140,143] Gabapentin seems to be effective for both SUNCT and SUNA.[144] In patients where lamotrigine is ineffective, gabapentin and topiramate are recommended as second-line agents.[72,155]

Similar to cluster headache, SUNCT may also respond to steroids.[72] A case of SUNCT responsive to verapamil has been described,[156]

in sharp contrast to past reports of a possible worsening of SUNCT secondary to verapamil.[157] Intravenous lidocaine may be needed in patients with a high frequency of attacks or as transitional therapy, but the effect is inconsistent.[142,144]

Surgery

Surgical treatments for SUNCT/SUNA are not sufficiently validated and rely on case reports or small series.[144] Hypothalamic stimulation has been used successfully in a number of patients with SUNCT.[144] Cases of SUNCT associated with trigeminal nerve compression and with a vascular malformation in the cerebellopontine angle have been reported.[158] Moreover, case reports have appeared in which surgical microvascular decompression and percutaneous trigeminal ganglion compression were performed for SUNCT, just as for trigeminal neuralgia.[159,160] In a series of nine patients with SUNCT/SUNA, immediate and complete relief was obtained in six. This was sustained for a mean follow-up of 22 months.[161] In other case series, 75% of patients subsequently treated with microvascular decompression achieved complete pain relief lasting up to 31 months; others were treated by glycerol or radiofrequency rhizotomy and gamma knife radiosurgery with reasonable outcomes.[154] For drug-refractory cases, microvascular decompression may be an option.

Hemicrania Continua

Clinical and neuroimaging findings suggest that hemicrania continua belongs with the TACs[2,162] (Table 11-8). Hemicrania continua has a chronic unremitting pattern and is considered a chronic daily headache, together with chronic (transformed) migraine, chronic tension-type headache, and new daily persistent headache (see chapters 8 and 10).

Patients with hemicrania continua often suffer from misdiagnosis, and the correct diagnosis often takes up to 5 to 7 years and more than four physicians[163,164]; even 12-year delays have been reported.[165] About one-third of patients with hemicrania continua consulted a dentist, and 20% received a diagnosis of dental pain.[163] Misdiagnosis in hemicrania continua

Table 11-8   **Diagnostic criteria for hemicrania continua***

Diagnostic criteria	Notes
A. Unilateral headache fulfilling criteria B through D	Unlike other TACs or migraine, no sleep association is reported.
B. Present for > 3 months, with exacerbations of moderate or greater intensity	Rare cases of remission are reported.

C. Either or both of the following:
  1. At least one of the following symptoms or signs, ipsilateral to the headache:
    a. Conjunctival injection and/or lacrimation
    b. Nasal congestion and/or rhinorrhea
    c. Eyelid edema
    d. Forehead and facial sweating
    e. Forehead and facial flushing
    f. Sensation of fullness in the ear
    g. Miosis and/or ptosis
  2. A sense of restlessness or agitation or aggravation of the pain by movement
	During exacerbation, hemicrania continua is distinctly similar to migraine.

D. Responds absolutely to therapeutic doses of indomethacin	Some cases have been reported secondary to analgesic and ergot abuse and may not be reversible.
E. Not better accounted for by another *International Classification of Headache Disorders,* third edition diagnosis	

*Reproduced with permission from the International Headache Society.

has been attributed to its relative rarity, the paucity of autonomic signs, medication overuse, and the distinct similarities to migraine during exarcebations.[163,164]

Clinical features

Clinical example

Case 11-4 (Figs 11-6 and 11-7) is an excellent example of a patient with hemicrania continua with good long-term follow-up. The pain is constant and has mild autonomic and migrainous features that become very prominent during exacerbations. Indomethacin is consistently effective. Failed treatments included amitriptyline, propranolol, and carbamazepine.

Location

Pain is generally felt in the frontal and temporal regions and periorbitally.[166] Some patients (18%) will describe a distinct ocular sensation mimicking a foreign body (or sand) that may accompa-

ny or precede the headaches.[167] Pain location around the teeth has been reported by 20% of patients.[166] The vast majority of cases are unilateral with no definite side preponderance noted, and few bilateral cases have been reported.[162,167] Although very rare, pain can also change sides.

Quality

Pain is described as throbbing in about one-third to two-thirds of patients and may be a constant feature of the pain or appear as pain intensity increases.[166–168] Other common pain descriptors include dull and pressure-like, whereas in exacerbations descriptions of stabbing and throbbing pain are common.[168] Exacerbations are also distinguishable in that they are totally disabling in about 40% of patients.[168] In addition, many patients report a sharp pain similar to the condition of jabs and jolts.[168]

Severity is graded as moderate (VAS 4 to 6) by most patients[164,168,169] and is characterized in many patients (74%) by fluctuations or exacerbations (VAS 8 to 9) in pain severity.[164,167]

A 30-year-old woman with hemicrania continua.

Present complaint: Continuous pain on the right side of the face and head (see Fig 11-6). The intensity of the pain is usually moderate (5 to 6 on a VAS) with occasional exacerbations (VAS of 7 to 8) that do not have a jabs-and-jolts quality. A throbbing, pressure-like quality is associated with the pain. The pain sometimes awakens her from sleep, usually in the early morning.

History of present complaint: Pain began approximately 2 years previously as a continuous headache. No accompanying autonomic or systemic signs were evident. Pain was also felt unilaterally intraorally in the maxillary first and second molar area. Dental treatment has been ineffective in relieving the pain. Acetaminophen in doses of 1 or 2 g per day has provided partial relief. No abnormal findings were noted on neurologic; ear, nose, and throat; and dental examinations. Hematologic and biochemical blood screenings were within normal limits. Computerized scanning of the head, paranasal sinuses, and temporomandibular joints and dental radiographs showed no pathology. Doppler examination of carotid blood flow was clinically normal. Past treatments have included propranolol, diazepam, ergotamine combinations, and intensive physiotherapy with no significant improvement. Diclofenac sodium had initially reduced pain intensity but became ineffective within approximately 10 days.

Physical examination: Mild masticatory and neck muscle tenderness ipsilateral to the pain with no limitation of mouth opening or neck movements.

Relevant medical history: None.

Diagnosis: Chronic daily headache; hemicrania continua.

Diagnostic and treatment considerations: The referral pattern caused confusion with dental pain, and the muscle tenderness falsely indicated a musculoskeletal disorder. Pain description is typical of a chronic daily headache. Because of the combination of musculoskeletal and vascular-type features, treatment was initiated with amitriptyline starting at 10 mg and increasing to 35 mg at bedtime. Four weeks later, the patient was seen again and had no change in pain frequency or intensity. The salient features of the pain were as follows:

- Unilateral, including half of the head and face
- Continuous, with a throbbing, sometimes pressure-like quality
- Fluctuating, from moderate to severe
- Not accompanied by autonomic signs
- Able to wake the patient

These features suggested a diagnosis of hemicrania continua. The patient began indomethacin 75 mg daily in three doses and reduced the amitriptyline to 10 mg daily. At her next review appointment 3 weeks later, the patient reported significant reduction in pain intensity and frequency on 50 mg indomethacin (see Fig 11-7). Relief began rapidly, and within 2 days she was essentially pain free. Gastrointestinal symptoms had been avoided with omeprazole 20 mg daily. The patient had continued pain relief and reported that any attempt to reduce the dose resulted in headaches.

Long-term review: The patient did not present for follow-up for about 6 months. She had attempted to stop the indomethacin because she wanted to get pregnant. All such attempts induced headache recurrence, however. Three months previously, she had visited a neurologist's clinic and had been treated with intramuscular steroids with no improvement. A further trial with propranolol slow release (80 mg) followed by carbamazepine (200 to 800 mg) had provided no pain relief. Without indomethacin, the patient reported that she still suffered moderate headaches (VAS 5 to 6) that rapidly responded to initiation of therapy (VAS 0 to 2). About 7 weeks before her visit, she began experiencing severe exacerbations of unilateral headaches (VAS 9 to 10) accompanied by nausea and ipsilateral autonomic signs (lacrimation, nasal congestion, eyelid edema). These attacks could last 36 to 48 hours. During the first 3 weeks, she suffered one attack. Subsequently, they became weekly (see Fig 11-7). The patient was instructed to cease the carbamazepine and reinitiate indomethacin 25 mg three times daily. Over a period of 11 weeks, the patient continued to take indomethacin and reported substantial improvement in baseline pain. The exacerbations became less frequent, shorter in duration, and less intense (see Fig 11-7).

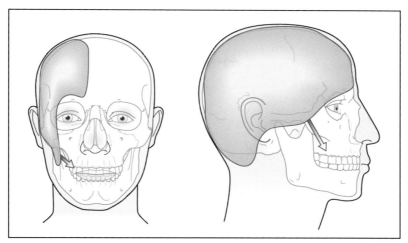

Fig 11-6 Pain location for the patient described in Case 11-4. Pain was located in the frontal, temporal, occipital, and periauricular regions on one side. Pain radiated intra-orally, usually to the ipsilateral maxillary first and second molars.

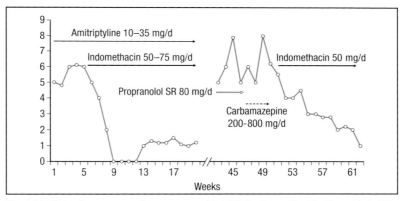

Fig 11-7 Pain diary representing mean weekly VAS for the patient in Case 11-4. After initial diagnosis and indomethacin treatment, there was rapid improvement (weeks 1 to 19). The patient was then lost to follow-up for about 6 months. The pain returned, and treatment with propranolol and carbamazepine was unsuccessful (weeks 43 to 50). Re-instatement of indomethacin was successful (week 52).

Temporal pattern

Two forms of hemicrania continua have been described: remitting and continuous. The remitting form is characterized by headache that can last for some days followed by a pain-free period lasting 2 to 15 days. This pattern is initially present in about half of patients; in the rest, pain is continuous from onset.[166–168] One-third of remitting cases become continuous after a mean duration of 7.8 years.[167,168]

Nocturnal attacks were reported in up to half of patients, and some patients report that if they wake up for other reasons, the pain is invariably present.[167,168]

Although hemicrania continua is characterized by continuous pain, about half of patients report daily exacerbations, and the rest suffer these several times per week.[164,169] Exacerbations often result in severe pain (VAS 9) lasting 30 minutes to 10 hours and even up to 2 to 5 days.[167–169] During an exacerbation, the features of hemicrania continua in most patients (≈70%) are indistinguishable from those of migraine.[163,168]

Precipitating or aggravating factors

A variety of factors, such as bending over, menses, strong odors, and stress, have been reported to provoke or worsen the pain.[167,168] These factors are reminiscent of migraine but are not consistent features of hemicrania continua. Some patients may clearly identify alcohol as a provoking or aggravating factor.[167,168]

Physical and laboratory findings

Hemicrania continua is not usually accompanied by notable pathology or other abnormalities.[167] In most published cases of hemicrania continua, computerized scanning of the head, neurologic and other physical examination, hematology, and serum biochemistry were all clinically normal. However, the clinician must be aware that cases of hemicrania continua secondary to pathology or systemic disease have been reported.[41]

Accompanying phenomena

A paucity of autonomic signs usually accompany the continuous pain.[170] However, during exacerbation, autonomic signs commonly appear singly or in various combinations, though they are still relatively mild.[166,169] This strengthens the hypothesis that activation of autonomic signs is dependent on pain severity. The most common signs, which present in 30% to 60% of patients, are photophobia, nausea, conjunctival injection, phonophobia, and tearing.[166,167] During exacerbations, up to 60% of patients display such qualities as photophobia, phonophobia, nausea, and, more rarely, vomiting.[165,168] Hemicrania continua with aura has also been described, further linking hemicrania continua to migraine pathophysiology.[171] More rarely (15% to 18% of patients), nasal stuffiness or rhinorrhea, vomiting, or ptosis may also be reported.[167] Restlessness and agitation may be reported in up to two-thirds of patients.[166,169] These features establish the hemicrania continua phenotype as straddling TACs and migraine.

Epidemiology

Prevalence of hemicrania continua may not be as low as previously thought and, although unconfirmed by indomethacin challenge, may reach 1%.[119,172] Most cases reported are female (female-male ratio, 2 to 2.8:1) with a mean age of onset of 28 to 33 years (range, 5 to 67 years).[167,168,173] No significant difference was observed in mean onset age between the remitting and continuous types.[167]

Symptomatic hemicrania continua

Three cases of hemicrania continua complicated or caused by medication abuse have been reported.[167] Two patients abused ergotamine and one acetaminophen; cessation of the drug eliminated or reduced headaches. Hemicrania continua secondary to a mesenchymal tumor in the sphenoid bone has also been reported.[167]

Some patients with hemicrania continua report a history of mild to moderate head trauma and surgery.[174,175] The patients met the IHS criteria for chronic posttraumatic headache and displayed clinical signs typical of hemicrania continua. Furthermore, treatment with indomethacin, with doses up to 200 mg daily, was successful in all patients.

Treatment

Indomethacin is usually totally effective in hemicrania continua and is included as part of its definition. In the vast majority (68%) of reported cases, patients have indeed responded to indomethacin.[168] The results are dramatic with a rapid onset of relief occurring within hours or 1 or 2 days, often with a dose response.[167] When 50 mg of indomethacin was given intramuscularly to 12 patients with hemicrania continua, complete pain relief occurred within an average of 73 minutes and lasted for 13 hours; this has been proposed as the diagnostic Indotest. However, the occurrence of indomethacin-resistant hemicrania continua is a possibility, although it may be a reflection of inadequate dosing. In indomethacin-resistant patients, topiramate has emerged as a useful alternative,[176-178] and reports suggest a role for occipital nerve stimulation.[179]

Other nonsteroidal anti-inflammatory drugs are less effective, although aspirin, ibuprofen, piroxicam-beta-cyclodextrin, diclofenac, COX-2 inhibitors, and acetaminophen have provided partial relief.[126,163,167] Piroxicam-beta-cyclodextrin is inferior to indomethacin in hemicrania continua, but its better tolerability may offer a good alternative for selected patients.[180] Triptans seem ineffective in hemicrania continua,[163] and only SC sumatriptan (6 mg) has partial but clinically doubtful efficacy.

Differential Diagnosis of TACs

Although the TACs are distinctive syndromes, delayed diagnosis or misdiagnosis seem relatively common.[163,181] The most common misdiagnoses for cluster headache remain migraine, sinusitis, dental/jaw problems, and trigeminal neuralgia. Because of its milder clinical phenotype, hemicrania continua can be a challenging diagnosis. In one series, about 80% of patients consulted neurologists and one-third attended dentists.[163] Migraine was the most common misdiagnosis followed by cluster headache, sinus headache, and dental pain. More than a third of patients had been subjected to ineffective invasive treatments, including dental extractions, sinus/deviated septum surgery, temporomandibular joint surgery, and cervical spine surgery. In paroxysmal hemicrania, the most common misdiagnoses are migraine, cluster headache, and dental problems.[112,181]

Substantial overlap exists for some of the ostensibly distinct diagnostic features.[182–184] Furthermore, descriptions of patients with co-existing headaches and reports of possible transformation of diagnoses within individual patients suggest common pathophysiologic mechanisms with a spectrum of clinical expression.[185–188] All of the cases of coexisting TACs described in a recent review involve the presence of cluster headache, and most of the patients had paroxysmal hemicrania or hemicrania continua.[187] Most of the patients suffered both headache types on the same side, but in the vast majority the headache types occurred subsequently rather than at the same time.[187]

In this section, the differential diagnosis of TACs is reviewed. The pain history and pain diary remain central to accurate diagnosis, and indeed, it is the overall combination of signs, symptoms, and behavior that lead an astute clinician to the correct diagnosis.

Within the TACs

Considerable overlap exists among the TACs in quality, location, and temporal patterns (Figs 11-8 and 11-9 and Tables 11-9 and 11-10; see also Cases 11-1 to 11-4). This stresses the importance of accurate intakes and the use of real-time pain diaries as follow-up.

The pain origin and patterns of referral are particularly similar in TACs and are characterized by orbital and periorbital pain that may radiate to the frontal and temporal regions (see Fig 11-8 and Cases 11-1 to 11-3). In 63% of patients with cluster headache, pain is orbital.[192] However, in SUNCT, pain may occur anywhere in the head, and 95% of patients with paroxysmal hemicrania report pain at sites outside the orbital region.[192]

The temporal pattern for each headache is clearly defined in the IHS classification.[1] Examine Cases 11-1 to 11-4; these are classic cases, and the differences in duration and frequency are striking. The plotting of information from pain diaries is sometimes invaluable in diagnosing complicated cases (see Fig 11-2).

A prolonged SUNCT attack may be just as lengthy as a short paroxysmal hemicrania attack, which similarly may, at the other end of the spectrum, overlap with short cluster headache attacks (see Fig 11-9 and Table 11-9). Relatively short migraine attacks[193] may occur, and when a patient suffers from chronic migraine with autonomic features, differentiation from TACs or hemicrania continua may be difficult.[184]

Similar overlap within the TACs is also evident with headache frequency (see Fig 11-9 and Table 11-9). Although high frequency is characteristic of paroxysmal hemicrania, frequent cluster headache may be confusing.[192] Additionally, migraine attacks may cluster or behave cyclically and overlap with more sustained cluster headache attacks.[194] Indeed, the typical clustering or seasonal pattern of cluster headache is often observed in other headaches, including hemicrania continua and

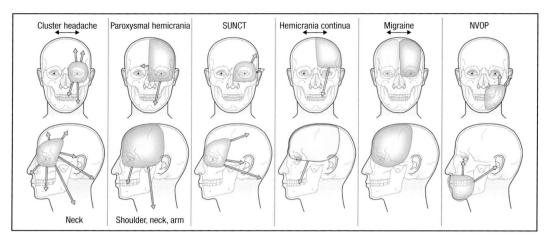

Fig 11-8 Pain location in TACs and neurovascular orofacial pain (NVOP). The TACs are characterized by orbital and periorbital pain. In paroxysmal hemicrania and hemicrania continua, large adjacent areas are affected. In SUNCT, it is now recognized that any ipsilateral trigeminal region may be involved. Migraine is largely unilateral but may be bilateral in up to 30% of patients (marked in the figure by a *lighter shaded area* contralaterally). NVOP is characterized by its location in the lower two-thirds of the face, and intraoral and perioral areas are frequently involved as primary sites. A *double-headed arrow* above a diagram indicates that side shift occurs in that specific headache type.

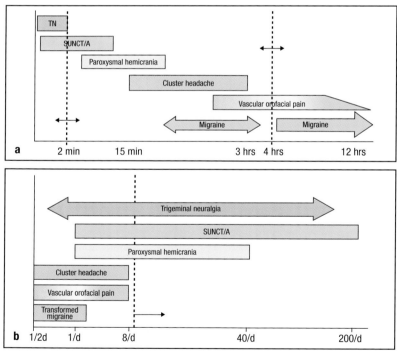

Fig 11-9 Duration *(a)* and frequency *(b)* in neurovascular headaches and trigeminal neuralgia. The IHS clearly defines pain duration and frequency, but there is considerable overlap. Duration overlap occurs particularly in headaches lasting from 2 minutes to 4 hours. Beyond these limits *(dotted lines in a)*, diagnosis is relatively limited. Note that migraines may occasionally last less than 4 hours *(orange double-headed arrow in a)* and that cluster headache has been reported to last up to 48 hours. The short-lasting headaches (trigeminal neuralgia [TN], SUNCT, paroxysmal hemicrania) are very frequent (more than eight per day; *dotted line in b*) with considerable overlap. Similarly, the long-lasting headaches overlap in the frequency of attacks. Trigeminal neuralgia *(purple double-headed arrow in b)* is often triggered but is usually of high frequency.

Table 11-9 **Typical clinical features in unilateral headaches with autonomic signs**

Parameter	Migraine	CH	CPH	SUNCT	NVOP	HC	TN
Demographics							
Onset age (years)	20 to 30	30 to 40*	30 to 40	40 to 50	40 to 50	30 to 40	50 to 60
Gender ratio (M:F)	1:3	5:1	1:2	9:1	1:3	1:2	1:2
Family history	60%	0.8% to 7%	None	Unknown	Unknown	Unknown	Unclear
Prevalence per 1,000	100 to 150	3	0.3 to 2.1	Rare	Rare	Rare	0.043
Pain duration	4 h to 3 d	15 min to 3 h	2 to 30 min	5 to 240 s	45 min to 12 h	Days	<120 s (preTN)
Sleep association	REM, III/IV	REM	REM	–	+	+	+/–
Awakens subjects	+	+	+	–	+	+	–
Time/frequency	Early morning	51%	33%	< 2%	35%	30% to 50%	–
Frequency	1 to 4/mo	½ to 8/d	5 to 40/d	3 to 200/d	Chronic	Chronic	↑†
Changes sides	Yes	May	Rare	No	Yes	No	No
Intensity	++	+++	++	++++	++	+/++	++++
Paroxysmal	+	+	+	+	+	–	+
Throbbing	++	+ (30%)	+/–	–	++	–‡	– (preTN)
Location	Forehead	Orbital	Upper	Orbital	Lower	Half	II>III>I
Remission	Pregnancy	Months to years	Unusual	+/–	–/Unknown	–	Weeks to years
Triggering							
Touch	–	–	–	+	–	–	++
Neck	–	–	+ (10%)	+	–	–	–
Alcohol	Delayed	+	+/–	+/–	–	+	–
Others (eg, foods, stress)	+	–	–	–	–	+	–

*Onset in women differs.
†Usually related to triggering events but of normally high frequency.
‡Increased during exacerbations.
CH, cluster headache; CPH, chronic paroxysmal hemicrania; NVOP; neurovascular orofacial pain; HC, hemicrania continua; TN, trigeminal neuralgia; M:F, male to female; preTN, pretrigeminal neuralgia.

paroxysmal hemicrania.[117,118,195] Most cases of paroxysmal hemicrania are characterized by chronic patterns that will differentiate them from the predominantly episodic nature of cluster headache.[192]

TACs may often occur with no or little autonomic signs and, conversely, autonomic signs may occur with no headache.[196] However, the presence of autonomic signs is common in all TACs, and differences rely more on their number and intensity. Across all TACs, lacrimation is the sign most often reported and is also observed in selected cases of trigeminal neuralgia, making it of poor predictive value (Fig 11-10).

TACs are different in their response to therapy (see Table 11-10), and clinicians often rely on this as a final endorsement of the diagnosis. For example, response to abortive oxygen, lithium, or verapamil would suggest a diagnosis of cluster headache. A positive indomethacin re-

Table 11-10	Accompanying signs and treatment response in unilateral headaches with autonomic signs*						
Parameter	Migraine	CH	CPH	SUNCT/A	NVOP	HC	TN
Autonomic signs	+	+++	++	+++	+/–	+/–†	+/–
Lacrimation	41%‡	84% to 91%	62%	+	10%	12% to 53%	5% to 31%
Conjunctival injection	‡	58% to 77%	36%	+	7%	12% to 32%	Unknown
Nasal congestion	14%§	48% to 72%	42%	+	7%	9% to 21%	Unknown
Rhinorrhea	§	43% to 72%	36%	+	7%	10% to 12%	Unknown
Flushing	+	–	–	–	+	2.9%	+
Ptosis/miosis	–	57% to 74%	–	–	–	2% to 28%	–
Ocular + nasal	46%‖						
Systemic signs	> 80%	24% to 56%	–	–	38%	50%	–
Treatment response							
Analgesics	+	+/–	–	–	+	–	–
Carbamazepine	–	–	–	–	Unknown	–	++
Valproic acid	+	+/–	–	–	Unknown	–	–
Lamotrigine	–	–	–	+	Unknown	–	+/–
Indomethacin	–	–	++	–	–	++	–
Sumatriptan	++	++	+/–	–	+	–	–
Amitriptyline	+	–	–	–	+	–	–
Steroids	–	+	–	–	Unknown	–	–
Beta-blockers	+	–	–	–	+	–	–
Ca²⁺-blockers	+	+	+ (cases)	–	–	–	–

*Data compiled from multiple studies.[4,14,56,57,95,140,144,163,167,168,189–191]
†Autonomic signs in HC refer to baseline and exacerbation studies.[168]
‡Specific ocular symptoms and §specific nasal symptoms: Numbers for migraine were reported together.[189]
‖Combination of all ocular and nasal symptoms in patients with migraine.[189]
   CH, cluster headache; CPH, chronic paroxysmal hemicrania; NVOP; neurovascular orofacial pain; HC, hemicrania continua; TN, trigeminal neuralgia.

sponse is considered highly indicative that the patient suffers from paroxysmal hemicrania or hemicrania continua.[197]

Based on initial grouping by duration and frequency, the clinician is often able to reach an accurate working diagnosis (Fig 11-11). In unclear TAC cases, it has been suggested that a trial of indomethacin is indicated.[198] However, because of the low prevalence of paroxysmal hemicrania and hemicrania continua, the best approach is to instigate indomethacin treatment in patients with five or more attacks daily and/or with attack duration less than 30 minutes.[198]

Migraine

Migraine is associated with a number of signs thought to be of high positive predictive value, such as aura, occasional hemiplegia, nausea, vomiting, photophobia, and phonophobia.[199] However, cluster headache with some of these

signs has been reported,[14,32] and similarly, exacerbations of hemicrania continua often present with migrainous-type features.[168,171] Specifically, photophobia or phonophobia occurs in up to 60% and nausea and vomiting in about 30% of patients with cluster headache, and some patients report an auralike preheadache phase.[200] Paroxysmal hemicrania may also present with migrainous features, but vomiting is very rare.[112]

Rarely, cluster headache may last for up to 48 hours,[6] so if accompanied by mild migrainous features, it would be a challenging diagnosis. Two clear extremes in duration are diagnostically significant: 2 minutes or less and 4 hours or more (see Fig 11-9a).

Distinguishing features of cluster headache as opposed to migraine are strict pain unilaterality and ipsilateral autonomic signs. However, a considerable number of patients with cluster headache report side shift within and between clusters.[5] Moreover, around half of migraineurs

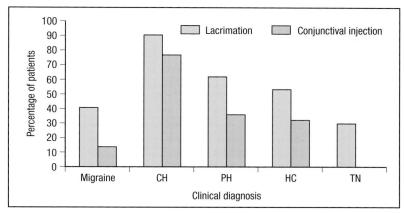

Fig 11-10 Percentage of patients with various craniofacial pain syndromes who report lacrimation or conjunctival injection. Although these signs are considered of high diagnostic value, they are clearly nonspecific in appearance. CH, cluster headache; PH, paroxysmal hemicrania; HC, hemicrania continua; TN, trigeminal neuralgia.

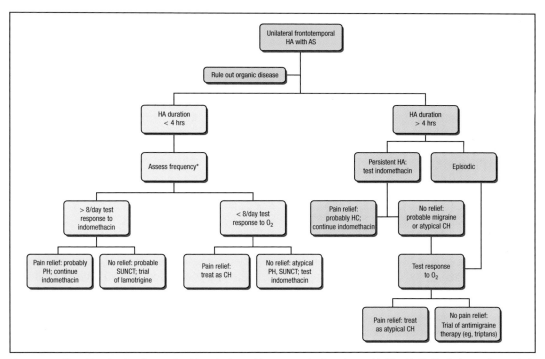

Fig 11-11 Algorithm for the diagnosis of headaches with autonomic signs (use with Fig 11-9). Preliminary diagnosis is based on location and accompanying autonomic signs. This is followed by duration, frequency, and treatment response, particularly to oxygen and indomethacin.* Bear in mind that facial pain with high frequency may also be trigeminal neuralgia with autonomic signs. HA, headache; AS, autonomic signs; O_2, oxygen; HC, hemicrania; CH, cluster headache; PH, paroxysmal hemicrania.

report lacrimation, which may be severe and side-locked in about 15% of patients.[22,189] Unilateral migraine may therefore be confusing; the location and accompanying autonomic signs are common features with TACs.[184] Although unilateral autonomic signs in migraine have been documented,[189,201] they seem to be usually bilateral, whereas in TACs they are strictly unilateral.[22,28] A lower-half headache with autonomic signs could be a lower cluster headache, lower-half migraine,[202] or neurovascular orofacial pain.[203] If the presence of autonomic signs is combined with duration, a headache accompanied by bilateral autonomic signs lasting more than 4 hours is highly likely to be migraine.[184,204] Patients with migraine usually seek out a dark quiet place; in contrast, patients with cluster headache exhibit extreme restlessness.

Dental pain

Referral patterns and pain quality in TACs often mimic dental pain, and at times, TACs may primarily present in intraoral or unusual facial sites.[12] Thus, cluster headache and paroxysmal hemicrania have been misdiagnosed as dental pain, which has led to unnecessary dental interventions.[5,6,10] In paroxysmal hemicrania, pain may be throbbing (30%) and may mimic the presentation of pulpitis, but it is not evoked.[190]

Ocular pain

Ocular pain is most commonly associated with redness and inflammation; however, eye pain can also occur in the absence of grossly visible pathology. Superficial eye pain is experienced as a foreign body sensation, most often caused by disorders of the eyelids, conjunctiva, or cornea, and is most commonly associated with redness and inflammation. The rich innervation of the cornea, conjunctiva, and periocular region means that even minor problems, such as a superficial corneal abrasion, can result in severe pain that is completely out of proportion to the scope and risk of the injury.[205] If the basic eye history is nonspecific, and the basic eye examinations are normal, then the likelihood of an intraocular cause for the pain is diminished but not excluded completely.[206]

Pain in the eye can be the first sign of a number of threatening conditions. Many of these

conditions, such as intermittent angle closure glaucoma, carotid artery dissection, idiopathic intracranial hypertension, and giant cell arteritis, can lead to permanent vision loss or blindness.[207] Thus, deep pain, often described as aching or throbbing, may be serious and demands examination. Pain associated with such changes as visual loss, change in color vision, change in visual field, or double vision should prompt the clinician to request an urgent ophthalmologic opinion.[205]

Temporomandibular disorders

Some patients with TACs suffer from ipsilateral masticatory muscle tenderness, and although confusing, this is consistent with findings in other primary neurovascular-type headaches, such as migraine, particularly chronic migraine (see chapter 10). Patients with hemicrania continua may also describe pain that refers to the jaw, ear, and mastoid and could be confused with pain arising from temporomandibular disorders (TMDs). However, although hemicrania continua and TMDs are both continuous, TMDs rarely wake the patient from sleep and are not throbbing in character. Up to 10% of patients with paroxysmal hemicrania have pain triggered by neck movement, which causes diagnostic confusion with musculoskeletal pain syndromes.

Sinus headache

Pain radiation to the midface region, over the maxillary sinuses, is common in TACs. These patients would likely see ear, nose, and throat surgeons who may erroneously diagnose these as sinus pathology[208] (see chapter 7). About one-fifth of patients with cluster headache may be misdiagnosed and treated for sinus headache,[6,14] but this occurs less frequently in paroxysmal hemicrania and hemicrania continua.[163,208]

Trigeminal neuralgia

The most challenging differential diagnosis is between trigeminal neuralgia and SUNCT; distinguishing trigeminal neuralgia from other TACs should not be difficult. Seeing as cluster headache and trigeminal neuralgia are such distinct entities, the reasons underlying their misdiagnosis are unclear.[10] One confusing early presentation of trigeminal neuralgia is long-lasting, throbbing pain (termed *pretrigeminal neuralgia*; see chapter 12).

Trigeminal neuralgia affecting the ophthalmic, maxillary, or mandibular branch accompanied by ipsilateral lacrimation has been reported.[209] Indeed, the sole presence of lacrimation in this type of trigeminal neuralgia versus the multiple autonomic signs in SUNCT may be a distinct diagnostic feature.[209]

Triggering is a particular feature of trigeminal neuralgia but may also occur in SUNCT and even in paroxysmal hemicrania. In most patients, however, the trigger in SUNCT is not responsive to local anesthetic block and there is no refractory period (see Paliwal et al[210]). The attack duration in trigeminal neuralgia is, on average, 10 times shorter than in SUNCT.[211]

SUNCT is distinguished by resistance to classical antineuralgic therapy.[140] Triggering of short, severe pain attacks may be observed in paroxysmal hemicrania, and the high frequency of SUNCT/SUNA and paroxysmal hemicrania attacks may cause confusion with trigeminal neuralgia. Nocturnal attacks are common in paroxysmal hemicrania but not in trigeminal neuralgia, although they do occur.[191]

Combination syndromes

The co-occurrence of cluster headache and trigeminal neuralgia in the same patients is termed *cluster-tic syndrome*. Trigeminal neuralgia has been reported to occur ipsilaterally in 4.5% of a large series of patients with cluster headache.[212] This high prevalence suggests that comorbidity is not by chance. Moreover, in most patients, trigeminal neuralgia attacks were intimately related to cluster headache activity. Neck movements may precipitate pain in cluster-tic syndrome (40%), and an atypical form of the syndrome has been described with very short attacks that make cluster-tic syndrome disturbingly similar to paroxysmal hemicrania and even SUNCT. Some patients with cluster-tic syndrome may enjoy improvement in pain related to cluster headache and trigeminal neuralgia after cluster headache treatment.[212]

Paroxysmal hemicrania has been associated with trigeminal neuralgia in a chronic paroxysmal hemicrania-tic syndrome.[213,214] Mixed attacks have also been described and may cause confusion with SUNCT; however, the chronic paroxysmal hemicrania-tic syndrome components are individually responsive to treatment.[213]

Cervicogenic headache

Cervicogenic headache is a unilateral headache that originates in the neck or back of the head and spreads anteriorly to the frontotemporal area (see chapter 14). Pain in cervicogenic headache is usually episodic but may become chronic and accompanied by mild autonomic signs. These clinical signs are similar to those seen in hemicrania continua. However, in cervicogenic headache, there are additional signs referable to the neck, including restricted motion, occipital nerve tenderness, and radiologic signs of neck pathology that follow a history of trauma (eg, whiplash).

Pathophysiology of TACs

The three major features of cluster headache and most TACs are trigeminal pain, rhythmicity, and autonomic signs. The overlap in pain duration, frequency, therapeutic responses, and other features suggest a common pathophysiology. A schematic summary of cluster headache pathophysiology is shown in Fig 11-12.

Pain

Fundamental to the pathophysiology of neurovascular headaches is the trigeminovascular system (described in chapter 10). The distribution of pain in TACs implicates activity of the trigeminal nerve, particularly the ophthalmic branch. A peripheral origin of the pain is supported by some data, including findings of pain improvement after nerve section in patients with cluster headache.[215] However, the results are inconsistent and often last for a short time only.[215–217]

An inflammatory process, initiating nociceptor activation, was thought to be involved in cluster headache. This could occur at any peripheral site, but the cavernous sinus was an attractive target. Within the cavernous sinus, the trigeminal nerve and autonomic nerves are together, so this is a prime site for a pathophys-

SSN

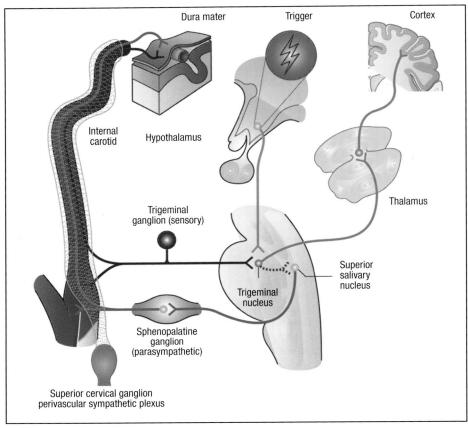

Fig 11-12 Pain and autonomic mechanisms of cluster headache and a schematic representation of the major areas involved. Neuroimaging studies implicate the hypothalamus as central to the pathogenesis of cluster headache. Trigeminal activation will result in neurogenic inflammation at peripheral sites (vasodilation, plasma extravasation, pain, swelling). At the brainstem level, connections exist to the superior salivary nucleus, which is therefore stimulated with subsequent activation of the parasympathetic nervous system, leading to autonomic signs (vasodilation, tearing, rhinorrhea); this is termed the *trigeminoparasympathetic reflex*. Researchers believe vasodilation causes neuropraxic injury to the perivascular sympathetic plexus (grid), inducing sympathetic dysfunction that is clinically observed as ptosis and miosis.

iologic process in cluster headache. A lesion at this site could induce trigeminal pain and parasympathetic and sympathetic characteristics, as seen in cluster headache. Early evidence for increased blood flow or lesions in the cavernous sinus during cluster headache suggested that this area may be the origin of pain.[218,219] However, studies have failed to show pathologic changes in the area of the cavernous sinus, and orbital phlebography studies demonstrate identical results in a number of other headache types, including SUNCT, migraine, tension-type headache, and paroxysmal hemicrania.[218,219]

Patients with cluster headache demonstrate significantly increased interleukin-2 receptors.[220] Elevated interleukin-2 receptors indicate T-cell and immune activation during cluster headache. Interleukin-2 is known to activate the hypothalamus and stimulate the release of corticotropin-releasing factor, potentially acting as a link between immune activation, cluster headache, hypothalamic activation, and hormonal imbalances.[220,221]

Peripheral nerve activation explains pain and, when it affects the trigeminal nerve, may initiate reflex autonomic manifestations. Nociceptor activation was thought to originate from dilated blood vessels that stimulate trigeminal afferents directly (see chapter 10). However, it seems likely that the vascular changes are an epiphenomenon of activation of the trigemino-vascular system.[97,222] Trigeminal and autonomic activation, as evidenced by increased levels of CGRP and vasoactive intestinal polypeptide (VIP) in the cranial circulation, are present in chronic paroxysmal hemicrania. Similar neuropeptide changes, including increased levels of NO, are seen in cluster headache and suggest a shared underlying pathophysiology within TACs.[223,224] Moreover, successful treatment with indomethacin normalizes levels of CGRP and VIP in chronic paroxysmal hemicrania, and oxygen administration reverses the elevation of CGRP in cluster headache.[225,226]

Observed ptosis and miosis, which are suggestive of sympathetic dysfunction, may be secondary to neuropraxic effects of carotid edema on the sympathetic plexus or may signify a generalized sympathetic dysfunction.[221] Indeed, a dysfunction in the central control of the autonomic system in cluster headache and paroxysmal hemicrania has been proposed.[111] However, autonomic dysfunction as a driving force in cluster headache does not explain pain that may occur in cluster headache with no autonomic signs and vice versa.

Moreover, case descriptions of continued tearing with no pain in patients with cluster headache after surgical section of the trigeminal nerve establish the role of central mechanisms in the TAC phenotype.[216] For example, a 59-year-old man with a 14-year history of left-sided cluster headache underwent surgical section of the ipsilateral trigeminal root but continued to suffer from both headaches and autonomic signs.[97] The patient also continued to respond to sumatriptan in spite of nerve sectioning. Clearly, in this patient, central nervous system structures only were necessary to induce cluster headache and express the full phenotype and therapeutic response, so it seems that pain need not originate peripherally. Current thinking is that primary headaches occur with no substantial peripheral pathology.[33,227]

Moreover, it is clear that pain distribution in TACs involves not only other branches of the trigeminal nerve but also extratrigeminal regions, such as the ear, neck, shoulder, and arm.[15,110,111,113,141,228] This suggests that the trigeminal nerve is not the most important or sole origin of pain and raises questions about a peripheral source.

Pain and the hypothalamus

The trigeminal system has a two-way connection to the hypothalamus via the trigeminohypothalamic tract.[102,229] Structural connections have been identified between the hypothalamus and the medullary dorsal reticular nucleus, a supraspinal system that gives origin to a descending projection that facilitates pain perception and other major structures involved in the affective and cognitive aspects of pain.[230] Accumulating data therefore indicate involvement of the hypothalamic ventricular nucleus in antinociception,[231] and studies with orexins—hypothalamic peptides located in the posterior hypothalamus—establish that the posterior hypothalamus is a modulator of trigeminal nucleus caudalis activity.[65,232,233] The orexins are neuropeptides found exclusively in the hypothalamus. The orexinergic system projects to areas involved in nociception and autonomic regulation, including the hypothalamus, periacqueductal gray, and spinal cord.[233] Although circumstantial, many lines of evidence indicate a role for the orexinergic system in the pathophysiology of cluster headache.[65,233]

The hypothalamus is therefore a prime candidate to initiate and manage the TACs. However, hypothalamic stimulation does not induce cluster headache attacks[101,234,235] and will not abort an ongoing attack.[236] Current thinking suggests that the hypothalamus plays a prime role in terminating attacks so that hypothalamic dysfunction may act in a permissive manner.[219,229] Activation from brain areas other than the hypothalamus may be a primary event triggering headache; for example, a nociceptive stimulus to the rat cortex induces trigeminal activation and plasma extravasation[237] (see chapter 10).

A role for the hypothalamus in TACs is supported by functional and morphometric neuroimaging. During TACs, but not in experimentally induced pain, there is marked activation of the hypothalamus—ipsilateral or contralateral to pain in cluster headache, contralateral to pain in paroxysmal hemicrania, contralateral or bilateral to pain in SUNCT, and contralateral to pain in hemicrania continua.[222,238–244] Activation in mi-

P.213

graine is seen largely in brainstem structures. In hemicrania continua, on the other hand, activation of the posterior hypothalamus is paralleled by activation in the dorsal rostral pons, an overlap of TAC and migraine symptomatology.[238,245] Studies with magnetic resonance spectroscopy demonstrate specifically impaired metabolic activity of the hypothalamus of patients with cluster headache, which indicates neuronal dysfunction.[246,247] Within headaches and interictally, positron emission tomography morphometric studies reveal a significant structural difference (increased volume) in the inferior posterior hypothalamus of patients with cluster headache. The morphometric and functional images identify the same area in the inferior posterior hypothalamus.[248]

Some of the reported hypothalamic changes are not specific to TACs and are found in other craniofacial and spinal pain syndromes.[230] This is not surprising given the connection of the hypothalamus mentioned earlier. The activity and potential pathophysiologic role of the posterior hypothalamus has been translated into a therapeutic approach in the form of deep brain stimulation to these sites.

Dysfunction of the descending pain modulatory system has been suggested in the pathophysiology of headaches.[249,250] Involvement of the opioid system and other top-down controls has been demonstrated in cluster headache.[251,252] These studies are supported by imaging findings of significant structural changes in pain modulation areas of patients with cluster headache.[253] Neurophysiologic testing of patients with cluster headache confirms defective supraspinal controls and facilitated temporal processing of pain, but whether these are a cause or a result of pain is unclear.[254]

Rhythmicity and the hypothalamus

The periodicity and sleep association in TACs suggest involvement of central sites that help control the human biologic clock. In humans, these are located in the anterior hypothalamic gray, an area termed the *suprachiasmatic nucleus.* Hypothalamic regulation of the endocrine system involves rhythmic and phasic homeostatic modulation of the hypophyseal hormones and melatonin. In cluster headache, changes have been observed in melatonin, cortisol,

P.130

follicular-stimulating hormone, luteinizing hormone, and thyroid-stimulating hormone.[221,255] Testosterone was an attractive target, as cluster headache is mostly a male disease, and lowered concentrations of testosterone in men with cluster headache were the first indications of hypothalamic involvement.[221] However, other studies have found lowered levels only in chronic cluster headache, and this may be a secondary effect. Melatonin is produced by the pineal gland, which receives sympathetic innervation from the hypothalamus and autonomic centers of the thoracic spinal cord, the sympathetic cervical plexus, and the carotid plexus. The principal external stimulus for the rhythmic production of melatonin is light intensity. This input reaches the suprachiasmatic nucleus of the hypothalamus via a direct pathway from the retina. In humans, melatonin levels are low during the day and increase during the hours of darkness. Studies of melatonin in patients with cluster headache found that 24-hour production was reduced and its pattern altered during the cluster period compared with clinically normal subjects. This finding links to descriptions of cluster headache variations with daylight hours, which partly explains the seasonal timing of active cluster periods. Twenty-four-hour cortisol production was also significantly increased in the cluster period, indicating hypothalamic-pituitary-adrenal axis hyperactivity. More recently, it was suggested that sympathetic dysfunction may affect hypothalamic function and result in the downstream effects along the hypothalamic axes.[221]

Autonomic signs and the trigeminoparasympathetic reflex

The blood vessels of craniofacial tissues are innervated by three sets of nerves: the cranial parasympathetic, the superior cervical sympathetic, and the trigeminal sensory nerves. Cranial parasympathetic fibers arise in the superior salivary nucleus and innervate part of the craniofacial structures via the oculomotor, facial, glossopharyngeal, or vagal nerves. These efferents synapse in the ciliary, pterygopalatine, submandibular, lingual, or otic ganglia, and postganglionic fibers project to specific craniofacial targets, such as the lacrimal, nasal mucosa, and salivary glands, as well as the craniofacial vasculature. Parasympathetic stimulation induces lacrimation and rhinorrhea, as observed in TACs. Elevated plasma VIP levels confirm the activity of the parasympathetic system in cluster headache and chronic paroxysmal hemicrania; in migraine, this occurs only if autonomic signs are present.

Painful experimental stimuli in areas innervated by trigeminal nerve divisions 1 and 2 will cause ipsilateral lacrimation and local sweating, signs similar to those observed in TACs.[256] After trigeminal nerve stimulation, decreased carotid artery resistance was observed, an effect blocked by trigeminal section. These effects are largely considered secondary to initiation of a parasympathetic reflex via trigeminal nerve activation—the trigeminoparasympathetic reflex (TPR). In TACs, the afferent limb of the TPR is the ophthalmic branch of the trigeminal nerve and the efferent is the facial nerve. Stimulation of the facial nerve and of parasympathetic fibers induces increased regional cerebral blood flow, which confirms the efferent role of the parasympathetic nervous system in the TPR. Existence of a TPR is established by anatomical and functional connections at the brainstem level between the trigeminal complex and the superior salivary nucleus.[257]

Interruption of the efferent branch of the TPR by sectioning the facial nerve produces an 80% reduction of vascular dilation. The remaining effect may be induced by antidromic activation of trigeminal neurons and neurogenic inflammatory effects. These two processes—TPR and neurogenic inflammation—are thought to be central to the pathophysiology of neurovascular headaches and occur simultaneously. Neurogenic inflammation is extensively described in chapter 10.

The autonomic system is regulated by hypothalamic nuclei acting through the nucleus tractus solitarius.[258] Specifically, the TPR is also actively modulated by higher centers, including the hypothalamus.[258] Intravenous injection of a gamma-aminobutyric acid (GABA) antagonist elicits a parasympathetic response similar to a reflex and supports the existence of a tonically active GABA-mediated inhibition of the TPR.[259] Furthermore, electrical stimulation of the anterior hypothalamus attenuates lip vasodilation in response to lingual nerve stimulation, an effect abolished by administration of a GABA antagonist.[259] This confirms a role for hypothalamic modulation of TPR in all branches of the trigeminal nerve. The TPR may therefore be pathologically disinhibited in TACs.

Neuropathic mechanisms

Attacks of paroxysmal hemicrania and SUNCT may be mechanically activated, often with a short latency, thereby implicating neurogenic transmission.[140] In paroxysmal hemicrania, 10% of patients report a clear trigger mechanism, usually neck movement, and patients with SUNCT demonstrate trigeminal neuralgia-like triggers.[111,148] Moreover, reports of successful microvascular decompression therapy in cluster headache and SUNCT, which is also successful in trigeminal neuralgia, suggests that in some patients neuropathic mechanisms may be involved.[159] Furthermore, initiation of cluster headache by traumatic events, such as head injury and dental extractions, suggests a role for nerve injury in the etiology of TACs.[42,43]

Taken together, the data suggest that cluster headache and other TACs are conditions for which the pathophysiologic basis is in the hypothalamic gray matter that drives the initiation of the clinical phenotype. The involvement of peripheral mechanisms is unclear.

References

1. Headache Classification Committee of the International Headache Society. The International Classification of Headache Disorders, 3rd edition (beta version). Cephalalgia 2013;33:629–808.
2. Vincent MB. Hemicrania continua. Unquestionably a trigeminal autonomic cephalalgia. Headache 2013;53:863–868.
3. Sahler K. Hemicrania continua: Functional imaging and clinical features with diagnostic implications [epub ahead of print 10 April 2013]. Headache doi:10.1111.head.12095.
4. Benoliel R, Elishoov H, Sharav Y. Orofacial pain with vascular-type features. Oral Surg Oral Med Oral Pathol Oral Radiol Endod 1997;84:506–512.
5. Bahra A, Goadsby PJ. Diagnostic delays and mis-management in cluster headache. Acta Neurol Scand 2004;109:175–179.
6. van Vliet JA, Eekers PJ, Haan J, Ferrari MD. Features involved in the diagnostic delay of cluster headache. J Neurol Neurosurg Psychiatry 2003;74:1123–1125.

7. Dodick DW, Rozen TD, Goadsby PJ, Silberstein SD. Cluster headache. Cephalalgia 2000;20:787–803.
8. Torelli P, Manzoni GC. Pain and behaviour in cluster headache. A prospective study and review of the literature. Funct Neurol 2003;18:205–210.
9. Rozen TD, Fishman RS. Cluster headache in the United States of America: Demographics, clinical characteristics, triggers, suicidality, and personal burden. Headache 2012;52:99–113.
10. Van Alboom E, Louis P, Van Zandijcke M, Crevits L, Vakaet A, Paemeleire K. Diagnostic and therapeutic trajectory of cluster headache patients in Flanders. Acta Neurol Belg 2009;109:10–17.
11. Klapper JA, Klapper A, Voss T. The misdiagnosis of cluster headache: A nonclinic, population-based, Internet survey. Headache 2000;40:730–735.
12. Gaul C, Christmann N, Schroder D, et al. Differences in clinical characteristics and frequency of accompanying migraine features in episodic and chronic cluster headache. Cephalalgia 2012;32:571–577.
13. Black DF, Bordini CA, Russell D. Symptomatology of cluster headache. In: Olesen J, Goadsby PJ, Ramadan NM, Tfelt-Hansen P, Welch KMA (eds). The Headaches, ed 3. Philadelphia: Lippincott Williams & Wilkins, 2006:789–796.
14. Bahra A, May A, Goadsby PJ. Cluster headache: A prospective clinical study with diagnostic implications. Neurology 2002;58:354–361.
15. Cademartiri C, Torelli P, Cologno D, Manzoni GC. Upper and lower cluster headache: Clinical and pathogenetic observations in 608 patients. Headache 2002;42:630–637.
16. Sjöstrand C, Waldenlind E, Ekbom K. A follow-up study of 60 patients after an assumed first period of cluster headache. Cephalalgia 2000;20:653–657.
17. Marmura MJ, Pello SJ, Young WB. Interictal pain in cluster headache. Cephalalgia 2010;30:1531–1534.
18. Lee YJ, Chen YT, Ou SM, et al. Temperature variation and the incidence of cluster headache periods: A nationwide population study. Cephalalgia 2014;34:656–663.
19. Xie Q, Huang Q, Wang J, Li N, Tan G, Zhou J. Clinical features of cluster headache: An outpatient clinic study from China. Pain Med 2013;14:802–807.
20. Torelli P, Cologno D, Cademartiri C, Manzoni GC. Possible predictive factors in the evolution of episodic to chronic cluster headache. Headache 2000;40:798–808.
21. Sances G, Tassorelli C, Pucci E, Ghiotto N, Sandrini G, Nappi G. Reliability of the nitroglycerin provocative test in the diagnosis of neurovascular headaches. Cephalalgia 2004;24:110–119.
22. Lai TH, Fuh JL, Wang SJ. Cranial autonomic symptoms in migraine: Characteristics and comparison with cluster headache. J Neurol Neurosurg Psychiatry 2009;80:1116–1119.
23. Martins IP, Gouveia RG, Parreira E. Cluster headache without autonomic symptoms: Why is it different? Headache 2005;45:190–195.
24. Torelli P, Cologno D, Cademartiri C, Manzoni GC. Application of the International Headache Society Classification Criteria in 652 cluster headache patients. Cephalalgia 2001;21:145–150.
25. Goadsby PJ, Matharu MS, Boes CJ. SUNCT syndrome or trigeminal neuralgia with lacrimation. Cephalalgia 2001;21:82–83.
26. Zidverc-Trajkovic J, Podgorac A, Radojicic A, Sternic N. Migraine-like accompanying features in patients with cluster headache. How important are they? Headache 2013;53:1464–1469.
27. Siow HC, Young WB, Peres MF, Rozen TD, Silberstein SD. Hemiplegic cluster. Headache 2002;42:136–139.
28. Goadsby PJ. Lacrimation, conjunctival injection, nasal symptoms... cluster headache, migraine and cranial autonomic symptoms in primary headache disorders — what's new? J Neurol Neurosurg Psychiatry 2009;80:1057-1058.
29. Irimia P, Cittadini E, Paemeleire K, Cohen AS, Goadsby PJ. Unilateral photophobia or phonophobia in migraine compared with trigeminal autonomic cephalalgias. Cephalalgia 2008;28:626–630.
30. Chervin RD, Zallek SN, Lin X, Hall JM, Sharma N, Hedger KM. Timing patterns of cluster headaches and association with symptoms of obstructive sleep apnea. Sleep Res Online 2000;3:107–112.
31. Raimondi E. Premonitory symptoms in cluster headache. Curr Pain Headache Rep 2001;5:55–59.
32. Langedijk M, van der Naalt J, Luijckx GJ, De Keyser J. Cluster-like headache aura status. Headache 2005;45:80–81.
33. Ekbom K, Hardebo JE. Cluster headache: Aetiology, diagnosis and management. Drugs 2002;62:61–69.
34. Cittadini E, Matharu MS. Symptomatic trigeminal autonomic cephalalgias. Neurologist 2009;15:305–312.
35. Favier I, van Vliet JA, Roon KI, et al. Trigeminal autonomic cephalgias due to structural lesions: A review of 31 cases. Arch Neurol 2007;64:25–31.
36. Edvardsson B. Symptomatic cluster headache: A review of 63 cases. Springerplus 2014;3:64.
37. Levy MJ, Jäger HR, Powell M, Matharu MS, Meeran K, Goadsby PJ. Pituitary volume and headache: Size is not everything. Arch Neurol 2004;61:721–725.
38. Levy MJ, Matharu MS, Meeran K, Powell M, Goadsby PJ. The clinical characteristics of headache in patients with pituitary tumours. Brain 2005;128(Pt 8):1921–1930.
39. Goadsby PJ. Trigeminal autonomic cephalalgias. Continuum (Minneap Minn) 2012;18:883–895.
40. Matharu MS, Boes CJ, Goadsby PJ. Management of trigeminal autonomic cephalgias and hemicrania continua. Drugs 2003;63:1637–1677.
41. Trucco M, Mainardi F, Maggioni F, Badino R, Zanchin G. Chronic paroxysmal hemicrania, hemicrania continua and SUNCT syndrome in association with other pathologies: A review. Cephalalgia 2004;24:173–184.
42. Peñarrocha M, Bandrés A, Peñarrocha MA, Bagán JV. Relationship between oral surgical and endodontic procedures and episodic cluster headache. Oral Surg Oral Med Oral Pathol Oral Radiol Endod 2001;92:499–502.
43. Sörös P, Frese A, Husstedt IW, Evers S. Cluster headache after dental extraction: Implications for the pathogenesis of cluster headache? Cephalalgia 2001;21:619–622.

44. Sarlani E, Schwartz AH, Greenspan JD, Grace EG. Facial pain as first manifestation of lung cancer: A case of lung cancer-related cluster headache and a review of the literature. J Orofac Pain 2003;17:262–267.

45. Carter DM. Cluster headache mimics. Curr Pain Headache Rep 2004;8:133–139.

46. Ekbom K, Svensson DA, Träff H, Waldenlind E. Age at onset and sex ratio in cluster headache: Observations over three decades. Cephalalgia 2002;22:94–100.

47. Tonon C, Guttmann S, Volpini M, Naccarato S, Cortelli P, D'Alessandro R. Prevalence and incidence of cluster headache in the Republic of San Marino. Neurology 2002;58:1407–1409.

48. Robbins MS, Lipton RB. The epidemiology of primary headache disorders. Semin Neurol 2010;30:107–119.

49. Fischera M, Marziniak M, Gralow I, Evers S. The incidence and prevalence of cluster headache: A meta-analysis of population-based studies. Cephalalgia 2008;28:614–618.

50. May A. Cluster headache: Pathogenesis, diagnosis, and management. Lancet 2005;366:843–855.

51. Rozen TD, Fishman RS. Female cluster headache in the United States of America: What are the gender differences? Results from the United States Cluster Headache Survey. J Neurol Sci 2012;317:17–28.

52. Rozen TD, Niknam RM, Shechter AL, Young WB, Silberstein SD. Cluster headache in women: Clinical characteristics and comparison with cluster headache in men. J Neurol Neurosurg Psychiatry 2001;70:613–617.

53. Mariani R, Capuano A, Torriero R, et al. Cluster headache in childhood: Case series from a pediatric headache center. J Child Neurol 2014;29:62–65.

54. Zidverc-Trajkovic J, Markovic K, Radojicic A, Podgorac A, Sternic N. Cluster headache: Is age of onset important for clinical presentation? Cephalalgia 2014;34:664–670.

55. Schürks M. Genetics of cluster headache. Curr Pain Headache Rep 2010;14:132–139.

56. Leone M, Russell MB, Rigamonti A, et al. Increased familial risk of cluster headache. Neurology 2001;56:1233–1236.

57. Russell MB. Epidemiology and genetics of cluster headache. Lancet Neurol 2004;3:279–283.

58. El Amrani M, Ducros A, Boulan P, et al. Familial cluster headache: A series of 186 index patients. Headache 2002;42:974–977.

59. Schuh-Hofer S, Meisel A, Reuter U, Arnold G. Monozygotic twin sisters suffering from cluster headache and migraine without aura. Neurology 2003;60:1864–1865.

60. Lipton RB, Bigal ME. Migraine: Epidemiology, impact, and risk factors for progression. Headache 2005;45(1, suppl):S3–S13.

61. Haan J, van Vliet JA, Kors EE, et al. No involvement of the calcium channel gene (CACNA1A) in a family with cluster headache. Cephalalgia 2001;21:959–962.

62. Sjöstrand C, Giedratis V, Ekbom K, Waldenlind E, Hillert J. CACNA1A gene polymorphisms in cluster headache. Cephalalgia 2001;21:953–958.

63. Sjöstrand C, Modin H, Masterman T, Ekbom K, Waldenlind E, Hillert J. Analysis of nitric oxide synthase genes in cluster headache. Cephalalgia 2002;22:758–764.

64. Rainero I, Rivoiro C, Gallone S, et al. Lack of association between the 3092 T-C clock gene polymorphism and cluster headache. Cephalalgia 2005;25:1078–1081.

65. Bartsch T, Levy MJ, Knight YE, Goadsby PJ. Differential modulation of nociceptive dural input to [hypocretin] orexin A and B receptor activation in the posterior hypothalamic area. Pain 2004;109:367–378.

66. Rainero I, Gallone S, Valfré W, et al. A polymorphism of the hypocretin receptor 2 gene is associated with cluster headache. Neurology 2004;63:1286–1288.

67. Tfelt-Hansen PC, Jensen RH. Management of cluster headache. CNS Drugs 2012;26:571–580.

68. Law S, Derry S, Moore RA. Triptans for acute cluster headache. Cochrane Database Syst Rev 2013;7.

69. Tyagi A, Matharu M. Evidence base for the medical treatments used in cluster headache. Curr Pain Headache Rep 2009;13:168–178.

70. May A, Leone M, Afra J, et al. EFNS guidelines on the treatment of cluster headache and other trigeminal-autonomic cephalalgias. Eur J Neurol 2006;13:1066–1077.

71. Ferrari A, Zappaterra M, Righi F, et al. Impact of continuing or quitting smoking on episodic cluster headache: A pilot survey. J Headache Pain 2013;14:48.

72. Pareja JA, Alvarez M. The usual treatment of trigeminal autonomic cephalalgias. Headache 2013;53:1401–1414.

73. Rozen TD. Inhaled oxygen for cluster headache: Efficacy, mechanism of action, utilization, and economics. Curr Pain Headache Rep 2012;16:175–179.

74. Rozen TD. High oxygen flow rates for cluster headache. Neurology 2004;63:593.

75. Akerman S, Holland PR, Lasalandra MP, Goadsby PJ. Oxygen inhibits neuronal activation in the trigeminocervical complex after stimulation of trigeminal autonomic reflex, but not during direct dural activation of trigeminal afferents. Headache 2009;49:1131–1143.

76. Centonze V, Bassi A, Causarano V, et al. Sumatriptan overuse in episodic cluster headache: Lack of adverse events, rebound syndromes, drug dependence and tachyphylaxis. Funct Neurol 2000;15:167–170.

77. van Vliet JA, Bahra A, Martin V, et al. Intranasal sumatriptan in cluster headache: Randomized placebo-controlled double-blind study. Neurology 2003;60:630–633.

78. Rossi P, Lorenzo GD, Formisano R, Buzzi MG. Subcutaneous sumatriptan induces changes in frequency pattern in cluster headache patients. Headache 2004;44:713–718.

79. Paemeleire K, Evers S, Goadsby PJ. Medication-overuse headache in patients with cluster headache. Curr Pain Headache Rep 2008;12:122–127.

80. Bahra A, Gawel MJ, Hardebo JE, Millson D, Breen SA, Goadsby PJ. Oral zolmitriptan is effective in the acute treatment of cluster headache. Neurology 2000;54:1832–1839.

81. Hedlund C, Rapoport AM, Dodick DW, Goadsby PJ. Zolmitriptan nasal spray in the acute treatment of cluster headache: A meta-analysis of two studies. Headache 2009;49:1315–1323.

82. Antonaci F, Costa A, Candeloro E, Sjaastad O, Nappi G. Single high-dose steroid treatment in episodic cluster headache. Cephalalgia 2005;25:290–295.

83. Ashkenazi A, Schwedt T. Cluster headache—acute and prophylactic therapy. Headache 2011;51:272–286.

84. Shapiro RE. Corticosteroid treatment in cluster headache: Evidence, rationale, and practice. Curr Pain Headache Rep 2005;9:126–131.

85. Mir P, Alberca R, Navarro A, et al. Prophylactic treatment of episodic cluster headache with intravenous bolus of methylprednisolone. Neurol Sci 2003;24:318–321.

86. Ambrosini A, Vandenheede M, Rossi P, et al. Suboccipital injection with a mixture of rapid- and long-acting steroids in cluster headache: A double-blind placebo-controlled study. Pain 2005;118:92–96.

87. Dodick DW. Suboccipital steroid injections for cluster headache. Lancet Neurol 2011;10:867–869.

88. Lambru G, Abu Bakar N, Stahlhut L, et al. Greater occipital nerve blocks in chronic cluster headache: A prospective open-label study. Eur J Neurol 2014;21:338–343.

89. Gantenbein AR, Lutz NJ, Riederer F, Sándor PS. Efficacy and safety of 121 injections of the greater occipital nerve in episodic and chronic cluster headache. Cephalalgia 2012;32:630–634.

90. Ambrosini A, Vandenheede M, Rossi P, et al. Suboccipital injection with a mixture of rapid- and long-acting steroids in cluster headache: A double-blind placebo-controlled study. Pain 2005;118:92–96.

91. Kinney MA, Wilson JL, Carmichael SW, De Ruyter ML, Fulgham JR. Prolonged facial hypesthesia resulting from greater occipital nerve block. Clin Anat 2003;16:362–365.

92. Peres MF, Stiles MA, Siow HC, Rozen TD, Young WB, Silberstein SD. Greater occipital nerve blockade for cluster headache. Cephalalgia 2002;22:520–522.

93. Cohen AS, Matharu MS, Goadsby PJ. Electrocardiographic abnormalities in patients with cluster headache on verapamil therapy. Neurology 2007;69:668–675.

94. Förderreuther S, Mayer M, Straube A. Treatment of cluster headache with topiramate: Effects and side-effects in five patients. Cephalalgia 2002;22:186–189.

95. Leone M. Chronic cluster headache: New and emerging treatment options. Curr Pain Headache Rep 2004;8:347–352.

96. Leone M, May A, Franzini A, et al. Deep brain stimulation for intractable chronic cluster headache: Proposals for patient selection. Cephalalgia 2004;24:934–937.

97. Matharu MS, Goadsby PJ. Persistence of attacks of cluster headache after trigeminal nerve root section. Brain 2002;125(Pt 5):976–984.

98. Hong J, Roberts DW. The surgical treatment of headache. Headache 2014;54:409–429.

99. Martelletti P, Jensen RH, Antal A, et al. Neuromodulation of chronic headaches: Position statement from the European Headache Federation. J Headache Pain 2013;14:86.

100. Tepper SJ, Stillman MJ. Cluster headache: Potential options for medically refractory patients (when all else fails). Headache 2013;53:1183–1190.

101. Leone M, Franzini A, Proietti Cecchini A, Bussone G. Success, failure, and putative mechanisms in hypothalamic stimulation for drug-resistant chronic cluster headache. Pain 2013;154:89–94.

102. May A, Leone M, Boecker H, et al. Hypothalamic deep brain stimulation in positron emission tomography. J Neurosci 2006;26:3589–3593.

103. Magis D, Schoenen J. Advances and challenges in neurostimulation for headaches. Lancet Neurol 2012;11:708–719.

104. Burns B, Watkins L, Goadsby PJ. Treatment of intractable chronic cluster headache by occipital nerve stimulation in 14 patients. Neurology 2009;72:341–345.

105. Magis D, Gerardy PY, Remacle JM, Schoenen J. Sustained effectiveness of occipital nerve stimulation in drug-resistant chronic cluster headache. Headache 2011;51:1191–1201.

106. Schytz HW, Barløse M, Guo S, et al. Experimental activation of the sphenopalatine ganglion provokes cluster-like attacks in humans. Cephalalgia 2013;33:831–841.

107. Schoenen J, Jensen RH, Lantéri-Minet M, et al. Stimulation of the sphenopalatine ganglion (SPG) for cluster headache treatment. Pathway CH-1: A randomized, sham-controlled study. Cephalalgia 2013;33:816–830.

108. Pipolo C, Bussone G, Leone M, Lozza P, Felisati G. Sphenopalatine endoscopic ganglion block in cluster headache: A reevaluation of the procedure after 5 years. Neurol Sci 2010;31(1, suppl):S197–S199.

109. Peñarrocha-Diago M, Boronat A, Peñarrocha-Oltra D, Ata-Ali J, Bagan JV, Peñarrocha-Diago M. Clinical course of patients with episodic cluster headache treated with corticosteroids in proximity to the sphenopalatine ganglion: A preliminary study of 23 patients. Med Oral Patol Oral Cir Bucal 2012;17:e477–e482.

110. Boes CJ, Dodick DW. Refining the clinical spectrum of chronic paroxysmal hemicrania: A review of 74 patients. Headache 2002;42:699–708.

111. Boes CJ, Vincent M, Russell D. Chronic paroxysmal hemicrania. In: Olesen J, Goadsby PJ, Ramadan NM, Tfelt-Hansen P, Welch KMA (eds). The Headaches, ed 3. Philadelphia: Lippincott Williams & Wilkins, 2006:815–822.

112. Prakash S, Belani P, Susvirkar A, Trivedi A, Ahuja S, Patel A. Paroxysmal hemicrania: A retrospective study of a consecutive series of 22 patients and a critical analysis of the diagnostic criteria. J Headache Pain 2013;14:26.

113. Cittadini E, Matharu MS, Goadsby PJ. Paroxysmal hemicrania: A prospective clinical study of 31 cases. Brain 2008;131(Pt 4):1142–1155.

114. Bingel U, Weiller C. An unusual indomethacin-sensitive headache: A case of bilateral episodic paroxysmal hemicrania without autonomic symptoms? Cephalalgia 2005;25:148–150.

115. Matharu MS, Goadsby PJ. Bilateral paroxysmal hemicrania or bilateral paroxysmal cephalalgia, another novel indomethacin-responsive primary headache syndrome? Cephalalgia 2005;25:79–81.

116. Sarlani E, Schwartz AH, Greenspan JD, Grace EG. Chronic paroxysmal hemicrania: A case report and review of the literature. J Orofac Pain 2003;17:74–78.

117. Siow HC. Seasonal episodic paroxysmal hemicrania responding to cyclooxygenase-2 inhibitors. Cephalalgia 2004;24:414–415.

118. Veloso GG, Kaup AO, Peres MF, Zukerman E. Episodic paroxysmal hemicrania with seasonal variation: Case report and the EPH-cluster headache continuum hypothesis. Arq Neuropsiquiatr 2001;59:944–947.

119. Sjaastad O, Bakketeig LS. The rare, unilateral headaches. Vågå Study of headache epidemiology. J Headache Pain 2007;8:19–27.

120. Blankenburg M, Hechler T, Dubbel G, Wamsler C, Zernikow B. Paroxysmal hemicrania in children—Symptoms, diagnostic criteria, therapy and outcome. Cephalalgia 2009;29:873–882.

121. Mariano da Silva H, Benevides-Luz I, Santos AC, Bordini CA, Campaner L, Speciali JG. Chronic paroxysmal hemicrania as a manifestation of intracranial parotid gland carcinoma metastasis—A case report. Cephalalgia 2004;24:223–227.

122. Antonaci F, Costa A, Ghirmai S, Sances G, Sjaastad O, Nappi G. Parenteral indomethacin (the INDOTEST) in cluster headache. Cephalalgia 2003;23:193–196.

123. Pareja JA, Caminero AB, Franco E, Casado JL, Pascual J, Sánchez del Río M. Dose, efficacy and tolerability of long-term indomethacin treatment of chronic paroxysmal hemicrania and hemicrania continua. Cephalalgia 2001;21:906–910.

124. Rozen TD. Can indomethacin act as a disease modifying agent in hemicrania continua? A supportive clinical case. Headache 2009;49:759–761.

125. Goadsby PJ, Cittadini E, Cohen AS. Trigeminal autonomic cephalalgias: Paroxysmal hemicrania, SUNCT/SUNA, and hemicrania continua. Semin Neurol 2010;30:186–191.

126. Peres MF, Silberstein SD. Hemicrania continua responds to cyclooxygenase-2 inhibitors. Headache 2002;42:530–531.

127. Porta-Etessam J, Cuadrado M, Rodríguez-Gómez O, García-Ptacek S, Valencia C. Are Cox-2 drugs the second line option in indomethacin responsive headaches? J Headache Pain 2010;11:405–407.

128. Rozen TD. LASH syndrome: A third reported case twelve years after the first. Headache 2012;52:1433–1438.

129. Sjaastad O, Vincent M. Indomethacin responsive headache syndromes: chronic paroxysmal hemicrania and hemicrania continua. How they were discovered and what we have learned since. Funct Neurol 2010;25:49–55.

130. Rozen TD. Indomethacin-responsive TACs (paroxysmal hemicrania, hemicrania continua, and LASH): Further proof of a distinct spectrum of headache disorders. Headache 2013;53:1499–1500.

131. Summ O, Andreou AP, Akerman S, Goadsby PJ. A potential nitrergic mechanism of action for indomethacin, but not of other COX inhibitors: Relevance to indomethacin-sensitive headaches. J Headache Pain 2010;11:477–483.

132. Summ O, Evers S. Mechanism of action of indomethacin in indomethacin-responsive headaches. Curr Pain Headache Rep 2013;17:327.

133. Buzzi MG, Sakas DE, Moskowitz MA. Indomethacin and acetylsalicylic acid block neurogenic plasma protein extravasation in rat dura mater. Eur J Pharmacol 1989;165:251–258.

134. Bakken IJ, Vincent MB, White LR, Cappelen J, Skaanes KO, Sjaastad O. Low concentrations of lithium and cyclooxygenase inhibitors enhance endothelin-1 (ET-1)-induced contractions in human temporal artery, but not in porcine ophthalmic artery. Headache 1992;32:475–479.

135. Neeb L, Hellen P, Boehnke C, et al. IL-1ß stimulates COX-2 dependent PGE_2 synthesis and CGRP release in rat trigeminal ganglia cells. PLoS One 2011;6:e17360.

136. Ventura-Martínez R, Déciga-Campos M, Díaz-Reval MI, González-Trujano ME, López-Muñoz FJ. Peripheral involvement of the nitric oxide-cGMP pathway in the indomethacin-induced antinociception in rat. Eur J Pharmacol 2004;503:43–48.

137. Hrabák A, Vercruysse V, Káhan IL, Vray B. Indomethacin prevents the induction of inducible nitric oxide synthase in murine peritoneal macrophages and decreases their nitric oxide production. Life Sci 2001;68:1923–1930.

138. Akerman S, Williamson DJ, Kaube H, Goadsby PJ. The effect of anti-migraine compounds on nitric oxide-induced dilation of dural meningeal vessels. Eur J Pharmacol 2002;452:223–228.

139. Akerman S, Holland PR, Summ O, Lasalandra MP, Goadsby PJ. A translational in vivo model of trigeminal autonomic cephalalgias: Therapeutic characterization. Brain 2012;135(Pt 12):3664–3675.

140. Pareja JA, Cuadrado ML. SUNCT syndrome: An update. Expert Opin Pharmacother 2005;6:591–599.

141. Cohen AS, Matharu MS, Goadsby PJ. Short-lasting unilateral neuralgiform headache attacks with conjunctival injection and tearing (SUNCT) or cranial autonomic features (SUNA)—A prospective clinical study of SUNCT and SUNA. Brain 2006;129(Pt 10):2746–2760.

142. Williams MH, Broadley SA. SUNCT and SUNA: Clinical features and medical treatment. J Clin Neurosci 2008;15:526–534.

143. Matharu MS, Cohen AS, Boes CJ, Goadsby PJ. Short-lasting unilateral neuralgiform headache with conjunctival injection and tearing syndrome: A review. Curr Pain Headache Rep 2003;7:308–318.

144. Pareja JA, Alvarez M, Montojo T. SUNCT and SUNA: Recognition and treatment. Curr Treat Options Neurol 2013;15:28–39.

145. Pareja JA, Caminero AB, Sjaastad O. SUNCT syndrome: Diagnosis and treatment. CNS Drugs 2002;16:373–383.

146. Montes E, Alberca R, Lozano P, Franco E, Martínez-Fernández E, Mir P. Statuslike SUNCT in two young women. Headache 2001;41:826–829.

147. Pareja JA, Sjaastad O. SUNCT syndrome in the female. Headache 1994;34:217–220.

148. Laín AH, Caminero AB, Pareja JA. SUNCT syndrome; Absence of refractory periods and modulation of attack duration by lengthening of the trigger stimuli. Cephalalgia 2000;20:671–673.

149. Matharu MS, Cohen AS, Goadsby PJ. SUNCT syndrome responsive to intravenous lidocaine. Cephalalgia 2004;24:985–992.

150. D'Andrea G, Granella F. SUNCT syndrome: The first case in childhood. Short-lasting unilateral neuralgiform headache attacks with conjunctival injection and tearing. Cephalalgia 2001;21:701–702.

151. Gantenbein AR, Goadsby PJ. Familial SUNCT. Cephalalgia 2005;25:457–459.

152. Putzki N, Nirkko A, Diener HC. Trigeminal autonomic cephalalgias: A case of post-traumatic SUNCT syndrome? Cephalalgia 2005;25:395–397.

153. Chitsantikul P, Becker WJ. SUNCT, SUNA and pituitary tumors: Clinical characteristics and treatment. Cephalalgia 2013;33:160–170.

154. Favoni V, Grimaldi D, Pierangeli G, Cortelli P, Cevoli S. SUNCT/SUNA and neurovascular compression: New cases and critical literature review. Cephalalgia 2013;33:1337–1348.

155. Lambru G, Matharu MS. SUNCT and SUNA: Medical and surgical treatments. Neurol Sci 2013;34(1, suppl):S75–S81.

156. Narbone MC, Gangemi S, Abbate M. A case of SUNCT syndrome responsive to verapamil. Cephalalgia 2005;25:476–478.

157. Jiménez-Huete A, Franch O, Pareja JA. SUNCT syndrome: Priming of symptomatic periods and worsening of symptoms by treatment with calcium channel blockers. Cephalalgia 2002;22:812–814.

158. Köseoglu E, Karaman Y, Kücük S, Arman F. SUNCT syndrome associated with compression of trigeminal nerve. Cephalalgia 2005;25:473–475.

159. Lagares A, Gómez PA, Pérez-Nuñez A, Lobato RD, Ramos A. Short-lasting unilateral neuralgiform headache with conjunctival injection and tearing syndrome treated with microvascular decompression of the trigeminal nerve: Case report. Neurosurgery 2005;56:E413.

160. Morales-Asín F, Espada F, López-Obarrio LA, Navas I, Escalza I, Iñiguez C. A SUNCT case with response to surgical treatment. Cephalalgia 2000;20:67–68.

161. Williams M, Bazina R, Tan L, Rice H, Broadley SA. Microvascular decompression of the trigeminal nerve in the treatment of SUNCT and SUNA. J Neurol Neurosurg Psychiatry 2010;81:992–996.

162. Charlson RW, Robbins MS. Hemicrania continua. Curr Neurol Neurosci Rep 2014;14:436.

163. Rossi P, Faroni J, Tassorelli C, Nappi G. Diagnostic delay and suboptimal management in a referral population with hemicrania continua. Headache 2009;49:227–234.

164. Cortijo E, Guerrero AL, Herrero S, et al. Hemicrania continua in a headache clinic: Referral source and diagnostic delay in a series of 22 patients. J Headache Pain 2012;13:567–569.

165. Moura LM, Bezerra JM, Fleming NR. Treatment of hemicrania continua: Case series and literature review. Rev Bras Anestesiol 2012;62:173–187.

166. Prakash S, Golwala P. A proposal for revision of hemicrania continua diagnostic criteria based on critical analysis of 62 patients. Cephalalgia 2012;32:860–868.

167. Benoliel R, Robinson S, Eliav E, Sharav Y. Hemicrania continua. J Orofac Pain 2002;16:317–325.

168. Peres MF, Silberstein SD, Nahmias S, et al. Hemicrania continua is not that rare. Neurology 2001;57:948–951.

169. Cittadini E, Goadsby PJ. Hemicrania continua: A clinical study of 39 patients with diagnostic implications. Brain 2010;133(Pt 7):1973–1986.

170. Rapoport AM, Bigal ME. Hemicrania continua: Clinical and nosographic update. Neurol Sci 2003;24(2, suppl):S118–S121.

171. Peres MF, Siow HC, Rozen TD. Hemicrania continua with aura. Cephalalgia 2002;22:246–248.

172. Obermann M, Katsarava Z. Epidemiology of unilateral headaches. Expert Rev Neurother 2008;8:1313–1320.

173. Nappi G, Perrotta A, Rossi P, Sandrini G. Chronic daily headache. Expert Rev Neurother 2008;8:361–384.

174. Evans RW, Lay CL. Posttraumatic hemicrania continua? Headache 2000;40:761–762.

175. Lay CL, Newman LC. Posttraumatic hemicrania continua. Headache 1999;39:275–279.

176. Brighina F, Palermo A, Cosentino G, Fierro B. Prophylaxis of hemicrania continua: Two new cases effectively treated with topiramate. Headache 2007;47:441–443.

177. Camarda C, Camarda R, Monastero R. Chronic paroxysmal hemicrania and hemicrania continua responding to topiramate: Two case reports. Clin Neurol Neurosurg 2008;110:88–91.

178. Matharu MS, Bradbury P, Swash M. Hemicrania continua: Side alternation and response to topiramate. Cephalalgia 2006;26:341–344.

179. Burns B, Watkins L, Goadsby PJ. Treatment of hemicrania continua by occipital nerve stimulation with a bion device: Long-term follow-up of a crossover study. Lancet Neurol 2008;7:1001–1012.

180. Sjaastad O, Antonaci F. A piroxicam derivative partly effective in chronic paroxysmal hemicrania and hemicrania continua. Headache 1995;35:549–550.

181. Viana M, Tassorelli C, Allena M, Nappi G, Sjaastad O, Antonaci F. Diagnostic and therapeutic errors in trigeminal autonomic cephalalgias and hemicrania continua: A systematic review. J Headache Pain 2013;14:14.

182. Buzzi MG, Formisano R. A patient with cluster headache responsive to indomethacin: Any relationship with chronic paroxysmal hemicrania? Cephalalgia 2003;23:401–404.

183. Fuad F, Jones NS. Paroxysmal hemicrania and cluster headache: Two discrete entities or is there an overlap? Clin Otolaryngol Allies Sci 2002;27:472–479.

184. Kaup AO, Mathew NT, Levyman C, Kailasam J, Meadors LA, Villarreal SS. 'Side locked' migraine and trigeminal autonomic cephalgias: Evidence for clinical overlap. Cephalalgia 2003;23:43–49.

185. Centonze V, Bassi A, Causarano V, Dalfino L, Centonze A, Albano O. Simultaneous occurrence of ipsilateral cluster headache and chronic paroxysmal hemicrania: A case report. Headache 2000;40:54–56.

186. Lisotto C, Mainardi F, Maggioni F, Zanchin G. Hemicrania continua with contralateral episodic cluster headache: A case report. Cephalalgia 2003;23:929–930.

187. Totzeck A, Diener HC, Gaul C. Concomitant occurrence of different trigeminal autonomic cephalalgias: A case series and review of the literature. Cephalalgia 2014;34:231–235.

188. Maggioni F, Manara R, Mampreso E, Viaro F, Mainardi F, Zanchin G. Trigeminal neuralgia and trigeminal-autonomic cephalalgias: A continuum or simple co-existence? Cephalalgia 2010;30:752–756.

189. Barbanti P, Fabbrini G, Pesare M, Vanacore N, Cerbo R. Unilateral cranial autonomic symptoms in migraine. Cephalalgia 2002;22:256–259.

190. Benoliel R, Sharav Y. Paroxysmal hemicrania. Case studies and review of the literature. Oral Surg Oral Med Oral Pathol Oral Radiol Endod 1998;85:285–292.

191. Benoliel R, Eliav E, Sharav Y. Self-reports of pain-related awakenings in persistent orofacial pain patients. J Orofac Pain 2009;23:330–338.

192. Zidverc-Trajkovic J, Pavlovic AM, Mijajlovic M, Jovanovic Z, Sternic N, Kostic VS. Cluster headache and paroxysmal hemicrania: Differential diagnosis. Cephalalgia 2005;25:244–248.

193. Stewart WF, Lipton RB, Kolodner K. Migraine disability assessment (MIDAS) score: Relation to headache frequency, pain intensity, and headache symptoms. Headache 2003;43:258–265.

194. Salvesen R, Bekkelund SI. Migraine, as compared to other headaches, is worse during midnight-sun summer than during polar night. A questionnaire study in an Arctic population. Headache 2000;40:824–829.

195. Peres MF, Stiles MA, Oshinsky M, Rozen TD. Remitting form of hemicrania continua with seasonal pattern. Headache 2001;41:592–594.

196. Leone M, Rigamonti A, Bussone G. Cluster headache sine headache: Two new cases in one family. Cephalalgia 2002;22:12–14.

197. Boes C. Differentiating paroxysmal hemicrania from cluster headache. Cephalalgia 2005;25:241–243.

198. Matharu MS, Goadsby PJ. Trigeminal autonomic cephalgias. J Neurol Neurosurg Psychiatry 2002;72(2, suppl):ii19–ii26.

199. Smetana GW. The diagnostic value of historical features in primary headache syndromes: A comprehensive review. Arch Intern Med 2000;160:2729–2737.

200. Schürks M, Kurth T, de Jesus J, Jonjic M, Rosskopf D, Diener HC. Cluster headache: Clinical presentation, lifestyle features, and medical treatment. Headache 2006;46:1246–1254.

201. Obermann M, Yoon MS, Dommes P, et al. Prevalence of trigeminal autonomic symptoms in migraine: A population-based study. Cephalalgia 2007;27:504–509.

202. Peñarrocha M, Bandrés A, Peñarrocha M, Bagán JV. Lower-half facial migraine: A report of 11 cases. J Oral Maxillofac Surg 2004;62:1453–1456.

203. Benoliel R, Birman N, Eliav E, Sharav Y. The International Classification of Headache Disorders: Accurate diagnosis of orofacial pain? Cephalalgia 2008;28:752–762.

204. Dora B. Migraine with cranial autonomic features and strict unilaterality. Cephalalgia 2003;23:561–562.

205. Waldman CW, Waldman SD, Waldman RA. Pain of ocular and periocular origin. Med Clin North Am 2013;97:293–307.

206. Lee AG, Al-Zubidi N, Beaver HA, Brazis PW. An update on eye pain for the neurologist. Neurol Clin 2014;32:489–505.

207. Ringeisen AL, Harrison AR, Lee MS. Ocular and orbital pain for the headache specialist. Curr Neurol Neurosci Rep 2011;11:156–163.

208. Eross E, Dodick D, Eross M. The Sinus, Allergy and Migraine Study (SAMS). Headache 2007;47:213–224.

209. Pareja JA, Barón M, Gili P, et al. Objective assessment of autonomic signs during triggered first division trigeminal neuralgia. Cephalalgia 2002;22:251–255.

210. Paliwal VK, Singh P, Kumar A, Rahi SK, Gupta RK. Refractory periods in SUNCT. J Headache Pain 2012;13:503.

211. Pareja JA, Cuadrado ML, Caminero AB, Barriga FJ, Barón M, Sánchez-del-Río M. Duration of attacks of first division trigeminal neuralgia. Cephalalgia 2005;25:305–308.

212. Wilbrink LA, Weller CM, Cheung C, Haan J, Ferrari MD. Cluster-tic syndrome: A cross-sectional study of cluster headache patients. Headache 2013;53:1334–1340.

213. Boes CJ, Matharu MS, Goadsby PJ. The paroxysmal hemicrania-tic syndrome. Cephalalgia 2003;23:24–28.

214. Zukerman E, Peres MF, Kaup AO, Monzillo PH, Costa AR. Chronic paroxysmal hemicrania-tic syndrome. Neurology 2000;54:1524–1526.

215. Jarrar RG, Black DF, Dodick DW, Davis DH. Outcome of trigeminal nerve section in the treatment of chronic cluster headache. Neurology 2003;60:1360–1362.

216. Lin H, Dodick DW. Tearing without pain after trigeminal root section for cluster headache. Neurology 2005;65:1650–1651.

217. Black DF, Dodick DW. Two cases of medically and surgically intractable SUNCT: A reason for caution and an argument for a central mechanism. Cephalalgia 2002;22:201–204.

218. Iacovelli E, Coppola G, Tinelli E, Pierelli F, Bianco F. Neuroimaging in cluster headache and other trigeminal autonomic cephalalgias. J Headache Pain 2012;13:11–20.

219. Matharu M, May A. Functional and structural neuroimaging in trigeminal autonomic cephalalgias. Curr Pain Headache Rep 2008;12:132–137.

220. Empl M, Förderreuther S, Schwarz M, Müller N, Straube A. Soluble interleukin-2 receptors increase during the active periods in cluster headache. Headache 2003;43:63–68.

221. Stillman M, Spears R. Endocrinology of cluster headache: Potential for therapeutic manipulation. Curr Pain Headache Rep 2008;12:138–144.

222. May A, Büchel C, Turner R, Goadsby PJ. Magnetic resonance angiography in facial and other pain: Neurovascular mechanisms of trigeminal sensation. J Cereb Blood Flow Metab 2001;21:1171–1176.

223. Costa A, Ravaglia S, Sances G, Antonaci F, Pucci E, Nappi G. Nitric oxide pathway and response to nitroglycerin in cluster headache patients: Plasma nitrite and citrulline levels. Cephalalgia 2003;23:407–413.

224. D'Amico D, Ferraris A, Leone M, et al. Increased plasma nitrites in migraine and cluster headache patients in interictal period: Basal hyperactivity of L-arginine-NO pathway? Cephalalgia 2002;22:33–36.

225. Goadsby PJ, Edvinsson L. Neuropeptide changes in a case of chronic paroxysmal hemicrania—Evidence for trigemino-parasympathetic activation. Cephalalgia 1996;16:448–450.

226. Goadsby PJ, Edvinsson L. Human in vivo evidence for trigeminovascular activation in cluster headache. Neuropeptide changes and effects of acute attacks therapies. Brain 1994;117(Pt 3):427–434.

227. Goadsby PJ, Lipton RB, Ferrari MD. Migraine—Current understanding and treatment. N Engl J Med 2002;346:257–270.

228. Prakash S, Patell R. Paroxysmal hemicrania: An update. Curr Pain Headache Rep 2014;18:407.

229. Leone M, Bussone G. Pathophysiology of trigeminal autonomic cephalalgias. Lancet Neurol 2009;8:755–764.

230. Holle D, Katsarava Z, Obermann M. The hypothalamus: Specific or nonspecific role in the pathophysiology of trigeminal autonomic cephalalgias? Curr Pain Headache Rep 2011;15:101–107.

231. Miranda-Cardenas Y, Rojas-Piloni G, Martínez-Lorenzana G, et al. Oxytocin and electrical stimulation of the paraventricular hypothalamic nucleus produce antinociceptive effects that are reversed by an oxytocin antagonist. Pain 2006;122:182–189.

232. Leone M, Franzini A, D'Andrea G, Broggi G, Casucci G, Bussone G. Deep brain stimulation to relieve drug-resistant SUNCT. Ann Neurol 2005;57:924–927.

233. Holland PR, Goadsby PJ. Cluster headache, hypothalamus, and orexin. Curr Pain Headache Rep 2009;13:147–154.

234. Bartsch T, Pinsker MO, Rasche D, et al. Hypothalamic deep brain stimulation for cluster headache: Experience from a new multicase series. Cephalalgia 2008;28:285–295.

235. Schoenen J, Di Clemente L, Vandenheede M, et al. Hypothalamic stimulation in chronic cluster headache: A pilot study of efficacy and mode of action. Brain 2005;128(Pt 4):940–947.

236. Leone M, Franzini A, Broggi G, Mea E, Cecchini AP, Bussone G. Acute hypothalamic stimulation and ongoing cluster headache attacks. Neurology 2006;67:1844–1845.

237. Bolay H, Reuter U, Dunn AK, Huang Z, Boas DA, Moskowitz MA. Intrinsic brain activity triggers trigeminal meningeal afferents in a migraine model. Nat Med 2002;8:136–142.

238. Matharu MS, Cohen AS, McGonigle DJ, Ward N, Frackowiak RS, Goadsby PJ. Posterior hypothalamic and brainstem activation in hemicrania continua. Headache 2004;44:747–761.

239. May A, Bahra A, Büchel C, Turner R, Goadsby PJ. Functional magnetic resonance imaging in spontaneous attacks of SUNCT: Short-lasting neuralgiform headache with conjunctival injection and tearing. Ann Neurol 1999;46:791–794.

240. May A, Bahra A, Büchel C, Frackowiak RS, Goadsby PJ. PET and MRA findings in cluster headache and MRA in experimental pain. Neurology 2000;55:1328–1335.

241. Matharu MS, Cohen AS, Frackowiak RS, Goadsby PJ. Posterior hypothalamic activation in paroxysmal hemicrania. Ann Neurol 2006;59:535–545.

242. May A, Bahra A, Büchel C, Frackowiak RS, Goadsby PJ. Hypothalamic activation in cluster headache attacks. Lancet 1998;352:275–278.

243. May A, Kaube H, Büchel C, et al. Experimental cranial pain elicited by capsaicin: A PET study. Pain 1998;74:61–66.

244. Cohen AS. Short-lasting unilateral neuralgiform headache attacks with conjunctival injection and tearing. Cephalalgia 2007;27:824–832.

245. Afridi SK, Matharu MS, Lee L, et al. A PET study exploring the laterality of brainstem activation in migraine using glyceryl trinitrate. Brain 2005(Pt 4);128:932–939.

246. Lodi R, Pierangeli G, Tonon C, et al. Study of hypothalamic metabolism in cluster headache by proton MR spectroscopy. Neurology 2006;66:1264–1266.

247. Wang SJ, Lirng JF, Fuh JL, Chen JJ. Reduction in hypothalamic 1H-MRS metabolite ratios in patients with cluster headache. J Neurol Neurosurg Psychiatry 2006;77:622–625.

248. May A, Ashburner J, Büchel C, et al. Correlation between structural and functional changes in brain in an idiopathic headache syndrome. Nat Med 1999;5:836–838.

249. Holland PR. Modulation of trigeminovascular processing: Novel insights into primary headache disorders. Cephalalgia 2009;29(3, suppl):1–6.

250. Moulton EA, Burstein R, Tully S, Hargreaves R, Becerra L, Borsook D. Interictal dysfunction of a brainstem descending modulatory center in migraine patients. PLoS One 2008;3:e3799.

251. Sprenger T, Ruether KV, Boecker H, et al. Altered metabolism in frontal brain circuits in cluster headache. Cephalalgia 2007;27:1033–1042.

252. Sprenger T, Willoch F, Miederer M, et al. Opioidergic changes in the pineal gland and hypothalamus in cluster headache: A ligand PET study. Neurology 2006;66:1108–1110.

253. Yang FC, Chou KH, Fuh JL, et al. Altered gray matter volume in the frontal pain modulation network in patients with cluster headache. Pain 2013;154:801–807.

254. Perrotta A, Serrao M, Ambrosini A, et al. Facilitated temporal processing of pain and defective supraspinal control of pain in cluster headache. Pain 2013;154:1325–1332.

255. Leone M, Bussone G. A review of hormonal findings in cluster headache. Evidence for hypothalamic involvement. Cephalalgia 1993;13:309–317.

256. Frese A, Evers S, May A. Autonomic activation in experimental trigeminal pain. Cephalalgia 2003;23:67–68.

257. Knight YE, Classey JD, Lasalandra MP, et al. Patterns of fos expression in the rostral medulla and caudal pons evoked by noxious craniovascular stimulation and periaqueductal gray stimulation in the cat. Brain Res 2005;1045:1–11.

258. Goadsby PJ. Trigeminal autonomic cephalalgias. Pathophysiology and classification. Rev Neurol (Paris) 2005;161:692–695.

259. Izumi H. Nervous control of blood flow in the orofacial region. Pharmacol Ther 1999;81:141–161.

Neuropathic Orofacial Pain

Rafael Benoliel, BDS
Gary M. Heir, DMD
Eli Eliav, DMD, MSc, PhD

Neuropathic pain is defined as pain "arising as a direct consequence of a lesion or disease affecting the somatosensory system."[1,2] This current definition includes two important changes from the previous definition of pain "initiated by a primary lesion or dysfunction of the nervous system": The word *dysfunction* has been replaced with *disease*, and it has been specified that the lesion or disease affects the somatosensory system. Neuropathic pain may appear after a physical insult, an infection, or a disease process affecting the peripheral or central nervous system. Although neuropathic pain may be due to ongoing disease, a healed injury may leave the nervous system in a pathologic state as in painful posttraumatic neuropathies. Often, no clear initiating cause is identifiable. This chapter describes the clinical features, pathophysiology, and differential diagnosis of neuropathic orofacial pain (Table 12-1); some cranial neuralgias are not described or appear in other chapters (Table 12-2). For a description of nonpainful neuropathies, see Smith and Cutrer.[3]

Table 12-1	Painful cranial neuropathies and other facial pains (IHS section 13)*

Level 1	Level 2	Level 3
13.1 Trigeminal neuralgia	13.1.1 Classical trigeminal neuralgia	13.1.1.1 Classical trigeminal neuralgia, purely paroxysmal 13.1.1.2 Classical trigeminal neuralgia with concomitant persistent facial pain
	13.1.2 Painful trigeminal neuropathy	13.1.2.1 Painful trigeminal neuropathy attributed to acute herpes zoster 13.1.2.2 Postherpetic trigeminal neuropathy 13.1.2.3 Painful posttraumatic trigeminal neuropathy 13.1.2.4 Painful trigeminal neuropathy attributed to multiple sclerosis plaque 13.1.2.5 Painful trigeminal neuropathy attributed to space-occupying lesion 13.1.2.6 Painful trigeminal neuropathy attributed to other disorder
13.2 Glossopharyngeal neuralgia		
13.3 Nervus intermedius (facial nerve) neuralgia	13.3.1 Classical nervus intermedius neuralgia 13.3.2 Nervus intermedius neuropathy attributed to herpes zoster	
13.4 Occipital neuralgia		
13.5 Optic neuritis		
13.6 Headache attributed to ischemic ocular motor nerve palsy		
13.7 Tolosa-Hunt syndrome		
13.8 Paratrigeminal oculosympathetic (Raeder) syndrome		
13.9 Recurrent painful ophthalmoplegic neuropathy		
13.10 Burning mouth syndrome		
13.11 Persistent idiopathic facial pain		
13.12 Central neuropathic pain	13.12.1 Central neuropathic pain attributed to multiple sclerosis 13.12.2 Central post-stroke pain	

*Reproduced with permission from the International Headache Society.

Clinical Approach to Neuropathic Pain

Symptomatology of neuropathic pain may include touch-evoked or stimulus-dependent pain that may be constant or intermittent. Additionally, there may be spontaneous or stimulus-independent pain.[4] Sensory symptoms may be positive (eg, hyperalgesia) and/or negative (eg, numbness), and these should be assessed and recorded using accepted terminology.[5] Some of these signs and symptoms (eg, thermal/mechanical allodynia) are frequently associated with neuropathic pain.[6]

Quantitative sensory testing provides data that is extremely valuable for the long-term follow-up of patients (see chapter 3). The mapping of affected areas and photographic documentation should form part of the patient

Table 12-2	Pain entities not covered in this chapter	
Diagnosis	**Comments**
13.1.2.6 Painful trigeminal neuropathy attributed to other disorder	See chapter 14.
13.3 Nervus intermedius (facial nerve) neuralgia	See chapter 7.
13.5 Optic neuritis	Often a manifestation of multiple sclerosis. Pain may precede impairment of vision. Head pain occurs in about 90% of patients with optic neuritis. Pain with eye movement is very common (90%) when there is an orbital segment enhancement in cranial magnetic resonance imaging, whereas in the absence of enhancement, 70% of patients will have no pain.
13.6 Headache attributed to ischemic ocular motor nerve palsy	Unilateral frontal and/or periorbital pain caused by and associated with other symptoms and/or clinical signs of ischemic paresis of the ipsilateral third, fourth, or fifth cranial nerves. Most ocular motor nerve palsies are painful, whether diabetes is present or not. Motor nerve palsy can occur before or concurrently with the onset of diplopia. Pain is most frequent in palsies affecting the third nerve, less so in the sixth nerve, and least in the fourth nerve.
13.7 Tolosa-Hunt syndrome	See chapter 14.
13.8 Paratrigeminal oculosympathetic (Raeder) syndrome	See chapter 14.
13.9 Recurrent painful ophthalmoplegic neuropathy	See chapter 14.
13.12.1 Central neuropathic pain attributed to multiple sclerosis	See chapter 14.

evaluation and follow-up. When an advanced quantitative sensory testing apparatus is unavailable, a simple pin, blunt instruments, warmed and cooled implements, and cotton wool may be used to test sensory function. More recently, sensory testing protocols have been introduced to examine changes in temporal summation and pain modulation (see chapter 3).

Epidemiology

Accurate data on the prevalence of neuropathic pain are lacking, partly because of inconsistent definitions and clinical criteria. A best estimate for the population prevalence of neuropathic pain is between 6.9% and 10.0%.[7] Increased life expectancy and disease survival rates will increase the prevalence of age-associated neuropathic pain syndromes. Neuropathic pain and its treatment lead to impaired quality of life, reduced employment, low productivity, and ex-

tensive usage of health care facilities.[8,9] Treatment of chronic neuropathies often requires long-term prescription medications that have significant side effects.[8] The use of nonsteroidal analgesics and opioids is particularly common, whereas use of antiepileptic drugs and tricyclic antidepressants (TCAs) are relatively uncommon.[8] This is surprising in view of the higher effectiveness of antiepileptic drugs and TCAs in neuropathic pain, and it suggests that patients may not be seeking treatment or are inadequately managed. Patients often turn to alternative medicine, and many report the use of vitamins and supplements[8] (see chapter 17).

Trigeminal Neuralgia

Trigeminal neuralgia is an excruciating, short-lasting, unilateral facial pain with clear classification criteria (Table 12-3). The diagnostic criteria published by the International Headache Society

Table 12-3 | **Diagnostic criteria for classical trigeminal neuralgia***

Diagnostic criteria	Notes
A. At least three attacks of unilateral facial pain fulfilling criteria B and C	Classical trigeminal neuralgia may be preceded by a period of atypical continuous pain, termed *pretrigeminal neuralgia* in the literature.
B. Occurring in one or more divisions of the trigeminal nerve with no radiation beyond the trigeminal distribution	Pain is mostly unilateral and does not cross the midline. It is very rarely bilateral, which may indicate disease (eg, multiple sclerosis). Most patients suffer pain in the distribution of the second or third division or both. Pain may be accompanied by spasm of the facial muscles. Periods of remission lasting from days to years may occur.
C. Pain has at least three of the following four characteristics: 1. Recurring in paroxysmal attacks lasting from a fraction of a second to 2 minutes 2. Severe intensity 3. Electric shock–like, shooting, stabbing, or sharp in quality 4. Precipitated by innocuous stimuli to the affected side of the face	Attack duration, distribution, and so on may vary between patients but are highly consistent within cases (ie, attacks are stereotyped in the individual patient). Precipitating stimuli are termed *triggers*, and these are usually mechanical (touch, wind, shaving), but they may also be temperature and taste. Trigger points may change location within the same patient. Some attacks may be, or may appear to be, spontaneous, but at least three must be precipitated in this way to meet this criterion. Mild autonomic symptoms, such as lacrimation and/or redness of the eye, may be present. A short gap between trigger and pain may be observed (latency). After an attack, a refractory period occurs where pain cannot be triggered.
D. No clinically evident neurologic deficit	Sensory testing may reveal mild deficits in the distribution of the trigeminal nerve. Hypoesthesia or hypoalgesia in the affected trigeminal region always indicates axonal damage. When either is present, there is trigeminal neuropathy, and extensive diagnostic workup is necessary to exclude symptomatic cases. Some patients have hyperalgesia in the painful region, which should not necessarily lead to a diagnosis of trigeminal neuropathy because it may reflect the patient's increased attention to the painful side.
E. Not better accounted for by another *International Classification of Headache Disorders,* third edition diagnosis	Other causes are ruled out by history, physical examination, and special investigations. Classical trigeminal neuralgia is caused by neurovascular compression, most frequently by the superior cerebellar artery. Imaging (preferably magnetic resonance imaging) should be done to exclude secondary causes and, in most patients, to demonstrate neurovascular compression of the trigeminal nerve.

*Reproduced with permission from the International Headache Society.

(IHS) classify classical trigeminal neuralgia (CTN, previously known as *idiopathic* or *primary trigeminal neuralgia*), which is now subdivided into those that are purely paroxysmal and those with concomitant persistent pain (Table 12-4). The classification abandons the diagnosis of symptomatic trigeminal neuralgia and introduces the term *painful trigeminal neuropathy*, bringing the classification in line with accepted neurologic terminology. The subgroup "painful trigeminal neuropathy" is subdivided according to etiologic factors and includes viral infection, trauma, multiple sclerosis (MS), space-occupying lesions, and other disorders (such as systemic diseases)[10] (see Table 12-1). The vast majority (> 85%) of patients with trigeminal neuralgia are diagnosed as having CTN.[11]

Clinical features of CTN

The diagnosis of CTN is based on a thorough history and characteristic clinical signs and symptoms. Clinical signs may vary depending on the stage at which a patient seeks treatment. In primary care, undiagnosed patients are common and are typically emotionally distressed and in severe pain. After initial diagnosis and treatment, patients may be symptomless but still visit specialist centers to request a second opinion. Relapsed patients with CTN in active treatment tend to return to their treating physician and are usually suffering from less severe pain. Each case demands careful history-taking to enable adequate management.

Table 12-4	Diagnostic criteria for classical trigeminal neuralgia, purely paroxysmal, and classical trigeminal neuralgia with concomitant persistent facial pain*
Diagnostic criteria	**Notes**
Classical trigeminal neuralgia, purely paroxysmal (13.1.1.1)	
A. Recurrent attacks of unilateral facial pain fulfilling criteria 13.1.1 classical trigeminal neuralgia (see Table 12-3)	
B. No persistent facial pain between attacks	
C. Not better accounted for by another *International Classification of Headache Disorders,* third edition diagnosis	Usually responsive, at least initially, to pharmacotherapy (especially carbamazepine or oxcarbazepine).
Classical trigeminal neuralgia with concomitant persistent facial pain (13.1.1.2)	
A. Recurrent attacks of unilateral facial pain fulfilling criteria 13.1.1 classical trigeminal neuralgia (see Table 12-3)	
B. Persistent facial pain of moderate intensity in the affected area.	
C. Not better accounted for by another *International Classification of Headache Disorders,* third edition diagnosis	Seen in about 30% of patients. Previously used terms: *persistent facial pain, atypical trigeminal neuralgia, trigeminal neuralgia type 2*. Central sensitization may account for the persistent facial pain. Neurovascular compression on MRI is less likely to be demonstrated. Responds poorly to conservative treatment and to neurosurgical interventions. Less likely to be triggered by innocuous stimuli.

*Reproduced with permission from the International Headache Society.

Most patients with CTN report characteristic paroxysmal attacks of pain. Some, however, have a history of concomitant background pain, which may account for up to 30% of patients with CTN. This condition is also known as *atypical* or *type 2 trigeminal neuralgia*.[12,13]

Classical trigeminal neuralgia, purely paroxysmal

The elderly patient described in Case 12-1 had a typical history of purely paroxysmal CTN with an onset some days previously.

Location. CTN is a unilateral facial pain syndrome.[14] Though bilateral pain has been reported in 1% to 5% of patients, one side usually precedes the onset of pain on the contralateral side by years.[15–17] Reviews of case series suggest that the right side is involved more often; however, this finding is inconsistent, and as no correlation has been found with age, sex, or handedness, the clinical significance is doubtful. Pain location is usually described according

to the major branches of the trigeminal nerve; 36% to 42% of patients report pain in one branch. In 16% to 18% of patients, the singly affected nerve will be the maxillary or the mandibular branch, whereas the ophthalmic nerve is affected singly in only about 2% of patients. Most commonly, the maxillary and mandibular branches are affected together (35%), and all three branches are involved in 14% of patients. The jaws are therefore involved in most patients, which explains why they often seek help from dentists. Pain radiation is within the dermatome of origin.

Although the location, intensity, and triggers of CTN vary across patients, they are highly stereotyped within individual patients with CTN; that is, each attack is similar in location, duration, and intensity.

Quality. Pain in CTN is most often described as paroxysmal, shooting, sharp, piercing, stabbing, or electrical in nature (70% to 95% of patients).[13,18] Pain severity in CTN is extreme; ratings are 9 or 10 on a 10-cm visual analog scale (VAS).[19,20]

CASE 12-1

An 81-year-old woman with CTN, purely paroxysmal.

Present complaint: Pain for the previous 3 months that has been increasing in frequency and severity. The pain occurs spontaneously or after touch over the lower left face. Eating or drinking can also induce pain.

History of present complaint: Similar pain had occurred for short periods of time about a year ago and 2 years ago with no treatment.

Physical examination: Cranial nerves are intact. The patient is edentulous. The panoramic radiograph showed no pathology (not shown). Pain was easily triggered by lightly touching the patient's face. The resulting pain lasted for less than 2 minutes and was excruciating (Fig 12-1).

Relevant medical history: Healthy.

Diagnosis: CTN, purely paroxysmal.

Diagnostic and treatment considerations: The presentation is typical of CTN. The prevalence of CTN increases with age and is therefore not a surprising event in an octogenarian. Treatment was with carbamazepine titrated slowly from 100 to 200 mg/day and increased until response (in this case, 600 mg/day). The patient was pain free within 72 hours. Computed tomographic brain imaging revealed no pathology. Liver function tests remained normal during follow-up, and carbamazepine levels were within the therapeutic range. Some months later, there was breakthrough pain, and the carbamazepine dose was increased to 800 mg/day, which provided pain relief.

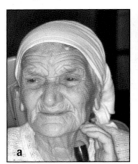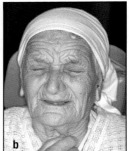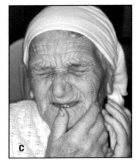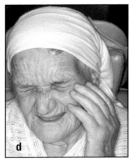

Fig 12-1 Case 12-1. *(a to d)* A patient with a recent onset of severe trigeminal pain; signs and symptoms were typical of trigeminal neuralgia. Attacks could be reproduced (triggered) in the clinic by gently touching the lower lip. Response to pharmacotherapy with carbamazepine was very rapid, and the patient was pain free by 72 hours. Note the guarding position of the patient's hand, the rapid onset of pain (8 seconds from *a* to *d*), and the accompanying facial tic.

Triggering

The diagnostic criteria for CTN include the premise that pain may be precipitated by light or innocuous touch in trigger areas or may be initiated by trigger factors. A short gap between stimulation of a trigger area and pain onset may be observed and is termed latency. CTN attacks are often spontaneous, and trigger areas are not always present or clinically identifiable; 40% to 50% of patients with CTN may not report a clear trigger.[13] Trigger-like areas may also be detected in about 9% of other orofacial pain syndromes, so this is suggestive but not pathognomonic.[13] Trigger areas in CTN are usually in the distribu- tion of the affected trigeminal branch, particularly around the lips, but may be extratrigeminal,[19] multiple, and even change location. The triggering stimuli are innocuous and include talking (76%), chewing (74%), touch (65%), temperature (cold 48%, heat 1%), wind, and shaving.[19] Data suggest that intraoral CTN triggers and pain are more often associated with the gingivae.[18,19] The triggering of CTN-like pain by gustatory stimuli is an interesting phenomenon that has been described as both primary and secondary (postsurgical) syndromes. The initiation of pain by sweet or salty foods is usually associated with dental pathology, so these patients present a difficult diagnosis (see chapter 6).

Trigger factors are distinct from trigger areas and include noise, lights, and stress.[19] These may also occur in up to 60% of other patients with orofacial pain,[13] but the rapid, severe, electric shock–like pain that occurs in CTN should distinguish it from other pain syndromes.

Temporal pattern. Individual attacks are characterized by a rapid onset and peak (see Fig 12-1) and then subside; overall, an attack lasts 10 seconds to 2 minutes.[21] This is followed by a refractory period that has a duration related to the intensity of the CTN attack; during this time, pain is impossible or extremely difficult to trigger. Attacks occur mostly during the day, but there are reports of nocturnal CTN.[22,23]

CTN may begin abruptly or via a rarer preceding syndrome, termed *pretrigeminal neuralgia*, which is described later in this chapter.[24] Long-term follow-up of patients with CTN reveals that there are well-defined periods of pain attacks variably followed by periods of remission that may last weeks to years. The median active period is reported at about 49 days, followed by remission of some months (36% of patients), weeks (16%), or even days (16%). Only 6% of patients may look forward to remissions of more than a year, and about 20% may suffer from incessant attacks. After a first attack of CTN, it has been calculated that 65% of patients will suffer a second attack within 5 years and 77% within 10 years.

CTN is a progressive disease with a poor prognosis.[25] About 90% of persons with CTN report increased attack frequency and severity.[19,26] Furthermore, initial response to carbamazepine is around 70%, but by 5 to 16 years the response rate is around 20%, and 44% of patients require drug combinations or alternative medication. Long-term follow-up of oxcarbazepine-treated patients demonstrated a high failure rate, which resulted in a need for surgery.[26] Supporting the progressive nature of CTN is the fact that microvascular decompression (MVD) has a significantly reduced prognosis in long-standing CTN (> 7 years).[27]

Associated sensory and motor signs. Sensory disturbances such as hypoesthesia have been documented in CTN. These may be more readily detected using sophisticated examination techniques[28–30] (see chapter 3) but may go

unnoticed in gross examinations. Reflex and evoked potential studies reveal nociceptive fiber dysfunction in CTN.[31] After successful MVD, nerve-conduction properties return to normal, but clinical improvement is often delayed.[32] However, more recently, examination of large series of patients with CTN revealed sensory abnormalities in around 30%.[33] The authors suggest that clinically detected sensory abnormalities should form part of the spectrum of CTN.[33]

Accompanying the pain of CTN is a classic contraction of the facial musculature, hence the use of the terms *tic douloureux* and *tic convulsif* (see Fig 12-1). Hemifacial spasm, probably secondary to vascular compression of the facial nerve root, is found in about 1% of patients with CTN and is more frequent in those with vertebrobasilar artery compression.

Accompanying autonomic signs. Characteristically, lacrimation is not considered a sign of neuropathic-type pain (see chapters 10 and 11). However, lacrimation and rhinorrhea have been reported in CTN. Lacrimation has been described in ophthalmic, maxillary, and mandibular CTN.[34–36] This presentation is diagnostically challenging (see the following sections and chapter 11). The appearance of lacrimation in CTN is inconsistent; it occurs in about a quarter of patients and seems to correlate with increasing pain severity (see chapter 11, the trigeminal-autonomic reflex). The presence of lacrimation may indicate a poorer prognosis for surgery.[35] Evidence of autonomic activity in CTN is found in reports of facial flushing (vasodilation), increased salivation, and swelling.[35,37]

Investigations. No specific diagnostic tests are available for CTN. A thorough clinical evaluation and adequate radiographs (bitewings, full-mouth periapicals, panoramic) of oral structures are essential to rule out pathology. A cranial nerve examination should be routine. Published evidence indicates that all patients with CTN undergo imaging (computed tomography or magnetic resonance imaging [MRI]) at least once during diagnosis and therapy.[38] Imaging techniques, such as magnetic resonance tomographic angiography (MRTA), may indicate neurovascular compression (see pathophysiology), and electrophysiologic testing offers promise in diagnosing symptomatic patients with

CTN. More sophisticated techniques, such as three-dimensional MRI with constructive interference in steady-state sequence, has shown superiority over MRTA in detecting venular compressions.[39]

All patients who are to be treated with anticonvulsants need baseline and follow-up of hematologic, electrolyte, and liver function tests (see chapter 16). Additionally, anticonvulsants increase the risk for suicidality, so careful follow-up of patients, particularly of at-risk persons, with close collaboration with the family physician should be maintained. In patients of Asian origin who are to be treated with carbamazepine, HLA-B*1502 testing to assess the risk of Stevens-Johnson syndrome or toxic epidermal necrolysis is recommended by the US Food and Drug Administration (see chapter 17). Patients at risk for these conditions with carbamazepine also carry an increased risk with other antiepileptic drugs.

Quality of life. The severity and progressive nature of CTN has resulted in patients committing suicide; however, CTN of itself does not alter life expectancy. Quality of life is much reduced in patients with CTN either as a direct effect of the pain or secondary to drug side effects.[19,40] These patients are often depressed and anxious[41] and need support and understanding; successful surgical treatment often relieves these negative emotions.

Features of CTN with concomitant persistent facial pain

The new subclassification of CTN with concomitant persistent facial pain is a welcome change and will aid in the study of the pathophysiology, natural history, and treatment responses of this subgroup of patients. This classification is based on findings that 35% to 49% of patients with CTN describe two types of pain: paroxysmal attacks of short sharp pain superimposed on a dull background pain of varying duration.[17,22] Background pain may be described as dull, throbbing, and burning,[12] of varying intensity, and with a mean VAS score of 4.6.[17] Some of these patients with CTN who have persistent pain also report longer attacks of paroxysmal pain. Continuous pain may be triggered in about 50% of patients, typically by chewing,

cold wind, talking, touch, or tooth brushing.[17] In one recent series, bilateral pain was significantly more common in CTN with background pain.[17] Patients with CTN and background pain are younger and more often females than those with purely paroxysmal CTN.[17]

The etiology of the persistent pain is unclear, but a faulty pain-modulation system or central sensitization have been proposed.[42,43] Patients with CTN with persistent pain experienced no experimental induction of conditioned pain modulation, which suggests a deficient descending inhibitory system.[43] Additionally, they had more tender points relative to control subjects and subjects with purely paroxysmal CTN, indicating central sensitization extending beyond the trigeminal system.[43] Central facilitation of trigeminal nociceptive processing was observed in patients with CTN with concomitant persistent facial pain, indicating overactivation of central sensory transmission.[44]

Some indications suggest that concomitant background facial pain is a clinical predictor of poorer treatment response, both pharmacologic and surgical.[12,17,45–47] Nearly half of these patients have clinical sensory loss,[17] and this is a negative predictor for the long-term outcome of MVD[48] and gamma knife surgery.[49] MVD provided absolute postoperative pain relief in CTN for 80% to 87% of patients and for 47% to 79% of those with CTN with background pain.[47,48] Long-term follow-up (> 5 years) revealed excellent results in 75% to 80% of patients with paroxysmal CTN but only in 35% to 54% of those with CTN with persistent facial pain.[47,48] The presence of background pain is also a negative prognostic factor in patients treated by rhizotomy.[50] In contrast, other centers reported no differences in surgical or gamma knife outcomes,[51,52] and this may be related to different inclusion criteria. The clear definition of such a subclassification is therefore clearly advantageous.

Pretrigeminal neuralgia

An early form of CTN, termed *pretrigeminal neuralgia*, has been reported in 18% of patients with CTN and is characterized by a dull continuous pain in one of the jaws that lasts from days to years.[24] As the process continues, pretrigeminal neuralgia becomes more typical with characteristic flashes of pain. Thermal stimuli may

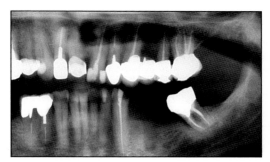

Fig 12-2 Patient diagnosed with left-sided trigeminal neuralgia who had undergone extensive dental treatment (multiple root canal therapies, extractions) in the maxillary and mandibular quadrants aimed at relieving the pain.

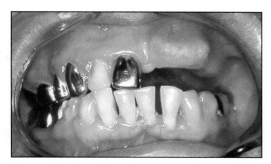

Fig 12-3 Patient with a history of misdiagnosed CTN. The pain was felt within the teeth in the maxillary left quadrant. Over a period of 5 years, the quadrant was made edentulous. When arriving at the pain clinic, the patient was diagnosed with CTN and a traumatic neuropathy.

cause triggering at a relatively higher rate, and a throbbing quality to pretrigeminal neuralgia pain is sometimes present, mimicking dental pathology. Indeed, these qualities, combined with the success of regional anesthesia, have led to misdiagnosis. Pretrigeminal neuralgia is, however, highly responsive to anticonvulsant therapy, and careful dental assessment should help differentiate it. The authors' clinical experience confirms that there are patients with highly atypical features that respond to carbamazepine and eventually develop into CTN. However, the lack of clear and consistent diagnostic criteria makes this a problematic entity to recognize; it is usually diagnosed when all other possibilities are exhausted or in retrospect once CTN develops.

CTN comorbidity

Combination syndromes

Trigeminal neuralgia most often occurs as a single pain syndrome. However, it has been reported rarely to occur with cluster headache and with paroxysmal hemicrania; these are termed *cluster-tic syndrome* and *chronic paroxysmal hemicrania-tic syndrome*, respectively (see differential diagnosis and chapter 11).

Hypertension

The presence of hypertension has been found to increase the risk of CTN by a factor of 2.1 in females and 1.5 in males.[18,53,54] The presence of hypertension in these cases has been linked with arterial compression of the ventrolateral

aspect of the rostral medulla in the region of the glossopharyngeal and vagus nerve roots.

Other neuralgias

Around 10% of patients with glossopharyngeal neuralgia may suffer comorbid CTN.[55] The two forms of neuralgia may occur simultaneously, which suggests some pathophysiologic association.

Differential diagnosis

Dental

CTN mimics dental pain, and up to a quarter of patients will initially consult a dentist.[18] Indeed, CTN is often misdiagnosed, and 33% to 65% of patients may undergo unwarranted dental interventions (Fig 12-2); up to 12% may be eventually rendered edentulous.[18,19] The number of patients with CTN who undergo extensive and misguided dental interventions suggests that many dentists are unaware of the features of CTN and pretrigeminal neuralgia. Invasive dental treatment must not be performed when no positive anamnestic, clinical, and radiographic signs indicate it. The patient depicted in Fig 12-3 had CTN. She felt pain in the maxillary left quadrant, and despite no overt pathology, dentists she consulted proceeded to extract all the teeth in that quadrant over a period of 5 years. By the time the authors saw her, she had signs and symptoms of CTN together with those of a traumatic neuropathy with allodynia and hyperalgesia. Management was extremely

Table 12-5	Typical clinical features of unilateral headaches relevant to the differential diagnosis of trigeminal neuralgia			
Parameter	**Paroxysmal hemicrania**	**Cluster-tic syndrome**	**SUNCT**	**Trigeminal neuralgia**
Age (years)	30 to 40	40 to 50	40 to 50	50 to 60
Pain duration (minutes)	2 to 30	< 45	< 4	< 2 (more in preTN)
Severity	++	+++	++	++++
Paroxysmal	+	+	+	+
Throbbing	+/–	+	–	– (+ in preTN)
Location	Hemicrania	Orbital	Orbital	Vb>Vc>Va
Wakes the patient	+	+/–	–	–
Frequency (no./24 h)	15	6 to 40	20 to 80	Triggering*
Triggering				
Touch	–	+	+	+
Neck	+	+ (40%)	+	–
Alcohol	+/–	+	+/–	–
Autonomic signs	+	+	+	+/–
Response to				
Carbamazepine	–	+/–	–	++
Indomethacin	++	–	–	–
Steroids	–	+/–	–	–
Lamotrigine	–	–	+	+/–

*Usually related to triggering events, but of normally high frequency.
preTN, pretrigeminal neuralgia; Va, trigeminal dermatomes ophthalmic; Vb trigeminal dermatomes maxillary; Vc trigeminal dermatomes mandibular.

difficult, and although the paroxysmal attacks of pain were eventually controlled, the patient continued to suffer from chronic pain.

SUNCT and cluster-tic syndrome

The differential diagnosis of CTN with lacrimation includes short-lasting unilateral neuralgiform headache attacks with conjunctival injection and tearing (SUNCT) and an atypical (shorter) cluster-tic syndrome (Table 12-5 and Fig 12-4). SUNCT syndrome is extensively discussed in chapter 11 and combines characteristics of neuralgiform pain with vascular-type signs, such as lacrimation.

Mechanical precipitation of attacks are a hallmark of CTN but are also seen in SUNCT.[56] Refractory periods are considered typical of CTN but are very rare in patients with SUNCT.[56] Supraorbital nerve blockade has been relatively unsuccessful in SUNCT,[56] whereas nerve blocks are effective in patients with CTN with lacrimation. CTN will initially respond to carbamazepine, whereas SUNCT syndrome is characterized by resistance to a wide range of drugs from its onset.[56] Neuroimaging studies suggest that SUNCT is related to the trigeminal autonomic cephalalgias[57] (see chapter 11), and the absence of trigeminal sensory pathway abnormalities would support the view that it is not a neuropathic type of pain.[58]

In cluster-tic syndrome, both cluster headache and CTN usually appear on the same side, and both respond favorably to carbamazepine therapy. Most patients with cluster-tic syndrome are females, and although onset may be at any age, it seems slightly more common between the ages of 40 and 50 years. Chronic paroxysmal hemicrania–tic syndrome has been reported.[59,60] The classic characteristics of both pain entities occur together on the same side and may be controlled with indomethacin.

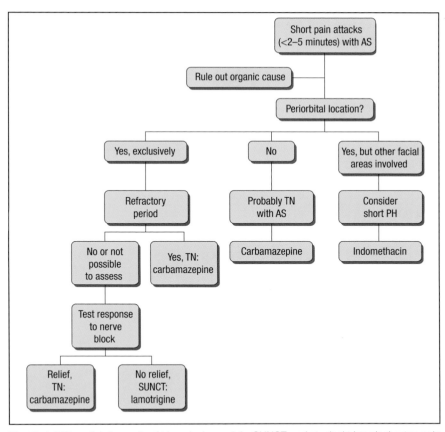

Fig 12-4 Differential diagnosis of trigeminal neuralgia, SUNCT, and atypical trigeminal autonomic cephalalgias. AS, autonomic signs; TN, trigeminal neuralgia; PH, paroxysmal hemicrania.

Epidemiology

Lifetime prevalence figures suggest around 70 cases of trigeminal neuralgia per 100,000 population, making it a rare condition.[61] The crude annual incidence of trigeminal neuralgia is 4.3 to 8 per 100,000, and it is higher in women (5.7) than in men (2.5). Recent data analysis suggests 12.6 to 28.9/100,000 person-years.[7] However, in persons older than 80 years, men have a very high incidence of 45/100,000.[61,62] Peak incidence begins at 50 to 60 years old and increases with age: 17.5/100,000 in 60- to 69-year-olds and 25.9/100,000 in those older than 80 years. Trigeminal neuralgia is extremely rare in children.

Treatment

CTN is a progressive disease, and eventually, dose escalation or addition of drugs to obtain synergism is common. The improved morbidity rates of neurosurgical techniques such as MVD, coupled with high efficacy rates, suggests that many patients may benefit from surgery, possibly at an earlier stage. At present, medical management is the basis for many patients with CTN; even for surgical candidates, medical therapy is essential preoperatively and is often needed postoperatively, albeit in reduced doses.[12]

Table 12-6	Drugs commonly used in the treatment of trigeminal neuralgia				
Drug	**Initial dose (mg)**	**Target dose (mg)***	**Dose increase (titration)***	**Schedule**	**Evidence†**
Carbamazepine	100 to 200	1,200	100 to 200 mg every 2 days	Three or four times per day	A
Carbamazepine controlled release	200 to 400	1,200	Usually transferred from regular format at equivalent dose	Two times per day	A
Oxcarbazepine	300	1,200 to 2,400	300 to 600 mg/week	Three times per day	B
Baclofen	5 to 15	30 to 60	5 mg every 3 days	Three times per day	A
Clonazepam	0.25 to 0.5	1 to 4	0.25 mg/week	Bedtime	
Gabapentin	300	900 to 2,400	300 mg every 1 or 2 days	Three times per day	B
Pregabalin	150	300 to 600	50 mg every 2 or 3 days	Two or three times per day	
Lamotrigine	25	400 to 600	25 to 50 mg/week	One or two times per day	A‡
Topiramate	25	100	25 mg/week	Two times per day	

*Titrate according to response and side effects.
†Evidence for efficacy rated A (best) or B (moderate).
‡Evidence for efficacy based on study using lamotrigine as add-on therapy.

Pharmacologic

Table 12-6 outlines drugs commonly used to treat trigeminal neuralgia. Carbamazepine is highly efficacious in CTN and is usually the first drug tested. The number needed to treat (NNT) for any pain relief for carbamazepine in CTN is 1.9 and for significant effectiveness is 2.6.[63,64] The success of carbamazepine in CTN has been extrapolated to serve as a diagnostic test. However, up to 30% of patients may be initially resistant, and up to 50% become refractory to carbamazepine therapy.[13] Serum levels of carbamazepine are useful to assess compliance and, in the elderly, to verify drug absorption; however, there seems to be no clinically significant correlation with response.[65] Oxcarbazepine, a carbamazepine derivative, is efficacious in CTN and has fewer side effects other than hyponatremia, but patients also develop resistance.[26] Baclofen has been successfully used in CTN, and some recommend it as first-line therapy. Because of its low side-effect profile, baclofen may be titrated to relatively high doses (80 mg/day) with an NNT of 1.4. Moreover, a strong synergistic effect with carbamazepine and phenytoin is reported, making baclofen suitable for combined therapy. Phenytoin was the first drug for CTN; it is prescribed at 150 to 200 mg twice daily but has a relatively low success rate (25%). Side effects such as drowsiness and dizziness occur in 10% of patients, even at low doses. Gingival hyperplasia is a common dental complication of phenytoin. Phenytoin is synergistic with carbamazepine and is therefore still used as add-on therapy. Clonazepam, at doses ranging from 3 to 8 mg daily, may provide some relief in CTN, but side effects are very common and limiting. The newer anticonvulsants have fewer side effects and have been shown to be effective for some patients as monotherapy or add-on therapy. Gabapentin has not been rigorously tested in CTN but may be useful in selected patients.[66] Pregabalin (150 to 600 mg/day) significantly improved pain in 60% to 70% of patients with CTN after 8 weeks.[46,67] Concomitant background facial pain was a clinical predictor of poorer treatment response.[46] Whether topiramate is effective for CTN is unclear.[68,69] Lamotrigine is effective as add-on therapy but has significant side effects.[70]

Based on the current evidence, the authors initiate therapy with carbamazepine and transfer patients at the earliest opportunity to the controlled-release formulation, which has fewer side effects. If carbamazepine causes troublesome side effects, the dose is reduced, and baclofen is added. Alternatively, oxcarbazepine or add-on therapy with lamotrigine may be tried. In refractory cases, drug combinations, as described earlier, should be tried. Gabapentin is probably the most promising of the new drugs[71] and is currently available in slow-release formulation in many countries. Pregabalin,[67] topiramate,[72] or even the older anticonvulsants valproate and phenytoin may be tried in recalcitrant cases[73,74] (see Table 12-6). It is important to appreciate that breakthrough pain may occur in successfully treated patients and may require temporary dose adjustment; in extreme cases, in-patient care with intravenous phenytoin may be needed.[74] Medically resistant patients who are physically able to withstand neurosurgery, particularly those with typical CTN, are prime candidates for surgery.

Alternative and future pharmacotherapy for CTN. Some non-antiepileptic or new drugs show promise in the management of CTN.[75] Pimozide is a centrally acting dopamine D2 receptor antagonist with evidence of efficacy that is greater than that of carbamazepine at 6 weeks.[76] Up to 83% of participants reported adverse effects, but these effects did not lead to withdrawal. Tizanidine is an alpha-2 adrenergic receptor agonist that is structurally related to clonidine and increases presynaptic inhibition of motor neurons. In a small trial, tizanidine was well tolerated, but the clinical effects were inferior to those of carbamazepine.[77] A later study revealed that patients experienced recurrence of trigeminal neuralgia within 1 to 3 months.[78]

Levetiracetam is an antiepileptic whose mechanism may involve inhibition of voltage-dependent N-type calcium channels, facilitation of gamma-aminobutyric acid (GABA)-ergic inhibitory transmission, reduction of delayed rectifier potassium current, and/or binding to synaptic proteins that modulate neurotransmitter release. Patients with refractory CTN were treated with levetiracetam (3 to 4 g/day) as add-on therapy and experienced a 62.4% reduction in the number of daily attacks. However, seven of the 23 patients withdrew from the study because of side effects.[79] The results in patients with central pain due to multiple sclerosis or painful polyneuropathy were

disappointing, and therefore the potential of levetiracetam in neuropathic pain management is unclear.[80,81] Lacosamide is a functionalized amino acid whose precise antiepileptic mechanism is unknown. However, it enhances sodium-channel inactivation, normalizes activation thresholds, decreases pathophysiologic neuronal activity, and is beneficial in animal models of neuropathic pain.[82] Lacosamide has a modest effect in painful diabetic neuropathy, but increasing dosages induced significant side effects with little clinical benefit.[83] Early clinical findings suggest some benefit for patients with refractory CTN.[84] Ziconotide is a nonopioid analgesic agent approved for intrathecal administration for severe, chronic pain in appropriate patients who are refractory to other treatments. Ziconotide is derived from the venom of a fish-eating cone snail, and it selectively targets the N-type voltage-sensitive calcium channel. This reduces pro-nociceptive neurotransmitter release (glutamate, calcitonin gene–related peptide, substance P) from nociceptive afferents. Ziconotide on its own or in combination has been used for neuropathic pain in various studies.[85,86] The drug has a narrow therapeutic window and a number of disturbing side effects, including nystagmus, confusional state, and nausea.[86] Although the intrathecal route complicates delivery, successful use in CTN has been reported.[87,88]

Surgical

The decision to opt for surgery is based on response to and side effects from medical treatment, the patient's age and profession, and the surgical facilities and expertise available. The candidate must be in a physical condition that will allow safe general anesthesia and neurosurgery. Patients require concise and clear explanations of the alternative neurosurgical procedures. The neurosurgical approach to CTN is described in chapter 13.

Surgery may be aimed peripherally at the affected branch or centrally at the trigeminal ganglion or the nerve root. Any surgical procedure seems to have a better prognosis when carried out as a first procedure, particularly on patients with purely paroxysmal CTN; in MVD, the best effects are obtained when performed within 7 years of CTN onset.[27] The changing trend in neurosurgical options in the United States was studied in a 20-year retrospective analysis.[89] The use of MVD nearly doubled from 1988 to 2008, whereas rhizotomy decreased to under one-tenth. Use of radiosurgery, introduced in the early 1990s, peaked in 2004 but has since declined. However, few quality trials have examined neurosurgical procedures for trigeminal neuralgia, particularly comparative studies that may aid in making individual choices.[90]

Peripheral procedures

Local anesthetics. Nerve blocks may provide some hours of absolute pain relief in CTN, and the authors have used these to permit patients to be involved in important personal activities. Within a hospital setting, continuous infusion of local anesthetic may be feasible but depends on the nerve branches involved.[91] This may be useful for pain control in patients scheduled to undergo neurosurgery for CTN and are resistant or suffer unbearable side effects to pharmacotherapy. One such case is described in the literature.[92]

Occipital nerve block with lidocaine and dexamethasone has been used in eight patients with trigeminal neuralgia. Response, which was defined as a reduction of at least 50% of the original pain, was obtained in 50% of these patients. The mechanism underlying this effect is unclear, but given that side effects are mild and the procedure is minimally invasive, it may be worth a trial.

Neurectomy. Early success rates for neurectomy are conflicting (50% to 80%) and involve relatively small series with short-term follow-up.[93,94] Moreover, peripheral neurectomy may lead to neuropathic pain and is therefore not recommended.

However, there has been renewed interest in this procedure, probably because it is so simple and relatively cheap. In 28 patients followed up for more than 3 years, only two (6.66%) reported recurrence.[95] This suggests that neurectomy is well tolerated and has few complications. One series of 36 patients examined remission times after repeat procedures (85 neurectomies on the infraorbital and mandibular nerves).[96] After the first operation, recurrence mainly appeared in the period between 12 and 18 months, and after the second operation, recurrence was

mainly between 9 and 12 months. Based on their data, the authors do not recommend repeating the surgery more than three times.

In the absence of adequate neurosurgical facilities, neurectomy may be a useful option. In 14 elderly patients with CTN who were still experiencing pain after carbamazepine therapy, neurectomy provided relief for 15 to 24 months in cases where neurectomy was done alone.[97] In cases where peripheral neurectomy was followed with obturation of the foramen with a stainless steel screw, none of the patients had painful symptoms at the 2-year follow-up.

Pterygopalatine fossa segment neurectomy of the maxillary nerve through the maxillary sinus was recently evaluated in 26 patients. Pain relief was accompanied by anesthesia or paresthesia in the operated side of the maxillary nerve dermatome. After a mean follow-up period of 2 years, 73% had an excellent response, 19% had a good response, 8% had a fair response, and none had a poor response. This technique provides an option for selected patients suffering from maxillary nerve CTN.

Cryotherapy. Median duration of pain relief after cryotherapy is about 6 months, which is significantly shorter than in thermocoagulation or MVD.[98] When pain recurred after cryotherapy, it affected the same sites as previously in 80% of patients. Repeated cryotherapy of mental and long buccal nerves, but not of infraorbital nerves, gave more prolonged pain relief than initial cryotherapy. One-third of patients undergoing cryotherapy suffered atypical facial pain after treatment, making this procedure extremely problematic.[98]

Sensation of the treated area returns 4 to 8 months after cryotherapy, and pain relief lasts at least 6 months.[99] In most cases, pain recurs within 6 to 12 months, but it is possible to repeat the procedure.[98,99]

Alcohol. Alcohol injections have been used but are painful, and fibrosis makes repeat injections technically difficult. Complications may include full-thickness skin or mucosal ulceration, cranial nerve palsies, herpes zoster reactivation, and bony necrosis.[93]

Median time for total pain control after the first alcohol block was 13 to 19 months in 68 peripheral alcohol injections.[100] These results suggest that peripheral alcohol nerve blocks may have a place in the temporary management of CTN, particularly in the elderly, the medically compromised, and those unwilling to undergo more extensive surgery. Postinjection neuropathic pain has been reported.

Peripheral glycerol. A 60% success rate at 24 months after peripheral glycerol injection has been reported, but others report pain relapse by 7 months.[100,101] Reinjection is possible, however, with reportedly good results.[101]

Summary. In summary, high recurrence and complication rates in peripheral procedures give no benefit over ganglion-level procedures. Moreover, all peripheral procedures aim at inducing nerve damage and carry the risk of developing neuropathic pain. Peripheral procedures should be reserved for emergency use or in patients with significant medical problems that make other procedures unsafe.[93]

Central procedures

Percutaneous trigeminal rhizotomy. Three techniques are available: radiofrequency, glycerol injection, or balloon compression (see chapter 13). The basis of these techniques is that controlled heat (69°C to 90°C), a neurotoxin, or ischemic and mechanical damage, respectively, will selectively ablate nociceptors (Aδ, C) while sparing mechanoreceptors (Aβ). However, patients often experience sensory loss of all fibers. Advantages of percutaneous techniques include shorter procedure duration and minimal anesthesia risk. These modalities give approximately equal initial pain relief (around 90%) but are each associated with different rates of recurrence and complications[102–107] (Figs 12-5 and 12-6).

Overall, radiofrequency rhizolysis consistently provides the highest rates of pain relief but is associated with high frequencies of facial and corneal numbness.[111] Radiofrequency allows for somatotopic nerve mapping and selective division lesioning, and it also provides pain relief in up to 97% of patients initially and 58% at 5 years.[106] Multiple treatments improve outcomes but also increase morbidity. Glycerol offers similar pain-free outcomes of 90% at 6 months and 54% at 3 years, but complication rates have been reported as higher (25% versus 16%)[106] and lower (11% versus 23%)[112] compared with balloon compression. This suggests that these procedures may be surgeon sensitive. Median time to recurrence was 21 months for the balloon procedure and 16 months for the glycerol procedure.[112]

Microvascular decompression. The MVD procedure is based on the hypothesis that contact between the intracerebral arteries and the trigeminal nerve root may allow pulsatile stimulation to cause chronic demyelination that may lead to trigeminal neuralgia. Thus, separating them may offer a permanent cure. The relatively high surgical morbidity (10%) reported in 1996 declined to about 0.3% to 3% in 2003, making MVD a safer option; mortality, however, remains a risk.[109] Complication rates are lowest in high-volume hospitals and when the surgeon performs a large number of MVDs yearly.[109] Long-term follow-up reveals that after 10 years, 30% to 40% of patients who underwent MVD will experience a relapse. Notwithstanding, in the long term, MVD seems the most cost-effective surgical approach to CTN,[113,114] but see Fransen.[115] A literature review on surgical modalities for CTN concludes that MVD is associated with the lowest rate of pain recurrence and the highest rate of patient satisfaction.[116] Patient satisfaction with MVD is particularly high when performed as a first intervention for CTN.[117]

Gamma knife. Gamma knife stereotactic radiosurgery (GKS) is a minimally invasive technique that precisely delivers radiosurgical doses of 70 to 90 Gy to the trigeminal nerve root at the point of vascular compression. The technique relies on accurate MRI mapping and sequencing. If no compressing vessels are identified, the site of exit of the trigeminal nerve from the pons or other preselected position on the trigeminal nerve is treated.

In a comparison of GKS with glycerol rhizotomy, it was concluded that despite greater facial numbness and a higher failure rate, glycerol provided more rapid pain relief than GKS. Indeed, in some reports, GKS is associated with delay before pain relief.[118] The percentage of patients who become pain free after GKS often increases over time (~ 24 months), which suggests that the procedure has cumu-

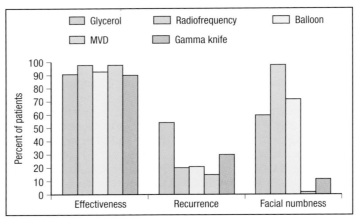

Fig 12-5 Effectiveness, recurrence, and side effects of surgical and radiofrequency interventions used in the treatment of trigeminal neuralgia.

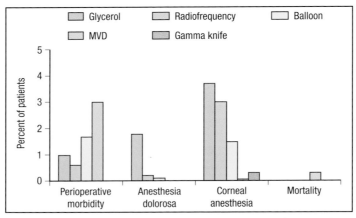

Fig 12-6 Complications and side effects of surgical and radiofrequency interventions used in the treatment of trigeminal neuralgia. (Data from Henson et al,[108] Kalkanis et al,[109] and Lim and Ayiku.[110])

lative effects.[119,120] GKS shows better long-term pain relief with less treatment-related morbidity than glycerol rhizotomy and thus may be indicated for patients who are poor candidates for MVD.[108,110] Although posterior fossa surgery (MVD or partial nerve section) was shown to be superior to GKS over a mean follow-up duration of about 2 years,[110,121] there are reports that GKS may be the procedure of choice for recurrent CTN.[122] Insufficient data are available at present to assess the long-term outcomes or complications of GKS, particularly the unknown effects of radiation in the area of the trigeminal

root. With GKS, better outcomes are associated with higher dosages; however, they also induce higher rates of sensory loss.[49]

Summary

Trigeminal neuralgia has a good initial response to almost all treatments but a predictable relapse of up to 40% to 50% over 15 years. Periods of pain relief are shortest for peripheral procedures, intermediate for drug therapy or rhizotomies, and longest for MVD. Accumulating evidence suggests that for healthy patients with typical CTN, surgery should be performed sooner rather than later; 7 years seems the current cutoff point, and beyond that the success of MVD declines. Because gamma knife radiosurgery centers and gamma knife units are still rare, the choice of treatment technique is restricted to percutaneous and MVD techniques. MVD remains the treatment of choice for CTN, in spite of the risks it entails.[123]

CTN is distressing, and the education of the patient's partners and close family is essential. TNA: The Facial Pain Association (www. tna-support.org) is an excellent resource and publishes an interesting layperson's guide to trigeminal neuralgia: *Striking Back!*

Pathophysiology of CTN

Several lines of evidence point to compression of the trigeminal root at or near the dorsal root entry zone (DREZ) by a blood vessel as a major causative or contributing factor.[12,32] The DREZ is the point where the peripheral and central myelin sheaths of Schwann cells and astrocytes meet. The compression is often arterial but may be venous or combined.[124] Imaging methods and surgical observations confirm a high rate of vascular compression of the nerve in patients with CTN.

This concept receives wide support from imaging and correlated surgical findings[125–127] and ultrastructural analysis of neuronal tissue[128,129] that confirm neurovascular compression in many patients with resultant clear histologic damage to neurons and their myelin sheaths. Biopsy specimens of trigeminal roots demonstrate pathologic changes such as axonal loss and demyelination.[32,128] Within zones of demyelination, groups of axons were often closely apposed without an intervening glial process. The location of the zone of demyelination matches the point of vascular indentation and extends about 2 mm in each direction.[32] Juxtaposed axons have also been demonstrated in patients with MS and CTN. Using the nociceptive blink reflex and pain-related evoked potentials, impairment of the trigeminal nociceptive system due to demyelination and/or axonal dysfunction on the symptomatic side was located close to the DREZ in the brainstem.[44] The trigeminal ganglion of patients with CTN demonstrates degenerative hypermyelination and microneuromata with no significant damage to neuronal soma; the initiating event, however, is unclear.

MVD of the nerve leads to prolonged pain relief in more than 90% of patients[109,130] (see chapter 13) and reversal of sensory loss in many patients.[131] The outcome is often related to the presence and degree of neurovascular compression.[132,133] Moreover, MVD results in sustained pain relief for about 10 years in ~70% of patients with CTN.[15,134] Further support is obtained from cadaver studies, where 91% of those with CTN had a vessel in contact with the trigeminal nerve adjacent to the brainstem, most with a demonstrable groove.[135] Grooving or deformation of the nerve is considered essential for the induction of pain.

Volumetric assessment of the affected trigeminal nerve in patients with CTN shows it to be significantly reduced.[136,137] This reflects atrophy of the nerve, which is often seen during surgery. Nerve degeneration, neuroinflammation, and edema have also been confirmed on diffusion tensor imaging.[138–140]

Reduced gray matter volume was observed in a cohort of patients with CTN,[141] similar to those described in other nerve injury models. The reduction of gray matter in some areas correlated with longer disease duration, which suggests that these structures have a possible role in the long-term changes associated with CTN, such as increased pain and resistance to pharmacotherapy. Microstructural alteration in white matter has also been shown in CTN, and it is proposed that this is possibly a reactive change to damage at the level of the root entry zone.[140]

A case-control functional MRI study examined patients with CTN before and after MVD surgery.[142] Activation of the sensory cortex by tactile stimuli at trigeminal and extratrigeminal sites was examined, and similar patterns were found in patients with CTN and control subjects before and after surgery. However, both groups displayed significantly reduced activation. This change suggests widespread alteration in somatosensory processing in patients with CTN. An earlier study investigated the changes in opioid receptor binding in patients with CTN before and after successful surgical treatment.[143] Significant increases in binding capacity were noted after surgery, which suggests decreased endogenous opioids and greater receptor occupancy.

These studies support a pathophysiologic model involving nerve injury but suggest that central nervous system structures have a significant contribution in the complex pathophysiology of CTN. In a study examining how triggering pain in CTN affects central nervous system structures,[144] evidence was found for pathologic hyperexcitability of the trigeminal nociceptive system. The pain neuromatrix showed significant activation during nonpainful stimulation of the trigger zone, which suggests a state of persistent sensitization of the trigeminal nociceptive system in CTN.[144] This finding supports the involvement of central mechanisms in the triggering phenomenon of CTN.

Intriguingly, the pain trigger in CTN is often innocuous stimulation. How is the trigeminal system altered so that light mechanical touch results in pain? After nerve injury, an increased proportion of neurons have subthreshold oscillations (pacemaker activity) that bring them close to their firing threshold. These neurons often generate ectopic discharges spontaneously or after external stimuli.[145] Ectopic discharges, termed *afterdischarge*, often last a number of seconds. Stimulation of the peripheral nerve (particularly Aβ fibers) or the dorsal root produces a transient depolarization in passive neighboring C-fiber neurons in the same ganglion.[146] In experimental setups, about 90% of neurons sampled responded with this cross-depolarization. In injured nerves, cross-depolarization leads to prolonged activity in neighboring neurons (crossed afterdischarge). These findings demonstrate a mechanism by which afferent nociceptors could be stimulated by activity in low-threshold mechanoreceptors, particularly after nerve injury. The *ignition hypothesis* was formulated based on these findings.[147] According to the hypothesis, injury renders axons and axotomized somata hyperexcitable, which in turn results in synchronized afterdischarge activity, cross-excitation of nociceptors, and pain paroxysms. Central nervous system neuroplasticity will no doubt occur in the presence of such peripheral changes and will ultimately affect the clinical phenotype and response to therapy. Although the ignition hypothesis explains many of the phenomena in CTN, it awaits definitive proof.

Furthermore, some studies do not support the involvement of neurovascular compression in the pathophysiology of CTN. Neurovascular contact is reported in pain-free control subjects and no neurovascular contact in a significant number of patients with CTN.[135,148–151] The finding of anatomical changes within the nerve in addition to neurovascular contact greatly increases specificity and positive predictive value.[151] Moreover, up to 14% of cadavers of persons with no history of CTN demonstrate vascular contacts, albeit with minimal grooving.[135,148] These studies indicate that other mechanisms beyond neurovascular compression may be involved. Alternatively, this may indicate that certain subjects are prone to develop pain after neurovascular compression, while others are resistant, which is similar to what occurs in traumatic neuropathies. The predisposition may be genetic, as evidenced by familial clusters of CTN.

Despite findings indicating dysfunction of the trigeminal system, patients with CTN do not always have clinically detectable neurosensory dysfunction. When present, any dysfunction is mild and primarily involves touch and thermal sensation. The findings are usually in the symptomatic division but may occur in the other two ipsilateral trigeminal branches, which suggests central mechanisms.[30] Sensory changes are reversed after successful MVD, a finding that supports neurovascular compression as the source of neuronal damage and pain. Brainstem reflexes are usually normal in CTN, but not in trigeminal neuralgia, due to systemic disease or regional pathology and are therefore useful for diagnosis. Patients with symptomatic trigeminal neuralgia usually have abnormal laser-evoked potentials (LEPs), but only a proportion of patients with CTN showed this abnormality[28]; thus, brainstem reflexes are more consistent in distinguishing CTN from symptomatic trigeminal neuralgia. In terms of elucidating neuronal dysfunction in CTN, LEPs are obviously superior. Indeed, the finding that some CTN patients have abnormal LEPs indicates a dysfunction of nociceptive fibers or of central nervous system pathways evoked by nociceptive afferent stimulation. Nociceptive fiber dysfunction may be a peripheral mechanism for the establishment of trigger points (pain induced by innocuous stimuli) in CTN.

The data therefore suggest several pathophysiologic subgroups of CTN that share a common clinical phenotype. Patients with neurovascular compression and signs of clear

Table 12-7	Diagnostic criteria for painful trigeminal neuropathy attributed to acute herpes zoster*	
Diagnostic criteria	**Notes**	
A. Unilateral head and/or facial pain lasting < 3 months and fulfilling criterion C		
B. Either or both of the following: 1. Herpetic eruption has occurred in the territory of a trigeminal nerve branch or branches 2. Varicella zoster virus DNA has been detected in the cerebrospinal fluid by polymerase chain reaction	Facial herpes zoster mostly affects the ophthalmic branch. Ophthalmic herpes may be associated with third, fourth, and sixth cranial nerve palsies. Involvement of the geniculate ganglion causes an eruption in the external auditory meatus and may also present with facial palsy (Ramsay Hunt syndrome; see chapter 7). In about 10% of patients, particularly the immunocompromised, the typical eruption may be caused by herpes simplex.	
C. Evidence of causation demonstrated by both of the following: 1. Pain preceded the herpetic eruption by < 7 days 2. Pain is located in the distribution of the same trigeminal nerve branch or branches	Prodrome of pain occurs in about 75% of patients. Pain is usually burning, stabbing/shooting, tingling, or aching and accompanied by cutaneous allodynia.	
D. Not better accounted for by another *International Classification of Headache Disorders,* third edition diagnosis	Herpes zoster is common in immunocompromised patients, occurring in about 10% of those with lymphoma and 25% of those with Hodgkin disease.	

*Reproduced with permission from the International Headache Society.

nerve damage may form one group, while patients lacking neurovascular compression may form a second group. However, no studies appear to correlate the degree of neurovascular compression (as shown by imaging) with neurophysiologic and psychophysical tests. Finally, in about 30% of patients with CTN, a constant background pain accompanies paroxysmal pain. It is possible that central mechanisms may be more involved in these patients. One study showed no differences in central nervous system structures in CTN patients with or without concomitant continuous pain,[141] but further imaging, neurophysiologic, and psychophysical studies are needed on these subgroups.

Discussion has been ongoing on whether SUNCT is a neuropathic pain related to trigeminal neuralgia or to the trigeminal autonomic cephalalgias. Imaging studies suggest that this condition is related to the trigeminal autonomic cephalalgias,[57] and the absence of trigeminal sensory pathway abnormalities would support the view that it is not a neuropathic type of pain.[58]

Painful trigeminal neuropathy

Painful trigeminal neuropathy is a new classification grouping that disposes of symptomatic

trigeminal neuralgia as a diagnosis.[10] Because most symptomatic trigeminal neuralgias are accompanied by sensory changes, these became neuropathies. Some interpret the term *neuralgia* to include paroxysmal-type qualities, which most symptomatic-type neuropathic pains are not, and the new terminology eradicates this ambiguity. Additionally, the more common etiologies for painful trigeminal neuropathies are now individually classified (see Table 12-1).

Painful trigeminal neuropathy attributed to acute herpes zoster

Acute herpes zoster (HZ), or shingles, is a reactivation of latent varicella virus infection that may occur decades after the primary infection. HZ is a disease of the dorsal root ganglion and therefore induces a dermatomal vesicular eruption. The exact mechanisms underlying viral reactivation and the subsequent appearance of acute HZ are unknown. In immunocompromised patients, the clinical presentation may be more severe, with numerous vesicles that take longer to heal. In these patients, herpes simplex may mimic a typical zoster infection.

Diagnosis of HZ is based on the clinical presentation (Table 12-7), as described in detail in

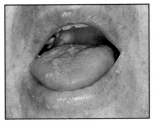
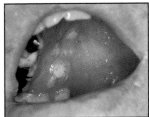
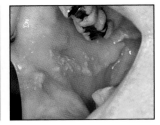

Fig 12-7 Patient with acute HZ in whom intact vesicles are apparent on the lips *(a)*. Most of the intraoral vesicles have ruptured, leaving ulcerations. The tongue and circumoral region *(a)*, palate *(b)*, and buccal mucosa *(c)* were all affected.

the following section.[10] The clinical features important to the diagnosis include a painful prodrome, a unilateral dermatomal distribution, a vesicular or popular eruption, history of a rash in the same distribution, and pain.[152] Definitive diagnosis may be obtained by identifying viral DNA from vesicular fluid or the cerebrospinal fluid using polymerase chain reaction.[153] More recently, the future identification of HZ DNA in saliva has been described as a possible and certainly less invasive diagnostic test.[153]

Clinical features

Location. The most common location for HZ is the thoracic region followed by the lumbar region. Trigeminal and cervical nerves are affected in 8% to 28% and 13% to 23% of patients, respectively. The ophthalmic branch is affected in more than 80% of the trigeminal cases, particularly in elderly men, and may cause sight-threatening keratitis. The vesicles and pain are dermatomal and unilateral and will appear intraorally when the maxillary or mandibular branches of the trigeminal nerve are affected (Fig 12-7).

Quality and severity. Pain is usually described as constant, but in one series more than a quarter of patients reported superimposed lancinating pains. In some patients, evoked (stimulus-dependent) pain may be the prominent feature. Descriptors of pain at rash onset include burning (26%), stabbing (15%), shooting (15%), tingling (10%), and aching (9%).[154] Pain may be moderate to severe (VAS 6.2), but up to 25% of patients are pain free.[155] High pain severity correlates with an increased incidence of postherpetic neuropathy (PHN).[155]

Temporal pattern. The timeline of acute HZ is critical in its diagnosis[152]; it begins with a prodrome of pain, headache, itching, and malaise.[156–158] Pain usually precedes the acute stage by 2 or 3 days (< 7 days) and may continue for up to 3 to 6 months with varying intensity.[157]

Associated signs. The acute stage is characterized by a red macopapular rash that develops into a vesicular eruption over a period of 3 to 5 days; these usually dry out over a further 7 to 10 days. Complete healing may take 1 month. Mechanical allodynia and disturbed sensory thresholds are often seen, and these usually spread to adjacent dermatomes and may also occur bilaterally.

Very rarely, dermatomal pain occurs with no rash and is termed *zoster sine herpete*. This entity cannot be accurately established based on the clinical presentation and requires evidence of concurrent viral reactivation.[159] Motor weakness may occur but is usually transient.

Epidemiology. Since the introduction of the varicella vaccination in 1995, the annual incidence of HZ has decreased by about 75%.[160] Currently, about 0.3% of people will develop HZ every year, and its incidence increases steadily with age from 0.06% between ages 15 to 19 years to 1% in persons over the age of 80 years.[160] In contrast to varicella, HZ does not follow a seasonal pattern and does not generally appear in epidemics. The overall lifetime risk of HZ is about 30% but is more than 50% in patients over the age of 80 years.[160]

Thus, HZ may occur in young patients but is less frequent. The question arises if and when

| Table 12-8 | Oral antiviral drugs used in the treatment of HZ that may also reduce incidence of postherpetic neuropathy |

Table 12-8 — Oral antiviral drugs used in the treatment of HZ that may also reduce incidence of postherpetic neuropathy

Drug	Dosage (mg)	Times daily	Duration (days)*	Notes
Aciclovir	800	5	7 to 10	Side effects may include rash, headache, nausea, vomiting, dizziness, and abdominal pain. Patients must maintain fluid intake to prevent renal drug deposition. May require dose adjustment in persons with renal dysfunction and in the elderly. Precautions must be taken for patients who are immunocompromised, as cases of severe thrombotic thrombocytopenia purpura have been reported. Pregnancy category B.
Valaciclovir	1,000	3	7	
Famciclovir	250 to 500†	3	7	Most common side effects are headache, paresthesia, nausea, and vomiting. Pregnancy category B. Elimination is impaired in patients with renal dysfunction.
Brivudine	125	1	7	Most common side effect is nausea. Severe interaction with 5-fluorouracil and other 5-fluoropyrimidines. Contraindicated in pregnancy.

*Longer treatment schedules are not associated with increased benefit.
†Recommended dosage in the United States.

this should be interpreted as a sign of underlying immunosuppressive disease. Proposed criteria for further investigation include HIV risk factors, confluent dermatomal rash, multiple dermatomal involvement, and renewal of lesions after 6 days.[160]

Treatment. Therapy is directed at controlling pain, accelerating healing, and reducing the risk of complications, such as dissemination, PHN, and local secondary infection.[157] When antivirals are initiated early (< 72 hours from onset of rash), particularly in patients older than 50 years, they decrease rash duration, pain severity, and incidence of PHN.[155,161] However, a recent meta-analysis found that oral aciclovir does not reduce the incidence of PHN significantly, and there was insufficient evidence to determine the effect of other antivirals.[162] Table 12-8 summarizes antiviral medications and dosages for the treatment of HZ. Based on pain resolution, valaciclovir (1,000 mg three times per day) is more efficacious than aciclovir (800 mg five times per day). Famciclovir (500 mg three times per day) is also an effective and well-tolerated therapy and has the advantage of reduced frequency of dosing. A direct head-to-head comparison of famciclovir and valaciclovir showed that the two drugs were therapeutically equivalent in healing rate and pain resolution.

Brivudine is licensed in some European countries for the early treatment of HZ in adults with immunocompetence. Brivudine (125 mg daily) has a mixed efficacy profile versus aciclovir (800 mg five times per day) but overall is superior.[163] Compared with famciclovir (250 mg three times per day), brivudine is as effective on pain and rash and has similar tolerability. Severe drug interactions have been reported between brivudine and 5-fluorouracil and other 5-fluoropyrimidines. Clearly, brivudine should not be administered concomitantly with 5-fluorouracil or its derivatives (capecitabine, floxuridine, and flucytosine).[163] Novel anti-HZ drugs have recently been evaluated in clinical trials and offer improved efficacy, reduced daily doses, and fewer side effects.[164]

When administered systemically within 72 hours of rash onset, corticosteroids have a clinically significant benefit on acute pain and quality-of-life outcomes but no demonstrable effect on PHN.[163] Fever and pain should be controlled initially by analgesics, such as acetaminophen, but opioids are effective for stronger pain. Amitriptyline and gabapentin will provide analgesia (see chapter 16); amitriptyline may also shorten illness duration and the incidence of PHN. However, amitriptyline is associated with significant cardiovascular effects that are problematic in the elderly, so nortriptyline or desipramine is preferred.

Amitriptyline- P. 589

Varicella vaccine. Vaccinating at-risk persons such as the elderly and infirm may be an efficacious technique to prevent HZ and PHN. An investigational zoster vaccine was 60% effective in reducing the incidence of PHN among older adults.[165] Additionally, the vaccine has been shown to be safe and partially effective in younger subjects with a 70% efficacy, and the recommendation is to vaccinate persons over the age of 50 years.[166] The vaccine has been further shown to reduce the duration and severity of PHN.[167] The vaccine is cleared in the United States for use in patients aged 50 years or older. Issues with the varicella vaccine include increased overall health care costs, particularly the cost of administration and implementation in the elderly population.[164] In addition, the efficacy of the vaccine seems to decrease with age, but changes to the vaccine may overcome this.[164]

Live vaccines cannot be dispensed to immunosuppressed persons, a group at high risk for infection. In these patients, an immune globulin preparation should be considered for postexposure prophylaxis.[164] VariZIG (Emergent BioSolutions) is currently the only varicella zoster immune globulin preparation available in the United States through an investigational new drug expanded access protocol. The period after exposure to varicella zoster virus during which a patient may receive VariZIG has been extended from 4 to 10 days.[168] Ideally, the drug should be administered as soon as possible after exposure, as there are indications of increased varicella incidence with increasing time between exposure and administration of the immune globulin.

Pathophysiology. Viral replication induces epithelial cell degeneration characterized by ballooning and followed by invasion of giant cells. Rarely, necrosis and bleeding may be observed. The vesicles subsequently become cloudy as polymorphonucleocytes, fibrin, and degenerated cells appear; subsequently, these rupture and release infectious contents.

Inflammation around the nerve trunk, including lymphocytic infiltration of the nerve root, and subsequent nerve damage underlie the pain in HZ. HZ affects one ganglion causing focal necrosis of neuronal cell bodies and satellite cells.[169] Viral DNA is found in most thoracic and trigeminal ganglial cells examined, and

infected dorsal root ganglion cells demonstrate cell degeneration and satellitosis. Spread within the spinal cord involves adjacent segments (bilaterally) and accounts for the distribution of sensory changes and hyperalgesia observed. In severe cases, the spinal ventral horn may be involved with resultant paralysis.

Postherpetic neuropathy

Several risk factors for persistent pain have emerged, including advanced age, severe prodromal pain, severe acute pain, and severe rash.[158,170] Of these, age older than 50 years and intense pain were independently shown to predict PHN 3 months after HZ infection.[170,171] The incidence of PHN is estimated at 3.9 to 42.0/100,000 person-years,[7] but the specific incidence of PHN in the trigeminal region is unclear.

A lack of consensus exists as to when acute HZ becomes PHN, and a number of definitions have been proposed, including persistent pain beginning at variable times after rash onset or disappearance as well as pain that persists 30 days, 90 days, or more after the onset of HZ rash.[163] Alternative views hold that pain associated with HZ (termed *zoster-associated pain*) should be viewed as a continuum until it resolves, if it does. This view, however, fails to differentiate acute pain from PHN, which seems to have a distinct pathophysiology. This has led to the suggestion that pain occurring after HZ infection be classified into three phases: acute HZ, subacute HZ, and PHN.[152] Thus, pain lasting less than 30 days is acute HZ, pain lasting more than 120 days is PHN, and subacute pain is anything in between. This classification is in line with evidence supporting the finding that acute HZ and PHN have different pathophysiologies[172] and reconciles the different reports of pain duration after acute HZ.

Persistent pain 3 months after acute HZ is more common in elderly patients and ranges from 0.3% in those younger than 44 years to 9% in persons aged 75 years and older.[169] Depending on individual patient characteristics, a proportion (5% to 40%) of patients with acute HZ will report pain 6 months after initial onset, but by 1 year, only 5% to 10% continue to suffer pain.[152,165] Few studies have investigated persistence of pain beyond 6 months, however. In patients older than 60 years, 5% have been

Table 12-9 **Diagnostic criteria for postherpetic neuropathy***

Diagnostic criteria	Notes
A. Unilateral head and/or facial pain persisting or recurring for ≥ 3 months and fulfilling criterion C	After acute HZ, PHN is more prevalent in the elderly.
B. History of acute HZ affecting a trigeminal nerve branch or branches	The first division of the trigeminal nerve is most commonly affected, but the second and third divisions may also be involved.
C. Evidence of causation demonstrated by both of the following: 1. Pain developed in temporal relation to the acute HZ 2. Pain is located in the distribution of the same trigeminal nerve branch or branches	Typically, the pain is burning and itching. Itching of affected areas may be very prominent and very bothersome. Sensory abnormalities and allodynia are usually present in the territory involved. Pale or light purple scars may be present as sequelae of the herpetic eruption.
D. Not better accounted for by another *International Classification of Headache Disorders,* third edition diagnosis	PHN is usually more common in patients older than 60 years.

*Reproduced with permission from the International Headache Society.

reported to suffer some pain for more than 1 year.[165] In a further study on patients 50 years and older, 6% suffered persisting pain at 1 year.[170] One long-term follow-up study (3.9 years) showed that once they were pain free at 6 months, no patients relapsed, and most continued to improve.[173] Why there is such discrepancy in the reported duration of pain is unclear.[152] Table 12-9 outlines the diagnostic criteria for PHN according to the IHS classification.

Clinical features

Location. Trigeminal PHN usually affects the ophthalmic branch (22%) of the trigeminal nerve.

Quality. The qualitative descriptors used for PHN include burning, throbbing, stabbing, shooting, or sharp. The presence of burning pain is significantly higher in patients who did not receive antiviral therapy in the acute HZ stage. Most patients with PHN describe a constant deep burning or aching pain with superimposed paroxysmal, lancinating pain and allodynia.

Itching of affected areas is present in 30% to 50% of patients and is more common in trigeminal dermatomes.[174] This has been termed *postherpetic itch*, and indeed, it may often be subjectively graded as worse than pain.[169]

Although postherpetic itch is usually mild to moderate, it may be very prominent and extremely bothersome; if accompanied by anesthesia, it may lead to self-injury from persistent scratching.[174]

Severity. PHN is usually severe (VAS ratings of 8) but is characterized by fluctuations from moderate background pain to excruciating, superimposed lancinating pains. Pain associated with PHN may be of low intensity and not clinically meaningful. The definition of clinically meaningful may be dependent on the VAS score (usually ≥ 3 of 10 is suggested), active pain pharmacotherapy, or active follow-up due to pain. Each of these gives different epidemiologies for significant pain associated with PHN. However, this should be defined by what the patient thinks is significant and how it affects his or her quality of life.[152,169]

Temporal pattern. The temporal pattern is variable; some patients complain of constant pain and others of paroxysmal pain as the leading symptom.[175] Most patients with PHN will have some degree of constant, burning pain.

Associated signs. Pale, sometimes red or purple scars may remain in the affected area, and

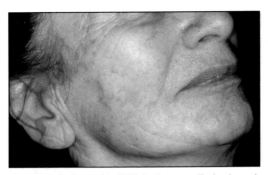

Fig 12-8 Patient with PHN in the mandibular branch of the trigeminal nerve. The area anterior to the ear and lateral to the mouth shows purplish scars that were very sensitive to touch.

these are usually hypoesthetic or anesthetic. Paradoxically, these areas may exhibit allodynia and hyperalgesia (Fig 12-8).

As in other neuropathic pains, PHN is characterized by a heterogenous mix of sensory signs and symptoms.[175] Most patients with PHN suffer from allodynia and exhibit deficits for temperature and pinprick sensation.

Treatment. Early treatment of established PHN seems to improve prognosis. Ophthalmic PHN per se seems to have the worst prognosis. Evidence-based treatment options for PHN include TCAs, gabapentin, pregabalin, opioids, and topical lidocaine or capsaicin patches[176,177] (see chapters 15 and 16). As a group, TCAs are effective in PHN (NNT, 2.6). Amitriptyline has been the most extensively studied TCA, but the evidence points to little difference among TCAs. TCAs may be contraindicated in the elderly, and nortriptyline and desipramine are safer alternatives. Gabapentin (NNT, 4.4) and pregabalin (NNT, 3.3 to 4.93) are of proven efficacy in PHN and safer in elderly patients.[176,177] Tramadol is a reasonable alternative, with an NNT of 4.8.[176,177] The NNT for opioids in PHN is around 2.7, and some patients may prefer opioids to TCAs. Lidocaine patches (NNT around 4) are useful, particularly in the presence of allodynia, and have significantly fewer side effects than systemic drugs.[178–180] Low-concentration capsaicin creams seem to offer minimal relief.[181] Capsaicin 8% is efficacious and safe, and one application may provide pain relief for up to 3 months, with an NNT of 8.8.[182] High-

er concentrations of capsaicin (10% and 20%) are currently under investigation.[183] A capsaicin patch is not recommended for use in the trigeminal system, and extreme care is required around the eyes.[184] Clearly, first-line therapy is TCAs, antiepileptics, and topicals, with opioids and tramadol as second line.[176,177]

Postherpetic itch is extremely difficult to treat and does not respond to antihistamines. Only local anesthetics provide any relief, albeit temporary.

More invasive modalities for PHN include epidural and intrathecal steroids, sympathetic and sensory nerve blocks, spinal cord stimulation, and a variety of neurosurgical techniques.[185,186] The most promising surgical intervention seems to be DREZ lesion (see chapter 13), which provides relief in 59% of patients. Central nervous system stimulation may also provide pain relief.

Pathophysiology. PHN, which is considered to be pathophysiologically separate from acute HZ, is a neuropathic pain syndrome resulting from viral-induced nerve injury. Scarring of sensory ganglia and peripheral nerve damage with loss of large myelinated fibers are commonly found in patients with PHN.[169] Two processes have been suggested: peripherally generated pain by irritable nociceptors and centrally generated pain secondary to nerve injury.[187] The clinical phenotype will be affected by the degree that each process plays in individual patients.

Skin biopsies from affected and contralateral sites demonstrate bilateral peripheral nerve damage. PHN occurred in the patients with the least epidermal neurites remaining after acute HZ, which suggests pain secondary to nerve injury.[169] It is interesting to note that cutaneous innervation in patients with PHN shows no recovery at all by 6 months.[188] Moreover, even after 7.7 years, reinnervation was not apparent, which indicates that recovery of sensory function and anatomical reinnervation of the skin is not a requirement for resolution of pain and allodynia.[173] In patients with trigeminal PHN, the intensity of the constant, burning pain correlated with neurophysiologic abnormalities in the Aδ fibers and C fibers, whereas paroxysmal pain correlated with Aβ-fiber dysfunction.[175] This suggests that although the constant pain is related to the pain/thermal pathways, the paroxysmal pain is related to abnormal impulses generated in demyelinated Aβ fibers.[189]

The virus is not usually recovered from the spinal cord of patients with PHN, which suggests that an infective process is not actively involved at this stage. Atrophy of the spinal dorsal horn is present in patients with PHN but not in patients who had acute HZ but did not develop PHN.[169] Postmortem examination of a patient with ophthalmic PHN revealed severe peripheral nerve pathology that also involved the contralateral side.[190] However, the trigeminal ganglion and trigeminal root were unaffected. PHN is possibly a disease that progresses from the periphery to central structures. Ongoing activity in peripheral nociceptors has been shown to be important in the early stages (< 1 year) of PHN, whereas central mechanisms may become prominent in later stages.[191]

Painful traumatic trigeminal neuropathy

Damage or disease to the sensory nervous system may induce sensory changes (neuropathy) that may, in some cases, be accompanied by pain (painful neuropathy).

Neural damage or disease can induce pain originating in a peripheral nerve (peripheral neuropathy), in a ganglion (ganglionopathy), in a dorsal root (radiculopathy), or from the central nervous system (central neuropathic pain). This section focuses on pain resulting from injury to the peripheral branch of the trigeminal neuron. The outcome of pain resulting from damage to the cell soma at the level of the trigeminal ganglion is covered in the section on complications of rhizotomy for the treatment of trigeminal neuralgia. Similarly, pain arising as a consequence of damage to the dorsal root is usually a result of neurosurgery. Although injury at the level of the peripheral branch of the neuron may leave the cell soma and its central branch (nerve root) intact, damage at the level of the trigeminal ganglion may potentially kill the afferent completely, thus deafferenting the area. Injury to the dorsal root is also different and potentially cuts all peripheral input to the central nervous system. Clearly, each of these injuries needs to be studied individually.

Probably the most common precipitating event is trauma, but infection (AIDS), metabolic abnormalities (diabetes), malnutrition, vascular abnormalities (trigeminal neuralgia), infarction (central post-stroke pain), neurotoxins, radiation, and autoimmune disease are also implicated. In orofacial pain clinics, reported onset most often has a clear association with craniofacial or oral trauma,[192] but pain may begin after minor dental interventions, such as nerve blocks, root canal therapy, and third-molar extractions.[193-197] It is of utmost importance to stress that the occurrence of iatrogenic painful traumatic trigeminal neuropathy (PTTN) or other posttraumatic neuropathies, such as complex regional pain syndrome (CRPS), does not in most cases reflect on the quality of the surgical intervention.[198]

Various terms describing PTTN abound in the literature, including *phantom tooth pain*, *atypical odontalgia*, and *atypical facial pain*; these probably also reflect traumatic neuropathies. Orofacial CRPS is a further posttraumatic entity for which the occurrence in the orofacial region is unclear (discussed later).

Epidemiology of traumatic trigeminal neuropathies. In general, traumatic injuries to the trigeminal nerve largely result in no residual deficit or in a nonpainful neuropathy. A small number of patients, as discussed later, develop a painful neuropathy.

Macrotrauma. After zygomatic complex fractures, residual, mild hypoesthesia of the infraorbital nerve is common, but chronic neuropathic pain developed in only 1 of 30 patients (3.3%) followed up for 6 months.[192] This compares with about 5% to 17% in other body regions.[199,200]

Implants. Dental implants pose a risk of neuropathy secondary to direct or indirect neuronal trauma. Table 12-10 outlines a proposed classification of post-implant neuropathy. Common neuronal complications after implant insertion are damage to adjacent nerves, altered sensory perception, and possibly pain.[201-203] The incidence of neurosensory disturbance ranges from 0.6% to 36%.[204-209] The damage can be direct, occurring during site preparation and/or implant placement, or indirect, caused by bleeding and pressure buildup around the nerve or a perineural inflammatory response.

Table 12-10 | **Proposed classification of post-implant neuropathy**

Nerve injury	Timing	Pain	Notes
Type I	Clear operative or imaging evidence of major nerve injury	Immediate	May be nonpainful (majority) or painful. Inferior alveolar nerve is usually involved. Injury occurs during surgical preparation and/or implant placement.
Type II	No operative or imaging evidence of major nerve injury	Immediate	Presumed injury to smaller nerve fibers.
		Delayed	Usually begins when the implant is loaded.

The authors' experience with post-implant PTTN has resulted in the identification of four interrelated groups:

1. The classic group is where there is obvious injury to a nerve, usually the inferior alveolar nerve. Injury may occur during the preparation of the implant site and is usually caused by the surgical bur. With modern equipment, thermal damage as a result of inadequate cooling and/or use of inappropriately high rotation speeds is unlikely, but this is a possibility. The injury is therefore most likely caused by the rotational forces of the surgical bur. In some cases, the preparation progresses without incident, but placement of the implant may impinge on the nerve trunk to a variable degree,[210,211] particularly if the implant is over-inserted into soft bone. All of these cases are usually accompanied by an immediate postoperative complaint of significant sensory dysfunction in the lower lip. The neuropathy is presumably due to inflammation and direct physical damage that is specific to the bur or the implant. Research shows that the character of the injury seems to be significant in terms of the resultant neuropathy.[212]

2. Often there is no history of intraoperative injury and no evidence that the implant itself caused damage, but there is proximity between the implant and the nerve trunk. Mild injury to the neurovascular bundle possibly occurs during preparation and is accompanied by bleeding and/or perineural inflammation. In a nerve that is encased, as in the inferior alveolar canal, or located in a tightly closed space, as in other trigeminal branches, the local inflammatory mediators and pressure buildup may cause secondary nerve damage. Indirect evidence of this type of neuronal damage is found in animal models of trigeminal perineural inflammation.[213]

3. Many implants associated with persistent pain are not in the vicinity of a large nerve trunk. This is true of most of the implants placed in the maxilla. In these cases, there is often no clinical complaint of sensory dysfunction. Theoretically, these cases may be caused by direct injury to small nerve branches, and as in all traumatic neuropathies, inflammation is involved. The underlying mechanism may be similar to that occurring in pain after endodontic procedures. If these cases are carefully examined (and are truly neuropathic), a variety of sensory aberrations are identified in the area of the implant: hypoalgesia, hyperalgesia (pinprick with a dental probe), allodynia (touching, pressing gently), and temporal or summation.

4. In this final group, all is well until the implants are loaded. The surgical history, postoperative period, and healing are uneventful. On loading, the patients complain of ongoing pain and sensitivity to mechanical (chewing, brushing) and often thermal stimuli. Radiographs usually show good osseointegration. Often, once initiated, the pain will remain even if the restoration is removed. The implants are all biologically intact, and the underlying mechanism is probably neuropathic, though this is unclear. There is evidence of extensive peri-implant innervation,[214] so theoretically, neuropathic-type pain may originate from here.

Mandibular third molars. Third-molar extractions are associated with transient hypoesthesia.[215] Disturbed sensation may remain in

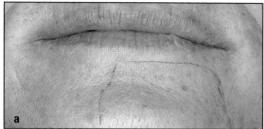

Fig 12-9 Case involving pain and neurosensory deficit after dental implants. *(a)* Area of pain and disturbed sensation. *(b)* Initial implant placement. Inset is a computed tomography section of an implant that is causing nerve damage. *(c)* Implants in the affected quadrant were removed, but no change in pain or numbness was achieved.

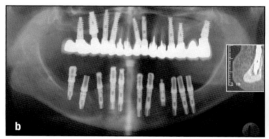

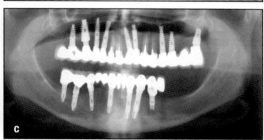

the lingual or inferior alveolar nerve for varying periods and has been found in 0.3% to 1% of patients.[216] However, follow-up of more than 1,900 patients failed to identify any cases of neuropathic pain.[217,218] Lingual nerve damage is rarer than inferior alveolar nerve injuries[219–221] but may commonly occur in certain extraction techniques, particularly with nerve retraction, and may reach 4%.[222] Complaints of tongue dysesthesia after injury may remain in a small group of patients (0.5%) and are variably correlated with the presence of histologic chronic inflammation, which suggests that the use of anti-inflammatory agents may be beneficial at late stages.[222,223] In a group of patients with extraction-related iatrogenic lesions to the mandibular branches of the trigeminal nerve, comorbid pain was present in about 70%.[195] The prognosis for nonpainful neuropathies secondary to dental interventions is reasonably good, and most patients report improvement.[224]

Root canal therapy. Nonpainful sensory changes related to endodontics are probably common and underreported. Nerve injury may be a result of apical infection or inflammation,[225,226] accidental injection of hypochlorite,[227–229] and extrusion of filling materials,[230,231] which may cause chemical injury in addition to the physical insult. Persistent pain after successful endodontic treatment was found to occur in 3% to 13% of patients,[193,232,233] whereas surgical endodontics resulted in chronic neuropathic pain in 5% of patients.[234] Factors significantly associated with persistent pain were long duration of preoperative pain, marked symptomatology from the tooth, previous chronic pain problems or a history of painful treatment in the orofacial region, and female sex.[235,236] The fact that preoperative pain parameters are important suggests that some form of sensitization may occur that predisposes a person to chronic pain. In all invasive dental procedures, there is also the possibility of nerve damage due to needle or local anesthetic injury.[237]

Clinical features of posttraumatic trigeminal neuropathies. In the patient presented in Fig 12-9, chronic neuropathic pain occurred after nerve injury from dental implants. The left mental nerve region (marked by a *black line* in Fig 12-9a) was hypoesthetic to electrical and thermal stimuli, which indicated frank nerve damage. The implants were impinging on the inferior alveolar nerve (Fig 12-9b). Removal of the implants (Fig 12-9c) did not improve the paresthesia or the pain.

The onset of neuropathic pain and its characteristics after identical injuries vary from patient to patient. Such variability is probably due to a combination of environmental, psychosocial, and genetic factors. A further con-

Table 12-11	Diagnostic criteria for painful traumatic trigeminal neuropathy*	
Diagnostic criteria	**Notes**
A. Unilateral facial and/or oral pain fulfilling criterion C	
B. History of an identifiable traumatic event to the trigeminal nerve, with clinically evident positive (hyperalgesia, allodynia) and/or negative (hypoesthesia, hypoalgesia) signs of trigeminal nerve dysfunction	Traumatic event may be mechanical, chemical, thermal, or caused by radiation.
C. Evidence of causation demonstrated by both of the following: 1. Pain is located in the distribution of the same trigeminal nerve	
2. Pain has developed within 3 to 6 months of the traumatic event	Pain duration varies widely from paroxysmal to constant and may be mixed. Specifically following radiation-induced injury, neuropathy may appear after more than 3 months.
D. Not better accounted for by another *International Classification of Headache Disorders,* third edition diagnosis	*Note:* Most trigeminal nerve injuries do not result in pain.

*Reproduced with permission from the International Headache Society.

sideration is that, relative to spinal nerves, the trigeminal nerve may show subtle differences in the pathophysiologic events that may lead to pain.[222,238]

Location. Pain is unilateral and may be precisely located to the dermatome of the affected nerve with demonstrable sensory dysfunction, particularly if a major nerve branch has been injured. The pain may be diffuse and spread across dermatomes but rarely, if ever, crosses the midline. Bilateral pain may occur in more extensive injuries where multiple nerves have been injured. Table 12-11 outlines the diagnostic criteria for PTTN.

Quality. Pain is of moderate to severe intensity (VAS 5 to 8) and is usually described as burning or shooting.[194,195,239–241]

Triggering. Cases of PTTN in which there is a clear triggering mechanism have been seen but are relatively rare.[239] In the authors' experience, these are usually not accompanied by a latency or refractory period. More often there is severe allodynia or a positive Tinel sign (pain upon percussion over the nerve).[194]

Temporal pattern. Pain is usually continuous, lasting most of the day and present on most days.[239] Paroxysmal pain may be spontaneous or triggered by touch or function.[194]

Associated sensory and motor signs. Painful neuropathies may present with a clinical phenotype involving combinations of spontaneous and evoked pain as well as positive (eg, dysesthesia) and negative symptomatology (eg, numbness).[239,240,242] Hyperalgesia and other sensory changes may be found in extratrigeminal sites, which suggests more extensive changes in central somatosensory processing.[243–245] Thermal modalities are usually preserved.[245,246]

Accompanying signs. Patients may complain of a feeling of swelling, foreign body, hot or cold, local redness, or flushing.[194,239]

Investigations. Sensory testing should be performed, preferably with quantitative and dynamic assessment[242,243] (see chapter 3). Imaging may be needed to assess the degree of injury from a dental implant or to detect foreign bodies and sequestra. The choice of plain radiography or cone beam computed tomography depends entirely on the patient. With trauma, patients should be carefully assessed to detect fractures and other injuries. Reviewing previous (preoperative) radiographs may be useful. The area of disturbed sensation should be mapped

> **Box 12-1** **Budapest Criteria for CRPS**
>
> 1. Continuing pain that is disproportionate to any inciting event.
> 2. Must report at least one symptom in three of the four following categories:
>   - Sensory: reports of hyperesthesia and/or allodynia
>   - Vasomotor: reports of temperature asymmetry and/or skin color changes and/or skin color asymmetry
>   - Sudomotor/edema: reports of edema and/or sweating changes and/or sweating asymmetry
>   - Motor/trophic: reports of decreased range of motion and/or motor dysfunction (weakness, tremor, dystonia) and/or trophic changes (hair, nail, skin)
> 3. Must display at least one sign at time of evaluation in two of more of the following categories:
>   - Sensory: evidence of hyperalgesia (to pinprick) and/or allodynia (to light touch and/or deep somatic pressure and/or joint movement)
>   - Vasomotor: evidence of temperature asymmetry and/or skin color changes and/or skin color asymmetry
>   - Sudomotor/edema: evidence of edema and/or sweating changes and/or sweating asymmetry
>   - Motor/trophic: evidence of decreased range of motion and/or motor dysfunction (weakness, tremor, dystonia) and/or trophic changes (hair, nail, skin)
> 4. There is no other diagnosis that better explains the signs and symptoms.

and photographed for future reference. More advanced electrophysiologic techniques will show distinct abnormalities but are not usually available in primary care.[247,248]

History. Onset age is typically around 45 to 50 years, and patients are usually women.[196,239,240,246] Patients often have undergone multiple treatment modalities aimed at eliminating pain, often including pharmacotherapy, occlusal adjustments, and surgery.[240]

Quality of life. PTTN is associated with a substantial psychosocial burden.[240] Patients with more severe pain demonstrate elevated levels of depression and pain catastrophizing as well as substantially reduced quality of life and coping efficacy levels.[249] The intensity of the pain is a good predictor for quality-of-life measures and emotional problems such as depression but not anxiety.

Prognosis. Long-term follow-up indicates that about one-third of patients report improvement.[224,240] In spite of this, about half reported the same or worsened pain, and most were still experiencing some degree of pain even at an average of 13 years after onset.[240]

Blunt macrotrauma. Chronic pain that continues after blunt macrotrauma (eg, road traffic accidents) may be difficult to diagnose as there may be no tangible physical signs. The problem is confounded by the fact that the severity of the original injury may have no bearing on the intensity of the resultant persistent pain, and significant disability may occur even after minor trauma. Moreover, major trauma often induces more than one pain syndrome in the same patient (see chapter 14).

Complex regional pain syndrome

CRPSs are chronic, painful neuropathic disorders that develop as a disproportionate consequence to injury, although up to 10% of patients report a spontaneous onset.[250] The incidence of CRPS is unclear but seems to increase with age and affects women more than men.[250,251] The International Association for the Study of Pain (IASP) classification has a low interrater reliability and low specificity (0.41), which contributes to overdiagnosis.[252] More recently, improved criteria (the Budapest Criteria) have been proposed and validated with similar sensitivity (0.99) to the IASP's but with improved specificity (0.79)[251,253] (Box 12-1). The Budapest Criteria expand the required signs and symptoms to include sensory, vasomotor, sudomotor/edema, and motor/trophic characteristics. Three subtypes have been defined: *(1)* CRPS I, previously known as *reflex sympathet-*

ic dystrophy; *(2)* CRPS II, previously known as *causalgia*; and, more recently, *(3)* CRPS-NOS (not otherwise specified) to allow the inclusion of patients who do not meet all the criteria.[254] They are characterized by spontaneous pain accompanied by allodynia and hyperalgesia that are not limited to dermatomal regions.[255] Although considered a type of traumatic neuropathy, CRPS is distinguished by significant autonomic, trophic, and motor changes. Some of the specific signs that significantly differentiate CRPS from non-CRPS neuropathic pain include regional changes in skin color, temperature, sweating, motor function, edema, and thermal allodynia.[251]

CRPS I may develop as a consequence of remote or relatively minor local trauma. The most common causes are surgery, fractures, crush injuries, and sprains.[256] Injections, local infection, and burns have even been implicated.[257] These result in minor or no identifiable nerve lesion with disproportionate pain. However, subsequent surgical attempts at treatment of the injury may be more important than the original injury. The less frequent form, CRPS II is characterized by a substantiated injury to a major nerve, most often after high-velocity missile trauma or surgery. Distinguishing between CRPS I and CRPS II is often difficult, and the need for such a subdivision is questionable.[257]

CRPS in the orofacial region. Some question the existence of CRPS in the craniofacial region. The cases reported have relied on cervical sympathectomy, clonidine, guanethidine, and stellate ganglion blockade to confirm CRPS.[258] Because sympathetic involvement is not essential, this has probably prevented the identification of more cases.[259] However, other CRPS features, such as trophic and motor changes, are not usually observed in PTTN. The other criteria listed are distinctly similar to those described in PTTN and, indeed, other neuropathic pain cases. The particular clinical phenotype may reflect the trigeminal system's differential response to trauma.[222]

Clinical features

Pain. The major distinguishing characteristic of CRPS is the disproportionate severity of the syndrome relative to the injury and its nonder-

matomal spread. Over time, patients typically report spread of pain beyond the injury site.[250]

Pain is usually of a burning or pricking character felt deep within the most distal part of the affected limb.[260] Particularly in CRPS I, pain is described as deep, dull, and aching.[257]

Temporal pattern. Pain can be spontaneous or evoked by physical and emotional stimuli. Three-quarters of patients will describe pain at rest, and movement or joint pressure will elicit or worsen pain.[261]

CRPS usually begins in the single affected limb distal to the injury. The signs and symptoms subsequently spread to the contralateral limb, head, and neck and may eventually involve the whole body.

Sensory disturbances. Patients with CRPS have a heterogenous mixture of sensory loss and gain in the affected region.[257] Hyperalgesia to cold is more common in patients with CRPS II.[261] Other sensory abnormalities include allodynia and hyperalgesia that are not restricted to nerve territories.[262] Paresthesias are rare, but about one-third will complain of a foreign, neglect-type feeling in the affected limb.

Reduced sensitivity to thermal and mechanical stimuli is usually present and may spread to involve the adjacent body quadrant or even half of the body, which suggests central sensitization.[263,264] These patients usually suffer more severe pain and longer illness than patients with localized sensory abnormalities.[263]

Motor signs. Weakness and limited range of motion of the affected site are observed in more than three-quarters of patients and may initially be due to guarding behavior.[257,261] Contraction and fibrosis may be seen, and tremor occurs in up to half of patients.[261] In CRPS II, focal dystonia (abnormal muscle tone) or myoclonus (involuntary muscle contraction) may be observed.

Autonomic disturbances. Patients usually present with a warm red and swollen extremity, known as *warm CRPS*. Over time, atrophic changes appear in skin, nails, and muscles. During the acute stage, more than 80% of patients have edema, which subsequently decreases over time to about 40% of patients.[257] Initially, there is cutaneous vasodilation, and the skin appears red; in the chronic stages, this may subsequently reverse into vasoconstriction and result in cold, bluish skin, termed *cold CRPS*.[261,265] Most patients with CRPS report that the limb feels cold, and this increases over time.[257] However, differences in skin temperature may occur at any stage (usually > 1°C). Increased sweating is observed in more than half of patients. Trophic changes include thin and shiny skin and altered hair and nail growth; there are also reports of muscle and bone atrophy (osteoporotic or osteopenic).

Treatment and prognosis. Therapy should be aimed at restoring function and reducing pain. Depending on the disease stage and symptomatology, steroids and sympathetic blocks may be indicated. Antidepressants and anticonvulsants may relieve neuropathic pain components, and opioids should be tried if these fail.[261,266,267] Graded motor imagery may also be of use in patients.[268] Resolution may occur during the first year (74% of patients) and seems to decrease during the first 6 years (36% of patients).[250,257] CRPS severely affects quality of life, and there is a significant personal burden of disease and disability that is often related to pain intensity.[250,269]

Treatment of painful traumatic trigeminal neuropathies

The inescapable progression of events after nerve or extensive tissue damage suggests that intervention is most effective within a specific time frame. Prevention is a primary objective but is not always attainable, so early treatment is essential.

Strategies for preventing neuropathic pain. The reasons why some patients develop persistent postsurgical (or injury) pain while others do not remain unclear. Some of the factors involved are known and may be grouped under three overlapping phases.[270] The preoperative phase includes risk factors specific to each patient, such as psychosocial parameters, genetically controlled pain-modulatory mechanisms, presence of related preoperative pain (ie, painful surgical site), and comorbidities (eg, pain, obesity, and sleep disorders).[271] The intraoperative phase involves surgery-dependent factors

such as technique, associated nerve and tissue injury, and the efficacy of analgesic regimens. The delayed postoperative phase involves the patient's coping ability, postoperative pain intensity, healing with scar formation, and the possible addition of such confounding factors as chemotherapy.[270,272]

Preventive analgesia, previously referred to as *preemptive analgesia*, aims to avert persistent postsurgical pain. The current term shifts the focus of possible strategies from solely before the surgery to all stages. Indeed, the timing of preventive interventions may be preoperative, intraoperative, and postoperative and usually involves various modalities. Although many studies on preventive analgesia have demonstrated reduced acute postsurgical pain, no solid data indicate that the incidence of persistent pain can be reduced.[273]

Preoperative opioids reduce postoperative pain, but in the head and neck, parenteral or oral delivery is needed.[274] However, it is unclear whether opioids prevent persistent pain. Data support the use of perioperative gabapentin and pregabalin to reduce the incidence of persistent postsurgical pain,[272] but this needs confirmation in further studies. From the available data, 1,200 mg of gabapentin should be administered 2 hours preoperatively and continued postoperatively. Pregabalin should be used at 300 mg administered 2 hours preoperatively and continued for 1 to 5 days.[272] Pregabalin has emerged as a more promising drug, possibly because of its better absorption.

Success in preventing the injury-associated afferent barrage and resultant central sensitization by using local anesthetic blocks during surgery has been inconsistent, although theoretically well based. Preoperative anesthetic blocks result in less postoperative pain compared with no local anesthesia, but no protocol has as yet received wide acceptance.[275,276] Local anesthetics have a strongly positive effect in suppressing postoperative pain scores and analgesic consumption, but it is unclear whether this also prevents chronic pain.[277]

Recent work suggests that it may be possible to identify at-risk patients by testing their pain-modulatory capacity.[278–280] The findings may eventually translate to chairside screening tests to predict the development of persistent pain after surgery (see chapter 3).

Lack of success in preventive strategies may be partly a result of weak study design, including inadequate management of the initial sensory barrage and insufficient treatment duration.[275,276] For the present, it would seem wise to provide a preventive program in selected procedures and patients. At a minimum, this would include preoperative and perioperative analgesics, deep local or regional anesthesia, and excellent postoperative analgesic cover.

Strategies for established painful traumatic trigeminal neuropathies. Not enough controlled trials are available on the treatment of neuropathic pain induced by peripheral nerve injury to calculate NNTs. The NNTs for drugs are largely similar across different neuropathic pains,[281] but from the authors' clinical experience, traumatic neuropathies are possibly the most recalcitrant.[282] Notwithstanding, NNTs may be extrapolated from efficacy studies in painful polyneuropathies, postherpetic neuropathy, mixed neuropathic pain, and central pain syndromes. Based on these, the mainstays of neuropathic pain treatment remain antiepileptic drugs and TCAs[176,177,281] (see chapter 16).

In contrast to the traditional 50% pain reduction for clinical significance, research has shown that about a 30% reduction represents meaningful pain relief for patients with neuropathic pain.[283] Therapy of neuropathic pain with any one of the established drug groups (antidepressants, anticonvulsants, opioids) leads to improved quality of life, sleep, and mood. However, pain intensity is reduced by 20% to 40% in only a subset of responders and is usually accompanied by significant side effects, particularly at the higher doses often required in neuropathic pain.[284–287]

Analgesic trials with antidepressants reveal that drugs with mixed serotonin and norepinephrine (eg, amitriptyline and nortriptyline) or serotonin and norepinephrine reuptake inhibitors (SNRIs; eg, venlafaxine and duloxetine) are superior to the selective serotonin reuptake inhibitors (SSRIs).[288,289] Calculations of the NNTs show that TCAs such as amitriptyline benefit approximately every other patient (NNT, 2.1) who is suffering from painful polyneuropathies.[281] The more novel antidepressant drugs, the SNRIs are effective in the treatment of painful polyneuropathy (NNT, 5). Because SNRIs have fewer side effects than the TCAs, they are attractive aternatives[281] (see chapter 16).

Anticonvulsant drugs are extremely heterogenous in their efficacy for painful neuropathies.[70,290] Carbamazepine and oxcarbazepine are efficacious in painful polyneuropathies (NNT, 3.7) but have more side effects than pregabalin (NNT, 4.5) or gabapentin (NNT, 6.4).[281] As a group, the anticonvulsant drugs are inferior to the antidepressants in the management of painful polyneuropathies. For trigeminal neuralgia, however, anticonvulsants remain the drugs of choice, particularly carbamazepine or oxcarbazepine.[291,292] Based on the efficacy of pregabalin and gabapentin in other peripheral neuropathies, they may also be good options in traumatic neuropathy. The sodium channel-blocking agent mexilitene may be useful in traumatic neuropathies but has been largely ineffective in other neuropathic pains.[281]

Opioid prescription practices have been under intense scrutiny, and clinicians are often reluctant to use them. Opioids have been clearly shown to improve painful polyneuropathies (NNT, 2.6) but have a specifically weaker effect on traumatic neuropathies (NNT, 5).[281] Tramadol is also a useful alternative (NNT, 4.9) for painful polyneuropathies.

Because neuropathic pain involves multiple and complex mechanisms, the use of drugs with different modes and sites of action may theoretically lead to improved efficacy and fewer side effects. The combination of duloxetine and pregabalin in the treatment of diabetic peripheral neuropathy provides no significant advantage over high-dose monotherapy.[293] However, most secondary end points consistently favored combination therapy. Researchers noted that 60 mg/day of duloxetine was superior to 300 mg/day of pregabalin. Similarly, combined nortriptyline and gabapentin was more efficacious than either drug given alone for diabetic polyneuropathy or postherpetic neuralgia.[294] In patients with painful diabetic neuropathy who did not respond to gabapentin monotherapy, the addition of venlafaxine in a double-blind fashion resulted in significant pain improvement.[295] These studies support the combination of an antidepressant (TCA or SNRI) with gabapentin or pregabalin. Treatment with an oxycodone-gabapentin mix is better than gabapentin alone in the treatment of diabetic

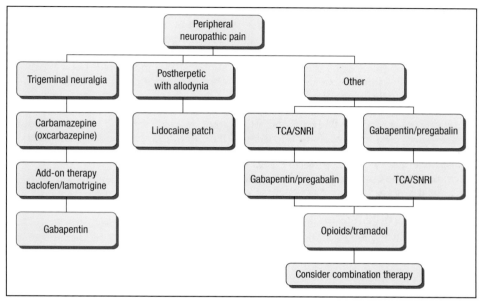

Fig 12-10 Treatment algorithm for peripheral neuropathic pain. The choice between TCAs or SNRIs versus the use of gabapentin or pregabalin is based on the medical profile and other patient-based variables (profession, comorbidities). TCAs are more effective than gabapentin/pregabalin but have significantly more side effects. SNRIs have not been as extensively tested as TCAs but seem less effective for neuropathic pain. Patients initiated on gabapentin or pregabalin who are not responding to treatment may not be medically suitable for second-line therapy with TCAs/SNRIs. In these cases, the patient is transferred directly to opioids singly or together with gabapentin.[295]

neuropathy.[296] Alternatively, gabapentin may be combined with morphine to achieve significant analgesia in patients with neuropathic pain (PHN and diabetic neuropathy) at a lower dose than each drug separately.[297] Meta-analysis, however, demonstrates a lack of evidence to support the recommendation of any one specific drug combination for neuropathic pain.[298] Only the gabapentin and opioid combination was significantly superior to gabapentin alone.[298] Yet this combination also produced significantly more frequent side effects.

Based on current evidence and the authors' clinical experience, TCAs/SNRIs or gabapentin/pregabalin would be the first drugs indicated in painful peripheral neuropathy[176,177,281] (Fig 12-10). The excellent NNTs for TCAs are counterbalanced by the excellent side-effect profile of the newer anticonvulsants and SNRIs. In patients started on amitriptyline who have problematic side effects, imipramine, desipramine, duloxetine, or venlafaxine should be tried. If these fail or are contraindicated, the anticonvulsants gabapentin and pregabalin offer the best chances for success. Similarly, in patients started on gabapentin/pregabalin, treatment failure is an indication for a trial of TCAs or SNRIs. Alternatively, if both of these avenues are only partly successful, combination therapy with their counterparts should be considered, that is, SNRI or TCA with gabapentin or pregabalin.[281] Third-line monotherapy or add-on therapy may be attained with opioids or tramadol (see also chapters 15 and 16).

The authors have tested this protocol in an open study on a cohort of patients with PTTN.[282] Only 11% of the patients achieved at least a 50% reduction in pain intensity, and higher pain-intensity scores were associated with a significantly reduced response to therapy. This is in line with response rates of other, similar painful neuropathies[281] and underpins the need for new drugs and other treatment options targeting chronic neuropathic pain.

Topical treatments carry the benefit of minimal side effects, but affected areas are not always amenable to treatment.[299] Evidence-based topicals include lidocaine or capsaicin (low and high concentrations) patches and locally injected botulinum toxin A (see chapter 16). Individually prescribed topical formulations are also in use.[299] Cannabinoids are increasingly being applied for the treatment of neuropathic pain[281] and have NNTs of 3 to 5 in peripheral and central neuropathic pain[300,301] (see chapter 16).

Cognitive-behavioral therapy. Neuropathic pain is associated with comorbid anxiety and depression. This would suggest that cognitive-behavioral or other psychosocial therapy might be beneficial. The findings of a meta-analysis did not show a significant effect of cognitive-behavioral therapy on pain intensity and quality-of-life measures.[302]

Surgery. The role of surgery in the management of nonpainful neuropathies is well established and improves level of sensation in injured patients.[303–305] Surgery is marginally more successful in inferior alveolar nerve injuries than in lingual nerve injuries,[306,307] but the presence of a neuroma is a negative prognostic factor.[308,309] Case series with repair within 1 year of injury show good success rates, as measured by sensory recovery.[304,309–312] About 50% of patients who undergo repair will recover with complete sensory function by 7 months.[308]

The efficacy of surgery for painful trigeminal neuropathies is unclear. In the authors' clinical experience, most patients who have undergone peripheral surgical procedures (exploration, further apicoectomies) for traumatic trigeminal neuropathy end up with more pain. One case series describes surgical intervention for a number of patients with PTTN.[313] Surgeries included exploration, release of scar tissue, decompression, and neuroma excision and showed good success rates. Unless there are specific indications, the authors advise patients with painful traumatic neuropathies not to undergo further surgery, but this has not been rigorously tested. In cases where surgery is aimed at nerve repair (larger branches such as the lingual nerve) and restoration of sensation, there seems to be no contraindication, and there may be improve-

ment in pain, but no rigorous trials have been published to the authors' knowledge. Some painful trigeminal neuropathies have been treated with peripheral glycerol injections with some success, but there have been no prospective controlled trials.

Anecdotal evidence suggests that central procedures may be useful for recalcitrant cases.[314,315] The authors suggest that the primary choice of operation should be minimally invasive, such as computed tomography–guided percutaneous trigeminal tractotomy-nucleotomy (surgical division of the descending fibers of the trigeminal tract in the medulla), which effectively ablates pathways that carry sensation from the face. Trigeminal DREZ operation (surgical damage to a portion of neurons in the trigeminal nerve root at the brainstem level) may be subsequently performed if the initial treatment fails.[315]

Offending implants: Remove and treat or leave? Some clinicians believe that by decompressing an injured nerve, healing may be encouraged, avoiding neuropathy and pain. This may be achieved by removing the implant completely or alternatively by shortening it so there is no nerve-to-implant contact. Additionally, anti-inflammatory drugs may achieve indirect decompression.

No prospective studies indicate whether removing an implant is better than leaving it as is. Each situation needs to be weighed according to the degree of nerve injury, type of injury, and time elapsed since insertion (see Fig 12-9 and Case 12-2). These cases were managed differently based on the time of presentation and the patients' preferences. The authors' clinical experience and published case reports suggest that if the implants are removed or replaced early after placement ($<$ 24 to 48 hours), there is a reduced incidence of neuropathy and pain.[313,316] Before performing total resections of nerve bundles, such as the inferior alveolar nerve, an oral surgery consult is advisable to discuss the possibility of microsurgical repair.

Management of early nerve injury and neuritis should also include pharmacotherapy, if the patient is medically fit. The authors use steroids at suitable doses (discussed later). The situation is different for offending implants that have osseointegrated, as the collateral damage in

A 61-year-old woman with PTTN.

CASE 12-2

Present complaint: Numbness in the left side of the lower lip for the previous 24 hours.

History of present complaint: The patient had undergone insertion of two dental implants the previous day in the mandibular left quadrant under local anesthetic (inferior alveolar nerve block). The numbness associated with the local anesthetic had worn off. She now felt her tongue, but the lip numbness persisted. She contacted her surgeon, who referred her immediately to the authors' center.

Physical examination: Sensory deficit was found in the left mental nerve dermatome to all modalities. The other cranial nerves were intact. The patient had no complaint of associated pain. Intraorally, a surgical wound with silk sutures was visible. A periapical radiograph showed possible impingement of the distal implant into the inferior alveolar canal. A cone beam computed tomographic image clearly showed impingement of the distal implant onto the inferior alveolar nerve (Fig 12-11). Quantitative sensory testing with electrical stimuli revealed significantly increased detection thresholds across all stimulation modalities, indicating nerve injury.

Relevant medical history: Healthy.

Diagnosis: Painful traumatic trigeminal neuropathy.

Diagnostic and treatment considerations: The patient was disappointed that the implant would be lost, compromising her long-term prosthodontic plans to restore the mandibular left posterior region. Therefore, the authors offered to insert a new but shorter implant, though she was warned that this approach may negatively affect her nerve healing and prognosis. However, the patient insisted, so the surgeon removed the offending implant, carefully irrigated the wound site, and replaced the implant. So as to reduce the effects of the inflammatory insult, the patient was treated with dexamethasone for 7 days, during which time she reported significant improvement.

Long-term review: The patient was reviewed regularly and at the 3-month recall reported mild sensations of itching and burning in the left mental nerve dermatome. A diagnosis of PTTN was established, and she was prescribed amitriptyline 10 mg at night. At recall, there was significant improvement, and after 6 months of therapy, the patient was pain free. Amitriptyline was continued for a further 3 months then tapered slowly and stopped. Quantitative sensory testing was performed 90, 180, and 360 days later and revealed improved thresholds. Although quantitative sensory testing showed almost full recovery by 360 days, the patient complained that her lip never quite felt "normal."

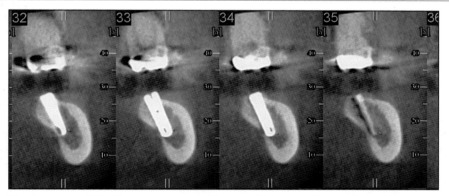

Fig 12-11 Case 12-2. Cone beam computed tomographic image of the mandibular left quadrant of the patient who presented with reports of a numb chin. An implant is impinging on the inferior alveolar nerve *(red dot)*.

removing these can be significant. The authors have not seen any such cases improve. In these cases, removal of the implants must be weighed against the potential dental handicap of losing those implants. Use of anti-inflammatory drugs does not seem to be indicated. In patients with neuropathic pain, however, pharmacotherapy should be offered.

Treating neuritis. In the orofacial region, dental and other invasive procedures can generate temporary perineural inflammation, usually asymptomatic. However, misplaced implants or periapical inflammation can induce classic symptoms, as described earlier. Other conditions, such as temporomandibular joint pathologies,[317] paranasal sinusitis,[318] or early malignancies,[319] can induce symptomatic perineural inflammation, pain, and abnormal sensations.

The involvement of inflammation in a clinical painful neuropathy is a clear indication for anti-inflammatory therapy. In mild cases or in cases where surgical or endodontic therapy is planned to further relieve inflammation, the authors use standard nonsteroidal anti-inflammatory drugs (NSAIDs; eg, naproxen 500 mg twice a day, ibuprofen 400 mg three times a day). In severe cases with marked pain and/or sensory changes, or in milder cases where adjuvant therapy is impractical, the use of steroids may be warranted (prednisone 40 to 60 mg initially then tapered over 7 to 10 days, dexamethasone 12 to 16 mg initially then similarly tapered). Tapering is aimed at reducing side effects from consistently high dosages. Experimental data show that early dexamethasone relieves neuropathic pain.[320]

Patients often report facial flushing, dyspepsia, and sleeplessness with steroid use, so treatment should be as short as possible. Antacids may be coprescribed. If treatment is successful, patients may be transferred to an NSAID with an antacid and treatment continued for a further 7 to 10 days.

On the treatment of CRPS. Although similar to traumatic neuropathies, the accompanying signs in CRPS often dictate a different treatment approach. These treatment avenues include rehabilitation (muscle spasm), bisphosphonates (to relieve pain in CRPS), sympathetic blocks, and surgical nerve decompression.[257]

Pathophysiology of painful traumatic neuropathies

The pathophysiology of painful inflammatory or traumatic neuropathies involves a cascade of events in nervous system function (Fig 12-12). These events include alterations in functional, biochemical, and physical characteristics of neurons and glia on a background of genetic sensitivity[321–328] (see also chapter 2). In the subsequent section, various selected aspects of these events are examined.

Peripheral sensitization: Tissue injury and inflammation. Peripheral sensitization is a common result of tissue inflammation. This is initiated by inflammatory bioactive molecules produced in response to a variety of stimuli and tissue injury that may directly activate or indirectly sensitize nociceptors. These changes develop rapidly but are reversible. As a result, nociceptors display altered neurophysiologic activity that may be spontaneous or stimulus induced. Peripheral sensitization is characterized by hyperalgesia and/or allodynia.

Even perineural inflammation with no axonal nerve damage (neuritis) of the nerve trunk elevates spontaneous activity and induces mechanosensitivity in myelinated axons.[329] Thus, the presence of inflammation can induce ectopic activity and spontaneous pain. Data show that inflammation anywhere along a nerve can be a source of pain in the organ supplied by the nerve.[330,331] Inflammation may affect nerve function by secretion of mediators, such as cytokines, or as a result of direct pressure induced by edema.[332] Both processes can induce nerve damage if allowed to persist.[333] Clinical studies have revealed that neuritis is characterized by tactile allodynia that originates in myelinated nerve fibers.[334]

Nerve injury and ectopic activity. If, as a consequence of trauma or severe inflammation, neuronal tissue is injured (eg, transection), cell death may ensue. However, if the proximal stump survives, healing involves disorganized sprouting of nerve fibers that form a neuroma. Neuroma formation is often dependent on the degree of nerve damage and always occurs when the perineurium is cut. Milder injuries, such as nerve constriction or compression, may also cause regions of neuroma formation and focal demyelination. These regions are characterized by ectopic discharge, partially caused by upregulation of specific sodium and calcium channels and downregulation of potassium channels. Ectopic activity is also seen in the cell bodies of injured nerves in the dorsal root or

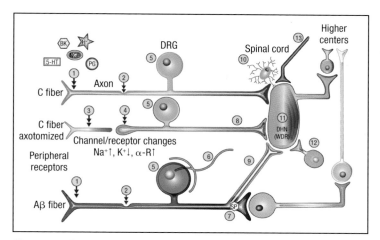

Fig 12-12 Peripheral and central nervous system changes in chronic pain. Peripheral sensitization: Tissue damage (1) releases inflammatory mediators— for example, bradykinin (BK), nerve growth factor (NGF), serotonin (5-HT), prostaglandins (PG), and protons (H+). This inflammatory soup of bioactive molecules induces increased sensitivity of peripheral nociceptors leading to allodynia and hyperalgesia. Axonal injury (2)—for example, transection, crush or chronic pressure, and inflammation—induces increases in sodium (Na+) and α-adrenoreceptors (α-R), initiating ectopic activity and increased sensitivity. Axotomy results in death of the distal part of the nerve (3), and if the proximal section survives, there is healing with neuroma formation (4). Some of the neurons will die, however. This activity leads to altered gene expression in the neuronal cell bodies located in the ganglia (DRG) (5). Nerve injury may lead to sympathetic nerve fiber sprouting (6), particularly around the larger DRG cells. The modulating effects of satellite glial cells in DRGs have recently been demonstrated. Aβ fibers undergo a phenotypic change (7) and express neurotransmitters associated with nociceptors—for example, substance P (SP). Injury-induced C-fiber degeneration (8) may result allowing Aβ fibers to sprout from deep to superficial dorsal horn layers (9), augmenting allodynia. Primary afferents and dorsal horn neurons activate glial cells in the dorsal horn (10), and these compromise opioid analgesia and enhance dorsal-horn-neuron and primary afferent activity and excitability. Persistent nociceptive input results in the sensitization of wide dynamic range (WDR) dorsal horn neurons (DHN; 11), excitation of adjacent neurons (central sensitization), and activation of glial cells. Glutamate-induced excitotoxicity reduces the number of inhibitory interneurons, augmenting excitation (12). Persistent pain initiates descending modulation, which in pathologic states tends toward facilitation (13).

trigeminal ganglia. These phenomena partly explain spontaneous neuropathic pain. Additionally, ectopic activity in neuromas is enhanced by mechanical and chemical stimulation; this explains the pain experienced when injured areas and neuromas are touched. Experiments have shown that trigeminal nerve neuromas (in myelinated and unmyelinated axons) are less active than sciatic nerve neuromas. Similarly, mechanosensitivity and acute injury discharge in trigeminal neuromas were minimal, which suggests the relative resistance of the trigeminal nerve to trauma-induced hyperactivity.

Phenotypic changes. Neuropeptide expression is altered in trigeminal ganglion after nerve injury, which suggests functional modification. For example, Aβ fibers usually transmit innocuous stimuli, but when catalyzed by inflammation or injury, a phenotypic change results in the expression of substance P.[324] Thus, Aβ fibers acquire the ability to induce painful sensations in response to peripheral stimulation and may underlie the phenomenon of allodynia.

Novel sensitivity to catecholamines. Patients may report increased pain, characterized by increased sympathetic activity, during periods of stress or anxiety. This may be due to upregulation of alpha-adrenoreceptors in the dorsal root ganglion and the site of injury, which induces sensitivity to circulating catecholamines. Additionally, basketlike sprouting of sympathetic fibers occurs around the neuronal cell bodies within the dorsal root ganglion, augmenting sensory-sympathetic interactions. This phenomenon has not, however, been experimentally detected in the trigeminal ganglion and may explain the relative rarity of sympathetically maintained craniofacial pain.[238]

Central sensitization. Central changes or plasticity is triggered by the barrage of activity from primary afferents transmitted to dorsal horn neurons (DHNs). Repeated primary nociceptive afferent input increasingly depolarizes DHNs, resulting in amplified responses, a phenomenon termed *windup*. Prolonged DHN depolarization ultimately results in the phosphorylation and sensitization of the *N*-methyl-D-aspartate–type glutamate receptor (NMDA-R), a calcium channel normally blocked by a magnesium ion. NMDA-R activation removes the magnesium ion plug and allows calcium ions into the DHN, initiating a variety of intracellular events. Although NMDA-R activation will not elicit nociception in and of itself, it enhances neuronal excitability and is thought to be important in establishing central sensitization. In addition to NMDA-R, other calcium channels (L-, P-, and N-type) are activated by repeated pain stimuli that lead to increases in intracellular calcium and DHN hypersensitivity, which manifests as hypersensitivity and/or allodynia.

Hypersensitivity may activate adjacent DHNs directly (possibly by diffusion of neurotransmitters) and by unmasking of silent inter-DHN connections. This increases the receptive field so that pain is felt in areas not normally innervated by the involved peripheral nerve. Clinically, sensitivity of uninjured areas in the vicinity of the injury is detectable as secondary hyperalgesia. This condition, termed *central sensitization*, accounts for increased pain and spread to adjacent structures in patients with severe facial pain. The early changes in neuronal excitability are activity dependent and are thus

amenable to therapy by controlling peripheral nociceptive input. However, with continuing stimuli, long-term changes are initiated in the dorsal root ganglion cells and DHNs; these changes involve modified gene expression and transcription as well as downregulation of repressor mechanisms, resulting in further excitability. Even minor injury such as third-molar extraction induced signs of central sensitization that lasted a week or more.[335] This was characterized by hyperalgesia, temporal summation, and abnormal aftersensation.

Some months after nerve injury, neuronal death is observed, mainly in C fibers. Withdrawal of injured C-fiber terminals from laminae I and II may allow sprouting of Aβ fibers from deeper laminae, augmenting pain induced by light touch.[336] Nerve injury–induced excitotoxic cell death is thought to deplete inhibitory interneurons and increase pain, although this does not seem necessary to allow development of persistent pain.[337] Supraspinal modification of peripheral signals is an essential part of balanced nociception, and in inflammatory or neuropathic pain states, there is evidence for decreased inhibition with increased facilitation.

The aforementioned events show how the progressive malfunctioning of the nervous system establishes conditions for chronic pain and increases the difficulty of therapeutic interventions.

Glial and satellite glial cells. Research implicates spinal cord glial cells in normal development, connectivity, and plasticity of the central nervous system.[321] Additionally, glial cells have been shown to play an important role in the initiation and maintenance of chronic pain. Glia express receptors and transporter proteins for many neurotransmitters, so they are well equipped to participate in pain modulation. In response to neuronal signals, glia are able to release excitatory molecules, including proinflammatory cytokines, glutamate, nitric oxide, and prostaglandins, which enhance DHN hyperexcitability and neurotransmitter release from primary afferents.[321,338] Glia have been shown to compromise the efficacy of opioid analgesia. Bacteria and viruses also activate glial cells, and this may explain the pain and allodynia often associated with some systemic infections. Because glial cells are involved in pathologic pain but not in acute nociceptive responses, they are an attractive therapeutic target. In a similar fashion, peripherally situated satellite glial cells (in sensory ganglia such as trigeminal ganglion) are thought to be able to interact with neurons and may play a role in changes after nerve injury.[339,340]

Studies on central neuroimaging. In neuropathic pain, imaging has enabled the identification of brain areas involved in sensory, emotional, cognitive, and modulatory processes.[341] Neuropathic pain originating from nerve injury may result in a decrease in contralateral thalamic gray volume[342] as well as cortical reorganization.[343] Thalamic gray matter changes were positively correlated with the time span after the injury. These findings implicate the thalamus in trigeminal neuropathic pain induced by peripheral injury.

Changes in cortical thickness of patients with trigeminal neuropathic pain frequently colocalize and correlate with experimental allodynia-induced functional activations. The changes in cortical thickness suggest a dynamic functionally driven plasticity of the brain.[344] The structural changes correlate with pain duration, age at onset, pain intensity, and cortical activity and may be specific targets for evaluating therapeutic interventions. Sensory processing in patients with trigeminal neuropathic pain is associated with distinct activation patterns consistent with sensitization within and outside the primary sensory pathway,[345] and both sensory and emotional circuits display changes. The data points to the possibility that a signature or fingerprint diagnostic may be identified for neuropathic pain.[344,345]

Contribution of macrotrauma. In macrotrauma, direct penetrating injuries around the face and scalp may damage peripheral nerves, and if these subsequently become painful, they behave much like PTTN. Similarly, direct damage to the temporomandibular joints and regional muscles may induce musculoskeletal pain (see chapters 8 and 9). Such macrotrauma has the added dangers of accelerating/decelerating injuries and blunt blows to the cranium. These have a common effect of exerting widespread shearing within the central nervous system, which may lead to extensive axonal injury, commonly known as *diffuse axonal injury*[346,347] (see also chapter 14).

Pathophysiology of CRPS. In addition to the sequence of events that follow nerve injury, as described earlier, research has suggested that particular processes are important in CRPS. Immobilization is commonly used for the treatment of injured or fractured limbs and jaws. Research has shown that immobilization on its own may induce CRPS-like syndromes.[257] Mechanisms responsible for sensory abnormalities in CRPS include sensitization of primary afferent nociceptors and spinothalamic tract neurons, disinhibition of central nociceptive neurons, and reorganization of thalamocortical somatosensory maps.[348] Neurogenic inflammation can explain the presence of edema, increased blood flow and skin temperature, and the early trophic changes observed.[257,349] Evidence exists for upregulated neuropeptide release and their impaired inactivation (exaggerated response) in patients with CRPS.[261] Concomitant release of neuropeptides centrally would induce sensitization. The role of psychiatric disorders in CRPS is unclear.[257]

Although adrenergic mechanisms appear to be involved in CRPS,[257] the link between nociceptive neuronal and postganglionic sympathetic activity is inconsistent, and sympathetic blocks sometimes modify the syndrome and sometimes not.[350] Proposed adrenergic mechanisms in CRPS include adrenergic excitation of sensitized nociceptors in the CRPS-affected limb and interaction between processes within the central nervous system that modulate nociception and emotional responses.[348] Central mechanisms could involve adrenergic facilitation of nociceptive transmission in the dorsal horn or thalamus and/or depletion of bulbospinal opioids or tolerance to their effects.[348]

Functional imaging studies provide evidence that the central nervous system plays an important role in CRPS. Reorganization of central somatosensory and motor networks has been shown to lead to altered central processing of tactile and nociceptive stimuli as well as altered cerebral organization of movement.[351] Structural changes include decreased gray-matter volume in several regions. Pain duration was associated with decreased gray matter in the left dorsolateral prefrontal cortex. Pain intensity was positively correlated with left posterior hippocampus and left amygdala volumes and was negatively correlated with the bilateral dorsolateral prefrontal cortex.[352] Mislocalization of tactile stimuli, changes in size and organization of the somatosensory map, changes in motor cortex representation, and body-perception disturbances have been described.[353] These findings may explain some of the clinical signs and symptoms in the CRPS and seem to be closely related to pain intensity.[354]

Interestingly, research has shown that some patients have immunoglobulin G serum autoantibodies directed against and activating autonomic receptors.[355] Some respond to treatment with immunoglobulins, and serum immunoglobulin G transferred to mice elicits abnormal behavior. These results suggest that in some cases, CRPS is associated with an autoantibody-mediated autoimmune process.[355]

Familial CRPS has been described,[356] and indeed, genetic susceptibility may explain why some patients develop CRPS while others do not. Accumulating data indicate a significant association with human leukocyte antigen-related alleles.[357,358]

Painful trigeminal neuropathy attributed to multiple sclerosis plaque

Multiple sclerosis (MS) is a common disabling disease affecting persons between the ages of 20 and 40 years. The typical MRI picture includes periventricular lesions in the cerebral hemispheres or infratentorially. Spinal cord lesions are also extremely common. The neuropathology is characterized by perivenous inflammation, neuronal demyelination, and ultimately gliosis. Cerebrospinal fluid demonstrates positive oligoclonal bands and an elevated immunoglobulin G index and synthesis rate. Evoked potentials aid in the diagnosis of MS but may be abnormal in other inflammatory conditions of the central nervous system. Patients with MS often present with paresthesias, numbness, motor weakness, and a painful optic neuritis with visual blurring. More than half of patients with MS will report some type of pain during the course of their disease.[359,360] More than a quarter will suffer central pain that is bilateral, constant, aching, burning, or pricking. Nonfacial pain may be a presenting symptom of

MS in 5.5% of cases, alone or in combination with other signs.

Trigeminal neuralgia in MS may be due to demyelination of the trigeminal nerve. Additionally, findings of neurovascular compression of the nerve root and positive outcome of MVD for these patients suggests that vascular malformations may also contribute to the appearance of trigeminal neuralgia in MS.[361] MS increases the risk of developing trigeminal neuralgia by a factor of 20. Clinical signs predictive of MS in patients with trigeminal neuralgia are bilateral pain (14% in MS) and young age.[362] Very rarely does trigeminal neuralgia herald the onset of MS; this was observed in only 0.3% of patients with MS. Usually, trigeminal neuralgia develops in a person diagnosed with MS, on average about 12 years after the onset of MS, and it occurs in 1.5% to 7.9% of patients with MS.[359,360,363] The diagnostic criteria for painful trigeminal neuropathy attributed to MS plaque are outlined in Table 12-12.

Painful trigeminal neuropathy attributed to space-occupying lesion

Trigeminal nerve dysfunction has been observed in 33% of patients with middle and posterior cranial fossa tumors but was the presenting symptom in only 13%.[364] About 10% of patients with intracranial tumors suffered from trigeminal neuralgia–like symptomatology. Pain may mimic trigeminal neuralgia, persistent idiopathic facial pain, and temporomandibular disorders.[365] Posterior fossa tumors and meningiomas are most likely to cause trigeminal neuralgia–like symptoms.[364,366] Cerebellopontine angle tumors (eg, acoustic neuromas; see chapter 13) may also cause trigeminal neuralgia, and this diagnosis is more likely when the patient is young and suffers pain in more than one trigeminal branch. In patients with trigeminal neuralgia who are under the age of 29 years, the prevalence of intracranial tumor or MS is extremely high (almost 100%) but subsequently decreases with increasing age.[367] Specifically, 10% to 13.4% of patients with trigeminal neuralgia may suffer from intracranial tumors, and MRI is the most sensitive diagnostic technique.[368] Most of these patients are usually younger than expected for cases of trigeminal neuralgia and develop subtle or frank neurolog-

Table 12-12	Diagnostic criteria for painful trigeminal neuropathy attributed to MS plaque*	
Diagnostic criteria		**Notes**
A. Head and/or facial pain with the characteristics of classical trigeminal neuralgia with or without concomitant persistent facial pain but not necessarily unilateral		Current studies indicate that about 7% of patients with MS have pain similar to classical trigeminal neuralgia. May be bilateral.
B. MS has been diagnosed		
C. An MS plaque affecting the trigeminal nerve root has been demonstrated by MRI or by routine electrophysiologic studies (blink reflex or trigeminal-evoked potentials) indicating impairment of the affected trigeminal nerve(s)		Usually more resistant to pharmacologic interventions than classical trigeminal neuralgia.
D. Not better accounted for by another *International Classification of Headache Disorders,* third edition diagnosis		*Note:* Symptoms of trigeminal neuralgia are very rarely a presenting feature of MS.

*Reproduced with permission from the International Headache Society.

Table 12-13	Diagnostic criteria for painful trigeminal neuropathy attributed to space-occupying lesion*	
Diagnostic criteria		**Notes**
A. Unilateral head and/or facial pain with the characteristics of 13.1.1 classical trigeminal neuralgia with or without concomitant persistent facial pain and fulfilling criterion C		
B. A space-occupying lesion and contact between the lesion and the affected trigeminal nerve have been demonstrated by imaging		Needs brain imaging.
C. Pain has developed after contact occurred between the lesion and the trigeminal nerve or led to its discovery		Patients usually have clinically detectable sensory signs or electrophysiologic abnormalities.
D. Not better accounted for by another *International Classification of Headache Disorders,* third edition diagnosis		

*Reproduced with permission from the International Headache Society.

ic deficits, but 2% had CTN with no significant sensory aberration. A reduced corneal reflex and hypoesthesia were typical of cranial masses. GKS has recently been used to treat benign intracranial tumors.[369,370] However, although tumor control is successful, symptoms such as facial pain do not always resolve. The diagnostic criteria for painful trigeminal neuropathy attributed to space-occupying lesion are outlined in Table 12-13.

Glossopharyngeal Neuralgia

Glossopharyngeal neuralgia is a rare condition that is similar in presentation to trigeminal neuralgia.[10] Glossopharyngeal neuralgia affects the throat or preauricular area corresponding to the distribution of auricular and pharyngeal branches of the vagus and glossopharyngeal nerves.[371,372] This accounts for the alternative term used: *vagoglossopharyngeal neuralgia.*[373] The characteristic pain location may send affected persons to other medical specialists,

Table 12-14 Diagnostic criteria for glossopharyngeal neuralgia*

Diagnostic criteria	Notes
A. At least three attacks of unilateral pain fulfilling criteria B and C	May co-occur with CTN.
B. Pain is located in the posterior part of the tongue, tonsillar fossa, pharynx, beneath the angle of the mandible, and/or in the ear	In the distributions of the auricular and pharyngeal branches of the vagus nerve as well as branches of the glossopharyngeal nerve. Before its development, unpleasant sensations can be experienced in affected areas for weeks to several months.
C. Pain has at least three of the following four characteristics: 1. Recurring in paroxysmal attacks lasting from a few seconds to 2 minutes 2. Severe intensity 3. Shooting, stabbing, or sharp in quality 4. Precipitated by swallowing, coughing, talking, or yawning	Less severe than CTN. In rare cases, attacks of pain are associated with vagal symptoms, such as cough, hoarseness, syncope, and/or bradycardia. Some distinguish among pharyngeal, otalgic, and vagal subtypes of neuralgia and suggest using the term *vagoglossopharyngeal neuralgia* when pain is accompanied by asystole, convulsions, and syncope.
D. No clinically evident neurologic deficit	Imaging may show neurovascular compression of the glossopharyngeal nerve.
E. Not better accounted for by another *International Classification of Headache Disorders,* third edition diagnosis	Reports exist of secondary glossopharyngeal neuropathy caused by neck trauma, MS, tonsillar or regional tumors, cerebellopontine angle tumors, and Arnold-Chiari malformation.

*Reproduced with permission from the International Headache Society.

such as otolaryngologists. Although similarities with trigeminal neuralgia are prominent, glossopharyngeal neuralgia is characterized by a milder natural history, and most patients go into remission. However, because of its location and features, glossopharyngeal neuralgia is a difficult diagnosis, and adequate treatment is often delayed for some years.[374]

Clinical features

Location

The glossopharyngeal (ninth) nerve has two main sensory branches: *(1)* the auricular (tympanic), which supplies the mastoid, auricle, and external meatus, and *(2)* the pharyngeal, which innervates the pharyngeal mucosa. The pharyngeal branches, together with vagal (tenth) afferents, also innervate the base of the tongue, the tonsils, and the soft palate. Pain distribution is therefore in the posterior part of the tongue, tonsillar fossa, pharynx, and the angle of the mandible and/or the ear.[375] Based on location

and referral patterns, two glossopharyngeal neuralgia variants—pharyngeal and tympanic—have been described.[371] Pain in pharyngeal glossopharyngeal neuralgia is usually located in the pharynx, tonsil, soft palate, or posterior tongue base and radiates upward to the inner ear or the angle of the mandible; however, it may involve the eye, nose, maxilla, or shoulder and even the tip of the tongue (Table 12-14).

Tympanic glossopharyngeal neuralgia is characterized by pain that remains confined to or markedly predominates in the ear but may subsequently radiate to the pharynx; these cases may pose serious differential diagnostic dilemmas vis-à-vis geniculate neuralgia (discussed later).

The left side is usually affected more often than the right, but the clinical significance of this is unclear.[374] Bilaterality is more common than in trigeminal neuralgia.

Quality and severity. Pain is usually described as sharp, stabbing, shooting, or lancinating. Some patients may report a scratching or foreign-body sensation in the throat. An atypical form with prominent burning and long-lasting pain has also been described. Attacks of glossopharyngeal neuralgia are commonly mild but may vary in intensity to excruciating. Features of pain attacks are stereotyped within patients. Usually, there is no warning sign of an oncoming attack, but some patients report pre-attack discomfort in the throat or ear.

Triggering. Typically, glossopharyngeal neuralgia trigger areas are located in the tonsillar region and posterior pharynx and are activated by swallowing, chewing, talking, coughing, and/or yawning.[376,377] Sneezing, clearing the throat, touching the gingiva or oral mucosa, blowing the nose, and rubbing the ear or around it often also trigger pain.[376] Topical analgesia to trigger areas will eliminate both trigger and pain.

Temporal pattern

Pain usually lasts 8 to 50 seconds[371] but may continue for a few minutes. Atypical cases with pain paroxysms lasting 4 to 40 minutes and cases with longer-lasting attacks consisting of continuous series of paroxysms have been described. Frequency of paroxysms may be 5 to 12 every hour but may occasionally reach 150 to 200 attacks per day. After an individual attack, a refractory period occurs during which further stimuli are incapable of inducing pain.

Attacks may occur in clusters lasting weeks to months, then relapse for up to a number of years. Spontaneous remissions were noted in 74% of patients, but 17% had no periods of pain relief. In two-thirds of patients, there may be only one attack, and the average annual recurrence rate for a second episode is low (3.6%).

Associated signs

In 10% of patients with glossopharyngeal neuralgia, excessive activation of the vagal nerve may lead to bradycardia, syncope, and cardiac arrest.[371,378] Uncontrollable coughing has been reported in 8% of patients. The pain paroxysms may also be associated with disturbed salivation. Rarely, pain may radiate to the eye and cause lacrimation.

Investigations

The relative rarity of glossopharyngeal neuralgia has prevented high-quality studies on the predictive value of special tests. Imaging of the head and neck to rule out pathology is indicated. An electrocardiogram should be performed before and after treatment. Preoperative MRTA is recommended to locate possible neurovascular contacts.

Differential diagnosis

The most common differential diagnosis is trigeminal neuralgia, particularly when the pain spreads to trigeminal dermatomes. Moreover, the co-occurrence of trigeminal neuralgia and glossopharyngeal neuralgia is common and expected to occur in 10% to 12% of patients with glossopharyngeal neuralgia. Bradycardia, clustering of attacks, and, very rarely, spread to the eye with lacrimation may cause confusion with cluster headache (see chapter 11).

Symptomatic glossopharyngeal neuralgia

A significant association between glossopharyngeal neuralgia and MS has been reported.[376] Regional infectious or inflammatory processes may mimic glossopharyngeal neuralgia. Tonsillar carcinoma invading the parapharyngeal space and other regional tumors (tongue, oropharyngeal) may cause glossopharyngeal neuralgia. Posttraumatic glossopharyngeal neuralgia is relatively rare but has been reported.[379] Cerebellopontine angle or pontine lesions may cause glossopharyngeal neuralgia–like symptoms.[380]

Epidemiology

Glossopharyngeal neuralgia is extremely rare and estimated at 0.2 to 0.4/100,000 person-years.[7] Mean age at onset is 64 years, and glossopharyngeal neuralgia is more common in men and in patients older than 50 years (57%); however, it may also occur in younger patients. Age-specific rates increase slightly with age, peaking at around 40 to 60 years.

(handwritten: ⊙ RAMSAY Hunt Syndrome p. 165, p. 1)

Treatment

Therapy for glossopharyngeal neuralgia has largely been based on treatments successful in trigeminal neuralgia. Life-threatening arrhythmias may require cardiac pacing.

Pharmacologic

Carbamazepine is usually successful and is the favored medication.[381] Alternatives include baclofen, oxcarbazepine, gabapentin, lamotrigine, and phenytoin.[382]

Surgical

(handwritten: PAROXYSMAL p. 12 ▲)

Patients with glossopharyngeal neuralgia who were successfully treated with anticonvulsants may become resistant, in which case there is a clear indication for surgery.[383] Glycerol injection may be suitable for older patients who are not good neurosurgical candidates.[384] More recently, MVD and GKS[385] have been successfully applied to patients with glossopharyngeal neuralgia.[55,372,386,387] MVD induced immediate and complete relief of pain in 80% to 95% of patients with glossopharyngeal neuralgia and produced stable long-term results.[374,388] Permanent neurologic deficits are rare (about 10%) and may include mild hoarseness and/or dysphagia or facial nerve paresis (see the earlier discussion of MVD and chapter 13). Section of the glossopharyngeal nerve, the upper rootlets of the vagus nerve, and the fifth cranial nerve (if trigeminal neuralgia was also present) has provided pain relief in more than 50% of patients.[372]

Pathophysiology

The pathophysiology of glossopharyngeal neuralgia is uncertain but is considered to probably be secondary to compression of the nerve root by a blood vessel. Patients with glossopharyngeal neuralgia demonstrate nerve compression on MRI and on surgical exposure,[372,387,389] and nerve biopsy shows variable myelin damage and patches of demyelinated axons in close membrane-to-membrane apposition to one another.[390] These morphologic changes are similar to those observed in patients with trigeminal neuralgia and suggest a shared pathophysiologic process.

Nervus Intermedius (Facial Nerve) Neuralgia

The intermedius nerve is a small sensory branch of the facial nerve that innervates the skin overlying the mastoid process and the external meatus. The cell bodies of the sensory afferents are located in the geniculate ganglion; hence, the alternative term for nervus intermedius neuralgia is *geniculate neuralgia*. *(handwritten: P.)*

Nervus intermedius neuralgia is centered directly in the ear and often felt deep within the ear.[10,391] Pain is described as sharp and stabbing, paroxysmal, and lasting seconds to minutes. The condition may, however, have a gradual onset and a persistent nature.[10,391] A trigger point in the posterior wall of the auditory canal may be present but is difficult to verify. Nervus intermedius neuralgia is extremely rare and has an uncertain pathogenesis, but it may occur secondary to HZ infection. When it presents together with facial palsy, ipsilateral loss of taste, and herpetic vesicles in the auditory canal, the condition is termed *nervus intermedius neuropathy attributed to herpes zoster* (historically termed *Ramsay Hunt syndrome*; see chapter 7).[10]

The exact mechanisms in nervus intermedius neuralgia are unclear at present. One study has shown nonspecific myelin sheath delamination.[391]

Treatment

Anticonvulsant pharmacotherapy should be tried, the same as for trigeminal neuralgia. In resistant cases or in patients with intolerable side effects, surgery may be necessary. Findings indicate that excision of the nervus intermedius and geniculate ganglion is an effective, definitive treatment for intractable geniculate neuralgia that can be routinely performed without causing facial paralysis.[391] The greater petrosal nerve is usually sectioned so that the ipsilateral eye remains tearless.[391] In some patients, nervus intermedius neuralgia may be accompanied by symptoms suggestive of trigeminal neuralgia and/or glossopharyngeal neuralgia, and these cases are managed by combined nerve section and MVD.

Occipital Neuralgia

Occipital neuralgia is a paroxysmal, shooting, or stabbing pain in the dermatomes of the major and/or lesser or third occipital nerves. On examination, tenderness to pressure over the course of the occipital nerves can be observed. A positive Tinel sign (pain upon percussion over the nerve) can be present. No data are available about the prevalence or incidence of this condition. Most often, trauma or irritation of affected nerves causes the neuralgia.

Clinical features

Location

Unilateral or bilateral pain in the suboccipital region that radiates over the vertex and posterior part of the scalp is characteristic of occipital neuralgia. The major occipital nerve is more frequently the source of pain (90% of patients) than the minor occipital (10% of patients) nerve, and both nerves are involved in 8.7% of patients.[392] The pain of occipital neuralgia may reach the fronto-orbital area through trigeminocervical interneuronal connections in the trigeminal spinal nuclei.[393]

Quality. The quality of the pain is mostly shooting or stabbing.[392]

Triggering. Trigger points may be identified at the emergence of the greater occipital nerve or in the area of distribution of C2.[392]

Temporal pattern. Constant pain can persist between the paroxysms.

Associated features

The condition may be accompanied by diminished sensation or dysesthesia in the affected area and is commonly associated with tenderness over the involved nerve(s). Vision impairment/ocular pain (67% of patients), tinnitus (33%), dizziness (50%), nausea (50%), and congested nose (17%) can be present because of connections with cranial nerves VIII, IX, and X as well as the cervical sympathicus.[394]

Investigations

Imaging studies of the cervical spine are necessary to exclude underlying pathologic conditions.

Differential diagnosis

Occipital neuralgia must be distinguished from occipital referral of pain arising from the atlantoaxial or upper zygapophyseal joints or from tender trigger points in neck muscles or their insertions. Tumors, infection, and congenital anomalies (Arnold-Chiari malformation) should be ruled out. Occipital neuralgia accompanied by nausea and nasal congestion can be mistaken for migraine (may be comorbid[395]), cluster headache, and even hemicrania continua in milder attacks. Other structures may cause similar pain, such as the upper cervical facet joints (C2-C3), osteoarthritis of the atlanto-occipital or atlantoaxial joint, giant cell arteritis, and tumors of the cervical spinal column.

Treatment

Initial therapy consists of a single infiltration of the nerves with local anesthetic and corticosteroids.[396] The infiltration sites of the nervus occipitalis major and minor are determined by external landmarks.[392] A 22-gauge needle is introduced until bone contact or paresthesia is obtained. Subsequently, the needle is slightly withdrawn, and the local anesthetic and corticosteroids are injected.[392]

Should injection of local anesthetic and corticosteroids fail to provide lasting relief, pulsed radiofrequency treatment of the occipital nerves can be considered. No evidence supports use of pulsed radiofrequency treatment of the C2 dorsal root ganglion. As such, this should only be done in a clinical trial setting. The reported effects of botulinum toxin A injections are contradictory. Subcutaneous occipital nerve stimulation can be considered if prior therapy with corticosteroid infiltration or pulsed radiofrequency treatment failed or provided only short-term relief.

Table 12-15 | **Diagnostic criteria for BMS***

Diagnostic criteria	Notes
A. Oral pain fulfilling criteria B and C	Usually bilateral and of fluctuating intensity.
B. Recurring daily for > 2 hours per day for more than 3 months	The condition has a high menopausal female prevalence, and some studies show comorbid psychosocial and psychiatric disorders.
C. Pain has both of the following characteristics: 1. Burning quality 2. Felt superficially in the oral mucosa	The most common site is the tip of the tongue. Subjective dryness of the mouth, dysesthesia, and altered taste may be present. Concomitant complaints may include dry mouth, paresthesia, and taste disturbance.
D. Oral mucosa is of normal appearance, and clinical examination, including sensory testing, is normal	Erosive or ulcerative mucosal diseases commonly induce burning. Sensory abnormalities may be detected using advanced techniques but are not usually clinically apparent.
E. Not better accounted for by another *International Classification of Headache Disorders,* third edition diagnosis	Whether secondary BMS is attributed to a local (candidiasis, lichen planus, hyposalivation) or systemic disorder (medication induced, anemia, deficiencies of vitamin B12 or folic acid, Sjögren's syndrome, diabetes) is a matter for debate.

*Reproduced with permission from the International Headache Society.

Burning Mouth Syndrome

~p. 98

Burning mouth syndrome (BMS) is a poorly understood pain condition that is most probably neuropathic with a central component. The condition is also known as *stomatodynia*, *oral dysesthesia*, or *stomatopyrosis* and is characterized by a burning mucosal pain with no major visible signs. BMS is often accompanied by dysgeusia and xerostomia, thus the use of the term *syndrome*. Some investigators argue against the term *BMS* altogether, and there is no indication that this is indeed a syndrome. The term *burning mouth disorder* has been suggested as a reasonable alternative until more information is available regarding etiology.[397] Although clear diagnostic criteria have been proposed (Table 12-15), these should be field-tested and validated. Future classifications of BMS should include criteria of oral pain or dysesthesia of a burning quality with no major paroxysmal character that lasts longer than 3 months or has a recurrent pattern. Symptoms should be present during most of the day, and clinical and/or radiographic examination should not reveal any obvious cause.

BMS may be subclassified into *(1)* primary BMS, or essential/idiopathic BMS, for which a neuropathologic cause is likely, and *(2)* secondary BMS, which results from local or systemic pathologic conditions.[398] By definition, primary BMS cannot be attributed to any systemic or local cause.[397] Although there has been much discussion about the terminology, in the authors' opinion there is currently no better classification system.

BMS is unfortunately characterized by resistance to a wide range of treatments and is one of the most challenging management problems in the field of orofacial pain.

Epidemiology

Due to vague criteria, the exact prevalence of BMS is unclear. However, it seems that BMS is most common in postmenopausal women, and reported prevalence rates in general populations vary from 0.7% to 15%.[399] In a countrywide survey of US residents aged 18 years and older, BMS-like symptoms were reported by 0.7% of all adults: 0.8% by women and 0.6% by men. In middle-aged and elderly women, BMS was reported by 4.6%. In Europe, the population prevalence of BMS has been estimated to be 13% to 15%,[400] but in one study about half had an oral disease that could cause symptoms. In men, no BMS was found in patients under the age of 40 years. In the 40- to 49-year-old age group, a prevalence of 0.7% was found, which increased to 3.6% in the 50- to 69-year-old age group.[401] In women, no BMS was found in patients under the age of 30 years. In the 30- to 39-year-old age group, the prevalence was 0.6%, which increased to 12.2% in the 50- to 69-year-old age group.

Clinical features

Location

The tongue, usually the anterior two-thirds, is the primary location of the burning complaint in most patients.[402,403] However, usually more than one site is involved, and in addition to the tongue, the hard palate, lips, and gingivae are frequently involved.

Quality and severity. The pain intensity with BMS varies from mild to severe; VAS scores are reported to range from 3 to 7 but may reach 8 to 10.[403–407] The most common terms used to describe the pain quality are burning and hot.

Temporal pattern

BMS typically has a spontaneous onset and lasts from months to several years.[397,399,408] Although a chronic unremitting pattern is usual, spontaneous remission of BMS has been reported in 3% of patients about 5 years after onset.[409,410] The pain pattern may be irregular, and reports suggest that many patients experience intermittent pain.[407] In general, pain intensity increases from the morning to the evening.[407]

Associated signs

More than two-thirds of patients complain of altered taste sensation (dysgeusia) accompanying the burning sensation. In many cases, it is described as a spontaneous metallic taste. Comorbid gastrointestinal problems may be prevalent and require early attention and referral.[402] A possible association with anxiety, depression, and personality disorders is also described in the literature, particularly in postmenopausal women,[398] but it is unclear if pain initiated the psychologic disorder or vice versa.[411,412] Approximately 21% of patients with BMS presented personality profiles that indicated a likelihood of significant psychologic distress requiring further evaluation by a relevant health professional.[413] However, as a group, patients with BMS have shown no evidence for significant clinical depression, anxiety, and somatization.[413] Moreover, patients with BMS report fewer disruptions in normal activities as a result of their pain relative to other patients with chronic pain.[413] This suggests that although a minority of patients with BMS suffer significant distress, the vast majority cope better than most patients with chronic pain.[413] Certainly, BMS significantly affects quality of life.[414] Patients with BMS demonstrate characteristics common among those with chronic pain conditions, including significantly higher adverse early life experiences compared with healthy controls, depression, anxiety, cancer phobia, gastrointestinal problems, and chronic fatigue.[415] Patients with BMS report sleep disturbances, but these may be related to levels of depression and anxiety.[416,417]

Secondary BMS

An oral and perioral burning sensation accompanying local or systemic factors or diseases is classified as secondary BMS.[398] Local factors and diseases known to induce secondary BMS include oral candidiasis, galvanism, lichen planus, allergies, hyposalivation, and xerostomia.[418] Systemic disorders known to induce secondary BMS include hormonal changes, nutritional abnormalities (eg, vitamin B12, folic acid, or iron deficiencies), diabetes mellitus, drugs (directly or indirectly), autoimmune diseases, and emotional stress.[398] Successful treatment aimed at the primary disease will usually (but not invariably) alleviate the burning sensation in patients with secondary BMS.[404]

Treatment

Disappointingly few evidence-based treatments are available for BMS. Patients with the condition usually report undergoing numerous special tests in the search for an underlying but elusive physical cause. Additionally, these patients may have been examined by numerous clinicians and received many, largely unsuccessful therapies. Although there is no one accepted treatment for BMS, this condition should be treated as a neuropathic pain. As such, outcomes should be assessed across a wider range of measures.[419]

Topical therapies may be useful, particularly in elderly, medically compromised patients. Topical clonazepam (sucking and spitting 1 mg three times daily for 2 weeks) was effective in reducing pain intensity in a subgroup of patients with BMS, and there was some carryover effect at 6 months.[405] Mouthwashes with 0.15% benzydamine or lactoperoxidase are ineffective in patients with BMS.[420] Topical anesthetics may decrease or increase pain, so this is not a predictable mode of therapy. Stimulation of salivary flow may be effective in some patients.[421]

Reduction in pain may occur after treatment with benzodiazepines or low-dose TCAs.[422–424] Some evidence suggests that systemic clonazepam affects BMS symptoms.[423,425] In one study, the combined use of topical and systemic clonazepam (sucking and swallowing around 0.5 mg three times per day) showed promising results.[403] Studies suggest that a 2-month course of 600 mg daily of alpha lipoic acid may be effective[426,427]; however, these results were recently contradicted.[428–430] Systemic capsaicin (0.25% capsule, three per day for 30 days) demonstrated beneficial effects in reducing BMS pain intensity.[406] However, the sample size was small, the study duration was short, and significant gastric pain was reported by more than 30% of patients.[406] One single-blind study compared the atypical antipsychotic amisulpride to the SSRIs paroxetine and sertraline.[431] The results suggest that all of these may be equally effective treatments for BMS and confirm previous work on SSRIs. However, amisulpride had a shorter response time and was associated with better compliance within the first week of treatment compared with SSRIs. Therapy-resistant BMS has been associated with underlying psychologic distress, and these patients in particular may benefit from cognitive-behavioral therapy, which has been successfully supplemented with alpha lipoic acid.[432]

Treatment may offer relief in 42% to 60% of patients, depending on the modalities used.[410]

Evidence-based management of BMS is therefore based on topical clonazepam, a systemic SSRI, alpha lipoic acid, and cognitive-behavioral therapy.[433,434] Widespread clinical practice for BMS and for neuropathic pains would support a trial for selected patients using topical therapy such as lidocaine, doxepin, or capsaicin. Similarly, systemic therapies would include TCAs, SNRIs and SSRIs, anticonvulsants, opioids, and benzodiazepines.

Pathophysiology

Various regional and local phenomena have been associated with idiopathic BMS, including reduced parotid gland function,[435] altered salivary composition (but not salivary flow rate reduction),[436] and epithelial changes in the tongue.[437] Patients with BMS generally exhibit greater vasoreactivity, which suggests involvement of the autonomic nervous system.[438]

Although its pathophysiology may involve hormonal[439] and psychosocial factors, BMS is considered a neuropathic pain state. Studies indicate that BMS may be a common clinical phenotype for various dysfunctions affecting the peripheral and central nervous systems, which are reviewed later in this chapter.

A decreased tolerance to heat pain and increased detection thresholds to warming and heat pain were the first indications that BMS might be a neuropathic pain.[440,441] Subsequently, a number of studies confirmed altered, mostly elevated, thermal detection threshold[436,442–444] and decreased tolerance to heat pain.[436] However, the sensory profile of patients with BMS is heterogenous and suggests different mechanisms in different patient populations. Quantitative sensory testing profiles in some of these patients indicate a loss of small fibers.[442,444] Epithelial small-fiber loss has been confirmed by tongue biopsy in various studies, although these are small studies with unclear criteria.[445–447] Immunocytochemistry has also shown upregulation of nerve growth factor, purinergic, sodium, and vanilloid receptors, as in other neuropathic pain states.[446,448]

Approximately 70% of patients with BMS report dysgeusia, which suggests an association between BMS and malfunction of the gustatory system.[449] In support of this suggestion, many patients with BMS report reduced burning during eating, and the anterior two-thirds of the tongue, the area most commonly affected by BMS, has a large number of taste buds. Hypothetically, taste-fiber activity tonically inhibits lingual nerve activity under normal conditions. Damage to the chorda tympani could thus disinhibit the somatosensory system, intensifying trigeminal nerve sensations, including pain, which is perceived by the patient as a constant burning sensation.[450,451] Quantitative sensory testing methodology was used to examine this hypothesis. Electrical stimulation to the tongue can induce one of two sensations: tingling or taste. Electrical taste/tingling ratio and taste-detection thresholds were significantly higher in patients with BMS compared with healthy control subjects, which indicates a dysfunction of Aδ fibers of the chorda tympani.[450,451] Moreover, patients who had experienced BMS for a prolonged time had an increased electric taste/tingling detection threshold ratio, suggesting progressive neural damage.

Presynaptic dopaminergic function was reported to be significantly decreased in the right putamen of patients with BMS compared with controls[452] (see chapter 11). This finding supports observations indicating decreased dopaminergic activity in patients with BMS,[453] and the results were replicated in a further study that indicated a decline in endogenous dopamine levels in the putamen in patients with BMS.[454] Together, these findings provide direct evidence of the involvement of the nigrostriatal dopaminergic system in BMS. A preliminary study performed in the authors' laboratory demonstrated that patients with BMS exhibit reduced conditioned pain modulation compared with matched healthy controls.

Patients with BMS display greater signal changes in the right anterior cingulate cortex and bilateral precuneus[455] as well as less volumetric activation throughout the entire brain compared with control subjects. These findings suggest that brain hypoactivity may be an important feature in the pathophysiology of BMS. Overall, patients with BMS display brain-activation patterns similar to those of patients with other neuropathic pain conditions and appear to process thermal painful stimulation to the trigeminal nerve in a manner that is qualitatively and quantitatively different from that found in pain-free persons.

Current evidence supports two main theories: (1) a sensory neuropathy that is probably both peripheral and central or (2) a neuropathic imbalance between the gustatory and sensory systems.

Taste sensation of the anterior two-thirds of the tongue is supplied by the chorda tympani nerve, a branch of the facial nerve. Other sensory modalities, such as mechanical and thermal sensations, are supplied by the lingual nerve, a branch of the mandibular division of the trigeminal nerve. Inhibitory influences between the two systems are thought to maintain a sensory balance in the tongue. Hypothetically, altered chorda tympani dysfunction can disrupt the equilibrium with the lingual nerve, leading to lingual nerve hyperfunction and burning sensation.

Burning mouth syndrome and taste

Data suggest that persons who suffer from BMS are likely to be supertasters (ie, they can taste the bitter compound phenylthiocarbamide) and have large numbers of fungiform papillae; these are innervated mostly (75%) by the trigeminal and partly (25%) by the chorda tympani nerve.[456] BMS and supertasting may result from hyperactivity of the sensory component of the trigeminal nerve after loss of central inhibition as a result of damage to the chorda tympani.[456,457] Indeed, hypofunction of the chorda tympani nerve was demonstrated using an electrogustatory test in patients with BMS.[458] The detection threshold for sweet taste is higher in patients with BMS, which suggests an altered taste sensation. Topical anesthetic applied to the tongue reduced dysgeusia but affected the pain component differentially: pain decreased, increased, or remained unchanged in subgroups of patients. Furthermore, in a study on patients with BMS, lower intensity ratings to salt and sweet stimuli were reported and are consistent with damage to the taste pathway.[459] However, this was found in female but not male subjects. Patients with BMS have decreased gustatory and somatosensory (in response to capsaicin) perception compared with healthy control subjects.[460] Although this was a small sample, the disorder duration was related to the capsaicin threshold, which suggests that the disorder may be progressive.

Based on these accumulating data, it has been suggested that BMS involves central and peripheral nervous system pathologies induced by damage to the taste system at the level of the chorda tympani nerve.[461] This damage results in reduced inhibition of the trigeminal nerve, which in turn leads to an intensified response to oral irritants and eventually to neuropathic pain. The exact mechanisms and interactions, however, are obscure and the evidence unclear.

Burning mouth syndrome as a painful neuropathy

BMS as a sensory neuropathy is suggested by findings that sensory threshold in the tongue was significantly higher in patients than in control subjects. Sensory assessment in patients with BMS revealed reduced thermal pain tolerance and elevated pain-detection thresholds. These patients perceived significantly more pain from mechanical stimulation that lasted longer and was described more intricately than in control subjects.[444] Additionally, patients with BMS have significantly elevated thermal sensory thresholds, decreased pain scores for tonic heat pain, and an increased level of somatization.[436] Taken together, these data suggest the presence of sensory nerve damage and indicate strong affective/motivational components to BMS. Patients with this condition have a significantly lower density of epithelial nerve fibers in the anterior two-thirds of the tongue, and this has some correlation with the duration of symptoms. Epithelial and subpapillary nerve fibers showed diffuse morphologic changes that reflect axonal degeneration and suggest a trigeminal small-fiber sensory neuropathy.[445] Combining quantitative sensory testing and blink reflex recordings in patients with BMS suggests the existence of several diagnostic subgroups.[442] About a fifth of patients may have trigeminal neuropathy or brainstem pathology, and a further fifth had increased excitability of the blink reflex with deficient habituation of one of its components. In about three-fourths of the patients, one or more sensory thresholds were abnormal, most with hypoesthesia. These findings indicate neuronal dysfunction, as only 10% of patients with BMS had clinically normal test findings. Altered blink reflex and/or thermal hypoesthesia was found in 89% of patients with BMS.[442,462] Applying a local anesthetic solution on the tongue of these patients reduced phantom dysgeusia but did not reduce the burning sensation, and the pain was aggravated in 40% of patients.[459]

Overall, these changes reflect a regional small-fiber idiopathic neuropathy that affects central and peripheral sensory and autonomic pathways and that results in disturbed oral sensation and inconsistently altered salivary secretion. The findings support the definition of BMS as an oral dysesthesia or neuropathic pain.

Central dysfunction of pain-modulatory systems in BMS has been confirmed by further studies. In patients with BMS, presynaptic dysfunction of the nigrostriatal dopaminergic system, which is involved in central pain modulation, has been shown by positron emission tomography.[454] A recent functional imaging study suggests that hypoactivity of the thalamus and brain may be involved in BMS, but this was a small and heterogenous sample.[455]

Based on collective evidence, it has been suggested that BMS can be divided into three subgroups.[463] The first subgroup (50% to 65% of patients) is characterized by peripheral small-diameter fiber neuropathy of intraoral mucosa. The second subgroup (20% to 25%) consists of patients with subclinical lingual, mandibular, or trigeminal system pathology that can be dissected with careful neurophysiologic examination but is clinically indistinguishable from the other two subgroups. The third subgroup (20% to 40%) fits the concept of central pain that may be related to hypofunction of dopaminergic neurons in the basal ganglia.

Physiologic levels of estrogens are neuroprotective in the nigrostriatal dopaminergic system so that their decline with menopause may partly explain the age and sex predilection of this disorder.[464] Moreover, findings suggest that estrogen receptors found in trigeminal neurons modulate nociceptive responses and may offer a valuable link in explaining the female preponderance observed in BMS patient populations.[465]

Table 12-16	Diagnostic criteria for persistent idiopathic facial pain*	
Diagnostic criteria	**Notes**
A. Facial and/or oral pain fulfilling criteria B and C	This is the current term for what was previously termed *atypical facial pain* or its intraoral counterpart, *atypical odontalgia*.
B. Recurring daily for > 2 hours per day for more than 3 months	It can have sharp exacerbations and is aggravated by stress.
C. Pain has both of the following characteristics: 1. Poorly localized and not following the distribution of a peripheral nerve	
2. Dull, aching, or nagging quality	Pain may be described as deep or superficial. With time, it may spread to a wider area of the craniocervical region.
D. Clinical neurologic examination is normal	A continuum seems to exist from persistent idiopathic facial pain induced by insignificant trauma to PTTN caused obviously by significant insult to the peripheral nerves. Persistent idiopathic facial pain may be initiated by a minor operation or injury to the face, jaws, teeth, or gums without any demonstrable local cause. However, psychophysical or neurophysiologic tests may demonstrate sensory abnormalities.
E. A dental cause has been excluded by appropriate investigations	The term *atypical odontalgia* has been applied to a continuous pain in one or more teeth or in a tooth socket after extraction in the absence of any usual dental cause. This is thought to be a subform of persistent idiopathic facial pain, although it is more localized, the mean age at onset is younger, and the sex predilection is more balanced.
F. Not better accounted for by another *International Classification of Headache Disorders,* third edition diagnosis	Persistent idiopathic facial pain may be comorbid with other pain conditions, such as chronic widespread pain and irritable bowel syndrome. In addition, it presents with high levels of psychiatric comorbidity and psychosocial disability.

*Reproduced with permission from the International Headache Society.

Persistent Idiopathic Facial Pain

The IHS criteria for persistent idiopathic facial pain include the presence of daily or near-daily pain that is initially confined but may subsequently spread (Table 12-16). The pain is not associated with sensory loss and cannot be attributed to any other pathologic process. This is a rather loose definition that may allow the classification of a large number of chronic facial pain disorders. The historical counterparts of persistent idiopathic facial pain include atypical facial pain and atypical odontalgia.

The diagnosis of atypical facial pain was essentially used when no other diagnosis was feasible and has therefore tended to include a heterogenous group of patients. Some patients with atypical facial pain responded to triptans, which suggests migraine-like mechanisms,

whereas triptans were ineffective in another study. As knowledge and diagnostic skills accumulated, many patients with atypical facial pain were classified as having chronic myofascial pain, traumatic neuropathy, pretrigeminal neuralgia or atypical trigeminal neuralgia, facial migraine, or neurovascular orofacial pain. Much of the collected data on atypical facial pain represents a neuropathic condition, and many patients demonstrate some degree of sensory dysfunction.

Clinical features

Pain is usually poorly localized, radiating, and mostly unilateral, although up to 40% of patients may describe bilateral pain. Atypical facial pain is commonly described as burning, throbbing, and often stabbing. Severity is mild to severe and rated approximately 7 on a VAS.[466] Most patients report long-lasting (years) chronic daily pain, although there have been reports of pain-free periods. Pain onset is often associated with surgical or other invasive procedures,[467] Although there should be no sensory deficits, these have been reported in many patients.[246] Often persistent idiopathic facial pain may coexist with other chronic orofacial pain syndromes, such as chronic myalgia.[468] The lack of a clear pathophysiologic basis[469] precludes the establishment of a treatment protocol. Some authors claim success with treatments aimed at the regional musculoskeletal system.[470] The use of TCAs, anticonvulsants, and low-level laser therapy may be beneficial; in addition, considering the chronicity and resulting distress,[471] behavioral interventions are indicated.[472–476]

Atypical Odontalgia

The IASP defines *atypical odontalgia* as a severe throbbing pain in the tooth without major pathology. The question whether atypical odontalgia is a neurovascular or neuropathic syndrome is a source of controversy, and some consider it to be a subentity of atypical facial pain. The incidence of pain that is pulsatile, episodic, and migrating suggests that this may be a vascular-type pain. However, many patients with atypical odontalgia present with neuropathic symptomatology, such as continuous, burning pain, and many report trauma as the initiating event. Indeed, atypical odontalgia has been referred to as *phantom toothache*, which supports a neuropathic etiology. This has led most researchers to conclude that it is a neuropathic syndrome.[477–479] However, it is also possible that the patient populations were totally different across studies and included patients with localized neuropathic and neurovascular syndromes. Patients with neurovascular or other undiagnosed orofacial pain (see chapter 10) may metamorphose into and coexist with trigeminal neuropathy as a result of nerve injury from repeated dental interventions aimed at pain relief. This theory is supported by findings that patients with chronic orofacial pain undergo extensive but often misguided surgical interventions.[480,481] Surgical intervention clearly exacerbated pain in 55% of surgically treated patients. A multidisci-

plinary group of experts concluded that most of these patients had been misdiagnosed—many had more than one diagnosis—and were subsequently mistreated.[480] Gross misdiagnosis, leading to serious sequelae and delay of necessary treatment, occurred in 5% of patients.[480]

The term *atypical odontalgia* is therefore ambiguous and should not be used.[482] Patients with a neuropathic-type pain after surgery or other trauma should be diagnosed as having PTTN (discussed earlier). Those with a neurovascular-type pain should be diagnosed as having neurovascular orofacial pain (discussed in chapter 10).

Seasoned clinicians are aware that a number of patients with intraoral pain do not fall clearly into any diagnostic category. These patients usually have persistent pain in the dentoalveolar region and have been grouped into a diagnosis of *persistent dentoalveolar pain*,[483,484] which, in many ways, seems the local counterpart of persistent idiopathic facial pain, similar to the relationship between atypical odontalgia and atypical facial pain.

Central Causes of Facial Pain

Central pain may be caused by direct damage, as in stroke and spinal cord trauma, or secondary to centrally occurring diseases, such as epilepsy, Parkinson disease, and MS (described earlier). Anesthesia dolorosa, sometimes termed *deafferentation pain* (see discussion on the true meaning of the term in chapter 2), denotes pain after lesions of the nervous system and is associated with decreased sensation.

Central post-stroke pain

Central post-stroke pain (CPSP) is characterized by constant or paroxysmal pain accompanied by sensory abnormalities, decreased perception, and often allodynia (Table 12-17). It is important to note that after a stroke, many patients are unable to self-report their pain and other symptoms,[485] which possibly leads to underestimation.

Table 12-17 Diagnostic criteria for central post-stroke pain*

Diagnostic criteria	Notes
A. Facial and/or head pain fulfilling criterion C	
B. Ischemic or hemorrhagic stroke has occurred	Diagnosis is often made retrospectively in a patient with a history of stroke and facial pain that started afterward. Central post-stroke pain is attributed to a lesion of the ascending projections of the trigeminal nuclei. Cervical spinothalamic pathways and cortical processing may also play a significant role. Therefore, symptoms may also involve the trunk and limbs of the affected side.
C. Evidence of causation demonstrated by both of the following: 1. Pain has developed within 6 months after the stroke	
2. Imaging (usually MRI) has demonstrated a vascular lesion in an appropriate site	Craniocervical pain after a thalamic lesion is part of a hemisyndrome. With lateral medullary lesions, hemifacial pain may occur in isolation but is more often accompanied by crossed hemidysesthesia. Pain and sensory disturbance are resistant to therapy.
D. Not better accounted for by another *International Classification of Headache Disorders,* third edition diagnosis	

*Reproduced with permission from the International Headache Society.

Clinical features

Location. Unilateral facial pain is common in brainstem lesions, particularly lateral medullary infarcts.[486] Facial pain is mostly reported periorbitally. Ipsilaterally, sensory dysfunction and corneal reflexes were abolished in all patients with facial pain. Facial pain was highly correlated to lesions of the lower medulla.[486]

Quality. The most common pain descriptors for CPSP are burning, aching, pricking, stinging, and lacerating.[487] Burning pain is most common, except among patients with thalamic stroke, who described lacerating pain more often.

Severity. Intensity is usually moderate to severe and increased by external stimuli, most commonly movement, light touch, and cold.[486]

Temporal pattern. According to IHS criteria, symptom onset must be within 6 months of a stroke to be classified as CPSP (see Table 12-17). However, although pain onset is usually within 1 month (range, 3 to 6 months),

it may take up to 6 years.[487] A gradual onset seems most common.[487]

Pain frequency is mostly constant but may be paroxysmal.[486] However, persistent pain with superimposed attacks was reported by 25% of patients, while 42% had only paroxysmal pain lasting seconds to minutes.[486]

Associated signs. Motor impairment and a variety of sensory symptoms may occur, depending on the extent and location of the lesion. Symptoms include pain and/or dysesthesia in half of the face, associated with loss of sensation to pinprick, temperature, and/or touch.[487] Dysesthesia is the most common abnormal sensation and may be evoked or constant.[488] Sensory dysfunction that correlates with the presence of pain occurs in more than half of patients, and thermal sensory impairment is present in most.[486] Muscle spasticity is present in about 60% of patients with CPSP.

Treatment. Amitriptyline is effective in CPSP, as is the anticonvulsant lamotrigine, and these should be considered first.[66,489,490] Gabapentin is a good second choice.[489] Short-term relief may be obtained with intravenous lignocaine or propofol.[489] Post-stroke patients are often not good candidates for TCAs, and therefore anticonvulsants are indicated.[491]

Pathophysiology

Damage to pain pathways in the thalamus was thought to initiate CPSP, hence the alternative term *thalamic pain*. CPSP is often linked with lesions of the ventrocaudal thalamic nuclei and particularly within the ventroposterior inferior nucleus. Later studies suggested that spinothalamic pathways and cortical processing play a significant role in CPSP.[489] However, many patients with post-stroke damage to spinothalamic pathways do not develop pain, so other factors must be involved. The pain of CPSP is thought to occur because of ectopic activity in damaged circuits induced by the stroke and an imbalance in facilitatory and inhibitory pathways.

Epidemiology

CPSP is quite common: 8.4% to 11% of all post-stroke patients and 25% of brainstem infarct patients develop pain over a 6- to 12-month follow-up period.[488,492] In post-stroke patients, CPSP was reported in the head in 1.68% to 6.4%, in both the head and extremities in a further 0.36% to 2%, and in the hemibody with the face in 26%.[487,492]

References

1. Treede RD, Jensen TS, Campbell JN, et al. Neuropathic pain: Redefinition and a grading system for clinical and research purposes. Neurology 2008;70:1630–1635.
2. Jensen TS, Baron R, Haanpaa M, et al. A new definition of neuropathic pain. Pain 2011;152:2204–2205.
3. Smith JH, Cutrer FM. Numbness matters: A clinical review of trigeminal neuropathy. Cephalalgia 2011;31:1131–1144.
4. Dworkin RH, Backonja M, Rowbotham MC, et al. Advances in neuropathic pain: Diagnosis, mechanisms, and treatment recommendations. Arch Neurol 2003;60:1524–1534.
5. International Association for the Study of Pain (IASP). IASP Taxonomy. Updated 22 May 2012. Accessed 12 December 2014. http://www.iasp-pain.org/Taxonomy?navItemNumber=576.
6. Rasmussen PV, Sindrup SH, Jensen TS, Bach FW. Symptoms and signs in patients with suspected neuropathic pain. Pain 2004;110:461–469.
7. Van Hecke O, Austin SK, Khan RA, Smith BH, Torrance N. Neuropathic pain in the general population: A systematic review of epidemiological studies. Pain 2013;155:654–662.
8. McDermott AM, Toelle TR, Rowbotham DJ, Schaefer CP, Dukes EM. The burden of neuropathic pain: Results from a cross-sectional survey. Eur J Pain 2006;10:127–135.
9. Meyer-Rosberg K, Kvarnström A, Kinnman E, Gordh T, Nordfors LO, Kristofferson A. Peripheral neuropathic pain—A multidimensional burden for patients. Eur J Pain 2001;5:379–389.
10. Headache Classification Subcommittee of the International Headache Society (IHS). The International Classification of Headache Disorders, 3rd edition (beta version). Cephalalgia 2013;33:629–808.
11. Gronseth G, Cruccu G, Alksne J, et al. Practice parameter: The diagnostic evaluation and treatment of trigeminal neuralgia (an evidence-based review): Report of the Quality Standards Subcommittee of the American Academy of Neurology and the European Federation of Neurological Societies. Neurology 2008;71:1183–1190.
12. Nurmikko TJ, Eldridge PR. Trigeminal neuralgia—Pathophysiology, diagnosis and current treatment. Br J Anaesth 2001;87:117–132.
13. Sato J, Saitoh T, Notani K, Fukuda H, Kaneyama K, Segami N. Diagnostic significance of carbamazepine and trigger zones in trigeminal neuralgia. Oral Surg Oral Med Oral Pathol Oral Radiol Endod 2004;97:18–22.
14. Siegenthaler A, Haug M, Eichenberger U, Suter MR, Moriggl B. Block of the superior cervical ganglion, description of a novel ultrasound-guided technique in human cadavers. Pain Med 2013;14:646–649.
15. Kuncz A, Voros E, Barzo P, et al. Comparison of clinical symptoms and magnetic resonance angiographic (MRA) results in patients with trigeminal neuralgia and persistent idiopathic facial pain. Medium-term outcome after microvascular decompression of cases with positive MRA findings. Cephalalgia 2006;26:266–276.
16. Tacconi L, Miles JB. Bilateral trigeminal neuralgia: A therapeutic dilemma. Br J Neurosurg 2000;14:33–39.
17. Maarbjerg S, Gozalov A, Olesen J, Bendtsen L. Concomitant persistent pain in classical trigeminal neuralgia—Evidence for different subtypes. Headache 2014;54:1173–1183.
18. de Siqueira SR, Nóbrega JC, Valle LB, Teixeira MJ, de Siqueira JT. Idiopathic trigeminal neuralgia: Clinical aspects and dental procedures. Oral Surg Oral Med Oral Pathol Oral Radiol Endod 2004;98:311–315.
19. Bowsher D. Trigeminal neuralgia: A symptomatic study of 126 successive patients with and without previous interventions. Pain Clinic 2000;12:93–98.
20. Reddy VK, Parker SL, Patrawala SA, Lockney DT, Su PF, Mericle RA. Microvascular decompression for classic trigeminal neuralgia: Determination of minimum clinically important difference in pain improvement for patient reported outcomes. Neurosurgery 2013;72:749–754.

21. Pareja JA, Barón M, Gili P, et al. Objective assessment of autonomic signs during triggered first division trigeminal neuralgia. Cephalalgia 2002;22:251–255.

22. Benoliel R, Eliav E, Sharav Y. Self-reports of pain-related awakenings in persistent orofacial pain patients. J Orofac Pain 2009;23:330–338.

23. Devor M, Wood I, Sharav Y, Zakrzewska JM. Trigeminal neuralgia during sleep. Pain Pract 2008;8:263–268.

24. Fromm GH, Graff-Radford SB, Terrence CF, Sweet WH. Pre-trigeminal neuralgia. Neurology 1990;40:1493–1495.

25. Zakrzewska JM, Lopez BC. Trigeminal neuralgia. Clin Evid 2004:1880–1890.

26. Zakrzewska JM, Patsalos PN. Long-term cohort study comparing medical (oxcarbazepine) and surgical management of intractable trigeminal neuralgia. Pain 2002;95:259–266.

27. Broggi G, Ferroli P, Franzini A, Servello D, Dones I. Microvascular decompression for trigeminal neuralgia: Comments on a series of 250 cases, including 10 patients with multiple sclerosis. J Neurol Neurosurg Psychiatry 2000;68:59–64.

28. Cruccu G, Leandri M, Iannetti GD, et al. Small-fiber dysfunction in trigeminal neuralgia: Carbamazepine effect on laser-evoked potentials. Neurology 2001;56:1722–1726.

29. Maier C, Baron R, Tölle TR, et al. Quantitative sensory testing in the German Research Network on Neuropathic Pain (DFNS): Somatosensory abnormalities in 1236 patients with different neuropathic pain syndromes. Pain 2010;150:439–450.

30. Sinay VJ, Bonamico LH, Dubrovsky A. Subclinical sensory abnormalities in trigeminal neuralgia. Cephalalgia 2003;23:541–544.

31. Cruccu G, Biasiotta A, Galeotti F, Iannetti GD, Truini A, Gronseth G. Diagnostic accuracy of trigeminal reflex testing in trigeminal neuralgia. Neurology 2006;66:139–141.

32. Love S, Coakham HB. Trigeminal neuralgia: Pathology and pathogenesis. Brain 2001;124:2347–2360.

33. Maarbjerg S, Sørensen MT, Gozalov A, Bendtsen L, Olesen J. Field-testing of the ICHD-3 beta diagnostic criteria for classical trigeminal neuralgia. Cephalalgia 2015;35:291–300.

34. Benoliel R, Sharav Y. Trigeminal neuralgia with lacrimation or SUNCT syndrome? Cephalalgia 1998;18:85–90.

35. Simms HN, Honey CR. The importance of autonomic symptoms in trigeminal neuralgia. Clinical article. J Neurosurg 2011;115:210–216.

36. Sjaastad O, Pareja JA, Zukerman E, Jansen J, Kruszewski P. Trigeminal neuralgia. Clinical manifestations of first division involvement. Headache 1997;37:346–357.

37. Nurmikko TJ, Haggett CE, Miles J. Neurogenic vasodilation in trigeminal neuralgia. In: Devor M, Rowbotham MC, Wiesenfeld-Hallin Z (eds). Progress in Pain Research and Management [Proceedings of the 9th World Congress of Pain, 22–27 Aug 1999, Vienna, Austria]. Seattle, WA: IASP, 2000:747–755.

38. Goh BT, Poon CY, Peck RH. The importance of routine magnetic resonance imaging in trigeminal neuralgia diagnosis. Oral Surg Oral Med Oral Pathol Oral Radiol Endod 2001;92:424–429.

39. Yoshino N, Akimoto H, Yamada I, et al. Trigeminal neuralgia: Evaluation of neuralgic manifestation and site of neurovascular compression with 3D CISS MR imaging and MR angiography. Radiology 2003;228:539–545.

40. Zakrzewska JM. Consumer views on management of trigeminal neuralgia. Headache 2001;41:369–376.

41. Mačianskytė D, Janužis G, Kubilius R, Adomaitienė V, Ščiupokas A. Associations between chronic pain and depressive symptoms in patients with trigeminal neuralgia. Medicina (Kaunas) 2011;47:386–392.

42. Hu WH, Zhang K, Zhang JG. Atypical trigeminal neuralgia: A consequence of central sensitization? Med Hypotheses 2010;75:65–66.

43. Leonard G, Goffaux P, Mathieu D, Blanchard J, Kenny B, Marchand S. Evidence of descending inhibition deficits in atypical but not classical trigeminal neuralgia. Pain 2009;147:217–223.

44. Obermann M, Yoon MS, Ese D, et al. Impaired trigeminal nociceptive processing in patients with trigeminal neuralgia. Neurology 2007;69:835–841.

45. Haines SJ, Chittum CJ. Which operation for trigeminal neuralgia? Pract Neurol 2003;3:30–35.

46. Obermann M, Yoon MS, Sensen K, Maschke M, Diener HC, Katsarava Z. Efficacy of pregabalin in the treatment of trigeminal neuralgia. Cephalalgia 2008;28:174–181.

47. Zhang H, Lei D, You C, Mao BY, Wu B, Fang Y. The long-term outcome predictors of pure microvascular decompression for primary trigeminal neuralgia. World Neurosurg 2013;79:756–762.

48. Tyler-Kabara EC, Kassam AB, Horowitz MH, et al. Predictors of outcome in surgically managed patients with typical and atypical trigeminal neuralgia: Comparison of results following microvascular decompression. J Neurosurg 2002;96:527–531.

49. Young B, Shivazad A, Kryscio RJ, St Clair W, Bush HM. Long-term outcome of high-dose gamma knife surgery in treatment of trigeminal neuralgia. J Neurosurg 2013;119:1166–1175.

50. Degn J, Brennum J. Surgical treatment of trigeminal neuralgia. Results from the use of glycerol injection, microvascular decompression, and rhizotomia. Acta Neurochir (Wien) 2010;152:2125–2132.

51. Sandel T, Eide PK. Long-term results of microvascular decompression for trigeminal neuralgia and hemifacial spasms according to preoperative symptomatology. Acta Neurochir (Wien) 2013;155:1681–1692.

52. Brisman R. Constant face pain in typical trigeminal neuralgia and response to gamma knife radiosurgery. Stereotact Funct Neurosurg 2013;91:122–128.

53. Katusic S, Beard CM, Bergstralh E, Kurland LT. Incidence and clinical features of trigeminal neuralgia, Rochester, Minnesota, 1945–1984. Ann Neurol 1990;27:89–95.

54. Pan SL, Yen MF, Chiu YH, Chen LS, Chen HH. Increased risk of trigeminal neuralgia after hypertension: A population-based study. Neurology 2011;77:1605–1610.

55. Gaul C, Hastreiter P, Duncker A, Naraghi R. Diagnosis and neurosurgical treatment of glossopharyngeal neuralgia: Clinical findings and 3-D visualization of neurovascular compression in 19 consecutive patients. J Headache Pain 2011;12:527–534.

56. Pareja JA, Cuadrado ML. SUNCT syndrome: An update. Expert Opin Pharmacother 2005;6:591–599.

57. Matharu M, May A. Functional and structural neuroimaging in trigeminal autonomic cephalalgias. Curr Pain Headache Rep 2008;12:132–137.

58. Truini A, Barbanti P, Galeotti F, Leandri M, Cruccu G. Trigeminal sensory pathway function in patients with SUNCT. Clin Neurophysiol 2006;117:1821–1825.

59. Boes CJ, Matharu MS, Goadsby PJ. The paroxysmal hemicrania-tic syndrome. Cephalalgia 2003;23:24–28.

60. Goadsby PJ, Lipton RB. Paroxysmal hemicrania-tic syndrome. Headache 2001;41:608–609.

61. MacDonald BK, Cockerell OC, Sander JW, Shorvon SD. The incidence and lifetime prevalence of neurological disorders in a prospective community-based study in the UK. Brain 2000;123:665–676.

62. Zakrzewska JM. Trigeminal neuralgia. Clin Evid 2003;(9):1490–1498.

63. Wiffen P, Collins S, McQuay H, Carroll D, Jadad A, Moore A. Anticonvulsant drugs for acute and chronic pain. Cochrane Database Syst Rev 2005;(3).

64. Wiffen PJ, McQuay HJ, Moore RA. Carbamazepine for acute and chronic pain. Cochrane Database Syst Rev 2005;(3).

65. Umino M, Ohwatari T, Shimoyama K, Nagao M. Long-term observation of the relation between pain intensity and serum carbamazepine concentration in elderly patients with trigeminal neuralgia. J Oral Maxillofac Surg 1993;51:1338-1344.

66. Saarto T, Wiffen PJ. Antidepressants for neuropathic pain. Cochrane Database Syst Rev 2005;(3).

67. Pérez C, Navarro A, Saldaña MT, Martínez S, Rejas J. Patient-reported outcomes in subjects with painful trigeminal neuralgia receiving pregabalin: Evidence from medical practice in primary care settings. Cephalalgia 2009;29:781–790.

68. Gilron I, Booher SL, Rowan JS, Max MB. Topiramate in trigeminal neuralgia: A randomized, placebo-controlled multiple crossover pilot study. Clin Neuropharmacol 2001;24:109–112.

69. Zvartau-Hind M, Din MU, Gilani A, Lisak RP, Khan OA. Topiramate relieves refractory trigeminal neuralgia in MS patients. Neurology 2000;55:1587–1588.

70. Wiffen PJ, Derry S, Moore RA. Lamotrigine for chronic neuropathic pain and fibromyalgia in adults. Cochrane Database Syst Rev 2013;12.

71. Solaro C, Messmer Uccelli M, Uccelli A, Leandri M, Mancardi GL. Low-dose gabapentin combined with either lamotrigine or carbamazepine can be useful therapies for trigeminal neuralgia in multiple sclerosis. Eur Neurol 2000;44:45–48.

72. Wang QP, Bai M. Topiramate versus carbamazepine for the treatment of classical trigeminal neuralgia: A meta-analysis. CNS Drugs 2011;25:847–857.

73. Cheshire WP Jr. Defining the role for gabapentin in the treatment of trigeminal neuralgia: A retrospective study. J Pain 2002;3:137–142.

74. Sindrup SH, Jensen TS. Pharmacotherapy of trigeminal neuralgia. Clin J Pain 2002;18:22–27.

75. Zhang J, Yang M, Zhou M, He L, Chen N, Zakrzewska JM. Non-antiepileptic drugs for trigeminal neuralgia. Cochrane Database Syst Rev 2013;12.

76. Lechin F, van der Dijs B, Lechin ME, et al. Pimozide therapy for trigeminal neuralgia. Arch Neurol 1989;46:960–963.

77. Vilming ST, Lyberg T, Lataste X. Tizanidine in the management of trigeminal neuralgia. Cephalalgia 1986;6:181–182.

78. Fromm GH, Aumentado D, Terrence CF. A clinical and experimental investigation of the effects of tizanidine in trigeminal neuralgia. Pain 1993;53:265–271.

79. Mitsikostas DD, Pantes GV, Avramidis TG, et al. An observational trial to investigate the efficacy and tolerability of levetiracetam in trigeminal neuralgia. Headache 2010;50:1371–1377.

80. Falah M, Madsen C, Holbech JV, Sindrup SH. A randomized, placebo-controlled trial of levetiracetam in central pain in multiple sclerosis. Eur J Pain 2012;16:860–869.

81. Holbech JV, Otto M, Bach FW, Jensen TS, Sindrup SH. The anticonvulsant levetiracetam for the treatment of pain in polyneuropathy: A randomized, placebo-controlled, cross-over trial. Eur J Pain 2011;15:608–614.

82. Hao JX, Stöhr T, Selve N, Wiesenfeld-Hallin Z, Xu XJ. Lacosamide, a new anti-epileptic, alleviates neuropathic pain-like behaviors in rat models of spinal cord or trigeminal nerve injury. Eur J Pharmacol 2006;553:135–140.

83. Hearn L, Derry S, Moore RA. Lacosamide for neuropathic pain and fibromyalgia in adults. Cochrane Database Syst Rev 2012;2.

84. Joshi S, Cohen J. Lacosamide as adjunctive therapy for refractory trigeminal neuralgia [abstract]. Neurology 2012;78.

85. Wallace MS, Rauck RL, Deer T. Ziconotide combination intrathecal therapy: Rationale and evidence. Clin J Pain 2010;26:635–644.

86. Rauck RL, Wallace MS, Burton AW, Kapural L, North JM. Intrathecal ziconotide for neuropathic pain: A review. Pain Pract 2009;9:327–337.

87. Michiels WB, McGlthlen GL, Platt BJ, Grigsby EJ. Trigeminal neuralgia relief with intrathecal ziconotide. Clin J Pain 2011;27:352–354.

88. Lux EA. Case report: Successful treatment of a patient with trigeminal neuropathy using ziconotide. Anesth Analg 2010;110:1195–1197.

89. Wang DD, Ouyang D, Englot DJ, et al. Trends in surgical treatment for trigeminal neuralgia in the United States of America from 1988 to 2008. J Clin Neurosci 2013;20:1538–1545.

90. Zakrzewska JM, Akram H. Neurosurgical interventions for the treatment of classical trigeminal neuralgia. Cochrane Database Syst Rev 2011;(9).

91. Ilfeld BM. Continuous peripheral nerve blocks: A review of the published evidence. Anesth Analg 2011;113:904–925.

92. Umino M, Kohase H, Ideguchi S, Sakurai N. Long-term pain control in trigeminal neuralgia with local anesthetics using an indwelling catheter in the mandibular nerve. Clin J Pain 2002;18:196–199.

93. Peters G, Nurmikko TJ. Peripheral and gasserian ganglion-level procedures for the treatment of trigeminal neuralgia. Clin J Pain 2002;18:28–34.

94. Freemont AJ, Millac P. The place of peripheral neurectomy in the management of trigeminal neuralgia. Postgrad Med J 1981;57(664):75–76.

95. Agrawal SM, Kambalimath DH. Peripheral neurectomy: A minimally invasive treatment for trigeminal neuralgia. A retrospective study. J Maxillofac Oral Surg 2011;10:195–198.

96. Cerovic R, Juretic M, Gobic MB. Neurectomy of the trigeminal nerve branches: Clinical evaluation of an "obsolete" treatment. J Craniomaxillofac Surg 2009;37:388–391.

97. Ali FM, Prasant M, Pai D, Aher VA, Kar S, Safiya T. Peripheral neurectomies: A treatment option for trigeminal neuralgia in rural practice. J Neurosci Rural Pract 2012;3:152–157.

98. Zakrzewska JM. Cryotherapy for trigeminal neuralgia: A 10 year audit. Br J Oral Maxillofac Surg 1991;29:1–4.

99. Pradel W, Hlawitschka M, Eckelt U, Herzog R, Koch K. Cryosurgical treatment of genuine trigeminal neuralgia. Br J Oral Maxillofac Surg 2002;40:244–247.

100. Fardy MJ, Zakrzewska JM, Patton DW. Peripheral surgical techniques for the management of trigeminal neuralgia—Alcohol and glycerol injections. Acta Neurochir (Wien) 1994;129:181–184.

101. Erdem E, Alkan A. Peripheral glycerol injections in the treatment of idiopathic trigeminal neuralgia: Retrospective analysis of 157 cases. J Oral Maxillofac Surg 2001;59:1176–1180.

102. Ammori MB, King AT, Siripurapu R, Herwadkar AV, Rutherford SA. Factors influencing decision-making and outcome in the surgical management of trigeminal neuralgia. J Neurol Surg B Skull Base 2013;74:75–81.

103. Nanjappa M, Kumaraswamy SV, Keerthi R, et al. Percutaneous radiofrequency rhizotomy in treatment of trigeminal neuralgia: A prospective study. J Maxillofac Oral Surg 2013;12:35–41.

104. Montano N, Papacci F, Cioni B, Di Bonaventura R, Meglio M. The role of percutaneous balloon compression in the treatment of trigeminal neuralgia recurring after other surgical procedures. Acta Neurol Belg 2013;114:59–64.

105. Reddy VK, Parker SL, Lockney DT, Patrawala SA, Su PF, Mericle RA. Percutaneous stereotactic radiofrequency lesioning for trigeminal neuralgia: Determination of minimum clinically important difference in pain improvement for patient reported outcomes. Neurosurgery 2014;74:262–266.

106. Cheng JS, Lim DA, Chang EF, Barbaro NM. A review of percutaneous treatments for trigeminal neuralgia. Neurosurgery 2014;10(Suppl 1):25–33.

107. Xu-Hui W, Chun Z, Guang-Jian S, et al. Long-term outcomes of percutaneous retrogasserian glycerol rhizotomy in 3370 patients with trigeminal neuralgia. Turk Neurosurg 2011;21:48–52.

108. Henson CF, Goldman HW, Rosenwasser RH, et al. Glycerol rhizotomy versus gamma knife radiosurgery for the treatment of trigeminal neuralgia: An analysis of patients treated at one institution. Int J Radiat Oncol Biol Phys 2005;63:82–90.

109. Kalkanis SN, Eskandar EN, Carter BS, Barker FG 2nd. Microvascular decompression surgery in the United States, 1996 to 2000: Mortality rates, morbidity rates, and the effects of hospital and surgeon volumes. Neurosurgery 2003;52:1251–1261.

110. Lim JNW, Ayiku L. The clinical efficacy and safety of stereotactic radiosurgery (gamma knife) in the treatment of trigeminal neuralgia: National Institute for Clinical Excellence (NICE), 2004.

111. Lopez BC, Hamlyn PJ, Zakrzewska JM. Systematic review of ablative neurosurgical techniques for the treatment of trigeminal neuralgia. Neurosurgery 2004;54:973–982.

112. Kouzounias K, Lind G, Schechtmann G, Winter J, Linderoth B. Comparison of percutaneous balloon compression and glycerol rhizotomy for the treatment of trigeminal neuralgia. J Neurosurg 2010;113:486–492.

113. Pollock BE, Ecker RD. A prospective cost-effectiveness study of trigeminal neuralgia surgery. Clin J Pain 2005;21:317–322.

114. Parmar M, Sharma N, Modgill V, Naidu P. Comparative evaluation of surgical procedures for trigeminal neuralgia. J Maxillofac Oral Surg 2013;12:400–409.

115. Fransen P. Cost-effectiveness in the surgical treatments for trigeminal neuralgia. Acta Neurol Belg 2012;112:245–247.

116. Tatli M, Satici O, Kanpolat Y, Sindou M. Various surgical modalities for trigeminal neuralgia: Literature study of respective long-term outcomes. Acta Neurochir (Wien) 2008;150:243–255.

117. Zakrzewska JM, Lopez BC, Kim SE, Coakham HB. Patient reports of satisfaction after microvascular decompression and partial sensory rhizotomy for trigeminal neuralgia. Neurosurgery 2005;56:1304–1311.

118. Jawahar A, Wadhwa R, Berk C, et al. Assessment of pain control, quality of life, and predictors of success after gamma knife surgery for the treatment of trigeminal neuralgia. Neurosurg Focus 2005;18:E8.

119. Loescher AR, Radatz M, Kemeny A, Rowe J. Stereotactic radiosurgery for trigeminal neuralgia: Outcomes and complications. Br J Neurosurg 2012;26:45–52.

120. Tuleasca C, Carron R, Resseguier N, et al. Patterns of pain-free response in 497 cases of classic trigeminal neuralgia treated with Gamma Knife surgery and followed up for least 1 year. J Neurosurg 2012;117(suppl 1):181–188.

121. Pollock BE. Comparison of posterior fossa exploration and stereotactic radiosurgery in patients with previously nonsurgically treated idiopathic trigeminal neuralgia. Neurosurg Focus 2005;18:E6.

122. Sanchez-Mejia RO, Limbo M, Cheng JS, Camara J, Ward MM, Barbaro NM. Recurrent or refractory trigeminal neuralgia after microvascular decompression, radiofrequency ablation, or radiosurgery. Neurosurg Focus 2005;18:E12.

123. Pagni CA, Fariselli L, Zeme S. Trigeminal neuralgia. Non-invasive techniques versus microvascular decompression. It is really available any further improvement? Acta Neurochir Suppl 2008;101:27–33.

124. Matsushima T, Huynh-Le P, Miyazono M. Trigeminal neuralgia caused by venous compression. Neurosurgery 2004;55:334–337.

125. Benes L, Shiratori K, Gurschi M, et al. Is preoperative high-resolution magnetic resonance imaging accurate in predicting neurovascular compression in patients with trigeminal neuralgia? A single-blind study. Neurosurg Rev 2005;28:131–136.

126. Cha J, Kim ST, Kim HJ, et al. Trigeminal neuralgia: assessment with T2 VISTA and FLAIR VISTA fusion imaging. Eur Radiol 2011;21:2633–2639.

127. Chen J, Guo ZY, Yang G, et al. Characterization of neurovascular compression in facial neuralgia patients by 3D high-resolution MRI and image fusion technique. Asian Pac J Trop Med 2012;5:476–479.

128. Devor M, Govrin-Lippmann R, Rappaport ZH. Mechanism of trigeminal neuralgia: An ultrastructural analysis of trigeminal root specimens obtained during microvascular decompression surgery. J Neurosurg 2002;96:532–543.

129. Love S, Hilton DA, Coakham HB. Central demyelination of the Vth nerve root in trigeminal neuralgia associated with vascular compression. Brain Pathol 1998;8:1–11.

130. Zhong J, Li ST, Zhu J, et al. A clinical analysis on microvascular decompression surgery in a series of 3000 cases. Clin Neurol Neurosurg 2012;114:846–851.

131. McLaughlin MR, Jannetta PJ, Clyde BL, Subach BR, Comey CH, Resnick DK. Microvascular decompression of cranial nerves: Lessons learned after 4400 operations. J Neurosurg 1999;90:1–8.

132. Han-Bing S, Wei-Guo Z, Jun Z, Ning L, Jian-Kang S, Yu C. Predicting the outcome of microvascular decompression for trigeminal neuralgia using magnetic resonance tomographic angiography. J Neuroimaging 2010;20:345–349.

133. Leal PR, Hermier M, Froment JC, Souza MA, Cristino-Filho G, Sindou M. Preoperative demonstration of the neurovascular compression characteristics with special emphasis on the degree of compression, using high-resolution magnetic resonance imaging: A prospective study, with comparison to surgical findings, in 100 consecutive patients who underwent microvascular decompression for trigeminal neuralgia. Acta Neurochir (Wien) 2010;152:817–825.

134. Barker FG 2nd, Jannetta PJ, Babu RP, Pomonis S, Bissonette DJ, Jho HD. Long-term outcome after operation for trigeminal neuralgia in patients with posterior fossa tumors. J Neurosurg 1996;84:818–825.

135. Hamlyn PJ. Neurovascular relationships in the posterior cranial fossa, with special reference to trigeminal neuralgia. 2. Neurovascular compression of the trigeminal nerve in cadaveric controls and patients with trigeminal neuralgia: Quantification and influence of method. Clin Anat 1997;10:380–388.

136. Horínek D, Brezová V, Nimsky C, et al. The MRI volumetry of the posterior fossa and its substructures in trigeminal neuralgia: A validated study. Acta Neurochir (Wien) 2009;151:669–675.

137. Kress B, Schindler M, Rasche D, et al. MRI volumetry for the preoperative diagnosis of trigeminal neuralgia. Eur Radiol 2005;15:1344–1348.

138. Leal PR, Roch JA, Hermier M, Souza MA, Cristino-Filho G, Sindou M. Structural abnormalities of the trigeminal root revealed by diffusion tensor imaging in patients with trigeminal neuralgia caused by neurovascular compression: A prospective, double-blind, controlled study. Pain 2011;152:2357–2364.

139. Herweh C, Kress B, Rasche D, et al. Loss of anisotropy in trigeminal neuralgia revealed by diffusion tensor imaging. Neurology 2007;68:776–778.

140. DeSouza DD, Hodaie M, Davis KD. Abnormal trigeminal nerve microstructure and brain white matter in idiopathic trigeminal neuralgia. Pain 2014;155:37–44.

141. Obermann M, Rodriguez-Raecke R, Naegel S, et al. Gray matter volume reduction reflects chronic pain in trigeminal neuralgia. Neuroimage 2013;74:352–358.

142. Blatow M, Nennig E, Sarpaczki E, et al. Altered somatosensory processing in trigeminal neuralgia. Hum Brain Mapp 2009;30:3495–3508.

143. Jones AK, Kitchen ND, Watabe H, et al. Measurement of changes in opioid receptor binding in vivo during trigeminal neuralgic pain using [11C] diprenorphine and positron emission tomography. J Cereb Blood Flow Metab 1999;19:803–808.

144. Moisset X, Villain N, Ducreux D, et al. Functional brain imaging of trigeminal neuralgia. Eur J Pain 2011;15:124–131.

145. Liu CN, Michaelis M, Amir R, Devor M. Spinal nerve injury enhances subthreshold membrane potential oscillations in DRG neurons: Relation to neuropathic pain. J Neurophysiol 2000;84:205–215.

146. Amir R, Devor M. Functional cross-excitation between afferent A- and C-neurons in dorsal root ganglia. Neuroscience 2000;95:189–195.

147. Devor M, Amir R, Rappaport ZH. Pathophysiology of trigeminal neuralgia: The ignition hypothesis. Clin J Pain 2002;18:4–13.

148. Hamlyn PJ. Neurovascular relationships in the posterior cranial fossa, with special reference to trigeminal neuralgia. 1. Review of the literature and development of a new method of vascular injection-filling in cadaveric controls. Clin Anat 1997;10:371–379.

149. Miller JP, Acar F, Hamilton BE, Burchiel KJ. Radiographic evaluation of trigeminal neurovascular compression in patients with and without trigeminal neuralgia. J Neurosurg 2009;110:627–632.

150. Peker S, Dincer A, Necmettin Pamir M. Vascular compression of the trigeminal nerve is a frequent finding in asymptomatic individuals: 3-T MR imaging of 200 trigeminal nerves using 3D CISS sequences. Acta Neurochir (Wien) 2009;151:1081–1088.

151. Antonini G, Di Pasquale A, Cruccu G, et al. Magnetic resonance imaging contribution for diagnosing symptomatic neurovascular contact in classical trigeminal neuralgia: A blinded case-control study and meta-analysis. Pain 2014;155:1464–1471.

152. Dworkin RH, Gnann JW Jr, Oaklander AL, Raja SN, Schmader KE, Whitley RJ. Diagnosis and assessment of pain associated with herpes zoster and postherpetic neuralgia. J Pain 2008;9(1, suppl):S37–S44.

153. Gershon AA, Gershon MD. Pathogenesis and current approaches to control of varicella-zoster virus infections. Clin Microbiol Rev 2013;26:728–743.

154. Goh CL, Khoo L. A retrospective study of the clinical presentation and outcome of herpes zoster in a tertiary dermatology outpatient referral clinic. Int J Dermatol 1997;36:667–672.

155. Dworkin RH, Nagasako EM, Johnson RW, Griffin DR. Acute pain in herpes zoster: The famciclovir database project. Pain 2001;94:113–119.

156. Haanpaa M, Laippala P, Nurmikko T. Pain and somatosensory dysfunction in acute herpes zoster. Clin J Pain 1999;15:78–84.

157. Volpi A, Gross G, Hercogova J, Johnson RW. Current management of herpes zoster: The European view. Am J Clin Dermatol 2005;6:317–325.

158. Jung BF, Johnson RW, Griffin DR, Dworkin RH. Risk factors for postherpetic neuralgia in patients with herpes zoster. Neurology 2004;62:1545–1551.

159. Dworkin RH, Johnson RW, Breuer J, et al. Recommendations for the management of herpes zoster. Clin Infect Dis 2007;44(suppl 1):S1–S26.

160. Gershon AA, Gershon MD, Breuer J, Levin MJ, Oaklander AL, Griffiths PD. Advances in the understanding of the pathogenesis and epidemiology of herpes zoster. J Clin Virol 2010;48(suppl 1):S2–S7.

161. Schmader K. Herpes zoster in older adults. Clin Infect Dis 2001;32:1481–1486.

162. Chen N, Li Q, Yang J, Zhou M, Zhou D, He L. Antiviral treatment for preventing postherpetic neuralgia. Cochrane Database Syst Rev 2014;2.

163. Whitley RJ, Volpi A, McKendrick M, Wijck A, Oaklander AL. Management of herpes zoster and post-herpetic neuralgia now and in the future. J Clin Virol 2010;48(suppl 1):S20–S28.

164. Andrei G, Snoeck R. Advances in the treatment of varicella-zoster virus infections. Adv Pharmacol 2013;67:107–168.

165. Oxman MN, Levin MJ, Johnson GR, et al. A vaccine to prevent herpes zoster and postherpetic neuralgia in older adults. N Engl J Med 2005;352:2271–2284.

166. Schmader KE, Levin MJ, Gnann JW Jr, et al. Efficacy, safety, and tolerability of herpes zoster vaccine in persons aged 50–59 years. Clin Infect Dis 2012;54:922–928.

167. Oxman MN, Levin MJ. Vaccination against herpes zoster and postherpetic neuralgia. J Infect Dis 2008;197(suppl 2):S228–S236.

168. Center for Disease Control and Prevention. FDA approval of an extended period for administering VariZIG for postexposure prophylaxis of varicella. Morb Mortal Wkly Rep 2012;61:212.

169. Opstelten W, McElhaney J, Weinberger B, Oaklander AL, Johnson RW. The impact of varicella zoster virus: Chronic pain. J Clin Virol 2010;48(suppl 1):S8–S13.

170. Bouhassira D, Chassany O, Gaillat J, et al. Patient perspective on herpes zoster and its complications: An observational prospective study in patients aged over 50 years in general practice. Pain 2012;153:342–349.

171. Coen PG, Scott F, Leedham-Green M, et al. Predicting and preventing post-herpetic neuralgia: Are current risk factors useful in clinical practice? Eur J Pain 2006;10:695–700.

172. Oaklander AL. Mechanisms of pain and itch caused by herpes zoster (shingles). J Pain 2008;9(1, suppl):S10–S18.

173. Reda H, Greene K, Rice FL, Rowbotham MC, Petersen KL. Natural history of herpes zoster: Late follow-up of 3.9 years (n=43) and 7.7 years (n=10). Pain 2013;154:2227–2233.

174. Oaklander AL, Bowsher D, Galer B, Haanpää M, Jensen MP. Herpes zoster itch: Preliminary epidemiologic data. J Pain 2003;4:338–343.

175. Truini A, Galeotti F, Haanpää M, et al. Pathophysiology of pain in postherpetic neuralgia: A clinical and neurophysiological study. Pain 2008;140:405–410.

176. Attal N, Cruccu G, Baron R, et al. EFNS guidelines on the pharmacological treatment of neuropathic pain: 2010 revision. Eur J Neurol 2010;17:1113.

177. Dworkin RH, O'Connor AB, Audette J, et al. Recommendations for the pharmacological management of neuropathic pain: An overview and literature update. Mayo Clin Proc 2010;85(3, suppl):S3–S14.

178. Wolff RF, Bala MM, Westwood M, Kessels AG, Kleijnen J. 5% lidocaine-medicated plaster vs other relevant interventions and placebo for post-herpetic neuralgia (PHN): A systematic review. Acta Neurol Scand 2011;123:295–309.

179. Baron R, Mayoral V, Leijon G, Binder A, Steigerwald I, Serpell M. 5% lidocaine medicated plaster versus pregabalin in post-herpetic neuralgia and diabetic polyneuropathy: An open-label, non-inferiority two-stage RCT study. Curr Med Res Opin 2009;25:1663–1676.

180. Hans G, Sabatowski R, Binder A, Boesl I, Rogers P, Baron R. Efficacy and tolerability of a 5% lidocaine medicated plaster for the topical treatment of post-herpetic neuralgia: Results of a long-term study. Curr Med Res Opin 2009;25:1295–1305.

181. Derry S, Moore RA. Topical capsaicin (low concentration) for chronic neuropathic pain in adults. Cochrane Database Syst Rev 2012;9.

182. Derry S, Sven-Rice A, Cole P, Tan T, Moore RA. Topical capsaicin (high concentration) for chronic neuropathic pain in adults. Cochrane Database Syst Rev 2013;2.

183. Peppin JF, Pappagallo M. Capsaicinoids in the treatment of neuropathic pain: A review. Ther Adv Neurol Disord 2014;7:22–32.

184. Sayanlar J, Guleyupoglu N, Portenoy R, Ashina S. Trigeminal postherpetic neuralgia responsive to treatment with capsaicin 8 % topical patch: A case report. J Headache Pain 2012;13:587–589.

185. Watson CP, Oaklander AL. Postherpetic neuralgia. Pain Practice 2002;2:295–307.

186. Wu CL, Raja SN. An update on the treatment of postherpetic neuralgia. J Pain 2008;9(1, suppl):S19–S30.

187. Nurmikko TJ, Haanpää M. Treatment of postherpetic neuralgia. Curr Pain Headache Rep 2005;9:161–167.

188. Petersen KL, Rice FL, Farhadi M, Reda H, Rowbotham MC. Natural history of cutaneous innervation following herpes zoster. Pain 2010;150:75–82.

189. Baron R. Mechanisms of postherpetic neuralgia—We are hot on the scent. Pain 2008;140:395–396.

190. Dostrovsky JO. Trigeminal postherpetic neuralgia postmortem: Clinically unilateral, pathologically bilateral. In: Devor M, Rowbotham MC, Wiesenfeld-Hallin Z (eds). Progress in Pain Research and Management Series, vol 16 [Proceedings of the 9th World Congress on Pain, 22–27 Aug 1999, Vienna, Austria]. Seattle: IASP, 2000:733–739.

191. Pappagallo M, Oaklander AL, Quatrano-Piacentini AL, Clark MR, Raja SN. Heterogenous patterns of sensory dysfunction in postherpetic neuralgia suggest multiple pathophysiologic mechanisms. Anesthesiology 2000;92:691–698.

192. Benoliel R, Birenboim R, Regev E, Eliav E. Neurosensory changes in the infraorbital nerve following zygomatic fractures. Oral Surg Oral Med Oral Pathol Oral Radiol Endod 2005;99:657–665.

193. Polycarpou N, Ng YL, Canavan D, Moles DR, Gulabivala K. Prevalence of persistent pain after endodontic treatment and factors affecting its occurrence in cases with complete radiographic healing. Int Endod J 2005;38:169–178.

194. Renton T, Yilmaz Z. Profiling of patients presenting with posttraumatic neuropathy of the trigeminal nerve. J Orofac Pain 2011;25:333–344.

195. Renton T, Yilmaz Z, Gaballah K. Evaluation of trigeminal nerve injuries in relation to third molar surgery in a prospective patient cohort. Recommendations for prevention. Int J Oral Maxillofac Surg 2012;41:1509–1518.

196. Peñarrocha MA, Peñarrocha D, Bagán JV, Peñarrocha M. Post-traumatic trigeminal neuropathy. A study of 63 cases. Med Oral Patol Oral Cir Bucal 2012;17:e297–e300.

197. Renton T, Adey-Viscuso D, Meechan JG, Yilmaz Z. Trigeminal nerve injuries in relation to the local anaesthesia in mandibular injections. Br Dent J 2010;209:e15.

198. Turner-Stokes L, Goebel A. Complex regional pain syndrome in adults: Concise guidance. Clin Med 2011;11:596–600.

199. Beniczky S, Tajti J, Timea Varga E, Vecsei L. Evidence-based pharmacological treatment of neuropathic pain syndromes. J Neural Transm 2005;112:735–749.

200. Macrae WA. Chronic pain after surgery. Br J Anaesth 2001;87:88–98.

201. Ardekian L, Dodson TB. Complications associated with the placement of dental implants. Oral Maxillofac Surg Clin North Am 2003;15:243–249.

202. Schmidt R, Schmelz M, Forster C, Ringkamp M, Torebjörk E, Handwerker H. Novel classes of responsive and unresponsive C nociceptors in human skin. J Neurosci 1995;15:333–341.

203. Renton T, Thexton A, Hankins M, McGurk M. Quantitative thermosensory testing of the lingual and inferior alveolar nerves in health and after iatrogenic injury. Brit J Oral Maxillofac Surg 2003;41:36–42.

204. Albrektsson T. A multicenter report on osseointegrated oral implants. J Prosthet Dent 1988;60:75–84.

205. Albrektsson T, Dahl E, Enbom L, et al. Osseointegrated oral implants. A Swedish multicenter study of 8139 consecutively inserted Nobelpharma implants. J Periodontol 1988;59:287–296.

206. Gregg JM. Neuropathic complications of mandibular implant surgery: Review and case presentations. Ann R Australas Coll Dent Surg 2000;15:176–180.

207. Higuchi KW, Folmer T, Kultje C. Implant survival rates in partially edentulous patients: A 3-year prospective multicenter study. J Oral Maxillofac Surg 1995;53:264–268.

208. Lazzara R, Siddiqui AA, Binon P, et al. Retrospective multicenter analysis of 3i endosseous dental implants placed over a five-year period. Clin Oral Implants Res 1996;7:73–83.

209. Haas DA, Lennon D. A 21 year retrospective study of reports of paresthesia following local anesthetic administration. J Can Dent Assoc 1995;61:319–320;323–316;329–330.

210. Juodzbalys G, Wang HL, Sabalys G. Injury of the inferior alveolar nerve during implant placement: A literature review. J Oral Maxillofac Res 2011;2:e1.

211. Juodzbalys G, Wang HL, Sabalys G, Sidlauskas A, Galindo-Moreno P. Inferior alveolar nerve injury associated with implant surgery. Clin Oral Implants Res 2013;24:183–190.

212. Zeltser R, Beilin B, Zaslansky R, Seltzer Z. Comparison of autotomy behavior induced in rats by various clinically-used neurectomy methods. Pain 2000;89:19–24.

213. Benoliel R, Wilensky A, Tal M, Eliav E. Application of a pro-inflammatory agent to the orbital portion of the rat infraorbital nerve induces changes indicative of ongoing trigeminal pain. Pain 2002;99:567–578.

214. Huang Y, Jacobs R, Van Dessel J, Bornstein MM, Lambrichts I, Politis C. A systematic review on the innervation of peri-implant tissues with special emphasis on the influence of implant placement and loading protocols [epub ahead of print 6 February 2014]. Clin Oral Implants Res doi: 10.1111/clr.12344.

215. Barron RP, Benoliel R, Zeltser R, Eliav E, Nahlieli O, Gracely RH. Effect of dexamethasone and dipyrone on lingual and inferior alveolar nerve hypersensitivity following third molar extractions: Preliminary report. J Orofac Pain 2004;18:62–68.

216. Valmaseda-Castellon E, Berini-Aytes L, Gay-Escoda C. Inferior alveolar nerve damage after lower third molar surgical extraction: A prospective study of 1117 surgical extractions. Oral Surg Oral Med Oral Pathol Oral Radiol Endod 2001;92:377–383.

217. Berge TI. Incidence of chronic neuropathic pain subsequent to surgical removal of impacted third molars. Acta Odontol Scand 2002;60:108–112.

218. Valmaseda-Castellon E, Berini-Aytes L, Gay-Escoda C. Lingual nerve damage after third lower molar surgical extraction. Oral Surg Oral Med Oral Pathol Oral Radiol Endod 2000;90:567–573.

219. Gomes AC, Vasconcelos BC, de Oliveira e Silva ED, da Silva LC. Lingual nerve damage after mandibular third molar surgery: A randomized clinical trial. J Oral Maxillofac Surg 2005;63:1443–1446.

220. Queral-Godoy E, Figueiredo R, Valmaseda-Castellon E, Berini-Aytes L, Gay-Escoda C. Frequency and evolution of lingual nerve lesions following lower third molar extraction. J Oral Maxillofac Surg 2006;64:402–407.

221. Robert RC, Bacchetti P, Pogrel MA. Frequency of trigeminal nerve injuries following third molar removal. J Oral Maxillofac Surg 2005;63:732–735.

222. Fried K, Bongenhielm U, Boissonade FM, Robinson PP. Nerve injury-induced pain in the trigeminal system. Neuroscientist 2001;7:155–165.

223. Vora AR, Loescher AR, Boissonade FM, Robinson PP. Ultrastructural characteristics of axons in traumatic neuromas of the human lingual nerve. J Orofac Pain 2005;19:22–33.

224. Pogrel MA, Jergensen R, Burgon E, Hulme D. Long-term outcome of trigeminal nerve injuries related to dental treatment. J Oral Maxillofac Surg 2011;69:2284–2288.

225. Von Ohle C, El Ayouti A. Neurosensory impairment of the mental nerve as a sequel of periapical periodontitis: Case report and review. Oral Surg Oral Med Oral Pathol Oral Radiol Endod 2010;110:e84–e89.

226. Ozkan BT, Celik S, Durmus E. Paresthesia of the mental nerve stem from periapical infection of mandibular canine tooth: A case report. Oral Surg Oral Med Oral Pathol Oral Radiol Endod 2008;105:e28–e31.

227. Singh PK. Root canal complications: 'The hypochlorite accident.' SADJ 2010;65:416–419.

228. Motta MV, Chaves-Mendonca MA, Stirton CG, Cardozo HF. Accidental injection with sodium hypochlorite: Report of a case. Int Endod J 2009;42:175–182.

229. Witton R, Henthorn K, Ethunandan M, Harmer S, Brennan PA. Neurological complications following extrusion of sodium hypochlorite solution during root canal treatment. Int Endod J 2005;38:843–848.

230. López-López J, Estrugo-Devesa A, Jané-Salas E, Segura-Egea JJ. Inferior alveolar nerve injury resulting from overextension of an endodontic sealer: Non-surgical management using the GABA analogue pregabalin. Int Endod J 2012;45:98–104.

231. Gambarini G, Plotino G, Grande NM, et al. Differential diagnosis of endodontic-related inferior alveolar nerve paraesthesia with cone beam computed tomography: A case report. Int Endod J 2011;44:176–181.

232. Marbach JJ, Hulbrock J, Hohn C, Segal AG. Incidence of phantom tooth pain: An atypical facial neuralgia. Oral Surg Oral Med Oral Pathol 1982;53:190–193.

233. Lobb WK, Zakariasen KL, McGrath PJ. Endodontic treatment outcomes: Do patients perceive problems? J Am Dent Assoc 1996;127:597–600.

234. Campbell RL, Parks KW, Dodds RN. Chronic facial pain associated with endodontic therapy. Oral Surg Oral Med Oral Pathol 1990;69:287–290.

235. Klasser GD, Kugelmann AM, Villines D, Bradford JR. The prevalence of persistent pain after nonsurgical root canal. Quintessence Int 2011;42:259–269.

236. Nixdorf DR, Moana-Filho EJ, Law AS, McGuire LA, Hodges JS, John MT. Frequency of persistent tooth pain after root canal therapy: A systematic review and meta-analysis. J Endod 2010;36:224–230.

237. Renton T, Adey-Viscuso D, Meechan JG, Yilmaz Z. Trigeminal nerve injuries in relation to the local anaesthesia in mandibular injections. Brit Dent J 2010;209:e15.

238. Benoliel R, Eliav E, Tal M. No sympathetic nerve sprouting in rat trigeminal ganglion following painful and non-painful infraorbital nerve neuropathy. Neurosci Lett 2001;297:151–154.

239. Benoliel R, Zadik Y, Eliav E, Sharav Y. Peripheral painful traumatic trigeminal neuropathy: Clinical features in 91 cases and proposal of novel diagnostic criteria. J Orofac Pain 2012;26:49–58.

240. Pigg M, Svensson P, Drangsholt M, List T. Seven-year follow-up of patients diagnosed with atypical odontalgia: A prospective study. J Orofac Pain 2013;27:151–164.

241. Baad-Hansen L, Leijon G, Svensson P, List T. Comparison of clinical findings and psychosocial factors in patients with atypical odontalgia and temporomandibular disorders. J Orofac Pain 2008;22:7–14.

242. Svensson P, Baad-Hansen L, Pigg M, et al. Guidelines and recommendations for assessment of somatosensory function in oro-facial pain conditions—A taskforce report. J Oral Rehabil 2011;38:366–394.

243. Baad-Hansen L, Pigg M, Ivanovic SE, et al. Chairside intraoral qualitative somatosensory testing: Reliability and comparison between patients with atypical odontalgia and healthy controls. J Orofac Pain 2013;27:165–170.

244. Baad-Hansen L, Pigg M, Ivanovic SE, et al. Intraoral somatosensory abnormalities in patients with atypical odontalgia—A controlled multicenter quantitative sensory testing study. Pain 2013;154:1287–1294.

245. List T, Leijon G, Svensson P. Somatosensory abnormalities in atypical odontalgia: A case-control study. Pain 2008;139:333–341.

246. Siqueira SR, Siviero M, Alvarez FK, Teixeira MJ, Siqueira JT. Quantitative sensory testing in trigeminal traumatic neuropathic pain and persistent idiopathic facial pain. Arq Neuropsiquiatr 2013;71:174–179.

247. Baad-Hansen L, List T, Kaube H, Jensen TS, Svensson P. Blink reflexes in patients with atypical odontalgia and matched healthy controls. Exp Brain Res 2006;172:498–506.

248. Jaaskelainen SK. The utility of clinical neurophysiological and quantitative sensory testing for trigeminal neuropathy. J Orofac Pain 2004;18:355–359.

249. Smith JG, Elias LA, Yilmaz Z, et al. The psychosocial and affective burden of posttraumatic neuropathy following injuries to the trigeminal nerve. J Orofac Pain 2013;27:293–303.

250. Marinus J, Moseley GL, Birklein F, et al. Clinical features and pathophysiology of complex regional pain syndrome. Lancet Neurol 2011;10:637–648.

251. Harden RN, Bruehl S, Perez RS, et al. Validation of proposed diagnostic criteria (the "Budapest Criteria") for complex regional pain syndrome. Pain 2010;150:268–274.

252. Merskey H, Bogduk N. Classification of Chronic Pain: Descriptions of Chronic Pain Syndromes and Definition of Pain Terms. Seattle: IASP, 1994.

253. Harden RN, Bruehl SP. Diagnosis of complex regional pain syndrome: Signs, symptoms, and new empirically derived diagnostic criteria. Clin J Pain 2006;22:415–419.

254. Hauser J, Hsu B, Nader ND. Inflammatory processes in complex regional pain syndromes. Immunol Invest 2013;42:263–272.

255. Janig W, Baron R. Experimental approach to CRPS. Pain 2004;108:3–7.

256. Bruehl S. An update on the pathophysiology of complex regional pain syndrome. Anesthesiology 2010;113:713–725.

257. Borchers AT, Gershwin ME. Complex regional pain syndrome: A comprehensive and critical review. Autoimmun Rev 2014;13:242–265.

258. Melis M, Zawawi K, al-Badawi E, Lobo Lobo S, Mehta N. Complex regional pain syndrome in the head and neck: Review of the literature. J Orofac Pain 2002;16:93104.

259. Heir GM, Nasri-Heir C, Thomas D, et al. Complex regional pain syndrome following trigeminal nerve injury: Report of 2 cases. Oral Surg Oral Med Oral Pathol Oral Radiol Endod 2012;114:733–739.

260. Baron R, Wasner G. Complex regional pain syndromes. Curr Pain Headache Rep 2001;5:114–123.

261. Birklein F. Complex regional pain syndrome. J Neurol 2005;252:131–138.

262. Maleki J, Le Bel AA, Bennett GJ, Schwartzman RJ. Patterns of spread in complex regional pain syndrome, type I (reflex sympathetic dystrophy). Pain 2000;88:259–266.

263. Rommel O, Malin JP, Zenz M, Janig W. Quantitative sensory testing, neurophysiological and psychological examination in patients with complex regional pain syndrome and hemisensory deficits. Pain 2001;93:279–293.

264. Verdugo RJ, Bell LA, Campero M, et al. Spectrum of cutaneous hyperalgesias/allodynias in neuropathic pain patients. Acta Neurol Scand 2004;110:368–376.

265. Wasner G, Schattschneider J, Baron R. Skin temperature side differences—A diagnostic tool for CRPS? Pain 2002;98:19–26.

266. Harden RN, Oaklander AL, Burton AW, et al. Complex regional pain syndrome: Practical diagnostic and treatment guidelines, 4th edition. Pain Med 2013;14:180–229.

267. O'Connell NE, Wand BM, McAuley J, Marston L, Moseley GL. Interventions for treating pain and disability in adults with complex regional pain syndrome. Cochrane Database Syst Rev 2013;4.

268. Daly AE, Bialocerkowski AE. Does evidence support physiotherapy management of adult complex regional pain syndrome Type One? A systematic review. Eur J Pain 2009;13:339–353.

269. van Velzen GA, Perez RS, van Gestel MA, et al. Health-related quality of life in 975 patients with complex regional pain syndrome type 1. Pain 2014;155:629–634.

270. Wu CL, Raja SN. Treatment of acute postoperative pain. Lancet 2011;377(9784):2215–2225.

271. Johansen A, Schirmer H, Stubhaug A, Nielsen CS. Persistent post-surgical pain and experimental pain sensitivity in the Tromso study: Comorbid pain matters. Pain 2014;155:341–348.

272. Clarke H, Bonin RP, Orser BA, Englesakis M, Wijeysundera DN, Katz J. The prevention of chronic postsurgical pain using gabapentin and pregabalin: A combined systematic review and meta-analysis. Anesth Analg 2012;115:428–442.

273. Dworkin RH, McDermott MP, Raja SN. Preventing chronic postsurgical pain: How much of a difference makes a difference? Anesthesiology 2010;112:516–518.

274. McGreevy K, Bottros MM, Raja SN. Preventing chronic pain following acute pain: Risk factors, preventive strategies, and their efficacy. Eur J Pain Suppl 2011;5:365–372.

275. Kelly DJ, Ahmad M, Brull SJ. Preemptive analgesia I: Physiological pathways and pharmacological modalities. Can J Anaesth 2001;48:1000–1010.

276. Kelly DJ, Ahmad M, Brull SJ. Preemptive analgesia II: Recent advances and current trends. Can J Anaesth 2001;48:1091–1101.

277. Barreveld A, Witte J, Chahal H, Durieux ME, Strichartz G. Preventive analgesia by local anesthetics: The reduction of postoperative pain by peripheral nerve blocks and intravenous drugs. Anesth Analg 2013;116:1141–1161.

278. Yarnitsky D, Crispel Y, Eisenberg E, et al. Prediction of chronic post-operative pain: Pre-operative DNIC testing identifies patients at risk. Pain 2008;138:22–28.

279. Weissman-Fogel I, Granovsky Y, Crispel Y, et al. Enhanced presurgical pain temporal summation response predicts post-thoracotomy pain intensity during the acute postoperative phase. J Pain 2009;10:628–636.

280. Landau R, Kraft JC, Flint LY, et al. An experimental paradigm for the prediction of Post-Operative Pain (PPOP). J Vis Exp 2010;(35).

281. Finnerup NB, Sindrup SH, Jensen TS. The evidence for pharmacological treatment of neuropathic pain. Pain 2010;150:573–581.

282. Haviv Y, Zadik Y, Sharav Y, Benoliel R. Painful traumatic trigeminal neuropathy: An open study on the pharmacotherapeutic response to stepped treatment. J Oral Facial Pain Headache 2014;28:52–60.

283. Sindrup SH, Jensen TS. Antidepressants in the treatment of neuropathic pain. In: Hanson PT, Fields HL, Hill RG, Marchettini P (eds). Neuropathic pain: Pathophysiology and Treatment, vol 21. Seattle: IASP, 2001:169–183.

284. Duhmke RM, Cornblath DD, Hollingshead JR. Tramadol for neuropathic pain. Cochrane Database Syst Rev 2004;(2).

285. Eisenberg E, McNicol ED, Carr DB. Efficacy and safety of opioid agonists in the treatment of neuropathic pain of nonmalignant origin: Systematic review and meta-analysis of randomized controlled trials. JAMA 2005;293:3043–3052.

286. McQuay HJ, Tramer M, Nye BA, Carroll D, Wiffen PJ, Moore RA. A systematic review of antidepressants in neuropathic pain. Pain 1996;68:217–227.

287. Rowbotham MC, Goli V, Kunz NR, Lei D. Venlafaxine extended release in the treatment of painful diabetic neuropathy: A double-blind, placebo-controlled study. Pain 2004;110:697–706.

288. Lunn MP, Hughes RA, Wiffen PJ. Duloxetine for treating painful neuropathy, chronic pain or fibromyalgia. Cochrane Database Syst Rev 2014;1.

289. Moore RA, Derry S, Aldington D, Cole P, Wiffen PJ. Amitriptyline for neuropathic pain and fibromyalgia in adults. Cochrane Database Syst Rev 2012;12.

290. Wiffen PJ, Derry S, Moore RA, et al. Antiepileptic drugs for neuropathic pain and fibromyalgia—An overview of Cochrane reviews. Cochrane Database Syst Rev 2013;11.

291. Cruccu G, Truini A. Refractory trigeminal neuralgia. Non-surgical treatment options. CNS Drugs 2013;27:91–96.

292. Zakrzewska JM, McMillan R. Trigeminal neuralgia: The diagnosis and management of this excruciating and poorly understood facial pain. Postgrad Med J 2011;87(1028):410–416.

293. Tesfaye S, Wilhelm S, Lledo A, et al. Duloxetine and pregabalin: High-dose monotherapy or their combination? The "COMBO-DN study"—A multinational, randomized, double-blind, parallel-group study in patients with diabetic peripheral neuropathic pain. Pain 2013;154:2616–2625.

294. Gilron I, Bailey JM, Tu D, Holden RR, Jackson AC, Houlden RL. Nortriptyline and gabapentin, alone and in combination for neuropathic pain: A double-blind, randomised controlled crossover trial. Lancet 2009;374(9697):1252–1261.

295. Simpson DA. Gabapentin and venlafaxine for the treatment of painful diabetic neuropathy. J Clin Neuromusc Disease 2001;3:53–62.

296. Hanna M, O'Brien C, Wilson MC. Prolonged-release oxycodone enhances the effects of existing gabapentin therapy in painful diabetic neuropathy patients. Eur J Pain 2008;12:804–813.

297. Gilron I, Bailey JM, Tu D, Holden RR, Weaver DF, Houlden RL. Morphine, gabapentin, or their combination for neuropathic pain. N Engl J Med 2005;352:1324–1334.

298. Chaparro LE, Wiffen PJ, Moore RA, Gilron I. Combination pharmacotherapy for the treatment of neuropathic pain in adults. Cochrane Database Syst Rev 2012;7.

299. Heir G, Karolchek S, Kalladka M, et al. Use of topical medication in orofacial neuropathic pain: A retrospective study. Oral Surg Oral Med Oral Pathol Oral Radiol Endod 2008;105:466–469.

300. Lynch ME, Cesar-Rittenberg P, Hohmann AG. A double-blind, placebo-controlled, crossover pilot trial with extension using an oral mucosal cannabinoid extract for treatment of chemotherapy-induced neuropathic pain. J Pain Symptom Manage 2014;47:166–173.

301. Wilsey B, Marcotte T, Deutsch R, Gouaux B, Sakai S, Donaghe H. Low-dose vaporized cannabis significantly improves neuropathic pain. J Pain 2013;14:136–148.

302. Wetering EJ, Lemmens KM, Nieboer AP, Huijsman R. Cognitive and behavioral interventions for the management of chronic neuropathic pain in adults—A systematic review. Eur J Pain 2010;14:670–681.

303. Ziccardi VB. Microsurgical techniques for repair of the inferior alveolar and lingual nerves. Atlas Oral Maxillofac Surg Clin North Am 2011;19:79–90.

304. Ziccardi VB, Steinberg MJ. Timing of trigeminal nerve microsurgery: A review of the literature. J Oral Maxillofac 2007;65:1341–1345.

305. Farole A, Jamal BT. A bioabsorbable collagen nerve cuff (NeuraGen) for repair of lingual and inferior alveolar nerve injuries: A case series. J Oral Maxillofac Surg 2008;66:2058–2062.

306. Pogrel MA. The results of microneurosurgery of the inferior alveolar and lingual nerve. J Oral Maxillofac Surg 2002;60:485–489.

307. Ziccardi VB, Rivera L, Gomes J. Comparison of lingual and inferior alveolar nerve microsurgery outcomes. Quintessence Int 2009;40:295–301.

308. Susarla SM, Kaban LB, Donoff RB, Dodson TB. Functional sensory recovery after trigeminal nerve repair. J Oral Maxillofac Surg 2007;65:60–65.

309. Susarla SM, Kaban LB, Donoff RB, Dodson TB. Does early repair of lingual nerve injuries improve functional sensory recovery? J Oral Maxillofac Surg 2007;65:1070–1076.

310. Caissie R, Goulet J, Fortin M, Morielli D. Iatrogenic paresthesia in the third division of the trigeminal nerve: 12 years of clinical experience. J Can Dent Assoc 2005;71:185–190.

311. Rutner TW, Ziccardi VB, Janal MN. Long-term outcome assessment for lingual nerve microsurgery. J Oral Maxillofac Surg 2005;63:1145–1149.

312. Strauss ER, Ziccardi VB, Janal MN. Outcome assessment of inferior alveolar nerve microsurgery: A retrospective review. J Oral Maxillofac Surg 2006;64:1767–1770.

313. Renton T, Yilmaz Z. Managing iatrogenic trigeminal nerve injury: A case series and review of the literature. Int J Oral Maxillofac Surg 2012;41:629–637.

314. Bullard DE, Nashold BS Jr. The caudalis DREZ for facial pain. Stereotact Funct Neurosurg 1997;68:168–174.

315. Kanpolat Y, Savas A, Ugur HC, Bozkurt M. The trigeminal tract and nucleus procedures in treatment of atypical facial pain. Surg Neurol 2005;64(2, suppl):S96–S100.

316. Renton T, Dawood A, Shah A, Searson L, Yilmaz Z. Post-implant neuropathy of the trigeminal nerve. A case series. Br Dent J 2012;212:e17.

317. Eliav E, Teich S, Nitzan D, et al. Facial arthralgia and myalgia: Can they be differentiated by trigeminal sensory assessment? Pain 2003;104:481–490.

318. Benoliel R, Quek S, Biron A, Nahlieli O, Eliav E. Trigeminal neurosensory changes following acute and chronic paranasal sinusitis. Quintessence Int 2006;37:437–443.

319. Eliav E, Teich S, Benoliel R, et al. Large myelinated nerve fiber hypersensitivity in oral malignancy. Oral Surg Oral Med Oral Pathol Oral Radiol Endod 2002;94:45–50.

320. Han SR, Yeo SP, Lee MK, Bae YC, Ahn DK. Early dexamethasone relieves trigeminal neuropathic pain. J Dent Res 2010;89:915–920.

321. Salter MW, Beggs S. Sublime microglia: Expanding roles for the guardians of the CNS. Cell 2014;158:15–24.

322. Lee MC, Tracey I. Imaging pain: A potent means for investigating pain mechanisms in patients. Br J Anaesth 2013;111:64–72.

323. von Hehn CA, Baron R, Woolf CJ. Deconstructing the neuropathic pain phenotype to reveal neural mechanisms. Neuron 2012;73:638–652.

324. Nitzan-Luques A, Devor M, Tal M. Genotype-selective phenotypic switch in primary afferent neurons contributes to neuropathic pain. Pain 2011;152:2413–2426.

325. Devor M. Ectopic discharge in Abeta afferents as a source of neuropathic pain. Exp Brain Res 2009;196:115–128.

326. Woolf CJ, Salter MW. Neuronal plasticity: Increasing the gain in pain. Science 2000;288(5472):1765–1769.

327. Mogil JS. Pain genetics: Past, present and future. Trends Genet 2012;28:258–266.

328. Salter MW. Deepening understanding of the neural substrates of chronic pain. Brain 2014;137:651–653.

329. Eliav E, Benoliel R, Tal M. Inflammation with no axonal damage of the rat saphenous nerve trunk induces ectopic discharge and mechanosensitivity in myelinated axons. Neurosci Lett 2001;311:49–52.

330. Benoliel R, Eliav E, Tal M. Strain-dependent modification of neuropathic pain behaviour in the rat hindpaw by a priming painful trigeminal nerve injury. Pain 2002;97:203–212.

331. Chacur M, Milligan ED, Gazda LS, et al. A new model of sciatic inflammatory neuritis (SIN): Induction of unilateral and bilateral mechanical allodynia following acute unilateral peri-sciatic immune activation in rats. Pain 2001;94:231–244.

332. Zelenka M, Schäfers M, Sommer C. Intraneural injection of interleukin-1beta and tumor necrosis factor-alpha into rat sciatic nerve at physiological doses induces signs of neuropathic pain. Pain 2005;116:257–263.

333. Eliav E, Tal M, Benoliel R. Experimental malignancy in the rat induces early hypersensitivity indicative of neuritis. Pain 2004;110:727–737.

334. Eliav E, Gracely RH, Nahlieli O, Benoliel R. Quantitative sensory testing in trigeminal nerve damage assessment. J Orofac Pain 2004;18:339–344.

335. Juhl GI, Jensen TS, Norholt SE, Svensson P. Central sensitization phenomena after third molar surgery: A quantitative sensory testing study. Eur J Pain 2008;12:116–127.

336. Tan AM, Chang YW, Zhao P, Hains BC, Waxman SG. Rac1-regulated dendritic spine remodeling contributes to neuropathic pain after peripheral nerve injury. Exp Neurol 2011;232:222–233.

337. Polgár E, Hughes DI, Arham AZ, Todd AJ. Loss of neurons from laminas I-III of the spinal dorsal horn is not required for development of tactile allodynia in the spared nerve injury model of neuropathic pain. J Neurosci 2005;25:6658–6666.

338. Vallejo R, Tilley DM, Vogel L, Benyamin R. The role of glia and the immune system in the development and maintenance of neuropathic pain. Pain Pract 2010;10:167–184.

339. Dublin P, Hanani M. Satellite glial cells in sensory ganglia: Their possible contribution to inflammatory pain. Brain Behav Immun 2007;21:592–598.

340. Hanani M. Satellite glial cells in sensory ganglia: From form to function. Brain Res Rev 2005;48:457–476.

341. Borsook D, Becerra L. How close are we in utilizing functional neuroimaging in routine clinical diagnosis of neuropathic pain? Curr Pain Headache Rep 2011;15:223–229.

342. Draganski B, Moser T, Lummel N, et al. Decrease of thalamic gray matter following limb amputation. Neuroimage 2006;31:951–957.

343. Flor H, Denke C, Schaefer M, Grüsser S. Effect of sensory discrimination training on cortical reorganisation and phantom limb pain. Lancet 2001;357(9270):1763–1764.

344. Da Silva AF, Becerra L, Pendse G, Chizh B, Tully S, Borsook D. Colocalized structural and functional changes in the cortex of patients with trigeminal neuropathic pain. PLoS One 2008;3:e3396.

345. Becerra L, Morris S, Bazes S, et al. Trigeminal neuropathic pain alters responses in CNS circuits to mechanical (brush) and thermal (cold and heat) stimuli. J Neurosci 2006;26:10646–10657.

346. Inglese M, Makani S, Johnson G, et al. Diffuse axonal injury in mild traumatic brain injury: A diffusion tensor imaging study. J Neurosurg 2005;103:298–303.

347. Povlishock JT, Katz DI. Update of neuropathology and neurological recovery after traumatic brain injury. J Head Trauma Rehabil 2005;20:76–94.

348. Drummond PD. Sensory disturbances in complex regional pain syndrome: Clinical observations, autonomic interactions, and possible mechanisms. Pain Med 2010;11:1257–1266.

349. Weber M, Birklein F, Neundorfer B, Schmelz M. Facilitated neurogenic inflammation in complex regional pain syndrome. Pain 2001;91:251–257.

350. Stanton TR, Wand BM, Carr DB, Birklein F, Wasner GL, O'Connell NE. Local anaesthetic sympathetic blockade for complex regional pain syndrome. Cochrane Database Syst Rev 2013;8.

351. Schwenkreis P, Maier C, Tegenthoff M. Functional imaging of central nervous system involvement in complex regional pain syndrome. AJNR Am J Neuroradiol 2009;30:1279–1284.

352. Barad MJ, Ueno T, Younger J, Chatterjee N, Mackey S. Complex regional pain syndrome is associated with structural abnormalities in pain-related regions of the human brain. J Pain 2014;15:197–203.

353. Swart CM, Stins JF, Beek PJ. Cortical changes in complex regional pain syndrome (CRPS). Eur J Pain 2009;13:902–907.

354. Bolwerk A, Seifert F, Maihofner C. Altered resting-state functional connectivity in complex regional pain syndrome. J Pain 2013;14:1107–1115.

355. Goebel A, Blaes F. Complex regional pain syndrome, prototype of a novel kind of autoimmune disease. Autoimmun Rev 2013;12:682–686.

356. Shirani P, Jawaid A, Moretti P, et al. Familial occurrence of complex regional pain syndrome. Can J Neurol Sci 2010;37:389–394.

357. van Rooijen DE, Roelen DL, Verduijn W, et al. Genetic HLA associations in complex regional pain syndrome with and without dystonia. J Pain 2012;13:784–789.

358. de Rooij AM, Florencia Gosso M, Haasnoot GW, et al. HLA-B62 and HLA-DQ8 are associated with complex regional pain syndrome with fixed dystonia. Pain 2009;145:82–85.

359. Osterberg A, Boivie J, Thuomas KA. Central pain in multiple sclerosis–prevalence and clinical characteristics. Eur J Pain 2005;9:531–542.

360. Foley PL, Vesterinen HM, Laird BJ, et al. Prevalence and natural history of pain in adults with multiple sclerosis: Systematic review and meta-analysis. Pain 2013;154:632–642.

361. Ariai MS, Mallory GW, Pollock BE. Outcomes after microvascular decompression for patients with trigeminal neuralgia and suspected multiple sclerosis. World Neurosurg 2014;81:599–603.

362. De Simone R, Marano E, Brescia Morra V, et al. A clinical comparison of trigeminal neuralgic pain in patients with and without underlying multiple sclerosis. Neurol Sci 2005;26(2, suppl):S150–S151.

363. Danesh-Sani SA, Rahimdoost A, Soltani M, Ghiyasi M, Haghdoost N, Sabzali-Zanjankhah S. Clinical assessment of orofacial manifestations in 500 patients with multiple sclerosis. J Oral Maxillofac Surg 2013;71:290–294.

364. Bullitt E, Tew JM, Boyd J. Intracranial tumors in patients with facial pain. J Neurosurg 1986;64:865–871.

365. Moazzam AA, Habibian M. Patients appearing to dental professionals with orofacial pain arising from intracranial tumors: A literature review. Oral Surg Oral Med Oral Pathol Oral Radiol Endod 2012;114:749–755.

366. Puca A, Meglio M, Vari R, Tamburrini G, Tancredi A. Evaluation of fifth nerve dysfunction in 136 patients with middle and posterior cranial fossae tumors. Eur Neurol 1995;35:33–37.

367. Yang J, Simonson TM, Ruprecht A, Meng D, Vincent SD, Yuh WT. Magnetic resonance imaging used to assess patients with trigeminal neuralgia. Oral Surg Oral Med Oral Pathol Oral Radiol Endod 1996;81:343–350.

368. Nomura T, Ikezaki K, Matsushima T, Fukui M. Trigeminal neuralgia: Differentiation between intracranial mass lesions and ordinary vascular compression as causative lesions. Neurosurg Rev 1994;17:51–57.

369. Park SH, Kano H, Niranjan A, Flickinger JC, Lunsford LD. Stereotactic radiosurgery for cerebellopontine angle meningiomas. J Neurosurg 2014;120:708–715.

370. Baschnagel AM, Cartier JL, Dreyer J, et al. Trigeminal neuralgia pain relief after gamma knife stereotactic radiosurgery. Clin Neurol Neurosurg 2014;117:107–111.

371. Blumenfeld A, Nikolskaya G. Glossopharyngeal neuralgia. Curr Pain Headache Rep 2013;17:343.

372. Rey-Dios R, Cohen-Gadol AA. Current neurosurgical management of glossopharyngeal neuralgia and technical nuances for microvascular decompression surgery. Neurosurg Focus 2013;34:e8.

373. Kandan SR, Khan S, Jeyaretna DS, Lhatoo S, Patel NK, Coakham HB. Neuralgia of the glossopharyngeal and vagal nerves: Long-term outcome following surgical treatment and literature review. Br J Neurosurg 2010;24:441–446.

374. Patel A, Kassam A, Horowitz M, Chang YF. Microvascular decompression in the management of glossopharyngeal neuralgia: Analysis of 217 cases. Neurosurgery 2002;50:705–710.

375. Teixeira MJ, de Siqueira SR, Bor-Seng-Shu E. Glossopharyngeal neuralgia: Neurosurgical treatment and differential diagnosis. Acta Neurochir (Wien) 2008;150:471–475.

376. Minagar A, Sheremata WA. Glossopharyngeal neuralgia and MS. Neurology 2000;54:1368–1370.

377. Olesen J, Bousser MG, Diener HC, et al. The International Classification of Headache Disorders, 2nd edition. Cephalalgia 2004;24(suppl 1):24–150.

378. Esaki T, Osada H, Nakao Y, et al. Surgical management for glossopharyngeal neuralgia associated with cardiac syncope: Two case reports. Br J Neurosurg 2007;21:599–602.

379. Webb CJ, Makura ZG, McCormick MS. Glossopharyngeal neuralgia following foreign body impaction in the neck. J Laryngol Otol 2000;114:70–72.

380. Huynh-Le P, Matsushima T, Hisada K, Matsumoto K. Glossopharyngeal neuralgia due to an epidermoid tumour in the cerebellopontine angle. J Clin Neurosci 2004;11:758–760.

381. Singh PM, Dehran M, Mohan VK, Trikha A, Kaur M. Analgesic efficacy and safety of medical therapy alone vs combined medical therapy and extraoral glossopharyngeal nerve block in glossopharyngeal neuralgia. Pain Med 2013;14:93–102.

382. Rozen TD. Trigeminal neuralgia and glossopharyngeal neuralgia. Neurol Clin 2004;22:185–206.

383. Martínez-González JM, Martínez-Rodríguez N, Calvo-Guirado JL, Brinkmann JC, Dorado CB. Glossopharyngeal neuralgia: A presentation of 14 cases. J Oral Maxillofac Surg 2011;69:e38–e41.

384. Yue WL, Zhang Y. Treatment for glossopharyngeal neuralgia with peripheral glycerol injection: Our experience in twenty-one older patients. Clin Otolaryngol 2013;38:533–535.

385. Pollock BE, Boes CJ. Stereotactic radiosurgery for glossopharyngeal neuralgia: Preliminary report of 5 cases. J Neurosurg 2011;115:936–939.

386. Stieber VW, Bourland JD, Ellis TL. Glossopharyngeal neuralgia treated with gamma knife surgery: Treatment outcome and failure analysis. Case report. J Neurosurg 2005;102(suppl 1):155–157.

387. Xiong NX, Zhao HY, Zhang FC, Liu RE. Vagoglossopharyngeal neuralgia treated by microvascular decompression and glossopharyngeal rhizotomy: Clinical results of 21 cases. Stereotact Funct Neurosurg 2012;90:45–50.

388. Sampson JH, Grossi PM, Asaoka K, Fukushima T. Microvascular decompression for glossopharyngeal neuralgia: Long-term effectiveness and complication avoidance. Neurosurgery 2004;54:884–889.

389. Fischbach F, Lehmann TN, Ricke J, Bruhn H. Vascular compression in glossopharyngeal neuralgia: Demonstration by high-resolution MRI at 3 tesla. Neuroradiology 2003;45:810–811.

390. Devor M, Govrin-Lippmann R, Rappaport ZH, Tasker RR, Dostrovsky JO. Cranial root injury in glossopharyngeal neuralgia: Electron microscopic observations. Case report. J Neurosurg 2002;96:603–606.

391. Pulec JL. Geniculate neuralgia: Long-term results of surgical treatment. Ear Nose Throat J 2002;81:30–33.

392. Vanelderen P, Lataster A, Levy R, Mekhail N, van Kleef M, Van Zundert J. 8. Occipital neuralgia. Pain Pract 2010;10:137–144.

393. Mason JO 3rd, Katz B, Greene HH. Severe ocular pain secondary to occipital neuralgia following vitrectomy surgery. Retina 2004;24:458–459.

394. Kuhn WF, Kuhn SC, Gilberstadt H. Occipital neuralgias: Clinical recognition of a complicated headache. A case series and literature review. J Orofac Pain 1997;11:158–165.

395. Sahai-Srivastava S, Zheng L. Occipital neuralgia with and without migraine: Difference in pain characteristics and risk factors. Headache 2011;51:124–128.

396. Ashkenazi A, Levin M. Three common neuralgias. How to manage trigeminal, occipital, and postherpetic pain. Postgrad Med 2004;116(3):16–18.

397. Rhodus NL, Carlson CR, Miller CS. Burning mouth (syndrome) disorder. Quintessence Int 2003;34:587–593.

398. Scala A, Checchi L, Montevecchi M, Marini I, Giamberardino MA. Update on burning mouth syndrome: Overview and patient management. Crit Rev Oral Biol Med 2003;14:275–291.

399. Zakrzewska JM, Forssell H, Glenny AM. Interventions for the treatment of burning mouth syndrome. Cochrane Database Syst Rev 2005;(1).

400. Femiano F. Statistical survey of afferent pathologies during a 5-year study in the oral pathology Department at the Second University of Naples [in Italian]. Minerva Stomatol 2002;51:73–78.

401. Bergdahl M, Bergdahl J. Burning mouth syndrome: Prevalence and associated factors. J Oral Pathol Med 1999;28:350–354.

402. Netto FO, Diniz IM, Grossmann SM, de Abreu MH, do Carmo MA, Aguiar MC. Risk factors in burning mouth syndrome: A case-control study based on patient records. Clin Oral Investig 2011;15:571–575.

403. Amos K, Yeoh SC, Farah CS. Combined topical and systemic clonazepam therapy for the management of burning mouth syndrome: A retrospective pilot study. J Orofac Pain 2011;25:125–130.

404. Danhauer SC, Miller CS, Rhodus NL, Carlson CR. Impact of criteria-based diagnosis of burning mouth syndrome on treatment outcome. J Orofac Pain 2002;16:305–311.

405. Gremeau-Richard C, Woda A, Navez ML, et al. Topical clonazepam in stomatodynia: A randomised placebo-controlled study. Pain 2004;108:51–57.

406. Petruzzi M, Lauritano D, De Benedittis M, Baldoni M, Serpico R. Systemic capsaicin for burning mouth syndrome: Short-term results of a pilot study. J Oral Pathol Med 2004;33:111–114.

407. Forssell H, Teerijoki-Oksa T, Kotiranta U, et al. Pain and pain behavior in burning mouth syndrome: A pain diary study. J Orofac Pain 2012;26:117–125.

408. Rhodus NL, Fricton J, Carlson P, Messner R. Oral symptoms associated with fibromyalgia syndrome. J Rheumatol 2003;30:1841–1845.

409. Sardella A, Lodi G, Demarosi F, Bez C, Cassano S, Carrassi A. Burning mouth syndrome: A retrospective study investigating spontaneous remission and response to treatments. Oral Dis 2006;12:152–155.

410. Rodríguez-de Rivera-Campillo E, López-López J. Evaluation of the response to treatment and clinical evolution in patients with burning mouth syndrome. Med Oral Patol Oral Cir Bucal 2013;18:e403–e410.

411. Al Quran FA. Psychological profile in burning mouth syndrome. Oral Surg Oral Med Oral Pathol Oral Radiol Endod 2004;97:339–344.

412. Maina G, Albert U, Gandolfo S, Vitalucci A, Bogetto F. Personality disorders in patients with burning mouth syndrome. J Personal Disord 2005;19:84–93.

413. Carlson CR, Miller CS, Reid KI. Psychosocial profiles of patients with burning mouth syndrome. J Orofac Pain 2000;14:59–64.

414. Ni Riordain R, Moloney E, O'Sullivan K, McCreary C. Burning mouth syndrome and oral health-related quality of life: Is there a change over time? Oral Dis 2010;16:643–647.

415. Lamey PJ, Freeman R, Eddie SA, Pankhurst C, Rees T. Vulnerability and presenting symptoms in burning mouth syndrome. Oral Surg Oral Med Oral Pathol Oral Radiol Endod 2005;99:48–54.

416. Adamo D, Schiavone V, Aria M, et al. Sleep disturbance in patients with burning mouth syndrome: A case-control study. J Orofac Pain 2013;27:304–313.

417. Chainani-Wu N, Madden E, Silverman S Jr. A case-control study of burning mouth syndrome and sleep dysfunction. Oral Surg Oral Med Oral Pathol Oral Radiol Endod 2011;112:203–208.

418. Vitkov L, Weitgasser R, Hannig M, Fuchs K, Krautgartner WD. Candida-induced stomatopyrosis and its relation to diabetes mellitus. J Oral Pathol Med 2003;32:46–50.

419. Dworkin RH, Turk DC, Farrar JT, et al. Core outcome measures for chronic pain clinical trials: IMMPACT recommendations. Pain 2005;113:9–19.

420. Femiano F. Burning mouth syndrome (BMS): An open trial of comparative efficacy of alpha-lipoic acid (thioctic acid) with other therapies. Minerva Stomatol 2002;51:405–409.

421. de Souza FT, Amaral TM, dos Santos TP, et al. Burning mouth syndrome: A therapeutic approach involving mechanical salivary stimulation. Headache 2012;52:1026–1034.

422. Pinto A, Sollecito TP, DeRossi SS. Burning mouth syndrome. A retrospective analysis of clinical characteristics and treatment outcomes. NY State Dent J 2003;69(3):18–24.

423. Ko JY, Kim MJ, Lee SG, Kho HS. Outcome predictors affecting the efficacy of clonazepam therapy for the management of burning mouth syndrome (BMS). Arch Gerontol Geriatr 2012;55:755–761.

424. Silvestre-Rangil J, Silvestre FJ, Tamarit-Santafe C, Bautista D. Burning mouth syndrome: Correlation of treatment to clinical variables of the disease. Med Oral Patol Oral Cir Bucal 2011;16:e890–e894.

425. Heckmann SM, Kirchner E, Grushka M, Wichmann MG, Hummel T. A double-blind study on clonazepam in patients with burning mouth syndrome. Laryngoscope 2012;122:813–816.

426. Femiano F, Gombos F, Scully C. Burning mouth syndrome: The efficacy of lipoic acid on subgroups. J Eur Acad Dermatol Venereol 2004;18:676–678.

427. Femiano F, Scully C. Burning mouth syndrome (BMS): Double blind controlled study of alpha-lipoic acid (thioctic acid) therapy. J Oral Pathol Med 2002;31:267–269.

428. Carbone M, Pentenero M, Carrozzo M, Ippolito A, Gandolfo S. Lack of efficacy of alpha-lipoic acid in burning mouth syndrome: A double-blind, randomized, placebo-controlled study. Eur J Pain 2009;13:492–496.

429. Cavalcanti DR, da Silveira FR. Alpha lipoic acid in burning mouth syndrome—A randomized double-blind placebo-controlled trial. J Oral Pathol Med 2009;38:254–261.

430. López-Jornet P, Camacho-Alonso F, Leon-Espinosa S. Efficacy of alpha lipoic acid in burning mouth syndrome: A randomized, placebo-treatment study. J Oral Rehabil 2009;36:52–57.

431. Maina G, Vitalucci A, Gandolfo S, Bogetto F. Comparative efficacy of SSRIs and amisulpride in burning mouth syndrome: A single-blind study. J Clin Psychiatry 2002;63:38–43.

432. Femiano F, Gombos F, Scully C. Burning mouth syndrome: Open trial of psychotherapy alone, medication with alpha-lipoic acid (thioctic acid), and combination therapy. Med Oral 2004;9:8–13.

433. de Moraes M, do Amaral Bezerra BA, da Rocha Neto PC, de Oliveira Soares AC, Pinto LP, de Lisboa Lopes Costa A. Randomized trials for the treatment of burning mouth syndrome: An evidence-based review of the literature. J Oral Pathol Med 2012;41:281–287.

434. Buchanan JA, Zakrzewska JM. Burning mouth syndrome. Clin Evid (Online) 2010;2010.

435. Lamey PJ, Murray BM, Eddie SA, Freeman RE. The secretion of parotid saliva as stimulated by 10% citric acid is not related to precipitating factors in burning mouth syndrome. J Oral Pathol Med 2001;30:121–124.

436. Granot M, Nagler RM. Association between regional idiopathic neuropathy and salivary involvement as the possible mechanism for oral sensory complaints. J Pain 2005;6:581–587.

437. Wandeur T, de Moura SA, de Medeiros AM, et al. Exfoliative cytology of the oral mucosa in burning mouth syndrome: A cytomorphological and cytomorphometric analysis. Gerodontology 2011;28:44–48.

438. Heckmann SM, Heckmann JG, Hilz MJ, et al. Oral mucosal blood flow in patients with burning mouth syndrome. Pain 2001;90:281–286.

439. Dias Fernandes CS, Salum FG, Bandeira D, Pawlowski J, Luz C, Cherubini K. Salivary dehydroepiandrosterone (DHEA) levels in patients with the complaint of burning mouth: A case-control study. Oral Surg Oral Med Oral Pathol Oral Radiol Endod 2009;108:537–543.

440. Svensson P, Bjerring P, Arendt-Nielsen L, Kaaber S. Sensory and pain thresholds to orofacial argon laser stimulation in patients with chronic burning mouth syndrome. Clin J Pain 1993;9:207–215.

441. Grushka M, Sessle BJ, Howley TP. Psychophysical assessment of tactile, pain and thermal sensory functions in burning mouth syndrome. Pain 1987;28:169–184.

442. Forssell H, Jaaskelainen S, Tenovuo O, Hinkka S. Sensory dysfunction in burning mouth syndrome. Pain 2002;99:41–47.

443. Gremeau-Richard C, Dubray C, Aublet-Cuvelier B, Ughetto S, Woda A. Effect of lingual nerve block on burning mouth syndrome (stomatodynia): A randomized crossover trial. Pain 2010;149:27–32.

444. Ito M, Kurita K, Ito T, Arao M. Pain threshold and pain recovery after experimental stimulation in patients with burning mouth syndrome. Psychiatry Clin Neurosci 2002;56:161–168.

445. Lauria G, Majorana A, Borgna M, et al. Trigeminal small-fiber sensory neuropathy causes burning mouth syndrome. Pain 2005;115:332–337.

446. Yilmaz Z, Renton T, Yiangou Y, et al. Burning mouth syndrome as a trigeminal small fibre neuropathy: Increased heat and capsaicin receptor TRPV1 in nerve fibres correlates with pain score. J Clin Neurosci 2007;14:864–871.

447. Beneng K, Yilmaz Z, Yiangou Y, McParland H, Anand P, Renton T. Sensory purinergic receptor P2X3 is elevated in burning mouth syndrome. Int J Oral Maxillofac Surg 2010;39:815–819.

448. Beneng K, Renton T, Yilmaz Z, Yiangou Y, Anand P. Sodium channel Na v 1.7 immunoreactivity in painful human dental pulp and burning mouth syndrome. BMC Neurosci 2010;11:71.

449. Formaker BK, Frank ME. Taste function in patients with oral burning. Chemical Senses 2000;25:575–581.

450. Nasri-Heir C, Gomes J, Heir GM, et al. The role of sensory input of the chorda tympani nerve and the number of fungiform papillae in burning mouth syndrome. Oral surgery, oral medicine, oral pathology, oral radiology, and endodontics 2011;112:65–72.

451. Eliav E, Kamran B, Schaham R, Czerninski R, Gracely RH, Benoliel R. Evidence of chorda tympani dysfunction in patients with burning mouth syndrome. J Am Dent Assoc 2007;138:628–633.

452. Jaaskelainen SK, Rinne JO, Forssell H, et al. Role of the dopaminergic system in chronic pain—A fluorodopa-PET study. Pain 2001;90:257–260.

453. Boras VV, Savage NW, Brailo V, Lukac J, Lukac M, Alajbeg IZ. Salivary and serum levels of substance P, neurokinin A and calcitonin gene related peptide in burning mouth syndrome. Med Oral Patol Oral Cir Bucal 2010;15:e427–e431.

454. Hagelberg N, Forssell H, Rinne JO, et al. Striatal dopamine D1 and D2 receptors in burning mouth syndrome. Pain 2003;101:149–154.

455. Albuquerque RJ, de Leeuw R, Carlson CR, Okeson JP, Miller CS, Andersen AH. Cerebral activation during thermal stimulation of patients who have burning mouth disorder: An fMRI study. Pain 2006;122:223–234.

456. Femiano F. Damage to taste system and oral pain: Burning mouth syndrome. Minerva Stomatol 2004;53:471–478.

457. Grushka M, Epstein JB, Gorsky M. Burning mouth syndrome and other oral sensory disorders: A unifying hypothesis. Pain Res Manag 2003;8:133–135.

458. Eliav E, Gracely RH, Nahlieli O, Benoliel R. Evidence for chorda tympani dysfunction in burning mouth syndrome patients. J Am Dent Assoc 2007;138:628–633.

459. Formaker BK, Frank ME. Taste function in patients with oral burning. Chem Senses 2000;25:575–581.

460. Just T, Steiner S, Pau HW. Oral pain perception and taste in burning mouth syndrome. J Oral Pathol Med 2010;39:22–27.

461. Bartoshuk LM, Snyder DJ, Grushka M, Berger AM, Duffy VB, Kveton JF. Taste damage: Previously unsuspected consequences. Chem Senses 2005;30(suppl 1):i218–i219.

462. Jaaskelainen SK, Forssell H, Tenovuo O. Abnormalities of the blink reflex in burning mouth syndrome. Pain 1997;73:455–460.

463. Jaaskelainen SK. Pathophysiology of primary burning mouth syndrome. Clin Neurophysiol 2012;123:71–77.

464. Gajjar TM, Anderson LI, Dluzen DE. Acute effects of estrogen upon methamphetamine induced neurotoxicity of the nigrostriatal dopaminergic system. J Neural Transm 2003;110:1215–1224.

465. Puri V, Cui L, Liverman CS, et al. Ovarian steroids regulate neuropeptides in the trigeminal ganglion. Neuropeptides 2005;39:409–417.

466. Agostoni E, Frigerio R, Santoro P. Atypical facial pain: Clinical considerations and differential diagnosis. Neurol Sci 2005;26 Suppl 2:S71–S74.

467. Nobrega JC, Siqueira SR, Siqueira JT, Teixeira MJ. Diferential diagnosis in atypical facial pain: A clinical study. Arq Neuropsiquiatr 2007;65:256–261.

468. Evans RW, Agostoni E. Persistent idiopathic facial pain. Headache 2006;46:1298–1300.

469. Lang E, Kaltenhauser M, Seidler S, Mattenklodt P, Neundorfer B. Persistent idiopathic facial pain exists independent of somatosensory input from the painful region: Findings from quantitative sensory functions and somatotopy of the primary somatosensory cortex. Pain 2005;118:80–91.

470. Didier H, Marchetti C, Borromeo G, Tullo V, Bussone G, Santoro F. Persistent idiopathic facial pain: Multidisciplinary approach and assumption of comorbidity. Neurol Sci 2010;31(suppl 1):S189–S195.

471. Sardella A, Demarosi F, Barbieri C, Lodi G. An up-to-date view on persistent idiopathic facial pain. Minerva Stomatol 2009;58:289–299.

472. Volcy M, Rapoport AM, Tepper SJ, Sheftell FD, Bigal ME. Persistent idiopathic facial pain responsive to topiramate. Cephalalgia 2006;26:489–491.

473. Cornelissen P, van Kleef M, Mekhail N, Day M, van Zundert J. Evidence-based interventional pain medicine according to clinical diagnoses. 3. Persistent idiopathic facial pain. Pain Pract 2009;9:443–448.

474. Klasser G. Management of persistent idiopathic facial pain. J Can Dent Assoc 2013;79:d71.

475. Yang HW, Huang YF. Treatment of persistent idiopathic facial pain (PIFP) with a low-level energy diode laser. Photomed Laser Surg 2011;29:707–710.

476. Nguyen CT, Wang MB. Complementary and integrative treatments: Atypical facial pain. Otolaryngol Clin North Am 2013;46:367–382.

477. Baad-Hansen L, List T, Kaube H, Jensen TS, Svensson P. Blink reflexes in patients with atypical odontalgia and matched healthy controls. Exp Brain Res 2006;172:498–506.

478. Melis M, Lobo SL, Ceneviz C, et al. Atypical odontalgia: A review of the literature. Headache 2003;43:1060–1074.

479. Vickers ER, Cousins MJ. Neuropathic orofacial pain part 1—Prevalence and pathophysiology. Aust Endod J 2000;26:19–26.

480. Israel HA, Ward JD, Horrell B, Scrivani SJ. Oral and maxillofacial surgery in patients with chronic orofacial pain. J Oral Maxillofac Surg 2003;61:662–667.

481. Merrill RL. Intraoral neuropathy. Curr Pain Headache Rep 2004;8:341–346.

482. Benoliel R. Atypical odontalgia: Quo vadis? Quintessence Int 2013;44:383.

483. Durham J, Exley C, John MT, Nixdorf DR. Persistent dentoalveolar pain: The patient's experience. J Orofac Pain 2013;27:6–13.

484. Nixdorf DR, Drangsholt MT, Ettlin DA, et al. Classifying orofacial pains: A new proposal of taxonomy based on ontology. J Oral Rehabil 2012;39:161–169.

485. Smith JH, Bottemiller KL, Flemming KD, Michael Cutrer F, Strand EA. Inability to self-report pain after a stroke: A population-based study. Pain 2013;154:1281–1286.

486. Fitzek S, Baumgärtner U, Fitzek C, et al. Mechanisms and predictors of chronic facial pain in lateral medullary infarction. Ann Neurol 2001;49:493–500.

487. Klit H, Finnerup NB, Jensen TS. Clinical characteristics of central poststroke pain. In: Henry JL, Panju A, Yashpal K (eds). Central Neuropathic Pain: Focus on Poststroke Pain. Seattle: IASP, 2007:27–41.

488. Nicholson BD. Evaluation and treatment of central pain syndromes. Neurology 2004;62(5, suppl):S30–S36.

489. Frese A, Husstedt IW, Ringelstein EB, Evers S. Pharmacologic treatment of central post-stroke pain. Clin J Pain 2006;22:252–260.

490. Vestergaard K, Andersen G, Gottrup H, Kristensen BT, Jensen TS. Lamotrigine for central poststroke pain: A randomized controlled trial. Neurology 2001;56:184–190.

491. Finnerup NB, Otto M, McQuay HJ, Jensen TS, Sindrup SH. Algorithm for neuropathic pain treatment: An evidence based proposal. Pain 2005;118:289–305.

492. Hansen AP, Marcussen NS, Klit H, Andersen G, Finnerup NB, Jensen TS. Pain following stroke: A prospective study. Eur J Pain 2012;16:1128–1136.

Neurosurgical Aspects of Orofacial Pain

Zvi Harry Rappaport, MD

Neurosurgical therapy is considered for the treatment of patients with orofacial pain when more conservative measures are deemed to have failed or when the pain is a symptom of a neurosurgical disease process. Data also support the improved prognosis of early surgical intervention in suitable cases (see chapter 12). Establishing the appropriate diagnosis is of paramount importance before considering surgical therapy because the type of procedure chosen and the likely success of the outcome are diagnosis dependent.[1] From a neurosurgical point of view, the temporal pattern of the pain and its anatomical distribution are important features in diagnosis. The temporal pattern may be divided into paroxysmal pain, paroxysmal superimposed on a constant pain, and continuous pain without paroxysms. For paroxysmal pain, successful treatment is more likely with surgery than medical therapy. Similarly, anatomical distribution affects outcome. If the pain is localized to known anatomical distribution, surgery can be directed to the appropriate structure. Diffuse non-anatomical or bilateral pain syndromes do not offer a successful surgical target. Finally, a sensory facial examination is of prognostic importance. Sensory hypoesthesia in the background of pain is detrimental to surgical outcome, unless a structural compressive lesion is present.

According to these principles, it is clear that trigeminal neuralgia, glossopharyngeal neuralgia, and the nervus intermedius are the main diagnoses that respond to surgical therapy. Surgery has a limited role, however, in ill-defined atypical facial pain syndromes. Neuropathic pain may be symptomatic of a mass lesion or vascular disease that requires life-saving intervention. When these are treated neurosurgically, the pain is usually, but not always, ameliorated.

Intracranial Sources

Vascular

Vascular compression of cranial nerves has emerged as the leading treatable etiology for orofacial neuralgic pain.[2,3] Pathologic studies have demonstrated changes in myelination within the compressed nerve root[4,5] that are compatible with a neurophysiologic understanding of the pain mechanism.[6] However, other rarer vascular causes of facial pain have also been described. These include arteriovenous malformations,[7,8] dural arteriovenous fistulae,[7] and intracavernous aneurysms.[9] These lesions can be visualized by magnetic resonance imaging (MRI) or magnetic resonance angiography. Cerebral vasculitis may be associated with headache, but it is rarely associated with facial pain.[10] Carotid and vertebral artery dissections occur mainly in the neck, but they may also be intracranial in location. Pain phenomena include Raeder paratrigeminal neuralgia, facial paresthesia, and orbital pain.[11–13] Associated neurologic signs, such as Horner syndrome, cranial nerve findings, and transient ischemic attacks, may suggest the correct diagnosis. Primary neurovascular craniofacial pain is discussed in chapters 10 and 11.

Neoplastic

Incidence

Intracranial tumors give rise to orofacial pain when they involve the trigeminal or glossopharyngeal roots. Approximately 7% of patients with trigeminal neuralgia suffer from a mass lesion along the course of the nerve root (secondary trigeminal neuralgia). Therefore, a brain imaging study should be performed on patients suffering from trigeminal pain before embarking on a therapeutic program.[14] The younger the patient, the more likely that a tumor or multiple sclerosis is causing the trigeminal symptoms. In patients with trigeminal neuralgia who are younger than 40 years, these etiologies may represent the majority.[15] In the series by Goh et al,[14] the average age of patients with trigeminal neuralgia secondary to tumors was 53 years.

Tumor types

Although typical trigeminal neuralgia is possible in this context, most cases of facial pain secondary to mass lesions cause some degree of facial numbness. Typical lesions that cause trigeminal pain include meningiomas[16]; schwannomas, such as trigeminal and acoustic neuromas[17–19]; and epidermoid cysts.[20,21] Meningiomas involving the trigeminal root are the most frequently encountered mass lesion causing trigeminal symptomatology; acoustic neuromas are the second most frequent. The tumor should be resected with the usual microneurosurgical techniques. Pain relief can be achieved in most patients.[18] When the tumor intimately involves the trigeminal root and has already caused hypoesthesia, neuropathic pain may persist after resection of the lesion.[16] Trigeminal pain due to circumscribed tumors in strategic locations, such as the cavernous sinus or the petrous apex, may respond favorably to radiosurgery.[22]

Other

Inflammatory lesions of the cavernous sinus cause intraorbital and supraorbital pain.[23] Associated ocular signs allow for anatomical localization and diagnosis. Pachymeningitis[24] and sarcoidosis[25] can involve the trigeminal root and its branches, giving rise to facial pain. Finally, in malignant disease both leptomeningeal carcinomatosis[26] and sellar and parasellar metastases are associated with facial pain and neurologic symptomatology.[27] Neurosurgical biopsy of the lesion may be required to arrive at the correct diagnosis.

Neurosurgical Interventions for Orofacial Pain

Trigeminal neuralgia

Of all the chronic pain syndromes, trigeminal neuralgia is one of the most gratifying to treat because virtually all patients respond to drug therapy (eg, carbamazepine) at least initially (see chapter 12). Approximately half of the patients will eventually require neurosurgical intervention, however, because of drug intolerance, side effects, or drug failure. Three categories of interventional therapy are available: peripheral neurectomy, percutaneous rhizotomy, and microvascular root decompression or rhizotomy via a craniotomy approach. Stimulation of the trigeminal root is an investigational procedure, but it is not commonly used in cases of refractory facial pain.[28] Stereotactic radiosurgery for the treatment of trigeminal neuralgia has been introduced more recently and has the advantage of being noninvasive and thus suitable for patients with significant comorbidities or who are taking anticoagulants. The treatment does have a longer latency period until pain relief sets in, however, and a somewhat lower success rate than other ablative procedures.[29,30]

As mentioned previously, it is important to classify the type of pain pattern in order to estimate the likelihood of success for the surgical procedure. Type I trigeminal neuralgia consists mostly of shocklike, episodic pain attacks. Good outcomes are expected in a high percentage of patients treated surgically. Patients with type II trigeminal neuralgia suffer mostly from constant pain and have a lower success rate. For example, after microvascular decompression (MVD), 84% of patients with type I trigeminal neuralgia will have an excellent or good outcome compared with 54% of patients with type II.[31] The pain type is the best predictor of outcome after this procedure and must be considered when selecting patients for intervention.

Peripheral neurectomy

In fragile elderly patients, peripheral neurectomy, especially of the supraorbital and infraorbital nerves, provides effective pain relief lasting for approximately 12 months.[32,33] Local dense anesthesia, the development of dysesthesia, and the rather rapid return of pain in most treated patients make this procedure unattractive for patients with a longer life expectancy.

Percutaneous trigeminal rhizotomy

Three methods are commonly used for percutaneous trigeminal rhizotomy: radiofrequency (RF) rhizolysis,[34–36] retrogasserian glycerol injection,[37–40] and trigeminal root balloon compression.[41] A percutaneous puncture of the foramen

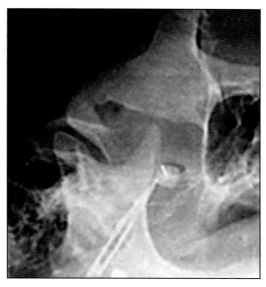

Fig 13-1 An oblique submental fluoroscopic view of the foramen ovale, which is visualized between the coronoid process of the mandible and the maxillary sinus. The needle used for the puncture is seen within the foramen.

ovale is performed under fluoroscopic guidance by inserting a spinal needle or guide with an indwelling stylet at a point approximately 3 cm lateral to the angle of the mouth (Fig 13-1). Partial damage to the nerve root and ganglion is achieved chemically or by heating with an RF electrode introduced through the guide, injecting glycerol through the needle, or performing compression with a balloon catheter inserted through the guide.

RF rhizolysis is the most established of the three percutaneous procedures. The end point of the procedure is to produce an area of decreased sensation in the painful area of the face. Patient cooperation during the stimulation testing procedure is important and is not readily obtained in some elderly patients. The recurrence rate is lower than for the other two procedures; however, the incidence of painful dysesthesia is greater. For ophthalmic branch neuralgia, the risk of corneal hypoesthesia is somewhat higher than with the alternative procedures.[42,43]

Glycerol rhizolysis does not require patient cooperation and has a lower incidence of facial dysesthesia. As glycerol rhizolysis has a higher recurrence rate (70% of patients remain pain

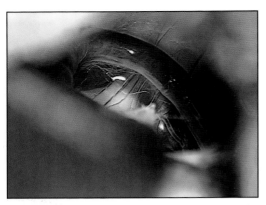

Fig 13-2 A view of the right trigeminal root through the operating microscope. An arterial loop of the superior cerebellar artery has been lifted off the root. The root has a bandlike grayish discoloration where it had been compressed close to its entrance to the brainstem.

free at the 1-year follow-up) than RF rhizolysis, repeat procedures may be necessary, but they increase the risk of subsequent dysesthesia.[44]

Balloon compression of the trigeminal root has a success rate between that of the other two procedures but results in a higher incidence of masticator muscle dysfunction. As a large-bore needle must be used for insertion, general anesthesia may be required, making it less appealing in the author's view.[45]

All three procedures are ablative. As in any procedure that damages the nervous system, the danger of developing dysesthesia and de-afferentation pain exists. For younger patients who have no significant medical risks, an MVD procedure may be more appropriate for the long term because it treats the structural cause of the pain-producing pathology without damaging the nerve root.[35,36,46]

Microvascular decompression

Many cases of trigeminal neuralgia are caused by vascular compression of the entry zone of the trigeminal root at the pons.[47] Other causes of trigeminal neuralgia, such as tumors compressing the trigeminal root (7% of patients) or multiple sclerosis (2% of patients), must be excluded, however, by performing an MRI scan before surgery. Using specific three-dimensional sequences, such as time-of-flight magnetic resonance angiography and

T2-driven equilibrium protocol, the vascular conflict can be visualized in a high percentage of patients,[48,49] allowing for a more targeted surgical approach.

The operation is performed under general anesthesia. A linear incision is made behind the ear on the side of the pain. A 20-mm craniotomy is performed at the angle between the transverse and sigmoid sinuses. Following the dural opening, the operative microscope is brought into the field and cerebrospinal fluid is allowed to egress. Cerebellar retraction is not needed if the patient is well anesthetized and properly positioned. The arachnoid over the trigeminal root is opened, and the root is carefully examined for possible arterial contacts. Arterial loops that knuckle into the root will frequently cause local discoloration of the root, implying secondary demyelination[4] (Fig 13-2). The vessel loop is moved from the root and kept at a distance by a shredded Teflon felt pledget. In about 10% of patients, no arterial contact is found despite diligent exploration. If a significant venous contact is present, a venous decompression typically provides pain relief.[50] Larger veins should not be coagulated because it is impossible to predict the presence of compensatory collaterals. No significant vascular contact is found on exploration in about 16% of patients.[51] In this situation, the trigeminal nerve fibers may be separated from each other by combing them with a micro-hook.[52] The patient can usually be discharged from the hospital 2 or 3 days after surgery (Case 13-1).

The advantage of MVD is that it resolves the causative pathology and stops the pain without causing nerve root damage. Sensory deafferentation phenomena are thereby avoided. The initial success rate is in the order of 90%, and the recurrence rate is around 2% per year,[53–55] with a 73% probability of cure at 15 years after surgery. These outcome results are better than those obtained in percutaneous rhizotomy. The outcome depends on the zeal and skill with which the surgeon can find the offending artery. In cases where no definite arterial compression is visualized, a topographically appropriate partial sensory rhizotomy has been suggested.[56–58] Newer techniques of rhizotomy, such as a partial crush of the root or internal neurolysis (combing) may lead to an acceptable level of

Trigeminal neuralgia treated by an MVD procedure.

CASE 13-1

Present complaint: A 49-year-old woman complained of daily, severe, knifelike pain attacks in the right side of her face. A trigger point was identified around the angle of the mouth from which the pain shot up to the temple on the same side. The attacks could be continuous for several hours. Speaking and chewing triggered attacks. The patient had recently increased her dosage of carbamazepine to 1,000 mg with the addition of baclofen 10 mg three times a day, but there was no effect on pain severity. As a result of the daily attacks, she had stopped working and refused to leave the house, except for frequenting the hospital's emergency department, where she received injections of narcotics.

History of present complaint: Five years ago, the patient underwent a root canal procedure in her right maxilla. She remembers suffering from intermittent pain in the area for several months afterward. The pain subsided spontaneously, but 18 months ago she suddenly developed the painful attacks from which she now suffers. At the time, they were less frequent, were limited in duration, and occurred over a smaller area of her face. She was prescribed carbamazepine 200 mg twice a day, which relieved her attacks for 2 months only. After the pain resumed, her dosage was gradually elevated to the present level. Two months ago, baclofen was added without effect.

Physical examination: Her physical and neurologic examinations, including facial sensation, were normal. During the examination, she had a painful attack. She winced on the right side of her face and became immobile for several seconds. Pressing her right cheek seemed to lessen the intensity of the pain.

Diagnostic examinations: A cranial MRI scan was performed. Nonspecific bright spots of white matter were seen in the cerebrum on the T2 scan. In the posterior fossa, the right trigeminal root was crossed by a vessel shadow at its entrance to the brainstem (Fig 13-3). A diagnostic evaluation for multiple sclerosis was negative.

Treatment considerations: The patient was referred for neurosurgical consultation. She refused to consider increasing her medication levels because they made her groggy. Considering her age and the positive MRI scan, an MVD procedure was recommended.

Operation: The patient was operated on under general anesthaesia in the supine position with her head turned to the left. Surgical exposure for MVD was performed as described earlier. The cerebellum was gently retracted to allow visualization of the upper cerebellopontine angle. The arachnoid over the trigeminal nerve was opened while preserving the petrosal vein intact. An artery was seen crossing and indenting the trigeminal root at its entry site into the brainstem. The artery was lifted off the nerve. A grayish discoloration of the nerve root was visible at the site of the vascular contact (see Fig 13-2). A small fluff of Teflon felt was inserted between the nerve root and the artery to prevent renewed contact. The wound was closed in a routine fashion. The operation was performed in 90 minutes.

Postoperative follow-up: The patient woke up from surgery without facial pain. She had an uncomplicated postoperative course and remained neurologically intact. Her medications were not renewed. She was discharged from the hospital after 48 hours. Seven years after surgery, she remained pain free.

dysesthesia while relieving the pain.[52,59] These results for MVD surgery refer to patients with typical trigeminal neuralgia.

When atypical features are present, such as a poorly defined trigger zone, a background of burning pain, or sensory loss, only about half the patients achieve a long-term satisfactory outcome.[31,60]

The morbidity of the surgery should be within 4%. This low morbidity and virtually zero mortality are achieved by limiting the operation to patients younger than 75 years who do not suffer from major systemic diseases. In older, high-risk patients percutaneous procedures would be more appropriate.[46] If the pain recurs after a successful MVD procedure, repeat MRI imaging should be performed. If no vascular compression is demonstrated, treatment options include re-exploration with internal neurolysis or a percutaneous rhizotomy.

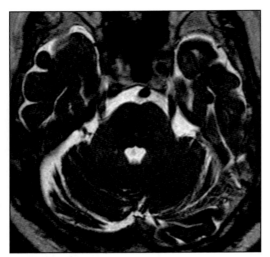

Fig 13-3 Case 13-1. A T2 MRI axial scan of the posterior fossa at the level of the trigeminal roots. A vessel is seen crossing the right trigeminal root, though the left trigeminal root is free of a vascular contact.

Stereotactic radiosurgery

In recent years, stereotactic radiosurgery has become a popular technique for the treatment of trigeminal neuralgia because of its relative noninvasiveness. This has made it an appropriate choice for high-risk patients, including those requiring anticoagulation therapy. The technique is also appropriate for patients for whom other surgical techniques have failed. The procedure involves the fixation of a stereotactic frame to the head of the patient under local anesthesia, MRI imaging while the patient is in the frame, and computer simulation of the radiosurgical treatment. Thus, the technique is more cumbersome, more labor intensive, and more expensive than the percutaneous ablative procedures. The onset of pain relief has a latency of several weeks; therefore, the technique is not desirable for patients with severe pain.[61] Recently, longer-term follow-up studies have shown that the effectiveness of the procedure is dose dependent. After a high radiation dose of 90 Gy, 70% of patients were pain free without or with medication for at least 2 years after treatment. However, 33% of patients suffered from facial numbness with this higher treatment

dose.[62] Freedom from pain, however, seems to decline notably over the years, limiting the appeal of this technique as a first-line therapy.[63]

Timing and choice of neurosurgical procedure in trigeminal neuralgia

Trigeminal neuralgia responds readily to medical therapy. Invasive therapy should only be considered after an adequate trial of medication has failed. If the patient stops responding to carbamazepine or suffers from side effects that affect quality of life, the medication may be switched to gabapentin or pregabalin, occasionally in combination with baclofen. If the patient remains symptomatic despite medical therapy, invasive therapy should be considered sooner rather than later. Chronic compression of the trigeminal nerve root may, over time, lead to neuropathic pain or atypical trigeminal neuralgia, which is less responsive to any type of therapy.[60,64]

The general consensus among neurosurgeons is that MVD is the procedure of choice in non-elderly and medically low-risk patients.[36,46,65] Modern high-tesla MRI scanners can often delineate the relevant artery compressing the trigeminal root[48,66] (see Fig 13-3). The high rates of long-term pain relief and the absence of neuropathic disturbances that accompany destructive procedures of the root make this procedure especially attractive for younger patients.

In the elderly or medically infirm, palliative percutaneous rhizolysis should be performed. Practitioners do not agree about which of the three commonly used procedures—retrogasserian glycerol injection, RF rhizolysis, or balloon compression—is preferred.[34,36,39,42] The author prefers glycerol rhizolysis because of its technical simplicity and because it does not require patient cooperation as RF rhizolysis does. After the glycerol procedure, some 40% of patients have sustained pain relief without noticeable hypoesthesia, whereas in the RF procedure, sensory loss is the end point of the thermal lesion in all patients. The trade-off is that after glycerol rhizolysis, only about 55% of patients are pain free at 5 years, compared with about 10% to 15% after RF rhizolysis. The ease of performing a repeat glycerol injection when pain recurs, however, outweighs the increased incidence of hypoesthesia and dysesthesia after the more aggressive RF rhizolysis. Because these two procedures are typically effective, there is little need for the balloon compression technique, which requires deeper sedation of the patient due to the large-bore needle used and has a higher incidence of serious side effects without providing notably better outcomes.

Trigeminal neuralgia secondary to multiple sclerosis

The incidence of trigeminal neuralgia in patients with multiple sclerosis is 2%. Although for most patients with multiple sclerosis the neuralgia is associated with reduction of facial sensation, at the beginning of the disease hypoesthesia may be absent. In the absence of typical neurologic symptomatology early in the course of the disease, an MRI image is pathognomonic of multiple sclerosis. After failure of medical therapy, the interventional options are similar to those for typical trigeminal neuralgia. If the MRI scan shows a typical vascular loop compressing the trigeminal root, an MVD procedure may be considered.[67–69] Given that only 50% of patients have long-term postoperative pain relief, a partial sensory rhizotomy should be added to the procedure unless the vessel pathology is very prominent.

More commonly, one of the percutaneous trigeminal rhizolysis procedures is chosen as a first-line option. Although treatment failures accumulate over time in most patients, significant pain relief can be obtained over a meaningful time frame. Balloon compression has been reported to have the highest initial pain-free response, followed by radiofrequency and glycerol rhizolysis.[70–72]

Glossopharyngeal neuralgia

Glossopharyngeal neuralgia is about 100 times more rare than trigeminal neuralgia. Its clinical manifestations, however, are more variable. Generally, pain is felt unilaterally in the throat region while swallowing or speaking. Autonomic manifestations, such as syncope or bradycardia leading even to asystole, are the most dramatic manifestations of the syndrome. Surgical therapy in patients who are medically refractory can be expected to lead to good results in a high percentage of patients. Classically, a

glossopharyngeal open rhizotomy is performed with the addition of an upper-third vagal rhizotomy. Complications include difficulty swallowing with or without hoarseness.[43] In the 1970s, percutaneous RF rhizotomy via the pars nervosa of the jugular foramen gained popularity and became the procedure of choice. Bradycardia and vocal cord paralysis are the risks of this procedure.[73] As with trigeminal neuralgia, MVD has been successful in relieving glossopharyngeal neuralgia pain, as the vascular etiology and pathologic picture have been found to be similar.[5] Some authors routinely perform a rhizotomy after vascular decompression.[73] Others have found that this is not necessary and have achieved long-term pain relief in more than 75% of patients with minimal permanent side effects.[53,74–76] These authors emphasize a careful search for the offending artery, which, when found, obviates the need for rhizotomy. Percutaneous computed tomography–guided RF trigeminal tractotomy-nucleotomy has more recently been described as useful for complex cases.[77] Very few centers, however, have experience with this technique.

Geniculate neuralgia

Geniculate neuralgia involves the sensory distribution of the seventh cranial nerve (facial nerve) via the nervus intermedius (of Wrisberg). The painful attacks are centered within the ear canal and are sharp and stabbing in nature. A dull background pain may persist for several hours after an attack.[78] Affected patients tend to be younger than those suffering from trigeminal and glossopharyngeal neuralgia. When seen together with hemifacial spasm, the term *tic convulsive* has been used.[79] The established surgical therapy is to section the nervus intermedius via a middle fossa approach[78] or in conjunction with an MVD of the adjacent cranial nerves.[80] A favorable outcome may be expected in up to 90% of patients.

Trigeminal autonomic cephalalgias

Of the trigeminal autonomic cephalalgias (see chapter 11), chronic cluster headaches that are unresponsive to medication have attracted surgical therapeutic attempts. RF ablation of the sphenopalatine ganglion has been useful in episodic cluster headaches but unsuccessful in patients with chronic headache.[81] Trigeminal rhizotomy may lead to corneal anesthesia and has an inconsistent beneficial effect.[82] Whether sectioning of the nervus intermedius improves outcome is doubtful,[82,83] though combining it with MVD of the trigeminal root has shown beneficial results.[84]

Percutaneous RF trigeminal rhizotomy is a less invasive procedure and has been successfully used to treat pain around the eye. Major pain in the malar and temporal areas responded poorly.[85] Considering the disabling consequences of the accompanying corneal hypoesthesia, glycerol trigeminal rhizolysis may be the initial invasive procedure of choice.[86] Glycerol trigeminal rhizolysis has also been successfully applied in the treatment of short-lasting unilateral neuralgiform headache attacks with conjunctival injection and tearing (SUNCT).[87]

Broggi et al[88] have summarized their experience in treating chronic trigeminal autonomic cephalalgias with electrical stimulation of the posterior hypothalamus. Of 16 patients with chronic cluster headaches, 10 were completely pain free over the 5-year follow-up period, as was the single patient with SUNCT. The same procedure failed completely in three patients with atypical facial pain. Because this procedure is relatively low risk and reversible, it provides an attractive treatment modality, if these results can be duplicated by others.

Atypical facial pain

Atypical facial pain is a poorly defined clinical entity that has a large variety of potential causes (see chapter 12) and is one of the most difficult chronic pain entities to treat. Consequently, patients have been subjected to a large variety of surgical procedures ranging from local neurectomies to cerebral ablative procedures.[43] Success rates have varied greatly, which reflects the lack of homogeneity of the patient population. Surgical procedures should not be performed if the pathophysiology of the pain syndrome remains obscure. In cases of trigeminal neuropathic pain, stimulation of the trigeminal root via a transoval percutaneously implanted electrode has shown some success, relieving pain in about half of the treated patients.[28] Movement and breakage of the elec-

trode during mastication limits the technical success rate of the procedure. Thus, it has had very limited popularity.

RF lesions to the entry zone of the nucleus caudalis dorsal root have been advocated for otherwise intractable facial pain syndromes. A posterior fossa craniotomy and upper cervical laminectomy are performed, and thermal lesions of the nucleus are made from the level of the obex down to the C2 level of the spinal cord.[89–90] Given the high incidence of neurologic complications (ipsilateral arm ataxia due to spinocerebellar tract injury and ipsilateral lower limb weakness from the pyramidal tract), this procedure should be reserved for pain secondary to malignancy only.

Percutaneous trigeminal tractotomy-nucleotomy is performed under computed tomography guidance by inserting an RF electrode between the occiput and the lamina of C1 into the posterolateral spinal cord. The technique has a lower incidence of undesirable neurologic side effects compared with open procedures but also more limited applicability.[77] In a recent series of 17 patients with atypical facial pain treated by this method, only 7 were deemed to have had a good long-term response.[91] The categorization of the pain type that shows the best response is as yet unclear, and the surgical experience is as yet quite limited. However, the technique remains an interesting option for severe cases.

Motor cortex stimulation has been used over the past several years in a variety of central pain conditions.[92] The motor cortex is visualized on an MRI scan transferred to a neuronavigation system in the operating room. A limited craniotomy is performed over the appropriate area, and the position of the motor cortex is confirmed by intraoperative electrical stimulation. The electrode is then implanted at this site and attached to a supraclavicular generator. For atypical facial pain, the electrode would be implanted over the facial motor cortex.[93] In a series reported by Brown and Pilitsis in 2005,[94] motor cortex stimulation was applied in 10 patients with facial pain due to postherpetic neuralgia, surgical trigeminal injury, and a medullary infarct. After trial stimulation, eight systems were implanted. At a mean follow-up of 10 months, patients had a 75% decrease in their pain, which had been present for a mean of 6 years. In their literature review, the authors found that 29 of 38 (76%) patients with neuropathic facial pain treated with motor cortex stimulation achieved greater than 50% pain relief. Monsalve[95] provided the most up-to-date literature review in 2012. He found a total of 118 patients who underwent a trial of motor cortex stimulation for chronic facial neuropathic pain; 100 patients underwent internalization of the stimulation system and had an 84% success rate.[95] However, no randomized controlled studies in chronic facial pain have as yet been reported. The procedure must therefore still be classified as experimental and should be performed by specialized centers as part of a research protocol. These encouraging results, if more widely confirmed, will open a therapeutic window for a difficult class of patients.

Conclusion

Structural lesions of the central and peripheral nervous system are not infrequent causes of orofacial pain that may be relieved by neurosurgical intervention. Paroxysmal pain in an anatomical neural distribution, such as in trigeminal neuralgia, is the type of pain most responsive to neurosurgical procedures. Destructive lesions of the nervous system may be required in the more diffuse chronic pain conditions, but these entail potential complications and have a lower success rate. Electrical stimulation is an attractive alternative that has the advantage of being reversible. The role of such procedures as motor cortex stimulation in the treatment of intractable chronic orofacial pain syndromes and deep brain stimulation for chronic trigeminal autonomic cephalalgias is still under investigation.

References

1. Burchiel KJ. A new classification for facial pain. Neurosurgery 2003;53:1164–1166.
2. Møller AR. Vascular compression of cranial nerves. I. History of the microvascular decompression operation. Neurol Res 1998;20:727–731.
3. Møller AR. Vascular compression of cranial nerves: II: Pathophysiology. Neurol Res 1999;21:439–443.
4. Devor M, Govrin-Lippmann R, Rappaport ZH. Mechanism of trigeminal neuralgia: An ultrastructural analysis of trigeminal root specimens obtained during microvascular decompression surgery. J Neurosurg 2002;96:532–543.
5. Devor M, Govrin-Lippmann R, Rappaport ZH, Tasker RR, Dostrovsky JO. Cranial root injury in glossopharyngeal neuralgia: Electron microscopic observations. Case report. J Neurosurg 2002;96:603–606.
6. Devor M, Amir R, Rappaport ZH. Pathophysiology of trigeminal neuralgia: The ignition hypothesis. Clin J Pain 2002;18:4–13
7. Ito M, Sonokawa T, Mishina H, Iizuka Y, Sato K. Dural arteriovenous malformation manifesting as tic douloureux. Surg Neurol 1996;45:370–375.
8. Karibe H, Shirane R, Jokura H, Yoshimoto T. Intrinsic arteriovenous malformation of the trigeminal nerve in a patient with trigeminal neuralgia: Case report. Neurosurgery 2004;55:1433.
9. Linskey ME, Sekhar LN, Hirsch WL Jr, Yonas H, Horton JA. Aneurysms of the intracavernous carotid artery: Natural history and indications for treatment. Neurosurgery 1990;26:933–937.
10. Younger DS. Headaches and vasculitis. Neurol Clin 2004;22:207–228.
11. Selky AK, Pascuzzi R. Raeder's paratrigeminal syndrome due to spontaneous dissection of the cervical and petrous internal carotid artery. Headache 1995;35:432–434.
12. Saeed AB, Shuaib A, Al-Sulaiti G, Emery D. Vertebral artery dissection: Warning symptoms, clinical features and prognosis in 26 patients. Can J Neurol Sci 2000;27:292–296.
13. Mainardi F, Maggioni F, Dainese F, Amistà P, Zanchin G. Spontaneous carotid artery dissection with cluster-like headache. Cephalalgia 2002;22:557–559.
14. Goh BT, Poon CY, Peck RH. The importance of routine magnetic resonance imaging in trigeminal neuralgia diagnosis. Oral Surg Oral Med Oral Pathol Oral Radiol Endod 2001;92:424–429.
15. Yang J, Simonson TM, Ruprecht A, Meng D, Vincent SD, Yuh WT. Magnetic resonance imaging used to assess patients with trigeminal neuralgia. Oral Surg Oral Med Oral Pathol Oral Radiol Endod 1996;81:343–350.
16. Samii M, Carvalho GA, Tatagiba M, Matthies C. Surgical management of meningiomas originating in Meckel's cave. Neurosurgery 1997;41:767–774.
17. Dolenc VV. Frontotemporal epidural approach to trigeminal neurinomas. Acta Neurochir (Wien) 1994;130:55–65.
18. Barker FG, Jannetta PJ, Babu RP, Pomonis S, Bissonette DJ, Jho HD. Long-term outcome after operation for trigeminal neuralgia in patients with posterior fossa tumors. J Neurosurg 1996;84:818–825.
19. Matsuka Y, Fort ET, Merrill RL. Trigeminal neuralgia due to an acoustic neuroma in the cerebellopontine angle. J Orofac Pain 2000;14:147–151.
20. Rappaport ZH. Epidermoid tumour of the cerebellopontine angle as a cause of trigeminal neuralgia. Neurochirurgia (Stuttg) 1985;28:211–212.
21. Meng L, Yuguang L, Feng L, Wandong S, Shugan Z, Chengyuan W. Cerebellopontine angle epidermoids presenting with trigeminal neuralgia. J Clin Neurosci 2005;12:784–786
22. Pollock BE, Iuliano BA, Foote RL, Gorman DA. Stereotactic radiosurgery for tumor-related trigeminal pain. Neurosurgery 2000;46:576–582.

23. Förderreuther S, Straube A. The criteria of the International Headache Society for Tolosa-Hunt syndrome need to be revised. J Neurol 1999;246:371–377.

24. Yamamoto T, Goto K, Suzuki A, Nakamura N, Mizuno Y. Long-term improvement of idiopathic hypertrophic cranial pachymeningitis by lymphocytapheresis. Ther Apher 2000;4:313–316.

25. Quinones-Hinojosa A, Chang EF, Khan SA, McDermott MW. Isolated trigeminal nerve sarcoid granuloma mimicking trigeminal schwannoma: Case report. Neurosurgery 2003;52:700–705.

26. Lee O, Cromwell LD, Weider DJ. Carcinomatous meningitis arising from primary nasopharyngeal carcinoma. Am J Otolaryngol 2005;26:193–197.

27. Yi HJ, Kim CH, Bak KH, Kim JM, Ko Y, Oh SJ. Metastatic tumors in the sellar and parasellar regions: Clinical review of four cases. J Korean Med Sci 2000;15:363–367.

28. Young RF. Electrical stimulation of the trigeminal nerve root for the treatment of chronic facial pain. J Neurosurg 1995;83:72–78.

29. McNatt SA, Yu C, Giannotta SL, Zee CS, Apuzzo ML, Petrovich Z. Gamma knife radiosurgery for trigeminal neuralgia. Neurosurgery 2005;56:1295–1301.

30. Sheehan J, Pan HC, Stroila M, Steiner L. Gamma knife surgery for trigeminal neuralgia: Outcomes and prognostic factors. J Neurosurg 2005;102:434–441.

31. Miller JP, Magill ST, Acar F, Burchiel KJ. Predictors of long-term success after microvascular decompression for trigeminal neuralgia. J Neurosurg 2009;110:620–626.

32. Oturai AB, Jensen K, Eriksen J, Madsen F. Neurosurgery for trigeminal neuralgia: Comparison of alcohol block, neurectomy, and radiofrequency coagulation. Clin J Pain 1996;12:311–315.

33. Murali R, Rovit RL. Are peripheral neurectomies of value in the treatment of trigeminal neuralgia? An analysis of new cases and cases involving previous radiofrequency gasserian thermocoagulation. J Neurosurg 1996;85:435–437.

34. Moraci A, Buonaiuto C, Punzo A, Parlato C, Amalfi R. Trigeminal neuralgia treated by percutaneous thermocoagulation. Comparative analysis of percutaneous thermocoagulation and other surgical procedures. Neurochirurgia (Stuttg) 1992;35:48–53.

35. Taha JM, Tew JM Jr. Comparison of surgical treatments for trigeminal neuralgia: Reevaluation of radiofrequency rhizotomy. Neurosurgery 1996;38:865–871.

36. Broggi G, Ferroli P, Franzini A, Galosi L. The role of surgery in the treatment of typical and atypical facial pain. Neurol Sci 2005;26(2, suppl):S95–S100.

37. Gomori JM, Rappaport ZH. Transovale trigeminal cistern puncture: Modified fluoroscopically guided technique. AJNR Am J Neuroradiol 1985;6:93–94.

38. Jho HD, Lunsford LD. Percutaneous retrogasserian glycerol rhizotomy. Current technique and results. Neurosurg Clin N Am 1997;8:63–74.

39. Kondziolka D, Lunsford LD. Percutaneous retrogasserian glycerol rhizotomy for trigeminal neuralgia: Technique and expectations. Neurosurg Focus 2005;18:e7.

40. Pollock BE. Percutaneous retrogasserian glycerol rhizotomy for patients with idiopathic trigeminal neuralgia: A prospective analysis of factors related to pain relief. J Neurosurg 2005;102:223–228.

41. Brown JA, Gouda JJ. Percutaneous balloon compression of the trigeminal nerve. Neurosurg Clin N Am 1997;8:53–62.

42. Sweet WH. Percutaneous methods for the treatment of trigeminal neuralgia and other faciocephalic pain: Comparison with microvascular decompression. Semin Neurol 1988;8:272–279.

43. Gybels JM, Sweet WH. Neurosurgical Treatment of Persistant Pain: Physiological and Pathological Mechanisms of Human Pain. Basel: Karger, 1989.

44. Rappaport ZH, Gomori JM. Recurrent trigeminal cistern glycerol injections for tic douloureux. Acta Neurochir (Wien) 1988;90:31–34.

45. Fraioli B, Esposito V, Guidetti B, Cruccu G, Manfredi M. Treatment of trigeminal neuralgia by thermocoagulation, glycerolization, and percutaneous compression of the gasserian ganglion and/or retrogasserian rootlets: Long-term results and therapeutic protocol. Neurosurgery 1989;24:239–245.

46. Rappaport ZH. The choice of therapy in medically intractable trigeminal neuralgia. Isr J Med Sci 1996;32:1232–1234.

47. Haines SJ, Jannetta PJ, Zorub DS. Microvascular relations of the trigeminal nerve. An anatomical study with clinical correlation. J Neurosurg 1980;52:381–386.

48. Miller JP, Acar F, Hamilton B, Burchiel KJ. Preoperative visualization of neurovascular anatomy in trigeminal neuralgia. J Neurosurg 2008;108:477–482.

49. Leal PR, Hermier M, Souza MA, Cristino-Filho G, Froment JC, Sindou M. Visualization of vascular compression of the trigeminal nerve with high-resolution 3T MRI: A prospective study comparing preoperative imaging analysis to surgical findings in 40 consecutive patients who underwent microvascular decompression for trigeminal neuralgia. Neurosurgery 2011;69:15–25.

50. Matsushima T, Huynh-Le P, Miyazono M. Trigeminal neuralgia caused by venous compression. Neurosurgery 2004;55:334–337.

51. Lee A, McCartney S, Burbidge C, Raslan AM, Burchiel KJ. Trigeminal neuralgia occurs and recurs in the absence of neurovascular compression. J Neurosurg 2014;120:1048–1054.

52. Jie H, Xuanchen Z, Deheng L, et al. The long-term outcome of nerve combing for trigeminal neuralgia. Acta Neurochir 2013;155:1703–1708.

53. Sindou M, Mertens P. Microsurgical vascular decompression (MVD) in trigeminal and glosso-vago-pharyngeal neuralgias. A twenty year experience. Acta Neurochir Suppl (Wien) 1993;58:168–170.

54. Barker FG 2nd, Jannetta PJ, Bissonette DJ, Larkins MV, Jho HD. The long-term outcome of microvascular decompression for trigeminal neuralgia. N Engl J Med 1996;334:1077–1083.

55. Sindou M, Leston J, Decullier E, Chapuis F. Microvascular decompression for primary trigeminal neuralgia: Long-term effectiveness and prognostic factors in a series of 362 consecutive patients with clear-cut neurovascular conflicts who underwent pure decompression. J Neurosurg 2007;107:1144–1153.

56. Bederson JB, Wilson CB. Evaluation of microvascular decompression and partial sensory rhizotomy in 252 cases of trigeminal neuralgia. J Neurosurg 1989;71:359–367.

57. Klun B. Microvascular decompression and partial sensory rhizotomy in the treatment of trigeminal neuralgia: Personal experience with 220 patients. Neurosurgery 1992;30:49–52.

58. Delitala A, Brunori A, Chiappetta F. Microsurgical posterior fossa exploration for trigeminal neuralgia: A study on 48 cases. Minim Invasive Neurosurg 2001;44:152-156.

59. Zakrzewska JM, Lopez BC, Kim SE, Coakham HB. Patient reports of satisfaction after microvascular decompression and partial sensory rhizotomy for trigeminal neuralgia. Neurosurgery 2005;56:1304–1311.

60. Tyler-Kabara EC, Kassam AB, Horowitz MH, et al. Predictors of outcome in surgically managed patients with typical and atypical trigeminal neuralgia: Comparison of results following microvascular decompression. J Neurosurg 2002;96:527–531.

61. Henson CF, Goldman HW, Rosenwasser RH, et al. Glycerol rhizotomy versus gamma knife radiosurgery for the treatment of trigeminal neuralgia: An analysis of patients treated at one institution. Int J Radiat Oncol Biol Phys 2005;63:82–90.

62. Young B, Shivazad A, Kryscio RA, St Clair W, Bush HM. Long-term outcome of high-dose γ knife surgery in treatment of trigeminal neuralgia. J Neurosurg 2012;119:1166–1175.

63. Dhople AA, Adams JR, Maggio WW, Naqvi SA, Regine WF, Kwok Y. Long-term outcomes of Gamma Knife radiosurgery for classic trigeminal neuralgia: Implications for treatment and critical review of the literature. J Neurosurg 2009;111:351–358.

64. Li ST, Pan Q, Liu N, Shen F, Liu Z, Guan Y. Trigeminal neuralgia: What are the important factors for good operative outcomes with microvascular decompression. Surg Neurol 2004;62:400–404.

65. Javadpour M, Eldridge PR, Varma TR, Miles JB, Nurmikko TJ. Microvascular decompression for trigeminal neuralgia in patients over 70 years of age. Neurology 2003;60:520.

66. Vörös E, Palkó A, Horváth K, Barzó P, Kardos L, Kuncz A. Three-dimensional time-of-flight MR angiography in trigeminal neuralgia on a 0.5-T system. Eur Radiol 2001;11:642–647.

67. Resnick DK, Jannetta PJ, Lunsford LD, Bissonette DJ. Microvascular decompression for trigeminal neuralgia in patients with multiple sclerosis. Surg Neurol 1996;–46:358–361.

68. Eldridge PR, Sinha AK, Javadpour M, Littlechild P, Varma TR. Microvascular decompression for trigeminal neuralgia in patients with multiple sclerosis. Stereotact Funct Neurosurg 2003;81:57–64.

69. Broggi G, Ferroli P, Franzini A, et al. Operative findings and outcomes of microvascular decompression for trigeminal neuralgia in 35 patients affected by multiple sclerosis. Neurosurgery 2004;55:830–838.

70. Berk C, Constantoyannis C, Honey CR. The treatment of trigeminal neuralgia in patients with multiple sclerosis using percutaneous radiofrequency rhizotomy. Can J Neurol Sci 2003;30:220–223.

71. Pickett GE, Bisnaire D, Ferguson GG. Percutaneous retrogasserian glycerol rhizotomy in the treatment of tic douloureux associated with multiple sclerosis. Neurosurgery 2005;56:537–545.

72. Mohammad-Mohammadi AM, Recinos PF, Lee JH, Elson P, Barnett GH. Surgical outcomes of trigeminal neuralgia in patients with multiple sclerosis. Neurosurgery 2013;73:941–950.

73. Taha JM, Tew JM Jr. Long-term results of surgical treatment of idiopathic neuralgias of the glossopharyngeal and vagal nerves. Neurosurgery 1995;36:926–930.

74. Resnick DK, Jannetta PJ, Bissonnette D, Jho HD, Lanzino G. Microvascular decompression for glossopharyngeal neuralgia. Neurosurgery 1995;36:64–68.

75. Kondo A. Follow-up results of using microvascular decompression for treatment of glossopharyngeal neuralgia. J Neurosurg 1998;88:221–225.

76. Rey-Dios R, Cohen-Gadol AA. Current neurosurgical management of glossopharyngeal neuralgia and technical nuances for microvascular decompression surgery. Neurosurg Focus 2013;34:e8.

77. Kanpolat Y, Savas A, Batay F, Sinav A. Computed tomography-guided trigeminal tractotomy-nucleotomy in the management of vagoglossopharyngeal and geniculate neuralgias. Neurosurgery 1998;43:484–489.

78. Pulec JL. Geniculate neuralgia: Long-term results of surgical treatment. Ear Nose Throat J 2002;81:30–33.

79. Yeh HS, Tew JM Jr. Tic convulsif, the combination of geniculate neuralgia and hemifacial spasm relieved by vascular decompression. Neurology 1984;34:682–683.

80. Lovely TJ, Jannetta PJ. Surgical management of geniculate neuralgia. Am J Otol 1997;18:512–517.

81. Sanders M, Zuurmond WW. Efficacy of sphenopalatine ganglion blockade in 66 patients suffering from cluster headache: A 12- to 70-month follow-up evaluation. J Neurosurg 1997;87:876–880.

82. Morgenlander JC, Wilkins RH. Surgical treatment of cluster headache. J Neurosurg 1990;72:866–871.

83. Rowed DW. Chronic cluster headache managed by nervus intermedius section. Headache 1990;30:401–406.

84. Lovely TJ, Kotsiakis X, Jannetta PJ. The surgical management of chronic cluster headache. Headache 1998;38:590–594.

85. Taha JM, Tew JM Jr. Long-term results of radiofrequency rhizotomy in the treatment of cluster headache. Headache 1995;35:193–196.

86. Hassenbusch SJ, Kunkel RS, Kosmorsky GS, Covington EC, Pillay PK. Trigeminal cisternal injection of glycerol for treatment of chronic intractable cluster headaches. Neurosurgery 1991;29:504–508.

87. Hannerz J, Linderoth B. Neurosurgical treatment of short-lasting, unilateral, neuralgiform hemicrania with conjuctival injection and tearing. Br J Neurosurg 2002;16:55–58.

88. Broggi G, Franzini A, Leone M, Bussone G. Update on neurosurgical treatment of chronic trigeminal autonomic cephalalgias and atypical facial pain with deep brain stimulation of posterior hypothalamus: Results and comments. Neurol Sci 2007;28(2, suppl):S138–S145.

89. Gorecki JP, Nashold BS Jr. The Duke experience with the nucleus caudalis DREZ operation. Acta Neurochir Suppl 1995;64:128–131.

90. Bullard DE, Nashold BS Jr. The caudalis DREZ for facial pain. Stereotact Funct Neurosurg 1997;68:168–174.

91. Kanpolat Y, Savas A, Ugur HC, Bozkurt M. The trigeminal tract and nucleus procedures in treatment of atypical facial pain. Surg Neurol 2005;64(suppl 2):S96–S100.

92. Tirakotai W, Riegel T, Sure U, et al. Image-guided motor cortex stimulation in patients with central pain. Minim Invasive Neurosurg 2004;47:273–277.

93. Rainov NG, Heidecke V. Motor cortex stimulation for neuropathic facial pain. Neurol Res 2003;25:157–61.

94. Brown JA, Pilitsis JG. Motor cortex stimulation for central and neuropathic facial pain: A prospective study of 10 patients and observations of enhanced sensory and motor function during stimulation. Neurosurgery 2005;56:290–297.

95. Monsalve GA. Motor cortex stimulation for facial chronic neuropathic pain: A review of the literature. Surg Neurol Int 2012;3(suppl 4):S290–S311.

Secondary Orofacial Pain and Headache: Systemic Diseases, Tumors, and Trauma

Sharon Elad, DMD, MSc

Herve Sroussi, DMD, PhD

Gary D. Klasser, DMD

Joel Epstein, DMD, MSD, FRCD(C), FDS RCS (Edin)

This chapter presents an overview of systemic diseases that may induce orofacial pain or headache. As clinicians, it is important to identify pain that may be secondary to systemic and remote disease processes and therefore amenable to therapy of the primary condition. This chapter reviews orofacial pain in cancer patients and extends the review on tumors that may cause headache or facial pain. Lastly, regional trauma is grouped as a secondary pain in this chapter (Box 14-1).

Orofacial Pain in Metabolic and Endocrine Disorders

Clinicians must be aware of the possibility that certain systemic metabolic disorders may cause facial pain, and this pain may even be the initial presentation of the disorder. Because the metabolic condition is systemic, the effects usually appear in multiple sites. The more common pain-inducing metabolic disorders that clinicians should note are diabetes, alcoholism, and nutritional neuropathies. The common hallmark of these disorders is involvement of peripheral nerves by alteration of the structure or function of myelin and axons due to metabolic pathway dysregulation. However, the exact mechanism by which a systemic condition can induce pain is still controversial (see also chapter 12). In most of these conditions, the pain associated with these metabolic polyneuropathies is customarily found in the extremities and not in the orofacial structures. However, even though pain in the facial region is rare, clinicians must appreciate the possibility that such neuropathies exist in order to direct therapy to the actual source of the condition.

- Orofacial Pain in Metabolic and Endocrine Disorders
- Orofacial Pain in Joint Disorders
- Orofacial Pain in Bone Disorders
- Orofacial Pain in Immunologically Mediated Diseases
- Orofacial Pain in Neurologic Disorders
- Orofacial Pain in Cardiovascular Diseases
- Orofacial Pain in Blood Disorders
- Orofacial Pain in Dialysis and Renal Disorders
- Orofacial Pain in Pulmonary Diseases
- Orofacial Pain in Patients with Cancer
- Orofacial Pain in Patients with HIV
- Aggregation disease
- Craniofacial Pain Related to Miscellaneous Medical Conditions

HIV, human immunodeficiency virus.

Diabetic neuropathy

Demyelination of peripheral nerves associated with diabetes may lead to neuropathic changes in the motor, autonomic, and sensory nervous systems. Up to 48% of persons with diabetes suffer from neuropathy.[1] The incidence of cranial nerve involvement ranges from 3% to 14%, and most of these are motor neuropathies.[2]

Diabetic polyneuropathy is multifactorial in etiology. Results from the Diabetes Control and Complications Trial demonstrated that hyperglycemia and insulin deficiency contribute to the development of diabetic neuropathy and that glycemic control lowers the risk of neuropathy by 60% over 5 years.[3] Researchers hypothesize that decreased bioavailability of systemic insulin in diabetes may contribute to more severe axonal atrophy or loss. Additionally, hyperglycemia may cause microvasculitis, which may lead to an ischemic injury and result in demyelination and axonal dystrophy.[4] Elevated endoneurial glucose, fructose, and sorbitol levels in diabetes are associated with neuronal degeneration and the severity of neuropathy.[5]

Involvement of the third, fourth, sixth, and seventh cranial nerves in diabetic neuropathies have been well documented.[6] The trigeminal (fifth cranial) nerve rarely appears to be involved in diabetes, although there are case reports.[7,8] In a case-control study involving 29 patients with type 2 diabetes, orofacial pain was reported by 55.2%, and 17.2% of patients had burning mouth syndrome. The authors observed a somatosensory impairment of the right maxillary branch of the trigeminal nerve, which suggests an asymmetric pattern, such as in distal body areas typical of this disease. Sensory loss at the trigeminal area was also observed based on poor control of glycemia and glycated hemoglobin.[9] Patients with diabetic neuropathy often complain of a sharp, shooting pain in the mandible and tongue with occasional involvement of the mucosa. Additionally, it has been found that peripheral polyneuropathies often cause subclinical damage to the trigeminal nerve (thus leading to an underreporting of such events). The mandibular branch is often affected, and patients complain of unilateral facial paresthesia or hypoesthesia in the mental nerve distribution, mandibular pain, and abnormal motor responses in facial or masticatory muscles.[7] The cramped anatomical route of nerves in the mandibular canal or below the internal pterygoid muscle and fascia may expose them to an increased risk of damage.[7] Primary treatment should be directed at the underlying metabolic condition. Symptoms of polyneuropathy may be treated with an approach similar to that of other neuropathic pain (see chapters 12 and 16).

Alcohol and nutritional neuropathy

Alcoholism, or addiction to alcohol, is a worldwide problem with enormous medical, social, and economic costs to the affected person and to society. People who engage in chronic alcohol consumption are at risk for a number of serious medical complications, including neurologic disorders.[10] Alcoholic polyneuropathy can be purely motor or purely sensory in its effects, although the most common clinical presentation is mixed. Persons with alcoholism frequently suffer from entrapment or pressure neuropathies, especially in the ulnar and peroneal nerves. Paresthesias, pain, and weakness are common, mainly in the extremities. Several reports appear in the literature that describe patients with alcoholism who have hearing loss, balance disturbances, and facial weakness related to degeneration of the eighth cranial nerve. Distal muscle weakness and atrophy are also common findings in the extremities but have not been reported from the orofacial region.[11]

The pathogenesis of alcoholic polyneuropathy is not fully understood.[12] Some believe that most associated medical disorders may be due to ethanol neurotoxicity.[13] Other reports suggest that malnutrition is the cause of most alcohol-related neurologic disorders; patients with alcoholism often obtain as much as 50% of their calories from ethanol, which allows serious nutritional deficiencies to develop, particularly for protein, thiamine, folate, and niacin.[14,15] Another possibility may be that alcohol consumption has direct negative effects on the gastrointestinal mucosa and pancreas that result in malabsorption of essential nutrients.[16] Neuropathy is characterized by axonal degeneration and demyelination, and evidence suggest that ethanol has a direct neurotoxic effect on the peripheral nerves.[17]

Hypothyroidism

Hypofunction of the thyroid gland is one of the most common endocrine disorders in older women and may be associated with headaches. Of 102 adult patients with hypothyroidism, 30% reported headaches 1 to 2 months after initial symptoms of hypothyroidism.[18] Headaches are usually bilateral, mild, nonpulsatile, and continuous, and there is a female preponderance and an association with a history of migraine in childhood. The headache is not associated with nausea or vomiting.[19] The condition has a good response to abortive salicylates, and administration of thyroid hormone usually leads to headache resolution. The pathophysiology of hypothyroidism-related headache may be due to an underlying metabolic or vascular process.[18]

Orofacial Pain in Joint Disorders

Polyarthritides are a group of disorders in which the articular surfaces become inflamed and that sometimes involve the temporomandibular joint (TMJ). The signs and symptoms in polyarthritides may be similar to those found in degenerative joint disease (osteoarthritis); however, the causative factors are different (see chapter 9). The polyarthritides include rheumatoid arthritis, psoriatic arthritis, ankylosing spondylitis, infectious arthritis, hyperuricemia, traumatic arthritis, Reiter syndrome, and neck-tongue syndrome. Differentiating among these various conditions is important as treatment modalities differ. As a general rule, systemic polyarthritides rarely involve the TMJ.

Rheumatoid arthritis

Rheumatoid arthritis is a systemic, chronic, inflammatory disease of unknown etiology. Factors associated with rheumatoid arthritis include the possibility of infectious triggers, genetic predisposition, and autoimmune response in that CD4p T cells stimulate the immune cascade, which leads to cytokine production such as tumor necrosis factor alpha and interleukin-1.[20,21] The disease affects the articular surfaces, including the synovial tissues, capsule, tendons, and ligaments. The inflammatory process leads to the secondary destruction of the articular cartilage and subchondral bone.[22] Rheumatoid arthritis has an insidious onset with periods of exacerbation and remission.

The prevalence in Western populations is 0.5% to 1%, and the female-male ratio is approximately 3:1.[23] The disease can occur at any age, though onset is usually between the ages of 25 and 50 years, and the incidence peaks in the fourth and fifth decades of life. Characteristically, rheumatoid arthritis affects small peripheral joints, such as those in the hands, wrists, and feet. Joint involvement in rheumatoid arthritis tends to be symmetric and more generalized in its clinical presentation compared with degenerative joint disease.[24] The prevalence of TMJ involvement in patients with rheumatic disease varies greatly, depending on the diagnostic criteria, the population studied, and the measures of assessment. Clinical involvement of the TMJ is present in approximately 50% of patients with rheumatoid arthritis and seems to correlate with disease duration and severity.[25] The most common clinical signs and symptoms in the orofacial region are bilateral, deep, dull, aching pain (exacerbated during function); tenderness and swelling in the preauricular regions; limitation of mandibular range of movement; stiffness in the TMJ upon awakening; intracapsular joint sounds (crepitus/clicking); and tenderness of the masticatory muscles.[22,24,26] As the disease progresses, limitation in opening may be worsened because of fibrous or bony ankylosis.[27,28] If greater destruction of the condyles occurs, the patient may develop a progressive Class II malocclusion with heavy posterior occlusal contacts and an anterior open bite caused by loss of ramus height.[24,29]

Approximately 50% to 80% of patients with rheumatoid arthritis have radiographic evidence of TMJ abnormalities.[30] The radiographic findings of the TMJ, although not evident in the early stages of the disease process, become more apparent with disease progression. Use of magnetic resonance imaging (MRI) and computed tomography reveal joint effusions, disc displacements, and condylar abnormalities, including erosions, flattening, sclerosis, subchondral cysts, and osteophytes.[31,32]

Symptomatic TMJs in patients with rheumatoid arthritis demonstrate a high frequency of synovial inflammation and connective tissue degeneration, similar to what is seen in patients with osteoarthritis but different from matched control subjects. Additionally, pronounced inflammatory and degenerative changes develop faster in rheumatoid arthritis than osteoarthritis.[33]

A pediatric form termed *juvenile rheumatoid arthritis* (the term commonly used in the United States), *juvenile idiopathic arthritis* (the term used mainly in pediatric rheumatology), or *juvenile chronic arthritis* occurs in patients under the age of 16 years. Prevalence estimates in the United States range from 0.2 to 0.5 cases per 1,000 children, and there is a predominance in females (female-male ratio of 2–3:1).[34]

Juvenile rheumatoid arthritis is characterized by two peaks of onset, one between the ages of 1 and 3 years and the other between the ages of 8 and 12 years.[35] The prevalence of TMJ involvement in patients with juvenile rheumatoid arthritis is variable because different methods are used in assessment,[36] and when present, it may lead to adverse effects on occlusion and facial growth.[37] Juvenile rheumatoid arthritis is subclassified into three categories: polyarticular (ie, multiple joints affected), pauciarticular or oligoarticular (ie, fewer than four joints affected),

and systemic, which features high fever, rash, and multiple organ involvement.[35] The International League of Associations for Rheumatology has a more extensive classification system (seven subtypes with specific exclusion and inclusion criteria) for juvenile idiopathic arthritis.[38] Although the TMJ may be involved in any of these categories, it is most often affected by the polyarticular form.[39] The clinical and radiographic features are similar to those observed in the adult form of the disease. A characteristic feature of advanced juvenile rheumatoid arthritis is a significant reduction in the dimensions of the lower third of the face caused by a combination of micrognathia and a Class II skeletal distortion termed *birdface deformity*. This is the result of destruction of the condylar growth site by the disease process.[40,41]

Psoriatic arthritis

Psoriatic arthritis is an inflammatory condition associated with psoriasis, which is a chronic, often pruritic dermatologic disease with a genetic component that affects 1% to 2% of the population. Associated arthritis affects approximately 6% of this population, making this a relatively uncommon condition.[42] Indeed, fewer than 40 cases of psoriatic arthritis affecting the TMJ have been reported.[43,44] However, clinical and radiographic findings associated with temporomandibular disorders (TMDs) in patients with generalized psoriatic arthritis seem to be more common than these case reports suggest.[45]

Psoriatic arthritis of the TMJ is often unilateral, of sudden onset, and episodic. Patients commonly complain of tenderness and pain in the preauricular region and the muscles of mastication, morning stiffness, fatigue, and tiredness in the jaws. Signs include joint crepitation, painful mandibular function, and a progressive decrease in interincisal opening.[44,46] Ankylosis of the joint has been reported in severe cases.[47,48] Spontaneous remission has also been reported.

Radiographic changes of the TMJs associated with psoriatic arthritis are quite common and include the following nonspecific findings: erosion, flattening, osteoporosis, limited range of motion, joint space narrowing, subchondral cysts, and ankylosis.[32]

Ankylosing spondylitis

Ankylosing spondylitis (Bechterew's disease), a chronic inflammatory disease of unknown etiology, is usually progressive and most often affects the sacroiliac joints and vertebral column. The main locus of pathology is the site where the ligaments and capsule insert into the bone and not the synovium.[49] This condition affects 1% to 2% of the white population and has a male-female prevalence ratio ranging from 6:1[50] to 2:1.[22] The affected male population demonstrates more involved joints and increased disease severity than the female population. Onset of the disease is usually between the ages of 16 and 40 years.[50] The prevalence of TMJ involvement is quite rare and ranges from 4% to 35%, depending on the diagnostic criteria used, the population studied, and the methods used to assess TMJ involvement.[51,52]

The clinical findings are similar to those of other arthritic conditions and include tenderness and/or pain in the masticatory muscles and TMJ, morning stiffness, fatigue in the jaws, limitation in mouth opening, and joint sounds.[50–53] Common radiographic signs consist of condylar erosions, flattening and sclerosis, flattening of the temporal bone, and joint space narrowing.[22,52–54]

Infectious arthritis

Infectious (septic) arthritis of the TMJ is a rare disease and is not frequently documented in the literature. The condition is an inflammatory reaction of the articular surfaces that results from bacterial invasion caused by a penetrating external injury and that spreads infection from adjacent structures (dental, parotid gland, or otic origins) or from bacteremia associated with systemic infection, such as tuberculosis, syphilis, and gonorrhea.[55,56] The most common bacteria involved with infectious arthritis are *Staphylococcus aureus*, *Neisseria gonorrhoeae*, and *Haemophilus influenza*.[57,58] Risk factors include diabetes mellitus, systemic lupus erythematosus, rheumatoid arthritis, other immunosuppressive diseases, or previous joint disease.[59] Patients often complain of limited and painful mouth opening with a warm, erythematous preauricular swelling. Mandibular deviation at rest to the contralateral side is due to joint effusion

and is often associated with a malocclusion.[57,60] Radiographically, the TMJ may appear clinically normal; however, with disease progression, there may be signs of erosion of the articular surfaces and bone destruction.[57,61] Bone scanning using technetium-99 phosphate has been used to detect physiologic bone changes earlier than radiographic anatomical changes; specificity is low but sensitivity is high, so a negative result strongly argues against an infectious arthritis.[62] If uncertain, white blood cell counts may provide helpful data on the presence or absence of infection. TMJ fibrosis and ankylosis resulting in impaired joint mobility and function are potential complications that usually occur in the later stages of the disease process.[61]

Hyperuricemia

Hyperuricemia (gout) comprises a heterogenous group of arthritic disorders characterized by the deposition or concentration of monosodium urate monohydrate crystals in joints and tendons (crystal arthritis).[63] The metatarsophalangeal joint (big toe) is involved in 90% of patients.[64] Gout progresses through four clinical phases: asymptomatic hyperuricemia, acute gouty arthritis, intercritical gout (intervals between acute attacks), and chronic tophaceous gout characterized by radiographically evident chalky deposits of sodium urate.[65] Pseudogout, another form of crystal arthritis, is due to the deposition of calcium pyrophosphate dihydrate crystals. Cases of pseudogout have been reported to affect the TMJ.[66] Gout is rare and affects at least 1% of the population in Western countries; peak incidence occurs in men 30 to 50 years old.[64]

Uric acid is the end product of purine metabolism and has no physiologic role. Humans genetically lack the enzyme uricase, which allows for the degradation of uric acid to the water-soluble and easily excreted product known as *allantoin*, thereby preventing uric acid accumulation. Elevated serum levels are a result of an overproduction and/or an underexcretion of uric acid. These mechanisms predispose a person to develop microcrystals that may precipitate in the synovium. Additionally, it may be caused by hematologic disorders or by the use of certain medications.[67]

Although the prevalence of gout has been increasing during the past two decades, involvement of the TMJ is very rare, and there are only 10 reports in the English-language literature.[68] If the TMJ is involved, the disease is usually confined to the joint space, which leads to pain and limitation of mouth opening.[69] However, a case where the disease process extended beyond the joint capsule into the pterygoid muscle with concomitant destruction of the head of the condyle, the temporal bone, and the greater wing of the sphenoid bone has been described.[69]

Reiter syndrome ~ p.258

Reiter syndrome, also known as *reactive arthritis*, was described in 1916 by Hans Reiter as a triad of arthritis, nongonococcal urethritis, and conjunctivitis, occurring concurrently or sequentially. More recently, Reiter syndrome has also been defined as a peripheral arthritis lasting longer than 1 month that is associated with urethritis, cervicitis, or diarrhea; additional features include mucocutaneous lesions, cardiac involvement, and central or peripheral nerve involvement.[70] Reactive arthritis refers to an acute nonpurulent (aseptic) arthritis initiated by a remote infection. Reiter syndrome is triggered by enteric or urogenital (venereal) infections. The bacteria implicated in the enteric form include *Shigella*, *Salmonella*, and *Yersinia* spp, whereas *Chlamydia* and *Mycoplasma* are associated with the urogenital type.[71]

Reiter syndrome is associated with human leukocyte antigen (HLA)-B27, although HLA-B27 is not always present in an affected person, particularly in the presence of HIV. The arthritis involved with this syndrome is usually in multiple joints, though the lower extremities are affected most often. The syndrome occurs mostly in men between the ages of 20 and 30 years.

Signs and symptoms of muscle and joint dysfunction in 52 men with Reiter syndrome were more frequent and severe than those in 52 matched control subjects with no general joint disease.[72] One-quarter of the Reiter syndrome group reported TMJ signs or symptoms, and the most characteristic were pain on function, tenderness to palpation, and pain when opening wide (15% of subjects). Tenderness to palpation of the masticatory muscles (19%) and stiffness/tiredness of the jaws in the morning were also reported.

Patients with Reiter syndrome more frequently display radiographic findings in the condyle (33%), and the most common finding is unilateral erosion (12%).[51]

Neck-tongue syndrome

Neck-tongue syndrome consists of the appearance of occipital or upper neck pain associated with an abnormal sensation on the ipsilateral side of the tongue. Pain is initiated by head rotation, usually to one side, and lasts some minutes.[73] Pain is usually sharp and radiates to the occipital, cervical, and lingual regions.[74,75] In the tongue, paresthesia, dysesthesia, or anesthesia may be reported, lasting from a few seconds to about 2 minutes.[76] This may or may not be preceded by tongue pain.[75,77] Patients may describe radicular symptoms and display restricted neck movements.[76] Although considered extremely rare, about 59 cases have been reported in the literature, and a prevalence of 0.22% has been estimated.[76,78]

Excessive range of movement of the atlantoaxial joint with impaction and stretching of the second cervical root (C2) is thought to underlie neck-tongue syndrome.[79] This in turn compresses proprioceptive fibers from the tongue that pass from the ansahypoglossi to the C2 ventral ramus.[75] Surgical findings confirm C2 nerve compression by the atlantoaxial joint.[74]

Spinal immobilization (soft collar), atlantoaxial fusion, or resection of the C2 spinal nerve may be needed; in uncomplicated cases, spinal manipulation may help.[74,80,81]

Orofacial Pain in Bone Disorders

Osteoporosis

Osteoporosis is the most common bone disease in humans and affects both men and women.[82] Osteoporosis may be diagnosed after a low-impact or fragility fracture. Low bone mineral density is best assessed by central dual-energy x-ray absorptiometry. Both nonpharmacologic therapy (calcium and vitamin D supplementation, weight-bearing exercise, and fall prevention) and pharmacologic treatments (antiresorptive and anabolic agents) may be helpful in the prevention and treatment of osteoporosis.

The literature suggests that osteoporosis is linked to TMDs[83,84] and atypical facial pain, and female hormones are implicated as a common risk factor.[85] This is based on the strong female prevalence in atypical facial pain and the physiologic and therapeutic modification of estrogen levels in patients with these pain conditions as well as in patients with osteoporosis.[86] The connection remains speculative (see also chapter 12).

Paget's disease

Paget's disease of bone is characterized by bone resorption in focal areas followed by excessive new bone formation, with eventual replacement of the normal bone marrow by vascular and fibrous tissue. The etiology of Paget's disease is not well understood; however, one gene linked to Paget's disease and several other susceptibility loci have been identified, and paramyxoviral gene products have been detected in Pagetic osteoclasts.[87] Because of the excessive bone formation in the craniofacial complex, neurologic deficits are common and include sensory changes in hearing, sight, and smell.[88–90] Comparison of oral status between patients with Paget's disease and healthy control subjects demonstrated that those with Paget's disease were more likely to report pain when opening the mouth.

Orofacial Pain in Immunologically Mediated Diseases

Immunologically mediated diseases are those with a prominent involvement of immunocytes and/or their products. In this section the presentation of orofacial pain in autoimmune diseases, allergy, and granulomatous and immune complex diseases is reviewed.

Systemic lupus erythematosus

Systemic lupus erythematosus (SLE) is a chronic autoimmune disease involving multiple organ systems. Characteristically, there is a state of immune hyperactivity and antibodies directed against cell nuclei. Autoantibodies, circulating immune complexes, and T lymphocytes all contribute to the expression of disease. Multisystem involvement appears as dermatologic, renal, central and peripheral nervous system, hematologic, musculoskeletal, cardiovascular, pulmonary, vascular endothelium, and gastrointestinal manifestations. Ninety percent of those suffering from SLE are women, and most (80%) are in their childbearing years. This led to the hypothesis that women who are exposed to estrogen-containing oral contraceptives or hormone replacement therapy have an increased risk of developing or exacerbating SLE[91–93]; however, other studies do not support this finding.[94,95]

TMJ involvement has been reported in SLE; one-third of patients had current complaints, and two-thirds had a history of severe symptoms from the TMJ.[96] Objective findings included locking or dislocation, tenderness to palpation, and pain on movement of the mandible in 22% of patients. Additionally, radiographic changes of the condyles, including flattening, erosions, osteophytes, and sclerosis were observed in 30% of patients. These findings were confirmed in a study that reported that 50.0% of patients with SLE experienced TMJ pain, 36.4% experienced TMJ sounds, and more than a quarter had difficulty opening their mouth.[97]

Trigeminal sensory neuropathy has been associated with SLE, most commonly facial numbness, paresthesia, dysesthesia, and pain; however, other cranial nerves may be involved.[98] Trigeminal neuropathy may be the initial feature of SLE or may follow disease onset, but it usually develops slowly.[98,99] Oral ulcerations have also been associated with SLE and may induce acute pain.[100]

Intractable headaches, so-called lupus headaches, have long been thought of as a common and characteristic manifestation of SLE. However, a controlled study showed that headache is not specifically related to SLE expression or severity.[101] Accepting the presence of headaches, even severe, as a neurologic manifestation of SLE in the absence of seizures or overt psychosis may result in overestimation of the disease status.[101] This approach was further supported by a recent meta-analysis.[102] Chronic pain in patients with SLE correlates with sleep disturbance, and 55% to 85% of these patients suffer from sleep disturbances.[103] Researchers suggest that mood disorder, which results in part from chronic pain, is a main contributing factor to sleep disorders in SLE.

Sjögren's syndrome

Sjögren's syndrome is a chronic, systemic autoimmune disorder of unknown etiology that affects the exocrine glands and is histologically characterized by a lymphocytic infiltrate of the affected glands.[104] The hallmark manifestations of Sjögren's syndrome are dryness of the mouth and eyes due to involvement of the salivary and lacrimal glands. In addition, Sjögren's syndrome may cause skin, nose, and vaginal dryness and may affect other organs of the body, including the kidneys, blood vessels, lungs, liver, pancreas, and brain. Sjögren's syndrome affects 1 to 4 million people in the United States, and patients are usually over the age of 40 years at diagnosis. Women are nine times more likely to have the condition than men. Primary Sjögren's syndrome occurs in people with no other rheumatologic disease. Secondary Sjögren's syndrome occurs in people who have another rheumatologic disease, most often SLE or rheumatoid arthritis and progressive systemic sclerosis (scleroderma).

The presence of dry mouth increases the risk for mucosal sensitivity and, because of impaired lubrication, often leads to secondary infection, mostly candidiasis.[105] Dry mouth also contributes to an increased risk of mucosal trauma, periodontal disease, and dental caries, which may lead to pain.[106,107] When interductal salivary flow rate is reduced, the cleansing effect of saliva is minimized, and retrograde infection with acute sialoadenitis may be associated with pain.

Distal, symmetric sensory neuropathy is present in 10% to 20% of patients with primary Sjögren's syndrome,[108] but there are reports of asymmetric neuropathies.[109] Isolated cranial nerve sensory neuropathy has been reported in a number of patients with Sjögren's syndrome,[110,111] including in the trigeminal nerve.[112] Trigeminal sensory neuropathy in Sjögren's syndrome is characterized by a slowly progressing, unilateral, or bilateral facial numbness or paresthesia, occasionally associated with

pain.[8] Independent of these reports of neuropathies in these patients, it does not seem that neuropathies are more common in patients with primary Sjögren's syndrome compared with healthy controls.[113] This also seems to be true of headaches, except for tension-type headaches, which may be more common in primary Sjögren's syndrome.[114] Headaches possibly relate more to the signs and symptoms of Sjögren's syndrome, such as dry eyes, than to the diagnosis.[115] The emotional aspects of pain in patients with the syndrome may significantly and negatively contribute to pain perception and reporting.[116] This is due in part to the fear of illness that is potentially associated with the reported pain. This may explain why patients with Sjögren's syndrome are more likely to report fatigue and pain than patients with SLE, whereas fibromyalgia is more often diagnosed in patients with SLE than with Sjögren's syndrome.[117]

Systemic sclerosis (scleroderma)

Systemic sclerosis is a multisystem connective tissue disorder of unknown etiology characterized by inflammation as well as vascular and fibrotic alterations in the skin, which becomes indurated and fixed to the underlying connective tissue.[118] The condition also involves various other internal organs, such as the gastrointestinal tract, heart, lungs, and kidneys, and causes fibrosis by the deposition of too much collagen. *Scleroderma* is a rather generic term that is used to describe a systemic as well as a localized cutaneous variant. The systemic form of scleroderma is classified as CREST syndrome, which is an acronym for the clinical manifestations: calcinosis, Raynaud phenomenon, esophageal dysmotility, sclerodactyly, and telangiectasia. This can be further subdivided into morphea scleroderma (a localized form of the disease) and linear scleroderma (a specific type of localized scleroderma). Diffuse systemic sclerosis, also known as *progressive systemic sclerosis*, is rare and carries a poor prognosis.[119] Women are affected more often than men, with a ratio of 3:1, and this tends to increase to 4:1 during the childbearing years; the highest onset of symptoms is between the ages of 30 and 50 years.[118]

The most characteristic orofacial manifestations are microstomia, resulting in limited mouth opening; mucogingival problems; fibrosis of the hard and soft palate; telangiectasis and chromatosis of the face and oral mucosa; xerostomia; dry eyes; widening of the periodontal ligament space; TMJ dysfunction; and trigeminal neuropathy.[120,121] These manifestations are either a direct result of the substitutions of normal tissues with collagen or the deposition of collagen around nerves or endothelial tissues.[122] TMJ noises and pain are extremely prevalent in scleroderma and may be experienced by more than 85% of patients.[97] Voice changes are also often reported in scleroderma, and patients report a significant decrease in quality of life.[123]

TMJ dysfunction is most often related to gross changes to the mandible, which include osteolytic activity and result in bone resorption of the coronoid process, condyles, angle of the mandible, and ramus.[119,120] These changes result in articular pain and swelling due to tendonitis and synovitis, with the accompanying radiographic changes described earlier.[124]

Trigeminal sensory neuropathy may involve all three branches and appears to be the most frequent orofacial phenomenon to precede this disorder.[98] Of 22 patients with scleroderma, 9 reported trigeminal neuropathy as the first symptom of the disorder.[125] The symptomatology consists of paresthesia, burning, and/or an intense sharp/stabbing pain that may be provoked by jaw use or movement, thus mimicking the presentation of trigeminal neuralgia.[118,126]

Mixed connective tissue disorder

The clinical findings in mixed connective tissue disorder often include Raynaud phenomenon, polyarthralgia or arthritis, lymphadenitis, cutaneous and mucosal lesions, and serositis in the form of pulmonary involvement. These features are commonly found in a number of different connective tissue diseases, including SLE, scleroderma, rheumatoid arthritis, and polymyositis. Thus, mixed connective tissue disorder is characterized by overlapping, nonspecific clinical features that may occur simultaneously or sequentially.[127]

The orofacial manifestations of these connective tissue disorders, although uncommon, include trigeminal sensory neuropathy and arthritis of the TMJ. The presence of trigeminal neuropathy has also been reported to include

both pain and numbness, and it appears that neurovascular headaches of mild to moderate severity are relatively common in this disorder.[98,127]

Patients with mixed connective tissue disorder demonstrate signs and symptoms of dysfunction of the masticatory system.[128] Masticatory muscle and TMJ tenderness, with associated clicking or crepitation, are common.[22] Radiographic changes of the TMJs were observed in 7 of 10 patients examined.[128] Moreover, in five of six patients with normal-appearing mucosa, histologic examination revealed chronic inflammation. Three of the 10 patients had clinically atrophic and erythematous oral mucosa; histologic examination again revealed chronic inflammation.

Mixed connective tissue disorder is often associated with secondary Sjögren's syndrome,[129] although this association does not influence the clinical course of mixed connective tissue disorder.[130] Suspicious cases of Sjögren's syndrome–like symptoms that are undiagnosed should be referred for medical assessment.

Antiphospholipid syndrome

The antiphospholipid syndrome (Hughes syndrome), first described in 1983, is a prothrombotic disease in which neurologic events feature prominently. Cerebrovascular accidents (CVAs), transient ischemic attacks, and headaches are important complications. Other neurologic symptoms, including diplopia, memory loss, ataxia, and multiple sclerosis–like features, are common.[131] Antiphospholipid syndrome is characterized by serum autoantibodies to phospholipids, which are deposited in small vessels and lead to intimal hyperplasia and acute thromboses, especially in cerebral, renal, pulmonary, cutaneous, and cardiac arteries. Antiphospholipid syndrome may be seen in isolation or associated with SLE or other connective tissue diseases, including Sjögren's syndrome.

Headache in antiphospholipid syndrome can vary from typical episodic migraine to an almost continuous incapacitating headache. Patient histories are often remarkably similar: teenagers with headaches that are frequently migrainous in character and temporally associated with premenstrual days. These headaches may subsequently disappear for 10 to 20 years only to return when the patient reaches the age of 30 to 40 years. Significantly, there is a strong family history of headaches or migraine in many of these patients, which suggests common genetic influences. Moreover, as in migraine with aura, some patients report headaches that are accompanied by visual or speech disturbance or by transient ischemic attacks.[131]

The association of migraine and antiphospholipid antibodies is controversial, and results vary widely. Some have reported association with lupus anticoagulant or anticardiolipin,[132,133] but others report no associations.[134] The difficulty in demonstrating a true association between anticardiolipin positivity and migraine stems in part from the high prevalence of migraine in the healthy population and the relatively low prevalence of anticardiolipin positivity in otherwise healthy people (see chapter 10). One of the major problems is that headaches, often nonmigrainous, have been loosely termed *migraine*, and these headaches may precede or accompany transient ischemic attacks or CVAs.[135] Antiphospholipid antibodies have also been detected in patients with transient neurologic symptoms, including migraine aura. Therefore, the controversy may be due in part to the inherent difficulty in distinguishing the transient focal neurologic events of migraine from transient ischemic attacks.[136] The available data suggest an association between the migraine-like *phenomena* and antiphospholipid antibodies but not between migraine *headache* and antiphospholipid antibodies.[137–141]

Anecdotal reports show that anticoagulation treatment is sometimes effective in reducing the number and the intensity of headache attacks in selected patients with antiphospholipid syndrome.[142] Similarly, memory loss often improves dramatically with appropriate warfarin dosage.[131,143]

Allergy

Orofacial allergic reactions may have a protean presentation in regard to acuity and spectrum of symptoms. The acute form of oral allergy, also known as *oral allergy syndrome*, is an uncommon variant of allergic reactions. The term refers to the combination of irritation, pruritus, and swelling of the lips, tongue, palate, and throat that is sometimes associated with other allergic features, such as rhinoconjunctivitis, asthma, urticaria-angioedema, and even anaphylactic shock. Symptoms usually develop within minutes but occasionally are delayed for more than an hour. They may include itching and burning of the lips, mouth, and throat; watery, itchy eyes; runny nose; and sneezing.

Most chronic forms of oral allergy are attributed to dental restorative materials. Gold is reported to cause itching, a burning pain sensation, and, at times, ulceration of the oral tissues adjacent to the gold restoration.[144] Immunologic-mediated lichenoid reactions have also been attributed to dental restorative materials and drugs.[145,146]

In the context of allergy and headache, an interdisciplinary consensus committee of the International Headache Society (IHS) and the American Academy of Otolaryngology-Head and Neck Surgery suggested that in patients with allergies and headaches, management of the allergies may reduce the frequency of the headaches. The mechanism for this may be related to reducing a trigger for the headache (ie, allergies) or by decreasing mucosal inflammation, which may be responsible for precipitating the headache. Patients with typical itchy eyes, itchy nose, and nasal congestion may benefit from an allergy evaluation.[147] This consensus meeting was part of an attempt to define conditions that lead to headaches of rhinogenic origin (see also chapter 7). This conclusion is supported by a previous study[148] that showed that the relationship between allergy and migraine can be based in part on an immunoglobulin E–mediated mechanism, with histamine release playing an important role.

Wegener's granulomatosis

Wegener's granulomatosis is an autoimmune disease that has a clinical predilection for the upper airways, lungs, and kidneys. Wegener's granulomatosis is a necrotizing granulomatous vasculitis characterized by the presence of antineutrophil cytoplasmic antibody. Neurologic involvement in this autoimmune disease is rare at onset. However, a case where headache was the initial, dominant presentation was reported.[149] The headache was migratory, throbbing, and accentuated by head movement; the symptoms disappeared when the treatment was directed at the underlying Wegener's granulomatosis. Two further cases have been published where the headache in Wegener's granulomatosis was described as a severe, lancinating, left-sided facial pain with green nasal discharge, postnasal drip, nasal obstruction, and photophobia, with the eventual development of hyperalgesia and allodynia.[150] The described pain was localized to the frontoethmoid area, extended retro-orbitally, and kept the patient awake at night. In the second case, hearing loss was also present. Unusual presentations of Wegener's granulomatosis include severe and bilateral facial palsy associated with ear pain[151] or meningitis.[152]

Neurosarcoidosis

Neurosarcoidosis is a multisystem granulomatous disease of unknown cause, most commonly affecting young adults. Sarcoid lesions are noncaseating epithelioid granulomas. Involvement of the central nervous system (CNS) is clinically evident in 5% and silent in 10% of patients with systemic sarcoidosis. It may occur at presentation in 10% to 30% of patients and more rarely is strictly confined to the CNS. Intracranial lesions are detectable by MRI.[153]

Headache and/or primary headaches are frequently reported in patients with neurosarcoidosis (30%) but rarely present as an initial symptom of the disease. However, occasional rare cases of headaches have been reported as a presenting symptom of sarcoidosis.[154,155] Headache character varies in relation to neuropathologic involvement; focal lesions, meningitis, cranial nerve palsies, and no typical characteristics of headache are known. Intractable headaches located occipitally and radiating frontally, with associated nausea and visual disturbances, have been reported in patients with isolated supratentorial tumor–like lesions.[156] Diffuse or bifrontal pain is a more typical symptom of leptomeningeal involvement, which may be associated with papilledema.[157] Other forms of cranial pain may be related to trigeminal or optic nerve involvement, and migraine has also been reported.[158]

Melkersson-Rosenthal syndrome

Melkersson-Rosenthal syndrome is an uncommon condition of uncertain pathogenesis and course. The classic triad of signs includes recurrent orofacial edema, recurrent facial nerve palsy, and lingua plica (fissured tongue). Seventy-five percent of all patients had labial swelling, 50% had facial edema, and 33% had Bell's palsy.[159] The condition produces nontender, persistent swelling of one or both lips and affects primarily young adults. Histologically, non-necrotizing granulomatous inflammation is seen.[160] Therefore, facial neuropathy involving facial palsy or symptomatic lip swelling should include Melkersson-Rosenthal syndrome as a differential diagnosis. Some authors suggest that Melkersson-Rosenthal syndrome is a variant of Crohn's disease.[161] Others have suggested a link between Hashimoto's thyroiditis and Melkersson-Rosenthal syndrome because of the common presence of antithyroperoxidase antibodies in both conditions.[162]

Giant cell arteritis

Giant cell arteritis (GCA), also referred to as *temporal arteritis*, is a chronic vasculitis of large- and medium-sized arteries. GCA is usually accompanied by head, face, or neck pain. The condition predominantly affects patients over the age of 50 years, typically in the seventh and eighth decades, and women are affected about twice as often as men.[163,164] The incidence is age related and rises from 2.3/100,000/year in 60-year-olds to 44.7/100,000/year in 90-year-olds.[165–169] GCA mainly affects whites, particularly people of Scandinavian or northern European descent, irrespective of their residence.[165,167–169] Additionally, genetic studies suggest an inherited component, and most point to an association with the HLA antigen system.[170]

The diagnosis of GCA relies on the presence of a swollen and tender scalp artery (usually the temporal artery) accompanied by an elevated erythrocyte sedimentation rate (ESR) and a rapid response (< 48 hours) to steroid therapy.[73] However, all of these factors may not always occur in a particular case, and definitive diagnosis is dependent on an artery biopsy demonstrating typical histopathology.

In relevant cases, an ESR is considered indicative of GCA, but ESRs < 40 mm/hour occur in up to 22.5% of patients, and clinically normal levels do not exclude diagnosis.[170,171] Constitutional symptoms are more common in patients with ESR > 100 mm/hour, and in patients with elevated ESR, disease activity correlates with ESR changes.[170,172] ESR is affected by sex, a number of autoimmune and hematologic disorders, malignancy, liver dysfunction, and use of anti-inflammatory drugs. Moreover, there is some disagreement as to the normal range of ESR. C-reactive protein has several advantages over ESR: It is unaffected by sex, age, plasma composition, and red cell morphology, and it has an accurately defined and accepted normal range. C-reactive protein is commonly used in conjunction with ESR for the diagnosis of GCA and significantly improves specificity.[173]

The diagnosis of GCA is dependent on temporal artery biopsy and should be performed in all patients, though up to 15% may have a negative biopsy.[170,174,175] The threat of blindness mandates that corticosteroid therapy not be delayed and that temporal artery biopsy be performed as soon as possible.[176–178] Because of the presence of skip lesions (discussed later), biopsy should include a length of at least 2.0 to 2.5 cm of artery, which should be serially sectioned every 1 mm. Sections should be stained with hematoxylin and eosin and with an elastin-specific stain. A negative biopsy in a clinically suspect patient may be an indication for a further, contralateral biopsy. Contralateral biopsy may be positive in up to 15% of patients after an initially negative ipsilateral result.[179,180]

Elevated platelet counts are commonly observed in GCA and promptly return to normal after steroid therapy. A number of other tests are more rarely used for the diagnosis and/or monitoring of GCA, including plasma viscosity, interleukin-6, fibrinogen, and liver function tests.[181]

Imaging techniques that may be useful include duplex ultrasonography, angiography, positron emission tomography, MRI, and computed tomography.[178] However, though most of these techniques are suitable for the assessment of large vessels, they are of limited value in the small cranial vessels. In expert hands with state-of-the-art equipment, ultrasonography is reliable (sensitivity, 88%; specificity, 99.5%) for the diagnosis of GCA, even in small vessels.[178] MRI has been shown to accurately detect areas of mural inflammation, even in the relatively small temporal artery.[182–184] MRI may therefore be a future possibility for diagnosis or to guide biopsy site selection.

GCA is well known for its variable clinical manifestations. The clinical signs are the result of damage to the arterial supply, which leads to tissue ischemia and injury. The most common presenting complaints include headache, scalp tenderness, jaw claudication, and arthralgia.[170,172,175,185] Jaw claudication may be expressed as tiredness and inefficient chewing, which lead to clinical similarities with TMDs. Uncommonly, areas with severe ischemia may necrose, including intraorally.

Patients with GCA may visit an orofacial pain clinic complaining primarily of pain, most commonly over the muscles of mastication, the TMJ, and the eye. Headache is present in 90% of patients and often localizes to the temple (ipsilateral or bilateral) and forehead, but location is highly variable.[178]

Pain quality may be throbbing, burning, boring, or lancinating and may vary from mild to severe. Head tenderness and allodynia, particularly over the temporal regions, may be marked. The temporal artery may be prominent, tender, or beaded, but these findings are inconsistent, and in more advanced cases the artery may not be easily located. Ophthalmoscopy may reveal anterior ischemic optic neuropathy with a pale and swollen optic disc.

Ocular involvement may occur in 14% to 70% of patients with GCA.[170] Transient visual disturbances, such as diplopia or ocular pain, are reported by 2% to 30% of patients.[185] Bilateral blindness has been reported in a third of patients and is usually the result of ischemic damage to the optic nerve, retina, or choroid.

Constitutional symptoms may include fever, weight loss, anorexia, and malaise. Additionally, alterations in mental status, including depression, dementia, confusion, and delusional thinking, have been reported.[170] Many of these symptoms are common in the elderly secondary to infectious, malignant, or age-related disease and may therefore be missed as a presenting sign of GCA. Typical clinical manifestations may be totally absent in up to 38% of patients who present solely with visual symptoms, termed *silent* or *occult GCA*.[170,186]

Concurrent symptoms commonly include proximal muscle ache, morning stiffness, and polymyalgia rheumatica, which is very common and affects 1 in every 130 persons over the age of 50 years and may be the presenting manifestation of GCA in up to 50% of patients.[172] Clinically, polymyalgia rheumatica is characterized by bilateral severe aching pain and morning stiffness of the neck, shoulder, and pelvic girdles. Women are more often affected, incidence increases with age, and there are signs of systemic inflammation, suggesting similarities with GCA.[187,188] Therefore, some consider polymyalgia rheumatica and GCA to be different phases of the same disease. However, polymyalgia rheumatica lacks the inflammatory infiltrate and vaso-occlusive ischemic manifestations of GCA. Polymyalgia rheumatica is often an isolated condition and does not demonstrate the strong HLA association seen in GCA.[166,189–192] Debate continues as to the precise nature of the comorbidity of polymyalgia rheumatica and GCA.[170]

The initial event that triggers the cascade of immune and inflammatory reactions underlying GCA has been suggested to be infective but remains unclear.[170] Current theory points to the activation of immature dendritic cells residing in the arterial wall. Activated dendritic cells then produce inflammatory cytokines and chemokines, which ultimately attract T cells and macrophages.[193,194] Many patients with GCA demonstrate signs of systemic inflammation. Interleukin-1 and interleukin-6 are considered to play a key role in the pathophysiology of GCA and induce the production of acute-phase proteins by the liver, fever, and myalgia.[170]

The aorta and its extracranial branches are specifically but not solely affected. In particular, the superficial temporal, ophthalmic, posterior ciliary, and vertebral arteries are commonly involved.[170] The central retinal and other branches of the external carotid artery are less commonly affected, whereas the intracranial arteries are spared.

In active disease, nodular inflammatory granulomatous reactions affect arteries with an elastic lamina; the distribution of disease correlates with the distribution of elastin.[195] Often, disease activity is variable within the same artery, which leads to _skip lesions_, that is, segments of inflamed regions adjacent to unaffected areas.[196–198] This is the rationale indicating that long sections of artery should be obtained as biopsy specimens.

Histopathology of affected arteries shows inflammation of the adventitia, media, and intima.

Also seen is predominant aggregation of CD4+ (T-helper/inducer) cells and a select group of T cells within the adventitial layer; these produce interferon gamma, which is thought to be the key regulating cytokine in GCA.[199] Macrophages are present in distinct functional groups throughout the arterial wall and induce a proinflammatory response in the adventitia and destruction of the media. Ischemic symptoms are probably secondary to narrowing of the lumen, but thrombosis is often present. Intimal thickening observed in GCA correlates with circulating levels of interferon gamma and is probably a healing response.[194,200,201]

GCA may run a self-limiting course lasting 2 to 4 years, but many patients require long-term therapy.[178,202–204] Because of the potentially severe effects, rapid and efficient treatment with corticosteroids is indicated.[170,178] Patients with suspected GCA should be rapidly assessed and referred for ophthalmologic examination and biopsy; however, steroid therapy should not be withheld.[176,178] Onset of visual loss after initial symptoms may be rapid and varies from weeks to months. The loss of vision in one eye usually indicates loss of vision in the second eye within 1 or 2 months.[170]

Recent recommendations suggest beginning with 60 to 80 mg of prednisone daily.[170,178] Patients with ocular involvement at presentation commonly receive very high initial doses (1,000 mg/day for 3 days). Resolution of systemic symptoms occurs within 24 to 72 hours, and the dose should be increased if necessary to attain symptomatic relief. The ESR normalizes only after several weeks. The effective dose should be maintained for 4 to 6 weeks and then tapered while closely monitoring clinical signs, ESR, and C-reactive protein. The dose is reduced by 10 mg per month, then 5 mg per month, and then 1 mg per month once a daily dose of 10 to 15 mg is attained.[170] Total treatment may span 1 or 2 years, and all dose adjustments should be accompanied by clinical and laboratory testing. Relapses are common, particularly in the first 18 months, and may be accurately predicted by changes in C-reactive protein levels.[170,205]

Patients on corticosteroids require expert medical management of side effects, including osteoporosis, depression, and gastrointestinal problems.[178] The incidence of serious effects associated with corticosteroid therapy is more than 50%.[205] For this reason, steroid-sparing drugs have been developed, but there is no consensus concerning their use for this condition. Patients taking aspirin before or at diagnosis demonstrate lower risk for visual loss.[206] However, aspirin may further increase gastrointestinal morbidity, so a proton pump inhibitor should therefore be prescribed.

Behçet's disease

Behçet's disease is a clinical triad of oral and genital ulceration and uveitis that affects young adult men, particularly in Turkey and Japan, and has an association to HLA-B5 and HLA-B51. Clinical features, such as arthralgia and vasculitis, suggest an immune complex–mediated basis, which is supported by findings of circulating immune complexes, but the antigen responsible has not been identified. Immunologic changes occur in Behçet's disease, including T-lymphocyte abnormalities, changes in serum complement, and increased polymorphonuclear motility. Mononuclear cells and natural killer cells may also be involved.[207,208]

Recurrent headache has been reported in more than 80% of patients with Behçet's disease.[209,210] Most fulfill the IHS criteria for migraine (see chapter 10) and have a higher than normal prevalence of visual sensory aura (52% of patients). In addition, 62% of patients showed moderate or severe disability according to the Migraine Disability Assessment Score.[209] Because the nervous system is involved in 5% of patients with Behçet's disease, headache appears to occur independently.[211] A much lower incidence of headache has been reported in patients with Behçet's disease (58%)[211]; however, migrainous headache was commonly associated with exacerbations of some of the systemic symptoms of the syndrome. Therefore, this form of headache is not specific for Behçet's disease but may be explained by a vascular headache triggered by the immunomediated disease activity in susceptible individuals.

Finally, a report indicated that patients with Behçet's disease may be more likely to be diagnosed with fibromyalgia, especially women.[212] The diagnosis of fibromyalgia in patients with Behçet's disease did not seem to affect the presence of oral ulcers but contributed to musculoskeletal pain, as would be expected.

Orofacial Pain in Neurologic Disorders

Headache associated with neurologic disorders is mainly observed in CVAs, multiple sclerosis, and changes in intracranial pressure (see also chapters 12 and 13). The IHS describes secondary headaches that may occur in patients affected by inflammatory diseases of the CNS, which are classified as headaches attributed to nonvascular intracranial disorders.[19] Headaches are frequently reported in patients with neurosarcoidosis (30%), Behçet's disease (55%), and acute disseminated encephalomyelitis (45% to 58%).[153]

Cerebrovascular accident

CVA, also known as *stroke*, is a syndrome of rapidly developing clinical signs and symptoms of focal and, at times, global disturbances of cerebral function lasting more than 24 hours or resulting in death within that time. When blood flow to the brain is interrupted for more than a few seconds, brain cells can die, causing infarction. The most common cause of CVA or stroke is cerebral atherosclerosis, which may lead to the main types of CVA: hemorrhagic (intracerebral or subarachnoid), thrombotic, or embolic. Rarely, strokes are secondary to other pathologies, such as carotid dissection, carotid stenosis, cocaine use, and syphilis.

In a prospective study involving 240 patients experiencing acute CVA, it was found that headache occurred in 38%. Headache patients were younger, and a history of tension-type headache was more significant in the headache group than in the nonheadache group. In patients with ischemic stroke, the incidence of headache was lower, and pain was shorter, more localized, and less intense compared with that in patients with hemorrhagic CVA.[213] The IHS has well-described criteria for headaches associated with cranial vascular disorders.[19]

The association between migraine and stroke remains controversial.[214,215] Epidemiologic studies suggest that migraine may be an independent risk factor for ischemic stroke in women younger than 45 years, and additional risk factors are cigarette smoking and oral contraceptive use.[216] The pathogenesis is not well understood but is thought to be related to common biochemical mechanisms between migraine and stroke. A classification of migraine-related stroke has been proposed that includes three major entities: coexisting stroke and migraine, stroke with clinical features of migraine, and migraine-induced stroke.[214] Coexisting stroke and migraine was proposed as an explanation for the relationship between stroke and migraine in patients affected by cardiac disease. In such a condition, a possible cause of ischemic stroke may be an increased propensity toward paradoxical cerebral emboli during migraine attacks when there is a condition of platelet hyperaggregation.

Stroke with clinical features of migraine stems from the hypothesis that in some arteriovenous malformations or neurologic diseases, circulation in the CNS may be affected by multiple minor infarcts, and the patient may present with migraine as a symptom of a minor infarct.

The concept of migraine-induced stroke is well represented by migrainous infarction, which is described as having one or more migraine aura symptoms associated with an ischemic brain lesion in the appropriate territory demonstrated by neuroimaging.[19] Interestingly, the condition mainly occurs in younger women in the posterior circulation, and most studies have shown a lack of association between migraine without aura and ischemic stroke.[217,218]

An association between multiple sclerosis and headache has been suggested.[219,220] In 137 patients with multiple sclerosis, 88 reported headache, 21 of whom developed headache after initiation of interferon treatment.[221] The prevalence of all headaches not due to interferon was 57.7%. Migraine was found in 25.0% of patients, tension-type headache in 31.9%, and cluster headache in only one patient. A significant correlation between migraine and relapsing-remitting multiple sclerosis was also found.[222] Some authors suggest that the mechanism for this is a serotoninergic link between multiple sclerosis and migraine headache.[223]

Intracranial pressure

Headache may be caused by raised intracranial pressure and intracranial hypotension.[224,225] Extremely high intracranial pressure commonly causes headache. Benign intracranial hypertension is a rare syndrome of increased intracranial pressure manifesting as headache, transient visual obscuration, and palsy of the sixth cranial nerve. In most patients, benign intracranial hypertension is idiopathic, but possible causes include tetracycline use, endocrine disorders such as obesity, hypoparathyroidism, hypervitaminosis A, and thyroid replacement. Cerebral edema, high cerebrospinal fluid outflow resistance, high cerebral venous pressure, or a combination of the three is thought to underlie benign intracranial hypertension. The management of benign intracranial hypertension includes symptomatic headache relief, removal of offending risk factors, and medical or surgical reduction of intracranial pressure. Spontaneous intracranial hypotension, characterized by postural headache, is rarer than benign intracranial hypertension. Diminished cerebrospinal fluid production, hyperabsorption, and cerebrospinal fluid leak are postulated mechanisms of spontaneous intracranial hypotension; cerebrospinal fluid pressure is typically less than 60 mm H_2O. Empiric treatment includes bed rest; administration of caffeine, corticosteroids, or mineralocorticoids; epidural blood patch; and epidural saline infusion.

Orofacial Pain in Cardiovascular Diseases

Orofacial pain in hypertension

Headache is generally regarded as a symptom of high blood pressure, in spite of conflicting opinions on their precise association. Most studies have shown that mild, chronic hypertension and headache are not associated.[226] Whether moderate hypertension predisposes a person to headache remains controversial, but there is little evidence. However, headaches caused by significant disturbances in arterial pressure are included in the IHS classification. The headaches that are associated with severe disturbance in arterial pressure were attributed to pheochromocytoma, malignant hypertension, preeclampsia and eclampsia, and acute pressor response to an exogenous agent.

Headache is common in hypertension and was present in 75% of patients with severe hypertension followed by the presence of chest pain and shortness of breath (62%) and dizziness (50%).[227,228] Mild or moderate hypertension may not be associated with headache, whereas severe hypertension and rapid change in blood pressure may be associated with headache.[229,230]

The potential impact of hypertension on facial pain has been evaluated, and conflicting results have been reported. Patients with periapical dental disease had blood pressure and pain recorded before and after nonsurgical endodontics. A significant correlation was observed between preoperative systolic blood pressure and posttreatment pain ($P < .05$), which suggests an interaction between the cardiovascular and trigeminal regulatory systems.[231] In a retrospective review of 84 patients with trigeminal neuralgia, hypertension was present in 37% compared with 32% of control subjects (not significant), which suggests that as both conditions are common in older adults, they likely represent coexisting conditions.[232]

The most common symptom of pheochromocytoma is a rapid-onset headache, which has been reported by up to 92% of patients with this condition.[233] The headache, which lasts less than an hour in most patients, is bilateral, severe, and throbbing, and it may be associated with nausea in 50% of patients. Paroxysms can begin spontaneously or be triggered by physical exertion, certain medications, emotional stress, changes in posture, and increases in intra-abdominal pressure.[226]

In malignant hypertension, the rate and extent of the increase in blood pressure are the most important factors in the development of acute cerebral syndrome. The presenting symptoms can be headache, nausea, and vomiting. Additional signs and symptoms include blurred vision, scintillating scotoma or visual loss, anxiety, and then decreased levels of consciousness until seizures begin.[226]

Preeclampsia occurs in up to 7% of pregnancies, and eclampsia is found in up to 0.3%. Some have suggested that headache in women with preeclampsia is strongly associated with the presence of abnormal cerebral perfusion pressure.[234] A strong association between migraine history and preeclampsia development, specifically the severe form of preeclampsia, has been shown.[235]

A sudden severe headache due to a rapid increase in blood pressure may occur in persons taking monoamine oxidase inhibitors concomitantly with drinking red wine, eating foods with high tyramine content (eg, cheese, chicken livers, or pickled herring), or taking sympathomimetic medications such as pseudoephedrine.[226] However, monoamine oxidase inhibitors are rarely used today in medical management.

Orofacial pain of cardiac origin

Ischemic heart disease may lead to the onset of painful symptoms usually located retrosternally or precordially with radiation to the left arm, left shoulder, and neck.[236] This symptom is termed *angina pectoris* and may be more rarely accompanied by referred pain to the back, right arm, epigastrium, head, and orofacial region.[237–240]

Stable angina pectoris is precipitated by effort, relieved by rest, and associated with coronary artery disease, whereas unstable angina pectoris is characterized by increasing pain frequency and/or duration and novel onset at rest or with minimal effort.[240] Atypical forms of angina pectoris may occur during sleep or at rest (eg, Prinzmetal's angina) or may not be associated with detectable coronary artery disease (eg, microvascular angina). Acute coronary syndrome describes the continuum from unstable angina pectoris at one end of the spectrum to myocardial infarction at the other end.[240]

Ischemic cardiac pain is usually described as variations of pressure-like descriptors (heavy, pressing, tight, squeezing) but may also be aching, sharp, burning/searing, or a burst-open feeling.[237,239] Accompanying manifestations will vary depending on whether the symptoms reflect stable/unstable angina pectoris or myocardial infarction. Patients commonly report accompanying sweating, weakness, nausea, dyspnea, and vomiting but may not report any manifestation other than pain.[237,239]

Pain referral to the orofacial region in angina pectoris or myocardial infarction has been variably reported from 4% to 18% of patients.[237–239] Headache associated with ischemic chest pain (cardiac cephalalgia) is defined by the IHS and requires the presence of head pain aggravated by exercise and accompanied by nausea. Evidence must exist for concomitant acute myocardial ischemia, and symptoms should resolve with effective cardiac therapy. Cardiac cephalalgia has been reported in 5.2% of one series of patients with myocardial infarction and usually accompanies chest symptoms.[237] In rarer instances, myocardial infarction pain may be primarily felt as headache (3.4% of patients), jaw pain (3.6%), or neck pain (8.4%).[237] Orofacial pain (8.3%) is more common in inferior myocardial infarction, and cardiac cephalalgia is more frequently reported (7.3%) in anterior myocardial infarction,[237] which suggests that anatomical factors influence the prevalence of pain referral. However, other studies have shown that women report a higher frequency of jaw pain associated with angina pectoris than do men, even after controlling for myocardial infarction severity and location.[239,241,242]

Reports of patients with headache and orofacial pain as the cardinal manifestation of ischemic heart disease have appeared in the literature.[243–251] Diagnosis is often dependent on the temporal profile, which may be suggestive of cardiac cephalalgia/orofacial pain. Typically, onset is in close proximity to exercise and subsides with rest or antianginal therapy. Rarely, as in unstable angina pectoris, pain may be felt at rest.[252] Pain may be moderate to severe and located in the neck, mandible (it may involve teeth and gums), unilaterally in the head, or even referring to the vertex. At-risk groups are patients older than 50 years with new-onset headache and risk factors for heart disease.

The mechanisms of referred pain in ischemic heart disease are unclear and may be multiple.[246,253,254] Convergence of sympathetic or vagal fibers that transduce cardiac pain with trigeminocervical pathways has been shown, and indeed, sympathectomy relieves angina pectoris in a subset of patients. Compromised cardiac function with impaired venous return may lead to increased intracranial pressure and subsequent pain. Cardiac ischemia may induce the release of a number of mediators that can cause distant pain.

Intracranial hypertension is associated with headache, which improves after diagnosis and effective treatment.[254] Diagnosis is critical, as treatment can avoid serious visual and CNS complications.[255]

Clinicians should be aware that migraine sufferers have an elevated incidence of vascular disease that may be critical to recognize. Patients with classic migraine with aura may have an increased risk of ischemic stroke and an association with cardiac disease that needs further evaluation. Once alerted, management of potential risk factors such as hypertension, tobacco use, and use of oral contraceptives may reduce cardiac risk.[256] A high prevalence of headache, particularly migraine, is seen in patients with atrial septal defects, which suggests benefits from atrial septal defect repair.[257,258] Furthermore, cardiac abnormalities are associated with a prolonged duration of migraine (> 10 years).[259] Associations have been shown between migraine headache and heart disease, and headache patients have increased cardiovascular disease risk factors.[260]

Vascular risk is known in women with migraine, particularly in the presence of smoking, hypertension, diabetes, thrombophilia, age over 35 years, and use of oral contraception.[261]

Though obtaining a history of prior cardiovascular disease and cardiovascular disease risk factors is appropriate in headache patients, testing for cardiovascular disease is not supported in the literature.[260]

Cervical artery dissection

Extracranial dissections of the internal carotid artery and vertebral artery are quite common, with an annual combined incidence of 5/100,000 persons; co-occurrences are termed *cervical artery dissections*.[262,263] The mean patient age is in the early 40s, and approximately 70% of patients are younger than 50 years.[263] Women, on average, are 5 years younger than men at the time of dissection and are more likely to have dissections in multiple vessels.[264] Spontaneous dissections occur with no history of trauma, whereas some patients report blunt trauma, particularly extension-flexion (whiplash) or rotation injuries to the neck.[263,265] Cervical artery dissections arise from a tear in the intima (inside-out theory) that allows blood to enter the artery wall under high pressure. The resulting intramural hematoma may compromise the lumen and lead to stenosis or may expand outward as an aneurismal dilation.[266] New evidence suggests that the pathologic process may begin with degenerative changes at the medial-adventitial border associated with neoangiogenesis of capillary vessels branching from the vasa vasorum in the adventitia (outside-in theory).[267,268]

The clinical presentation is varied and may consist of a single symptom or a combination of symptoms, such as pain, Horner syndrome, and neck tenderness. The most common presentation of cervical artery dissections is head, face, or neck pain with or without other signs, with up to 95% of patients reporting such pain in internal carotid artery dissection and 70% in vertebral artery dissection.[263,266,269–272] In internal carotid artery dissections, a unilateral headache may be the single symptom in 45% of patients and is ipsilateral to dissection with a steady or throbbing quality.[263,273] Frequently, pain occurs in the orbital, periorbital, and frontal regions and may commonly involve the cheek, angle of the mandible, jaw, and ear. Anterolateral neck pain occurs in 25% of patients. Other accompanying signs include diplopia, pulsatile tinnitus, tongue paresis, and dysgeusia.[266,274] In vertebral artery dissections, the headache is unilateral in two-thirds of patients and ipsilateral to the dissection. Pain is located in the posterior head and is rarely associated with facial pain. Posterior neck pain is noted in almost 50% of patients with vertebral artery dissections. Horner syndrome may be the presenting sign of internal carotid artery dissection in about half of patients with or without pain.[263,269,270,275]

Diagnosis is by angiography, Doppler, MRI, or magnetic resonance angiography, but false-negatives are possible. Treatment may include anticoagulation therapy, antiplatelet therapy, surgery, or placement of stents, and mortality from cervical artery dissection is low (5%); the prognosis for cervical artery dissections is considered to be very good in the vast majority of patients.[263,276,277] Pain resolves within 1 week but may last up to 5 weeks.[266] Recurrence is not uncommon, however, and is most frequent within the first 2 months after the initial event; 6% to 17% of patients will suffer a dissection in another vessel within 10 years.[263,278] Early recurrences of dissection in the weeks after the initial event could be a manifestation of a unique transient disorder, whereas late recurrences occurring several months or years later could indicate an underlying connective tissue weakness.[279,280]

Orofacial Pain in Blood Disorders

Disorders of the red blood cells may cause orofacial pain and headaches. Anemia, defined as a reduction in the oxygen-carrying capacity of the blood, is usually related to a decrease in the number of circulating red blood cells or to an abnormality in the red blood cell hemoglobin content. In some forms of hemoglobinopathies—thalassemia and sickle cell anemia—facial pain or headache may be present as part of the clinical presentation.

Thalassemias are autosomally dominant inherited disorders in which either alpha- or beta-globin chains are synthesized at a low rate, thereby lessening the production of hemoglobin A. The unaffected chains are produced in excess and precipitate within the erythrocytes to cause excessive erythrocyte fragility and hemolysis. Thalassemias are characterized by a hypochromic microcytic anemia and may be severe (major, homozygous) or mild (minor, heterozygous) and may affect beta-chains (beta thalassemia) or alpha-chains (alpha thalassemia).

In beta thalassemia, neurologic complications have been attributed to various factors, such as chronic hypoxia, bone marrow expansion, iron overload, and desferrioxamine neurotoxicity.[281] Cranial nerve palsies have been described in thalassemia due to the extramedullary hematopoiesis resulting in pressure on the nerves.[282,283] Thromboembolic events have been frequently reported in patients with beta thalassemia in association with such risk factors as diabetes, complex cardiopulmonary abnormalities, hypothyroidisim, liver function anomalies, and postsplenectomy thrombocytosis. A multicenter Italian study identified 32 patients with thromboembolic episodes in a total of 735 subjects with thalassemia. The researchers found great variation in localization of the thromboemboli, mainly in the CNS (16/32), with a clinical picture of headache, seizures, and hemiparesis.[284] Thalassemia major may present with multiple orofacial abnormalities. A study of 54 patients with thalassemia major identified dental/jaw pain in 40.0% and headache in 29.6%.[285] Anecdotally, patients with thalassemia may experience painful swelling of the parotid glands, with xerostomia caused by iron deposition, and a sore or burning tongue related to folate deficiency.[286]

In sickle cell anemia, amino acid substitution in the globin chain results in hemoglobin with a propensity to polymerize or precipitate, causing gross distortions in the shape of erythrocytes and membrane damage. The erythrocytes lose flexibility and sickle, which may cause microvascular occlusions. Painful crises that are usually due to infarction as a result of sickling are brought on by infection, dehydration, hypoxia, acidosis, or cold; cause severe pain and pyrexia; and may occur in the jaw. Orofacial pain during sickle-cell crises may occur, and dental care should be deferred until the crisis is managed and specific diagnosis of dental disease is made. Headaches, mental nerve paresthesia, and jaw pain have been reported in sickle-cell crises, probably because of the intensive extramedullary hematopoiesis or necrosis in the jaws.[287,288] Painful infarcts in the jaws may be mistaken for toothache or osteomyelitis. Pulpal symptoms are common in the absence of any obvious dental disease, and pulpal necrosis has sometimes resulted.[289,290] Skull infarction should be considered as a cause of new-onset headache located at the vertex in patients with sickle cell disease, especially if scalp edema is present.[291]

A study on the characteristics of headaches in children with sickle cell disease showed an incidence of 31.2% of frequent headaches (greater than once a week) with moderate average pain severity (5.8 on a scale of 0 to 10). Duration of headaches ranged from 30 minutes to several days (mean, 5 hours). Based on IHS criteria, 50.0% of children had headache symptoms consistent with tension-type headaches, 43.8% with migraines, and 6.2% with migraine with aura. Children with symptoms of migraine had significantly greater functional disability compared with children with symptoms of tension-type headaches.

The use of cytokines and growth factors, some with known toxicities, has become common in the treatment of hematologic disorders.[292] Granulocyte macrophage colony-stimulating factor (GM-CSF) is administered to prevent myelotoxicity or accelerate hematopoietic recovery after chemotherapy and has been reported to cause headache.[293] A common adverse event due to the ability of GM-CSF to increase hematopoiesis in bone marrow is bone pain with the potential involvement of the jaw. GM-CSF is increasingly used to mobilize hematopoietic stem cells to the peripheral blood in the healthy donor population, thereby exposing this group to potential adverse events presenting in the orofacial complex.

Orofacial Pain in Dialysis and Renal Disorders

Dialysis may induce severe headache as a result of overhydration and electrolyte shifts. About 70% of patients on hemodialysis complain of headache, and about 57% of patients experience headache during hemodialysis sessions.[294,295] The most prevalent features of dialysis headache include bilateralism; frontotemporal, occipital, or diffuse location; moderate to severe intensity; throbbing quality; and duration less than 4 hours.[296,297]

The IHS criteria for headache related to hemodialysis specify that the headaches must begin during hemodialysis and spontaneously terminate within 72 hours after the end of the hemodialysis session.[19] This headache commonly occurs in association with hypotension and dialysis disequilibrium syndrome. However, variations of headache related to hemodialysis may not follow these specific criteria.[295] The literature suggests that the dialysis protocol may also affect headache frequency.[298] Sporadic reports describe a complication of nephrotic syndrome that causes headache, specifically cerebral venous thrombosis.[299,300]

Alport syndrome is an unusual genetic disease that ultimately results in renal failure and has an associated high incidence of sensorineural hearing loss that may present as one of the first symptoms.[301] A case of a patient with Alport syndrome and TMJ involvement is described in the literature.[302] The patient had complaints of facial and joint pain that resembled TMD with headache, tinnitus, joint pain, and temporal swelling.

Orofacial Pain in Pulmonary Diseases

Chronic obstructive pulmonary disease is a chronic, slowly progressive irreversible disease characterized by breathlessness, wheezing, cough, and sputum production. About 30% of patients with moderate or severe, stable chronic obstructive pulmonary disease complain of headache, and 45.5% report sleep disorders. Significant risk factors include a family history of chronic obstructive pulmonary disease, presence of other systemic or sleep disorders (eg, snoring, bruxism), and laboratory data indicating chronic hypoxemia and airway obstruction.[303] This suggests a relationship between chronic hypoxemia and headache.

Asthma is a state of bronchial hyperreactivity that causes paroxysmal expiratory wheezing, dyspnea, and cough. Generalized reversible bronchial narrowing is caused by excessive bronchial smooth muscle tone, mucosal edema and congestion, and mucus hypersecretion with diminished ciliary clearance. Evidence for an association between migraine and asthma is based on a matched case-control study including a patient population of more than 5 million subjects.[304] However, the mechanism shared by migraine and asthma is unclear. Orofacial pain may be referred from the chest due to heart or lung disease via the vagus nerve and present as facial pain, and in some patients it may be an early manifestation of an occult cardiovascular or malignant disease.

Orofacial Pain in Patients with Cancer

Patients with oropharyngeal and head and neck cancer often experience pain and suffering that reduce quality of life. Additionally, oral manifestations of hematologic cancers and metastasis to the oral tissues may cause pain. Cancer therapy is well known to frequently induce painful oral complications. This oral pain has significant impact on the patients' well being and compliance with treatment.

Cancer pain reduces quality of life and increases anxiety and depression.[305–308] An esti-

mated 45% to 60% of all patients with cancer do not have adequate pain control,[309,310] possibly because of patient reluctance to report pain, practices of health care providers, preconceived fears of addiction, and the strict regulations regarding opioids.

The pathogenesis of oral cancer pain is not fully understood (Table 14-1). Many mediators have been implicated, including endothelin-1, proteases, and nerve growth factor. The evidence is weaker for the role of other mediators, such as protons, transient receptor potential vanilloid, substance P, calcitonin gene–related peptide, adenosine triphosphate, and bradykinin.[311]

Orofacial pain in patients with cancer can be classified according to the underlying pathophysiology (eg, nociceptive, inflammatory, infectious, neuropathic), the location of the tumor (local versus distant), the primary initiating agent (cancer or cancer therapy), or the relation between the onset of pain and the time of cancer treatment (before, during, or after cancer therapy). The following sections cover orofacial pain due to cancer, orofacial pain due to cancer therapy, and orofacial pain of noncancerous etiology in patients with cancer.

Orofacial pain due to cancer

Orofacial pain may occur in primary oropharyngeal and head and neck cancers, by way of local involvement of systemic cancers, and from metastases to the head and neck from distant tumors. The orofacial pain may also be referred from cancers at distant sites.

Pain in regional malignancy

Local regional cancers commonly causing pain in the head and neck include oral, oropharyngeal, sinus, nasopharyngeal, salivary gland, intracranial, and extracranial primary and metastatic tumors. Some reports state that pain is the initial complaint of oral cancer in 30% to 50% of patients,[312] and the reported incidence of pain is up to 85% in these patients when referred for cancer treatment.[313]

Of patients with advanced cancer, 75% to 90% experience significant pain,[314] and up to 85% of patients with head and neck cancer report pain at the time of diagnosis.[313,315,316] More

Table 14-1	Mechanisms of pain in malignant disease
Immediate affector	**Macroscopic and microscopic mechanism**
Pain due to cancer	
Mass pressure/ altered function	Mechanical nerve pain, nerve entrapment, hypoxia, movement dysfunction/TMD
Tumor invasion	Connective tissue, neurogenic pain, nerve invasion/dysfunction, vascular penetration
Barrier damage	Erythema/atrophy/erosion/ulceration
Inflammation/ neurogenic sensitization	Reactive oxygen species, cytokine release (eg, tumor necrosis factor), low pH, algesic compounds (prostaglandins, cyclo-oxygenase-2, bradykinin, norepinephrine, serotonin, substance P, calcitonin gene–related peptide), upregulation of peripheral opioid receptors
Pain due to treatment of malignant disease	
Surgery	Acute: surgical Chronic: fibrosis and change in function, nerve pain, inflammation
Radiation therapy	Barrier damage: reactive oxygen species, cytokine release (eg, tumor necrosis factor), low pH, algesic compounds (prostaglandins, cyclo-oxygenase-2, bradykinin, norepinephrine, serotonin, substance P, calcitonin gene–related peptide), upregulation of peripheral opioid receptors, response to secondary microbial irritation
Chemotherapy	Same as radiation therapy; in addition, mucosal toxicity and neuropathy
Tumor lysis	Same as radiation therapy

than three-fourths suffer from pain secondary to bone destruction and nerve injury[317,318] involving inflammatory and neuropathic mechanisms.[305,319] After treatment of head and neck cancer, 78% of patients reported pain in the head, face, or mouth; 54% in the cervical region or shoulder; and some at distant sites, including the chest (7%), lower back (7%), and limbs (5%).[320]

In patients with oral cancer pain, symptoms were nonspecific and included descriptions such as sore throat, pain on function (swallowing, chewing), and pain in the region of the tongue, mouth, teeth, and ear. Symptoms varied from mild discomfort to severe pain. Pain was found to be associated with advanced disease[321] and lesions located on the tongue.[322] Primary tumors to the jaw and infratemporal fossa may cause neurologic symptoms presenting as pain and numbness. Interestingly, excruciating pain after the first few bites (ie, first-bite syndrome) may be the presentation of a mass in the parotid region.[323]

Patients with nasopharyngeal cancer often report pain in the TMJ region and may be misdiagnosed as having a TMD.[324–326] In such cases, pain is described as dull and aching and resulting in a headache; earache; or jaw, midface, or neck discomfort.[324]

Systemic cancers such as leukemia may affect the head and neck area, causing pain and loss of function.[313,327] Infiltration of the leukemic cells into enclosed oral spaces creates pressure that causes pain. In addition, hematologic cancers cause oral pain indirectly by increasing the risk of secondary infections (fungal, bacterial, and viral) because of damaged mucosal barriers and possible myelosuppression.[328–330]

Lymphoma is a common neoplasm occurring in the oral region and accounting for 3.5% of oral malignancies.[331,332] Lymphoma may present as a firm rubbery mass associated with discomfort in approximately half of patients. Pressure from the mass on local structures can cause pain or neuropathy. Secondary inflammation may also contribute to the pain.

Multiple myeloma frequently presents as asymptomatic lytic bony lesions.[333] The less frequent extramedullary presentation varies greatly, ranging from a mass to an ulcer associated with pain, and may pose a diagnostic challenge.[333,334]

Metastasis to the jaw may present similarly. Bone pain results from structural damage, periosteal irritation, and nerve entrapment. Metastatic tumors to the jaw commonly arise from the breast, colon, prostate, thyroid, lung, and kidney.[335–338] Metastases to the jaw rarely

Table 14-2 **Estimated frequency of oropharyngeal mucositis**

Disease	Therapy	Percentage of patients with mucositis
Upper airway and digestive tract carcinoma	Radiotherapy alone	More than 80%
Intensive chemotherapy	Chemoradiotherapy	Up to 100%
	With hematopoietic stem cell transplantation rescue	Up to 75% with herpes simplex virus prophylaxis
Solid cancers of gastrointestinal system, genitourinary system, and breast	With neutropenia-inducing chemotherapy	Up to 50% of patients; ulcerative mucositis in up to 20% of patients

involve the soft tissues and usually occur in the posterior mandible, angle of the jaw, and ramus.[339] In up to 30% of patients, oral metastases are the first indication of a distant tumor.[339] Other orofacial malignancies, such as malignant melanoma and intraoral sarcomas, are rare but can present as a mass accompanied with discomfort.[340,341]

Orofacial pain or headache is reported in up to 6% of patients with intracranial tumors[342–347] (see also chapters 12 and 13). The presentation may be similar to that of trigeminal neuralgia, persistent facial pain, and TMDs. About 60% of these patients have sensory or motor function loss at presentation.[348]

Pain as an isolated symptom is an unreliable predictor of orofacial malignancy because pain quality and intensity are highly variable. However, the combination of numbness, pain, and swelling is highly predictive of malignancy, particularly in the presence of systemic signs (eg, weight loss, fatigue, anemia).

Pain secondary to malignancy at a distant site

Orofacial pain may arise from a distant, non-metastasized cancer, most commonly from the lungs,[349–351] due to activation of nociceptive pathways in mediastinal or head and neck structures.[351] Pain may occur due to invasion or compression of the vagus nerve,[352] and referred facial pain may be mediated by termination of vagal afferents in the spinal trigeminal nucleus.[353,354] In addition, the phrenic nerve may refer pain from the pleura and subdiaphragmatic areas to the head and neck.[355] Paraneoplastic processes resulting in peripheral neuropathies and cytokine production are common, partic-

ularly in lung cancer.[356–358] Typical presentations include unilateral dull aching pain (ipsilateral to the lung tumor), often located around the ear, jaw, and temporal regions; weight loss; hemoptysis; persistent cough; and chest wall pain.[351] Similar mechanisms may be associated with gastrointestinal and pancreatic cancers that present with orofacial pain.[359,360]

Peripheral neuropathy was found in 48% of patients with lung cancer before chemotherapy.[361] Neuromuscular dysfunction occurs in 30% of patients with diverse tumors, most commonly in ovarian, testicular, or bronchogenic cancers.[362] Often, these neuropathies are accompanied by detectable autoantibodies that aid in diagnosis.

Orofacial pain due to cancer therapy

Treatment-related orofacial pain may be acute during active therapy or delayed due to late complications of therapy. In this chapter, orofacial pain due to cancer therapy is presented according to etiology.

Pain due to conventional chemotherapy and radiotherapy

The most common acute oral side effect of cancer chemotherapy or radiotherapy is mucositis (Table 14-2). Oral mucositis pain results from tissue injury that causes the release of reactive oxygen species, proinflammatory cytokines, and neurotransmitters that activate nociceptive receptors. The severity of the pain is related to the degree of tissue damage and is modified by the emotional and sociocultural background of the patient.[363–366] Other factors that may influence the severity of mucositis pain are age, mucosal infection, type of treatment, and cumulative dose.[363,364,367]

In chemotherapy-induced mucositis, the sites most commonly involved are nonkeratinized (buccal and labial mucosa, ventral and lateral aspects of the tongue, soft palate, and floor of the mouth). Signs of mucositis appear approximately 6 to 10 days after treatment, although the biologic changes begin immediately.[368] Pain associated with mucositis is the most distressing symptom in patients undergoing aggressive neutropenia-inducing chemotherapy regimens.[369–371] Mucositis is also well documented in patients undergoing hematopoietic stem cell transplantation and is the most frequent serious side effect of therapy in the first 100 days.[372–374] Patients treated with high-dose cancer chemotherapy for solid malignancies, particularly of epithelial origin (eg, gastrointestinal and breast), suffer painful oral mucositis due to mucosal toxicity of chemotherapy, and prevalence and severity increase throughout successive courses of chemotherapy.[373,375]

Mucositis from radiation therapy typically affects nonkeratinized mucosa in the radiation field beginning at week 3 of therapy, peaking at weeks 5 to 6, and then remitting 4 to 8 weeks after therapy.[376,377] Mucositis pain is common (58% to 75% of patients) and interferes with daily activities in 33% to 60% of patients.[312,378–382] The incidence, severity, and duration of mucositis increase with use of combined chemoradiotherapy of head and neck cancer.[381–383] Mucosal symptoms continue for 6 to 12 months in up to a third of patients, even after clinical resolution of the mucosal lesion,[381–384] which suggests epithelial atrophy and/or neuropathy. Patients with mucosal pain before cancer therapy may experience more severe mucositis-associated pain during treatment, which suggests the establishment of sensitization.[385] Newer radiotherapy technologies allow reduction of the high-dose volume while increasing the area of low-dose exposure in the region treated.[386]

Pain due to oral mucositis has a dramatic impact on quality of life and frequently requires opioid analgesics, tube feeding, extended hospitalization, and unanticipated rehospitalization, and it may lead to the modification or interruption of cancer therapy.[375,377,387] Mucositis pain can be severe, preventing oral intake of food and medications and limiting verbal communication, which causes psychosocial distress. Oral mucosal pain can be exacerbated by comorbidities such as dry mouth and secondary mucosal infection (eg, candidiasis).[388] The breakdown of the epithelial barrier in mucositis produces a portal for opportunistic systemic infection.[375,387,389] Dry mouth may be secondary to dehydration or due to the effects of radiation therapy on salivary glands.

Acute mucosal injury may progress into chronic mucosal change, and symptoms range from mild sensitivity to severe, debilitating pain.[312,390] Associated signs may be mucosal atrophy, vascular change (telangiectasia), depapillation of the tongue, and dry mouth.

As the use of targeted therapies increases, more oral complications are reported, including pain. Stomatitis associated with the mammalian target of rapamycin inhibitor may affect more than 50% of patients and has a different presentation from conventional cytotoxic mucositis.[391,392] The pain from the oral ulcers was found to be severe enough to prompt a dosage reduction in 24% of patients.[391] As data accumulate, the pathophysiologies of pain-preventive approaches and pain-management techniques are expected to improve. Disruption of the oral mucosa barrier likely causes inflammation, and the areas become infected secondarily. Stomatitis and oral pain were also reported in patients treated with epidermal growth factor receptor inhibitors, such as cetuximab and erlotinib, and in those receiving imatinib, the tyrosine kinase inhibitor for platelet-derived growth factor receptor.[392,393]

Some neurotoxic cytotoxic agents (eg, vincristine, vinblastine, platinum derivatives, taxanes, cyclophosphamide, and thalidomide) may cause jaw pain and neuropathy.[394–398]

Soft tissue necrosis and osteonecrosis after radiation therapy are known complications that may be associated with pain.[399,400] The onset of symptoms is variable and may appear decades after radiation therapy.[399,401–403]

Pain due to surgical procedures

Surgical procedures result in acute orofacial pain and may ultimately lead to chronic pain involving inflammatory and neuropathic mechanisms. Adjuvant therapies may affect the severity and frequency of pain, and neck dissection may increase musculoskeletal dysfunction and cause neuropathic pain.[404] Radiation therapy may increase postsurgical fibrosis and dysfunction and result in posttraumatic neuropathy.

Orofacial pain after head and neck cancer therapy can develop due to secondary musculoskeletal syndromes (TMDs) or neuropathic syndromes. The impact may be severe if there is discontinuity of the jaw or if fibrosis of muscles and soft tissue occurs. Resection of the mandible to excise a tumor inevitably leads to sensory impairment; 50% of patients experience regional hyperalgesia or allodynia.[405] Two to 5 years after maxillectomy, approximately 90% of patients reported persistent pain.[406] Functional consequences are often secondary to pain and postsurgical fibrosis.[407]

Pain scores after head and neck cancer surgery were highest for oral cavity cancers followed by cancers of the larynx, oropharynx, and nasopharynx.[408] More than 50% of these patients experienced postoperative functional problems. For example, persistent impairment from moderate to severe pain was found in 34.3% of patients more than 6 months after surgery.[385] The most frequent sites of pain were the shoulder (31.0% to 38.5% of patients), neck (4.9% to 34.9%), TMJ (4.9% to 20.1%), oral cavity (4.2% to 18.7%), and other sites of the head and face (4.2% to 15.6%),[385,407] which reflects morbidity secondary to tumor and regional lymph node resection.[404,409] Despite the fact that more than 60% of patients reported pain, most of which was rated as severe, 75% of these patients were not taking analgesics.[385] In any event, analgesics and physiotherapy were found to be largely ineffective in the treatment of chronic pain in these patients.[407] At 54 to 60 months after surgery, a smaller proportion of reviewed patients (14.9%) had persistent pain,[407] which suggests gradual remission over time. In patients after cancer surgery, pain is characterized as acute and chronic. The acute pain lasts 1 or 2 months and gradually improves.[410–412] The chronic pain in survivors of head and neck cancer is often unrecognized and therefore untreated, though it may remain more than 3 years and is associated with functional problems.[411]

Orofacial pain of noncancerous etiology in patients with cancer

Orofacial pain of noncancerous causes occurs frequently during cancer treatment. Immunosuppression, surgery, and emotional stress contribute to increased risk for orofacial infections. Pain may be due to oral bacterial or fungal infection or due to reactivation of viral infections in the oral tissues. Postherpetic neuralgia may result in chronic pain in approximately 10% of patients, and pain may persist for years (see chapter 12). Pain may also be due to local dental disease (see chapter 6), and if it is due to infection, the pain may be more significant in patients who are myelosuppressed.[413,414]

Osteonecrosis of the jaws due to antiresorptive and antiangiogenic compounds occurs in approximately 7% (range, 0% to 27.5%) of patients treated with bisphosphonates, denosumab, sunitinib, and bevacizumab for oncology indications,[415] and it is associated with pain in most identified cases of necrosis.[416,417] Pain in patients with osteonecrosis of the jaws may be explained by secondary infection, local ischemia, or bone fracture. Neuropathy may develop when the lesion involved in osteonecrosis of the jaws is adjacent to the mandibular nerve.[418]

Oral graft-versus-host disease (GVHD) is a manifestation of systemic GVHD, secondary to allogeneic hematopoietic stem cell transplantation. Little information is known about acute oral GVHD. Chronic oral GVHD mimics a number of autoimmune disorders, including lichen planus, SLE, and systemic sclerosis and has a clinical presentation that includes mucosal erythema, atrophy, pseudomembranous ulceration, hyperkeratotic striae, plaques, and papules; these oral mucosa changes may cause pain.[419]

Treatment of orofacial pain in patients with cancer

Effective management of orofacial pain in patients with cancer requires comprehensive assessment of the multifactorial etiologies and treatment directed at these causative factors. Treatment of cancer-related pain is accomplished by effective treatment of the malignant disease. Treatment of head and neck cancer is beyond the scope of this book. For the management of oral complications in patients with cancer, the reader is referred to several systematic reviews.[420–431] Numerous studies regarding oral mucositis are described later, and principles of palliative care are relevant to all oral mucosal injuries.

Prevention of mucosal damage

Treating malignancies with minimal damage to healthy tissues is a goal of cancer therapy. However, because of poor cure rates in head and neck cancer, particularly in advanced disease, more intense radiation protocols with hyperfractionation, combined chemoradiotherapy, and radiation for recurrences increase the intensity, severity, and duration of mucositis. Patients receiving these intensive regimens are at a greater risk of mucositis, which then limits therapy.[375] Considerable effort is made to minimize mucositis, including radiation treatment planning (intensive modulated radiotherapy); changes in chemotherapy drugs, doses, or schedule of delivery; and effective prophylaxis and early treatment of emerging mucositis. According to the clinical practice guidelines for the management of oral mucositis developed by the Multinational Association of Supportive Care in Cancer (MASCC)/International Society of Oral Oncology (ISOO), several modalities are recommended for the prevention of oral mucositis. The guidelines are specific to the population of cancer patients. Prevention of oral mucositis indirectly reduces pain[423] (Table 14-3).

Basic oral care

The goal of basic oral care is to maintain oral health, reduce tissue irritation, and control dental plaque levels. Evidence suggests that good oral hygiene, which decreases the microbial load, may reduce the frequency and severity of oral mucositis and, therefore, of associated pain.[364,432] The MASCC/ISOO clinical practice guidelines suggest that an oral care protocol be implemented to prevent oral mucositis in all age groups and across all cancer treatment modalities.[424]

Topical approaches for mucosal pain relief

The oral mucosa is accessible for topical interventions, although the unpleasant taste, associated nausea, and diluting effects of saliva may limit compliance and effectiveness (see chapter 16). Topical anesthetics are used to treat pain from mucosal injury. Topical anesthetics have a limited duration of effect (15 to 30 minutes), may sting upon application to damaged mucosa, and suppress taste and the gag reflex. After lidocaine rinse, systemic absorption across ulcerated mucosal surfaces is increased compared with that for healthy persons; however, the difference is relatively minimal.[433] Topical anesthetics are often mixed with coating and antimicrobial agents, such as milk of magnesia, diphenhydramine, or nystatin (often called "magic mouthwash" or "oncology mouthwash").

The MASCC/ISOO guidelines for the management of oral mucositis include a few topical treatment modalities and present evidence that doxepin and morphine reduce pain[423] (see Table 14-3). Doxepin (a tricyclic antidepressant) 0.5% mouthrinse in patients with cancer results in analgesia and is maintained for at least 4 hours after a single application.[434] Topical morphine in a 0.2% mouthwash has been shown to be effective for relieving pain,[435] but there is concern about dispensing large volumes of the medication.

Coating agents have been promoted for managing pain from mucosal injury. Sucralfate was suggested for pain management, although it has not been shown to reduce oral mucositis.[436] Other coating agents, such as antacids and milk of magnesia, have not been shown to significantly reduce pain.

Nonpharmacologic local approaches for pain relief in patients with cancer include light therapy and cryotherapy.[423] Other agents mentioned in the MASCC/ISOO systematic review and additional guidelines may develop as data accumulate.[420–422,424–431,437]

Systemic medications

The World Health Organization (WHO) Pain Management Ladder has been recommended for managing pain in patients with cancer[310] (Box 14-2). Pain is reduced by following the WHO ladder to one-third of pretreatment intensity in 70% to 90% of patients[438,439]; therefore, 10% to 30% of patients with cancer do not achieve adequate pain control.[440] The WHO analgesic ladder assumes that pain progress-

Table 14-3 **MASCC/ISOO evidence-based clinical practice guidelines for mucositis secondary to cancer therapy**[423]

Intervention	Guideline
Recommendations in favor	
Cryotherapy	30 minutes of oral cryotherapy should be used to prevent oral mucositis in patients receiving bolus 5-fluorouracil chemotherapy.
Recombinant human keratinocyte growth factor-1	Recombinant human keratinocyte growth factor-1/palifermin should be used to prevent oral mucositis (at a dose of 60 μg/kg per day for 3 days before conditioning treatment and for 3 days after transplant) in patients receiving high-dose chemotherapy and total body irradiation, followed by autogenous stem-cell transplantation for a hematologic malignancy.
Low-level laser therapy	Low-level laser therapy (wavelength at 650 nm, power of 40 mW, and each square centimeter treated with the required time to a tissue energy dose of 2 J/cm^2) should be used to prevent oral mucositis in patients receiving hematopoietic stem-cell transplantation conditioned with high-dose chemotherapy, with or without total body irradiation.
Patient-controlled analgesia	Patient-controlled analgesia with morphine should be used to treat pain due to oral mucositis in patients undergoing hematopoietic stem-cell transplantation.
Benzydamine	Benzydamine mouthwash should be used to prevent oral mucositis in patients with head and neck cancer receiving moderate-dose radiation therapy (up to 50 Gy) without concomitant chemotherapy.
Suggestions in favor	
Oral care protocols	Oral care protocols should be used to prevent oral mucositis in all age groups and across all cancer treatment modalities.
Cryotherapy	Cryotherapy should be used to prevent oral mucositis in patients receiving high-dose melphalan, with or without total body irradiation, as conditioning for hematopoietic stem-cell transplantation.
Low-level laser therapy	Low-level laser therapy (wavelength around 632.8 nm) should be used to prevent oral mucositis in patients undergoing radiotherapy, without concomitant chemotherapy, for head and neck cancer.
Transdermal fentanyl	Transdermal fentanyl may be effective to treat pain due to oral mucositis in patients receiving conventional or high-dose chemotherapy, with or without total body irradiation.
Morphine mouthwash	0.2% morphine mouthwash may be effective to treat pain due to oral mucositis in patients receiving chemoradiation for head and neck cancer.
Doxepin mouthwash	0.5% doxepin mouthwash may be effective to treat pain due to oral mucositis.
Zinc	Systemic zinc supplements administered orally may be of benefit to prevent oral mucositis in patients with oral cancer who are receiving radiation therapy or chemoradiation.
Recommendations against	
PTA and BCoG	PTA and BCoG antimicrobial lozenges and PTA paste should not be used to prevent oral mucositis in patients receiving radiation therapy for head and cancer.
Iseganan	Iseganan antimicrobial mouthwash should not be used to prevent oral mucositis in patients receiving high-dose chemotherapy, with or without total body irradiation, for hematopoietic stem-cell transplantation (level of evidence II), or in patients receiving radiation therapy or concomitant chemoradiation for head and neck cancer.
Sucralfate mouthwash	Sucralfate mouthwash should not be used to prevent or treat oral mucositis in patients receiving chemotherapy for cancer or in patients receiving radiation therapy or concomitant chemoradiation for head and neck cancer.
Intravenous glutamine	Intravenous glutamine should not be used to prevent oral mucositis in patients receiving high-dose chemotherapy, with or without total body irradiation, for hematopoietic stem-cell transplantation.

Table 14-3 (cont)

Intervention	Guideline
Suggestions against	
Chlorhexidine mouthwash	Chlorhexidine mouthwash should not be used to prevent oral mucositis in patients receiving radiation therapy for head and neck cancer.
Granulocyte macrophage colony-stimulating factor mouthwash	Granulocyte macrophage colony-stimulating factor mouthwash should not be used to prevent oral mucositis in patients receiving high-dose chemotherapy for autologous or allogeneic stem-cell transplantation.
Misoprostol mouthwash	Misoprostol mouthwash should not be used to prevent oral mucositis in patients receiving radiation therapy for head and neck cancer.
Pentoxifylline	Systemic pentoxifylline, administered orally, should not be used to prevent oral mucositis in patients undergoing bone marrow transplantation.
Pilocarpine	Systemic pilocarpine, administered orally, should not be used to prevent oral mucositis in patients receiving radiation therapy for head and neck cancer (level of evidence III) or in patients receiving high-dose chemotherapy, with or without total body irradiation, for hematopoietic stem-cell transplantation.

PTA, polymyxin, tobramycin, amphotericin B; BCoG, bacitracin, clotrimazole, gentamicin.

Box 14-2 | **Steps in the management of orofacial pain in patients with cancer (based on the modified WHO pain ladder)**

1. Diagnose/treat cause
2. Topical therapy for mucosal pain
3. Nonopioid analgesics
4. Strong opioids
   - Adjunctive medications: centrally acting analgesics*
   - Adjunctive/complementary management†
5. Repeated assessment of effect and side effects

*For example, tricyclic antidepressants, gabapentin, antiseizure medications, antianxiety agents, muscle relaxants, and sleep-promoting medications.
†Physical therapy, acupuncture, and psychologic management.

---

es gradually, which may not be accurate. Furthermore, a meta-analysis has challenged the effectiveness of weak opioids (step II medications); no difference in effectiveness was seen between nonsteroidal anti-inflammatory medications (NSAIDs; step I) and weak opioids (step II) regarding pain management, but there were increased side effects from the weak opioids.[441,442] The strong opioids (step III), however, provide better pain control.[443] Therefore, a change in the WHO ladder has been discussed, where step I medications are used for mild pain, and the lowest effective doses of strong opioids are individually titrated (dose and administration route) to control more severe pain[444] (see Table 14-3). Transdermal fentanyl has become widely used in the management of oropharyn-

geal pain in patients with cancer.[445–447] Evidence supports the use of transdermal fentanyl for the management of oral mucositis pain.[423] Ideally, patients should be as close to pain free as possible with regular analgesics, and additional analgesics should be administered for breakthrough pain.[448–450] Daily assessment of pain levels and modification of pain medications according to the WHO ladder have been shown to improve pain control in patients with head and neck cancer who are receiving radiotherapy.[451]

Addiction to opioids is not a concern for patients with cancer. The focus should be on escalating to stronger opioids as needed and using adjuvant approaches to provide adequate pain relief. Tolerance and physical side effects, such as constipation, nausea, vomiting, and

---

Box 14-3   **Additional and complementary pain management techniques in oncology**

- Palliative radiation therapy
- Cold/moist heat applications
- Hypnosis
- Acupuncture
- Psychologic
  - Distraction techniques
  - Relaxation/imagery techniques
- Music therapy or drama therapy

- Counseling
- Cognitive-behavioral therapy
- Topical anesthetics/analgesics
- Adjunctive medications
  - Anxiolytics
  - Coanalgesics/centrally acting agents
    ° Anticonvulsants
    ° Antidepressants

---

mental clouding, may occur with opioid use and should be anticipated and managed prophylactically, if possible.

Improved pain control may be achieved with opioid substitution and rotation.[448,449,452] Parenteral opioids have been shown to provide improved analgesia for patients suffering from cancer pain who have not responded to oral opioids, which suggests that a change in route of administration can be effective. Administration of more than one opioid may also offer increased pain relief; for example, oxycodone used in addition to morphine and methadone may improve pain relief.[438]

NSAIDs for patients with cancer reduce the need for opioids, although they may lead to gastrointestinal discomfort.[453] Topical agents should be continued after systemic medications have been started.

Adjuvant medications, such as centrally acting pain medications (eg, tricyclic antidepressants, gabapentin) have been suggested.[438,454] Amitriptyline has been studied in a placebo-controlled trial in addition to morphine in neuropathic cancer pain. A limited additional analgesic effect was reported, but sleep improved. However, increased side effects including drowsiness, confusion, and dry mouth were observed.[448,449] Improved pain control from combining gabapentin with morphine was noted during wound dressing changes in patients with cancer[454] and may affect the neuropathic component of pain.[438]

Complementary pain management strategies

Complementary pain management techniques are presented in Box 14-3 (see also chapter 17). Hypnosis has been studied in randomized trials as a complementary method of pain control in patients with cancer. A variety of hypnotic techniques have been discussed, including vocal techniques, listening, and instrumental techniques, but there are no controlled studies of their impact on cancer pain.[438,455] Additional psychologic techniques, including counseling, distraction, relaxation, and other cognitive and behavioral training programs have been discussed.

Physical management of orofacial pain may include ice chips for oral cooling and cold compresses, notwithstanding that cryotherapy is an evidence-based preventive therapy for certain types of mucositis (see Table 14-3).

Complementary and alternative medicine, including acupuncture, transcutaneous nerve stimulation, group therapy, self-hypnosis, relaxation, imagery, cognitive-behavioral training, and massage therapy have been assessed for pain management in patients with advanced cancer and may reduce pain.[429,456] A controlled trial showed that relaxation and imagery improve pain in oral mucositis.[457]

Orofacial Pain in Patients with HIV

HIV-related headache

Headache is a common symptom in patients with human immunodeficiency virus (HIV) infection. Primary or secondary headache may be seen in 42% to 50% of patients,[458–460] although there is great variability in the reported incidence of primary headache in patients with HIV infection. Primary headache was found to occur in 2.8% of patients with HIV infection admitted to an HIV service over a 1-year period. This incidence was much higher than the incidence of headache among HIV-negative patients admitted to the neurology service (0.8%).[461] Others have reported the incidence of primary headache in HIV-positive patients to be as high as 38%.[460,462] The most prevalent types of primary headaches are tension-type headache and migraine (14% to 45.8% and 16% to 76%, respectively). Cluster headache is much less common (10%).[462,463] Identifiable, serious causes of headache are found in up to 82% of patients with HIV infection who presented with headache.[460,462]

TMDs may be associated with headache and cause facial pain and dysfunction. Patients with HIV infection often report chronic pain and pathologies targeting body joints during retroviral therapy, including TMDs.[464]

Because HIV is a neurotropic virus, it can be anticipated that neurologic complications in AIDS are common.[465,466] HIV crosses the blood-brain barrier,[466] infects macrophages and microglia in the CNS, and is a common cause of neurocognitive impairment.[467] The release of inflammatory mediators by HIV-infected microglia and macrophages and the concurrent neuronal damage play central roles in the HIV-related neuropathology.[468]

Secondary headaches in HIV patients have numerous causes, such as acute HIV meningitis and malignant disease. Head and neck and CNS cancer due to local primary cancer, systemic cancer, and metastatic disease may cause pain in HIV-positive persons.[469]

A chronic form of headache in HIV is associated with cerebrospinal pleocytosis. Headaches may be caused by neoplasms and opportunistic infections, resulting in meningitis (cryptococcal, tuberculous, or syphilitic), focal brain lesions (lymphoma, toxoplasmosis), or diffuse brain disease (cytomegalovirus, herpes simplex, progressive multifocal leukoencephalopathy).[465,470] Cryptococcal meningitis (39%) and CNS toxoplasmosis (16%) were the leading infectious etiologies for HIV headache.[460]

Facial pain may be caused by sinusitis, ocular pathology, and systemic infection and may be associated with diagnostic testing (eg, intracranial hypotension from diagnostic lumbar puncture).[465,470,471] Sinusitis due to deep mycotic

infection may present chronic pain until diagnosed and successfully treated. Affected patients usually have advanced HIV infection.[461] A correlation between the presence of headache and the degree of immunosuppression has been observed.[472] Nevertheless, HIV-related headaches can occur at any time during infection—at seroconversion, during the incubation period, in patients with symptomatic HIV infection, or after an AIDS-defining illness.[470] Investigators have suggested that progression of immunologic deficiency is related to a decrease in the frequency of migraine and an increase in the frequency of tension-type headache.[463]

The stage of disease also has a practical implication, as the value of computed tomography scan was shown to be highest for patients with CD4 counts less than 200 cells/μL.[466,473] The highest prevalence of positive scans was found in patients with advanced disease. This is in accordance with the fact that CD4 counts predict the relative risk of developing opportunistic infections and neoplasms, including those in the CNS. Thus, in the absence of significant immunosuppression, computed tomography or MRI is not suggested unless focal findings are present on neurologic examination. However, the headache frequency and characteristics may bear no relation to CD4 counts, cerebrospinal fluid parameters, cranial MRI abnormalities, the presence of sinusitis, or the use of zidovudine.

Treatment of head or facial pain is directed at the etiology when this is possible. Unfortunately, headaches in patients with HIV frequently do not respond to conventional management and carry a poor prognosis.[462]

HIV-related oral painful mucosal lesions

The oral cavity is a common site of painful lesions in patients who are seropositive for HIV[474,475] and is one of the most common sites of pain in the whole body.[459] A report of 157 HIV-positive people, 99 on highly active antiretroviral therapy (HAART) and 58 not on HAART, found greater risk of orofacial pain, oral lesions, and periodontal pockets for those on HAART and for those on long-term HAART than those on short-term treatment ($P < .05$).[476]

Oral candidiasis, the most common oral lesion identified, may cause an oral burning sensation. Other oral infections—fungal, viral, and bacterial—are well recognized and often result in local pain with possible systemic febrile episodes.

Patients with HIV may suffer from the major form of oral recurrent aphthous ulcers, which can result in considerable pain that affects oral function. Although recurrent aphthous ulcers are not etiologically related to a specific pathogen, secondary infection can occur at the lesion's site.[477]

Necrotizing gingivitis and necrotizing periodontitis can progress rapidly and can be extremely painful.[478] A more extensive form, necrotizing stomatitis, is also reported.[478,479] Recurrent herpetic simplex infections and herpes zoster can be of extended duration, involve keratinized and nonkeratinized mucosa, and result in persisting pain.

HIV-related neuropathy

Neurologic manifestations of HIV have been reported in the head and neck[480] but are rare.[481] Some cases of facial nerve dysfunction[482,483] and cases of recalcitrant headaches have been reported.[484] Peripheral neurologic symptoms have been recognized early in primary HIV infection[485,486] and later in the disease progression, mainly as a potential side effect of HIV antiviral medications.[487–489] Although often difficult to manage, peripheral neuropathy due to medications such as thalidomide may be improved if the suspected medication is discontinued.[490] Strong associations between neuropathies and opportunistic viral herpetic infections or thalidomide have been documented.[491–493]

Clinical management of neuropathic pain should be aggressive with a multidisciplinary, comprehensive approach similar to that for cancer-related pain.[484,493,494] Clinicians should address the etiology of the pain, whenever possible, especially in cases of the viral-related pain that still is commonly observed in HIV disease.[495]

Lyme disease has been reported in HIV-positive patients and is estimated to be more common than previously thought, with more severe symptoms in increasingly immunosuppressed patients and associated with CNS and neuropathologic symptoms.[496]

Aggregation Disease

Fabry disease

Fabry disease is a rare X-linked lysosomal storage disorder. Its annual reported incidence is 1 in 100,000, but this may be an underestimate. It is caused by a deficiency of the enzyme alpha-galactosidase A, which causes glycolipids, such as globotriaosylceramide, to accumulate in the vascular endothelium of several organs, including the skin, kidneys, nervous system, and heart, thereby triggering inflammation and fibrosis. These processes generally result in organ dysfunction, which is usually the first clinical evidence of Fabry disease. Evolving knowledge about the natural course of disease suggests that it is more appropriate to describe Fabry disease as a disease with a wide spectrum of heterogenously progressive clinical phenotypes. Most female heterozygotes develop symptoms due to as-yet undetermined mechanisms, and a high percentage of females develop vital organ involvement, including the kidneys, heart, and/or brain about a decade later than males.[497,498] One of the predominant signs of Fabry disease found in a cohort of young patients was acroparesthesia (paresthesia of the limbs and tips of other extremities due to nerve compression or polyneuritis).[499] Cranial nerve dysfunction resulting in facial paresthesia, odontogenic-like pain, trigeminal neuralgia, taste and smell impairment, or glossomotor dysfunction has been described.[500] Neurologic and psychologic changes, such as headache, recurrent vertigo, tinnitus, diminished level of activity, fatigue, and depression, have also been reported in patients with Fabry disease.[499] In patients with Fabry disease, it is noteworthy that there is an increased prevalence of cutaneous and mucosal angiokeratomas and telangiectasia as well as cysts or pseudocysts of the maxillary sinuses.[501,502]

Amyloidosis

Amyloid is an eosinophilic hyaline protein that pathologically accumulates within tissues in a number of diseases and is thus nonspecific. Amyloid has a characteristic fibrillar structure, seen on electron microscopy, that varies in different forms of amyloidosis but is in all cases associated with a nonfibrillar component termed *amyloid P*. The widespread lesions in amyloid disease and the possible involvement of virtually any system make this disorder protean in its manifestations. Systemically, amyloid is deposited mainly in the heart, skeletal muscle, and gastrointestinal tract, so that normal function of these organs is severely compromised. Orofacial manifestations may occur by amyloid deposits developing in the temporal arteries, mimicking the symptoms of temporal arteritis.[503] Other local complaints include burning pain in the oral cavity, especially on the tongue, which manifests as macroglossia or a firm tongue.[504] Additionally, the development of intraoral papules/nodules and xerostomia has been reported.[505,506]

Craniofacial Pain Related to Miscellaneous Medical Conditions

Medication-overuse headache

Medication-overuse headache (MOH) is a refractory chronic headache associated with medication management for pain.[507] The development of MOH is associated with frequency of use of medication and behavioral predispositions, including potential psychopathology and drug dependence. MOH affects quality of life and causes symptoms that may include daily and incapacitating headaches, insomnia, poor sleep, distress, and reduced functioning. Acetaminophen, combination analgesics (caffeine combinations), opioids, barbiturates, NSAIDs, and triptans are common classes of drugs implicated in MOH. Migraine seems to be the most common diagnosis leading to MOH.

MOH is associated with biochemical, structural, and functional brain changes. Relapse after detoxification is a challenge but can be addressed by scheduling expert and regular follow-up on an ongoing basis, using prophylactic pharmacotherapy, using abortive medication with minimal risk of MOH, withholding previously overused medication, and providing psychologic support.[507]

MOH appears to be due to increased excitability of neurons in the cerebral cortex and trigeminal system after medication overuse.[508,509] Prior chronic exposure to analgesics may increase susceptibility to evoked cortical-spreading depression. Cortical hyperexcitability may facilitate cortical spreading, and increased excitability of trigeminal neurons may facilitate peripheral and central sensitization. These changes may lead to altered central serotonin (5-hydroxytryptamine) and perhaps cannabinoid modulation, leading to a decrease in inhibitory control that may then lead to central sensitization. Low 5-hydroxytryptamine levels may also increase release of calcitonin gene–related peptide from the trigeminal ganglion and sensitize trigeminal nociceptors. This central modulation of the trigeminal system associated with chronic medication use may increase sensitivity to facial pain and headache.[508]

A systematic literature review of MOH included 27 studies.[510] The commonly used case definition for MOH was headache for at least 15 days per month with concurrent medication overuse of at least 3 months. A wide range of prevalence—0.5% to 7.2%—was observed due to variable definitions and criteria for drug overuse and persisting headache symptoms that may overlap symptoms.

NSAIDs may be associated with MOH and rebound headache. Inhibition of cyclooxygenase-1 and cyclooxygenase-2 may result in inhibition of synthesis of prostaglandins and may also increase risk of vascular complications, including stroke.[511]

The medical treatment of patients with chronic primary headache syndromes (chronic migraine, chronic tension-type headache, chronic cluster headache, hemicrania continua) is challenging.[512] When a definitive lack of responsiveness to conservative treatments is observed, consideration should be given to the potential for MOH. Approaches to management include discontinuing probable etiologic agent(s), potential trial of neurologically active agents such as valproic acid, and neuromodulation.[512] A total of 694 patients with MOH were treated by detoxification and prophylactic treatment.[513] Management resulted in a 58.4% reduction in headache days ($P < .001$) and a 57.1% reduction in disability score from baseline ($P < .001$). The number of patients with depression was reduced by 50.7%, and the number with anxiety was reduced by 27.1% (both

Table 14-4	ICHD-3 diagnostic criteria for Tolosa-Hunt syndrome

Diagnostic criteria

A. Unilateral headache fulfilling criterion C

B. Both of the following:
  1. Granulomatous inflammation of the cavernous sinus, superior orbital fissure, or orbit, demonstrated by MRI or biopsy
  2. Paresis of one or more of the ipsilateral third, fourth, and/or sixth cranial nerves

C. Evidence of causation demonstrated by both of the following:
  1. Headache has preceded paresis of the third, fourth, and/or sixth nerves by at least 2 weeks or developed with it
  2. Headache is localized around the ipsilateral brow and eye

D. Not better accounted for by another ICHD-3 diagnosis

$P < .001$) (see also chapter 10). The impact of treatment emphasizes the need for awareness of potential overuse of headache medications.

Tolosa-Hunt syndrome

Tolosa-Hunt syndrome is defined as unilateral orbital pain associated with paresis of one or more of the third, fourth, and/or sixth cranial nerves caused by a granulomatous inflammation in the cavernous sinus, superior orbital fissure, or orbit,[19] according to the *International Classification of Headache Disorders,* third edition (ICHD-3). Considering that the trigeminal nerve; internal carotid artery; the third, fourth, and sixth cranial nerves; and the autonomic nerves of the eye are intimately related in the cavernous sinus, lesions in this area can cause facial pain associated with a number of ocular signs depending on which nerves are affected.

Two reports laid the groundwork for the definition of this syndrome.[514,515] In large series, Tolosa-Hunt syndrome was reported to develop in the fifth decade on average; however, it affects people of all ages.[516–518] The diagnostic criteria for the syndrome were revised in 2013[19,518] (Table 14-4). Accordingly, Tolosa-Hunt syndrome is characterized by episodes of unilateral orbital pain persisting for weeks. Coinciding with the onset of pain, or closely following it, is paresis of one or more of the third, fourth, and sixth cranial nerves. Previously, the response to corticosteroids was considered a diagnostic criterion, but this was removed in the most recent ICHD classification. Debate continues in the literature regarding diagnostic criteria.[518]

Diagnosis is based on the clinical presentation, biopsy, and MRI demonstrating a granulomatous lesion.[19] The typical clinical presentation is pain in the orbital or retro-orbital area of severe and fluctuating intensity.[519,520] The pain is described as pressure, boring, or knifelike pain in the eye.[520] The third nerve is involved in most patients (90%) and the fourth nerve in 40%.[521] The incidence of identifiable lesions in the cavernous sinus increases with the number of nerves involved.[522] Often, there may be a reduced pupillary light reflex and ptosis suggestive of autonomic dysfunction. Periorbital hypoesthesia and a reduced corneal reflex are secondary to sensory dysfunction of the frontal branch of the ophthalmic nerve. Optic nerve involvement (reduced acuity) and involvement of the maxillary nerve suggest lesion enlargement.[521]

The typical MRI findings include T1 isointense and T2 hypointense focal-enhancing masses expanding the ipsilateral cavernous sinus.[523] Occasionally, lateral bulging of the anterior cavernous sinus contour and internal carotid artery narrowing are seen on the MRI.[524] Obtaining evidence of the granulomatous nature of the lesion is challenging,,[525] and occasionally no evidence of inflammation is observed on the imaging; therefore, the subclassifications *benign Tolosa-Hunt syndrome* and *granulomatous lesion–related Tolosa-Hunt syndrome* have been suggested.[526,527]

Clinical variations include involvement of other cranial nerves or bilateral involvement. Involvement of the fifth nerve (commonly the first division) or optic, seventh, or eighth nerve was reported, as well as sympathetic innervation

Table 14-5	ICHD-3 diagnostic criteria for cervicogenic headache

Diagnostic criteria

A. Unilateral headache fulfilling criterion C

B. Clinical, laboratory, and/or imaging evidence of a disorder or lesion within the cervical spine or soft tissues of the neck, known to be able to cause headache

C. Evidence of causation demonstrated by at least two of the following:
   1. Headache has developed in temporal relation to the onset of the cervical disorder or appearance of the lesion
   2. Headache has significantly improved or resolved in parallel with improvement in or resolution of the cervical disorder or lesion
   3. Cervical range of motion is reduced and headache is made significantly worse by provocative maneuvers
   4. Headache is abolished after diagnostic blockade of a cervical structure or its nerve supply

D. Not better accounted for by another ICHD-3 diagnosis

of the pupil. This presentation suggests that Tolosa-Hunt syndrome may be a presentation of a more widespread disorder.[19,528–530]

The differential diagnosis of the syndrome includes other vascular disorders, such as cavernous sinus thrombosis and giant cell arteritis of the temporal artery, diabetic neuropathy, and ophthlamoplegic migraine. Neoplastic and infectious processes in the region and infiltrative disorders such as SLE, lymphoma, sarcoidosis, and syphilis have also been associated with orbital pain.[531,532]

Treatment is with high-dose steroids (80 to 100 mg of prednisone daily) tapered over 7 to 14 days. Longer treatment is often needed to completely resolve the symptoms. Surgical excision may be necessary. Recurrence and resistant cases have been described, and there has been some success using experimental treatments.[533,534]

Cervicogenic headache

Musculoskeletal spine disease may be associated with cervicogenic headache. The clinical features of cervicogenic headache are nonspecific and often mimic migraines or tension-type headaches. Headaches may be unilateral or bilateral. Quality is nonthrobbing, is of moderate intensity, and may be continuous or intermittent. The headache is usually aggravated by neck movements, pressure on the neck, or awkward neck postures. Reduced cervical range of motion and pain referral to the ipsilateral shoulder and arm may also be observed. Autonomic

signs such as nausea, vomiting, phonophobia, photophobia, and edema or flushing around the eye may present, but much less than in migraine and tension-type headache. Provocation of the cervicogenic headache by digital pressure on neck muscles is suggestive of the diagnosis but not considered conclusive.[19] The ICHD-3 diagnostic criteria help differentiate cervicogenic headache from other headaches[19] (Table 14-5). Cervicogenic headache may or may not be accompanied by neck pain; however, it is clearly triggered by cervical structures,[535] and cervical lesions have been detected by neuroimaging techniques in some patients.

Although the neck is the origin of this headache, it has been suggested that the neck is not an independent headache generator.[535] Accordingly, the pathophysiology of cervicogenic headache includes local neck changes and a central predisposition that activates the trigeminovascular system and generates pain. Another hypothesis is that musculoskeletal problems in the neck cause headache by the mechanism of referred pain. The greater and lesser occipital branches of the sensory second cervical (C) root may refer pain to the back of the head. The sensory first cervical root may refer pain to the vertex or frontal region, but some consider this unlikely. Connections between C2 branches from the posterior fossa to branches of the ophthalmic nerve would refer pain to the front of the head.

Clearly, when an underlying organic disease is identified as the cause of the cervicogenic headache, treatment should be aimed at the source of the problem. Various treatment approaches have been examined: steroids,[536] manual therapy and physical therapy,[537–539] electrotherapy,[540] botulinum toxin injections,[541] cervical anesthetic blocks targeting distinct nerves or roots, and surgery. Physical therapy may decrease pain outcomes in patients with cervicogenic headache.[537] More studies are needed to determine the effectiveness of these treatments.

Craniofacial pain attributed to trauma or injury to the head and/or neck

Traumatic injury to the head is defined as structural or functional damage from the action of external forces on the head. These include striking the head, or using the head to strike an object, penetration of the head by a foreign body, forces generated from blasts or explosions, and other forces yet to be defined.[19]

Headache or facial pain that occurs de novo in close temporal relation to trauma or an existing pain disorder that becomes significantly worse may be classified as having headache attributed to trauma or injury (HATI). In the previous ICHD-2 classification, the equivalent term was *posttraumatic headache*.

According to the ICHD-3, HATI may be acute or persistent and may be subclassified according to the severity of the injury as mild or moderate to severe[19] (Table 14-6). Acute HATI occurs within 7 days and resolves within 3 months of injury; persistent HATI is diagnosed if pain persists beyond 3 months.

No criteria comparable with those of the IHS have been established for posttraumatic facial pain. Extrapolating from the ICHD criteria would allow the description "HATI" to be added to patients where the facial pain began in close temporal proximity to a traumatic event (< 7 days) and persists beyond 3 months.[542] The individual distribution of craniofacial posttraumatic pain may dictate the specialist a patient consults, but the etiologic events and mechanisms are probably similar. The authors therefore refer to HATI and/or facial pain as *craniofacial pain attributed to trauma or injury* (CFPATI) throughout the following section. Other entities within the scope of trauma-related oral pain, such as cracked tooth, barodontalgia (diving or flying), and dental trauma, are cov-

ered elsewhere in this textbook. Other types of trauma-related headaches, including headache attributed to whiplash, headache attributed to craniotomy, and headache attributed to radiosurgery of the brain, are discussed in the following sections.

CFPATI epidemiology and risk factors

Acute headache that occurs after trauma to the head or face region is relatively common and occurs in 30% to 90% of patients.[543–548] The number of patients that continue to suffer pain and develop chronic CFPATI is variable.[549] About a third of patients with head injury report persistent headache at 3 months, a quarter or more may still report pain 4 or 5 years after injury, and 11% suffer frequent headaches after 22 years of follow-up.[549–552] Most chronic CFPATI cases were caused by motor vehicle accidents, some by falls or assaults, and a minority by sports injuries.[542,553]

The long-term persistence of CFPATI is unrelated to physical variables associated with the trauma, such as severity or loss of consciousness.[552] The factors that significantly increased the persistence of CFPATI 22 years after trauma were female sex, high intensity of the acute CFPATI, and psychiatric comorbidity.[552]

CFPATI clinical features and comorbidity

CFPATI is diagnosed primarily based on the temporal relation between the trauma or injury and pain onset (see Table 14-6). The 7-day interval is arbitrary, but there is not enough evidence to support a longer interval. In reference to cases in which the latent period is longer, the ICHD-3 appendix lists "delayed-onset acute headache attributed to moderate or severe traumatic injury to the head" and "delayed-onset acute headache attributed to mild traumatic injury to the head."

The clinical features commonly resemble tension-type headache or migraine, and more than one disorder may occur concomitantly.[542–544,548,554–558] Migraine-type headaches seem to be more common after acceleration/deceleration injuries to the neck, that is, whiplash injuries to the cervical complex.[544] Musculoskeletal-type pain has also been re-

Table 14-6	ICHD-3 diagnostic criteria for headache attributed to traumatic injury to the head and/or neck

Acute ICHD code 5.1	Persistent ICHD code 5.2
Diagnostic criteria	
A. Any headache fulfilling criteria C and D	A. Any headache fulfilling criteria C and D
B. Traumatic injury to the head has occurred	B. Traumatic injury to the head has occurred
C. Headache is reported to have developed within 7 days after one of the following: 1. Injury to the head 2. Regaining consciousness after injury to the head 3. Discontinuation of medication(s) that impair ability to sense or report headache after injury to the head	C. Headache is reported to have developed within 7 days after one of the following: 1. Injury to the head 2. Regaining consciousness after injury to the head 3. Discontinuation of medication(s) that impair ability to sense or report headache after injury to the head
D. Either of the following: 1. Headache has resolved within 3 months after the injury to the head 2. Headache has not yet resolved but 3 months have not yet passed since the injury to the head	D. Headache persists for > 3 months after injury to the head
E. Not better accounted for by another ICHD-3 diagnosis	E. Not better accounted for by another ICHD-3 diagnosis
Subtypes	
Attributed to moderate or severe traumatic injury to the head	
A. Headache fulfilling criteria for 5.1 acute headache attributed to traumatic injury to the head	A. Headache fulfilling criteria 5.2 persistent headache attributed to traumatic injury to the head
B. Injury to the head associated with at least one of the following: 1. Loss of consciousness for > 30 minutes 2. Glasgow Coma Scale score < 13 3. Posttraumatic amnesia lasting > 24 hours 4. Alteration in level of awareness for > 24 hours 5. Imaging evidence of a traumatic head injury, such as intracranial hemorrhage and/or brain contusion	B. Injury to the head associated with at least one of the following: 1. Loss of consciousness for > 30 minutes 2. Glasgow Coma Scale score < 13 3. Posttraumatic amnesia lasting > 24 hours 4. Alteration in level of awareness for > 24 hours 5. Imaging evidence of a traumatic head injury, such as intracranial hemorrhage and/or brain contusion
Attributed to mild traumatic injury to the head	
A. Headache fulfilling criteria for 5.1 acute headache attributed to traumatic injury to the head	A. Headache fulfilling criteria 5.2 persistent headache attributed to traumatic injury to the head

B. Head injury fulfilling both of the following:
1. Associated with *none* of the following:
  a. Loss of consciousness for > 30 minutes
  b. Glasgow Coma Scale score < 13
  c. Posttraumatic amnesia lasting > 24 hours
  d. Altered level of awareness for > 24 hours
  e. Imaging evidence of a traumatic head injury, such as intracranial hemorrhage and/or brain contusion
2. Associated, immediately after head injury, with one or more of the following symptoms and/or signs:
  a. Transient confusion, disorientation, or impaired consciousness
  b. Loss of memory for events immediately before or after the head injury
  c. Two or more other symptoms suggestive of mild traumatic brain injury: nausea, vomiting, visual disturbances, dizziness and/or vertigo, impaired memory and/or concentration
	B. Head injury fulfilling both of the following:
	1. Associated with *none* of the following:
	  a. Loss of consciousness for > 30 minutes
	  b. Glasgow Coma Scale score < 13
	  c. Posttraumatic amnesia lasting > 24 hours
	  d. Altered level of awareness for > 24 hours
	  e. Imaging evidence of a traumatic head injury, such as intracranial hemorrhage and/or brain contusion
	2. Associated, immediately after head injury, with one or more of the following symptoms and/or signs:
	  a. Transient confusion, disorientation, or impaired consciousness
	  b. Loss of memory for events immediately before or after the head injury
	  c. Two or more other symptoms suggestive of mild traumatic brain injury: nausea, vomiting, visual disturbances, dizziness and/or vertigo, impaired memory and/or concentration

ported.[542,559,560] In rare cases, acute CFPATI could be clinically similar to cluster headaches, hemicrania continua, chronic paroxysmal hemicrania, and SUNCT syndrome (short-lasting unilateral neuralgiform headache attacks with conjunctival injection and tearing).[548]

When headache occurs in conjunction with symptoms of dizziness, fatigue, reduced ability to concentrate, insomnia, anxiety, personality changes, and irritability, post-concussion syndrome is considered.[19,561]

Chronic CFPATI may form part of a symptom complex termed *posttraumatic stress disorder* (PTSD), which includes psychologic, social, and cognitive impairments.[554,559,560,562–565] After orofacial injury, acute PTSD is particularly prominent and may persist with associated disabilities.[566,567] If PTSD becomes established, a multidisciplinary approach involving pain specialists, psychologist/psychiatrists, physiotherapists, social workers, family physicians, as well as cooperation from family members and coworkers, is required. Additionally, patients may be involved in litigation, and although there is no evidence to suggest that CFPATI is related to ongoing litigation,[543,568] a careful workup to exclude malingering should be performed.[569]

Posttraumatic sleep disturbances, mood disturbances, and psychosocial stressors may aggravate CFPATI. The overuse of abortive pain medications may contribute to the persistence of CFPATI (see the section on medication-overuse headache).

CFPATI pathophysiology

The pathophysiology of CFPATI is unclear and probably involves a number of mechanisms that interplay with the psychosocial capabilities and genotype of the patient to dictate who will or will not suffer chronic pain.[558] The role of trauma in some craniofacial pain syndromes, such as TMDs, is well established (see chapters 8 and 9). Direct injury to musculoskeletal structures may initiate changes that result in persistent pain in susceptible persons. The degree of brain injury is not consistently associated with the incidence or severity of pain. Thus, frank injury to brain tissue plays some part, but other factors are involved. Shear forces applied to the brain result in a phenomenon termed *diffuse axonal injury* (see chapter 12), which may

be involved in the initiation of some CFPATI symptoms.

CFPATI treatment

Symptomatic treatment includes the use of drugs relevant to the primary pain disorders (see chapters 8 through 12, 15, and 16) and usually requires additional modalities, such as physical therapy, trigger point injections, and occlusal splints (see chapters 8 and 9). Cognitive-behavioral therapy may be indicated (see chapter 4) and is successful in patients with persistent CFPATI.[570]

Other types of craniofacial pain attributed to trauma

Whiplash injury results from sudden and inadequately restrained acceleration/deceleration movements of the head with flexion/extension of the neck.[19] Whiplash most commonly occurs in the context of motor vehicle accidents. Headaches attributed to whiplash are subclassified into acute and persistent based on the duration of the pain (> 3 months is considered persistent).

Whether whiplash induces TMDs is unclear and is discussed in chapter 8. Acute pain occurring locally in the neck after whiplash injuries is relatively common.[549] Acute headache occurs after many whiplash injuries.[571] Additionally, whiplash may lead to chronic cervical pain with disability and may induce headache, as described later.[572] Whiplash-associated disorders have been defined and categorized[573]; subtype I includes cervical pain and tenderness, and type II has additional features of reduced range of motion and point tenderness. Whiplash-associated disorders I and II are referred to in this section as *chronic whiplash pain*. Types III and IV are associated with fractures and distinct neurologic signs and are beyond the scope of this book. Depending on culture and geographic distribution, up to 82% of patients continue to suffer from chronic pain after whiplash injury.[549,574,575] The persistence of pain is not consistently related to the degree of trauma or cervical pathology. Similarly, many patients with structural cervical lesions suffer no pain.[549]

A recent study identified a list of risk factors for persistent problems after acute whiplash injury: The significant variables included

Table 14-7	ICHD-3 diagnostic criteria for paratrigeminal oculosympathetic (Raeder) syndrome

Diagnostic criteria

A. Constant, unilateral headache fulfilling criterion C

B. Imaging evidence of underlying disease of either the middle cranial fossa or the ipsilateral carotid artery

C. Evidence of causation demonstrated by both of the following:
   1. Headache has developed in temporal relation to the onset of the underlying disorder
   2. Headache has either or both of the following features:
      a. Localized to the distribution of the ophthalmic division of the trigeminal nerve, with or without spread to the maxillary division
      b. Aggravated by eye movement

D. Ipsilateral Horner syndrome

E. Not better accounted for by another ICHD-3 diagnosis

high baseline pain intensity (> 5.5/10), report of headache at inception, less than postsecondary education, no seatbelt used during the accident, report of lower back pain at inception, high Neck Disability Index score (> 14.5/50), preinjury neck pain, report of neck pain at inception (regardless of intensity), high catastrophizing, female sex, whiplash-associated disorders grade II or III, or whiplash-associated disorder grade III alone.[576]

Diffuse axonal injury, as described earlier (see also chapter 12), may be involved in the initiation of chronic pain after whiplash injury. The role of litigation in persistence of chronic whiplash pain is unclear. However, one study has shown that when compensation for pain and suffering is eliminated, there is a decreased incidence and improved prognosis of whiplash injury.[577]

Structural lesions of the cervical spine should be assessed by an orthopedic surgeon or neurologist. Similarly, conservative treatment of chronic whiplash pain should be performed in cooperation with an orthopedic surgeon or neurologist and should involve the use of multimodal therapy/medication, physical therapy, soft collars, trigger point injections, and cognitive-behavioral therapy.

Other types of trauma-related headaches include *headache attributed to craniotomy*, which is defined as headache of less than 3 months' duration caused by surgical craniotomy. *Headache attributed to radiosurgery of the brain* is defined by its temporal relationship to radiosurgery. Similar to HATI, it is subclassified as acute if resolved within 3 months after radiosurgery and persistent if it lasts longer.

Paratrigeminal oculosympathetic syndrome

Paratrigeminal oculosympathetic syndrome (POSS), formerly known as *Raeder syndrome*, was originally described as trigeminal nerve dysfunction or pain accompanied by ocular sympathetic dysfunction[19] (Table 14-7). This was proposed to be the result of a lesion in the middle cranial fossa in the paratrigeminal area. The sympathetic nerve supply to the eye (oculosympathetic outflow) arises from the internal carotid plexus in the middle cranial fossa, medial to the trigeminal ganglion. A lesion in this area would induce trigeminal symptoms (paresthesia, pain) and sympathetic dysfunction of the eye—miosis or ptosis (Horner syndrome). POSS should appear with no alteration in forehead sweating; sympathetic innervation to the sweat glands is mediated by fibers that exit the carotid plexus before the middle cranial fossa and relatively laterally to the occulosympathetic outflow.[578] In some instances, however, the parasympathetic system reinnervates the sweat glands so that intact sweating does not signify a functional sympathetic innervation.[578] Although the original case had a paratrigeminal neoplasm, later cases were described with no organic pathology.[271] Thus, various subgroups were described that presented with a similar phenotype, that is, Horner syndrome with ipsilateral trigeminal pain/dysfunction.[271]

Patients with oculosympathetic loss, miosis or ptosis, or both, with normal forehead sweating and evidence of trigeminal involvement (either sensory change or neuralgic pain), are highly likely to have a lesion in the middle cranial fossa that is medial to the trigeminal ganglion (paratrigeminal). These patients should be classified as having POSS and should be thoroughly examined, including an MRI at baseline and further studies as needed.[578] In addition to paratrigeminal middle cranial fossa neoplasms, the most common differential diagnosis is pathology of the carotid artery, which would affect the sympathetic plexus. In particular, carotid artery dissection may occur with unilateral facial pain and Horner syndrome.[263] In support of a crucial role of the carotid artery in the etiology of POSS, a case report demonstrated that POSS-like symptoms could develop in a patient immediately after surgical manipulation of the carotid artery during an endovascular trapping of a carotid artery aneurysm.[579]

Conclusion

Orofacial pain in a medically complex patient represents a potentially challanging diagnosis and management. Underlying conditions and diseases may be the cause of pain or may represent comorbidities. If the etiology of the pain can be addressed, or if comorbid conditions can also be managed, better pain management can often be achieved. Pain practitioners must have broad knowledge and use high-level diagnositic skills. Often, a multimodal interdisciplinary team approoch is required for comprehensive patient care.

References

1. Dyck PJ, Davies JL, Wilson DM, Service FJ, Melton LJ 3rd, O'Brien PC. Risk factors for severity of diabetic polyneuropathy: Intensive longitudinal assessment of the Rochester Diabetic Neuropathy Study cohort. Diabetes Care 1999;22:1479–1486.

2. Irkeç C, Nazliel B, Yetkin I, Koçer B. Facial nerve conduction in diabetic neuropathy. Acta Neurol Belg 2001;101:177–179.

3. Tamborlane WV, Ahern J. Implications and results of the Diabetes Control and Complications Trial. Pediatr Clin North Am 1997;44:285–300.

4. Dyck PJ, Norell JE. Microvasculitis and ischemia in diabetic lumbosacral radiculoplexus neuropathy. Neurology 1999;53:2113–2121.

5. Dyck PJ, Zimmerman BR, Vilen TH, et al. Nerve glucose, fructose, sorbitol, myo-inositol, and fiber degeneration and regeneration in diabetic neuropathy. N Engl J Med 1988;319:542–548.

6. Eshbaugh CG, Siatkowski RM, Smith JL, Kline LB. Simultaneous, multiple cranial neuropathies in diabetes mellitus. J Neuroophthalmol 1995;15:219–224.

7. Cruccu G, Agostino R, Inghilleri M, Innocenti P, Romaniello A, Manfredi M. Mandibular nerve involvement in diabetic polyneuropathy and chronic inflammatory demyelinating polyneuropathy. Muscle Nerve 1998;21:1673–1679.

8. Urban PP, Forst T, Lenfers M, Koehler J, Connemann BJ, Beyer J. Incidence of subclinical trigeminal and facial nerve involvement in diabetes mellitus. Electromyogr Clin Neurophysiol 1999;39:267–272.

9. Arap A, Siqueira SR, Silva CB, Teixeira MJ, Siqueira JT. Trigeminal pain and quantitative sensory testing in painful peripheral diabetic neuropathy. Arch Oral Biol 2010;55:486–493.

10. de la Monte SM, Kril JJ. Human alcohol-related neuropathology. Acta Neuropathol 2014;127:71–90.

11. Preedy VR, Ohlendieck K, Adachi J, et al. The importance of alcohol-induced muscle disease. J Muscle Res Cell Motil 2003;24:55–63.

12. Chopra K, Tiwari V. Alcoholic neuropathy: Possible mechanisms and future treatment possibilities. Br J Clin Pharmacol 2012;73:348–362.

13. Charness ME, Simon RP, Greenberg DA. Ethanol and the nervous system. N Engl J Med 1989;321:442–454.

14. Mellion M, Gilchrist JM, de la Monte S. Alcohol-related peripheral neuropathy: Nutritional, toxic, or both? Muscle Nerve 2011;43:309–316.

15. Diamond I, Messing RO. Neurologic effects of alcoholism. West J Med 1994;161:279–287.

16. Stickel F, Hoehn B, Schuppan D, Seitz HK. Review article: Nutritional therapy in alcoholic liver disease. Aliment Pharmacol Ther 2003;18:357–373.

17. Mellion ML, Nguyen V, Tong M, Gilchrist J, de La Monte S. Experimental model of alcohol-related peripheral neuropathy. Muscle Nerve 2013;48:204–211.

18. Moreau T, Manceau E, Giroud-Baleydier F, Dumas R, Giroud M. Headache in hypothyroidism. Prevalence and outcome under thyroid hormone therapy. Cephalalgia 1998;18:687–689.

19. Headache Classification Committee of the International Headache Society (IHS). The International Classification of Headache Disorders, 3rd edition (beta version). Cephalalgia 2013;33:629–808.

20. Dodeller F, Schulze-Koops H. The p38 mitogen-activated protein kinase signaling cascade in CD4 T cells. Arthritis Res Ther 2006;8:205.

21. Dombrecht EJ, Aerts NE, Schuerwegh AJ, et al. Influence of anti-tumor necrosis factor therapy (Adalimumab) on regulatory T cells and dendritic cells in rheumatoid arthritis. Clin Exp Rheumatol 2006;24:31–37.

22. Helenius LM, Hallikainen D, Helenius I, et al. Clinical and radiographic findings of the temporomandibular joint in patients with various rheumatic diseases. A case-control study. Oral Surg Oral Med Oral Pathol Oral Radiol Endod 2005;99:455–463.

23. Symmons DP, Barrett EM, Bankhead CR, Scott DG, Silman AJ. The incidence of rheumatoid arthritis in the United Kingdom: Results from the Norfolk Arthritis Register. Br J Rheumatol 1994;33:735–739.

24. Laskin DM. The clinical diagnosis of temporomandibular disorders in the orthodontic patient. Semin Orthod 1995;1:197–206.

25. Gleissner C, Kaesser U, Dehne F, Bolten WW, Willershausen B. Temporomandibular joint function in patients with longstanding rheumatoid arthritis—I. Role of periodontal status and prosthetic care—A clinical study. Eur J Med Res 2003;8:98–108.

26. Yilmaz HH, Yildirim D, Ugan Y, et al. Clinical and magnetic resonance imaging findings of the temporomandibular joint and masticatory muscles in patients with rheumatoid arthritis. Rheumatol Int 2012;32:1171–1178.

27. Cunha CO, Pinto LM, de Mendonça LM, Saldanha AD, Conti AC, Conti PC. Bilateral asymptomatic fibrous-ankylosis of the temporomandibular joint associated with rheumatoid arthritis: A case report. Braz Dent J 2012;23:779–782.

28. Kobayashi R, Utsunomiya T, Yamamoto H, Nagura H. Ankylosis of the temporomandibular joint caused by rheumatoid arthritis: A pathological study and review. J Oral Sci 2001;43:97–101.

29. Marini I, Vecchiet F, Spiazzi L, Capurso U. Stomatognathic function in juvenile rheumatoid arthritis and in developmental open-bite subjects. ASDC J Dent Child 1999;66:30–35;12.

30. Larheim TA, Smith HJ, Aspestrand F. Rheumatic disease of the temporomandibular joint: MR imaging and tomographic manifestations. Radiology 1990;175:527–531.

31. Kretapirom K, Okochi K, Nakamura S, et al. MRI characteristics of rheumatoid arthritis in the temporomandibular joint. Dentomaxillofac Radiol 2013;42(4).

32. Manfredini D, Tognini F, Melchiorre D, Bazzichi L, Bosco M. Ultrasonography of the temporomandibular joint: Comparison of findings in patients with rheumatic diseases and temporomandibular disorders. A preliminary report. Oral Surg Oral Med Oral Pathol Oral Radiol Endod 2005;100:481–485.

33. Gynther GW, Holmlund AB, Reinholt FP, Lindblad S. Temporomandibular joint involvement in generalized osteoarthritis and rheumatoid arthritis: A clinical, arthroscopic, histologic, and immunohistochemical study. Int J Oral Maxillofac Surg 1997;26:10–16.

34. Gewanter HL, Roghmann KJ, Baum J. The prevalence of juvenile arthritis. Arthritis Rheum 1983;26:599–603.

35. Katz W (ed). Diagnosis and Management of Rheumatic Diseases. Philadelphia: Lippincott, 1988.

36. Twilt M, Mobers SM, Arends LR, ten Cate R, van Suijlekom-Smit L. Temporomandibular involvement in juvenile idiopathic arthritis. J Rheumatol 2004;31:1418–1422.

37. Walton AG, Welbury RR, Foster HE, Thomason JM. Juvenile chronic arthritis: A dental review. Oral Dis 1999;5:68–75.

38. Petty RE, Southwood TR, Manners P, et al. International League of Associations for Rheumatology classification of juvenile idiopathic arthritis: Second revision, Edmonton, 2001. J Rheumatol 2004;31:390–392.

39. Pedersen TK, Jensen JJ, Melsen B, Herlin T. Resorption of the temporomandibular condylar bone according to subtypes of juvenile chronic arthritis. J Rheumatol 2001;28:2109–2115.

40. Carvalho RT, Braga FS, Brito F, Capelli Júnior J, Figueredo CM, Sztajnbok FR. Temporomandibular joint alterations and their orofacial complications in patients with juvenile idiopathic arthritis. Rev Bras Reumatol 2012;52:907–911.

41. Beena JP. Juvenile idiopathic arthritis: Review of the literature and case report. J Dent Child (Chic) 2013;80:25–30.

42. Zhu JF, Kaminski MJ, Pulitzer DR, Hu J, Thomas HF. Psoriasis: Pathophysiology and oral manifestations. Oral Dis 1996;2:135–144.

43. Farronato G, Garagiola U, Carletti V, Cressoni P, Bellintani C. Psoriatic arthritis: Temporomandibular joint involvement as the first articular phenomenon. Quintessence Int 2010;41:395–398.

44. Dervis E. The prevalence of temporomandibular disorders in patients with psoriasis with or without psoriatic arthritis. J Oral Rehabil 2005;32:786–793.

45. Könönen M. Craniomandibular disorders in psoriatic arthritis. Correlations between subjective symptoms, clinical signs, and radiographic changes. Acta Odontol Scand 1986;44:369–375.

46. Koorbusch GF, Zeitler DL, Fotos PG, Doss JB. Psoriatic arthritis of the temporomandibular joints with ankylosis. Literature review and case reports. Oral Surg Oral Med Oral Pathol 1991;71:267–274.

47. Gogălniceanu D, Trandafir V, Chiriac R, Gogălniceanu P. Temporomandibular joint ankylosis. A possible complication in juvenile psoriatic rheumatism. Rev Med Chir Soc Med Nat Iasi 2005;109:652–659.

48. Miles DA, Kaugars GA. Psoriatic involvement of the temporomandibular joint. Literature review and report of two cases. Oral Surg Oral Med Oral Pathol 1991;71:770–774.

49. McGonagle D, Gibbon W, Emery P. Classification of inflammatory arthritis by enthesitis. Lancet 1998;352:1137-1140.

50. Locher MC, Felder M, Sailer HF. Involvement of the temporomandibular joints in ankylosing spondylitis (Bechterew's disease). J Craniomaxillofac Surg 1996;24:205–213.

51. Könönen M, Wenneberg B, Kallenberg A. Craniomandibular disorders in rheumatoid arthritis, psoriatic arthritis, and ankylosing spondylitis. A clinical study. Acta Odontol Scand 1992;50:281–287.

52. Ramos-Remus C, Major P, Gomez-Vargas A, et al. Temporomandibular joint osseous morphology in a consecutive sample of ankylosing spondylitis patients. Ann Rheum Dis 1997;56:103–107.

53. Arora P, Amarnath J, Ravindra SV, Rallan M. Temporomandibular joint involvement in ankylosing spondylitis. BMJ Case Rep 2013;2013.

54. Major P, Ramos-Remus C, Suarez-Almazor ME, Hatcher D, Parfitt M, Russell AS. Magnetic resonance imaging and clinical assessment of temporomandibular joint pathology in ankylosing spondylitis. J Rheumatol 1999;26:616–621.

55. Gayle EA, Young SM, McKenna SJ, McNaughton CD. Septic arthritis of the temporomandibular joint: Case reports and review of the literature. J Emerg Med 2013;45:674–678.

56. Okeson J. Diagnosis of temporomandibular disorders. In: Okeson J (ed). Management of Temporomandibular Disorders and Occlusion, ed 5. St Louis: Mosby, 2003:356.

57. Cai XY, Yang C, Zhang ZY, Qiu WL, Chen MJ, Zhang SY. Septic arthritis of the temporomandibular joint: A retrospective review of 40 cases. J Oral Maxillofac Surg 2010;68:731–738.

58. Hincapie JW, Tobon D, Diaz-Reyes GA. Septic arthritis of the temporomandibular joint. Otolaryngol Head Neck Surg 1999;121:836–837.

59. Klüppel LE, Bernabé FB, Primo BT, et al. Septic arthritis of the temporomandibular joint. J Craniofac Surg 2012;23:1752–1754.

60. Hekkenberg RJ, Piedade L, Mock D, Baker G, Freeman JL. Septic arthritis of the temporomandibular joint. Otolaryngol Head Neck Surg 1999;120:780–782.

61. Leighty SM, Spach DH, Myall RW, Burns JL. Septic arthritis of the temporomandibular joint: Review of the literature and report of two cases in children. Int J Oral Maxillofac Surg 1993;22:292–297.

62. Goldschmidt MJ, Butterfield KJ, Goracy ES, Goldberg MH. Streptococcal infection of the temporomandibular joint of hematogenous origin: A case report and contemporary therapy. J Oral Maxillofac Surg 2002;60:1347–1353.

63. Hamburger M, Baraf HS, Adamson TC 3rd, et al. 2011 Recommendations for the diagnosis and management of gout and hyperuricemia. Postgrad Med 2011;123(6, suppl):3–36.

64. Saag KG, Mikuls TR. Recent advances in the epidemiology of gout. Curr Rheumatol Rep 2005;7:235–241.

65. Harris MD, Siegel LB, Alloway JA. Gout and hyperuricemia. Am Fam Physician 1999;59:925–934.

66. Srinivasan V, Wensel A, Dutcher P, Newlands S, Johnson M, Vates GE. Calcium pyrophosphate deposition disease of the temporomandibular joint. J Neurol Surg Rep 2012;73:6–8.

67. Pittman JR, Bross MH. Diagnosis and management of gout. Am Fam Physician 1999;59:1799–1806;1810.

68. Bhattacharyya I, Chehal H, Gremillion H, Nair M. Gout of the temporomandibular joint: A review of the literature. J Am Dent Assoc 2010;141:979–985.

69. Barthélémy I, Karanas Y, Sannajust JP, Emering C, Mondié JM. Gout of the temporomandibular joint: pitfalls in diagnosis. J Craniomaxillofac Surg 2001;29:307–310.

70. Kataria RK, Brent LH. Spondyloarthropathies. Am Fam Physician 2004;69:2853–2860.

71. Dworkin MS, Shoemaker PC, Goldoft MJ, Kobayashi JM. Reactive arthritis and Reiter's syndrome following an outbreak of gastroenteritis caused by salmonella enteritidis. Clin Infect Dis 2001;33:1010–1014.

72. Könönen M. Signs and symptoms of craniomandibular disorders in men with Reiter's disease. J Craniomandib Disord 1992;6:247–253.

73. Headache Classification Subcommittee of the International Headache Society. The International Classification of Headache Disorders, 2nd edition. Cephalalgia 2004;24(suppl 1):24–150.

74. Elisevich K, Stratford J, Bray G, Finlayson M. Neck tongue syndrome: Operative management. J Neurol Neurosurg Psychiatry 1984;47:407–409.

75. Lance JW, Anthony M. Neck-tongue syndrome on sudden turning of the head. J Neurol Neurosurg Psychiatry 1980;43:97–101.

76. Sjaastad O, Bakketeig LS. Neck-tongue syndrome and related (?) conditions. Cephalalgia 2006;26:233–240.

77. Chedrawi AK, Fishman MA, Miller G. Neck-tongue syndrome. Pediatr Neurol 2000;22:397–399.

78. Wig S, Romanowski C, Akil M. An unusual cause of the neck-tongue syndrome. J Rheumatol 2009;36:857–858.

79. Bogduk N. An anatomical basis for the neck-tongue syndrome. J Neurol Neurosurg Psychiatry 1981;44:202–208.

80. Borody C. Neck-tongue syndrome. J Manipulative Physiol Ther 2004;27:e8.

81. Fortin CJ, Biller J. Neck tongue syndrome. Headache 1985;25:255–258.

82. Mauck KF, Clarke BL. Diagnosis, screening, prevention, and treatment of osteoporosis. Mayo Clin Proc 2006;81:662–672.

83. Gruber HE, Gregg J. Subchondral bone resorption in temporomandibular joint disorders. Cells Tissues Organs 2003;174:17–25.

84. Klemetti E, Vainio P, Kroger H. Craniomandibular disorders and skeletal mineral status. Cranio 1995;13:89–92.

85. Woda A, Pionchon P. A unified concept of idiopathic orofacial pain: Pathophysiologic features. J Orofac Pain 2000;14:196–212.

86. Pfaffenrath V, Rath M, Pöllmann W, Keeser W. Atypical facial pain—Application of the IHS criteria in a clinical sample. Cephalalgia 1993;13(12, suppl):8488.

87. Roodman GD, Windle JJ. Paget disease of bone. J Clin Invest 2005;115:200–208.

88. Bone HG. Nonmalignant complications of Paget's disease. J Bone Miner Res 2006;21(suppl 2):P64–P68.

89. Silverman SL. Paget disease of bone: Therapeutic options. J Clin Rheumatol 2008;14:299–305.

90. Wheeler TT, Alberts MA, Dolan TA, McGorray SP. Dental, visual, auditory and olfactory complications in Paget's disease of bone. J Am Geriatr Soc 1995;43:1384–1391.

91. Julkunen HA. Oral contraceptives in systemic lupus erythematosus: Side-effects and influence on the activity of SLE. Scand J Rheumatol 1991;20:427–433.

92. Skaer TL. Medication-induced systemic lupus erythematosus. Clin Ther 1992;14:496–506.

93. Sanchez-Guerrero J, Karlson EW, Liang MH, Hunter DJ, Speizer FE, Colditz GA. Past use of oral contraceptives and the risk of developing systemic lupus erythematosus. Arthritis Rheum 1997;40:804–808.

94. Mok CC, Lau CS, Wong RW. Use of exogenous estrogens in systemic lupus erythematosus. Semin Arthritis Rheum 2001;30:426–435.

95. Cooper GS, Dooley MA, Treadwell EL, St Clair EW, Gilkeson GS. Hormonal and reproductive risk factors for development of systemic lupus erythematosus: Results of a population-based, case-control study. Arthritis Rheum 2002;46:1830–1839.

96. Jonsson R, Lindvall AM, Nyberg G. Temporomandibular joint involvement in systemic lupus erythematosus. Arthritis Rheum 1983;26:1506–1510.

97. Aliko A, Ciancaglini R, Alushi A, Tafaj A, Ruci D. Temporomandibular joint involvement in rheumatoid arthritis, systemic lupus erythematosus and systemic sclerosis. Int J Oral Maxillofac Surg 2011;40:704–709.

98. Hagen NA, Stevens JC, Michet CJ Jr. Trigeminal sensory neuropathy associated with connective tissue diseases. Neurology 1990;40:891-896.

99. Shotts RH, Porter SR, Kumar N, Scully C. Longstanding trigeminal sensory neuropathy of nontraumatic cause. Oral Surg Oral Med Oral Pathol Oral Radiol Endod 1999;87:572–576.

100. Jorizzo JL, Salisbury PL, Rogers RS 3rd, et al. Oral lesions in systemic lupus erythematosus. Do ulcerative lesions represent a necrotizing vasculitis? J Am Acad Dermatol 1992;27:389–394.

101. Sfikakis PP, Mitsikostas DD, Manoussakis MN, Foukaneli D, Moutsopoulos HM. Headache in systemic lupus erythematosus: A controlled study. Br J Rheumatol 1998;37:300–303.

102. Mitsikostas DD, Sfikakis PP, Goadsby PJ. A meta-analysis for headache in systemic lupus erythematosus: The evidence and the myth. Brain 2004;127(Pt 5):1200–1209.

103. Palagini L, Tani C, Mauri M, et al. Sleep disorders and systemic lupus erythematosus. Lupus 2014;23:115–123.

104. Fox RI. Sjögren's syndrome. Lancet 2005;366:321–331.

105. Guggenheimer J, Moore PA. Xerostomia: Etiology, recognition and treatment. J Am Dent Assoc 2003;134:61–69.

106. Ahmadi E, Fallahi S, Alaeddini M, Hasani Tabatabaei M. Severe dental caries as the first presenting clinical feature in primary Sjögren's syndrome. Caspian J Intern Med 2013;4:731–734.

107. Felix DH, Luker J, Scully C. Oral medicine: 4. Dry mouth and disorders of salivation. Dent Update 2012;39:738–743.

108. Olney RK. Neuropathies associated with connective tissue disease. Semin Neurol 1998;18:63–72.

109. Denislic M, Meh D. Early asymmetric neuropathy in primary Sjögren's syndrome. J Neurol 1997;244:383–387.

110. Urban PP, Keilmann A, Teichmann EM, Hopf HC. Sensory neuropathy of the trigeminal, glossopharyngeal, and vagal nerves in Sjögren's syndrome. J Neurol Sci 2001;186:59–63.

111. Mori K, Iijima M, Koike H, et al. The wide spectrum of clinical manifestations in Sjögren's syndrome-associated neuropathy. Brain 2005;128(Pt 11):2518–2534.

112. Font J, Ramos-Casals M, de la Red G, et al. Pure sensory neuropathy in primary Sjögren's syndrome. Longterm prospective followup and review of the literature. J Rheumatol 2003;30:1552–1557.

113. Segal BM, Pogatchnik B, Henn L, Rudser K, Sivils KM. Pain severity and neuropathic pain symptoms in primary Sjögren's syndrome: A comparison study of seropositive and seronegative Sjögren's syndrome patients. Arthritis Care Res (Hoboken) 2013;65:1291–1298.

114. Tjensvoll AB, Harboe E, Gøransson LG, et al. Headache in primary Sjögren's syndrome: A population-based retrospective cohort study. Eur J Neurol 2013;20:558–563.

115. Koktekir BE, Celik G, Karalezli A, Kal A. Dry eyes and migraines: Is there really a correlation? Cornea 2012;31:1414–1416.

116. Segal BM, Pogatchnik B, Rhodus N, Sivils KM, McElvain G, Solid CA. Pain in primary Sjögren's syndrome: The role of catastrophizing and negative illness perceptions. Scand J Rheumatol 2014;43:234–241.

117. Iannuccelli C, Spinelli FR, Guzzo MP, et al. Fatigue and widespread pain in systemic lupus erythematosus and Sjögren's syndrome: Symptoms of the inflammatory disease or associated fibromyalgia? Clin Exp Rheumatol 2012;30(6, suppl):117—121.

118. Spackman GK. Scleroderma: What the general dentist should know. Gen Dent 1999;47:576–579.

119. Scardina GA, Messina P. Systemic sclerosis: Description and diagnostic role of the oral phenomena. Gen Dent 2004;52:42–47.

120. Chaffee NR. CREST syndrome: Clinical manifestations and dental management. J Prosthodont 1998;7:155–160.

121. Nagy G, Kovács J, Zeher M, Cziráak L. Analysis of the oral manifestations of systemic sclerosis. Oral Surg Oral Med Oral Pathol 1994;77:141–146.

122. Wood RE, Lee P. Analysis of the oral manifestations of systemic sclerosis (scleroderma). Oral Surg Oral Med Oral Pathol 1988;65:172–178.

123. Vitali C, Borghi E, Napoletano A, et al. Oropharyngolaryngeal disorders in scleroderma: Development and validation of the SLS scale. Dysphagia 2010;25:127–138.

124. Ramon Y, Samra H, Oberman M. Mandibular condylosis and apertognathia as presenting symptoms in progressive systemic sclerosis (scleroderma). Pattern of mandibular bony lesions and atrophy of masticatory muscles in PSS, presumably caused by affected muscular arteries. Oral Surg Oral Med Oral Pathol 1987;63:269–274.

125. Lecky BR, Hughes RA, Murray NM. Trigeminal sensory neuropathy. A study of 22 cases. Brain 1987;110(Pt 6):1463–1485.

126. Fischoff DK, Sirois D. Painful trigeminal neuropathy caused by severe mandibular resorption and nerve compression in a patient with systemic sclerosis: Case report and literature review. Oral Surg Oral Med Oral Pathol Oral Radiol Endod 2000;90:456–459.

127. Alfaro-Giner A, Peñarrocha-Diago M, Bagán-Sebastián JV. Orofacial manifestations of mixed connective tissue disease with an uncommon serologic evolution. Oral Surg Oral Med Oral Pathol 1992;73:441–444.

128. Konttinen YT, Tuominen TS, Piirainen HI, et al. Signs and symptoms in the masticatory system in ten patients with mixed connective tissue disease. Scand J Rheumatol 1990;19:363–373.

129. Alarcón-Segovia D. Symptomatic Sjögren's syndrome in mixed connective tissue disease. J Rheumatol 1984;11:582–583.

130. Ohtsuka E, Nonaka S, Shingu M, Yasuda M, Nobunaga M. Sjögren's syndrome and mixed connective tissue disease. Clin Exp Rheumatol 1992;10:339–344.

131. Hughes GR. Migraine, memory loss, and "multiple sclerosis." Neurological features of the antiphospholipid (Hughes') syndrome. Postgrad Med J 2003;79:81–83.

132. Levine SR, Joseph R, D'Andrea G, Welch KM. Migraine and the lupus anticoagulant. Case reports and review of the literature. Cephalalgia 1987;7:93–99.

133. Hogan MJ, Brunet DG, Ford PM, Lillicrap D. Lupus anticoagulant, antiphospholipid antibodies and migraine. Can J Neurol Sci 1988;15:420–425.

134. Alarcón-Segovia D, Delezé M, Oria CV, et al. Antiphospholipid antibodies and the antiphospholipid syndrome in systemic lupus erythematosus. A prospective analysis of 500 consecutive patients. Medicine (Baltimore) 1989;68:353–365.

135. Tzourio C, Kittner SJ, Bousser MG, Alpérovitch A. Migraine and stroke in young women. Cephalalgia 2000;20:190–199.

136. Sanna G, Bertolaccini ML, Cuadrado MJ, Khamashta MA, Hughes GR. Central nervous system involvement in the antiphospholipid (Hughes) syndrome. Rheumatology (Oxford) 2003;42:200–213.

137. Shuaib A, Barklay L, Lee MA, Suchowersky O. Migraine and anti-phospholipid antibodies. Headache 1989;29:42–45.

138. Tietjen GE. Migraine and antiphospholipid antibodies. Cephalalgia 1992;12:69–74.

139. Montalbán J, Cervera R, Font J, et al. Lack of association between anticardiolipin antibodies and migraine in systemic lupus erythematosus. Neurology 1992;42:681–682.

140. Tietjen GE, Day M, Norris L, et al. Role of anticardiolipin antibodies in young persons with migraine and transient focal neurologic events: A prospective study. Neurology 1998;50:1433–1440.

141. Verrotti A, Cieri F, Pelliccia P, Morgese G, Chiarelli F. Lack of association between antiphospholipid antibodies and migraine in children. Int J Clin Lab Res 2000;30:109–111.

142. Cuadrado MJ, Khamashta MA, Hughes GR. Migraine and stroke in young women. QJM 2000;93:317–318.

143. Cuadrado MJ, Khamashta MA, D'Cruz D, Hughes GR. Migraine in Hughes syndrome—Heparin as a therapeutic trial? QJM 2001;94:114–115.

144. van Loon LA, Bos JD, Davidson CL. Clinical evaluation of fifty-six patients referred with symptoms tentatively related to allergic contact stomatitis. Oral Surg Oral Med Oral Pathol 1992;74:572–575.

145. Issa Y, Duxbury AJ, Macfarlane TV, Brunton PA. Oral lichenoid lesions related to dental restorative materials. Br Dent J 2005;198:361–366.

146. Scully C, Bagan JV. Adverse drug reactions in the orofacial region. Crit Rev Oral Biol Med 2004;15:221–239.

147. Cady RK, Dodick DW, Levine HL, et al. Sinus headache: A neurology, otolaryngology, allergy, and primary care consensus on diagnosis and treatment. Mayo Clin Proc 2005;80:908–916.

148. Gazerani P, Pourpak Z, Ahmadiani A, Hemmati A, Kazemnejad A. A correlation between migraine, histamine and immunoglobulin e. Scand J Immunol 2003;57:286–290.

149. Lim IG, Spira PJ, McNeil HP. Headache as the initial presentation of Wegener's granulomatosis. Ann Rheum Dis 2002;61:571–572.

150. Makura ZG, Robson AK. Wegener's granulomatosis presenting as a temporal headache. J Laryngol Otol 1996;110:802–804.

151. Roszkowska A, Morawska-Kochman M, Temporale H, Sikorska-Żuk M, Krecicki T. Bilateral facial palsy in rapidly progressive course of Wegener's granulomatosis: A case report. Case Rep Otolaryngol 2013;2013.

152. Thiel G, Shakeel M, Ah-See K. Wegener's granulomatosis presenting as meningitis. J Laryngol Otol 2012;126:207–209.

153. La Mantia L, Erbetta A. Headache and inflammatory disorders of the central nervous system. Neurol Sci 2004;25(3 suppl):S148–S153.

154. Strub GM, Moore JE, Huang AT, Stevenson AW, Reiter ER. Chronic facial pain and Meckel cave masses as the initial presentation of neurosarcoidosis: A case report. Ear Nose Throat J 2013;92:558–565.

155. Curone M, Tullo V, Peccarisi C, Bussone G, D'Amico D. Headache as presenting symptom of neurosarcoidosis. Neurol Sci 2013;34(1, suppl):S183–S185.

156. Vannemreddy PS, Nanda A, Reddy PK, Gonzalez E. Primary cerebral sarcoid granuloma: The importance of definitive diagnosis in the high-risk patient population. Clin Neurol Neurosurg 2002;104:289–292.

157. Katz JM, Bruno MK, Winterkorn JM, Nealon N. The pathogenesis and treatment of optic disc swelling in neurosarcoidosis: A unique therapeutic response to infliximab. Arch Neurol 2003;60:426–430.

158. Dizdarević K, Dizdarević S, Dizdarević Z. Neurosarcoidosis presenting with transitory neurodeficit and generalized epileptic seizures associated with migraine [in Croatian]. Med Arh 1998;52:159–162.

159. Zimmer WM, Rogers RS 3rd, Reeve CM, Sheridan PJ. Orofacial manifestations of Melkersson-Rosenthal syndrome. A study of 42 patients and review of 220 cases from the literature. Oral Surg Oral Med Oral Pathol 1992;74:610–619.

160. Allen CM, Camisa C, Hamzeh S, Stephens L. Cheilitis granulomatosa: Report of six cases and review of the literature. J Am Acad Dermatol 1990;23:444–450.

161. Scully C, Cawson RA. Medical Problems in Dentistry, ed 5. Edinburgh: Elsevier, 2005.

162. Scagliusi P, Sisto M, Lisi S, Lazzari A, D'Amore M. Hashimoto's thyroiditis in Melkersson-Rosenthal syndrome patient: Casual association or related diseases? Panminerva Med 2008;50:255–257.

163. Gabriel SE, O'Fallon WM, Achkar AA, Lie JT, Hunder GG. The use of clinical characteristics to predict the results of temporal artery biopsy among patients with suspected giant cell arteritis. J Rheumatol 1995;22:93–96.

164. Nordborg C, Nordborg E, Petursdottir V. Giant cell arteritis. Epidemiology, etiology and pathogenesis. APMIS 2000;108:713–724.

165. Baldursson O, Steinsson K, Björnsson J, Lie JT. Giant cell arteritis in Iceland. An epidemiologic and histopathologic analysis. Arthritis Rheum 1994;37:1007–1012.

166. González-Gay MA, Garcia-Porrua C, Rivas MJ, Rodriguez-Ledo P, Llorca J. Epidemiology of biopsy proven giant cell arteritis in northwestern Spain: Trend over an 18 year period. Ann Rheum Dis 2001;60:367–371.

167. Gran JT, Myklebust G. The incidence of polymyalgia rheumatica and temporal arteritis in the county of Aust Agder, South Norway: A prospective study 1987–94. J Rheumatol 1997;24:1739–1743.

168. Machado EB, Michet CJ, Ballard DJ, et al. Trends in incidence and clinical presentation of temporal arteritis in Olmsted County, Minnesota, 1950–1985. Arthritis Rheum 1988;31:745–749.

169. Nordborg E, Bengtsson BA. Epidemiology of biopsy-proven giant cell arteritis (GCA). J Intern Med 1990;227:233–236.

170. Carroll SC, Gaskin BJ, Danesh-Meyer HV. Giant cell arteritis. Clin Experiment Ophthalmol 2006;34:159–173.

171. Salvarani C, Hunder GG. Giant cell arteritis with low erythrocyte sedimentation rate: Frequency of occurence in a population-based study. Arthritis Rheum 2001;45:140–145.

172. Gonzalez-Gay MA, Lopez-Diaz MJ, Barros S, et al. Giant cell arteritis: Laboratory tests at the time of diagnosis in a series of 240 patients. Medicine (Baltimore) 2005;84:277–290.

173. Hayreh SS, Podhajsky PA, Raman R, Zimmerman B. Giant cell arteritis: Validity and reliability of various diagnostic criteria. Am J Ophthalmol 1997;123:285–296.

174. Schmidt WA, Gromnica-Ihle E. What is the best approach to diagnosing large-vessel vasculitis? Best Pract Res Clin Rheumatol 2005;19:223–242.

175. Smetana GW, Shmerling RH. Does this patient have temporal arteritis? JAMA 2002;287:92–101.

176. Nordborg E, Nordborg C. Giant cell arteritis: Strategies in diagnosis and treatment. Curr Opin Rheumatol 2004;16:25–30.

177. Ray-Chaudhuri N, Kiné DA, Tijani SO, et al. Effect of prior steroid treatment on temporal artery biopsy findings in giant cell arteritis. Br J Ophthalmol 2002;86:530–532.

178. Schmidt WA. Current diagnosis and treatment of temporal arteritis. Curr Treat Options Cardiovasc Med 2006;8:145–151.

179. Danesh-Meyer HV, Savino PJ, Eagle RC Jr, Kubis KC, Sergott RC. Low diagnostic yield with second biopsies in suspected giant cell arteritis. J Neuroophthalmol 2000;20:213–215.

180. Ponge T, Barrier JH, Grolleau JY, Ponge A, Vlasak AM, Cottin S. The efficacy of selective unilateral temporal artery biopsy versus bilateral biopsies for diagnosis of giant cell arteritis. J Rheumatol 1988;15:997–1000.

181. Salvarani C, Cantini F, Boiardi L, Hunder GG. Laboratory investigations useful in giant cell arteritis and Takayasu's arteritis. Clin Exp Rheumatol 2003;21(6, suppl):S23–S28.

182. Bley TA, Uhl M, Venhoff N, Thoden J, Langer M, Markl M. 3-T MRI reveals cranial and thoracic inflammatory changes in giant cell arteritis. Clin Rheumatol 2007;26:448–450.

183. Bley TA, Warnatz K, Wieben O, et al. High-resolution MRI in giant cell arteritis with multiple inflammatory stenoses in both calves. Rheumatology (Oxford) 2005;44:954–955.

184. Bley TA, Weiben O, Uhl M, et al. Assessment of the cranial involvement pattern of giant cell arteritis with 3T magnetic resonance imaging. Arthritis Rheum 2005;52:2470–2477.

185. Hayreh SS. Masticatory muscle pain: An important indicator of giant cell arteritis. Spec Care Dentist 1998;18:60–65.

186. Keltner JL. Giant-cell arteritis. Signs and symptoms. Ophthalmology 1982;89:1101–1110.

187. Evans JM, Hunder GG. Polymyalgia rheumatica and giant cell arteritis. Rheum Dis Clin North Am 2000;26:493–515.

188. Salvarani C, Cantini F, Boiardi L, Hunder GG. Polymyalgia rheumatica and giant-cell arteritis. N Engl J Med 2002;347:261–271.

189. González-Gay MA. Giant cell arteritis and polymyalgia rheumatica: Two different but often overlapping conditions. Semin Arthritis Rheum 2004;33:289–293.

190. Martinez-Taboda VM, Bartolome MJ, Lopez-Hoyos M, et al. HLA-DRB1 allele distribution in polymyalgia rheumatica and giant cell arteritis: Influence on clinical subgroups and prognosis. Semin Arthritis Rheum 2004;34:454–464.

191. González-Gay MA, García-Porrúa C, Vázquez-Caruncho M. Polymyalgia rheumatica in biopsy proven giant cell arteritis does not constitute a different subset but differs from isolated polymyalgia rheumatica. J Rheumatol 1998;25:1750–1755.

192. Dababneh A, González-Gay MA, García-Porrúa C, Hajeer A, Thomson W, Ollier W. Giant cell arteritis and polymyalgia rheumatica can be differentiated by distinct patterns of HLA class II association. J Rheumatol 1998;25:2140–2145.

193. Ma-Krupa W, Jeon MS, Spoerl S, Tedder TF, Goronzy JJ, Weyand CM. Activation of arterial wall dendritic cells and breakdown of self-tolerance in giant cell arteritis. J Exp Med 2004;199:173–183.

194. Weyand CM, Goronzy JJ. Medium- and large-vessel vasculitis. N Engl J Med 2003;349:160–169.

195. Nordborg E, Nordborg C. The inflammatory reaction in giant cell arteritis: An immunohistochemical investigation. Clin Exp Rheumatol 1998;16:165–168.

196. Lie JT. Temporal artery biopsy diagnosis of giant cell arteritis: Lessons from 1109 biopsies. Anat Pathol 1996;1:69–97.

197. Poller DN, van Wyk Q, Jeffrey MJ. The importance of skip lesions in temporal arteritis. J Clin Pathol 2000;53:137–139.

198. Taylor-Gjevre R, Vo M, Shukla D, Resch L. Temporal artery biopsy for giant cell arteritis. J Rheumatol 2005;32:1279–1282.

199. Wagner AD, Björnsson J, Bartley GB, Goronzy JJ, Weyand CM. Interferon-γ-producing T cells in giant cell vasculitis represent a minority of tissue-infiltrating cells and are located distant from the site of pathology. Am J Pathol 1996;148:1925–1933.

200. Kaiser M, Weyand CM, Björnsson J, Goronzy JJ. Platelet-derived growth factor, intimal hyperplasia, and ischemic complications in giant cell arteritis. Arthritis Rheum 1998;41:623–633.

201. Kaiser M, Younge B, Björnsson J, Goronzy JJ, Weyand CM. Formation of new vasa vasorum in vasculitis. Production of angiogenic cytokines by multinucleated giant cells. Am J Pathol 1999;155:765–774.

202. Kyle V. Treatment of polymyalgia rheumatica/giant cell arteritis. Baillieres Clin Rheumatol 1991;5:485–491.

203. Kyle V, Hazleman BL. The clinical and laboratory course of polymyalgia rheumatica/giant cell arteritis after the first two months of treatment. Ann Rheum Dis 1993;52:847–850.

204. Swannell AJ. Polymyalgia rheumatica and temporal arteritis: Diagnosis and management. BMJ 1997;314:1329–1332.

205. Proven A, Gabriel SE, Orces C, O'Fallon WM, Hunder GG. Glucocorticoid therapy in giant cell arteritis: Duration and adverse outcomes. Arthritis Rheum 2003;49:703–708.

206. Nesher G, Berkun Y, Mates M, Baras M, Rubinow A, Sonnenblick M. Low-dose aspirin and prevention of cranial ischemic complications in giant cell arteritis. Arthritis Rheum 2004;50:1332–1337.

207. Yamashita N. Hyperreactivity of neutrophils and abnormal T cell homeostasis: A new insight for pathogenesis of Behçet's disease. Int Rev Immunol 1997;14:11–19.

208. Zierhut M, Mizuki N, Ohno S, et al. Immunology and functional genomics of Behçet's disease. Cell Mol Life Sci 2003;60:1903–1922.

209. Kidd D. The prevalence of headache in Behçet's syndrome. Rheumatology (Oxford) 2006;45:621–623.

210. Monastero R, Mannino M, Lopez G, et al. Prevalence of headache in patients with Behçet's disease without overt neurological involvement. Cephalalgia 2003;23:105–108.

211. Saip S, Siva A, Altintas A, et al. Headache in Behçet's syndrome. Headache 2005;45:911–919.

212. Melikoglu M, Melikoglu MA. The prevalence of fibromyalgia in patients with Behçet's disease and its relation with disease activity. Rheumatol Int 2013;33:1219–1222.

213. Arboix A, Massons J, Oliveres M, Arribas MP, Titus F. Headache in acute cerebrovascular disease: A prospective clinical study in 240 patients. Cephalalgia 1994;14:37–40.

214. Agostoni E, Fumagalli L, Santoro P, Ferrarese C. Migraine and stroke. Neurol Sci 2004;25(3, suppl):S123–S125.

215. Rothrock JF. Headaches due to vascular disorders. Neurol Clin 2004;22:21–37.

216. Tzourio C, Tehindrazanarivelo A, Iglésias S, et al. Case-control study of migraine and risk of ischaemic stroke in young women. BMJ 1995;310:830–833.

217. Wolf ME, Szabo K, Griebe M, et al. Clinical and MRI characteristics of acute migrainous infarction. Neurology 2011;76:1911–1917.

218. Laurell K, Lundström E. Migrainous infarction: Aspects on risk factors and therapy. Curr Pain Headache Rep 2012;16:255–260.

219. Tabby D, Majeed MH, Youngman B, Wilcox J. Headache in multiple sclerosis: Features and implications for disease management. Int J MS Care 2013;15:73–80.

220. Rolak LA, Brown S. Headaches and multiple sclerosis: A clinical study and review of the literature. J Neurol 1990;237:300–302.

221. D'Amico D, La Mantia L, Rigamonti A, et al. Prevalence of primary headaches in people with multiple sclerosis. Cephalalgia 2004;24:980–984.

222. Kister I, Caminero AB, Monteith TS, et al. Migraine is comorbid with multiple sclerosis and associated with a more symptomatic MS course. J Headache Pain 2010;11:417–425.

223. Sandyk R, Awerbuch GI. The co-occurrence of multiple sclerosis and migraine headache: The serotoninergic link. Int J Neurosci 1994;76:249–257.

224. Ramadan NM. Headache caused by raised intracranial pressure and intracranial hypotension. Curr Opin Neurol 1996;9:214–218.

225. Mokri B. Headaches caused by decreased intracranial pressure: Diagnosis and management. Curr Opin Neurol 2003;16:319–326.

226. Cortelli P, Grimaldi D, Guaraldi P, Pierangeli G. Headache and hypertension. Neurol Sci 2004;25(3, suppl):S132–S134.

227. Salkic S, Batic-Mujanovic O, Ljuca F, Brkic S. Clinical presentation of hypertensive crises in emergency medical services. Mater Sociomed 2014;26:12–16.

228. Lagman-Bartolome AM, Gladstone J. Metabolic headaches. Neurol Clin 2014;32:451–469.

229. Franklin MM, Allen W, Pickett S, Peters RM. Hypertensive symptom representations: A pilot study. J Am Assoc Nurse Pract 2015;27:48–53.

230. Assarzadegan F, Asadollahi M, Hesami O, Aryani O, Mansouri B, Beladi Moghadam N. Secondary headaches attributed to arterial hypertension. Iran J Neurol 2013;12(3):106–110.

231. King JW, Bair E, Duggan D, Maixner W, Khan AA. The relationship between resting arterial blood pressure and acute postoperative pain in endodontic patients. J Orofac Pain 2012;26:321–327.

232. Teruel A, Ram S, Kumar SK, Hariri S, Clark GT. Prevalence of hypertension in patients with trigeminal neuralgia. J Headache Pain 2009;10:199–201.

233. Mannelli M, Ianni L, Cilotti A, Conti A. Pheochromocytoma in Italy: A multicentric retrospective study. Eur J Endocrinol 1999;141:619–624.

234. Belfort MA, Saade GR, Grunewald C, et al. Association of cerebral perfusion pressure with headache in women with pre-eclampsia. Br J Obstet Gynaecol 1999;106:814–821.

235. Facchinetti F, Allais G, D'Amico R, Benedetto C, Volpe A. The relationship between headache and pre-eclampsia: A case-control study. Eur J Obstet Gynecol Reprod Biol 2005;121:143–148.

236. Eslick GD. Usefulness of chest pain character and location as diagnostic indicators of an acute coronary syndrome. Am J Cardiol 2005;95:1228–1231.

237. Culić V, Mirić D, Eterović D. Correlation between symptomatology and site of acute myocardial infarction. Int J Cardiol 2001;77:163–168.

238. Edmondstone WM. Cardiac chest pain: Does body language help the diagnosis? BMJ 1995;311:1660–1661.

239. Kosuge M, Kimura K, Ishikawa T, et al. Differences between men and women in terms of clinical features of ST-segment elevation acute myocardial infarction. Circ J 2006;70:222–226.

240. Theroux P. Angina pectoris. In: Goldman L, Ausellio D (eds). Cecil Textbook of Medicine, ed 22. Philadelphia: Saunders, 2004:389–400.

241. Granot M, Goldstein-Ferber S, Azzam ZS. Gender differences in the perception of chest pain. J Pain Symptom Manage 2004;27:149–155.

242. Løvlien M, Schei B, Gjengedal E. Are there gender differences related to symptoms of acute myocardial infarction? A Norwegian perspective. Prog Cardiovasc Nurs 2006;21:14–19.

243. de Oliveira Franco AC, de Siqueira JT, Mansur AJ. Bilateral facial pain from cardiac origin. A case report. Br Dent J 2005;198:679–680.

244. Durso BC, Israel MS, Janini ME, Cardoso AS. Orofacial pain of cardiac origin: A case report. Cranio 2003;21:152–153.

245. Stöllberger C, Finsterer J, Habitzl W, Kopsa W, Deutsch M. Toothache leading to emergency cardiac surgery. Intensive Care Med 2001;27:1100–1101.

246. Kreiner M, Okeson JP. Toothache of cardiac origin. J Orofac Pain 1999;13:201–207.

247. Sandler NA, Ziccardi V, Ochs M. Differential diagnosis of jaw pain in the elderly. J Am Dent Assoc 1995;126:1263–1272.

248. Batchelder BJ, Krutchkoff DJ, Amara J. Mandibular pain as the initial and sole clinical manifestation of coronary insufficiency: Report of case. J Am Dent Assoc 1987;115:710–712.

249. Graham LL, Schinbeckler GA. Orofacial pain of cardiac origin. J Am Dent Assoc 1982;104:47–48.

250. Tzukert A, Hasin Y, Sharav Y. Orofacial pain of cardiac origin. Oral Surg Oral Med Oral Pathol 1981;51:484–486.

251. Natkin E, Harrington GW, Mandel MA. Anginal pain referred to the teeth. Report of a case. Oral Surg Oral Med Oral Pathol 1975;40:678–680.

252. Gutiérrez-Morlote J, Pascual J. Cardiac cephalgia is not necessarily an exertional headache: Case report. Cephalalgia 2002;22:765–766.

253. Foreman RD. Mechanisms of cardiac pain. Annu Rev Physiol 1999;61:143–167.

254. Yri HM, Rönnbäck C, Wegener M, Hamann S, Jensen RH. The course of headache in idiopathic intracranial hypertension: A 12-month prospective follow-up study [epub ahead of print 29 July 2014]. Eur J Neurol doi: 10.1111/ene.12512.

255. Wakerley B, Tan M, Ting E. Idiopathic intracranial hypertension. Cephalalgia 2015;35:248–261.

256. Sacco S, Ricci S, Carolei A. Migraine and vascular diseases: A review of the evidence and potential implications for management. Cephalalgia 2012;32:785–795.

257. Riederer F, Baumgartner H, Sándor PS, Wessely P, Wöber C. Headache in 25 consecutive patients with atrial septal defects before and after percutaneous closure—A prospective case series. Headache 2011;51:1297–1304.

258. Kato Y, Hayashi T, Kobayashi T, Tanahashi N. Migraine prevalence in patients with atrial septal defect. J Headache Pain 2013;14:63.

259. Ekici B, Unal-Cevik I, Akgul-Ercan E, Morkavuk G, Yakut Y, Erkan AF. Duration of migraine is associated with cardiac diastolic dysfunction. Pain Med 2013;14:988–993.

260. Kirkham KE, Colon RJ, Solomon GD. The role of cardiovascular screening in headache patients. Headache 2011;51:331–337.

261. Nappi RE, Merki-Feld GS, Terreno E, Pellegrinelli A, Viana M. Hormonal contraception in women with migraine: Is progestogen-only contraception a better choice? J Headache Pain 2013;14:66.

262. Lee VH, Brown RD Jr, Mandrekar JN, Mokri B. Incidence and outcome of cervical artery dissection: A population-based study. Neurology 2006;67:1809–1812.

263. Mokri B. Headaches in cervical artery dissections. Curr Pain Headache Rep 2002;6:209–216.

264. Shah Q, Messé SR. Cervicocranial arterial dissection. Curr Treat Options Neurol 2007;9:55–62.

265. Rahme RJ, Aoun SG, McClendon J Jr, El Ahmadieh TY, Bendok BR. Spontaneous cervical and cerebral arterial dissections: Diagnosis and management. Neuroimaging Clin N Am 2013;23:661–671.

266. Biousse V, Mitsias P. Carotid or vertebral artery disease. In: Olesen J, Goadsby PJ, Ramadan NM, Tfelt-Hansen P, Welch KMA (eds). The Headaches, ed 3. Philadelphia: Lippincott Williams & Wilkins, 2006:911–918.

267. Völker W, Besselmann M, Dittrich R, et al. Generalized arteriopathy in patients with cervical artery dissection. Neurology 2005;64:1508–1513.

268. Völker W, Dittrich R, Grewe S, et al. The outer arterial wall layers are primarily affected in spontaneous cervical artery dissection. Neurology 2011;76:1463–1471.

269. Biousse V, Touboul PJ, D'Anglejan-Chatillon J, Lévy C, Schaison M, Bousser MG. Ophthalmologic manifestations of internal carotid artery dissection. Am J Ophthalmol 1998;126:565–577.

270. Hart RG, Easton JD. Dissections of cervical and cerebral arteries. Neurol Clin 1983;1:155–182.

271. Solomon S, Lustig JP. Benign Raeder's syndrome is probably a manifestation of carotid artery disease. Cephalalgia 2001;21:1–11.

272. Debette S, Leys D. Cervical-artery dissections: Predisposing factors, diagnosis, and outcome. Lancet Neurol 2009;8:668–678.

273. Evans RW, Mokri B. Headache in cervical artery dissections. Headache 2002;42:1061–1063.

274. Patel RR, Adam R, Maldjian C, Lincoln CM, Yuen A, Arneja A. Cervical carotid artery dissection: Current review of diagnosis and treatment. Cardiol Rev 2012;20:145–152.

275. Mokri B. Traumatic and spontaneous extracranial internal carotid artery dissections. J Neurol 1990;237:356–361.

276. Lyrer P, Engelter S. Antithrombotic drugs for carotid artery dissection. Cochrane Database Syst Rev 2010;(6).

277. Medel R, Starke RM, Valle-Giler EP, Martin-Schild S, El Khoury R, Dumont AS. Diagnosis and treatment of arterial dissections. Curr Neurol Neurosci Rep 2014;14:419.

278. Dittrich R, Nassenstein I, Bachmann R, et al. Polyarterial clustered recurrence of cervical artery dissection seems to be the rule. Neurology 2007;69:180–186.

279. Schievink WI. Spontaneous dissection of the carotid and vertebral arteries. N Engl J Med 2001;344:898–906.

280. Brandt T, Grond-Ginsbach C. Spontaneous cervical artery dissection: From risk factors toward pathogenesis. Stroke 2002;33:657–658.

281. Zafeiriou DI, Economou M, Athanasiou-Metaxa M. Neurological complications in beta-thalassemia. Brain Dev 2006;28:477–481.

282. Aarabi B, Haghshenas M, Rakeii V. Visual failure caused by suprasellar extramedullary hematopoiesis in beta thalassemia: Case report. Neurosurgery 1998;42:922–925.

283. To KW, Nadel AJ. Ophthalmologic complications in hemoglobinopathies. Hematol Oncol Clin North Am 1991;5:535–548.

284. Borgna Pignatti C, Carnelli V, Caruso V, et al. Thromboembolic events in beta thalassemia major: An Italian multicenter study. Acta Haematol 1998;99:76–79.

285. Hattab FN. Periodontal condition and orofacial changes in patients with thalassemia major: A clinical and radiographic overview. J Clin Pediatr Dent 2012;36:301–307.

286. Goldfarb A, Nitzan DW, Marmary Y. Changes in the parotid salivary gland of beta-thalassemia patients due to hemosiderin deposits. Int J Oral Surg 1983;12:115–119.

287. Mendes PH, Fonseca NG, Martelli DR, et al. Orofacial manifestations in patients with sickle cell anemia. Quintessence Int 2011;42:701–709.

288. Watanabe M, Saito N, Nadgir RN, et al. Craniofacial bone infarcts in sickle cell disease: Clinical and radiological manifestations. J Comput Assist Tomogr 2013;37:91–97.

289. O'Rourke C, Mitropoulos C. Orofacial pain in patients with sickle cell disease. Br Dent J 1990;169:130–132.

290. Demirbas Kaya A, Aktener BO, Unsal C. Pulpal necrosis with sickle cell anaemia. Int Endod J 2004;37:602–606.

291. Pari G, Schipper HM. Headache and scalp edema in sickle cell disease. Can J Neurol Sci 1996;23:224–226.

292. Vial T, Descotes J. Clinical toxicity of cytokines used as haemopoietic growth factors. Drug Saf 1995;13:371–406.

293. Hovgaard DJ, Nissen NI. Effect of recombinant human granulocyte-macrophage colony-stimulating factor in patients with Hodgkin's disease: A phase I/II study. J Clin Oncol 1992;10:390–397.

294. Antoniazzi AL, Corrado AP. Dialysis headache. Curr Pain Headache Rep 2007;11:297–303.

295. Antoniazzi AL, Bigal ME, Bordini CA, Tepper SJ, Speciali JG. Headache and hemodialysis: A prospective study. Headache 2003;43:99–102.

296. Antoniazzi AL, Bigal ME. Expert opinion: Headaches and hemodialysis. Headache 2009;49:463–466.

297. Göksan B, Karaali-Savrun F, Ertan S, Savrun M. Haemodialysis-related headache. Cephalalgia 2004;24:284–287.

298. Heidenheim AP, Leitch R, Kortas C, Lindsay RM. Patient monitoring in the London Daily/Nocturnal Hemodialysis Study. Am J Kidney Dis 2003;42(1, suppl):61–65.

299. Pillekamp F, Hoppe B, Roth B, Querfeld U. Vomiting, headache and seizures in a child with idiopathic nephrotic syndrome. Nephrol Dial Transplant 1997;12:1280–1281.

300. Chan KH, Cheung RT, Mak W, Au-Yeung KM, Ho SL. Cerebral venous thrombosis presenting as unilateral headache and visual blurring in a man with nephrotic syndrome. Hosp Med 2004;65:54–55.

301. Alves FR, de A Quintanilha Ribeiro F. Revision about hearing loss in the Alport's syndrome, analyzing the clinical, genetic and bio-molecular aspects. Braz J Otorhinolaryngol 2005;71:813–819.

302. Gingrass D. Temporomandibular joint degeneration in Alport's syndrome: Review of literature and case report. J Orofac Pain 1993;7:307–310.

303. Ozge A, Ozge C, Kaleagasi H, Yalin OO, Unal O, Ozgür ES. Headache in patients with chronic obstructive pulmonary disease: Effects of chronic hypoxaemia. J Headache Pain 2006;7:37–43.

304. Davey G, Sedgwick P, Maier W, Visick G, Strachan DP, Anderson HR. Association between migraine and asthma: Matched case-control study. Br J Gen Pract 2002;52:723–727.

305. Caraceni A, Portenoy RK. An international survey of cancer pain characteristics and syndromes. IASP Task Force on Cancer Pain. International Association for the Study of Pain. Pain 1999;82:263–274.

306. Portenoy RK, Payne D, Jacobsen P. Breakthrough pain: Characteristics and impact in patients with cancer pain. Pain 1999;81:129–134.

307. Epstein JB, Schubert MM. Oropharyngeal mucositis in cancer therapy. Review of pathogenesis, diagnosis, and management. Oncology (Huntingt) 2003;17:1767–1779.

308. Sonis ST. Oral mucositis in cancer therapy. J Support Oncol 2004;2(6, suppl):3–8.

309. de Wit R, van Dam F, Loonstra S, et al. The Amsterdam Pain Management Index compared to eight frequently used outcome measures to evaluate the adequacy of pain treatment in cancer patients with chronic pain. Pain 2001;91:339–349.

310. Meuser T, Pietruck C, Radbruch L, Stute P, Lehmann KA, Grond S. Symptoms during cancer pain treatment following WHO-guidelines: A longitudinal follow-up study of symptom prevalence, severity and etiology. Pain 2001;93:247–257.

311. Viet CT, Schmidt BL. Biologic mechanisms of oral cancer pain and implications for clinical therapy. J Dent Res 2012;91:447–453.

312. Epstein JB, Hong C, Logan RM, et al. A systematic review of orofacial pain in patients receiving cancer therapy. Support Care Cancer 2010;18:1023–1031.

313. Epstein JB, Stewart KH. Radiation therapy and pain in patients with head and neck cancer. Eur J Cancer B Oral Oncol 1993;29B:191–199.

314. Portenoy RK, Lesage P. Management of cancer pain. Lancet 1999;353:1695–1700.

315. Lam DK, Schmidt BL. Orofacial pain onset predicts transition to head and neck cancer. Pain 2011;152:1206–1209.

316. Foley KM, Inturrisi CE. Analgesic drug therapy in cancer pain: Principles and practice. Med Clin North Am 1987;71:207–232.

317. Coleman RE. How can we improve the treatment of bone metastases further? Curr Opin Oncol 1998;10(suppl 1):S7–S13.

318. Foley KM. Advances in cancer pain. Arch Neurol 1999;56:413–417.

319. Kanner R. Diagnosis and management of neuropathic pain in patients with cancer. Cancer Invest 2001;19:324–333.

320. Grond S, Zech D, Diefenbach C, Radbruch L, Lehmann KA. Assessment of cancer pain: A prospective evaluation in 2266 cancer patients referred to a pain service. Pain 1996;64:107–114.

321. Oliveira KG, von Zeidler SV, Podestá JR, et al. Influence of pain severity on the quality of life in patients with head and neck cancer before antineoplastic therapy. BMC Cancer 2014;14:39.

322. Cuffari L, Tesseroli de Siqueira JT, Nemr K, Rapaport A. Pain complaint as the first symptom of oral cancer: A descriptive study. Oral Surg Oral Med Oral Pathol Oral Radiol Endod 2006;102:56–61.

323. Diercks GR, Rosow DE, Prasad M, Kuhel WI. A case of preoperative "first-bite syndrome" associated with mucoepidermoid carcinoma of the parotid gland. Laryngoscope 2011;121:760–762.

324. Epstein JB, Jones CK. Presenting signs and symptoms of nasopharyngeal carcinoma. Oral Surg Oral Med Oral Pathol 1993;75:32–36.

325. Su CY, Lui CC. Perineural invasion of the trigeminal nerve in patients with nasopharyngeal carcinoma. Imaging and clinical correlations. Cancer 1996;78:2063–2069.

326. Wang CJ, Howng SL. Trigeminal neuralgia caused by nasopharyngeal carcinoma with skull base invasion—A case report. Kaohsiung J Med Sci 2001;17:630–632.

327. McGuire DB, Yeager KA, Dudley WN, et al. Acute oral pain and mucositis in bone marrow transplant and leukemia patients: Data from a pilot study. Cancer Nurs 1998;21:385–393.

328. Bergmann OJ, Andersen PL. Acute oral candidiasis during febrile episodes in immunocompromised patients with haematologic malignancies. Scand J Infect Dis 1990;22:353–358.

329. Bergmann OJ, Mogensen SC, Ellegaard J. Herpes simplex virus and intraoral ulcers in immunocompromised patients with haematologic malignancies. Eur J Clin Microbiol Infect Dis 1990;9:184–190.

330. Epstein JB, Polsky B. Oropharyngeal candidiasis: A review of its clinical spectrum and current therapies. Clin Ther 1998;20:40–57.

331. Epstein JB, Epstein JD, Le ND, Gorsky M. Characteristics of oral and paraoral malignant lymphoma: A population-based review of 361 cases. Oral Surg Oral Med Oral Pathol Oral Radiol Endod 2001;92:519–525.

332. Hoffman HT, Karnell LH, Funk GF, Robinson RA, Menck HR. The National Cancer Data Base report on cancer of the head and neck. Arch Otolaryngol Head Neck Surg 1998;124:951–962.

333. Witt C, Borges AC, Klein K, Neumann HJ. Radiographic manifestations of multiple myeloma in the mandible: A retrospective study of 77 patients. J Oral Maxillofac Surg 1997;55:450–453.

334. Epstein JB. Radiographic manifestations of multiple myeloma in the mandible: A retrospective study of 77 patients. J Oral Maxillofac Surg 1997;55:454–455.

335. Hirshberg A, Shnaiderman-Shapiro A, Kaplan I, Berger R. Metastatic tumours to the oral cavity—Pathogenesis and analysis of 673 cases. Oral Oncol 2008;44:743–752.

336. Cohen HV, Rosenheck AH. Metastatic cancer presenting as TMD. A case report. J N J Dent Assoc 1998;69(3):17–19.

337. Schreiber A, Kinney LA, Salman R. Large-cell lymphoma of the infratemporal fossa presenting as myofacial pain. J Craniomandib Disord 1991;5:286–289.

338. McClure SA, Movahed R, Salama A, Ord RA. Maxillofacial metastases: A retrospective review of one institution's 15-year experience. J Oral Maxillofac Surg 2013;71:178–188.

339. Hirshberg A, Buchner A. Metastatic tumours to the oral region. An overview. Eur J Cancer B Oral Oncol 1995;31B:355–360.

340. Gorsky M, Epstein JB. Melanoma arising from the mucosal surfaces of the head and neck. Oral Surg Oral Med Oral Pathol Oral Radiol Endod 1998;86:715–719.

341. Gorsky M, Epstein JB. Head and neck and intra-oral soft tissue sarcomas. Oral Oncol 1998;34:292–296.

342. Bhaya MH, Har-El G. Referred facial pain from intracranial tumors: A diagnostic dilemma. Am J Otolaryngol 1998;19:383–386.

343. Bullitt E, Tew JM, Boyd J. Intracranial tumors in patients with facial pain. J Neurosurg 1986;64:865–871.

344. Christiaans MH, Kelder JC, Arnoldus EP, Tijssen CC. Prediction of intracranial metastases in cancer patients with headache. Cancer 2002;94:2063–2068.

345. Luyk NH, Hammond-Tooke G, Bishara SN, Ferguson MM. Facial pain and muscle atrophy secondary to an intracranial tumour. Br J Oral Maxillofac Surg 1991;29:204–207.

346. Pfund Z, Szapáry L, Jászberényi O, Nagy F, Czopf J. Headache in intracranial tumors. Cephalalgia 1999;19:787–790.

347. Puca A, Meglio M, Tamburrini G, Vari R. Trigeminal involvement in intracranial tumours. Anatomical and clinical observations on 73 patients. Acta Neurochir (Wien) 1993;125:47–51.

348. Moazzam AA, Habibian M. Patients appearing to dental professionals with orofacial pain arising from intracranial tumors: A literature review. Oral Surg Oral Med Oral Pathol Oral Radiol 2012;114:749–755.

349. Abraham PJ, Capobianco DJ, Cheshire WP. Facial pain as the presenting symptom of lung carcinoma with normal chest radiograph. Headache 2003;43:499–504.

350. Eross EJ, Dodick DW, Swanson JW, Capobianco DJ. A review of intractable facial pain secondary to underlying lung neoplasms. Cephalalgia 2003;23:2–5.

351. Sarlani E, Schwartz AH, Greenspan JD, Grace EG. Facial pain as first manifestation of lung cancer: A case of lung cancer-related cluster headache and a review of the literature. J Orofac Pain 2003;17:262–267.

352. Bindoff LA, Heseltine D. Unilateral facial pain in patients with lung cancer: A referred pain via the vagus? Lancet 1988;1:812–815.

353. Contreras RJ, Beckstead RM, Norgren R. The central projections of the trigeminal, facial, glossopharyngeal and vagus nerves: An autoradiographic study in the rat. J Auton Nerv Syst 1982;6:303–322.

354. Gwyn DG, Leslie RA, Hopkins DA. Observations on the afferent and efferent organization of the vagus nerve and the innervation of the stomach in the squirrel monkey. J Comp Neurol 1985;239:163–175.

355. Goldberg HL. Chest cancer refers pain to face and jaw: A case review. Cranio 1997;15:167–169.

356. Amato AA, Collins MP. Neuropathies associated with malignancy. Semin Neurol 1998;18:125–144.

357. Antoine JC, Mosnier JF, Absi L, Convers P, Honnorat J, Michel D. Carcinoma associated paraneoplastic peripheral neuropathies in patients with and without anti-onconeural antibodies. J Neurol Neurosurg Psychiatry 1999;67:7–14.

358. Mallecourt C, Delattre JY. Paraneoplastic neuropathies [in French]. Presse Med 2000;29:447–452.

359. Daggett P, Nabarro J. Neurological aspects of insulinomas. Postgrad Med J 1984;60:577–581.

360. Littlewood T, Mandelli F. The effects of anemia in hematologic malignancies: More than a symptom. Semin Oncol 2002;29(3, suppl):40–44.

361. Teräväinen H, Larsen A. Some features of the neuromuscular complications of pulmonary carcinoma. Ann Neurol 1977;2:495–502.

362. Paul T, Katiyar BC, Misra S, Pant GC. Carcinomatous neuromuscular syndromes. A clinical and quantitative electrophysiological study. Brain 1978;101:53–63.

363. Chen SC, Lai YH, Huang BS, Lin CY, Fan KH, Chang JT. Changes and predictors of radiation induced oral mucositis in patients with oral cavity cancer during active treatment [Epub ahead of print Jan 10 2015]. Eur J Oncol Nurs doi:10.1016/j.ejon.2014.12.001.

364. Ohbayashi Y, Imataki O, Ohnishi H, et al. Multivariate analysis of factors influencing oral mucositis in allogeneic hematopoetic stem cell transplantation. Ann Hematol 2008;87:837–845.

365. Schulz-Kindermann F, Hennings U, Ramm G, Zander AR, Hasenbring M. The role of biomedical and psychosocial factors for the prediction of pain and distress in patients undergoing high-dose therapy and BMT/PBSCT. Bone Marrow Transplant 2002;29:341–351.

366. Dodd MJ, Dibble S, Miaskowski C, et al. A comparison of the affective state and quality of life of chemotherapy patients who do and do not develop chemotherapy-induced oral mucositis. J Pain Symptom Manage 2001;21:498–505.

367. Pederson C, Parran L, Harbaugh B. Children's perceptions of pain during 3 weeks of bone marrow transplant experience. J Pediatr Oncol Nurs 2000;17:22–32.

368. Sonis ST. The pathobiology of mucositis. Nat Rev Cancer 2004;4:277–284.

369. Epstein JB, Phillips N, Parry J, Epstein MS, Nevill T, Stevenson-Moore P. Quality of life, taste, olfactory and oral function following high-dose chemotherapy and allogeneic hematopoietic cell transplantation. Bone Marrow Transplant 2002;30:785–792.

370. Rubenstein EB, Peterson DE, Schubert M, et al. Clinical practice guidelines for the prevention and treatment of cancer therapy-induced oral and gastrointestinal mucositis. Cancer 2004;100(suppl 9):2026–2046.

371. Duncan GG, Epstein JB, Tu D, et al. Quality of life, mucositis, and xerostomia from radiotherapy for head and neck cancers: A report from the NCIC CTG HN2 randomized trial of an antimicrobial lozenge to prevent mucositis. Head Neck 2005;27:421–428.

372. Bellm LA, Epstein JB, Rose-Ped A, Martin P, Fuchs HJ. Patient reports of complications of bone marrow transplantation. Support Care Cancer 2000;8:33–39.

373. Stiff P. Mucositis associated with stem cell transplantation: Current status and innovative approaches to management. Bone Marrow Transplant 2001;27(suppl 2):S3–S11.

374. Vera-Llonch M, Oster G, Ford C, Lu J, Sonis S. Oral mucositis and outcomes of allogeneic hematopoietic stem-cell transplantation in patients with hematologic malignancies. Support Care Cancer 2007;15:491–496.

375. Elting LS, Cooksley C, Chambers M, Cantor SB, Manzullo E, Rubenstein EB. The burdens of cancer therapy. Clinical and economic outcomes of chemotherapy-induced mucositis. Cancer 2003;98:1531–1539.

376. Epstein JB, Robertson M, Emerton S, Phillips N, Stevenson-Moore P. Quality of life and oral function in patients treated with radiation therapy for head and neck cancer. Head Neck 2001;23:389–398.

377. Epstein JB, Silverman S Jr, Paggiarino DA, et al. Benzydamine HCl for prophylaxis of radiation-induced oral mucositis: Results from a multicenter, randomized, double-blind, placebo-controlled clinical trial. Cancer 2001;92:875-885.

378. McGuire DB, Altomonte V, Peterson DE, Wingard JR, Jones RJ, Grochow LB. Patterns of mucositis and pain in patients receiving preparative chemotherapy and bone marrow transplantation. Oncol Nurs Forum 1993;20:1493–1502.

379. Sonis ST, Elting LS, Keefe D, et al. Perspectives on cancer therapy-induced mucosal injury: Pathogenesis, measurement, epidemiology, and consequences for patients. Cancer 2004;100(9, suppl):1995–2025.

380. Trotti A, Bellm LA, Epstein JB, et al. Mucositis incidence, severity and associated outcomes in patients with head and neck cancer receiving radiotherapy with or without chemotherapy: A systematic literature review. Radiother Oncol 2003;66:253–262.

381. Bernier J, Domenge C, Ozsahin M, et al. Postoperative irradiation with or without concomitant chemotherapy for locally advanced head and neck cancer. N Engl J Med 2004;350:1945–1952.

382. Cooper JS, Pajak TF, Forastiere AA, et al. Postoperative concurrent radiotherapy and chemotherapy for high-risk squamous-cell carcinoma of the head and neck. N Engl J Med 2004;350:1937–1944.

383. List MA, Siston A, Haraf D, et al. Quality of life and performance in advanced head and neck cancer patients on concomitant chemoradiotherapy: A prospective examination. J Clin Oncol 1999;17:1020–1028.

384. Huang HY, Wilkie DJ, Chapman CR, Ting LL. Pain trajectory of Taiwanese with nasopharyngeal carcinoma over the course of radiation therapy. J Pain Symptom Manage 2003;25:247–255.

385. Gellrich NC, Schimming R, Schramm A, Schmalohr D, Bremerich A, Kugler J. Pain, function, and psychologic outcome before, during, and after intraoral tumor resection. J Oral Maxillofac Surg 2002;60:772–777.

386. Wang ZH, Zhang SZ, Zhang ZY, et al. Protecting the oral mucosa in patients with oral tongue squamous cell carcinoma treated postoperatively with intensity-modulated radiotherapy: A randomized study. Laryngoscope 2012;122:291–298.

387. Sonis ST, Oster G, Fuchs H, et al. Oral mucositis and the clinical and economic outcomes of hematopoietic stem-cell transplantation. J Clin Oncol 2001;19:2201–2205.

388. Epstein JB, Tsang AH, Warkentin D, Ship JA. The role of salivary function in modulating chemotherapy-induced oropharyngeal mucositis: A review of the literature. Oral Surg Oral Med Oral Pathol Oral Radiol Endod 2002;94:39–44.

389. Giles FJ, Miller CB, Hurd DD, et al. A phase III, randomized, double-blind, placebo-controlled, multinational trial of iseganan for the prevention of oral mucositis in patients receiving stomatotoxic chemotherapy (PROMPT-CT trial). Leuk Lymphoma 2003;44:1165–1172.

390. Fischer DJ, Klasser GD, Epstein JB. Cancer and orofacial pain. Oral Maxillofac Surg Clin North Am 2008;20:287–301.

391. Baselga J, Campone M, Piccart M, et al. Everolimus in postmenopausal hormone-receptor-positive advanced breast cancer. N Engl J Med 2012;366:520–529.

392. Watters AL, Epstein JB, Agulnik M. Oral complications of targeted cancer therapies: A narrative literature review. Oral Oncol 2011;47:441–448.

393. Boers-Doets CB, Epstein JB, Raber-Durlacher JE, et al. Oral adverse events associated with tyrosine kinase and mammalian target of rapamycin inhibitors in renal cell carcinoma: A structured literature review. Oncologist 2012;17:135–144.

394. McCarthy GM, Skillings JR. Jaw and other orofacial pain in patients receiving vincristine for the treatment of cancer. Oral Surg Oral Med Oral Pathol 1992;74:299–304.

395. Cella D, Peterman A, Hudgens S, Webster K, Socinski MA. Measuring the side effects of taxane therapy in oncology: The functional assesment of cancer therapy-taxane (FACT-taxane). Cancer 2003;98:822–831.

396. Forman AD. Peripheral neuropathy and cancer. Curr Oncol Rep 2004;6:20–25.

397. Hilkens PH, Pronk LC, Verweij J, Vecht CJ, van Putten WL, van den Bent MJ. Peripheral neuropathy induced by combination chemotherapy of docetaxel and cisplatin. Br J Cancer 1997;75:417–422.

398. Zadik Y, Vainstein V, Heling I, Neuman T, Drucker S, Elad S. Cytotoxic chemotherapy-induced odontalgia: A differential diagnosis for dental pain. J Endod 2010;36:1588–1592.

399. Epstein J, van der Meij E, McKenzie M, Wong F, Lepawsky M, Stevenson-Moore P. Postradiation osteonecrosis of the mandible: A long-term follow-up study. Oral Surg Oral Med Oral Pathol Oral Radiol Endod 1997;83:657–662.

400. Marx RE, Johnson RP. Studies in the radiobiology of osteoradionecrosis and their clinical significance. Oral Surg Oral Med Oral Pathol 1987;64:379–390.

401. Cramer CK, Epstein JB, Sheps SB, Schechter MT, Busser JR. Modified Delphi survey for decision analysis for prophylaxis of post-radiation osteonecrosis. Oral Oncol 2002;38:574–583.

402. McKenzie MR, Wong FL, Epstein JB, Lepawsky M. Hyperbaric oxygen and postradiation osteonecrosis of the mandible. Eur J Cancer B Oral Oncol 1993;29B:201–207.

403. Reuther T, Schuster T, Mende U, Kubler A. Osteoradionecrosis of the jaws as a side effect of radiotherapy of head and neck tumour patients—A report of a thirty year retrospective review. Int J Oral Maxillofac Surg 2003;32:289–295.

404. Terrell JE, Welsh DE, Bradford CR, et al. Pain, quality of life, and spinal accessory nerve status after neck dissection. Laryngoscope 2000;110:620–626.

405. Chow HT, Teh LY. Sensory impairment after resection of the mandible: A case report of 10 cases. J Oral Maxillofac Surg 2000;58:629–635.

406. Rogers SN, Lowe D, McNally D, Brown JS, Vaughan ED. Health-related quality of life after maxillectomy: A comparison between prosthetic obturation and free flap. J Oral Maxillofac Surg 2003;61:174–181.

407. Gellrich NC, Schramm A, Böckmann R, Kugler J. Follow-up in patients with oral cancer. J Oral Maxillofac Surg 2002;60:380–386.

408. Terrell JE, Nanavati K, Esclamado RM, Bradford CR, Wolf GT. Health impact of head and neck cancer. Otolaryngol Head Neck Surg 1999;120:852–859.

409. Taylor JC, Terrell JE, Ronis DL, et al. Disability in patients with head and neck cancer. Arch Otolaryngol Head Neck Surg 2004;130:764–769.

410. Bjordal K, Ahlner-Elmqvist M, Hammerlid E, et al. A prospective study of quality of life in head and neck cancer patients. Part II: Longitudinal data. Laryngoscope 2001;111:1440–1452.

411. Hammerlid E, Silander E, Hörnestam L, Sullivan M. Health-related quality of life three years after diagnosis of head and neck cancer—A longitudinal study. Head Neck 2001;23:113–125.

412. Hammerlid E, Taft C. Health-related quality of life in long-term head and neck cancer survivors: A comparison with general population norms. Br J Cancer 2001;84:149–156.

413. Schubert MM. Oral manifestations of viral infections in immunocompromised patients. Curr Opin Dent 1991;1:384–397.

414. Jones AC, Freedman PD, Phelan JA, Baughman RA, Kerpel SM. Cytomegalovirus infections of the oral cavity. A report of six cases and review of the literature. Oral Surg Oral Med Oral Pathol 1993;75:76–85.

415. Kuhl S, Walter C, Acham S, Pfeffer R, Lambrecht JT. Bisphosphonate-related osteonecrosis of the jaws—A review. Oral Oncol 2012;48:938–947.

416. Otto S, Schreyer C, Hafner S, et al. Bisphosphonate-related osteonecrosis of the jaws—Characteristics, risk factors, clinical features, localization and impact on oncological treatment. J Craniomaxillofac Surg 2012;40:303–309.

417. Miksad RA, Lai KC, Dodson TB, et al. Quality of life implications of bisphosphonate-associated osteonecrosis of the jaw. Oncologist 2011;16:121–132.

418. Zadik Y, Benoliel R, Fleissig Y, Casap N. Painful trigeminal neuropathy induced by oral bisphosphonate-related osteonecrosis of the jaw: A new etiology for the numb-chin syndrome. Quintessence Int 2012;43:97–104.

419. Kuten-Shorrer M, Woo SB, Treister NS. Oral graft-versus-host disease. Dent Clin North Am 2014;58:351–368.

420. Bowen JM, Elad S, Hutchins RD, Lalla RV. Methodology for the MASCC/ISOO mucositis clinical practice guidelines update. Support Care Cancer 2013;21:303–308.

421. Elad S, Bowen J, Zadik Y, Lalla RV. Development of the MASCC/ISOO clinical practice guidelines for mucositis: Considerations underlying the process. Support Care Cancer 2013;21:309–312.

422. Jensen SB, Jarvis V, Zadik Y, et al. Systematic review of miscellaneous agents for the management of oral mucositis in cancer patients. Support Care Cancer 2013;21:3223–3232.

423. Lalla RV, Bowen J, Barasch A, et al. MASCC/ISOO clinical practice guidelines for the management of mucositis secondary to cancer therapy. Cancer 2014;120:1453–1461.

424. McGuire DB, Fulton JS, Park J, et al. Systematic review of basic oral care for the management of oral mucositis in cancer patients. Support Care Cancer 2013;21:3165–3177.

425. Migliorati C, Hewson I, Lalla RV, et al. Systematic review of laser and other light therapy for the management of oral mucositis in cancer patients. Support Care Cancer 2013;21:333–341.

426. Peterson DE, Ohrn K, Bowen J, et al. Systematic review of oral cryotherapy for management of oral mucositis caused by cancer therapy. Support Care Cancer 2013;21:327–332.

427. Raber-Durlacher JE, von Bültzingslöwen I, Logan RM, et al. Systematic review of cytokines and growth factors for the management of oral mucositis in cancer patients. Support Care Cancer 2013;21:343–355.

428. Saunders DP, Epstein JB, Elad S, et al. Systematic review of antimicrobials, mucosal coating agents, anesthetics, and analgesics for the management of oral mucositis in cancer patients. Support Care Cancer 2013;21:3191–3207.

429. Yarom N, Ariyawardana A, Hovan A, et al. Systematic review of natural agents for the management of oral mucositis in cancer patients. Support Care Cancer 2013;21:3209–3221.

430. Nicolatou-Galitis O, Sarri T, Bowen J, et al. Systematic review of anti-inflammatory agents for the management of oral mucositis in cancer patients. Support Care Cancer 2013;21:3179–3189.

431. Nicolatou-Galitis O, Sarri T, Bowen J, et al. Systematic review of amifostine for the management of oral mucositis in cancer patients. Support Care Cancer 2013;21:357–364.

432. Borowski B, Benhamou E, Pico JL, Laplanche A, Margainaud JP, Hayat M. Prevention of oral mucositis in patients treated with high-dose chemotherapy and bone marrow transplantation: A randomised controlled trial comparing two protocols of dental care. Eur J Cancer B Oral Oncol 1994;30B:93–97.

433. Elad S, Cohen G, Zylber-Katz E, et al. Systemic absorption of lidocaine after topical application for the treatment of oral mucositis in bone marrow transplantation patients. J Oral Pathol Med 1999;28:170–172.

434. Epstein JB, Epstein JD, Epstein MS, Oien H, Truelove EL. Oral doxepin rinse: The analgesic effect and duration of pain reduction in patients with oral mucositis due to cancer therapy. Anesth Analg 2006;103:465–470.

435. Cerchietti LC, Navigante AH, Bonomi MR, et al. Effect of topical morphine for mucositis-associated pain following concomitant chemoradiotherapy for head and neck carcinoma. Cancer 2002;95:2230–2236.

436. Epstein JB, Wong FL. The efficacy of sucralfate suspension in the prevention of oral mucositis due to radiation therapy. Int J Radiat Oncol Biol Phys 1994;28:693–698.

437. Lalla RV. The MASCC/ISOO mucositis guidelines update: Introduction to the first set of articles. Support Care Cancer 2013;21:301–302.

438. Ripamonti C, Dickerson ED. Strategies for the treatment of cancer pain in the new millennium. Drugs 2001;61:955–977.

439. Zech DF, Grond S, Lynch J, Hertel D, Lehmann KA. Validation of World Health Organization guidelines for cancer pain relief: A 10-year prospective study. Pain 1995;63:65–76.

440. Larue F, Colleau SM, Brasseur L, Cleeland CS. Multicentre study of cancer pain and its treatment in France. BMJ 1995;310:1034–1037.

441. Eisenberg E, Berkey CS, Carr DB, Mosteller F, Chalmers TC. Efficacy and safety of nonsteroidal antiinflammatory drugs for cancer pain: A meta-analysis. J Clin Oncol 1994;12:2756–2765.

442. McNicol E, Strassels S, Goudas L, Lau J, Carr D. Nonsteroidal anti-inflammatory drugs, alone or combined with opioids, for cancer pain: A systematic review. J Clin Oncol 2004;22:1975–1992.

443. Benedetti C, Brock C, Cleeland C, et al. NCCN practice guidelines for cancer pain. Oncology (Williston Park) 2000;14(11):135–150.

444. Eisenberg E, Marinangeli F, Birkhahn J, Paladini A, Varrassi G. Time to Modify the WHO analgesic Ladder? Pain: Clin Updates 2005;13:1–4.

445. Sloan PA, Moulin DE, Hays H. A clinical evaluation of transdermal therapeutic system fentanyl for the treatment of cancer pain. J Pain Symptom Manage 1998;16:102–111.

446. Mystakidou K, Befon S, Tsilika E, Dardoufas K, Georgaki S, Vlahos L. Use of TTS fentanyl as a single opioid for cancer pain relief: A safety and efficacy clinical trial in patients naive to mild or strong opioids. Oncology 2002;62:9–16.

447. Menahem S, Shvartzman P. High-dose fentanyl patch for cancer pain. J Am Board Fam Pract 2004;17:388–390.

448. Coluzzi PH, Schwartzberg L, Conroy JD, et al. Breakthrough cancer pain: A randomized trial comparing oral transmucosal fentanyl citrate (OTFC) and morphine sulfate immediate release (MSIR). Pain 2001;91:123–130.

449. Lucas LK, Lipman AG. Recent advances in pharmacotherapy for cancer pain management. Cancer Pract 2002;10(suppl 1):S14–S20.

450. Payne R, Coluzzi P, Hart L, et al. Long-term safety of oral transmucosal fentanyl citrate for breakthrough cancer pain. J Pain Symptom Manage 2001;22(1):575–583.

451. Menzies K, Murray J, Wilcock A. Audit of cancer pain management in a cancer centre. Int J Palliat Nurs 2000;6:443–447.

452. Drake R, Longworth J, Collins JJ. Opioid rotation in children with cancer. J Palliat Med 2004;7:419–422.

453. Enting RH, Oldenmenger WH, van der Rijt CC, et al. A prospective study evaluating the response of patients with unrelieved cancer pain to parenteral opioids. Cancer 2002;94:3049–3056.

454. Devulder J, Lambert J, Naeyaert JM. Gabapentin for pain control in cancer patients' wound dressing care. J Pain Symptom Manage 2001;22:622–626.

455. Magill L. The use of music therapy to address the suffering in advanced cancer pain. J Palliat Care 2001;17:167–172.

456. Pan CX, Morrison RS, Ness J, Fugh-Berman A, Leipzig RM. Complementary and alternative medicine in the management of pain, dyspnea, and nausea and vomiting near the end of life. A systematic review. J Pain Symptom Manage 2000;20:374–387.

457. Syrjala KL, Donaldson GW, Davis MW, Kippes ME, Carr JE. Relaxation and imagery and cognitive-behavioral training reduce pain during cancer treatment: A controlled clinical trial. Pain 1995;63:189–198.

458. Berger JR, Stein N, Pall L. Headache and human immunodeficiency virus infection: A case control study. Eur Neurol 1996;36:229–233.

459. Norval DA. Symptoms and sites of pain experienced by AIDS patients. S Afr Med J 2004;94:450–454.

460. Lipton RB, Feraru ER, Weiss G, et al. Headache in HIV-1-related disorders. Headache 1991;31:518–522.

461. Brew BJ, Miller J. Human immunodeficiency virus-related headache. Neurology 1993;43:1098–1100.

462. Mirsattari SM, Power C, Nath A. Primary headaches in HIV-infected patients. Headache 1999;39:3–10.

463. Evers S, Wibbeke B, Reichelt D, Suhr B, Brilla R, Husstedt I. The impact of HIV infection on primary headache. Unexpected findings from retrospective, cross-sectional, and prospective analyses. Pain 2000;85:191–200.

464. Fiorentino PM, Piancino MG, Debernardi C, Attard N. Temporomandibular joint disorders during HIV infection: A case report. J Orofac Pain 2009;23:174–176.

465. Goldstein J. Headache and acquired immunodeficiency syndrome. Neurol Clin 1990;8:947–960.

466. Graham CB 3rd, Wippold FJ 3rd. Headache in the HIV patient: A review with special attention to the role of imaging. Cephalalgia 2001;21:169–174.

467. Dunfee R, Thomas ER, Gorry PR, Wang J, Ancuta P, Gabuzda D. Mechanisms of HIV-1 neurotropism. Curr HIV Res 2006;4:267–278.

468. Power C, Johnson RT. Neuroimmune and neurovirological aspects of human immunodeficiency virus infection. Adv Virus Res 2001;56:389–433.

469. Berretta M, Zanet E, Di Benedetto F, et al. Unusual presentation of metastatic hepatocellular carcinoma in an HIV/HCV coinfected patient: Case report and review of the literature. Tumori 2008;94:589–591.

470. Holloway RG, Kieburtz KD. Headache and the human immunodeficiency virus type 1 infection. Headache 1995;35:245–255.

471. Rinaldi R, Manfredi R, Azzimondi G, et al. Recurrent 'migrainelike' episodes in patients with HIV disease. Headache 1997;37:443–448.

472. Berger JR, Nath A. A careful neurologic examination should precede neuroimaging studies in HIV-infected patients with headache. AJNR Am J Neuroradiol 2000;21:441–442.

473. Gifford AL, Hecht FM. Evaluating HIV-infected patients with headache: Who needs computed tomography? Headache 2001;41:441–448.

474. Gillespie GM, Mariño R. Oral manifestations of HIV infection: A Panamerican perspective. J Oral Pathol Med 1993;22:2–7.

475. Patton LL, Phelan JA, Ramos-Gomez FJ, Nittayananta W, Shiboski CH, Mbuguye TL. Prevalence and classification of HIV-associated oral lesions. Oral Dis 2002;8(suppl 2):98–109.

476. Nittayananta W, Talungchit S, Jaruratanasirikul S, et al. Effects of long-term use of HAART on oral health status of HIV-infected subjects. J Oral Pathol Med 2010;39:397–406.

477. Kerr AR, Ship JA. Management strategies for HIV-associated aphthous stomatitis. Am J Clin Dermatol 2003;4:669–680.

478. Barr CE. Periodontal problems related to HIV-1 infection. Adv Dent Res 1995;9:147–151.

479. Barasch A, Gordon S, Geist RY, Geist JR. Necrotizing stomatitis: Report of 3 *Pseudomonas aeruginosa*-positive patients. Oral Surg Oral Med Oral Pathol Oral Radiol Endod 2003;96:136–140.

480. Milam SB, Rees TD, Leiman HI. An unusual cause of bilateral mental neuropathy in an AIDS patient. Report of a case. J Periodontol 1986;57:753–755.

481. Schiødt M. Less common oral lesions associated with HIV infection: Prevalence and classification. Oral Dis 1997;3(suppl 1):S208–S213.

482. Durham TM, Hodges ED, Swindels S, Green JG. Facial nerve paralysis related to HIV disease. Case report and dental considerations. Oral Surg Oral Med Oral Pathol 1993;75:37–40.

483. Belec L, Georges AJ, Bouree P, et al. Peripheral facial nerve palsy related to HIV infection: Relationship with the immunological status and the HIV staging in Central Africa. Cent Afr J Med 1991;37(3):88–93.

484. Penfold J, Clark AJ. Pain syndromes in HIV infection. Can J Anaesth 1992;39:724–730.

485. Ackerman Z, Zeltser R, Maayan S. AIDS and oropharyngeal candidiasis. Isr J Dent Sci 1989;2:162–166.

486. Denning DW. The neurological features of acute HIV infection. Biomed Pharmacother 1988;42:11–14.

487. Moyle GJ, Bouza E, Antunes F, et al. Zidovudine monotherapy versus zidovudine plus zalcitabine combination therapy in HIV-positive persons with CD4 cell counts 300–500 cells/mm³: A double-blind controlled trial. The M50003 Study Group Coordinating and Writing Committee. Antivir Ther 1997;2:229–236.

488. Kilbourne AM, Justice AC, Rabeneck L, Rodriguez-Barradas M, Weissman S. General medical and psychiatric comorbidity among HIV-infected veterans in the post-HAART era. J Clin Epidemiol 2001;54(1, suppl):S22–S28.

489. Nieuwkerk PT, Gisolf EH, Colebunders R, Wu AW, Danner SA, Sprangers MA. Quality of life in asymptomatic- and symptomatic HIV infected patients in a trial of ritonavir/saquinavir therapy. The Prometheus Study Group. AIDS 2000;14:181–187.

490. Elad S, Galili D, Garfunkel AA, Or R. Thalidomide-induced perioral neuropathy. Oral Surg Oral Med Oral Pathol Oral Radiol Endod 1997;84:362–364.

491. Chopra KF, Evans T, Severson J, Tyring SK. Acute varicella zoster with postherpetic hyperhidrosis as the initial presentation of HIV infection. J Am Acad Dermatol 1999;41:119–121.

492. Paterson DL, Georghiou PR, Allworth AM, Kemp RJ. Thalidomide as treatment of refractory aphthous ulceration related to human immunodeficiency virus infection. Clin Infect Dis 1995;20:250–254.

493. Brix Finnerup N, Hein Sindrup S, Staehelin Jensen T. Management of painful neuropathies. Handb Clin Neurol 2013;115:279–290.

494. Katz N. Neuropathic pain in cancer and AIDS. Clin J Pain 2000;16(suppl 2):S41–S48.

495. Gebo KA, Kalyani R, Moore RD, Polydefkis MJ. The incidence of, risk factors for, and sequelae of herpes zoster among HIV patients in the highly active antiretroviral therapy era. J Acquir Immune Defic Syndr 2005;40:169–174.

496. Bremell D, Säll C, Gisslén M, Hagberg L. Lyme neuroborreliosis in HIV-1 positive men successfully treated with oral doxycycline: A case series and literature review. J Med Case Rep 2011;5:465.

497. Tuttolomondo A, Pecoraro R, Simonetta I, Miceli S, Pinto A, Licata G. Anderson-Fabry disease: A multiorgan disease. Curr Pharm Des 2013;19:5974–5996.

498. Germain DP. Fabry disease. Orphanet J Rare Dis 2010;5:30.

499. Ries M, Ramaswami U, Parini R, et al. The early clinical phenotype of Fabry disease: A study on 35 European children and adolescents. Eur J Pediatr 2003;162:767–772.

500. Cable WJ, Kolodny EH, Adams RD. Fabry disease: Impaired autonomic function. Neurology 1982;32:498–502.

501. Shah SS, Kurago ZB. Unusual papillary lesion of the ventral tongue: Case report of solitary angiokeratoma of the oral cavity. N Y State Dent J 2013;79(3):46–49.

502. Baccaglini L, Schiffmann R, Brennan MT, Lancaster HE Jr, Kulkarni AB, Brahim JS. Oral and craniofacial findings in Fabry's disease: A report of 13 patients. Oral Surg Oral Med Oral Pathol Oral Radiol Endod 2001;92:415–419.

503. Ing EB, Woolf IZ, Younge BR, Bjornsson J, Leavitt JA. Systemic amyloidosis with temporal artery involvement mimicking temporal arteritis. Ophthalmic Surg Lasers 1997;28:328–331.

504. Elad S, Czerninski R, Fischman S, et al. Exceptional oral manifestations of amyloid light chain protein (AL) systemic amyloidosis. Amyloid 2010;17:27–31.

505. Aono J, Yamagata K, Yoshida H. Local amyloidosis in the hard palate: A case report. Oral Maxillofac Surg 2009;13:119–122.

506. Koloktronis A, Chatzigiannis I, Paloukidou N. Oral involvement in a case of AA amyloidosis. Oral Dis 2003;9:269–272.

507. Da Silva AN, Lake AE 3rd. Clinical aspects of medication overuse headaches. Headache 2014;54:211–217.

508. Srikiatkhachorn A, le Grand SM, Supornsilpchai W, Storer RJ. Pathophysiology of medication overuse headache—An update. Headache 2014;54:204–210.

509. Green AL, Gu P, De Felice M, Dodick D, Ossipov MH, Porreca F. Increased susceptibility to cortical spreading depression in an animal model of medication-overuse headache. Cephalalgia 2013;34:594–604.

510. Westergaard ML, Hansen EH, Glümer C, Olesen J, Jensen RH. Definitions of medication-overuse headache in population-based studies and their implications on prevalence estimates: A systematic review. Cephalalgia 2013;34:409–425.

511. Auriel E, Regev K, Korczyn AD. Nonsteroidal anti-inflammatory drugs exposure and the central nervous system. Handb Clin Neurol 2014;119:577–584.

512. Martelletti P, Jensen RH, Antal A, et al. Neuromodulation of chronic headaches: Position statement from the European Headache Federation. J Headache Pain 2013;14:86.

513. Bendtsen L, Munksgaard S, Tassorelli C, et al. Disability, anxiety and depression associated with medication-overuse headache can be considerably reduced by detoxification and prophylactic treatment. Results from a multicentre, multinational study (COMOESTAS project). Cephalalgia 2013;34:426–433.

514. Tolosa E. Periarteritic lesions of the carotid siphon with the clinical features of a carotid infraclinoidal aneurysm. J Neurol Neurosurg Psychiatry 1954;17:300–302.

515. Hunt WE, Meagher JN, Lefever HE, Zeman W. Painful opthalmoplegia. Its relation to indolent inflammation of the carvernous sinus. Neurology 1961;11:56–62.

516. Yeung MC, Kwong KL, Wong YC, Wong SN. Paediatric Tolosa-Hunt syndrome. J Paediatr Child Health 2004;40:410–413.

517. Pienczk-Reclawowicz K, Pilarska E, Lemka M, Konieczna S. Paediatric Tolosa-Hunt syndrome: The need for treatment guidelines and renewed criteria. Dev Med Child Neurol 2010;52:873–874.

518. Zhang X, Zhou Z, Steiner TJ, et al. Validation of ICHD-3 beta diagnostic criteria for 13.7 Tolosa-Hunt syndrome: Analysis of 77 cases of painful ophthalmoplegia. Cephalalgia 2014;34:624–632.

519. Gonzales GR. Pain in Tolosa-Hunt syndrome. J Pain Symptom Manage 1998;16:199–204.

520. Hannerz J. Pain characteristics of painful ophthalmoplegia (the Tolosa-Hunt syndrome). Cephalalgia 1985;5:103–106.

521. Bogduk N. Pain of cranial nerve and cervical nerve origin other than primary neuralgias. In: Olesen J, Goadsby PJ, Ramadan NM, Tfelt-Hansen P, Welch KMA (eds). The Headaches, ed 3. Philadelphia: Lippincott Williams & Wilkins, 2006:1043–1051.

522. Lin CC, Tsai JJ. Relationship between the number of involved cranial nerves and the percentage of lesions located in the cavernous sinus. Eur Neurol 2003;49:98–102.

523. Jain R, Sawhney S, Koul RL, Chand P. Tolosa-Hunt syndrome: MRI appearances. J Med Imaging Radiat Oncol 2008;52:447–451.

524. Schuknecht B, Sturm V, Huisman TA, Landau K. Tolosa-Hunt syndrome: MR imaging features in 15 patients with 20 episodes of painful ophthalmoplegia. Eur J Radiol 2009;69:445–453.

525. La Mantia L, Curone M, Rapoport AM, Bussone G. Tolosa-Hunt syndrome: Critical literature review based on IHS 2004 criteria. Cephalalgia 2006;26:772–781.

526. Hung CH, Chang KH, Chu CC, et al. Painful ophthalmoplegia with normal cranial imaging. BMC Neurol 2014;14:7.

527. Hung CH, Chang KH, Wu YM, et al. A comparison of benign and inflammatory manifestations of Tolosa-Hunt syndrome. Cephalalgia 2013;33:842–852.

528. Hunt WE, Brightman RP. The Tolosa-Hunt syndrome: A problem in differential diagnosis. Acta Neurochir Suppl (Wien) 1988;42:248–252.

529. Cerisola A, González G, Scavone C. Tolosa-Hunt syndrome preceded by facial palsy in a child. Pediatr Neurol 2011;44:61–64.

530. Nieri A, Bazan R, Almeida L, et al. Bilateral painful idiopathic ophthalmoplegia: A case report. Headache 2007;47:848–851.

531. Gladstone JP, Dodick DW. Painful ophthalmoplegia: Overview with a focus on Tolosa-Hunt syndrome. Curr Pain Headache Rep 2004;8:321–329.

532. La Mantia L, Erbetta A, Bussone G. Painful ophthalmoplegia: An unresolved clinical problem. Neurol Sci 2005;26(2, suppl):S79–S82.

533. Navi BB, Safdieh JE. Recurrent, alternating Tolosa-Hunt syndrome. Neurologist 2010;16:54–55.

534. O'Connor G, Hutchinson M. Tolosa-Hunt syndrome responsive to infliximab therapy. J Neurol 2009;256:660–661.

535. Vincent MB. Cervicogenic headache: The neck is a generator: Con. Headache 2010;50:706–709.

536. Tobin J, Flitman S. Occipital nerve blocks: When and what to inject? Headache 2009;49:1521–1533.

537. Racicki S, Gerwin S, Diclaudio S, Reinmann S, Donaldson M. Conservative physical therapy management for the treatment of cervicogenic headache: A systematic review. J Man Manip Ther 2013;21:113–124.

538. Chaibi A, Russell MB. Manual therapies for cervicogenic headache: A systematic review. J Headache Pain 2012;13:351–359.

539. Kay TM, Gross A, Goldsmith CH, et al. Exercises for mechanical neck disorders. Cochrane Database Syst Rev 2012;8.

540. Kroeling P, Gross A, Graham N, et al. Electrotherapy for neck pain. Cochrane Database Syst Rev 2013;8.

541. Linde M, Hagen K, Stovner LJ. Botulinum toxin treatment of secondary headaches and cranial neuralgias: A review of evidence. Acta Neurol Scand Suppl 2011;(191):50–55.

542. Benoliel R, Eliav E, Elishoov H, Sharav Y. Diagnosis and treatment of persistent pain after trauma to the head and neck. J Oral Maxillofac Surg 1994;52:1138–1147.

543. Evans RW. Post-traumatic headaches. Neurol Clin 2004;22:237–249.

544. Lew HL, Lin PH, Fuh JL, Wang SJ, Clark DJ, Walker WC. Characteristics and treatment of headache after traumatic brain injury: A focused review. Am J Phys Med Rehabil 2006;85:619–627.

545. Walker WC, Seel RT, Curtiss G, Warden DL. Headache after moderate and severe traumatic brain injury: A longitudinal analysis. Arch Phys Med Rehabil 2005;86:1793–1800.

546. Benoliel R, Birenboim R, Regev E, Eliav E. Neurosensory changes in the infraorbital nerve following zygomatic fractures. Oral Surg Oral Med Oral Pathol Oral Radiol Endod 2005;99:657–665.

547. Nicholson K, Martelli MF. The problem of pain. J Head Trauma Rehabil 2004;19:2–9.

548. D'Onofrio F, Russo A, Conte F, Casucci G, Tessitore A, Tedeschi G. Post-traumatic headaches: An epidemiological overview. Neurol Sci 2014;35(1, suppl):203–206.

549. Solomon S. Chronic post-traumatic neck and head pain. Headache 2005;45:53–67.

550. Edna TH, Cappelen J. Late post-concussional symptoms in traumatic head injury. An analysis of frequency and risk factors. Acta Neurochir (Wien) 1987;86:12–17.

551. Hillier SL, Sharpe MH, Metzer J. Outcomes 5 years post-traumatic brain injury (with further reference to neurophysical impairment and disability). Brain Inj 1997;11:661–675.

552. Nestvold K, Lundar T, Mowinckel P, Stavem K. Predictors of headache 22 years after hospitalization for head injury. Acta Neurol Scand 2005;112:13–18.

553. Young W, Packard RC, Ramadan N. Headaches associated with head trauma. In: Silberstein S, Lipton RB, Dalesio DJ (eds). Wolf's Headache and Other Head Pain, ed 7. New York: Oxford University, 2001:325–348.

554. Baandrup L, Jensen R. Chronic post-traumatic headache—A clinical analysis in relation to the International Headache Classification 2nd edition. Cephalalgia 2005;25:132–138.

555. Lane JC, Arciniegas DB. Post-traumatic headache. Curr Treat Options Neurol 2002;4:89–104.

556. Bettucci D, Aguggia M, Bolamperti L, Riccio A, Mutani R. Chronic post-traumatic headache associated with minor cranial trauma: A description of cephalalgic patterns. Ital J Neurol Sci 1998;19:20–24.

557. Haas DC. Chronic post-traumatic headaches classified and compared with natural headaches. Cephalalgia 1996;16:486–493.

558. Russo A, D'Onofrio F, Conte F, Petretta V, Tedeschi G, Tessitore A. Post-traumatic headaches: A clinical overview. Neurol Sci 2014;35(1, suppl):153–156.

559. De Leeuw R, Bertoli E, Schmidt JE, Carlson CR. Prevalence of traumatic stressors in patients with temporomandibular disorders. J Oral Maxillofac Surg 2005;63:42–50.

560. De Leeuw R, Bertoli E, Schmidt JE, Carlson CR. Prevalence of post-traumatic stress disorder symptoms in orofacial pain patients. Oral Surg Oral Med Oral Pathol Oral Radiol Endod 2005;99:558–568.

561. Maroon JC, Lepere DB, Blaylock RL, Bost JW. Post-concussion syndrome: A review of pathophysiology and potential nonpharmacological approaches to treatment. Phys Sportsmed 2012;40(4):73–87.

562. Stulemeijer M, van der Werf S, Bleijenberg G, Biert J, Brauer J, Vos PE. Recovery from mild traumatic brain injury: A focus on fatigue. J Neurol 2006;253:1041–1047.

563. Branca B. Neuropsychologic aspects of post-traumatic headache and chronic daily headache. Curr Pain Headache Rep 2006;10:54–66.

564. Tatrow K, Blanchard EB, Hickling EJ, Silverman DJ. Posttraumatic headache: Biopsychosocial comparisons with multiple control groups. Headache 2003;43:755–766.

565. Sherman JJ, Carlson CR, Wilson JF, Okeson JP, McCubbin JA. Post-traumatic stress disorder among patients with orofacial pain. J Orofac Pain 2005;19:309–317.

566. Aghabeigi B, Feinmann C, Harris M. Prevalence of post-traumatic stress disorder in patients with chronic idiopathic facial pain. Br J Oral Maxillofac Surg 1992;30:360–364.

567. Glynn SM, Asarnow JR, Asarnow R, et al. The development of acute post-traumatic stress disorder after orofacial injury: A prospective study in a large urban hospital. J Oral Maxillofac Surg 2003;61:785–792.

568. Mooney G, Speed J, Sheppard S. Factors related to recovery after mild traumatic brain injury. Brain Inj 2005;19:975–987.

569. Burgess JA, Dworkin SF. Litigation and post-traumatic TMD: How patients report treatment outcome. J Am Dent Assoc 1993;124(6):105–110.

570. Gurr B, Coetzer BR. The effectiveness of cognitive-behavioural therapy for post-traumatic headaches. Brain Inj 2005;19:481–491.

571. Di Stefano G, Radanov BP. Course of attention and memory after common whiplash: A two-years prospective study with age, education and gender pair-matched patients. Acta Neurol Scand 1995;91:346–352.

572. Cteé P, Cassidy JD, Carroll L. Is a lifetime history of neck injury in a traffic collision associated with prevalent neck pain, headache and depressive symptomatology? Accid Anal Prev 2000;32:151–159.

573. Spitzer WO, Skovron ML, Salmi LR, et al. Scientific monograph of the Quebec Task Force on whiplash-associated disorders: Redefining "whiplash" and its management. Spine 1995;20(8, suppl):S1–S73.

574. Barnsley L, Lord S, Bogduk N. Whiplash injury. Pain 1994;58:283–307.

575. Freeman MD, Croft AC, Rossignol AM, Weaver DS, Reiser M. A review and methodologic critique of the literature refuting whiplash syndrome. Spine 1999;24:86–96.

576. Walton DM, Macdermid JC, Giorgianni AA, Mascarenhas JC, West SC, Zammit CA. Risk factors for persistent problems following acute whiplash injury: Update of a systematic review and meta-analysis. J Orthop Sports Phys Ther 2013;43(2):31–43.

577. Cassidy JD, Carroll LJ, Côté P, Lemstra M, Berglund A, Nygren A. Effect of eliminating compensation for pain and suffering on the outcome of insurance claims for whiplash injury. N Engl J Med 2000;342:1179–1186.

578. Goadsby PJ. Raeder's syndrome [corrected]: Paratrigeminal paralysis of the oculopupillary sympathetic system. J Neurol Neurosurg Psychiatry 2002;72:297–299.

579. Tatsui CE, Prevedello DM, Koerbel A, Cordeiro JG, Ditzel LF, Araujo JC. Raeder's syndrome after embolization of a giant intracavernous carotid artery aneurysm: Pathophysiological considerations. Arq Neuropsiquiatr 2005;63:676–680.

Pharmacotherapy for Acute Orofacial Pain

15

Yair Sharav, DMD, MS
Rafael Benoliel, BDS

Prescription drugs are a mainstay of acute and chronic pain management, and one of the most widely used drug classes in the United States remains the opioids.[1] One study reported on the characteristics of 79.5 million prescriptions for opioid analgesics, which made up 39% of the estimated 201.9 million opioid prescriptions dispensed in the United States in 2009.[2] The main prescribers were primary care physicians (28.8%), followed by internists (14.6%), dentists (8.0%), and orthopedic surgeons (7.7%). Of importance is the finding that 56.4% (44.8 million) of opioid prescriptions were dispensed to patients who had already filled another opioid prescription within the previous month. Acetaminophen with oxycodone was the second most sold prescription drug in 2013 at 28.7 million, and oxycodone ranked 43rd at 3.4 million units sold.[3] Celecoxib, a selective nonsteroidal anti-inflammatory drug (NSAID) used for inflammation and pain associated with osteoarthritis, seems to be the highest-selling prescription NSAID, ranking 46th in 2013 at nearly 3 million units sold. NSAIDs are associated with multiple adverse effects, some severe. For example, current users of NSAIDs are estimated to be at a two to four times higher risk for acute renal failure.[4–6] The addiction potential of opioids is a serious problem, and oxycodone remains the most abused prescription drug in the United States.[7,8] These figures offer an insight into the scope of drug use for pain and problems associated with long-term use of some of these drugs.

This chapter presents a strategy for providing pharmacotherapy directed at relieving acute orofacial pain with maximum efficacy and minimal side effects. The spectrum of analgesic drug efficacy is rather narrow; some may be somewhat better than others, but mostly it will be the patient's profile (eg, general health, other drugs taken, pregnancy, age) and, hence, possible side effects that will dictate which drug to use. As stressed throughout this chapter, clinicians should think patient first and then drug. Ideally, an analgesic drug provides significant relief across all pain severities, has minimal side effects, has few drug interactions, and is convenient to administer (eg, single daily oral dose, pleasant tasting, and rapid absorption). However, ideal drugs do not exist, and when administering an analgesic, consideration should be given to pain severity, the patient's medical history, the patient's susceptibility to the various side effects (eg, gastrointestinal, cardiac, renal), and complex pharmacologic interactions with other medications that the patient may be taking.[9,10] One should be aware that patients may differ genetically in their response to analgesics,[11–13] so sex-specific benefits or adverse effects should be considered.[14,15] Orofacial pain practitioners need to thoroughly understand the different classes of analgesics and their mechanisms of actions and should also appreciate that drug actions and interactions change with a patient's age and medical status. This chapter reviews the clinical pharmacology of drugs typically used in the treatment of acute orofacial pain. First, the strategy of pharmacotherapy is introduced. The next sections describe the efficacy and side effects of recommended drugs and explain mechanisms of action. Finally, adverse effects are discussed under various conditions (eg, gastrointestinal and cardiovascular risk, asthma, pregnancy).

The pathogenesis of acute and chronic pain involves peripheral and central mechanisms of sensitization that are associated with plasticity in primary sensory and dorsal horn neurons. The local inflammatory response leads to heightened sensitivity and activity of local nociceptors and to distant effects at the level of the central nervous system (CNS).[16] A mechanism-based strategy for pain control with analgesics should have at least three major aims:

1. Prevent sensitization of peripheral nociceptors
2. Interrupt the neuronal transmission of nociceptive signals
3. Attenuate the nociceptive message in the spinal cord and other parts of the CNS

Acute pain is usually activated by tissue damage and subsequent inflammatory processes, so the initial strategy to attain analgesia would normally involve the use of anti-inflammatory drugs. However, a reduction in the inflammatory response may not be sufficient to obtain adequate analgesia. NSAIDs, including selective cyclooxygenase (COX-2) inhibitors, combine anti-inflammatory effects with analgesic actions on peripheral and central neural targets.

Pharmacotherapy Strategy for Acute Orofacial Pain

As stated, the aim of drug therapy for acute orofacial pain is to relieve pain at maximum efficacy *with minimal side effects*. In other words: think patient first, then drug. Therefore, the patient's medical history is the primary consideration when choosing an analgesic.

When efficacy, side effects, and cost are balanced, the evidence supports an oral analgesic treatment schedule that begins with acetaminophen (paracetamol) 500 to 1,000 mg for mild to moderate orofacial pain to be continued with 500 mg every 6 hours. Acetaminophen is, on average, a weaker analgesic than NSAIDs or COX-2 selective inhibitors but is often preferred because of its better tolerance.[17] Ibuprofen 400 mg four times a day or naproxen sodium 550 mg twice a day are efficient alternatives for short-term therapy. Ibuprofen in doses of 400 mg every 6 hours is the safest conventional, nonselective NSAID in terms of gastrointestinal side effects. Higher doses may offer somewhat greater analgesia but with more adverse effects. Other NSAIDs have failed to demonstrate consistently greater efficacy or safety than ibuprofen.[18] Recently, the use of 200 mg of ibuprofen together with 500 mg of acetaminophen has been recommended; the combination provides a very robust analgesic with minimal side effects that may be repeated every 4 to 6 hours.[19] Keeping ibuprofen at a low dose is meaningful as low-dose ibuprofen is least likely to increase cardiovascular risk, which was seen only with higher doses.[20] Naproxen has emerged as the safest NSAID in most studies when cardiovascular risks are considered.[10,21–24] Naproxen may be combined with a proton pump inhibitor as needed,[9,25] thereby providing excellent analgesia and gastrointestinal as well as cardiovascular safety. COX-2 inhibitors provide analgesia equal to that of traditional NSAIDs for many painful conditions but lack a better safety profile in acute pain treatment and are significantly more expensive.[18] However, celecoxib or etoricoxib should be considered in patients with a history of asthma or urticaria.[26–29] Cardiovascular risks need to be taken into account, bearing in mind that etoricoxib cannot be prescribed in the United States. For

Table 15-1	Pharmacotherapeutic strategy for the management of acute orofacial pain					
Pain intensity	Option	Healthy patient	Patient with GI limitations	Patient with CV limitations	Patient on anticoagulants	Patient with asthma, urticaria, or angioedema
Mild to moderate	1	Acetaminophen 500 mg	Acetaminophen 500 mg	Acetaminophen 500 mg	Acetaminophen 500 mg	COX-2 inhibitor*
	2	Ibuprofen 400 mg	COX-2 inhibitor	Naproxen sodium 500 mg	COX-2 inhibitor	Acetaminophen 500 mg[†]
	3	Naproxen sodium 550 mg	Naproxen/ ibuprofen with proton pump inhibitor			
Moderate to severe	1	Ibuprofen 400 to 600 mg	Oxycodone 5 mg; acetaminophen 325 mg	Oxycodone 5 mg; acetaminophen 325 mg	Oxycodone 5 mg; acetaminophen 325 mg	COX-2 inhibitor*
	2	Acetaminophen 500 mg/ ibuprofen 200 mg	Oxycodone 5 mg; acetaminophen 325 mg	Oxycodone 5 mg; acetaminophen 325 mg	Oxycodone 5 mg; acetaminophen 325 mg	COX-2 inhibitor*
	3	Oxycodone 5 mg; acetaminophen 325 mg	Dipryone 500 to 1,000 mg	Dipryone 500 to 1,000 mg	COX-2 inhibitor	Oxycodone 5 mg; acetaminophen 325 mg[†]

*There is a standard warning against use of COX-2 inhibitors in cases of asthma and urticaria. However, this warning could not be validated by several controlled studies that found rofecoxib, celecoxib, and etoricoxib safe in these circumstances.[28,33–38]
[†]Acetaminophen demonstrates cross-reactivity in aspirin-induced asthma but usually at doses higher than 500 mg.[33]
GI, gastrointestinal; CV, cardiovascular.

moderate to severe pain that does not respond to acetaminophen, and where ibuprofen or naproxen are contraindicated, the use of narcotics combined with acetaminophen is indicated. The combination of acetaminophen 325 mg plus oxycodone 5 mg every 4 to 6 hours or acetaminophen 650 mg plus oxycodone 10 mg every 8 to 10 hours gives good analgesia with minimal side effects.[30,31]

Sometimes patients prefer a certain analgesic because they think it works better for them, and unless the drug requested is contraindicated, the authors tend not to argue with patients' preferences. One should consider that males and females may differ in their response to NSAIDs and indeed females enjoy less analgesia with ibuprofen than do males.[14] Also, given the fact that patients may differ genetically in their response to analgesics, the patient may actually be right.[11–13] On the whole, the strategy described here is a good starting point when pain severity is the main lead. However, the patient's age, medical background, and habits (eg, smoking or alcohol consumption) as well as adverse drug interactions are foremost considerations to minimize side effects.[34] Table 15-1 provides guidance for the management of acute orofacial pain, which takes into consideration both pain severity and the patient's medical background. One should consider, however, that Table 15-1 does not take into consideration the frequently occurring situation that more than one medical limitation may persist in the same patient, posing an increased risk.[39] In these instances, the reader is advised to consult the relevant sections in this chapter. Table 15-2 summarizes the initial and maintenance doses and main medical contraindications for the common, single-formulation, non-opioid analgesics. Although the authors' aim is to equip the reader with the best pharmacotherapy tools for relieving acute orofacial

Table 15-2 Doses and medical considerations of common analgesics

Drug	Dose (mg)*	Maintenance dose (mg × dosages per day)	Medical considerations	Pregnancy† Category	Pregnancy† Comment	Effect on breastfeeding	Common side effects‡
Acetaminophen§	500 or 1,000	500 × 4 or 1,000 × 4	Renal insufficiency, dermatologic, alcohol, hypothermia	B	Avoid frequent use in third trimester	Minimal	Rash, hypothermia
Ibuprofen	400	400 × 4	Renal insufficiency, AIA, CIU, GI, asthma	B and C	DA; third	Minimal	CSE, stomatitis
Naproxen sodium	275 to 550	275 × 3 or 550 × 2	Renal insufficiency, liver disease, GI, asthma	C	DA; third	Minimal	CSE, stomatitis
Naproxen	250 to 500	250 × 3 or 500 × 2	Renal insufficiency, liver disease, GI, asthma	C	DA; third	Minimal	CSE, stomatitis
Etodolac	200 or 400	200 × 3 or 400 × 3	CV, GI, neurologic, asthma	C	DA	Unclear	CSE, malaise, flatulence
Etodolac extended or modified release	400 to 1,000	Once daily	CV, GI, neurologic, asthma	C	DA	Unclear	CSE, malaise, flatulence
Indomethacin	25 to 50	25 × 3 or 50 × 3	CV, GI, asthma, AIA	C	DA; third	Minimal	CSE, fatigue, depression
Diclofenac‖	25 to 50	25 × 3 or 4; 50 × 2 or 3	CV, GI, asthma, AIA	C	DA; third	Unclear	CSE, flatulence
Diclofenac standard release	100	Once daily	CV, GI, asthma, AIA	C	DA; third	Unclear	CSE, flatulence
Celecoxib	400	200 × 2	CIU, sulfa, prothrombotic	C	CI	CI	CSE, pharyngitis
Etoricoxib	120	60 × 2 or 120 × 1	CIU, CV, GI, prothrombotic	NS	CI	CI	CSE, taste disturbance, flatulence, fatigue
Dipryone	500 or 1,000	500 × 4 or 1,000 × 4	Hematologic, G6PD, liver disease	NS		Unclear	Rash, GI agranulocytosis, anemia

* For moderate to severe pain.

† According to the US and Australian food and drug administrations and to UK product labeling. DA indicates that use in late pregnancy may induce premature closure of the ductus arteriosus, and *third* indicates that use in third trimester may delay birth.

‡ CSE indicates risk for the common side effects for all NSAIDs: edema, GI complaints (abdominal pain, diarrhea, constipation, dyspepsia, heartburn, nausea, vomiting), rashes or pruritus, tinnitus, dizziness, somnolence, headache, and increased liver function tests.

§ Contraindicated in first and second trimesters of pregnancy unless the potential benefit to the patient outweighs the potential risk to the fetus.

‖ Diclofenac is also available in 50-mg and 75-mg formulations with 200 µg misoprostol, but this formulation is contraindicated during pregnancy.

AIA, aspirin-induced asthma; alcohol, abusers of alcohol (> three drinks daily); CIU, chronic idiopathic urticaria; CI, contraindicated; CV, cardiovascular; G6PD, glucose-6-phosphate dehydrogenase deficiency; GI, gastrointestinal; NS, not stated.

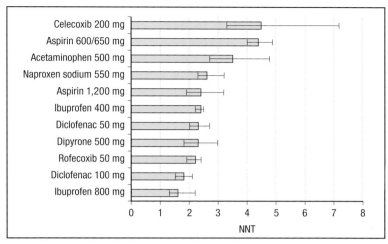

Fig 15-1 NNT for one patient to achieve at least 50% pain relief (95% CI) for non-opioid analgesics at usual recommended doses. (Data from Barden et al,[40–42] Collins et al,[43] and Mason et al.[44])

pain, this chapter does not by any means replace the need to also consult other comprehensive textbooks of pharmacology. Data are constantly accumulating, so it is important for clinicians to regularly review the evidence for risk-benefit ratios in individual drugs.

Commonly Used Analgesics for Acute Orofacial Pain

Efficacy of analgesics

The number needed to treat (NNT) represents the number of patients that would need to be treated to achieve one patient with at least 50% pain relief; the statistic describes the differences between active treatment and control and is a meaningful way to express the benefit of an active treatment over a control. Head-to-head comparisons of analgesic drugs are not common, so the NNT provides a useful way of comparing the relative efficacy of analgesics. The NNT can be used to help the clinician choose between two treatment options. If, for example, the NNT for drug A is lower than that for drug B, it suggests that it may be more effective and—all other things being equal—choosing A

rather than B would make sense. The ideal NNT would be 1, meaning that all the patients in the treatment group have improved but no patient in the control group has improved. In theory, the higher the NNT, the less effective the treatment, because more people need to receive the treatment to see a benefit in one person. However, the value of an NNT should be interpreted in light of its clinical connotation. Thus, an NNT of 2 to 5 would normally indicate an effective therapy for an analgesic for the treatment of acute pain. The relative efficacy of non-opioid analgesics is presented in Fig 15-1, and the relative efficacy of acetaminophen combined with opioids or tramadol is presented in Figs 15-2 and 15-3.

Acetaminophen (paracetamol)

Mode of action

Acetaminophen is generally considered to be a weak inhibitor of the synthesis of prostaglandins. Indeed, acetaminophen fails to inhibit the formation of prostaglandins in peripheral tissues and does not suppress the inflammation of rheumatoid arthritis. Acetaminophen depresses the nociceptive activity evoked in thalamic neurons by electrical stimulation of nociceptive afferents and presents evidence for a central analgesic effect that is independent of endogenous opioids.[48] COX-3, a splice vari-

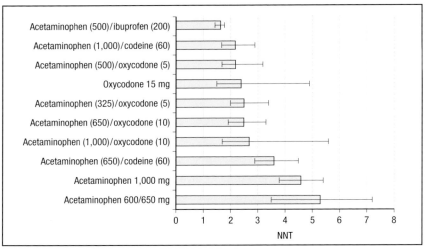

Fig 15-2 NNT for one patient to achieve at least 50% pain relief (95% CI) for acetaminophen and for acetaminophen combined with codeine or with oxycodone. (Data from Moore and Hersh,[19] Edwards et al,[30] and Weil et al.[45])

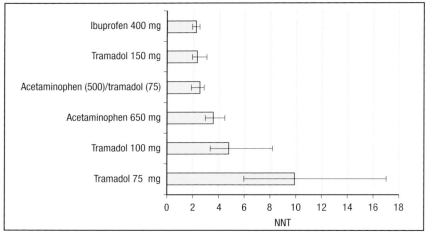

Fig 15-3 NNT for one patient to achieve at least 50% pain relief (95% CI) for acetaminophen, tramadol, and acetaminophen combined with tramadol compared with ibuprofen. (Data from Edwards et al,[30] Moore et al,[46] and Moore et al.[47])

ant of COX-1, has been suggested to be the target of acetaminophen action, but genomic and kinetic analysis indicates that this selective interaction is unlikely to be clinically relevant.[49] Considerable evidence suggests that the analgesic effect of acetaminophen is central and is due to activation of descending serotonergic pathways, but its primary site of action may still be inhibition of prostaglandin synthesis.[49] Evidence also suggests that the analgesic effect of acetaminophen is due to the indirect activation

of cannabinoid receptor type 1. In the brain and spinal cord, acetaminophen, after deacetylation to its primary amine (p-aminophenol), is conjugated with arachidonic acid to form N-arachidonoylphenolamine, a compound already known as an endogenous cannabinoid. This suggests that acetaminophen acts as a prodrug, the active one being a cannabinoid.[50,51]

Despite the similarities of acetaminophen to NSAIDs, the mode of action of acetaminophen has been uncertain; however, it is now generally accepted that it inhibits COX-1 and COX-2 through metabolism by the peroxidase function of these isoenzymes.[17] This results in inhibition of phenoxyl radical formation from a critical tyrosine residue essential for the activity of COX-1 and COX-2 and prostaglandin synthesis. Acetaminophen shows selectivity for inhibiting the synthesis of prostaglandins and related factors when low levels of arachidonic acid and peroxides are available, but conversely, it has little activity at substantial levels of arachidonic acid and peroxides. The result is that acetaminophen does not suppress the severe inflammation of rheumatoid arthritis and acute gout but does inhibit the lesser inflammation resulting from extraction of teeth.[17] Acetaminophen, NSAIDs, and selective COX-2 inhibitors all have central and peripheral effects. As is the case with the NSAIDs, including the selective COX-2 inhibitors, the analgesic effects of acetaminophen are reduced by inhibitors of many endogenous neurotransmitter systems, including serotonergic, opioid, and cannabinoid systems.[17]

Efficacy

The NNT over 4 to 6 hours after a single dose of acetaminophen 500 mg was 3.5 (confidence interval [CI], 2.7 to 4.8), and increasing doses up to 1,500 mg did not result in better NNTs in a systematic review of acetaminophen.[41] Adverse effects are generally mild and transient, and there are no statistically significant differences between acetaminophen 975/1,000 mg and placebo; similar ranges of efficacy were demonstrated with NNTs of 3.5 to 5.0 for 600 to 1,000 mg of acetaminophen.[46] Similarly, no differences were found in adverse effects between acetaminophen and placebo in a later Cochrane review.[45] Acetaminophen provided a statistically significant benefit over placebo after third-molar extraction for pain relief and pain intensity at 4 and 6 hours. Doses up to 1,000 mg and at 1,000 mg had statistically significant benefit over placebo with NNTs of 4 (CI, 3 to 4) and 3 (CI, 3 to 4), respectively, with an enhanced benefit for the higher dose ($P < .0001$). A qualitative review on head-to-head comparisons of acetaminophen and NSAIDs[52] found that of 15 dental studies, 8 showed that NSAIDs were superior to acetaminophen, 5 showed equal results, and 2 showed that acetaminophen was

superior to NSAIDs. NSAIDs therefore seem to be superior to acetaminophen in dental surgery in terms of pain scores and remedication. On the other hand, a crossover study of 36 patients who underwent surgical removal of bilateral third molars and acted as their own controls compared the effects of ibuprofen 600 mg four times per day with acetaminophen 1,000 mg four times per day; the investigators found no significant differences in pain scores or swelling between the two drugs.[53]

Acetaminophen is therefore a viable alternative to NSAIDs, especially because of the low incidence of adverse effects, and should be the preferred choice in high-risk patients[52] (see Table 15-1). For example, the sustained use of acetaminophen during oral anticoagulant therapy in itself does not provoke clinically relevant changes in international normalized ratios.[54] Furthermore, based on the data available to date, it still seems prudent to use NSAIDs only in those patients in whom there is good evidence of improved efficacy over acetaminophen.[55]

Clinical considerations

Initially, for mild to moderate pain, 500 to 1,000 mg of acetaminophen should be given followed by 500 mg orally every 4 hours, as needed, to a maximum of 4 g/day. (In June 2009, a joint advisory panel to the US Food and Drug Administration [FDA] cleared a preliminary recommendation reducing the maximum daily adult dose of acetaminophen products to less than 4,000 mg per day; however, a new maximum daily dose was not specified.) The hepatotoxicity of therapeutic doses of acetaminophen has prompted considerable debate. Much of the toxicity may result from overuse of combinations of acetaminophen with opioids (discussed later in this chapter), which are widely used, particularly in the United States.[56] The use of acetaminophen is contraindicated in persons who abuse alcohol (more than three alcoholic drinks per day). Moreover, the observation of elevated liver enzymes during high-dose therapy (4 g/day) is a significant concern in patients with liver disease.[57]

Common adverse effects include rash and hypothermia. On August, 1, 2013, the FDA issued a safety announcement stating that "Rarely, acetaminophen can cause serious, potentially fatal skin reactions, such as acute generalized exanthematous pustulosis (AGEP), Stevens-Johnson syndrome (SJS), and toxic epidermal necrolysis (TEN)."[58] Note that other drugs used to treat fever and pain (eg, NSAIDS, such as ibuprofen and naproxen) also carry a risk of serious skin reactions, which is already described in the warnings section of their drug labels. This information is not meant to alarm clinicians or patients, but because these rare but serious side effects can be fatal, clinicians and patients must be aware of the risks and understand how to react quickly to the initial symptoms of these conditions.

Acetaminophen is the analgesic of choice during pregnancy (pregnancy category B) or breastfeeding. Though it is excreted into breast milk, it is considered safe to breastfeeding neonates. Evidence suggests that the risk of asthma in later childhood might be increased with exposure to acetaminophen during pregnancy with an odds ratio (OR) of 1.21 (CI, 1.02 to 1.44).[59] The evidence was confirmed in a later study[60] that showed an adjusted incidence rate ratio of 1.35 (CI, 1.17 to 1.57) for exposure in any trimester of pregnancy. Frequent use of acetaminophen during the last trimester of pregnancy is contraindicated. The risk of preterm birth in women using acetaminophen during the third trimester of pregnancy was increased in mothers with preeclampsia (hazard ratio, 1.55; CI, 1.16 to 2.07) but not in women without preeclampsia (hazard ratio, 1.08; CI, 0.97 to 1.20). Tobacco smoking and coffee consumption did not modify the effect of acetaminophen in any consistent pattern. No association was found between acetaminophen use and risk of preterm complications, miscarriages, stillbirths, low birth weight, or small size for gestational age.[61] Exposure to acetaminophen for more than 4 weeks during pregnancy, especially during the first and second trimesters, may moderately increase the occurrence of cryptorchidism (hazard ratio, 1.33; CI, 1.00 to 1.77), a risk not associated with exposure to ibuprofen and acetylsalicylic acid.[62]

Conventional NSAIDs

The use of NSAIDs is advocated for the management of postoperative pain, and these drugs have been widely used for pain relief in dentistry. Prostaglandins represent one of the key chemicals involved in the sensitization of peripheral nociceptors, thereby contributing to the development of primary and subsequent secondary hyperalgesia. Prostaglandins are synthesized rather rapidly after tissue injury and appear in significant concentrations just 1 hour after trauma.[63] The prostaglandin E_2 (PGE_2) prostanoid is especially important in inflammatory pain, and levels of PGE_2 correlate with pain intensity levels after the extraction of impacted third molars.[64] The dental model for analgesic efficacy examines the effect of analgesics after surgical extraction of the third mandibular molar. This is a widely established model to induce postsurgical, inflammation-based, moderate to severe pain and a useful tool to examine the efficacy of analgesics.[65] This model is particularly relevant to the discussion of analgesic efficacy for acute orofacial pain, as there is evidence that NSAIDs may be more effective in dental surgery relative to, for example, orthopedic surgery.[52] Conventional NSAIDs typically inhibit prostaglandin production by both COX-1 and COX-2 enzyme systems (Fig 15-4; see later in this chapter). Even though significant advances in the understanding of COXs and prostaglandins and their involvement in pain production have led to the development of the specific COX-2 inhibitors, the nonselective NSAIDs have retained their position as analgesics of choice for the general population.[66] Important differences in adverse effects exist between different NSAIDs, in contrast to their similar beneficial effects.[66] The differences in side effects are most important in considering which NSAID to choose, such as the relative risks (RRs) of gastrointestinal ulceration compared with the potential increase in cardiovascular risk.[22] The evidence suggests that if one NSAID is unsatisfactory, then switching to another NSAID will not provide better analgesia. Likewise, doubling the therapeutic dose of an NSAID leads to only a small increase in effect, which may not be clinically relevant.[67] The dose-response curve saturates at high doses, and recommended dosages are close to providing a ceiling effect.[68] However, the incidence of adverse effects increases in an approximately linear fashion with the dose.[69] Thus, there is a ceiling effect on analgesic efficacy but not on adverse effects.

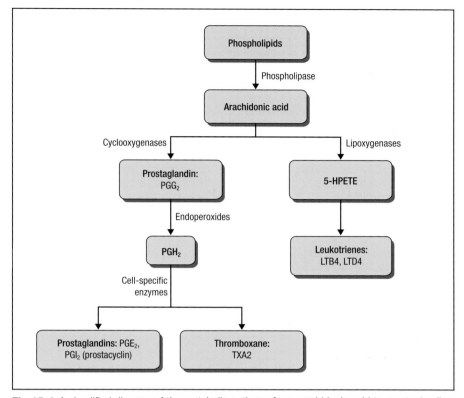

Fig 15-4 A simplified diagram of the metabolic pathway from arachidonic acid to prostaglandins, thromboxanes, and leukotrienes. The mechanisms of analgesia-associated adverse effects occur through the regulation of prostaglandin synthesis by anti-inflammatory drugs. Blocking the effect of COX-1 and COX-2 by aspirin or traditional NSAIDs inhibits the production of prostaglandins, in particular PGE_2, and causes analgesia. However, prostaglandins are needed for protection of the gastric mucosa and kidney blood perfusion, hence the deleterious effect on these organs as a possible side effect of NSAID administration. Blocking COX-1 activity also inhibits production of thromboxanes, which are needed for platelet aggregation and normal blood clotting. By blocking the COX pathway, more arachidonic acid 5-hydroperoxide (5-HPETE) is available for the lipoxygenase pathway, and more leukotrienes such as leukotriene B4 (LTB4) and LTD4 are produced. LTB4 induces neutrophil-dependent hyperalgesia; LTD4 is associated with sensitivity reactions. Selective inhibition of COX-2 minimally blocks the production of PGE_2 but selectively suppresses prostacyclin (prostaglandin $I_2[PGI_2]$) production (which has antithrombotic and antihypertensive effects) without affecting thromboxane A2 (TXA2) and could therefore predispose the patient (especially the elderly or those with other cardiovascular factors) to thromboembolic adverse effects and hypertension. Additionally, some leukotrienes increase gastric acid production that is unbalanced by the protective prostaglandins, leading to increased gastrointestinal side effects. PGG_2, prostaglandin G_2; PGH_2, prostaglandin H_2.

Therefore, general principles of NSAID use include the following:

- Use the lowest effective dose for the shortest possible duration.
- After observing initial response and side effects, titrate dose and frequency to meet the needs of the individual patient.

Ibuprofen

Ibuprofen is a prototypical NSAID and represents the gold standard against which new analgesic agents are evaluated for efficacy in acute orofacial pain.[70,71] Ibuprofen is one of the most commonly prescribed NSAIDs for dental pain, and this drug is widely available over the counter (ie, without prescription) around the world. A number of clinical trials have shown that ibuprofen is an effective analgesic in the control of postoperative dental pain.[72] Ibuprofen 400 mg is apparently the most suitable dose after third-molar surgery; a 200-mg dose did not differ from placebo, and there is little analgesic advantage in increasing the dose to 600 mg.[72] Ibuprofen 800 mg, however, is extremely effective in acute pain and may be indicated in moderate to severe cases (see Fig 15-1). The analgesic efficacies relative to placebo are similar for ibuprofen 400 mg (NNT, 2.4; CI, 2.3 to 2.6), diclofenac 50 mg (NNT, 2.3; CI, 2.0 to 2.7), and naproxen sodium 550 mg (NNT, 2.6; CI, 2.2 to 3.2).[43] Ibuprofen 400 mg, however, is superior to acetaminophen 500 mg (NNT, 3.5; CI, 2.7 to 4.8) and aspirin 600/650 mg (NNT, 4.4; CI, 4.0 to 4.9).[41,43,44] Overall, ibuprofen was associated with the lowest relative gastrointestinal risk of conventional NSAIDs. Indeed, ibuprofen has an excellent gastrointestinal safety profile that is not significantly different from placebo in dosages of 800 to 1,200 mg per day over 1 to 10 days' duration.[73] Other NSAIDs, such as ketoprofen and piroxicam, ranked highest for risk, and indomethacin, naproxen, sulindac, and aspirin occupied intermediate positions. Higher doses of ibuprofen (> 1,200 mg/day) were associated with RRs similar to those with naproxen and indomethacin.[69] In summary, extensive epidemiologic data on efficacy and safety support the use of 400 mg of ibuprofen first when choosing an NSAID.[69]

Recent evidence suggests that ibuprofen, particularly at high doses, increases risk for serious cardiovascular events.[21–23] Ibuprofen significantly increased major coronary events (RR, 2.22; CI, 1.10 to 4.48; $P = .0253$) but not major vascular events (RR, 1.44; CI, 0.89 to 2.33), whereas high-dose naproxen was associated with less vascular risk than other NSAIDs.[74]

Clinical considerations. For mild to moderate pain, 400 mg as an initial dose followed by 400 mg orally every 4 hours or as needed is effective, up to 2,400 mg/day. Strong pain may be treated with an 800-mg initial dose. Analgesic onset occurs within 30 minutes.[75]

Common side effects of ibuprofen include edema, gastrointestinal complaints (abdominal pain, diarrhea, constipation, dyspepsia, heart-burn, nausea, vomiting), rashes or pruritus, tinnitus, dizziness, somnolence, headache, and increased liver function tests. Rarer but serious side effects include cardiovascular events, gastrointestinal ulceration, anemia, agranulocytosis, leukopenia, hepatitis, and depression. Erythema multiforme or SJS has also been reported. Severe, even fatal anaphylactic-like reactions have been reported in patients who have experienced asthma, urticaria, or allergic-type reactions after taking aspirin or other nonsteroidal anti-inflammatory agents. Treatment of patients with renal impairment should be coordinated with the treating physician and initiated at the lowest recommended dosage. The patient must be monitored closely and the dosage reduced if necessary. Ibuprofen should be avoided in late pregnancy, particularly as it may cause premature closure of the ductus arteriosus (pregnancy category B and C but D from 30 weeks of gestation onward); as with all NSAIDs, ibuprofen may delay the onset of childbirth. The drug is excreted into breast milk, so breastfeeding is not recommended.

Ibuprofen and acetaminophen combined

Analgesic drug combinations and their rationale are discussed in detail later in this chapter in connection to acetaminophen combined with opioids or tramadol. However, because of mounting concerns regarding the misuse and abuse of prescribed opioids,[76] alternative combination analgesics that do not contain opioids have been advocated as a means for avoiding their potential adverse reactions and misuse.[19,77] Combining ibuprofen and acetaminophen appears to be an attractive combination, and the use of 200 mg of ibuprofen, together with 500 mg of acetaminophen, tested after third-molar extractions, provided a very robust analgesic (NNT, 1.6; CI, 1.4 to 1.8) with minimal side effects.[19] One should be aware of all the limitations associated with prescribing NSAIDs in patients with background restrictions, including gastrointestinal, cardiovascular, and renal concerns as well as those with hypersensitivities, such as asthma or urticaria. Also, as with all drug combinations, the patient should be aware of the maximum daily dose for each of the two drugs (3,000 mg for acetaminophen and 2,400 mg for ibuprofen). This is especially true for patients taking other medications that contain each of the two drugs; in particular, acetaminophen is used in many drug combinations.

Naproxen

Meta-analysis of six trials that compared naproxen sodium 550 mg with placebo gave an NNT of 2.6 (CI, 2.2 to 3.2).[44,78] Naproxen sodium is more suitable for treatment of acute pain than naproxen because of the earlier onset of analgesia (30 minutes versus 1 hour, respectively). The analgesic efficacy and onset are similar to that of ibuprofen 400 mg (see Fig 15-1), but naproxen produces a longer duration of analgesia. Weighted mean time to remedication for naproxen sodium 550 mg was 7.6 hours compared with 2.6 hours for placebo, and the effects of one dose last, on average, up to 7 hours.[44,78] The investigators concluded that naproxen sodium 440 to 550 mg and naproxen 400 mg administered orally are effective analgesics for the treatment of acute postoperative pain in adults. A low incidence of adverse events was found along with no significant difference between treatment and placebo, but reporting was inconsistent.[78] In an updated Cochrane review,[79] efficacy, duration of action, and associated adverse events of single-dose oral naproxen or naproxen sodium in acute postoperative pain in adults were assessed. Using 500/550 mg naproxen or naproxen sodium, the NNT for at least 50% pain relief over 4 to 6 hours was 2.7 (CI, 2.3 to 3.2). Median time to the use of rescue medication was 8.9 hours for naproxen 500/550 mg compared with 2 hours for placebo. Associated adverse events did not differ from placebo. Evidence suggests that naproxen may also be associated with fewer cardiovascular complications than other NSAIDs for short-term and long-term therapy. Investigators concluded that doses equivalent to 500 mg naproxen sodium and 400 mg naproxen administered orally provided effective analgesia to adults with moderate to severe acute postoperative pain.

Clinical considerations. For mild to moderate pain, an initial dose of naproxen sodium 550 mg will provide efficient and rapid analgesia. Maintenance of relief may be obtained with 275 mg of naproxen sodium orally every 6 to 8 hours or 550 mg every 12 hours as needed. The drug's long half-life may offer some advantages. Naproxen has emerged as the safest NSAID in most studies when cardiovascular risks are considered.[10,21-24] The drug may be combined with a proton pump inhibitor as needed[9,25] and provides excellent analgesia as well as gastrointestinal and cardiovascular safety. For naproxen sodium, doses should not exceed 1,350 mg/day initially, then 1,100 mg/day. Alternatively, to reduce sodium consumption, maintenance may be performed with naproxen 250 mg orally every 6 to 8 hours or 500 mg every 12 hours as needed.

Common side effects of naproxen include edema, gastrointestinal complaints (abdominal pain, diarrhea, constipation, dyspepsia, heartburn, nausea, vomiting), stomatitis, rashes or pruritus, tinnitus, dizziness, somnolence, headache, and increased liver function tests. Rarer but serious side effects include cardiovascular events, gastrointestinal ulceration, anemia, agranulocytosis, leukopenia, hepatitis, and depression. SJS has been reported as well as severe, even fatal anaphylactic-like reactions in patients who had experienced asthma, urticaria, or allergic-type reactions after taking aspirin or other nonsteroidal anti-inflammatory agents. Naproxen should be used only if absolutely necessary and with caution in patients with a history of asthma. Geriatric patients should not exceed 200 mg every 12 hours. Patients with liver disease or renal impairment may require dosage reduction and need to be monitored closely; such patients should be treated in conjunction with the treating physician. Naproxen should be avoided in late pregnancy, particularly as it may cause premature closure of the ductus arteriosus (Pregnancy category C but D if used for prolonged periods or near term). As with all NSAIDs, naproxen may delay the onset of childbirth and is possibly unsafe for breastfeeding. The effect on the infant is unknown, so clinicians should consider alternatives or weigh the risk versus benefit.

Etodolac

Etodolac, a pyrano-indoleacetic acid derivative, is a member of a class of NSAIDs that preferentially inhibit COX-2.[80] The FDA has cleared etodolac for treating acute pain in adults but not in children. Some studies have indicated a more rapid onset of analgesic action with etodolac 200 mg compared with aspirin 650 mg and significantly better analgesic efficacy[81]; however, other studies have not confirmed these findings.[82] The analgesic efficacy of etodolac 200 mg is comparable to that of acetaminophen 600 mg plus codeine 60 mg, and etodolac 400 mg is significantly superior to the latter combination.[83] A recent Cochrane review[84] reported on single-dose etodolac for acute postoperative pain in adults. Most participants had pain after dental extractions. For at least 50% of patients, pain relief over 4 to 6 hours was comparable with placebo. The NNT was 4.8 (CI, 3.5 to 7.8) for etodolac 100 mg and 3.3 (CI, 2.7 to 4.2) for etodolac 200 mg, compared with an NNT of 2.4 (CI, 2.3 to 2.6) for ibuprofen 400 mg and 2.6 (CI, 2.2 to 3.2) for naproxen sodium 550 mg.[43] Very limited information is available for the extended-release formulation, but it does not seem to offer improved benefits.

Researchers reported that etodolac possesses a more favorable therapeutic index, in terms of anti-inflammatory effects and gastric irritation, compared with other NSAIDs.[85] However, this favorable index could not be confirmed in a later study.[86] The semiselective NSAIDs, including etodolac, had a higher OR for upper gastrointestinal events, even after adjusting for various potential confounders (adjusted odds ratio [AOR], 3.63; CI, 3.08 to 4.28), followed by nonselective NSAIDs (AOR, 2.98; CI, 2.70 to 3.29) and COX-2 selective NSAIDs (AOR, 2.53; CI, 2.09 to 3.07). Therefore, etodolac does not seem to offer any gastrointestinal advantage over other NSAIDs. A systematic review of cardiovascular risks of NSAIDs[20] showed that the highest overall risks were seen with rofecoxib (AOR, 1.45; CI, 1.33 to 1.59) and diclofenac (AOR, 1.40; CI, 1.27 to 1.55), and the lowest risks were seen with ibuprofen (AOR, 1.18; CI, 1.11 to 1.25) and naproxen (AOR, 1.09; CI, 1.02 to 1.16). Of the less studied drugs, etoricoxib (AOR, 2.05; CI, 1.45 to 2.88), etodolac (AOR, 1.55; CI, 1.28 to 1.87), and indomethacin (AOR, 1.30; CI, 1.19 to 1.41) had the highest risks. These studies demonstrate that etodolac possesses a cardiovascular risk comparable with that of other COX-2 inhibitors, and gastrointestinal adverse events were not lower than those seen for nonselective NSAIDs.

Clinical considerations. Etodolac is also available in an extended (modified) release formulation. For mild to moderate acute pain, it is advisable to use the immediate-release formulation at 200 to 400 mg orally every 6 to 8 hours as needed up to a maximum of 1,200 mg/day. Maintenance can also be performed with the extended-release formulation; for adults weighing more than 50 kg, the recommendation is 800 to 1,200 mg every 24 hours.

Common side effects of etodolac include gastrointestinal complaints (abdominal pain, diarrhea, dyspepsia, flatulence, nausea) and malaise. Edema has been reported with the use of etodolac, so it should be avoided in patients with cardiovascular disease. Rarer but serious side effects include bronchospasm, cardiovascular events, gastrointestinal ulceration, anemia, agranulocytosis, leukopenia, hepatitis, and depression. SJS and toxic epidermal necrolysis have also been reported. As with other NSAIDs, etodolac should be avoided in late pregnancy as it may cause premature closure of the ductus arteriosus (pregnancy category C). Data on danger for breastfeeding infants is inadequate to assess risk, though caution is advised.

Diclofenac

A recent Cochrane review assessed single-dose oral diclofenac for the treatment of acute postoperative pain.[87] At 50 mg and 100 mg, NNTs for immediate-release diclofenac potassium were 2.1 (CI, 1.8 to 2.4) and 1.9 (CI, 1.7 to 2.2), respectively, which is significantly lower than for those same amounts of delayed-release diclofenac sodium: 6.7 (CI, 4.2 to 17) and 4.5 (CI, 3.2 to 7.7). Adverse events were reported at a similar rate to placebo, and there were no serious events.

Use of diclofenac in healthy persons was associated with an increased risk of cardiovascular death, similar to that of the selective COX-2 inhibitor rofecoxib (OR, 1.91; CI, 1.62 to 2.42), with a dose-dependent increase in risk compared with ibuprofen (OR, 1.29; CI, 1.02 to 1.63) or naproxen (OR, 0.84; CI. 0.50 to 1.42).[88] The incidence of stroke was increased with the use of rofecoxib (RR, 1.64; CI. 1.15 to 2.33) and diclofenac (RR, 1.27; CI, 1.08 to 1.48) but not with naproxen, ibuprofen, and celecoxib, which indicates an increased risk of stroke with the use of diclofenac.[89] In patients with prior myocardial infarction (MI), analyses of individual NSAIDs also showed that diclofenac was associated with the highest risk (RR, 3.26; CI, 2.57 to 3.86) for death from MI at days 1 to 7 of treatment, compared with NSAIDs overall (RR, 1.45; CI, 1.29 to 1.62).[90] Diclofenac is also known for its idiosyncratic liver injury, which may be associated with genetic susceptibility contributed by *UGT2B7*, *CYP2C8*, and *ABCC2* genotypes, which may promote the formation and accumulation of reactive diclofenac metabolites associated with diclofenac hepatotoxicity.[91] Most hepatic drug reactions occur in only a small proportion of persons, making them difficult to detect at the time of adverse drug reaction development; therefore, the prevalence of drug hepatotoxicity is poorly documented.[92]

Clinical considerations. Diclofenac is FDA cleared for rheumatoid arthritis and osteoarthritis, ankylosing spondylitis, inflammatory disorder of the eye, and refractive keratoplasty. In addition to standard (12.5, 25, 50, 75 mg) and slow-release (100 mg) formulations, diclofenac is available as 100-mg suppositories and a 1% topical gel (see chapter 16). For patients with gastrointestinal discomfort, diclofenac is available as a 50-mg or 75-mg formulation with 200 μg of misoprostol, a gastroprotective prostaglandin analog. Diclofenac is efficacious in acute pain; the analgesic efficacy of diclofenac 50 mg (NNT, 2.3; CI, 2.0 to 2.7) is similar to that of ibuprofen 400 mg or naproxen sodium 550 mg.[43] The drug may be prescribed as 25 to 50 mg three times daily or as a once-daily dosage of 100 mg of the slow-release formulation.

Diclofenac is usually well tolerated and has relatively few gastrointestinal side effects, although it may cause dyspepsia, nausea, abdominal pain, and constipation. However, gastrointestinal bleeding and perforation have been reported. Headache, dizziness, and drowsiness are common side effects. The drug is contraindicated in patients who have experienced asthma, urticaria, or allergic-type reactions after taking aspirin or other nonsteroidal anti-inflammatory agents; severe, even fatal anaphylactic-like reactions have also been reported. Recent evidence points to a significantly increased risk of serious cardiovascular events with diclofenac[21,23,93,94] (see the earlier discussion). Diclofenac has a cardiovascular risk very similar to that of rofecoxib, which was withdrawn from worldwide markets owing to cardiovascular toxicity, and it was suggested that diclofenac should be removed from the Essential Medicines Lists of the World Health Organization.[95] The drug has also been associated with fluid retention and edema. Increased liver function tests are commonly observed, but hepatitis is relatively uncommon, and idiosyncratic liver injury occurs rarely. SJS and toxic epidermal necrolysis have also been reported.

Diclofenac should be avoided in late pregnancy, particularly as it may cause premature closure of the ductus arteriosus (pregnancy category C), and as with all NSAIDS, it may delay the onset of childbirth. The diclofenac/misoprostol combination is contraindicated in pregnancy because misoprostol can induce uterus contraction. The risks of diclofenac for breastfeeding infants are unclear, so caution is advised.

Indomethacin

Currently, indomethacin is not used in routine dentistry or indeed for the control of any acute pain due to commonly occurring and significant side effects. However, its important diagnostic and therapeutic role in paroxysmal hemicrania and hemicrania continua mandates a brief review (a more extensive review is found in chapter 11). Indomethacin is FDA cleared for rheumatoid arthritis and osteoarthritis, gout, ankylosing spondylitis, patent ductus arteriosus, and acute shoulder pain. The drug's use for the treatment of patent ductus arteriosus has recently been challenged by the effectiveness of ibuprofen, which is as effective as indomethacin in closing a patent ductus arteriosus, causes fewer transient adverse effects on the kidney, and reduces the risk of necrotizing enterocolitis.[96]

Experimentally, indomethacin has been shown to block neurogenic inflammation.[97] Data from animal and human experiments have shown that intravenous indomethacin produces rapid, significant reductions (26% to 40%) in cerebral blood flow.[98] Indomethacin also possesses non–COX-based modes of action that may differentially modulate blood vessels.[99] An interaction between indomethacin and nitric oxide, which is involved in headache patho- genesis, has been proposed. Findings from an experimental pain model suggest that an inter- action between indomethacin and local nitric oxide synthesis is involved in the antinocicep- tive effects of indomethacin.[100]

Clinical considerations. Indomethacin is available in standard and slow-release formu- lations (75 mg) and as suppositories. Standard dosages are 25 to 50 mg two or three times dai- ly. Most patients with paroxysmal hemicrania will respond to 25 mg three times daily within 24 hours; however, therapy should be contin- ued for 3 days at 75 mg, followed, if needed, by 150 mg for a further 3 days to verify diagnosis (see chapter 11).

Adverse effects are probably more fre- quent with indomethacin than with most other NSAIDs. The most common are gastrointesti- nal disturbances (abdominal pain, constipation, diarrhea, dyspepsia, nausea, vomiting), head- ache, vertigo, dizziness, and lightheadedness. More serious but rarer events include gastro- intestinal perforation, ulceration, and bleeding. Rectal irritation and bleeding have been report- ed occasionally in patients who have received indomethacin suppositories. Other adverse ef- fects include depression, drowsiness, tinnitus, confusion, insomnia, edema and weight gain, hypertension, hematuria, and stomatitis. Indo- methacin may increase the risk of serious car- diovascular events and is to be avoided in at-risk patients.[21,94,101] Indomethacin is contraindicated in patients who have experienced asthma, ur- ticaria, or allergic-type reactions after taking aspirin or other nonsteroidal anti-inflammatory agents; severe, even fatal anaphylactic-like re- actions have been reported. Serious skin reac- tions, such as SJS and toxic epidermal necroly- sis, are rare. No dose adjustment is needed in persons with renal disease, but indomethacin should be used with caution in persons with hepatic disease; the elderly require a 25% dose reduction. A complaint of blurred vision may be an early symptom of indomethacin-related corneal deposits and warrants evaluation by an ophthalmologist; these effects are reversible.

Indomethacin should be avoided in late pregnancy, particularly as it may cause prema- ture closure of the ductus arteriosus (pregnancy category C). As with all NSAIDs, indomethacin may delay the onset of childbirth. Indomethacin enters breast milk and is not compatible with breastfeeding.

Selective COX-2 inhibitors (coxibs)

The documentation of significantly increased cardiovascular and renal risks with COX-2 inhib- itors has raised important issues relating to their continued use, particularly for chronic pain.[21,102] Moreover, the lack of any significant increase in analgesic efficacy of COX-2 inhibitors over the classic NSAIDs suggests that clinicians should probably stay with the well-researched, older NSAIDs such as ibuprofen and naproxen. Recent meta-analyses also show that adverse cardiovascular events associated with COX-2 inhibitors actually occur quite quickly after ini- tiation of therapy and not months afterward, as was initially claimed.[21] This raises the important question of whether COX-2 inhibitors should be used at all for pain control. Unless gastrointesti- nal complications outweigh cardiovascular ad- verse effects, the authors' approach has been to first use conventional NSAIDs, particularly ibuprofen or naproxen. Emerging evidence of cardiovascular safety suggests that naproxen is presently the drug of choice; combined with a proton pump inhibitor, naproxen provides gastrointestinal and cardiovascular safety.[9,25] However, the COX-2 inhibitors are still widely available and are extensively used, particularly in patients with gastrointestinal problems, as they provide the highest gastrointestinal safety profile, especially when combined with a pro- ton pump inhibitor.[103] In addition, COX-2 inhib- itors (eg, celecoxib, etoricoxib) are safe drugs for patients with aspirin-induced asthma or urticaria.[27,28,34]

Rofecoxib

Rofecoxib was voluntarily withdrawn from the market by the manufacturer in 2004 because of safety concerns related to an increased risk for cardiovascular events, including heart attack and stroke. However, rofecoxib's effectiveness for acute pain is excellent, and as one of the first selective COX-2 inhibitors, it deserves a brief review.

The NNT for rofecoxib 50 mg versus place- bo was found to be 2.2 (CI, 1.9 to 2.4)[42] with a median time to onset of analgesia of 34 minutes. After surgical extraction of third molars, rofecoxib 50 mg demonstrated significantly better analgesic efficacy and duration compared with celecoxib 400 mg,[104] enteric-coated diclofenac sodium (as a single 50-mg dose and three 50-mg doses),[105] and codeine/acetaminophen 60/600 mg.[106] The overall analgesic efficacy of rofecoxib 50 mg was similar to that of ibuprofen 400 mg but lasted significantly longer (up to 24 hours). A recent systematic review[20] indicated that the highest overall cardiovascular risks of all NSAIDs (nonselective or COX-2 selective) were seen with rofecoxib (RR, 1.45; CI, 1.33 to 1.59).

Celecoxib

Single-dose celecoxib 200 mg per day was compared with ibuprofen 1,200 mg and to placebo in patients with moderate or severe pain after surgical extraction of impacted third molars.[107] Time to meaningful relief was significantly shorter for ibuprofen compared with celecoxib, and the mean 4-, 8-, and 12-hour summed pain relief scores were significantly better for ibuprofen. Both active treatments were significantly more effective than placebo; they were well tolerated and displayed no differences in incidence or severity of adverse events. In other studies, ibuprofen 400 mg has been shown to be superior to celecoxib 200 mg.[104] The use of single-dose celecoxib for acute postoperative pain was updated in a recent Cochrane review.[108] The NNT for celecoxib 200 mg and 400 mg—compared with placebo for at least 50% of maximum pain relief over 4 to 6 hours—was 4.2 (CI, 3.4 to 5.6) and 2.5 (CI, 2.2 to 2.9), respectively. The median time to the use of rescue medication was 6.6 hours with celecoxib 200 mg, 8.4 hours with celecoxib 400 mg, and 2.3 hours with placebo. The authors[108] concluded that single-dose oral celecoxib is an effective analgesic for postoperative pain relief and that indirect comparison suggests that the 400-mg dose has similar efficacy to ibuprofen 400 mg. However, although celecoxib 200 mg is safe in terms of cardiovascular events, celecoxib 400 mg significantly increases the risk for serious cardiovascular events.[21] Also, a 2005 FDA alert stated that celecoxib has been associated with an increased risk of serious adverse cardiovas-

cular events in a long-term placebo-controlled trial. A recent meta-analysis[101] showed that the risk ratio for MI was lowest for naproxen (RR, 1.06; CI, 0.94 to 1.20), followed by celecoxib (RR, 1.12; CI, 1.00 to 1.24) and ibuprofen (RR, 1.14; CI, 0.98 to 1.31). However, for new users, the RRs were 0.85 (CI, 0.73 to 1.00) for naproxen, 1.20 (CI, 0.97 to 1.48) for ibuprofen, and 1.23 (CI, 1.00 to 1.52) for celecoxib. As for gastrointestinal adverse effects, a recent review[109] found that the combined incidence rates of clinically significant upper and lower gastrointestinal events were 0.3, 0.9, and 0.3 per 100 patient-years in the celecoxib, NSAIDs, and placebo groups, respectively. The time to incidence of these events was significantly longer with celecoxib than with NSAIDs (P = .0004). The investigators concluded that celecoxib is associated with a significantly lower risk of all clinically significant gastrointestinal events throughout the entire gastrointestinal tract.

Clinical considerations. For mild to moderate acute pain, an initial single dose of 400 mg orally should be administered plus one additional 200-mg dose as needed on the first day. Maintenance may be achieved with 200 mg twice a day as needed.

Common side effects of celecoxib include edema, gastrointestinal complaints (abdominal pain, diarrhea, dyspepsia, flatulence, and nausea), rash, dizziness, headache, insomnia, and respiratory problems (pharyngitis, sinusitis, and rhinitis). Rarer but serious side effects include cardiovascular events, gastrointestinal ulceration, anemia, increased liver function tests, and hepatitis. Erythema multiforme and SJS have also been reported. Celecoxib is contraindicated in patients with hypersensitivity to sulfonamides. Several reports indicate that celecoxib is safe for patients with aspirin-induced asthma or urticaria.[26-28] Celecoxib is in pregnancy category C, but many consider all COX-2 inhibitors to be contraindicated during pregnancy. Use during breastfeeding is contraindicated.

Etoricoxib

Etoricoxib, a novel COX-2 inhibitor with high selectivity for COX-2 (106 COX-2/COX-1 ratio compared with 35 for rofecoxib or 1.78 for ibuprofen), is as effective as ibuprofen and naproxen and more effective than acetaminophen for arthritis pain.[110] In patients recovering from extraction of two or more third molars, etoricoxib 120 mg and oxycodone/acetaminophen 10/650 mg achieved significant analgesia with a rapid onset, although the time was slightly faster for oxycodone/acetaminophen.[111] The peak effect was similar for both drugs. Oxycodone/acetaminophen treatment resulted in more frequent drug-related nausea and vomiting compared with etoricoxib treatment.[108] The duration of analgesic effect after third-molar extractions, defined as median time to rescue medication use, was more than 24 hours for etoricoxib 120 mg, 20.8 hours for naproxen sodium 550 mg, 3.6 hours for acetaminophen/codeine 600/60 mg, and 1.6 hours for placebo. All three active treatments had rapid onset of analgesia.[75] The median time to onset of analgesia for etoricoxib 120 to 240 mg is about 25 to 30 minutes.[75] No significant differences were found in the onset of analgesia between etoricoxib and ibuprofen. The duration of analgesic effect was more than 24 hours for etoricoxib 120 to 240 mg and 12.1 hours for etoricoxib 60 mg. The duration of effect was significantly longer with all four etoricoxib doses compared with ibuprofen. Etoricoxib 120 mg provided superior overall analgesic effect with a smaller percentage of patients experiencing nausea compared with both oxycodone/acetaminophen 10 mg/650 mg and codeine/acetaminophen 60 mg/600 mg.[112] Based on these placebo-controlled studies, the authors calculated a mean NNT of 1.6 for good to excellent pain relief at 8 hours using 120 mg of etoricoxib and an NNT of 1.4 using 180 mg of etoricoxib.[75,112] However, these attractive NNTs must be taken together with NNTs for the active controls in these studies, which were similarly low: 1.4 for 550 mg of naproxen sodium, 1.7 for 400 mg of ibuprofen, and 1.6 for an oxycodone 10 mg/acetaminophen 650 mg combination. A recent Cochrane review of single-dose etoricoxib for acute postoperative pain[110] reported at least 50% pain relief by 66% of patients with etoricoxib 120 mg and 12% with placebo, with an NNT of 1.8 (CI, 1.7 to 2.0). For dental studies only, the NNT was 1.6 (CI, 1.5 to 1.8). The authors concluded that single-dose oral etoricoxib produces high levels of good-quality pain relief after surgery and that adverse events did not differ from placebo.

The 120-mg dose is as effective as, or better than, other commonly used analgesics.

Clinical considerations. The optimal doses of etoricoxib have not been clearly established. An oral dose of 120 mg has been effective in acute pain after dental surgery with a rapid onset (25 to 30 minutes). No significant benefit is obtained at higher doses (180 or 240 mg). The drug's long half-life offers the possibility of once-daily dosing. As mentioned earlier,[113] it was concluded that single-dose oral etoricoxib produces high levels of good-quality pain relief after surgery, and adverse events did not differ from those with placebo. The 120-mg dose is as effective as, or better than, other commonly used analgesics.

Despite its excellent analgesic properties, etoricoxib is not available on the US market; in a 2007 nonapprovable letter, the FDA indicated that Merck would need to provide additional data in support of the benefit-to-risk profile for the proposed doses of Arcoxia (etoricoxib) to gain clearance. However, the drug is available in many other parts of the world, including Australia, Europe, South America, Singapore, and Israel. However, in the United Kingdom, it is recommended that the use of selective COX-2 inhibitors be limited to patients with good cardiovascular health and at high risk of developing serious gastrointestinal problems if given a nonselective NSAID.

Early data suggest that etoricoxib is indeed associated with thromboembolic events and increased cardiovascular risk.[93,94] In a later systematic review of community-based observations,[20] etoricoxib demonstrated high cardiovascular risk (RR, 2.05; CI, 1.45 to 2.88) compared with ibuprofen (RR, 1.40; CI, 1.27 to 1.55) and naproxen (RR, 1.18; CI, 1.11 to 1.25). A recent nationwide cohort study performed after the withdrawal of rofecoxib[114] revealed no significant association of coxib use with risk for MI, ischemic stroke, or heart failure. In contrast to these findings, coxib use was associated with an increased risk for a first episode of atrial fibrillation (RR, 1.16; CI, 1.05 to 1.29). A post hoc analysis for different coxibs revealed a significant association with incident atrial fibrillation for etoricoxib (RR, 1.35; CI, 1.19 to 1.54) but not for celecoxib (RR, 0.94; CI, 0.79 to 1.11).[114] In light of these findings, cardiovascular risks need to be taken into account when prescribing etoricoxib, bearing in mind that etoricoxib cannot be prescribed in the United States.

Adverse reactions to NSAIDs are commonly observed, particularly among patients with chronic urticaria or asthma. The identification of a safe and reliable alternative is a frequent problem in clinical practice. Etoricoxib seems to be a safe alternative for patients with well-demonstrated NSAID hypersensitivity.[35] In a study that included 77 patients who had experienced asthma induced by aspirin and at least one other NSAID drug,[34] each patient was challenged with placebo and three ascending doses of etoricoxib. None of the patients experienced any asthma signs, and the results confirm the lack of cross-reactivity between etoricoxib and aspirin in aspirin-exacerbated respiratory disease. Tolerance to etoricoxib was studied in 37 patients with urticaria and angioedema induced by NSAIDs.[29] Thirty-four patients tolerated etoricoxib treatment without adverse reactions, but a generalized urticarial rash developed in three patients (8%). The investigators concluded[29] that etoricoxib, like other COX-2 inhibitors, is a well-tolerated drug in most NSAID-sensitive patients. However, a previous challenge test in a safe environment may be necessary before prescribing the drug to such patients. Gastrointestinal effects (nausea, vomiting, diarrhea, flatulence, taste disturbances, decreased appetite), headache, dizziness, and fatigue have been reported but are relatively rare. Etoricoxib has not been categorized for use in pregnancy; however, many consider all COX-2 inhibitors to be contraindicated during pregnancy. Similarly, use during breastfeeding is contraindicated.

Valdecoxib

Valdecoxib was voluntarily withdrawn from the market in 2005 because of safety concerns over increased risk of cardiovascular events and reports of serious and potentially life-threatening skin reactions, including deaths. Valdecoxib is a new, highly selective COX-2 inhibitor with a rapid onset of action and significant analgesic properties. In patients with rheumatoid arthritis, valdecoxib at 10, 20, or 40 mg/day was significantly more effective than placebo and similar in efficacy to naproxen 500 mg twice daily; there were no significant differences in efficacy between the three dosages of valdecoxib.[115]

Patients undergoing oral surgery who received valdecoxib 40 mg experienced a significantly quicker onset of analgesia, significantly improved pain relief, and lower pain intensity compared with patients receiving rofecoxib 50 mg.[116] Valdecoxib, rofecoxib, and placebo were equally well tolerated.

Lumiracoxib

Lumiracoxib can be associated with severe liver injury[117] and therefore was withdrawn from the Australian, Canadian, and European markets in 2007 and withdrawn by the World Health Organization in 2011.

Lumiracoxib is a new coxib with even higher COX-2 selectivity (COX-2/COX-1 ratio, 700).[118] In patients with postoperative dental pain, lumiracoxib 100 mg was comparable to ibuprofen 400 mg, but lumiracoxib 400 mg was superior to both.[71] The NNT for 400 mg of lumiracoxib for postoperative pain in adults was 2.4 (CI, 2.1 to 2.8).[119]

Dual-acting NSAIDs

As discussed earlier, the standard NSAIDs and the newer selective COX-2 inhibitors are associated with a number of severe gastrointestinal, cardiovascular, and renal side effects. This is due to the inhibition of protective prostaglandins and the unchecked effects of specific leukotrienes on the gastric mucosa (NSAID mechanisms of action are discussed later in the chapter). Additionally, the proalgesic and proinflammatory effects of the leukotrienes are largely unaffected by these drugs. Drugs acting on both COX and lipoxygenase enzymes are an attractive option and are collectively referred to as *dual-acting NSAIDs*.[120] The dual-acting NSAIDs are still in the experimental stage but have shown promising results in animal models of pain and osteoarthritis.[121] Additionally, a series of lumiracoxib derivatives were designed to explore the influence of isosteric substitution on balancing COX-2 inhibition and thromboxane A2 (TXA2) prostanoid receptor antagonism,[122] which might contribute to the rational design of a new class of cardioprotective anti-inflammatory agents. All of these are still in a development stage and as yet are not available on the market.

NSAIDs: Conclusion

Significant advances in the understanding of COXs and prostaglandins have led to the development of the specific COX-2 inhibitors. Yet the nonselective NSAIDs remain a reliable class of analgesics because of their predictability and tolerability.[66] Important differences in adverse effects exist among different NSAIDs and, among other factors, depend on their selectivity for the different COXs, but the analgesic efficacy of NSAIDs and the newer COX-2 inhibitors seem similar. Thus, the differences in adverse events have a major effect on the considerations presented here; for example, reduction in ulcers with COX-2 inhibitors should be weighed against their potential increase in cardiovascular risk compared with the older NSAIDs.[22] The use of selective COX-2 inhibitors should be limited to patients with good cardiovascular health and at high risk of developing serious gastrointestinal problems if given a nonselective NSAID or when asthma or urticaria are present in patients with moderate to severe pain. Naproxen has emerged as the safest NSAID in most studies when cardiovascular risks are considered.[10,21–24] Naproxen may be combined with a proton pump inhibitor as needed,[9,25] providing excellent analgesia as well as gastrointestinal and cardiovascular safety. Obtaining the medical history of the patient is therefore mandatory and provides the most important consideration for selecting the proper analgesic.[10] Ibuprofen remains the analgesic gold standard against which new pain-relieving drugs are evaluated.[70,71] Ibuprofen 400 mg is considered the first-line NSAID based on its good safety profile, high efficacy, and low cost.[18] The evidence to date fails to demonstrate any therapeutic advantage of COX-2 inhibitors over ibuprofen in the treatment of acute dental pain.[123] Unless there is a specific contraindication to their use, short-term NSAIDs are effective for treating acute dental pain in ambulatory patients who generally experience a higher incidence of adverse effects after ingesting an opioid analgesic.[70,124]

Dipyrone

Dipyrone, the most widely used pyrazolone derivative, is a rapidly reversible inhibitor of COX.[125] Dipyrone possesses analgesic, antipyretic, anti-inflammatory, and spasmolytic properties and is often classified as peripherally acting. For example, it was found that dipyrone inhibited platelet aggregation and markedly decreased TXA2 synthesis, which is consistent with a competitive inhibitory effect of dipyrone on prostaglandin synthetase activity.[126] Some researchers have suggested that a central action is also involved in the analgesic effect of dipyrone and that this central action manifests itself by an activation of inhibition originating in the periaqueductal gray.[127] Dipyrone depresses pain-evoked potentials in thalamic neurons but less effectively than morphine.[128] Naloxone abolishes the depressant effects of morphine but not of dipyrone.[128] Thus, it appears that several mechanisms contribute to the analgesic effect of dipyrone, including the possibility that the effects of dipyrone result from antagonism of the pharmacologic effects of prostaglandins rather than from inhibition of their synthesis.[125] For a single oral dose of oral dipyrone 500 mg, the NNT was 2.3 (CI, 1.8 to 3.0),[129] which was confirmed in a Cochrane review update[130] with comparable results (NNT, 2.4; CI, 1.9 to 3.2).

Dipyrone is relatively safe for the gastrointestinal tract. Administered for 2 weeks, dipyrone has effects on the gastric and duodenal mucosa that are comparable to those of acetaminophen and placebo, though noticeable damage is detectable at a dosage of 3 g/day.[131] Dipyrone is comparable in this respect to acetaminophen and much safer than diclofenac.[132] Dipyrone inhibits platelet aggregation and markedly decreases TXA2 synthesis.[126]

Pyrazolone hypersensitivity associated with chronic asthma is similar to that of aspirin-induced asthma and probably involves prostaglandin inhibition and overproduction of cystenyl leukotrienes. Other patients may develop anaphylaxis, urticaria, and other forms of rash, and the hypersensitivity is due to immunologic mechanisms.[133] However, a mixed form is probably more common. Thus, of patients with dipyrone intolerance, 76% of those with asthma and 9% of those without asthma reacted with bronchospasm after ingestion of dipyrone, whereas urticaria developed in 26% of those with asthma and 65% of those without asthma.[134]

The use of dipyrone as an analgesic is controversial. The drug is used most commonly to treat postoperative pain, colic pain, cancer pain, and migraine, and in many countries (eg, Russia, Spain, Germany, and in many parts of South America and Africa), it is the most popular non-opioid first-line analgesic. In other countries (eg, the United States and the United Kingdom), it has been banned because of its association with blood dyscrasias such as agranulocytosis. Significant regional variability was found in the rate ratio estimate for the epidemiology of agranulocytosis due to the use of dipyrone.[135] In a recent study in Poland, where dipyrone is a common nonprescription product, estimates of the rate of agranulocytosis and aplastic anemia associated with metamizole (dipyrone) were 0.16 and 0.08 cases/million person-days of use, respectively.[136] Non–chemotherapy drug–induced agranulocytosis is considered a potentially life-threatening idiosyncratic blood dyscrasia that is thought to result from a partly elucidated immune and/or toxic damage on myelopoiesis, due to a multitude of drugs.[137] With improved intensive care treatment and alertness of physicians, the case fatality rate of the disorder has recently decreased to 5%.[137]

Clinical considerations

Dipyrone is effective for adults with moderate to severe postoperative pain, and single-dose oral dipyrone 500 mg was found to be of similar efficacy to ibuprofen 400 mg. The drug should be repeated at 6- to 8-hour intervals, not to exceed 4 g/day. Adverse effects were poorly reported, but the most common were drowsiness, gastric discomfort, and nausea. The risk to pregnant or lactating mothers is unclear, and use during pregnancy or for lactating women is not recommended.

Opioids

Opiates are drugs derived from opium and include morphine, codeine, and a wide variety of semisynthetic congeners derived from them as well as from thebaine, another component of opium. The term *opioid* is more inclusive, applying to all agonists and antagonists with morphine-like activity as well as to naturally occurring and synthetic opioid peptides. *Endorphin* is a generic term referring to the three families of endogenous opioid peptides: the enkephalins, dynorphins, and beta-endorphins.

Multiple opioid receptors

Evidence is convincing that there are three major classes of opioid receptors in the CNS, designated mu, kappa, and delta, as well as indications of subtypes within each class. Although the commonly prescribed opioids bind preferentially to the mu receptor, they associate with all three receptor types.[138] Morphine shows the greatest relative preference for the mu receptor. Codeine displays exceedingly poor binding to opioid receptors, which raises the possibility that it is a prodrug where the pharmacologically active species is morphine (discussed later). A similar situation probably applies to oxycodone, where the metabolite oxymorphone may be responsible for the pharmacologic effect. Alternatively, the intrinsic antinociceptive effect of oxycodone may be mediated via kappa receptors.[139]

Mechanisms and sites of opioid-induced analgesia

Opioid-induced analgesia is due to action at several sites within the CNS; both spinal and multiple supraspinal sites were identified. Peripherally, opioid receptors on the terminals of primary afferent nerves mediate inhibition of the release of neurotransmitters, including substance P. Morphine also antagonizes the effects of exogenously administered substance P by exerting postsynaptic inhibitory action on interneurons and on the output neurons of the spinothalamic tract that conveys nociceptive information to higher centers in the brain. Morphine selectively inhibits various nociceptive reflexes and induces profound analgesia without affecting other sensory modalities. Intrathecal administration of opioids can produce profound segmental analgesia without causing significant alteration of motor or sensory functions.[140]

Tramadol is a synthetic, centrally acting opioid analgesic. However, it only binds weakly to mu opioid receptors and with weak affinity to delta and kappa receptors. Tramadol-induced antinociception is mediated by the opioid mu receptor and additionally by non-opioid mechanisms[141] that include the inhibition of norepinephrine and serotonin pathways within the CNS.[142]

Efficacy for acute pain

Traditionally, opioids have been classified as weak and strong. Weak opioids include codeine, dihydrocodeine, dextropropoxyphene, and tramadol. Morphine, fentanyl, methadone, oxycodone, and buprenorphine are considered strong opioids.[143] The weak opioids are relatively poor analgesics on their own: codeine 30 mg (NNT, 16.7), tramadol 75 mg (NNT, 9.9), dextropropoxyphene 65 mg (NNT, 7.7).[144,145] In addition, codeine, a prodrug for morphine, is converted to morphine in the liver, but 8% to 10% of the population lacks the cytochrome P450 enzyme 2D6 (*CYP2D6*) for this conversion, a further limitation of the analgesic activity of codeine.[146] Evidence suggests that *CYP2D6* polymorphisms might influence pain sensitivity and clinical response to tramadol.[147]

Morphine is the gold standard for opioid therapy and only lately was replaced by oxycodone as the most used opioid worldwide.[143] Although oral morphine is fully absorbed, it has a limited and very variable oral bioavailability between 10% and 45% due to an extensive first-pass metabolism.[148] Oxycodone, a synthetic derivative of thebaine, has a higher bioavailability than morphine ($\approx$ 60%) and is available in a wide range of oral (including controlled-release preparations) and parenteral preparations. Oxycodone analgesic efficacy is comparable with that of morphine, with a median oxycodone/morphine dose ratio of 1:1.5, and controlled-release oxycodone is as safe and effective as controlled-release morphine.[149] The data also suggest that oxycodone has a reduced rate of hallucinations and itch compared with morphine.[149] Although there was no benefit for oxycodone 5 mg, a significant effect for oxycodone 15 mg relative to placebo was shown with an NNT of 2.4 (CI, 1.5 to 4.9) for moderate to severe postoperative pain.[30] A later

review demonstrated a poorer outcome for 15 mg oxycodone, in which the NNT for at least 50% pain relief was 4.6 (CI, 2.9 to 11).[31]

Adverse effects

For a patient to report an adverse effect with a single dose of oxycodone 15 mg compared with placebo, the number needed to harm (NNH) was 3.1 (CI, 1.8 to 11), but no increased adverse effects were shown for oxycodone 5 mg over placebo.[30] In a single-dose study, adverse events occurred more frequently with oxycodone combination therapy than placebo but were generally described as mild to moderate in severity and rarely led to withdrawal.[31] Use of any oral opioid for a period of up to 4 weeks produced higher rates of adverse events than did placebo. In more than 50% of patients, one or more adverse effects were reported. Dry mouth (25%), nausea (21%), constipation (15%), pruritis (12%), and dizziness (12%) were the most commonly reported adverse events. A substantial proportion of patients on opioids (22%) withdrew because of adverse events. Most side effects are reported at the initial stage of opioid use.[150]

Administration for chronic pain

As this chapter focuses on acute pain, the following discussion on opioids for chronic pain is quite limited. The development of the Analgesic Ladder by the World Health Organization in 1984 paved the way for a rational approach to the management of chronic cancer pain and legitimized the regular administration of oral opioids for these patients. However, opinions are even more divided about the use of opioids in patients with noncancer pain who have a normal expected life span. A 10-year follow-up study on opioid use for chronic pain revealed that dose escalation occurred in only a few patients, suggesting that pain-related tolerance is rare.[151] Physical dependence can be easily avoided by gradual reduction in dosage, but this is not to be confused with psychologic dependency. The risk of psychologic dependence to opioids when used in the management of chronic pain is low, unless there is a prior history of substance abuse, major personality disorder, or social disruption.[152] Opioid administration for nonmalignant chronic pain is largely reserved for resistant neuropathic pain syndromes (discussed in chapter 12).

Analgesic Drug Combinations

Combination pharmacotherapy is not new in medicine and is commonly used in the management of hypertension and other cardiovascular diseases. Clinical outcomes might be improved under certain conditions with the use of a combination of analgesics rather than reliance on a single agent. Combination analgesic formulations are an important and effective means of pain relief and could prove useful in treating the elderly and other groups of patients who often cannot tolerate NSAIDs, including the newer COX-2 inhibitors. A combination of systemic analgesics is most effective when the individual agents act through different mechanisms and result in synergistic pain control.[141] Combinations aim at taking advantage of such complementary modes and sites of action and reducing side effects. The combination of an NSAID with acetaminophen is a good example.[19,153] Moreover, drug combinations need not necessarily be synergistic to provide an improved risk-benefit ratio; additive or even subadditive analgesic effects, but with reduced side effects, may offer clinical benefits. NSAIDs clearly have an analgesic ceiling,[68] but the combination of two NSAIDs with different toxicity profiles would be advantageous in terms of side effects without significantly increasing analgesic potency. The combination of 75 mg of tramadol with 500 mg of acetaminophen (described later) provides equivalent analgesia to tramadol 150 mg but with reduced side effects. Future work may analyze the combinations of more than two analgesics with complementary modes of action.

Acetaminophen in combination with opioids

The combination of opioids with acetaminophen may enhance efficacy and reduce side effects. A good choice for moderate to strong acute orofacial pain when the use of opioids is indicated, especially when NSAIDs are not recommended, seems to be oral administration of a combination of acetaminophen with a weak opioid, such as tramadol or codeine, or a strong opioid, such as oxycodone (see Figs 15-2 and 15-3). The weak opioids are relatively poor analgesics on their own,[144,145] are more effective when combined with acetaminophen, and show synergistic efficacy; with lower opioid dosage, there are significantly fewer side effects.

Codeine and acetaminophen

In two systematic reviews on postoperative pain,[46,47] acetaminophen 1,000 mg had an NNT of 4.6 (CI, 3.8 to 5.4) compared with placebo, and acetaminophen 600/650 mg had an NNT of 5.3 (CI, 4.1 to 7.2). Acetaminophen 600/650 mg plus codeine 60 mg had an NNT of 3.6 (CI, 2.9 to 4.5). The combination of 1,000 mg of acetaminophen with 60 mg of codeine improves the NNT to 2.2 (CI, 1.7 to 2.9) (see Fig 15-2) with no significant increase in side-effect profile relative to lower acetaminophen dose–containing combinations. The RR estimates for acetaminophen 600/650 mg plus codeine 60 mg versus placebo showed a significant difference for drowsiness/somnolence (NNH, 11) and dizziness (NNH, 27) but no significant difference for nausea/vomiting.[46,47]

Clinical considerations. For mild to moderate pain, acetaminophen 300 to 1,000 mg (≤ 4,000 mg/day) with codeine 15 to 60 mg (≤ 360 mg/day) orally every 4 hours as needed is very effective. Common adverse effects of these combinations include lightheadedness, nausea, vomiting, dizziness, sedation, and dyspnea that may be severe. Codeine is in pregnancy category C and should be used with caution in breastfeeding. See earlier sections for acetaminophen.

Oxycodone and acetaminophen

Oxycodone is a strong opioid and is similar to morphine in its effects, with the exception of hallucinations, which occur, although rarely, with morphine. The efficacies of oxycodone 15 mg, oxycodone 5 mg plus acetaminophen 325 mg, and oxycodone 10 mg plus acetaminophen 650 mg were similar; the relative benefit estimates and NNTs were about 2.5 for each (see Fig 15-2). This indicates that the dose of oxycodone may be lowered when it is combined with acetaminophen with no loss of efficacy.[30]

Oxycodone 5 mg plus acetaminophen (325 mg, 500 mg, and 1,000 mg) was significantly more effective than placebo, with NNTs of 2.5 (CI, 2.0 to 3.4), 2.2 (CI, 1.7 to 3.2), and 3.9 (CI, 2.1 to 20), respectively, for moderate to severe postoperative pain over 4 to 6 hours.[30] For single-dose oxycodone 10 mg plus acetaminophen (650 mg or 1,000 mg), NNTs were 2.5 (CI, 2.0 to 3.3) and 2.7 (CI, 1.7 to 5.6), respectively, for moderate to severe postoperative pain over 4 to 6 hours (see Fig 15-2). Because the combination of oxycodone 10 mg with acetaminophen did not show a better NNT than oxycodone 5 mg plus acetaminophen (see Fig 15-2), and oxycodone 10 mg exhibited more adverse effects than 5 mg (whether on its own or combined with acetaminophen),[30] one should prefer the lower-dose combination. A recent Cochrane update review[31] indicated that oxycodone 10 mg plus acetaminophen 650 mg (NNT, 2.7; CI, 2.4 to 3.1) did not differ from the fixed-dose combination available on the market of acetaminophen 325 mg plus oxycodone 5 mg (NNT, 2.5; CI. 2.0 to 3.4), except that durations of effect were 10 hours with oxycodone 10 mg plus acetaminophen 650 mg and 4 hours with half that dose. Fewer participants needed rescue medication over 6 hours at the higher dose. Adverse events occurred more frequently with combination therapy than placebo but were generally described as mild to moderate in severity and rarely led to withdrawal.[31]

Clinical considerations. Using the oxycodone 5 mg/acetaminophen 325 mg combination as first choice for moderate to severe pain seems prudent. Dosing is every 4 to 6 hours, and the total daily dosage should not exceed 4,000 mg of acetaminophen and 60 mg of oxycodone. Common adverse effects include lightheadedness, pruritus, rash, constipation, nausea, and vomiting. Dizziness, sedation, and a dysphoric mood have also been reported. Headache and vomiting were also reported with oxycodone 10 mg plus acetaminophen 650 mg, but no adverse effects were severe in nature.[30] Oxycodone is in

pregnancy category B but is associated with infant risk during breastfeeding and is therefore contraindicated for lactating mothers.

Tramadol and acetaminophen

Tramadol is a synthetic, centrally acting analgesic that binds weakly to mu opioid receptors and inhibits norepinephrine and serotonin pathways within the CNS.[142] After third-molar extraction, a single oral dose of tramadol 75 mg plus acetaminophen 650 mg produces effective analgesia in moderate to severe pain (NNT, 2.6; CI, 2.3 to 3.0).[144] For tramadol 75 mg on its own, the equivalent NNT was 9.9 (CI, 6.0 to 17), and for acetaminophen 650 mg it was 3.6 (CI, 3.0 to 4.5).[144] In a meta-analysis of postsurgical pain, tramadol 50 mg, 100 mg, and 150 mg had NNTs of 7.1 (CI, 4.6 to 18), 4.8 (CI, 3.4 to 8.2), and 2.4 (CI, 2.0 to 3.1), respectively.[154] However, with the same doses of drug, postsurgical patients at large had more pain relief than those having dental surgery, and it was concluded that absolute ranking of analgesic performance should be done separately for dental pain.[154] A later study examined the tramadol/acetaminophen combination specifically for dental pain in 456 patients after third-molar extraction.[155] This study established the superiority of tramadol/acetaminophen 75 mg/650 mg over tramadol 100 mg in the treatment of acute pain after oral surgery. Adverse events occurred more frequently in the tramadol group than in the tramadol/acetaminophen group. Significantly more patients reported adverse effects with tramadol 75 mg or tramadol 75 mg plus acetaminophen 650 mg than with placebo; the NNHs for a patient to report any adverse effects were 5.0 (CI, 3.7 to 7.3) and 5.4 (4.0 to 8.2), respectively.

Clinical considerations. For moderate to severe pain after third-molar extraction, a single oral dose of tramadol 75 mg plus acetaminophen 650 mg produces effective analgesia. A fixed combination dose of 37.5 mg tramadol 325 mg acetaminophen, available on the market, can be repeated every 4 to 6 hours as needed. Maximum daily doses should not exceed 3,000 mg of acetaminophen and 300 mg of tramadol. In patients with pulmonary disease, regular monitoring of vital signs is indicated for higher doses or prolonged treatment.

Common adverse effects include nausea, dizziness, vomiting, excessive sweating, pruritus, rash, and slight weight loss. Confusion, headache, somnolence, tremor, anxiety, and fatigue are also commonly reported.

Withdrawal of tramadol, particularly if abrupt, may induce anxiety, insomnia, nausea, tremors, diaphoresis, and hallucinations. Slow tapering will minimize or alleviate these withdrawal symptoms. Tramadol is in pregnancy category C. The drug is excreted in breast milk in high concentration, so breastfeeding should be avoided.

NSAID drug combinations

NSAIDs and opioids

The combination of NSAIDs with opioids seems less successful than the combination of acetaminophen and opioids. Trials of combinations of an NSAID with an opioid have found no difference (4 of 14 articles), a statistically insignificant trend toward superiority (1 of 14 articles), or at most a slight but statistically significant advantage (9 of 14 articles) compared with either single entity.[156] In a recent Cochrane review,[157] no significant difference was found between ibuprofen 400 mg plus oxycodone 5 mg and ibuprofen 400 mg alone. The ibuprofen/oxycodone combination had a longer analgesic effect, and fewer participants needed rescue medication with ibuprofen plus oxycodone than with placebo or ibuprofen alone.

NSAIDs and acetaminophen

Several controlled clinical studies among patients with musculoskeletal conditions, dental pain, or postoperative pain have shown that combinations of acetaminophen and NSAIDs provide additive pain-relieving activity, thereby leading to dose-sparing effects and improved safety.[158] Analgesic activity of acetaminophen and NSAIDs was assessed in mice using the writhing test (abdominal constriction after acetic acid intraperitoneal injection). The isobolographic analysis of the various combinations of NSAIDs and acetaminophen resulted in synergistic interactions.[153] These synergistic interactions were confirmed later on in clinical studies, as indicated below.

Because of mounting concerns regarding the misuse and abuse of prescribed opioids,[76] alternative combination analgesics that do not contain opioids have been advocated as a means for avoiding their potential adverse reactions and misuse.[19,77] The fixed-dose combination ibuprofen 400 mg/acetaminophen 1,000 mg was significantly more effective than ibuprofen 400 mg ($P = .02$) and acetaminophen 1,000 mg ($P < .001$), and the fixed-dose combination ibuprofen 200 mg/acetaminophen 500 mg was significantly more effective than ibuprofen 200 mg ($P < .001$) and acetaminophen 500 mg ($P < .001$). The fixed-dose combination ibuprofen 200 mg/acetaminophen 500 mg was also significantly more effective than acetaminophen 1,000 mg ($P < .001$) but failed to reach statistical significance in comparison with ibuprofen 400 mg.[159] Combining ibuprofen and acetaminophen appears to be an attractive combination, and the use of 200 mg of ibuprofen together with 500 mg of acetaminophen, tested after third-molar extractions, provided a very robust analgesic (NNT, 1.6; CI, 1.4 to 1.8) with minimal side effects.[19] Keeping ibuprofen at a low dose is meaningful in terms of cardiovascular risk, as low-dose ibuprofen is least likely to increase cardiovascular risk, which was seen only with higher doses.[20] As with all drug combinations, the patient should be aware of the maximum daily dose for each of the two drugs (3,000 mg for acetaminophen and 2,400 mg for ibuprofen), especially when taking other medications that contain either of the two, in particular acetaminophen, which is used in many drug combinations. The authors believe there are not sufficient data to indicate whether reaching the daily maximum dose of the two drugs simultaneously is safe.

Mechanisms of Analgesia

Understanding the mechanisms of analgesia provides clinicians with the knowledge to better appreciate the underlying mechanisms of drug efficacy and, even more important, knowledge of the side effects of analgesic drugs.

The inflammatory soup

The term *inflammatory soup* refers to a mixture of bioactive molecules (bradykinin, histamine, prostaglandins, neurotrophins, and interleukins) produced in response to a variety of stimuli and tissue injury. These molecules may act peripherally on primary afferents by direct and/or indirect effects. Direct effects include activation of primary afferent nociceptors and sensitization of nociceptors that result in increasing responses to various stimuli. Indirect effects are mediated by leukocytes and the sympathetic nervous system. These effects may involve increased excitability of dorsal horn neurons, leading to altered descending pain-control mechanisms and adaptive changes in the thalamus, cortex, and higher centers.[160] The concomitant presence of such mediators as nerve growth factor, 5-hydroxytryptamine, interleukin-1, and bradykinin at sites of inflammation has led to the collective term *inflammatory soup*.[161] This soup synergistically activates peripheral nociceptors.[162] An important characteristic of inflammation is acidosis, and protons will directly and indirectly cause pain and hyperalgesia.[163] Protons directly activate sensory neurons, mainly through acid-sensing ion channels (ASICs).[164,165] The inflammatory soup also induces ASIC upregulation, increases ASIC-expressing neurons, and activates sensory neurons, which leads to increased excitability.[161] An additional receptor, the dorsal-root ASIC, is both proton sensitive and mechanosensitive.[166] Further synergism is observed via an interaction between mediators in the inflammatory soup and an acidic pH; enhanced effects are mutual, and a two-way intensification of experimental human pain has been reported.[167] Protons also induce a decrease in the activation threshold for other receptors and therefore an increase in pain.

Prostaglandins

Prostaglandins are synthesized by the constitutive enzyme COX-1 and its inducible isoform COX-2. COX-2 is induced in peripheral tissues by a number of inflammatory mediators, including cytokines and growth factors.[168] Neuronal effects of prostaglandins are mediated by a direct action on the nociceptors[169,170] and are not under the control of nerve growth factor.[171] Prostaglandins are prime examples of sensitizing agents, and specific subtypes (PGE$_2$ and prostaglandin I$_2$ [PGI$_2$]) have been found to mediate the hyperalgesia induced by bradykinin and noradrenaline.[172] Experimentally, PGE$_2$ will induce sensitization of multiple classes of cutaneous afferents, including C-polymodal nociceptors and A-delta high-threshold mechanonociceptors.[173]

COX-2 is upregulated in the spinal cord during peripheral inflammation, and COX-2 products contribute to the increased excitability of spinal cord neurons during persistent peripheral inflammation.[174] This suggests that prostaglandins are involved at various sites and at anatomical levels of the inflammatory-nociceptive pathway.[175] Therefore, it is not surprising that drugs acting on prostaglandins such as nonselective NSAIDs and selective COX-2 inhibitors are effective analgesic and anti-inflammatory drugs.

The diagram presented in Fig 15-4 is a highly simplified version of the metabolic pathway from arachidonic acid to prostaglandins, thromboxanes, and leukotrienes.[176] Arachidonic acid is a product of cell membrane phospholipids, and its formation may be enhanced by tissue injury. After the release of arachidonic acid, COX catalyzes a complex reaction that converts arachidonic acid to prostaglandin G$_2$ (PGG$_2$). In a second step, a peroxidase-catalyzed reaction converts PGG$_2$ to prostaglandin H$_2$ (PGH$_2$),[176] which then reacts with other enzymes, determined by the host tissue/cell, into different prostaglandins or thromboxanes. For example, PGH$_2$ in platelets is converted into TXA2, whereas in endothelial cells it will be converted into PGE$_2$ and PGI$_2$.[177,178] TXA2 is a powerful vasoconstrictor that stimulates platelet aggregation. PGE$_2$ and PGI$_2$ are vasodilators that affect renal glomerular filtration rate and possess gastroprotective properties.[179] Specific leukotrienes lead to vasoconstriction and increased acid secretion in gastric mucosa, while others lead to hypersensitivity reactions, such as edema and bronchospasm.[179] Additionally, leukotriene B4 is known to induce a number of proinflammatory effects. These have been implicated in chronic inflammation, tissue destruction, and inflammatory joint disease.[120]

Modes of action of NSAIDs

The blockade of the enzymatic effects of COX by aspirin or other NSAIDs inhibits the production of prostaglandins associated with nociception (in particular PGE_2), hence the analgesic effect of these drugs.[180] However, as described in detail later in this chapter, prostaglandins are essential for the normal function of many organs (eg, gastrointestinal system, kidneys), and their disruption is associated with serious side effects. Additionally, the production of thromboxanes is also blocked. TXA2 is associated with platelet aggregation, and blocking the production of TXA2 interferes with normal blood clotting. Blockade of the COX pathway increases the amount of arachidonic acid substrate available for the lipoxygenase pathway, thereby enhancing the production of leukotrienes. An excess of leukotrienes is associated with asthmatic attacks, urticaria, and other sensitivity reactions.[181] Evidence suggests that some NSAIDs, such as ibuprofen and indomethacin, exert part of their effect by COX-independent mechanisms.[182] These mechanisms probably involve inhibition of transcription factors mediated by alterations in the activity of cellular kinases.

COX isoforms

An important advance in prostaglandin research was the discovery that COX exists in various isoforms, primarily COX-1 and COX-2,[183] and recent evidence points to the existence of COX-3. The level of COX-1 in cells varies relatively over a narrow range (twofold to fourfold) and is considered a constitutive or housekeeping enzyme largely unrelated to inflammation. COX-1 maintains prostaglandin and thromboxane synthesis in the stomach, the kidney, endothelial cells, blood platelets, and other tissues. COX-2, however, is mostly an inducible enzyme and is considered part of the inflammatory process.[184] COX-2 is produced in monocytes, synovial cells, and fibroblasts after stimulation by cytokines and growth factors, and its expression is augmented 10- to 80-fold when cells are activated.[178] Less is known about COX-3, which is found in the cerebral cortex and cardiac tissue and appears to be involved in centrally mediated pain. The kinetics of COX-2 inhibition are different from that of COX-1. COX-1 inhibition is instantaneous and competitively reversible. COX-2 inhibition is time dependent, with selectivity developing over 15 to 30 minutes, and it is essentially irreversible.[185] Different genes encode these two enzymes, and experiments in mice have used stem-cell technology to knock out the genes for both COX-1 and COX-2, in separate experiments, to provide evidence of the role of each of these enzymes.[186,187] However, some of the results in these knockout mice were quite unexpected, stressing a possible constitutive role for COX-2. Thus, deletion of the COX-2 gene was associated with a shortened life span, infertility due to failure of ovarian development, and incomplete maturation of nephrons resulting in renal failure.[186] Also, the results of experimental inflammation were similar in mice lacking the COX-2 gene and control mice, which stresses the important role of COX-1 in inflammation.[186] Another surprising finding was that even though mice lacking COX-1 had gastric PGE levels that were only 1% of the levels of controls, they had no gastric pathology and were less susceptible to indomethacin-induced gastropathy than controls.[187]

Indeed, it was first assumed that drugs with COX-2 selectivity would spare physiologic prostaglandin synthesis and possess anti-inflammatory action with less or none of the typical adverse effects of NSAIDs on the gastrointestinal tract, kidneys, platelets, and lungs.[188] However, it became obvious that COX-1 has an important role in the inflammatory response, whereas COX-2 has fundamental constitutive roles. Animal experiments and clinical trials with specific COX-2 inhibitors have revealed that COX-2 is important for the normal function of many systems.[189,190] This is particularly true for the kidney, CNS, cardiovascular system, and reproductive system.

Moreover, human platelets and vascular endothelial cells process PGH_2 to produce TXA2 and prostacyclin (PGI_2), respectively.[191] COX-1 converts arachidonic acid to TXA2 (mostly from platelets), which induces platelet aggregation and vasoconstriction. COX-2 is responsible for the conversion of arachidonic acid to PGI_2, which inhibits platelet aggregation and induces vasodilation. Selective inhibition of COX-2 causes suppression of PGI_2 production without affecting TXA2 and predisposes a person to hypertension and increased thromboembolic risks, the so-called prothrombotic effect,[192,193]

Adverse Effects of Analgesics

NSAIDs interfere with the production of prostaglandins and thromboxanes and enhance the amount of leukotrienes. The main adverse effects of NSAID administration that are associated with inhibition of prostaglandins are gastrointestinal toxicity, cardiovascular risk, and renal failure. Inhibition of thromboxanes is associated with coagulation problems, and the surplus production of leukotrienes is mainly associated with hypersensitive reactions, such as asthma and urticaria. The selective COX-2 inhibitors gained widespread popularity, having analgesic and anti-inflammatory effects equivalent to those of the conventional NSAIDs, yet with reduced gastrointestinal side effects.[194–196]

Recently, COX-2 inhibitors have been shown to increase the risk of cardiovascular events, such as MI and ischemic stroke.[197] They are also intimately involved in prostaglandin-dependent renal homeostatic processes and therefore do not offer renal safety over that of NSAIDs.[198] In a very short time, COX-2 inhibitors have gone from the darlings to the pariahs of the pharmaceutical industry.[199] Furthermore, traditional NSAIDs, such as diclofenac and ibuprofen, have also been implicated in increased MI risk.[21,23] The risks and adverse effects of traditional NSAIDs and of the newer, more selective COX-2 inhibitors are detailed later in the chapter.

Gastrointestinal

Pathophysiology

Gastroduodenal mucosal injury develops when the deleterious effect of gastric acid overwhelms the normal defensive properties of the mucosa. Concepts about NSAID-induced gastroduodenal mucosal injury have evolved from a simple notion of topical injury to theories involving multiple mechanisms with both local and systemic effects. Topical injury caused by

NSAIDs contributes to the development of gastroduodenal mucosal injury, but the systemic effects of these agents appear to have the predominant role,[200] largely through the decreased synthesis of mucosal prostaglandins.[201] Aspirin, at a dose as low as 30 mg, is sufficient to suppress prostaglandin synthesis in the gastric mucosa.[202] Prostaglandin inhibition, in turn, leads to decreases in epithelial mucus production, secretion of bicarbonate, mucosal blood flow, epithelial proliferation, and mucosal resistance to injury.[203] The impairment in mucosal resistance permits injury by endogenous factors, including acid, pepsin, and bile salts, as well as by exogenous noxious agents.

Selective COX-2 inhibitors hold the promise of fewer adverse effects as far as the gastrointestinal tract and platelets are concerned.[195,196,204] However, despite the 50% reduction of symptomatic ulcers, perforations, and bleeding observed for rofecoxib,[194] the risk for serious gastrointestinal toxicity by selective COX-2 inhibitors is still within the 2% to 4% range for COX-nonselective NSAIDs. Furthermore, there is increasing evidence of the importance of COX-2 in the resolution of mucosal inflammation and ulcer healing.[205] COX-2 inhibitors are therefore contraindicated for use in patients with diagnosed and actively treated gastrointestinal ulcers.[118]

Epidemiology

According to prospective data, 13 of every 1,000 patients with rheumatoid arthritis who take NSAIDs for 1 year have a serious gastrointestinal complication. The risk in patients with osteoarthritis is somewhat lower (7.3 per 1,000 patients per year).[206] Mortality attributed to NSAID-related gastrointestinal toxic effects is 0.22% per year, with an annual RR of 4.21 compared with the risk for persons not using NSAIDs.[206] The severity of the NSAID-associated gastrointestinal injury is not to be underestimated; on average, 1 in 1,200 patients taking NSAIDs for at least 2 months will die of gastroduodenal complications who would not have died had they not taken NSAIDs. This extrapolates to about 2,000 deaths each year in the United Kingdom alone.[207] These figures are true for 1999, before the wide introduction of COX-2 inhibitors such as celecoxib or rofecoxib. However, the use of COX-2 inhibitors has declined dramatically in recent years because of their cardiovascular side effects, and traditional NSAIDs have maintained their wide use.[95] In a recent systematic review,[208] the RRs were studied for upper gastrointestinal complications associated with the use of individual NSAIDs, including selective COX-2 inhibitors, and individual NSAIDs were compared with non-use of NSAIDs. Pooled RRs were calculated for individual NSAIDs, including celecoxib (RR, 1.45; CI, 1.17 to 1.81), ibuprofen (RR, 1.84; CI, 1.54 to 2.20), diclofenac (RR, 3.34; CI, 2.79 to 3.99), naproxen (RR, 4.10; CI, 3.22 to 5.23), and indomethacin (RR, 4.14; CI, 2.91 to 5.90). The RRs for the use of high daily doses of NSAIDs versus non-use were two to three times higher than those associated with low daily doses.

Risk factors

The risk for adverse gastrointestinal events increases linearly with age.[209] Other risk factors that have been identified in multiple studies are higher doses of NSAIDs, (including the use of two or more NSAIDs); a history of gastroduodenal ulcer or gastrointestinal bleeding; concomitant use of corticosteroids; serious coexisting medical conditions; alcohol abuse; and concomitant use of anticoagulants, including aspirin.[103,210] However, many of these studies are based on univariate analysis and do not consider the interactions among multiple factors and coexisting conditions, so for medically complex patients the risk may be even higher.[34]

Clinical spectrum of injury

In most patients, NSAID-induced gastroduodenal mucosal injury is superficial and self-limiting. However, peptic ulcers develop in some patients, and they may lead to gastroduodenal hemorrhage, perforation, and death. After ingestion of an NSAID, ultrastructural damage to the gastric surface epithelium occurs within minutes, and gross, endoscopically detectable hemorrhages and erosions in the gastroduodenal epithelium occur within several hours.[211]

Prevention and management

At least 10% to 20% of patients have dyspeptic symptoms during NSAID therapy.[212] However, such symptoms are poorly correlated with the endoscopic appearance and severity of mucosal injury. Up to 40% of persons with endoscopic evidence of erosive gastritis are asymptomatic,[213] and as many as 50% of patients with dyspepsia have normal-appearing mucosa.[213] Histamine H_2-receptor antagonists improve dyspeptic symptoms but still permit a high risk of gastrointestinal complications.[34]

The concomitant use of antacid medication in susceptible persons or for long-term therapy is common practice. The proton pump inhibitor omeprazole and the PGE_1 analog misoprostol are commonly used for the treatment and prevention of NSAID-related gastroduodenal ulcers. However, omeprazole provided greater symptomatic relief and better healing of gastroduodenal ulcers in patients receiving ongoing NSAIDs.[214] A quality-of-life evaluation showed that patients receiving omeprazole had significantly greater improvement in scores on the Gastrointestinal Symptom Rating Scale than patients receiving misoprostol.[214] Additionally, based on a cost-effectiveness analysis, omeprazole is preferable to misoprostol.[215] Proton pump inhibitors represent a suitable means of preventing the development of gastroduodenal ulcers associated with the use of NSAIDs and appear to provide a safe and effective form of therapy for NSAID-associated dyspepsia.[9] A recent, updated Cochrane systematic review with data collected up to 2009[103] concluded that misoprostol and proton pump inhibitors are effective at preventing chronic NSAID-related endoscopic gastric and duodenal ulcers. However, lower doses of misoprostol are less effective and are still associated with diarrhea. In patients with previous gastrointestinal bleeds caused by an NSAID, a COX-2 inhibitor alone is equivalent to a traditional NSAID plus proton pump inhibitor, though both strategies have relatively high rebleeding rates. The greatest gastrointestinal safety profile in high-risk patients is therefore offered by the combination of a COX-2 inhibitor and a proton pump inhibitor,[103] and this is the standard recommended protocol.[9]

Cardiovascular

Risk for myocardial infarction and ischemic stroke

Although COX-2 inhibitors gained widespread popularity as effective anti-inflammatory and analgesic agents with reduced gastrointestinal side effects,[194–196] concerns over cardiovascular risk of selective COX-2 inhibitors were raised as early as 2001 and may outweigh any gain in gastrointestinal safety.[204] Increased risk was shown for certain vascular events: MI and ischemic stroke.[23,216] Rofecoxib was withdrawn from the market in 2004 after it was found that it doubled the risk of vascular events compared with placebo (RR, 1.92; CI, 1.19 to 3.11).[216] Death from cardiovascular causes, MI, stroke, or heart failure was also higher in patients taking celecoxib, another COX-2 inhibitor, 200 mg or 400 mg twice per day, compared with the placebo group (RR, 2.8; CI, 1.3 to 6.3).[217] MI, cardiac arrest, stroke, and pulmonary embolism were more frequent among the patients given the newer coxibs—valdecoxib and its prodrug parecoxib—than among those given placebo. A pooled analysis of these studies suggests that parecoxib/valdecoxib elevates the combined incidence of MI and stroke by threefold in these populations.[218] Valdecoxib was voluntarily withdrawn from the market in 2005 due to safety concerns of increased risk of cardiovascular events and reports of serious and potentially life-threatening skin reactions, including deaths.

Current users of any nonselective NSAIDs are estimated to have up to a twofold increase in risk of hospitalization for congestive heart failure, and an even greater risk exists for patients with preexisting heart disease.[23,210] The risk is dose dependent and higher during the first month of therapy.[23,219] Most frequently, NSAIDs used in clinical practice, except naproxen, are associated with an increased risk of acute MI at high doses or in persons with diagnosed coronary heart disease. For diclofenac and rofecoxib, the risk was increased at low and high doses.[101] Even short-term treatment with most NSAIDs was associated with increased risk of death and recurrent MI in patients with prior MI. Neither short- nor long-term treatment with NSAIDs is advised in this population.[90] In-

domethacin may increase the risk of serious cardiovascular events and is to be avoided in at-risk patients.[21,94,101] Evidence points out that, particularly at high doses, ibuprofen increased risk for serious cardiovascular events.[21–23] Ibuprofen significantly increased the risk for major coronary events (RR, 2·22; CI, 1.10 to 4.48; $P = .0253$) but not major vascular events (RR, 1.44; CI, 0.89 to 2.33), whereas high-dose naproxen is associated with less vascular risk than other NSAIDs.[220] Naproxen has emerged as the safest NSAID in most studies when cardiovascular risks are considered,[10,21–24] and it may be combined with a proton pump inhibitor as needed,[9,25] providing excellent analgesia as well as gastrointestinal and cardiovascular safety. In aspirin-treated patients with first-time MI, treatment with proton pump inhibitors was associated with an increased risk of adverse cardiovascular events but no increase in risk related to use of H2 receptor blockers.

A recent systematic review[20] demonstrated that among commonly used NSAIDs, naproxen (RR, 1.09; CI, 1.02 to 1.16) and low-dose ibuprofen (RR, 1.18; CI, 1.11 to 1.25) are least likely to increase cardiovascular risk. Ibuprofen risk was seen only with higher doses. Naproxen was risk-neutral at all doses. Diclofenac in doses available without prescription elevates risk (RR, 1.40; CI, 1.27 to 1.55). Of the less studied drugs, etoricoxib (RR, 2.05; CI, 1.45 to 2.88), etodolac (RR, 1.55; CI, 1.28 to 1.87), and indomethacin (RR, 1.30; CI, 1.19 to 1.41) had the highest risks. In pairwise comparisons, etoricoxib had a higher RR than ibuprofen (RR, 1.68; CI, 1.14 to 2.49) and naproxen (RR; CI, 1.16 to 2.64); etodolac was not significantly different from naproxen and ibuprofen. Naproxen had a significantly lower risk than ibuprofen, and low-dose ibuprofen (RR, 1.18; CI, 1.11 to 1.25) was least likely to increase cardiovascular risk. Ibuprofen risk was seen only with higher doses. The authors of the review concluded[20] that among widely used NSAIDs, naproxen and low-dose ibuprofen are least likely to increase cardiovascular risk. In 2013, the same authors[95] studied the extent to which evidence on cardiovascular risk with NSAIDs has translated into guidance and sales in 15 countries. They found that no preference was given to low-risk drugs and that diclofenac and etoricoxib accounted for 33.2% of market share and naproxen for less than 10%. They recommend that diclofenac should be removed from the Essential Medicine Lists. Etoricoxib is currently not available in the US market.

Hypertension

Patients with hypertension who are on NSAIDs are more susceptible to blood pressure increases than patients who are normotensive,[221] and they also demonstrate significantly increased rates of MI or cerebrovascular accident relative to patients who are normotensive.[222] Concomitant NSAID and antihypertensive treatment may induce clinically significant drug interactions. Indomethacin and piroxicam induce a greater hypertensive effect compared with alternative NSAIDs. A relatively greater antagonism is also found between NSAIDs and beta-blockers compared with other antihypertensives.[222] Fortunately, the cardiovascular risk of short-term use of most NSAIDs is minimal, and most serious side effects occur only after long-term use. Three classes of antihypertensive agents, however, can interact with NSAIDs: angiotensin-converting enzyme inhibitors, beta-blockers, and diuretics. The action of all these drugs is aided by renal prostaglandins. With the principal effect of NSAIDs being prostaglandin inhibition, the effectiveness of these agents may be diminished. This interaction usually takes approximately 7 to 8 days to occur. Therefore, NSAID use in a patient with hypertension who is on these medications should be limited to 4 to 6 days.[32]

Platelet effects and concomitant aspirin use

Human platelets and vascular endothelial cells process PGH_2 to produce TXA2 and PGI_2, respectively.[191] COX-1 converts arachidonic acid to TXA2 (mostly from platelets), which induces platelet aggregation and vasoconstriction. COX-2 is responsible for the conversion of arachidonic acid to PGI_2, which inhibits platelet aggregation and induces vasodilation. Selective inhibition of COX-2 suppresses PGI_2 production without affecting TXA2 and predisposes a patient to hypertension and increased thromboembolic risks, the so-called prothrombotic effect.[192,193]

The best-characterized mechanism of action of aspirin is related to its capacity to irreversibly inactivate COX-1 and COX-2. Because aspirin probably also inactivates COX-1 in relatively mature megakaryocytes, and only 10% of the platelet pool is replenished each day, once-daily dosing of aspirin is able to maintain virtually complete inhibition of platelet TXA2 production.[223] Vascular PGI_2 can be derived from COX-1 and COX-2,[224] and there is substantial residual COX-2-dependent PGI_2 biosynthesis in vivo at daily doses of aspirin in the range of 30 to 100 mg to maintain vascular homeostasis.[225] Experimental studies support the importance of PGI_2 in the prevention of arterial thrombosis.[226] Research has not established that more profound suppression of PGI_2 formation by higher doses of aspirin is sufficient to initiate or to predispose to thrombosis. However, one trial showed a significantly lower rate of vascular events in patients receiving 80 or 325 mg of aspirin compared with patients receiving 650 or 1,300 mg daily, which is consistent with an important role for PGI_2 in preventing thrombosis.[227]

In contrast to the irreversible effects of aspirin, traditional NSAIDs reversibly inhibit platelet aggregation and prolong bleeding time.[228] The regular administration of naproxen 500 mg twice a day can mimic the antiplatelet COX-1 effect of low-dose aspirin but does not decrease PGI_2 biosynthesis in vivo.[229] Rofecoxib and valdecoxib do not impair platelet aggregation, and rofecoxib does not alter the antiplatelet effect of aspirin.[230,231] Thus, in terms of bleeding, COX-2 inhibitors may be given more safely than traditional NSAIDs in the dental perioperative setting.

Aspirin is taken on a daily basis by a large number of patients, especially for cardioprotection.[229] Choosing an analgesic that does not interfere with aspirin's action or increase adverse events is important. For example, the use of NSAIDs in conjunction with aspirin may increase the risk of gastrointestinal complications. Moreover, ibuprofen and naproxen interfere with aspirin's ability to irreversibly acetylate platelet COX-1 and, theoretically, may reduce aspirin's protective antithrombotic effect.[229] Data from epidemiologic studies suggest that taking any NSAID may cancel aspirin's cardioprotective effects.[229] Treatment with NSAIDs, particularly ibuprofen or naproxen, should be avoided in patients taking concomitant low-dose aspirin.[10] Taking aspirin before ibuprofen or naproxen ingestion does not seem to resolve this interaction.[10,229] The use of COX-2 inhibitors in patients taking aspirin a priori defeats the very reason for prescribing COX-2 inhibitors: gastrointestinal safety. Preferentially using acetaminophen for these patients would therefore seem prudent.[229]

Selective serotonin reuptake inhibitor antidepressants decrease platelet serotonin storage and platelet function and may be associated with postsurgical bleeding. However, the frequency of oral bleeding complications after invasive dental treatment is low to negligible in patients taking selective serotonin reuptake inhibitor medications.[232]

American Heart Association statement

The American Heart Association released its latest scientific statement to aid clinicians in the selection of analgesics for patients with increased cardiovascular risk.[10] Their recommendations reiterate the conclusions summarized in detail at the beginning of this chapter. In brief, for patients with increased cardiovascular risk, acetaminophen or aspirin should be tried initially. Naproxen remains the NSAID with the most data indicating no increased risk for cardiovascular events and is therefore a logical second option; the use of gastroprotective agents should be considered in at-risk persons.[214] COX-2 inhibitors are contraindicated in patients with recent bypass surgery, unstable angina, previous MI, ischemic cerebrovascular events, or any other active atherosclerotic process, as they are associated with significantly increased risk for adverse cardiovascular events.[10] Additionally, COX-2 inhibitors may lead to impaired renal perfusion, sodium retention, and increased blood pressure, which contribute to increased cardiovascular risk. When NSAIDs are indicated, they should be used at the lowest dose for the shortest time, particularly COX-2 inhibitors.[10]

Renal

The kidney is the second most frequent target of serious adverse effects of NSAIDs related to inhibition of COX; it is estimated to affect 2 million patients annually in the United States alone.[233] The epidemiologic impact is substantial, and current users of NSAIDs are estimated to be two to four times more at risk for acute renal failure.[4–6] This risk is dose dependent and is highest (RR > 8) during the first month of therapy.[5,6] Indomethacin presented a higher RR for acute renal failure than the other conventional NSAIDs.[6] Other risk factors for acute renal failure are long drug half-life, male sex, increasing age, cardiovascular comorbidity, renal diseases, concomitant use of other nephrotoxic drugs, and any recent hospitalization.[5,6] The NSAID effect on acute renal failure is stronger among patients with a previous history of renal disease and in those with a history of gout or hyperuricemia. Among these patients, NSAID exposure increases the risk of acute renal failure by a factor of seven.[5,234]

The renal side effects of NSAIDs include reduction in renal blood flow and glomerular filtration rate, sodium/water retention, and hyperkalemia.[233] Animal experiments and clinical trials with preferential and specific COX-2 inhibitors revealed that COX-2 is the critical enzyme for sodium excretion and renin release and the likely antagonism of antidiuretic hormone; these are prime examples of a constitutive role for COX-2. Additionally, a significant role of COX-2 in nephrogenesis is suggested.[235] Furthermore, PGI_2 significantly influences the renal system of medically compromised patients, especially those with diabetes, peripheral vascular disease, or other causes of renal insufficiency. COX-2 inhibition decreases PGE_2 and PGI_2, modifiers of glomerular filtration in compromised kidneys, and causes sodium retention, promoting peripheral edema and hypertension as well as lower renal perfusion with renal ischemia.[236] The dose-dependent consequences of standard NSAIDs and COX-2 inhibitors on the kidney include elevated blood pressure, edema, and congestive heart failure in some compromised patients and in patients taking beta-adrenergic blocker drugs or angiotensin-converting enzyme inhibitors.[237] The risk is much higher in individuals who have a low perfusion state, as in congestive heart failure.[238]

At this stage, with regard to renal adverse events, it can be concluded that selective

COX-2 inhibitors do not offer a clinically relevant advantage over conventional NSAIDs.[118,232] The renal effect, however, seems to be related to individual COX-2 inhibitors and is not a class effect.[102,233] Rofecoxib has been found to significantly increase the risk for peripheral edema, hypertension, renal dysfunction, and arrhythmias, and increased dose and duration were associated with increased risk.[102] A multicenter study assessed renal function during dosing with etoricoxib 90 mg daily, celecoxib 200 mg twice daily, and naproxen 500 mg twice daily. Men and women 60 to 81 years old (n = 85) who were on a controlled, normal-sodium diet were treated for 15 days. No clinically meaningful between-treatment differences were found in urinary sodium excretion, creatinine clearance, body weight, or serum electrolytes during the 2 weeks of treatment. Systolic blood pressures were significantly higher in all the treatment groups than in the placebo group, and there were moderately greater increases for etoricoxib relative to other active treatments. Diastolic blood pressures were significantly higher than those in the placebo group for the etoricoxib and naproxen groups but not for the celecoxib group.[239] High-dose celecoxib (400 mg twice a day) was relatively well tolerated for 6 months[54] in persons with prostate cancer who participated in an oncologic trial. Renal functional reserve remained stable, and there were minor electrolyte alterations.[240] From these data, celecoxib seems to express somewhat more favorable results than other NSAIDs.

Hypersensitivity reaction

Aspirin and other NSAIDs have a well-known potential to exacerbate various forms of urticaria and asthma.[241,242] Aspirin sensitivity can be confirmed by drug challenge tests in 20% to 41% of patients with urticaria.[243] In contrast, the rate of aspirin sensitivity in the healthy population is about 1%.[244] Susceptible persons have cross-sensitivity to the entire class of drugs, regardless of their chemical structure. The most common clinical presentation is urticaria and angioedema. Current theories regarding the mechanisms of NSAID sensitivity in chronic idiopathic urticaria are largely inferred from studies of an analogous, well-defined clinical syndrome of aspirin-induced asthma,

which affects about 10% of adult patients with asthma.[242] Both syndromes affect middle-aged persons, and there is a female preponderance. Sensitivity to NSAIDs is present in only a subset of patients with asthma and chronic idiopathic urticaria. Although some NSAID-induced cutaneous eruptions are immunologic, in most cases the mechanism involves inhibition of COX. In aspirin-induced asthma the mechanism of sensitivity involves inhibition of COX-1.[245] At the biochemical level, aspirin-induced asthma is characterized by overproduction of leukotrienes and increased urinary excretion of leukotriene E_4.[246] The mechanism of sensitivity to NSAIDs in chronic idiopathic urticaria is also associated with overproduction of leukotrienes and mast cell activation and most likely depends on inhibition of COX-1.[247]

COX-2 inhibitors do not induce urticaria in patients with chronic idiopathic urticaria who are sensitive to NSAIDs. Etoricoxib, a second-generation COX-2 inhibitor, at 120-mg dosage was found to be safe in patients with NSAID drug–induced urticaria and angioedema[35,36] as well as in aspirin-induced asthma.[34] However, a previous challenge test in a safe environment may be necessary before prescribing the drug to such patients.[29] Celecoxib 200 mg was also safe in patients with aspirin-induced asthma[37,38] and in most patients with cutaneous reactions due to aspirin/NSAIDs intolerance.[28]

Cross-reactivity of patients with aspirin-induced asthma to acetaminophen is fairly prevalent, especially in doses greater than 1,000 mg. Thus, 34% of patients with aspirin-induced asthma reacted to acetaminophen in doses of 1,000 to 1,500 mg (CI, 20% to 49%). By contrast, none of the patients who did not have aspirin-induced asthma reacted to acetaminophen (CI, 0% to 14%). This difference was highly significant and supports the hypothesis that cross-sensitivity between aspirin and acetaminophen is unique in patients with aspirin-induced asthma. Investigators recommend that frequent (daily) or high doses of acetaminophen (1,000 mg or greater) should be avoided in patients with asthma who are aspirin sensitive.[248] Evidence suggests that the risk of asthma might be increased in later childhood with exposure to acetaminophen during pregnancy (OR, 1.21; CI, 1.02 to 1.44).[59] The evidence was confirmed in a later study[60] showing an adjusted incidence rate ratio of 1.35 (CI, 1.17 to 1.57) for exposure in any trimester of pregnancy. Daily acetaminophen use increases the risk of asthma by a factor of 2.38 (CI, 1.22 to 4.64).

Anaphylactic shock and urticaria/angioedema after a single dose of dipyrone has been reported.[249] All patients had positive skin tests to these drugs but no cross-reactivity with NSAIDs. Dipyrone-induced hypersensitivity reactions include skin rash with an intriguing geographic difference in frequency.[135] Respiratory asthma-like reactions with cross-reactivity in patients sensitive to aspirin have been reported more rarely.[135] Dipyrone has been clearly shown to cause agranulocytosis, but there is insufficient useful information to adequately quantify the risk. Most studies are old, methodologically weak, and small and use different definitions of agranulocytosis.[250] Absolute risks are the ones that are important when determining harm. Absolute risks of rare events after some drug treatments have been determined, but this is not possible for determining the risk of agranulocytosis with dipyrone, and uncertainty is likely to remain.[207,250]

The pathogenesis of agranulocytosis after the use of dipyrone (and other pyrazolones) is considered immunologic.[135] Conflicting data and regulations prevail worldwide as to the incidence of agranulocytosis after the use of pyrazolones in general and dipyrone in particular.[135] A multinational study found significant regional variability in the risk ratio for agranulocytosis after the use of dipyrone.[251] In Ulm, Berlin, and Barcelona, Spain, the risk ratio was 23.7, and the excess risk estimate connected with hospital admission for agranulocytosis from any dipyrone use in a 7-day period amounted to 1.1 cases per million users. In Israel and Budapest, Hungary, there was no evidence of increased risk associated with dipyrone use.[251] The reason for the geographic variation in the risk of dipyrone-induced agranulocytosis and rash is unclear.[135] In a recent study in Poland, where the drug is a common nonprescription product, estimates of the rate of agranulocytosis and aplastic anemia associated with metamizole (dipyrone) were 0.16 and 0.08 cases/million person-days of use, respectively.[136] Non–chemotherapy drug–induced agranulocytosis is considered a potentially life-threatening idio-syncratic blood dyscrasia that is thought to result from a partly elucidated immune response and/or toxic damage on myelopoiesis due to a multitude of drugs.[137] With improved intensive care treatment and alert physicians, the case fatality of the disorder has recently decreased to 5%.[137]

Considerations for Analgesic Use

Pregnancy and breastfeeding

Counseling pregnant women regarding the risks or safety of drug treatments is often complicated by a lack of information about the nature, magnitude, or even existence of a teratogenic risk in humans. The mean time for a treatment initially classified as having an undetermined risk to be assigned a more precise risk was 27 years (CI, 26 to 28 years). The lack of information needed to assess the safety of drug treatments during human pregnancy remains a serious public health problem.[252] NSAIDs and aspirin may affect fertility and increase the risk of early pregnancy loss. In the second trimester, their use is considered reasonably safe, but the drug has been associated with fetal cryptorchidism. In the third trimester, NSAIDs and aspirin are usually avoided because of significant fetal risks, such as renal injury, oligohydramnios, and constriction of the ductus arteriosus (with potential for persistent pulmonary hypertension in newborns), necrotizing enterocolitis, and intracranial hemorrhage. Maternal administration or ingestion of most NSAIDs results in low infant exposure via breast milk, such that both COX-1 and COX-2 inhibitors are generally considered safe, and preferable to aspirin, when breastfeeding.[253]

Use of NSAIDs during the first 20 weeks of pregnancy was associated with an 80% increased risk of miscarriage over non-use (RR, 1.8; CI, 1 to 3.2). Risk of miscarriage was highest when the drug was taken around the time of conception (RR, 5.6; CI, 2.3 to 13.7) or used for more than a week (RR, 8.1; CI, 2.8 to 23.4). Absolute risk of NSAID-associated miscarriage was 10% for any use, 35% for use around the time of conception, and 52% for use longer than 1 week.[254] However, prenatal use of acetaminophen and aspirin was not associated with increased risk of miscarriage, regardless of timing and duration of use.[254] In view of the aforementioned, warnings of drug effects on reproduction have been included in the product labeling of marketed NSAIDs and COX-2-specific inhibitors.[255]

Acetaminophen is the analgesic of choice during pregnancy or breastfeeding (pregnancy category B). However, the use of acetaminophen, but not aspirin, was positively associated with asthma and persistent wheezing in infants of mothers who took acetaminophen frequently (defined as most days or daily use) in late pregnancy.[256] The risk of asthma in later childhood might be increased with exposure to acetaminophen during pregnancy (OR, 1.21; CI, 1.02 to 1.44),[59] a finding confirmed in a later study[60] showing an adjusted incidence rate ratio of 1.35 (CI, 1.17 to 1.57) for exposure in any trimester of pregnancy. No association was found with hay fever, eczema, or skin-test positivity. The proportion of asthma attributable to acetaminophen use in late pregnancy, assuming a causal relation, was 7%.[256] The number of pregnant women taking frequent doses was very small, so the authors recommend that infrequent acetaminophen remains the analgesic of choice in pregnancy.[256] For specific analgesic use during pregnancy, consult the relevant section for each drug.

Pharmacogenomics

Genomic variations influence response to pharmacotherapy of pain. Polymorphisms of CYP2D6 influence metabolism of codeine, tramadol, hydrocodone, oxycodone, and tricyclic antidepressants. Blood concentrations of some NSAIDs depend on CYP2C9 and/or CYP2C8 activity. Genomic variants of these genes associate well with the side-effect profile of NSAIDs. Although pharmacogenetics as a diagnostic tool has the potential to improve patient therapy, well-designed studies are still needed to demonstrate superiority to conventional dosing regimens.[257] The modulation of CYP2D6 and CYP3A activities had clear effects on oxycodone pharmacodynamics, and these effects were dependent on CYP2D6 genetic polymorphism.[12]

Codeine is biotransformed by the highly polymorphic CYP2D6.[11] Ultrarapid metabolizers, that is, persons with multiple active copies of CYP2D6, can biotransform up to 50% more codeine into morphine than clinically normal persons can. These persons will have immediate pain relief from codeine but with a lot of adverse effects due to dizziness and constipation. In contrast, poor metabolizers, that is, persons who have no active CYP2D6 genes, convert almost no codeine into morphine and as a result may take multiple doses of codeine without attaining analgesia.[146] The enzyme catechol-O-methyltransferase (COMT) metabolizes catecholamine neurotransmitters involved in a number of physiologic functions, including pain perception. COMT genes possess functional polymorphisms contributing to interindividual variability in pain phenotypes, such as sensitivity to noxious stimuli, severity of clinical pain, and response to pain treatment. In humans, the haplotype coding for low COMT activity increased experimentally capsaicin-induced pain perception in women but not men.[15] The COMT single-nucleotide polymorphism was associated with a clinically meaningful pain outcome after third-molar extraction.[13] Notably, even though many studies investigated a possible role of the CYP2D6 polymorphisms on pain sensitivity, pharmacokinetics and pharmacodynamics of these drugs, the results of analgesia, and adverse effects are conflicting.[147]

References

1. Manchikanti L, Helm S 2nd, Fellows B, et al. Opioid epidemic in the United States. Pain Physician 2012;15(suppl 3):S9–S38.
2. Volkow ND, McLellan TA, Cotto JH, Karithanom M, Weiss SR. Characteristics of opioid prescriptions in 2009. JAMA 2011;305:1299–1301.
3. Drugs.com. US Pharmaceutical Sales—2013. Top 100 Drugs for 2013 by Units Sold. http://www.drugs.com/stats/top100/2013/units. Acessed 23 May 2015.
4. Evans JM, McGregor E, McMahon AD, et al. Non-steroidal anti-inflammatory drugs and hospitalization for acute renal failure. QJM 1995;88:551-557.
5. Henry D, Page J, Whyte I, Nanra R, Hall C. Consumption of non-steroidal anti-inflammatory drugs and the development of functional renal impairment in elderly subjects. Results of a case-control study. Br J Clin Pharmacol 1997;44:85–90.

6. Pérez Gutthann S, García Rodríguez LA, Raiford DS, Duque Oliart A, Ris Romeu J. Nonsteroidal anti-inflammatory drugs and the risk of hospitalization for acute renal failure. Arch Intern Med 1996;156:2433-2439.

7. Paulozzi LJ. Prescription drug overdoses: A review. J Safety Res 2012;43:283–289.

8. Genetic Engineering & Biotechnology News. Top 17 Abused Prescription Drugs of 2013. http://www.genengnews.com/insight-and-intelligenceand153/top-17-abused-prescription-drugs-of-2013/77899961/. Accessed 23 May 2015.

9. Abraham NS, Hlatky MA, Antman EM, et al. ACCF/ACG/AHA 2010 Expert Consensus Document on the concomitant use of proton pump inhibitors and thienopyridines: A focused update of the ACCF/ACG/AHA 2008 expert consensus document on reducing the gastrointestinal risks of antiplatelet therapy and NSAID use: A report of the American College of Cardiology Foundation Task Force on Expert Consensus Documents. Circulation 2010;122:2619–2633.

10. Antman EM, Bennett JS, Daugherty A, et al. Use of nonsteroidal antiinflammatory drugs: An update for clinicians: A scientific statement from the American Heart Association. Circulation 2007;115:1634–1642.

11. Lötsch J, Geisslinger G. Current evidence for a genetic modulation of the response to analgesics. Pain 2006;121:1–5.

12. Stamer UM, Zhang L, Book M, Lehmann LE, Stuber F, Musshoff F. CYP2D6 genotype dependent oxycodone metabolism in postoperative patients. PLoS One 2013;8(3).

13. Lee PJ, Delaney P, Keogh J, Sleeman D, Shorten GD. Catecholamine-o-methyltransferase polymorphisms are associated with postoperative pain intensity. Clin J Pain 2011;27:93–101.

14. Walker JS, Carmody JJ. Experimental pain in healthy human subjects: Gender differences in nociception and in response to ibuprofen. Anesth Analg 1998;86:1257–1262.

15. Belfer I, Segall SK, Lariviere WR, et al. Pain modality- and sex-specific effects of COMT genetic functional variants. Pain 2013;154:1368–1376.

16. Kuner R. Central mechanisms of pathological pain. Nat Med 2010;16:1258–1266.

17. Graham GG, Davies MJ, Day RO, Mohamudally A, Scott KF. The modern pharmacology of paracetamol: Therapeutic actions, mechanism of action, metabolism, toxicity and recent pharmacological findings. Inflammopharmacology 2013;21:201–232.

18. Sachs CJ. Oral analgesics for acute nonspecific pain. Am Fam Physician 2005;71:913–918.

19. Moore PA, Hersh EV. Combining ibuprofen and acetaminophen for acute pain management after third-molar extractions: Translating clinical research to dental practice. J Am Dent Assoc 2013;144:898–908.

20. McGettigan P, Henry D. Cardiovascular risk with non-steroidal anti-inflammatory drugs: Systematic review of population-based controlled observational studies. PLoS Med 2011;8(9).

21. McGettigan P, Henry D. Cardiovascular risk and inhibition of cyclooxygenase: A systematic review of the observational studies of selective and nonselective inhibitors of cyclooxygenase 2. JAMA 2006;296:1633–1644.

22. Jüni P, Reichenbach S, Egger M. COX 2 inhibitors, traditional NSAIDs, and the heart. BMJ 2005;330:1342–1343.

23. Kearney PM, Baigent C, Godwin J, Halls H, Emberson JR, Patrono C. Do selective cyclo-oxygenase-2 inhibitors and traditional non-steroidal anti-inflammatory drugs increase the risk of atherothrombosis? Meta-analysis of randomised trials. BMJ 2006;332:1302–1308.

24. McGettigan P, Lincz LF, Attia J, et al. The risk of coronary thrombosis with cyclo-oxygenase-2 inhibitors does not vary with polymorphisms in two regions of the cyclo-oxygenase-2 gene. Br J Clin Pharmacol 2011;72:707–714.

25. Lai KC, Chu KM, Hui WM, et al. Celecoxib compared with lansoprazole and naproxen to prevent gastrointestinal ulcer complications. Am J Med 2005;118:1271–1278.

26. Woessner KM, Simon RA, Stevenson DD. The safety of celecoxib in patients with aspirin-sensitive asthma. Arthritis Rheum 2002;46:2201–2206.

27. Kowalski ML, Makowska J. Use of nonsteroidal anti-inflammatory drugs in patients with aspirin hypersensitivity: Safety of cyclo-oxygenase-2 inhibitors. Treat Respir Med 2006;5:399–406.

28. Andri L, Falagiani P. Safety of celecoxib in patients with cutaneous reactions due to ASA-NSAIDs intolerance. Allergol Immunopathol (Madr) 2007;35(4):126-129.

29. Muratore L, Ventura M, Calogiuri G, et al. Tolerance to etoricoxib in 37 patients with urticaria and angioedema induced by nonsteroidal anti-inflammatory drugs. Ann Allergy Asthma Immunol 2007;98:168–171.

30. Edwards JE, Moore RA, McQuay HJ. Single dose oxycodone and oxycodone plus paracetamol (acetaminophen) for acute postoperative pain. Cochrane Database Syst Rev 2000;(4).

31. Gaskell H, Derry S, Moore RA, McQuay HJ. Single dose oral oxycodone and oxycodone plus paracetamol (acetaminophen) for acute postoperative pain in adults. Cochrane Database Syst Rev 2009;(3).

32. Haas DA. Adverse drug interactions in dental practice: Interactions associated with analgesics, Part III in a series. J Am Dent Assoc 1999;130:397–407.

33. Martín-García C, Hinojosa M, Berges P, et al. Safety of a cyclooxygenase-2 inhibitor in patients with aspirin-sensitive asthma. Chest 2002;121:1812–1817.

34. El Miedany Y, Youssef S, Ahmed I, El Gaafary M. Safety of etoricoxib, a specific cyclooxygenase-2 inhibitor, in asthmatic patients with aspirin-exacerbated respiratory disease. Ann Allergy Asthma Immunol 2006;97:105–109.

35. Viola M, Quaratino D, Gaeta F, Caruso C, Valluzzi R, Romano A. Etoricoxib tolerability in patients with hypersensitivity to nonsteroidal anti-inflammatory drugs. Int Arch Allergy Immunol 2007;143:103–108.

36. Sánchez-Borges M, Caballero-Fonseca F, Capriles-Hulett A. Safety of etoricoxib, a new cyclooxygenase 2 inhibitor, in patients with nonsteroidal anti-inflammatory drug-induced urticaria and angioedema. Ann Allergy Asthma Immunol 2005;95:154–158.

37. Celik G, Pasaoglu G, Bavbek S, et al. Tolerability of selective cyclooxygenase inhibitor, celecoxib, in patients with analgesic intolerance. J Asthma 2005;42:127–131.

38. Martín-García C, Hinojosa M, Berges P, Camacho E, García-Rodriguez R, Alfaya T. Celecoxib, a highly selective COX-2 inhibitor, is safe in aspirin-induced asthma patients. J Investig Allergol Clin Immunol 2003;13:20–25.

39. Wolfe MM, Lichtenstein DR, Singh G. Gastrointestinal toxicity of nonsteroidal antiinflammatory drugs. N Engl J Med 1999;340:1888–1899.

40. Barden J, Edwards JE, McQuay HJ, Moore RA. Single dose oral celecoxib for postoperative pain. Cochrane Database Syst Rev 2003;(2).

41. Barden J, Edwards J, Moore A, McQuay H. Single dose oral paracetamol (acetaminophen) for postoperative pain. Cochrane Database Syst Rev 2004;(1).

42. Barden J, Edwards J, Moore RA, McQuay HJ. Single dose oral rofecoxib for postoperative pain. Cochrane Database Syst Rev 2005;(1).

43. Collins SL, Moore RA, McQuay HJ, Wiffen PJ, Edwards JE. Single dose oral ibuprofen and diclofenac for postoperative pain. Cochrane Database Syst Rev 2000;(2).

44. Mason L, Edwards JE, Moore RA, McQuay HJ. Single dose oral naproxen and naproxen sodium for acute postoperative pain. Cochrane Database Syst Rev 2004;(4).

45. Weil K, Hooper L, Afzal Z, et al. Paracetamol for pain relief after surgical removal of lower wisdom teeth. Cochrane Database Syst Rev 2007;(3).

46. Moore A, Collins S, Carroll D, McQuay H, Edwards J. Single dose paracetamol (acetaminophen), with and without codeine, for postoperative pain. Cochrane Database Syst Rev 2000;(2).

47. Moore A, Collins S, Carroll D, McQuay H. Paracetamol with and without codeine in acute pain: A quantitative systematic review. Pain 1997;70:193–201.

48. Carlsson KH, Jurna I. Central analgesic effect of paracetamol manifested by depression of nociceptive activity in thalamic neurones of the rat. Neurosci Lett 1987;77:339–343.

49. Graham GG, Scott KF. Mechanism of action of paracetamol. Am J Ther 2005;12:46–55.

50. Ottani A, Leone S, Sandrini M, Ferrari A, Bertolini A. The analgesic activity of paracetamol is prevented by the blockade of cannabinoid CB1 receptors. Eur J Pharmacol 2006;531:280–281.

51. Bertolini A, Ferrari A, Ottani A, Guerzoni S, Tacchi R, Leone S. Paracetamol: New vistas of an old drug. CNS Drug Rev 2006;12:250–275.

52. Hyllested M, Jones S, Pedersen JL, Kehlet H. Comparative effect of paracetamol, NSAIDs or their combination in postoperative pain management: A qualitative review. Br J Anaesth 2002;88:199–214.

53. Bjornsson GA, Haanaes HR, Skoglund LA. A randomized, double-blind crossover trial of paracetamol 1000 mg four times daily vs ibuprofen 600 mg: Effect on swelling and other postoperative events after third molar surgery. Br J Clin Pharmacol 2003;55:405–412.

54. Gadisseur AP, Van Der Meer FJ, Rosendaal FR. Sustained intake of paracetamol (acetaminophen) during oral anticoagulant therapy with coumarins does not cause clinically important INR changes: A randomized double-blind clinical trial. J Thromb Haemost 2003;1:714–717.

55. Nikles CJ, Yelland M, Del Mar C, Wilkinson D. The role of paracetamol in chronic pain: An evidence-based approach. Am J Ther 2005;12:80–91.

56. Woodcock J. A difficult balance—pain management, drug safety, and the FDA. N Engl J Med 2009;361:2105–2107.

57. Watkins PB, Kaplowitz N, Slattery JT, et al. Aminotransferase elevations in healthy adults receiving 4 grams of acetaminophen daily: A randomized controlled trial. JAMA 2006;296:87–93.

58. US Food and Drug Administration. FDA Warns of Rare Acetaminophen Risk. http://www.fda.gov/ForConsumers/ConsumerUpdates/ucm363010.htm. Acessed 23 May 2015.

59. Eyers S, Weatherall M, Jefferies S, Beasley R. Paracetamol in pregnancy and the risk of wheezing in offspring: A systematic review and meta-analysis. Clin Exp Allergy 2011;41:482–489.

60. Andersen AB, Farkas DK, Mehnert F, Ehrenstein V, Erichsen R. Use of prescription paracetamol during pregnancy and risk of asthma in children: A population-based Danish cohort study. Clin Epidemiol 2012;4:33–40.

61. Rebordosa C, Kogevinas M, Bech BH, Sorensen HT, Olsen J. Use of acetaminophen during pregnancy and risk of adverse pregnancy outcomes. Int J Epidemiol 2009;38:706–714.

62. Jensen MS, Rebordosa C, Thulstrup AM, et al. Maternal use of acetaminophen, ibuprofen, and acetylsalicylic acid during pregnancy and risk of cryptorchidism. Epidemiology 2010;21:779–785.

63. Henman MC, Leach GD, Naylor IL. Production of prostaglandin-like materials by rat tail skin in response to injury [proceedings]. Br J Pharmacol 1979;66:448P.

64. Roszkowski MT, Swift JQ, Hargreaves KM. Effect of NSAID administration on tissue levels of immunoreactive prostaglandin E2, leukotriene B4, and (S)-flurbiprofen after extraction of impacted third molars. Pain 1997;73:339–345.

65. Norholt SE. Treatment of acute pain following removal of mandibular third molars. Use of the dental pain model in pharmacological research and development of a comparable animal model. Int J Oral Maxillofac Surg 1998;27(suppl 1):1–41.

66. Gotzsche PC. Musculoskeletal disorders. Non-steroidal anti-inflammatory drugs. Clin Evid 2005;(14):1498–1505.

67. Huskisson EC, Woolf DL, Balme HW, Scott J, Franklin S. Four new anti-inflammatory drugs: Responses and variations. Br Med J 1976;1:1048–1049.

68. Eisenberg E, Berkey CS, Carr DB, Mosteller F, Chalmers TC. Efficacy and safety of nonsteroidal antiinflammatory drugs for cancer pain: A meta-analysis. J Clin Oncol 1994;12:2756–2765.

69. Henry D, Lim LL, García Rodríguez LA, et al. Variability in risk of gastrointestinal complications with individual non-steroidal anti-inflammatory drugs: Results of a collaborative meta-analysis. BMJ 1996;312:1563–1566.

70. Dionne RA, Berthold CW. Therapeutic uses of non-steroidal anti-inflammatory drugs in dentistry. Crit Rev Oral Biol Med 2001;12:315–330.

71. Zelenakas K, Fricke JR Jr, Jayawardene S, Kellstein D. Analgesic efficacy of single oral doses of lumiracoxib and ibuprofen in patients with postoperative dental pain. Int J Clin Pract 2004;58:251–256.

72. Seymour RA, Ward-Booth P, Kelly PJ. Evaluation of different doses of soluble ibuprofen and ibuprofen tablets in postoperative dental pain. Br J Oral Maxillofac Surg 1996;34:110–114.

73. Kellstein DE, Waksman JA, Furey SA, Binstok G, Cooper SA. The safety profile of nonprescription ibuprofen in multiple-dose use: A meta-analysis. J Clin Pharmacol 1999;39:520–532.

74. Coxib and traditional NSAID Trialists' (CNT) Collaboration, Bhala N, Emberson J, et al. Vascular and upper gastrointestinal effects of non-steroidal anti-inflammatory drugs: Meta-analyses of individual participant data from randomised trials. Lancet 2013;382:769–779.

75. Malmstrom K, Kotey P, Coughlin H, Desjardins PJ. A randomized, double-blind, parallel-group study comparing the analgesic effect of etoricoxib to placebo, naproxen sodium, and acetaminophen with codeine using the dental impaction pain model. Clin J Pain 2004;20:147–155.

76. Denisco RC, Kenna GA, O'Neil MG, et al. Prevention of prescription opioid abuse: The role of the dentist. J Am Dent Assoc 2011;142:800–810.

77. Derry CJ, Derry S, Moore RA. Single dose oral ibuprofen plus paracetamol (acetaminophen) for acute postoperative pain. Cochrane Database Syst Rev 2013;6.

78. Mason L, Edwards JE, Moore RA, McQuay HJ. Single-dose oral naproxen for acute postoperative pain: A quantitative systematic review. BMC Anesthesiol 2003;3:4.

79. Derry C, Derry S, Moore RA, McQuay HJ. Single dose oral naproxen and naproxen sodium for acute postoperative pain in adults. Cochrane Database Syst Rev 2009;(1).

80. Riendeau D, Percival MD, Brideau C, et al. Etoricoxib (MK-0663): Preclinical profile and comparison with other agents that selectively inhibit cyclooxygenase-2. J Pharmacol Exp Ther 2001;296:558–566.

81. Gaston GW, Mallow RD, Frank JE. Comparison of etodolac, aspirin and placebo for pain after oral surgery. Pharmacotherapy 1986;6:199–205.

82. Hutton CE. The effectiveness of 100 and 200 mg etodolac (ultradol), aspirin, and placebo in patients with pain following oral surgery. Oral Surg Oral Med Oral Pathol 1983;56:575–580.

83. Mizraji M. Clinical response to etodolac in the management of pain. Eur J Rheumatol Inflamm 1990;10:35–43.

84. Tirunagari SK, Derry S, Moore RA, McQuay HJ. Single dose oral etodolac for acute postoperative pain in adults. Cochrane Database Syst Rev 2009;(3).

85. Martel RR, Klicius J. Comparison in rats of the anti-inflammatory and gastric irritant effects of etodolac with several clinically effective anti-inflammatory drugs. Agents Actions 1982;12:295–297.

86. Helin-Salmivaara A, Saarelainen S, Grönroos JM, Vesalainen R, Klaukka T, Huupponen R. Risk of upper gastrointestinal events with the use of various NSAIDs: A case-control study in a general population. Scand J Gastroenterol 2007;42:923–932.

87. Derry P, Derry S, Moore RA, McQuay HJ. Single dose oral diclofenac for acute postoperative pain in adults. Cochrane Database Syst Rev 2009;(2).

88. Fosbol EL, Folke F, Jacobsen S, et al. Cause-specific cardiovascular risk associated with nonsteroidal anti-inflammatory drugs among healthy persons. Circ Cardiovasc Qual Outcomes 2010;3:395–405.

89. Varas-Lorenzo C, Riera-Guardia N, Calingaert B, et al. Stroke risk and NSAIDs: A systematic review of observational studies. Pharmacoepidemiol Drug Saf 2011;20:1225–1236.

90. Schjerning Olsen AM, Fosbol EL, Lindhardsen J, et al. Duration of treatment with nonsteroidal anti-inflammatory drugs and impact on risk of death and recurrent myocardial infarction in patients with prior myocardial infarction: A nationwide cohort study. Circulation 2011;123:2226–2235.

91. Daly AK, Aithal GP, Leathart JB, Swainsbury RA, Dang TS, Day CP. Genetic susceptibility to diclofenac-induced hepatotoxicity: Contribution of UGT2B7, CYP2C8, and ABCC2 genotypes. Gastroenterology 2007;132:272–281.

92. Larrey D. Epidemiology and individual susceptibility to adverse drug reactions affecting the liver. Semin Liver Dis 2002;22:145–155.

93. Andersohn F, Suissa S, Garbe E. Use of first- and second-generation cyclooxygenase-2-selective nonsteroidal antiinflammatory drugs and risk of acute myocardial infarction. Circulation 2006;113:1950–1957.

94. Helin-Salmivaara A, Virtanen A, Vesalainen R, et al. NSAID use and the risk of hospitalization for first myocardial infarction in the general population: A nationwide case-control study from Finland. Eur Heart J 2006;27:1657–1663.

95. McGettigan P, Henry D. Use of non-steroidal anti-inflammatory drugs that elevate cardiovascular risk: An examination of sales and essential medicines lists in low-, middle-, and high-income countries. PLoS Med 2013;10:e1001388.

96. Ohlsson A, Walia R, Shah SS. Ibuprofen for the treatment of patent ductus arteriosus in preterm and/or low birth weight infants. Cochrane Database Syst Rev 2013;4.

97. Buzzi MG, Sakas DE, Moskowitz MA. Indomethacin and acetylsalicylic acid block neurogenic plasma protein extravasation in rat dura mater. Eur J Pharmacol 1989;165:251–258.

98. Slavik RS, Rhoney DH. Indomethacin: A review of its cerebral blood flow effects and potential use for controlling intracranial pressure in traumatic brain injury patients. Neurol Res 1999;21:491–499.

99. Quintana A, Raczka E, Quintana MA. Effects of indomethacin and diclofenac on cerebral blood flow in hypercapnic conscious rats. Eur J Pharmacol 1988;149:385–388.

100. Ventura-Martínez R, Déciga-Campos M, Díaz-Reval MI, González-Trujano ME, López-Munoz FJ. Peripheral involvement of the nitric oxide-cGMP pathway in the indomethacin-induced antinociception in rat. Eur J Pharmacol 2004;503:43–48.

101. Varas-Lorenzo C, Riera-Guardia N, Calingaert B, et al. Myocardial infarction and individual nonsteroidal anti-inflammatory drugs meta-analysis of observational studies. Pharmacoepidemiol Drug Saf 2013;22:559–570.

102. Zhang J, Ding EL, Song Y. Adverse effects of cyclooxygenase 2 inhibitors on renal and arrhythmia events: Meta-analysis of randomized trials. JAMA 2006;296:1619–1632.

103. Rostom A, Muir K, Dube C, Lanas A, Jolicoeur E, Tugwell P. Prevention of NSAID-related upper gastrointestinal toxicity: A meta-analysis of traditional NSAIDs with gastroprotection and COX-2 inhibitors. Drug Healthc Patient Saf 2009;1:47–71.

104. Malmstrom K, Fricke JR, Kotey P, Kress B, Morrison B. A comparison of rofecoxib versus celecoxib in treating pain after dental surgery: A single-center, randomized, double-blind, placebo- and active-comparator-controlled, parallel-group, single-dose study using the dental impaction pain model. Clin Ther 2002;24:1549–1560.

105. Chang DJ, Desjardins PJ, Chen E, et al. Comparison of the analgesic efficacy of rofecoxib and enteric-coated diclofenac sodium in the treatment of postoperative dental pain: A randomized, placebo-controlled clinical trial. Clin Ther 2002;24:490–503.

106. Chang DJ, Bird SR, Bohidar NR, King T. Analgesic efficacy of rofecoxib compared with codeine/acetaminophen using a model of acute dental pain. Oral Surg Oral Med Oral Pathol Oral Radiol Endod 2005;100:e74–e80.

107. Doyle G, Jayawardena S, Ashraf E, Cooper SA. Efficacy and tolerability of nonprescription ibuprofen versus celecoxib for dental pain. J Clin Pharmacol 2002;42:912–919.

108. Derry S, Moore RA. Single dose oral celecoxib for acute postoperative pain in adults. Cochrane Database Syst Rev 2012;3.

109. Moore A, Makinson G, Li C. Patient-level pooled analysis of adjudicated gastrointestinal outcomes in celecoxib clinical trials: Meta-analysis of 51,000 patients enrolled in 52 randomized trials. Arthritis Res Ther 2013;15:R6.

110. Cochrane DJ, Jarvis B, Keating GM. Etoricoxib. Drugs 2002;62:2637–2651.

111. Chang DJ, Desjardins PJ, King TR, Erb T, Geba GP. The analgesic efficacy of etoricoxib compared with oxycodone/acetaminophen in an acute postoperative pain model: A randomized, double-blind clinical trial. Anesth Analg 2004;99:807–815.

112. Malmstrom K, Ang J, Fricke JR, Shingo S, Reicin A. The analgesic effect of etoricoxib relative to that of acetaminophen analgesics: A randomized, controlled single-dose study in acute dental impaction pain. Curr Med Res Opin 2005;21:141–149.

113. Clarke R, Derry S, Moore RA. Single dose oral etoricoxib for acute postoperative pain in adults. Cochrane Database Syst Rev 2012;4.

114. Back M, Yin L, Ingelsson E. Cyclooxygenase-2 inhibitors and cardiovascular risk in a nation-wide cohort study after the withdrawal of rofecoxib. Eur Heart J 2012;33:1928–1933.

115. Ormrod D, Wellington K, Wagstaff AJ. Valdecoxib. Drugs 2002;62:2059–2071.

116. Fricke J, Varkalis J, Zwillich S, et al. Valdecoxib is more efficacious than rofecoxib in relieving pain associated with oral surgery. Am J Ther 2002;9:89–97.

117. Pillans PI, Ghiculescu RA, Lampe G, Wilson R, Wong R, Macdonald GA. Severe acute liver injury associated with lumiracoxib. J Gastroenterol Hepatol 2012;27:1102–1105.

118. Stichtenoth DO, Frolich JC. The second generation of COX-2 inhibitors: What advantages do the newest offer? Drugs 2003;63:33–45.

119. Roy YM, Derry S, Moore RA. Single dose oral lumiracoxib for postoperative pain in adults. Cochrane Database Syst Rev 2010;(7).

120. Bertolini A, Ottani A, Sandrini M. Dual acting anti-inflammatory drugs: A reappraisal. Pharmacol Res 2001;44:437–450.

121. Singh VP, Patil CS, Kulkarni SK. Anti-inflammatory effect of licofelone against various inflammatory challenges. Fundam Clin Pharmacol 2006;20:65–71.

122. Bertinaria M, Shaikh MA, Buccellati C, et al. Designing multitarget anti-inflammatory agents: Chemical modulation of the lumiracoxib structure toward dual thromboxane antagonists-COX-2 inhibitors. Chem Med Chem 2012;7:1647–1660.

123. Huber MA, Terezhalmy GT. The use of COX-2 inhibitors for acute dental pain: A second look. J Am Dent Assoc 2006;137:480–487.

124. Savage MG, Henry MA. Preoperative nonsteroidal anti-inflammatory agents: Review of the literature. Oral Surg Oral Med Oral Pathol Oral Radiol Endod 2004;98:146–152.

125. Brogden RN. Pyrazolone derivatives. Drugs 1986;32(4, suppl):60–70.

126. Eldor A, Zylber-Katz E, Levy M. The effect of oral administration of dipyrone on the capacity of blood platelets to synthesize thromboxane A2 in man. Eur J Clin Pharmacol 1984;26:171–176.

127. Carlsson KH, Helmreich J, Jurna I. Activation of inhibition from the periaqueductal grey matter mediates central analgesic effect of metamizol (dipyrone). Pain 1986;27:373–390.

128. Carlsson KH, Monzel W, Jurna I. Depression by morphine and the non-opioid analgesic agents, metamizol (dipyrone), lysine acetylsalicylate, and paracetamol, of activity in rat thalamus neurones evoked by electrical stimulation of nociceptive afferents. Pain 1988;32:313–326.

129. Edwards JE, Meseguer F, Faura C, Moore RA, McQuay HJ. Single-dose dipyrone for acute postoperative pain. Cochrane Database Syst Rev 2001;(3).

130. Edwards J, Meseguer F, Faura C, Moore RA, McQuay HJ, Derry S. Single dose dipyrone for acute postoperative pain. Cochrane Database Syst Rev 2010;(9).

131. Bianchi Porro G, Ardizzone S, Petrillo M, Caruso I, Montrone F. Endoscopic assessment of the effects of dipyrone (metamizol) in comparison to paracetamol and placebo on the gastric and duodenal mucosa of healthy adult volunteers. Digestion 1996;57:186–190.

132. Sánchez S, Martín MJ, Ortiz P, Motilva V, Alarcón de la Lastra C. Effects of dipyrone on inflammatory infiltration and oxidative metabolism in gastric mucosa: Comparison with acetaminophen and diclofenac. Dig Dis Sci 2002;47:1389–1398.

133. Czerniawska-Mysik G, Szczeklik A. Idiosyncrasy to pyrazolone drugs. Allergy 1981;36:381–384.

134. Karakaya G, Kalyoncu AF. Metamizole intolerance and bronchial asthma. Allergol Immunopathol (Madr) 2002;30:267–272.

135. Levy M. Hypersensitivity to pyrazolones. Thorax 2000;55(suppl 2):S72–S74.

136. Basak GW, Drozd-Sokolowska J, Wiktor-Jedrzejczak W. Update on the incidence of metamizole sodium-induced blood dyscrasias in Poland. J Int Med Res 2010;38:1374–1380.

137. Pontikoglou C, Papadaki HA. Idiosyncratic drug-induced agranulocytosis: The paradigm of deferiprone. Hemoglobin 2010;34:291–304.

138. Gourlay G (ed). Clinical Pharmacology of Opioids in the Treatment of Pain. Seattle: IASP, 2002.

139. Ross FB, Smith MT. The intrinsic antinociceptive effects of oxycodone appear to be kappa-opioid receptor mediated. Pain 1997;73:151–157.

140. Yaksh TL, Rudy TA. Narcotic analgestics: CNS sites and mechanisms of action as revealed by intracerebral injection techniques. Pain 1978;4:299–359.

141. Raffa RB. Pharmacology of oral combination analgesics: Rational therapy for pain. J Clin Pharm Ther 2001;26:257–264.

142. Scott LJ, Perry CM. Tramadol: A review of its use in perioperative pain. Drugs 2000;60:139–176.

143. Schug SA, Gandham N. Opioids: Clinical use. In: McMahon SB, Koltzenburg M (eds). Wall and Melzack's Textbook of Pain, ed 5. Philadelphia: Elsevier, 2006:443–457.

144. Edwards JE, McQuay HJ, Moore RA. Combination analgesic efficacy: Individual patient data meta-analysis of single-dose oral tramadol plus acetaminophen in acute postoperative pain. J Pain Symptom Manage 2002;23:121–130.

145. Collins SL, Edwards JE, Moore RA, McQuay HJ. Single dose dextropropoxyphene, alone and with paracetamol (acetaminophen), for postoperative pain. Cochrane Database Syst Rev 2000;(2).

146. VanderVaart S, Berger H, Sistonen J, et al. CYP2D6 polymorphisms and codeine analgesia in postpartum pain management: A pilot study. Ther Drug Monit 2011;33:425–432.

147. Zahari Z, Ismail R. Influence of cytochrome P450, family 2, subfamily D, polypeptide 6 (CYP2D6) polymorphisms on pain sensitivity and clinical response to weak opioid analgesics. Drug Metab Pharmacokinet 2014;29:29–43.

148. Gourlay GK, Cherry DA, Cousins MJ. A comparative study of the efficacy and pharmacokinetics of oral methadone and morphine in the treatment of severe pain in patients with cancer. Pain 1986;25:297–312.

149. Bruera E, Belzile M, Pituskin E, et al. Randomized, double-blind, cross-over trial comparing safety and efficacy of oral controlled-release oxycodone with controlled-release morphine in patients with cancer pain. J Clin Oncol 1998;16:3222–3229.

150. Moore RA, McQuay HJ. Prevalence of opioid adverse events in chronic non-malignant pain: Systematic review of randomised trials of oral opioids. Arthritis Res Ther 2005;7:R1046–R1051.

151. Jensen MK, Thomsen AB, Hojsted J. 10-year follow-up of chronic non-malignant pain patients: Opioid use, health related quality of life and health care utilization. Eur J Pain 2006;10:423–433.

152. Moulin D. Opioids in Chronic Non-Malignant Pain. Cambridge: Cambridge University, 1999.

153. Miranda HF, Puig MM, Prieto JC, Pinardi G. Synergism between paracetamol and nonsteroidal anti-inflammatory drugs in experimental acute pain. Pain 2006;121:22–28.

154. Moore A, Collins S, Carroll D, McQuay H. Paracetamol with and without codeine in acute pain: A quantitative systematic review. Pain 1997;70:193–201.

155. Fricke JR Jr, Hewitt DJ, Jordan DM, Fisher A, Rosenthal NR. A double-blind placebo-controlled comparison of tramadol/acetaminophen and tramadol in patients with postoperative dental pain. Pain 2004;109:250–257.

156. McNicol E, Strassels SA, Goudas L, Lau J, Carr DB. NSAIDS or paracetamol, alone or combined with opioids, for cancer pain. Cochrane Database Syst Rev 2005;(1).

157. Derry S, Derry CJ, Moore RA. Single dose oral ibuprofen plus oxycodone for acute postoperative pain in adults. Cochrane Database Syst Rev 2013;6.

158. Altman RD. A rationale for combining acetaminophen and NSAIDs for mild-to-moderate pain. Clin Exp Rheumatol 2004;22:110–117.

159. Mehlisch DR, Aspley S, Daniels SE, Southerden KA, Christensen KS. A single-tablet fixed-dose combination of racemic ibuprofen/paracetamol in the management of moderate to severe postoperative dental pain in adult and adolescent patients: A multicenter, two-stage, randomized, double-blind, parallel-group, placebo-controlled, factorial study. Clin Ther 2010;32:1033–1049.

160. Millan MJ. The induction of pain: An integrative review. Prog Neurobiol 1999;57:1–164.

161. Mamet J, Baron A, Lazdunski M, Voilley N. Proinflammatory mediators, stimulators of sensory neuron excitability via the expression of acid-sensing ion channels. J Neurosci 2002;22:10662–10670.

162. Kessler W, Kirchhoff C, Reeh PW, Handwerker HO. Excitation of cutaneous afferent nerve endings in vitro by a combination of inflammatory mediators and conditioning effect of substance P. Exp Brain Res 1992;91:467–476.

163. Steen KH, Issberner U, Reeh PW. Pain due to experimental acidosis in human skin: Evidence for non-adapting nociceptor excitation. Neurosci Lett 1995;199:29–32.

164. Ichikawa H, Sugimoto T. The co-expression of ASIC3 with calcitonin gene-related peptide and parvalbumin in the rat trigeminal ganglion. Brain Res 2002;943:287–291.

165. Julius D, Basbaum AI. Molecular mechanisms of nociception. Nature 2001;413(6852):203–210.

166. Price MP, McIlwrath SL, Xie J, et al. The DRASIC cation channel contributes to the detection of cutaneous touch and acid stimuli in mice. Neuron 2001;32:1071–1083.

167. Steen KH, Steen AE, Kreysel HW, Reeh PW. Inflammatory mediators potentiate pain induced by experimental tissue acidosis. Pain 1996;66:163–170.

168. Ballou LR, Botting RM, Goorha S, Zhang J, Vane JR. Nociception in cyclooxygenase isozyme-deficient mice. Proc Natl Acad Sci USA 2000;97:10272–10276.

169. Taiwo YO, Levine JD. Prostaglandin effects after elimination of indirect hyperalgesic mechanisms in the skin of the rat. Brain Res 1989;492:397–399.

170. Noda K, Ueda Y, Suzuki K, Yoda K. Excitatory effects of algesic compounds on neuronal processes in murine dorsal root ganglion cell culture. Brain Res 1997;751:348–351.

171. Southall MD, Vasko MR. Prostaglandin E(2)-mediated sensitization of rat sensory neurons is not altered by nerve growth factor. Neurosci Lett 2000;287:33–36.

172. Taiwo YO, Heller PH, Levine JD. Characterization of distinct phospholipases mediating bradykinin and noradrenaline hyperalgesia. Neuroscience 1990;39:523–531.

173. Martin HA, Basbaum AI, Kwiat GC, Goetzl EJ, Levine JD. Leukotriene and prostaglandin sensitization of cutaneous high-threshold C- and A-delta mechanonociceptors in the hairy skin of rat hindlimbs. Neuroscience 1987;22:651–659.

174. Seybold VS, Jia YP, Abrahams LG. Cyclo-oxygenase-2 contributes to central sensitization in rats with peripheral inflammation. Pain 2003;105:47–55.

175. Rueff A, Dray A. Sensitization of peripheral afferent fibres in the in vitro neonatal rat spinal cord-tail by bradykinin and prostaglandins. Neuroscience 1993;54:527–535.

176. Funk CD. Prostaglandins and leukotrienes: Advances in eicosanoid biology. Science 2001;294(5548):1871–1875.

177. Smith WL, Marnett LJ. Prostaglandin endoperoxide synthase: Structure and catalysis. Biochim Biophys Acta 1991;1083:1–17.

178. Smith WL, Meade EA, DeWitt DL. Interactions of PGH synthase isozymes-1 and -2 with NSAIDs. Ann NY Acad Sci 1994;744:50–57.

179. Brune K. Safety of anti-inflammatory treatment—New ways of thinking. Rheumatology (Oxford) 2004;43(suppl 1):i16–i20.

180. Vane JR. Inhibition of prostaglandin synthesis as a mechanism of action for aspirin-like drugs. Nat New Biol 1971;231:232–235.

181. Israel E, Fischer AR, Rosenberg MA, et al. The pivotal role of 5-lipoxygenase products in the reaction of aspirin-sensitive asthmatics to aspirin. Am Rev Respir Dis 1993;148:1447–1451.

182. Tegeder I, Pfeilschifter J, Geisslinger G. Cyclooxygenase-independent actions of cyclooxygenase inhibitors. Faseb J 2001;15:2057–2072.

183. Fu JY, Masferrer JL, Seibert K, Raz A, Needleman P. The induction and suppression of prostaglandin H2 synthase (cyclooxygenase) in human monocytes. J Biol Chem 1990;265:16737–16740.

184. Robinson DR. Regulation of prostaglandin synthesis by antiinflammatory drugs. J Rheumatol Suppl 1997;47:32–39.

185. Hawkey CJ. COX-2 inhibitors. Lancet 1999;353(9149):307–314.

186. Dinchuk JE, Car BD, Focht RJ, et al. Renal abnormalities and an altered inflammatory response in mice lacking cyclooxygenase II. Nature 1995;378(6555):406–409.

187. Langenbach R, Morham SG, Tiano HF, et al. Prostaglandin synthase 1 gene disruption in mice reduces arachidonic acid-induced inflammation and indomethacin-induced gastric ulceration. Cell 1995;83:483–492.

188. Vane J. Towards a better aspirin. Nature 1994;367(6460):215–216.

189. Crofford LJ, Lipsky PE, Brooks P, Abramson SB, Simon LS, van de Putte LB. Basic biology and clinical application of specific cyclooxygenase-2 inhibitors. Arthritis Rheum 2000;43:4–13.

190. Katori M, Majima M. Cyclooxygenase-2: Its rich diversity of roles and possible application of its selective inhibitors. Inflamm Res 2000;49:367–392.

191. Majerus PW. Arachidonate metabolism in vascular disorders. J Clin Invest 1983;72:1521–1525.

192. Fitzgerald GA. Coxibs and cardiovascular disease. N Engl J Med 2004;351:1709–1711.

193. Grosser T, Fries S, Fitzgerald GA. Biological basis for the cardiovascular consequences of COX-2 inhibition: Therapeutic challenges and opportunities. J Clin Invest 2006;116:4–15.

194. Bombardier C, Laine L, Reicin A, et al. Comparison of upper gastrointestinal toxicity of rofecoxib and naproxen in patients with rheumatoid arthritis. VIGOR Study Group. N Engl J Med 2000;343:1520–1528.

195. Silverstein FE, Faich G, Goldstein JL, et al. Gastrointestinal toxicity with celecoxib vs nonsteroidal anti-inflammatory drugs for osteoarthritis and rheumatoid arthritis: The CLASS study: A randomized controlled trial. Celecoxib Long-term Arthritis Safety Study. JAMA 2000;284:1247–1255.

196. Schnitzer TJ, Burmester GR, Mysler E, et al. Comparison of lumiracoxib with naproxen and ibuprofen in the Therapeutic Arthritis Research and Gastrointestinal Event Trial (TARGET), reduction in ulcer complications: Randomised controlled trial. Lancet 2004;364(9435):665–674.

197. Wong M, Chowienczyk P, Kirkham B. Cardiovascular issues of COX-2 inhibitors and NSAIDs. Aust Fam Physician 2005;34:945–948.

198. Brater DC, Harris C, Redfern JS, Gertz BJ. Renal effects of COX-2-selective inhibitors. Am J Nephrol 2001;21:1–15.
199. Brophy JM. Cardiovascular risk associated with celecoxib. N Engl J Med 2005;352:2648–2650.
200. Schoen RT, Vender RJ. Mechanisms of nonsteroidal anti-inflammatory drug-induced gastric damage. Am J Med 1989;86:449–458.
201. Lanza FL, Royer GL Jr, Nelson RS. Endoscopic evaluation of the effects of aspirin, buffered aspirin, and enteric-coated aspirin on gastric and duodenal mucosa. N Engl J Med 1980;303:136–138.
202. Lee M, Cryer B, Feldman M. Dose effects of aspirin on gastric prostaglandins and stomach mucosal injury. Ann Intern Med 1994;120:184–189.
203. Wolfe MM, Soll AH. The physiology of gastric acid secretion. N Engl J Med 1988;319:1707–1715.
204. Fitzgerald GA, Patrono C. The coxibs, selective inhibitors of cyclooxygenase-2. N Engl J Med 2001;345:433–442.
205. Wallace JL, Devchand PR. Emerging roles for cyclooxygenase-2 in gastrointestinal mucosal defense. Br J Pharmacol 2005;145:275–282.
206. Singh G, Triadafilopoulos G. Epidemiology of NSAID induced gastrointestinal complications. J Rheumatol Suppl 1999;56:18–24.
207. Tramèr MR, Moore RA, Reynolds DJ, McQuay HJ. Quantitative estimation of rare adverse events which follow a biological progression: A new model applied to chronic NSAID use. Pain 2000;85:169–182.
208. Castellsague J, Riera-Guardia N, Calingaert B, et al. Individual NSAIDs and upper gastrointestinal complications: A systematic review and meta-analysis of observational studies (the SOS project). Drug Saf 2012;35:1127–1146.
209. Longstreth GF. Epidemiology of hospitalization for acute upper gastrointestinal hemorrhage: A population-based study. Am J Gastroenterol 1995;90:206–210.
210. Hernández-Díaz S, García-Rodríguez LA. Epidemiologic assessment of the safety of conventional nonsteroidal anti-inflammatory drugs. Am J Med 2001;110(3, suppl):20S–27S.
211. Graham DY, Smith JL. Aspirin and the stomach. Ann Intern Med 1986;104:390–398.
212. Singh G, Ramey DR, Morfeld D, Shi H, Hatoum HT, Fries JF. Gastrointestinal tract complications of nonsteroidal anti-inflammatory drug treatment in rheumatoid arthritis. A prospective observational cohort study. Arch Intern Med 1996;156:1530–1536.
213. Larkai EN, Smith JL, Lidsky MD, Graham DY. Gastroduodenal mucosa and dyspeptic symptoms in arthritic patients during chronic nonsteroidal anti-inflammatory drug use. Am J Gastroenterol 1987;82:1153–1158.
214. Hawkey CJ, Karrasch JA, Szczepański L, et al. Omeprazole compared with misoprostol for ulcers associated with nonsteroidal antiinflammatory drugs. Omeprazole versus Misoprostol for NSAID-induced Ulcer Management (OMNIUM) Study Group. N Engl J Med 1998;338:727–734.
215. Eccles M, Freemantle N, Mason J. North of England evidence based guideline development project: Summary guideline for non-steroidal anti-inflammatory drugs versus basic analgesia in treating the pain of degenerative arthritis. The North of England Non-Steroidal Anti-Inflammatory Drug Guideline Development Group. BMJ 1998;317(7157):526–530.
216. Bresalier RS, Sandler RS, Quan H, et al. Cardiovascular events associated with rofecoxib in a colorectal adenoma chemoprevention trial. N Engl J Med 2005;352:1092–1102.
217. Solomon SD, McMurray JJ, Pfeffer MA, et al. Cardiovascular risk associated with celecoxib in a clinical trial for colorectal adenoma prevention. N Engl J Med 2005;352:1071–1080.
218. Furberg CD, Psaty BM, Fitzgerald GA. Parecoxib, valdecoxib, and cardiovascular risk. Circulation 2005;111:249.
219. Page J, Henry D. Consumption of NSAIDs and the development of congestive heart failure in elderly patients: An underrecognized public health problem. Arch Intern Med 2000;160:777–784.
220. Bhala N, Emberson J, Merhi A, et al. Vascular and upper gastrointestinal effects of non-steroidal anti-inflammatory drugs: Meta-analyses of individual participant data from randomised trials. Lancet 2013;382(9894):769–779.
221. Johnson AG, Nguyen TV, Day RO. Do nonsteroidal anti-inflammatory drugs affect blood pressure? A meta-analysis. Ann Intern Med 1994;121:289–300.
222. Johnson AG. NSAIDs and blood pressure. Clinical importance for older patients. Drugs Aging 1998;12:17–27.
223. Patrono C, Coller B, Dalen JE, et al. Platelet-active drugs: The relationships among dose, effectiveness, and side effects. Chest 2001;119(1, suppl):39S–63S.
224. McAdam BF, Catella-Lawson F, Mardini IA, Kapoor S, Lawson JA, Fitzgerald GA. Systemic biosynthesis of prostacyclin by cyclooxygenase (COX)-2: The human pharmacology of a selective inhibitor of COX-2. Proc Natl Acad Sci USA 1999;96:272–277.
225. Clarke RJ, Mayo G, Price P, Fitzgerald GA. Suppression of thromboxane A2 but not of systemic prostacyclin by controlled-release aspirin. N Engl J Med 1991;325:1137–1141.
226. Murata T, Ushikubi F, Matsuoka T, et al. Altered pain perception and inflammatory response in mice lacking prostacyclin receptor. Nature 1997;388(6643):678–682.
227. Taylor DW, Barnett HJ, Haynes RB, et al. Low-dose and high-dose acetylsalicylic acid for patients undergoing carotid endarterectomy: A randomised controlled trial. ASA and Carotid Endarterectomy (ACE) trial collaborators. Lancet 1999;353(9171):2179–2184.
228. Schafer AI. Effects of nonsteroidal anti-inflammatory therapy on platelets. Am J Med 1999;106(5, suppl):25S–36S.
229. Capone ML, Tacconelli S, Sciulli MG, et al. Clinical pharmacology of platelet, monocyte, and vascular cyclooxygenase inhibition by naproxen and low-dose aspirin in healthy subjects. Circulation 2004;109:1468–1471.

230. Leese PT, Talwalker S, Kent JD, Recker DP. Valdecoxib does not impair platelet function. Am J Emerg Med 2002;20:275–281.

231. Ouellet M, Riendeau D, Percival MD. A high level of cyclooxygenase-2 inhibitor selectivity is associated with a reduced interference of platelet cyclooxygenase-1 inactivation by aspirin. Proc Natl Acad Sci USA 2001;98:14583–14588.

232. Napenas JJ, Hong CH, Kempter E, Brennan MT, Furney SL, Lockhart PB. Selective serotonin reuptake inhibitors and oral bleeding complications after invasive dental treatment. Oral Surg Oral Med Oral Pathol Oral Radiol Endod 2011;112:463–467.

233. Sandhu GK, Heyneman CA. Nephrotoxic potential of selective cyclooxygenase-2 inhibitors. Ann Pharmacother 2004;38:700–704.

234. Whelton A, Stout RL, Spilman PS, Klassen DK. Renal effects of ibuprofen, piroxicam, and sulindac in patients with asymptomatic renal failure. A prospective, randomized, crossover comparison. Ann Intern Med 1990;112:568–576.

235. Stichtenoth DO, Frölich JC. COX-2 and the kidneys. Curr Pharm Des 2000;6:1737–1753.

236. Khan KN, Stanfield KM, Harris RK, Baron DA. Expression of cyclooxygenase-2 in the macula densa of human kidney in hypertension, congestive heart failure, and diabetic nephropathy. Ren Fail 2001;23:321–330.

237. Whelton A, White WB, Bello AE, Puma JA, Fort JG. Effects of celecoxib and rofecoxib on blood pressure and edema in patients > or =65 years of age with systemic hypertension and osteoarthritis. Am J Cardiol 2002;90:959–963.

238. Akinbamowo AO, Salzberg DJ, Weir MR. Renal consequences of prostaglandin inhibition in heart failure. Heart Fail Clin 2008;4:505–510.

239. Schwartz JI, Thach C, Lasseter KC, et al. Effects of etoricoxib and comparator nonsteroidal anti-inflammatory drugs on urinary sodium excretion, blood pressure, and other renal function indicators in elderly subjects consuming a controlled sodium diet. J Clin Pharmacol 2007;47:1521–1531.

240. Benson P, Yudd M, Sims D, Chang V, Srinivas S, Kasimis B. Renal effects of high-dose celecoxib in elderly men with stage D2 prostate carcinoma. Clin Nephrol 2012;78:376–381.

241. Stevenson DD, Sanchez-Borges M, Szczeklik A. Classification of allergic and pseudoallergic reactions to drugs that inhibit cyclooxygenase enzymes. Ann Allergy Asthma Immunol 2001;87:177–180.

242. Szczeklik A, Stevenson DD. Aspirin-induced asthma: Advances in pathogenesis and management. J Allergy Clin Immunol 1999;104:5–13.

243. Juhlin L. Recurrent urticaria: Clinical investigation of 330 patients. Br J Dermatol 1981;104:369–381.

244. Bigby M. Rates of cutaneous reactions to drugs. Arch Dermatol 2001;137:765–770.

245. Szczeklik A. The cyclooxygenase theory of aspirin-induced asthma. Eur Respir J 1990;3:588–593.

246. Christie PE, Tagari P, Ford-Hutchinson AW, et al. Urinary leukotriene E4 concentrations increase after aspirin challenge in aspirin-sensitive asthmatic subjects. Am Rev Respir Dis 1991;143:1025–1029.

247. Zembowicz A, Mastalerz L, Setkowicz M, Radziszewski W, Szczeklik A. Safety of cyclooxygenase 2 inhibitors and increased leukotriene synthesis in chronic idiopathic urticaria with sensitivity to nonsteroidal anti-inflammatory drugs. Arch Dermatol 2003;139:1577–1582.

248. Settipane RA, Schrank PJ, Simon RA, Mathison DA, Christiansen SC, Stevenson DD. Prevalence of cross-sensitivity with acetaminophen in aspirin-sensitive asthmatic subjects. J Allergy Clin Immunol 1995;96:480–485.

249. Szczeklik A, Gryglewski RJ, Czerniawska-Mysik G. Clinical patterns of hypersensitivity to nonsteroidal anti-inflammatory drugs and their pathogenesis. J Allergy Clin Immunol 1977;60:276–284.

250. Edwards JE, McQuay HJ. Dipyrone and agranulocytosis: What is the risk? Lancet 2002;360(9344):1438.

251. Risks of agranulocytosis and aplastic anemia. A first report of their relation to drug use with special reference to analgesics [editorial]. JAMA 1986;256:1749–1757.

252. Adam MP, Polifka JE, Friedman JM. Evolving knowledge of the teratogenicity of medications in human pregnancy. Am J Med Genet C Semin Med Genet 2011;157:175–182.

253. Bloor M, Paech M. Nonsteroidal anti-inflammatory drugs during pregnancy and the initiation of lactation. Anesth Analg 2013;116:1063–1075.

254. Li DK, Liu L, Odouli R. Exposure to non-steroidal anti-inflammatory drugs during pregnancy and risk of miscarriage: Population based cohort study. BMJ 2003;327:368.

255. Chan VS. A mechanistic perspective on the specificity and extent of COX-2 inhibition in pregnancy. Drug Saf 2004;27:421–426.

256. Shaheen SO, Newson RB, Henderson AJ, et al. Prenatal paracetamol exposure and risk of asthma and elevated immunoglobulin E in childhood. Clin Exp Allergy 2005;35:18–25.

257. Stamer UM, Zhang L, Stüber F. Personalized therapy in pain management: Where do we stand? Pharmacogenomics 2010;11:843–864.

Pharmacotherapy for Chronic Orofacial Pain

16

Rafael Benoliel, BDS

Yair Sharav, DMD, MS

Although clinicians would like to offer treatment that eradicates chronic pain, they are, at present, unable to do so. Clinicians are generally in the difficult situation of managing chronic pain. However, multimodality management affords many patients at least partial, but significant, improvement. A major component of most of these multimodality approaches includes the use of prescription drugs that offer significant relief, although sometimes with significant morbidity. These are a mainstay of pain management.

This chapter describes the mechanisms underlying drugs used in the prevention and management of recurrent or chronic pain in the head and neck. The indications and choice of drugs for specific clinical syndromes are described in chapters 8 through 12.

Treatment Approach

Ideally, drug selection is patient tailored and mechanism based, targeting specific pathophysiologic processes. However, many of the mechanisms involved are still unclear, and evidence implicates multiple mechanisms in the emergence of persistent pain. Current pain pharmacotherapy is largely the result of clinical observation, at times serendipitous, with double-blind randomized controlled trials (RCTs) following. The modes of action of the drugs clinicians use are often unclear.

In spite of accepted pharmacotherapy guidelines for many pain syndromes, similar conditions are often treated differently across practitioners,[1] and approaches depend on a physician's training and continuing education activities.[2] Moreover, the sex, age, ethnicity, and race of both the patient and the physician will significantly affect treatment approaches,[2,3] and substantial evidence needs to be presented to change a physician's established practices. National guidelines and treatment protocols that rely on evidence-based medicine help overcome treatment bias.[4]

Drug Prescription and Treatment Plan

Most of the drugs used for chronic pain have side effects, some of which affect quality of life. Combining drugs (usually of different drug classes) is indicated at times and depends on the suspected pain mechanisms, pain control achieved with a single drug, and other factors. Drug combinations are often used in the treatment of migraine (see chapter 10), neuropathic pain (see chapter 12), and acute pain (see chapters 6 and 15); specific combinations are therefore discussed in the chapters covering these entities. However, polypharmacy often significantly increases side effects and drug interactions, so there must be a clear gain in therapeutic efficacy to justify combinations. Additionally, treatment approaches to chronic or recurrent pain may be preventive or abortive and depend partly on pain frequency, associated disability, and patient preferences. Patients should be aware of the therapeutic aims (eg, 50% reduction in pain severity or frequency), which are often less ambitious than their own expectations. The management of chronic pain is a long process involving several drug trials over prolonged periods with multiple follow-up visits, all of which require patient cooperation. Pain diaries are an essential part of the assessment of treatment outcome in terms of pain severity, attack duration, and attack frequency and must be carefully documented.

Because chronic pain is a complex interaction of physical and emotional experiences, practitioners need to be aware of comorbidities such as depression, anxiety, sleeplessness, and drug abuse. Chronic pain management often requires patient referral to medical colleagues for the management of such comorbidities. Many patients will prefer not to take medications because of potential side effects and will instead opt for nonpharmacologic interventions. Some studies show that cognitive-behavioral therapy is effective in reducing pain experience and helping patients cope with chronic pain (see chapter 4). As described in chapter 17, pain patients are increasingly turning to complementary or alternative medicine for the management of pain. Basic knowledge of available modalities in addition to mainstream therapies is advantageous.

Assessing Drug Effects

Ideally, drugs should be effective across the widest range of patients, be easy to take, and have minimal side effects. To assess the efficacy of available drugs, clinicians require an easy tool. The results of RCTs are considered reliable evidence as they account for physician bias, the potent effects of placebo, and patient expectation. The perceived effect of an active drug must be balanced by that observed in the placebo arm of the trial; this may be an active drug, as in head-to-head studies, and not placebo (see also chapter 17). Additionally, because the end point of the trial often differs across studies, it should be clearly defined; a 50% reduction in pain severity is commonly used.

Randomized controlled trials

An increasing number of RCTs are failing to demonstrate a statistically significant superiority of well-recognized, approved analgesics relative to placebo.[5] How should this lack of analgesic superiority be interpreted? Improved study design, patient selection, and outcome measures have improved the validity of these RCTs, so it is possible that drugs thought to be efficacious are actually not. Conversely, various characteristics of clinical trials can compromise their ability to reveal efficacy. Often the effect of the placebo is weak, thereby strengthening the apparent effect of the drug studied. In other studies, the placebo effect is robust and challenges the effect of the active drug. When reports of analgesic efficacy can be assumed to be valid and designs are comparable, failures to demonstrate efficacy can be attributed to limitations in *assay sensitivity*, which has been defined as the ability of a clinical trial "to distinguish an effective treatment from a less effective or ineffective treatment."[5] Various recommendations on study design have been proposed to improve assay sensitivity.[6]

Meta-analyses and systematic reviews of RCTs further provide a way in which to assess effects across different populations, medical teams, countries, and time. These are more likely than individual trials to describe the true clinical effect of a drug.

Expressing drug efficacy

Statistics arising from RCTs are often difficult to interpret and apply in everyday practice. The number needed to treat (NNT) is a comfortable way of expressing the efficiency of a drug relative to placebo. The NNT indicates the number of patients that would need to be treated in order for one patient to obtain the desired outcome. Calculation of the NNT accounts for the effects of the placebo arm of the trial, so the placebo's effect may significantly change the NNT. It is essential to appreciate that NNTs are not strict rules but another well-based factor to be considered when deciding on the best treatment strategy for patients. The NNT is extremely useful to compare several drugs that have been assessed for the same outcome measure in patients with similar conditions. Using NNTs allows clinicians to rank interventions relative to one another and choose a specific drug based on efficacy (see chapters 10 through 15 and 17). However, NNTs need to be balanced against adverse events, costs, patient characteristics, expectations, and preferences.

For adverse events, the NNT becomes the number needed to harm (NNH), which reflects the number of patients that would need to be treated before one patient would suffer the studied side effect. NNTs and NNHs are collected for each RCT on a particular drug, and a mean is then calculated. Because the error is usually large and much overlap may exist between drugs, NNTs should ideally be given with 95% confidence intervals. NNTs are disease specific and cannot be compared across diagnoses. NNT (and NNH) must always specify the comparator, the therapeutic outcome, and the duration of treatment that is necessary to achieve that outcome. Therefore, clinicians search for drugs with low NNTs and high NNHs, both with compact confidence intervals.

In addition to scientific journals, excellent evidence-based databases are available (eg, Bandolier [http://www.medicine.ox.ac.uk/bandolier/], BMJ Clinical Evidence [http://www.clinicalevidence.com/ceweb/conditions/index.jsp], The Cochrane Collaboration [http://www.cochrane.org/index0.htm], and the National Institute for Health and Care Excellence [http://www.nice.org.uk]), although these generally require a subscription. Additionally, many professional bodies publish recommendations, although specific guidelines for the management of many orofacial pain syndromes are lacking at present.

Animal studies are also used to assess the efficacy of drugs in various pain states, both inflammatory and neuropathic. Often, however, the extrapolation of experimental findings from rodents to humans is disappointing, and drugs that were analgesic in rats often prove ineffective in humans. Notwithstanding, experimental data from rodent studies remain the backbone of what is understood about the mechanisms of drugs and the pathophysiology of chronic pain.

Systemic Drugs Used in the Management of Chronic Pain

In many cases, the US Food and Drug Administration (FDA) or other national agency controlling drug use does not list drugs used in the management of pain for such use. This accepted clinical practice, termed *off-label prescribing*, should always be based on solid evidence. In some countries and institutions, off-label usage requires prior approval.

This section provides a review of the major drug groups commonly used in the management of chronic orofacial pain: antidepressants, antiepileptic drugs, antihypertensives, muscle relaxants, and triptans. Additionally, a short overview is provided on the use of cannabinoids, *N*-methyl-D-aspartate (NMDA) antagonists, and botulinum toxin in the treatment of pain and headache. The large number of available drugs is impossible to completely review. Even within the drug groups selected for this chapter, the detailed pharmacology, drug interactions, and adverse effects are within the scope of clinical pharmacology texts that should form part of any practice or specialized clinic. Adverse effects and drug safety, particularly in pregnant and lactating women, are a major concern. This chapter provides an over-

Table 16-1	FDA pregnancy category definitions for drugs

Category	Description
A	Controlled studies in women fail to demonstrate a risk to the fetus in the first trimester and no evidence of a risk in later trimesters. The possibility of fetal harm appears remote.
B	Animal studies have not demonstrated a fetal risk, but risk remains unconfirmed in studies in pregnant women OR animal studies have shown an adverse effect that was not confirmed in controlled studies in women in the first trimester.
C	Studies in animals have revealed adverse effects on the fetus, but there are no controlled studies in pregnant women. Drugs should be given only if the potential benefit justifies the potential risk to the fetus.
D	Positive evidence of human fetal risk. Benefits from use in pregnant women may be acceptable despite the risk for life-threatening situations or serious disease.
X	Studies in animals or human beings have demonstrated fetal abnormalities. The risk of the use of the drug in women that are or may become pregnant clearly outweighs any possible benefit.

view of the prominent side effects for each drug described as well as guidelines for use in pregnancy (Table 16-1) and breastfeeding based on FDA and other recommendations.[7] However, as reports of adverse effects, particularly for the newer drugs, are constantly updated, the reader should refer to clinical pharmacology sources for updated information, including such databases as Micromedex (http://www.micromedex.com), Epocrates (http://www.epocrates.com), and RxList (http://www.rxlist.com), some at no cost. These sources provide all the necessary information and may offer software that examines possible drug interactions.

Several strategies are essential across all the drugs used in the management of pain. Needless to say, the medical status of the patient must be balanced with the pharmacologic profile of the intended drug, and possible interactions with other drugs must be explored. Therapy should be started at low doses and slowly titrated upward based on therapeutic response and side effects; this maximizes a patient's adherence to therapy and tends to minimize side effects. Drug therapy often exerts progressive effects over a period of weeks or months, so specific drugs should not be abandoned early. Careful supervision and scheduled laboratory tests for drug effects (eg, in carbamazepine therapy) are essential and reassure patients that they are being cared for competently.

Antidepressants

Antidepressants are effective for the treatment of neuropathic, musculoskeletal, and neurovascular type pains (Table 16-2; see also chapters 8 and 10 through 13). For some syndromes, these are the drugs of choice. The best evidence of pain relief in painful neuropathies is for tricyclic antidepressants (TCAs); amitriptyline, for example, has an NNT of 2.[8,9] Limited data are available on the analgesic effectiveness of selective serotonin reuptake inhibitors (SSRIs) and selective serotonin and norepinephrine reuptake inhibitors (SNRIs), but they are less effective than TCAs.

Tricyclic antidepressants

The TCAs were initially used for the treatment of depression. The advent of the newer antidepressants (SSRI, SNRI) with reduced side effects has largely shifted the use of TCAs to other problems, such as pain. Amitriptyline is probably the most frequently used TCA in chronic orofacial pain syndromes, and the newer SNRIs have been applied with some success in pain medicine. Human and experimental analgesic trials reveal that drugs with mixed serotonin (5-hydroxytryptamine [5-HT])/noradrenaline effects) (eg, imipramine and amitriptyline) and SNRIs (eg, venlafaxine) are superior to SSRIs (eg, fluoxetine or paroxetine).[10]

Table 16-2 Antidepressants

Drug	Initial dose (mg)	Target or maximum dose (mg)*	Dose increase (titration)*	Schedule	Taken with food	Pregnancy category	Breastfeeding	Medical contraindications	Drug interactions	Common side effects
Amitriptyline	10	35 to 50	10 mg/wk	Bedtime	No	C	Probably safe	Cardiac problems, diabetes, epilepsy, glaucoma, hepatic problems, psychiatric problems, thyroid problems, urinary retention	Anticoagulants, antidepressants, antihypertensives, carbamazepine, catecholamines, cimetidine, ergotamine, fluconazole, insulin, NSAIDs, sulfonylureas, thyroid hormones, triptans	Weight gain, bloating, constipation, xerostomia, asthenia, dizziness, headache, urinary retention, blurred vision, fatigue, somnolence
Imipramine	12.5	25 to 50	12.5 mg/wk	Bedtime	No	C	Unknown			
Venlafaxine	37.5	75 to 150	75 mg every 4 to 7 days	Two or three times per day	Yes	C other than the third trimester	Unknown	Cardiac problems, epilepsy, glaucoma, hepatic/renal problems, hypertension, hyperlipidemia, psychiatric problems	Antidepressants, erythromycin, fluconazole, NSAIDs, triptans	Hypertension, sweating, weight loss, constipation, loss of appetite, nausea, xerostomia, asthenia, dizziness, headache, insomnia or somnolence, tremor, nervousness, abnormal ejaculation, impotence
Venlafaxine extended release	37.5	75 to 225	75 mg every 4 to 7 days	Once daily						
Duloxetine	20 to 40	60 to 120	20 mg/wk	One or two times per day	No	C other than the third trimester	Unknown	Epilepsy, glaucoma, hepatic/renal problems, psychiatric problems	Antidepressants	Sweating, constipation, loss of appetite, nausea, xerostomia, diarrhea, gastritis, dizziness, insomnia or somnolence, blurred vision, dysuria, fatigue

*This is a rough guideline; clinicians should clinically titrate based on therapeutic response versus side effects.
NSAIDs, nonsteroidal anti-inflammatory drugs.

5-HT = SEROTONIN

Mode of action. At present, much of the research relates to TCAs, but as the newer drugs are investigated, their modes of action may become clearer. The major pharmacologic effect of TCAs is inhibition of 5-HT and noradrenaline reuptake. The modes of action of SNRIs in pain are at present unclear but probably involve some of the mechanisms of the TCAs. The importance of 5-HT and noradrenaline pathways in pain modulation suggests that antidepressants act by enhancing descending inhibitory controls. Indeed, 5-HT and noradrenaline antagonists and depletion of central 5-HT and noradrenaline will attenuate the analgesia obtained with TCAs.[11,12] However, the clinical effects of TCAs appear after a lag of days to weeks, and their pharmacologic effects occur within hours. Therefore, research suggests that the pharmacologic mechanisms, although important in themselves, also induce changes in gene expression that lead to modified formation of neuropeptides and receptors.

Indeed, chronic TCA administration modifies opioid receptor densities and increases endogenous brain opioid levels.[13,14] TCAs therefore enhance endogenous opioid effects (analgesia and neuronal inhibition) and will act synergistically with opioids in providing pain relief.[15] Additionally, TCAs have an NMDA antagonist effect that makes them useful in pain syndromes with characteristics of central sensitization.[16] TCAs possess sodium, calcium, and potassium channel–blocking properties.[17] The sodium channel–blocking properties of TCAs are robust; regional application of TCAs has an effect comparable with that of local anesthetics.[18] This will stabilize neurons, prevent peripheral sensitization, and may underlie the mechanisms of peripheral analgesia.[19] More recently, it has been shown that a number of antidepressants induce an upregulation of gamma-aminobutyric acid (GABA) receptor expression in the spinal cord.[20]

Other peripheral actions include the ability to block alpha-adrenergic receptors, which may be beneficial in sympathetically maintained pain syndromes. The enhancement of inhibitory GABA and opioid effects are also present peripherally, thereby increasing the analgesic effects of TCAs.[21] TCAs and other antidepressants have moderate anti-inflammatory actions that would augment analgesia.[22] Histamine and cholinergic receptor blockade is thought to augment the analgesic effects of TCAs but also causes many of the observed side effects.[23,24] Amitriptyline is thought to act antagonistically at cephalic blood-vessel 5-HT$_{2B/7}$ receptors; it downregulates 5-HT$_{2B}$ receptors, thus reducing vessel wall reactivity and vasodilation.[25] For many years, amitriptyline has therefore been in the front line of migraine prophylaxis (see chapter 10). Amitriptyline may be superior to other drugs when pain comorbidity includes myalgia, depression, or sleeplessness.

Drugs related to the dopaminergic, serotonergic, and adrenergic systems, such as antidepressants, have been shown to suppress or exacerbate bruxist activity in humans and animals.[26] However, there is insufficient evidence-based data to draw definite conclusions concerning the effects of specific drugs on bruxism.

Pharmacodynamics. A common clinical observation is the variability in side effects across patients. Some of this may be attributed to genetic variations in components of the monoamine neurotransmitter pathways and efflux transporters.[27] The presence of a single nucleotide polymorphism in a drug-metabolizing enzyme will result in one of four functional phenotypes: poor metabolizer, intermediate metabolizer, extensive metabolizer, or ultrarapid metabolizer.[27]

TCAs have a 50-fold interindividual variation in plasma concentrations with a standard dosing, which leads to significant potential for toxicity.[28] The major pathways of amitriptyline lead to the formation of nortriptyline, which is also an antidepressant.[29] Nortriptyline undergoes further metabolism by the *CYP2D6* gene to the corresponding inactive metabolite 10-hydroxynortriptyline, which then undergoes further metabolism via glucuronidation to facilitate renal elimination. For TCAs (and some SNRIs) for which CYP2D6-catalyzed metabolism is a major clearance mechanism, patients with a poor-metabolizer phenotype are at risk for adverse drug reactions or toxicity at regular doses because of the higher circulating plasma concentrations as well as clinically significant drug-drug interactions.[30] Patients with both the CYP2C19 extensive-metabolizer and the CYP2D6 intermediate/poor-metabolizer phenotypes are at particularly high risk for adverse events after amitriptyline and imipramine administration.[29] Conversely, those with the ultrarapid-metabolizer phenotype will require higher doses to achieve therapeutic plasma drug concentrations.[30]

Amitriptyline. Amitriptyline is FDA cleared for the treatment of depression but is used extensively off-label for migraine, tension-type headache, irritable bowel syndrome, polyneuropathy, fibromyalgia, postherpetic neuropathy, myofascial pain, and other chronic pain states. Nortriptyline, its active metabolite, has similar therapeutic effects but a milder side-effect profile.

Efficacy. Amitriptyline is effective in the management of many chronic orofacial pains and chronic tension-type headaches. In addition to reducing subjective pain parameters, amitriptyline induces a reduction of myofascial tenderness in the affected areas.[31] At doses of 25 to 125 mg, daily amitriptyline is beneficial in the management of painful neuropathies, such as painful diabetic neuropathy and postherpetic neuropathy with an overall NNT of 4.6.[9] The evidence points to a significant but selective effect on a small group of patients.

Clinical considerations. The analgesic effect of TCAs is independent of their antidepressant actions and may be attained at much lower doses[32,33]; 10 mg taken 1 or 2 hours before bedtime is the recommended initial dose. The long elimination half-life of amitriptyline (10 to 26 hours) allows for a once-daily schedule. The dose may be increased if necessary at a rate of 10 mg a week to a maximum of 35 to 50 mg. Chronic administration of 25 mg amitriptyline daily is not associated with significant reductions in a patient's processing or task-performing capacity.[34] Higher doses (> 100 mg) are prescribed to patients with headache and other chronic pain syndromes, but these are accompanied by significant side effects. Additionally, the danger of sudden death increases by 40% for 100 mg or more of amitriptyline or other equivalent TCA doses.[35] Analgesic effects may be observed at 1 week but may take up to several weeks. Therapy should be continued for 3 to 6 months before being slowly tapered and discontinued.

Adverse effects. Side effects at low doses are rare and not serious and usually include dry mouth, sedation, palpitations, nausea, and sweating. Other common effects include bloating, constipation, <u>asthenia</u>, dizziness, headache, blurred vision, fatigue, and somnolence. In patients taking 25 mg amitriptyline daily for 12 weeks, a mean weight gain of 3.2 kg has been reported.[36] Weight control should therefore be an integral part of patient management. Rarely, patients may feel anxiety or agitation, but adding a benzodiazepine (eg, 5 mg diazepam or 0.5 to 1 mg of slow-release alprazolam) may resolve this. This combination may, however, increase sedative effects. Possible contraindications for amitriptyline include urinary retention and narrow-angle glaucoma. TCAs decrease the convulsive threshold and thus are problematic in existing epileptic disorder. The use of TCAs with antiarrhythmics is contraindicated, and the presence of cardiovascular disorders requires a medical consult. In ongoing antidepressant therapy (eg, SSRIs) or in patients with depression or suicidal tendencies, TCAs are to be initiated only after consultation with the treating psychiatrist. TCAs possess antihyperglycemic effects and therefore may alter insulin or other hypoglycemic drug requirements in patients with diabetes. Carbamazepine increases the metabolism of TCAs and reduces effective plasma concentrations. Thyroid disease and thyroid hormones may interact with TCAs to increase receptor sensitivity to catecholamines.

TCAs and SSRIs increase the risk of upper gastrointestinal (GI) bleeding.[37] The amount of upper GI bleeding episodes in patients on amitriptyline and imipramine was 2.5 and 3.5 times more than expected. The use of TCAs with nonsteroidal anti-inflammatory drugs (NSAIDs) or aspirin increased risk of GI bleeding by 9.6 and 8.3, respectively. SSRI use was associated with a 3.6-times increased risk, and combined use with NSAIDs or low-dose aspirin increased the risk to 12.2 and 5.2 times, respectively.[37] Antidepressants without action on the serotonin receptor had no significant effect on the risk of upper GI bleeding. The increased risk disappeared after cessation of SSRI use. However, the risks of upper GI bleeding remained increased during periods when TCAs were stopped, which suggests that other mechanisms were involved.

Rare but serious side effects reported include myocardial infarction, cerebrovascular accident, orthostatic hypotension, and syncope. Rare hematologic events include agranulocytosis, aplastic anemia, leukopenia, thrombocytopenia, or pancytopenia. Similarly, decreased liver function and jaundice have been reported rarely.

Amitriptyline is in pregnancy category C (see Table 16-1); it is excreted into milk but with low resulting concentrations in breastfeeding neonates and is therefore probably safe for breastfeeding infants.

Venlafaxine/desvenlafaxine

Venlafaxine is a structurally novel SNRI antidepressant that is FDA cleared for the treatment of depression, generalized anxiety disorder, panic disorder, and social phobia. The drug's active metabolite, desvenlafaxine, has become available in an extended-release formulation that seems to have effects similar to those of the parent compound.[38] Both drugs are more potent inhibitors of the serotonin transporter. However, compared with venlafaxine, desvenlafaxine has a relatively greater effect on the norepinephrine transporter and a longer elimination half-life.

Efficacy. Venlafaxine extended release has shown promise in the prophylaxis of migraine and tension-type headache.[39] Moreover, in a double-blind RCT, venlafaxine extended release 150 mg provided significant prophylaxis for patients with migraine.[40] Benefits from the use of venlafaxine in patients with painful diabetic neuropathy or neuropathic pain of unknown cause have been reported.[41,42] Venlafaxine extended release at doses ranging from 150 to 225 mg had an NNT of 4.5 to 5.7 for moderate or 50% relief in painful diabetic neuropathy.[43,44] Venlafaxine (75 mg) was found to be modestly effective in the treatment of atypical facial pain.[45] No significant correlation was found between venlafaxine serum concentration and treatment response. Analgesia was independent of antidepressive or antianxiety effects, and adverse events were equally common with venlafaxine and placebo.

Clinical considerations. To minimize side effects, patients are often started on 37.5 mg daily for the first 4 to 7 days before increasing to 75 mg daily. If necessary, the dose may be increased to 150 mg daily after several weeks. Further increases, to a maximum daily dose of 225 mg, may be made at intervals of not less than 4 days. Extended-release preparations enable once-daily dosing. Desvenlafaxine should be initiated at 50 mg daily, and the maximum recommended dose is 100 mg daily.

Adverse effects. The most frequently reported adverse events with venlafaxine are nausea, headache, insomnia, somnolence, dry mouth, dizziness, constipation, sexual dysfunction (abnormal ejaculation or impotence), asthenia, sweating, tremor, and nervousness. Patients, especially the elderly, should be warned of the risk of dizziness or unsteadiness due to orthostatic hypotension. As with other antidepressants, venlafaxine may impair performance of skilled tasks, and, if affected, patients should not drive or operate machinery. Venlafaxine should be used with caution in patients with moderate to severe hepatic or renal impairment, and dosage adjustment may be necessary. A medical consult is indicated in patients with a recent history of myocardial infarction or unstable heart disease or whose condition might be exacerbated by an increase in heart rate. Because of the risk of dose-related hypertension, blood-pressure monitoring is advisable. Loss of appetite and weight loss are commonly reported.

Measurement of serum cholesterol levels should also be considered with long-term treatment. Venlafaxine should not be used when bleeding disorders are present. Because of an increased risk of relapse in patients with a history of hypomania, mania, or epilepsy, venlafaxine should also be used with caution and be discontinued in any patient with a history of developing a seizure. Patients with raised intraocular pressure or at risk of angle-closure glaucoma should be monitored closely. Patients who develop a rash, urticaria, or related allergic reaction with venlafaxine should be referred for medical consultation. Rare but serious side effects reported include hyponatremia and hepatitis.

Venlafaxine and desvenlafaxine are in pregnancy category C, but extreme caution is recommended in the third trimester. Low levels are detectable in about half of breastfeeding neonates, and the exact risk is unknown.

Duloxetine

Duloxetine is a new-generation SNRI that is FDA cleared for the treatment of major depressive disorder, generalized anxiety disorder, fibromyalgia, chronic musculoskeletal pain, and painful diabetic neuropathy. There is increased selectivity of the serotonin transporter, but duloxetine is more balanced than venlafaxine. Experimental data suggest that duloxetine has analgesic properties with an NNT in neuropathic pain of about 5.[46–48]

Efficacy. Clinical data have shown the effectiveness of duloxetine in the treatment of painful diabetic neuropathy and fibromyalgia.[48–50] In the treatment of depression, usual doses are 20 to 30 mg twice daily or 60 mg once daily.

Clinical considerations. The recommended dose for pain is 60 mg once daily taken irrespective of meal times. In cases where this dose causes considerable side effects, a lower starting dose is indicated. Whether doses higher than 60 mg are more effective is unclear, but 90 to 120 mg has also been successfully used, albeit with a higher dropout rate due to side effects.[48,50]

Adverse effects. The incidence of adverse effects in duloxetine therapy has largely been assessed in open studies, so the figures are unreliable. Insomnia, headache, and sleepiness are common; less frequent nervous system effects include dizziness, blurred vision, somnolence or fatigue, tremor, and agitation. GI effects are also relatively common and include loss of appetite, nausea, diarrhea or constipation, gastritis, and dry mouth; less frequently, anorexia and taste changes have been described. Increased daytime and nighttime sweating may occur. Duloxetine should not be used in patients with hepatic impairment. Dysuria is common, but no dosage adjustment is considered necessary in patients with mild to moderate renal impairment. Rare but serious side effects include worsening of depression, suicidal thoughts, and even suicide. Duloxetine is in pregnancy category C, but extreme caution is recommended in the third trimester. Because of a lack of data, the exact risk to breastfeeding neonates is unknown.

Antiepileptic drugs

Anticonvulsants or antiepileptic drugs (AEDs) have been extensively used in the management of neuropathic pain (eg, trigeminal neuralgia, diabetic neuropathy, and traumatic neuropathy) and, more recently, in the prophylaxis of neurovascular pains (Table 16-3). The AEDs consist of a number of heterogenous drugs with varied modes of action; most commonly, carbamazepine, gabapentin, and pregabalin are specifically used in the management of orofacial pain. Other agents assessed for pain include topiramate and lamotrigine. Experiments have found no correlation between antiepileptic activity and analgesic efficacy in neuropathic pain, which suggests multimodal mechanisms.[51] Different drugs possess different combinations of these modes of action (see Fig 16-1), and specific drugs may be more effective against particular expressions of neuropathic pain (eg, mechanohyperalgesia) or may modulate inflammatory components more than others.[52,53] In some cases, therefore, the combination of two AEDs may offer some benefit. Many of the modes of action of AEDs in pain are common across a wide variety of agents, and these are reviewed in this section.

In 2008, the FDA announced that all AEDs must carry a clear warning that their use increases risk of suicidal thoughts and behaviors (suicidality). These include AEDs commonly used for the management of pain: carbamazepine, oxcarbazepine, divalproex sodium, gabapentin, pregabalin, lamotrigine, and topiramate. The FDA also announced that valproate sodium and related products (ie, valproic acid and divalproex sodium) are contraindicated and should not be taken by pregnant women. The warning is specifically for its use in the prevention of migraines and does not cover its use for epilepsy and manic episodes. Some evidence suggests that these medications can cause decreased IQ scores in children whose mothers took them while pregnant.

Table 16-3 **Anticonvulsants**

Drug	Initial dose (mg)	Target or maximum dose (mg)*	Dose increase (titration)*	Schedule	Taken with food	Pregnancy category	Breastfeeding
Carbamazepine	100 to 200	1,200	100 to 200 mg every 2 days	Three or four times per day	Yes	D	Probably safe
Carbamazepine controlled release	400	1,200	Usually transfer from regular format to equivalent dose	Two times per day	No		
Oxcarbazepine	300	1,200 to 2,400	300 to 600 mg/wk	NA	No	C	NA
Sodium valproate	200 to 600	1,000 to 2,000	200 mg every 3 days	Two times per day	Yes	X†	Probably safe
Divalproex	250 to 500	500 to 1,000	250 mg/wk	One or two times per day			
Divalproex extended release	500	500 to 1,000	500 mg/wk	Once daily			
Clonazepam	0.25 to 0.5	1 to 4	0.25 mg/wk	Bedtime	No	D	Risk unclear
Gabapentin	300	900 to 2,400	300 mg every 1 or 2 days	Three times per day	No	C	Probably safe
Pregabalin	150	300	50 mg every 2 or 3 days	Two or three times per day	No	C	Risk unclear
Lamotrigine	25	400 to 600	25 to 50 mg/wk	One or two times per day	No	C	Risk unclear
Topiramate	25	100	25 mg/wk	Two or three times per day	No	C	Risk unclear
Duloxetine	20 to 40	60 to 120	20 mg/wk	One or two times per day	No	C other than the third trimester	Unknown

*This is a rough guideline; clinicians should clinically titrate based on therapeutic response versus side effects.
†FDA altered the drug category to X specifically for migraine; for epilepsy and manic episodes, the drug remains in category D.
BDZ, benzodiazepine; NA, not applicable; OCP, oral contraceptive pill.

Medical contraindications	Drug interactions	Common side effects
Bone marrow problems, cardiac problems, blood disorders, glaucoma	Alcohol, anticoagulants, BDZs, calcium-channel blockers, cimetidine/ omeprazole, doxycycline, erythromycin, OCP, SSRIs/ TCAs, tramadol	Hypertension, hypotension, lightheadedness, rash, pruritus, erythematous condition, nausea, vomiting, confusion, dizziness, nystagmus, somnolence, blurred vision, diplopia
Bone marrow problems, hepatic/renal problems, psychiatric problems	Alcohol, OCP	Abdominal pain, nausea, vomiting, ataxia, dizziness, headache, nystagmus, somnolence, tremor, diplopia, rhinitis, fatigue
Hepatic problems, urea disorders	Antiplatelets	Alopecia, weight gain, abdominal pain, diarrhea, loss of appetite, nausea, vomiting, asthenia, ataxia, dizziness, diplopia, headache
Hepatic/renal problems, psychiatric problems, glaucoma, respiratory problems	Alcohol	Salivation, ataxia, dizziness, somnolence, depression, respiratory depression
Renal problems	AEDs	Edema, myalgia, ataxia, dizziness, somnolence, tremor, mood swings, hostility, fatigue
NA	AEDs	Edema, weight gain, constipation, xerostomia, ataxia, dizziness, somnolence, blurred vision, diplopia
Hepatic/renal problems, cardiac problems, bone marrow problems, psychiatric problems	AEDs, OCP	Rash, nausea, vomiting, ataxia, dizziness, headache, somnolence, blurred vision, diplopia
Hepatic/renal problems, psychiatric problems, glaucoma, respiratory problems	AEDs, OCP, digoxin, valproate	Nausea, dizziness, asthenia, ataxia, tremor, paresthesia, nystagmus, glaucoma, diplopia, nervousness, fatigue
Epilepsy, glaucoma, hepatic/ renal problems, psychiatric problems	Antidepressants	Sweating, constipation, loss of appetite, nausea, xerostomia, diarrhea, gastritis, dizziness, insomnia or somnolence, blurred vision, dysuria, fatigue

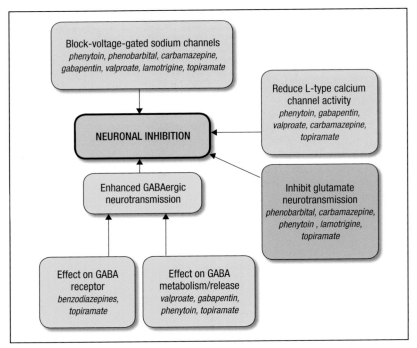

Fig 16-1 The modes of action of anticonvulsants.

Modes of action

The therapeutic effects of AEDs in headache, orofacial pain, and neuropathic pain are mediated by a reduction in neurogenic inflammation and central trigeminal activation, modulation of central nervous system effects, and enhancement of antinociceptive mechanisms.[54,55] At least in part, AEDs are analgesic by their ability to suppress neuronal excitability through a number of mechanisms[54,56] (Fig 16-1).Different AEDs possess varying combinations of these effects, and some of the newer drugs may have as yet undiscovered modes of action.

GABA effects. When GABA is released from the presynaptic terminal, it binds to at least two postsynaptic receptors. Activation of the GABA-A receptor induces an influx of chloride ions, and activation of GABA-B induces an inhibition of calcium channels or deactivation of potassium channels.[56] This effectively hyperpolarizes the postsynaptic neuron inhibiting activity. Some AEDs are able to facilitate GABA neurotransmission by increasing presynaptic GABA

levels and postsynaptic GABA-receptor function. The central analgesic actions of carbamazepine are partially mediated by GABAergic systems in the periaqueductal gray.[57] Valproate is thought to act by increasing brain levels of GABA, whereas benzodiazepines and barbiturates enhance postsynaptic GABA-receptor binding.

Sodium-channel blockade. A large number of AEDs act on sodium channels, probably via a prolongation in the recovery phase after channel activation. The effect is use- and voltage-dependent; that is, the number of channels inactivated increases with each additional stimulus and is more pronounced in excited neurons, leading to the modulation of neurotransmitter release. The stepwise blockade of sodium channels is an important facet of certain AEDs and limits side effects.

Glutamate. Glutamate is a major excitatory neurotransmitter, and its release is modulated by presynaptic sodium and calcium channels. After its release, glutamate binds to NMDA and non-NMDA receptors

(AMPA [α-amino-3-hydroxy-5-methyl-4-isoxazolepropionic], kainate, metabotropic) on the postsynaptic membrane. Activation of non-NMDA receptors induces an influx of sodium ions and depolarization and excitation of the neuron. This excitation ultimately leads to the activation of NMDA receptors (see chapters 3 and 13) and an influx of calcium ions, which leads to further excitation of the postsynaptic neuron. Glutamate exhibits excitotoxic properties by causing membrane depolarization and an influx of sodium and calcium. These ionic fluxes, under ischemic conditions, initiate the cascade of reactions that culminate in neuronal injury and death.[58,59] Thus, the control of glutamate release may offer protection from neuronal damage.

AEDs directly modulate glutamate effects by blockading excitatory receptors and altering glutamate metabolism or its release, and they indirectly modulate sodium and calcium channels that will affect glutamate release. Carbamazepine and phenytoin block NMDA receptors,[56] and gabapentin inhibits glutamate release in the spinal cord.[60] Experimental evidence suggests that inhibition of glutamate release by carbamazepine, oxcarbazepine, and lamotrigine is probably mediated via sodium-channel blockade.[61,62]

Calcium-channel blockade. Blockade of calcium channels modulates neurotransmitter release similar to the effect after sodium-channel blockade. AEDs act at the L-type calcium channels, which are involved in generating action potentials and intracellular calcium signals. At present, the effects of gabapentin are thought to be mediated primarily via this mechanism.

Effects of chronic therapy. Long-term valproate therapy has been shown to modulate the intracellular pathways that are strategically involved in the mediation of neurochemical changes and gene expression associated with chronic pain.[63] These processes lead to long-term neuroplasticity, neuronal sensitivity, and neuronal activity so that valproic acid may potentially be able to modify these changes. Additionally, valproic acid has been shown to induce the neuroprotective gene *BCL-2*, which suggests that it may be neuroprotective in traumatic neuropathies [63] Evidence exists

for the neuroprotective properties of valproic acid, topiramate, and lamotrigine in models of ischemic and traumatic neuronal injuries.[59,63] Topiramate has demonstrated neuroprotective properties in animal models of epilepsy[64] but not in a peripheral painful mononeuropathy.[65] In humans, topiramate showed some evidence of encouraging neuroregeneration in diabetic neuropathy,[66] but no further studies have published similar effects. Further research will elucidate the possible role of such mechanisms in the management of chronic pain syndromes.

Antiepileptic drug hypersensitivity syndrome

Occurrence of rash in patients taking anticonvulsants, particularly carbamazepine, is of concern as this may be a part of antiepileptic drug hypersensitivity syndrome (AHS). This syndrome, comprising fever, rash, lymphadenopathy, and, less commonly, hepatosplenomegaly and eosinophilia, has been associated with some AEDs, including carbamazepine.[67] These reactions usually occur within 30 days and require immediate withdrawal and alternative therapy. Cross-reactivity (75%) may occur with phenobarbital and phenytoin, so these drugs should be avoided. Hypertension or hypotension is also commonly reported.

Stevens-Johnson syndrome (SJS) or toxic epidermal necrolysis (TEN) often fulfills the diagnostic criteria for AHS (fever, rash, and some sign of systemic organ involvement), and it can be difficult to distinguish among them. The rashes from SJS and TEN begin as areas of macular erythema that can merge and develop into necrosis of the epidermal layer of the skin, which leads to desquamation. Both of these exfoliative rashes are usually accompanied by fever, and systemic organ involvement frequently occurs. If the symptomatology of a case of SJS or TEN associated with anticonvulsant drug use fulfills the requirements for AHS, then it should be considered AHS, and appropriate precautions should be taken with regard to avoiding other anticonvulsant drugs that may exhibit cross-sensitivity.

The overall estimated risk of SJS/TEN associated with carbamazepine is fairly low—1 to 6 per 10,000 new users—but is based on countries with mainly white populations.[68,69]

Reports of postmarketing adverse events have pointed to a 10-times higher rate of SJS/TEN in some Asian countries. Subsequent studies have shown that this increased risk of SJS/TEN was associated with HLA-B*1502, an inherited allelic variant of the *HLA-B* gene found almost exclusively in some persons across broad areas of Asia, including South Asian Indians.[70–72] HLA-B*1502 is largely absent in persons not of Asian origin and therefore has not been found to be a risk factor for SJS/TEN in whites.[73]

Carbamazepine

Carbamazepine is FDA cleared for the treatment of bipolar disorder, acute manic and mixed episodes, epilepsy (partial, generalized, mixed types), and trigeminal neuralgia.

Efficacy. Experiments found that carbamazepine elevates pain thresholds in rats[74] and suppresses neuronal activity in response to the application of bradykinin to tooth pulp[75] or spinal nerve injury.[76] Experimental data support the clinical observation that carbamazepine is generally ineffective in trigeminal traumatic neuropathies.[77] In addition to the modes of action described earlier (see Fig 16-1), carbamazepine also seems to exert analgesic effects via the adenosine system.[78]

In orofacial pain, carbamazepine is almost exclusively used for trigeminal neuralgia. Rarely, a therapeutic trial with carbamazepine is used in patients with posttraumatic neuropathy who exhibit a prominent lancinating/electrical and paroxysmal quality to their pain. The authors initiate therapy at 100 mg (half a tablet) in the evening (with food) and increase on alternate days by 100 to 200 mg in the morning, then at midday. In trigeminal neuralgia, therapeutic effects are observed at 48 to 72 hours. Final dose titration is based on response and side effects but may reach 1,200 mg/day or more; if side effects are prominent, a slower increase in dosage should be performed. When a positive response is observed without serious side effects, controlled-release carbamazepine should be initiated at a dose that is at least equivalent to the standard formulation. Controlled-release carbamazepine has fewer side effects and is taken on a twice-daily schedule with or without food, which makes it more convenient.

Adverse effects. Side effects such as light-headedness, confusion, dizziness, vertigo, blurred vision or diplopia, sedation (somnolence), vomiting, nystagmus, and nausea are very common and cause 5% to 20% of patients to request drug cessation. Skin rashes, sometimes pruritic, occur in up to 10% of patients. This may be an early sign of AHS, as described earlier.

Carbamazepine is a hepatic enzyme inducer, and transient elevation in liver enzymes may occur in 5% to 10% of patients. Carbamazepine therefore induces its own metabolism, as well as that of a number of other drugs, including some antibacterials (notably doxycycline), anticoagulants, and oral contraceptives. Erythromycin may cause substantial elevations of serum carbamazepine levels. Carbamazepine may diminish the activity of warfarin and other coumarins through increased metabolism.

Serious side effects are rarer but include cardiac arrhythmias, hepatitis, systemic lupus erythematosus, nephrotoxicity, acute renal failure, and angioedema. Carbamazepine should be avoided in patients with atrioventricular conduction abnormalities, blood disorders, or a history of bone marrow depression. Transient leukopenia is observed in 5% of patients and may become persistent in 2%. Aplastic anemia is a serious effect that may occur in 1 of 15,000 to 200,000 patients. Hyponatremia is observed in 4% to 22% of carbamazepine-treated patients and requires drug withdrawal; the mechanism is uncertain and may involve direct effects on the kidneys or increased secretion of antidiuretic hormone. Mild antimuscarinic properties of carbamazepine suggest that caution should be observed in patients with glaucoma or raised intraocular pressure. Scattered punctate lens opacities occur rarely during carbamazepine therapy.

Because of the side-effect profile of carbamazepine, baseline and periodic testing of patients should include liver function, differential blood count, serum electrolytes, serum iron and folic acid, eye examination, and renal function. Although the value of such testing has been questioned, it is generally routine in clinical practice. Additionally, plasma levels of carbamazepine are monitored to assess patient compliance and adequate drug absorption. No data are available on therapeutic ranges for carbamazepine in the treatment of trigeminal neuralgia, and the authors generally aim at maintaining therapeutic plasma concentrations as for epilepsy (4 to 12 µg/mL). Carbamazepine is classified as pregnancy category D, and the risk for breastfeeding neonates is probably acceptable.

Oxcarbazepine

Oxcarbazepine is a derivative of carbamazepine that is FDA cleared for the treatment of partial seizures.

Efficacy. Data from experiments on spinal and trigeminal pain suggest that oxcarbazepine is antinociceptive in inflammatory or neuropathic pain and reduces neuronal activity.[79,80] Initial dosage is 600 mg daily by mouth in two divided doses and may be increased thereafter, if necessary, in maximum increments of 600 mg daily at approximately weekly intervals. Maintenance doses are usually in the range of 600 to 1,200 mg daily (up to 2,400 mg) and are usually higher than carbamazepine doses for control of trigeminal neuralgia[81]; 300 mg of oxcarbazepine is approximately equivalent to 200 mg of carbamazepine.[82] Onset of action in trigeminal neuralgia has been reported to be about 24 to 48 hours.[81,82]

Adverse effects. Although adverse events are similar, there are indications that oxcarbazepine has significantly fewer nervous system side effects than carbamazepine. Common side effects include abdominal pain, nausea, vomiting, ataxia, dizziness, headache, nystagmus, somnolence, tremor, diplopia, rhinitis, and fatigue.

Hypersensitivity reactions such as skin rashes occur less frequently with oxcarbazepine than with carbamazepine but may be serious, such as in multiorgan hypersensitivity reaction, SJS, or TEN. Moreover, cross-sensitivity does occur, and about 25% to 30% of patients who are hypersensitive to carbamazepine may experience such reactions with oxcarbazepine. Dose-related hyponatremia has also been observed with oxcarbazepine and may even be more common (2.5% to 29.9%) than with carbamazepine.[83] Oxcarbazepine is in pregnancy category C, and although it is probably safe, the exact risk to breastfeeding neonates is unknown.

Valproate

Valproate is a broad term applied to a group of related compounds that include valproic acid, divalproex sodium, and sodium valproate. Divalproex sodium is a stable coordination complex that comprises sodium valproate and valproic acid in a 1:1 molar ratio. The group is FDA cleared for the treatment of seizures and acute mania as well as for migraine prophylaxis.

Efficacy. Valproates increase the brain levels of GABA.[84] In the trigeminal system, valproate decreases nociceptor-induced activity of second-order neurons (c-fos expression) and meningeal neurogenic inflammation.[85] The formats most frequently used are sodium valproate and divalproex (extended release). Divalproex is first-line therapy for migraine prohylaxis and is superior to amitriptyline.[86,87] Clinical use of valproates also includes the treatment of chronic daily headaches.[88]

Sodium valproate. The suggested initial oral dose for adults is 600 mg daily in two divided doses. This may be increased by 200 mg every 3 days to a usual range of 1 to 2 g daily (20 to 30 mg/kg daily); up to a maximum of 2.5 g daily may be necessary.

Valproic acid. Adults and children begin with an initial daily dose of 15 mg/kg (ie, 1,200 mg/day for an 80-kg adult) that is increased by 5 to 10 mg/kg at 1-week intervals. Valproic acid may be given in two to four divided doses. The maximum recommended dose of valproic acid in the United Kingdom is 30 mg/kg daily, whereas in the United States it is 60 mg/kg daily.

Divalproex sodium. The initial dose is 250 mg twice daily; a single 250-mg dose at bedtime may be tried, however, for patients with initial side effects. The usual maximum dose is 1 g/day. Extended-release tablets should be initiated with a 500-mg dose once daily for 1 week and may be increased to 1 g daily if needed. At 500 mg daily, divalproex sodium is effective in treating migraine, although some patients may need higher doses.[89] The extended-release form of divalproex sodium has comparable efficacy to the standard formulation, and adverse-effect rates are comparable with those of placebo.[90]

Adverse effects. Side effects with valproate therapy are very common and are often associated with too high a starting dose, increasing doses too rapidly, or concomitant use of other AEDs. The most frequently reported adverse effects are GI disturbances (abdominal pain, diarrhea, loss of appetite, nausea, vomiting), particularly at the start of therapy. Starting with low doses and advising patients to take medication with meals may minimize these. Enteric-coated formulations are available and may further reduce GI distress; in patients with gastric discomfort, adding an antacid (eg, omeprazole) is helpful.

Increased appetite may occur, but long-term (up to 6 years) studies of divalproex use revealed no hepatotoxicity and negligible weight gain.[88] Neurologic adverse effects include ataxia, dizziness, diplopia, tremor, sedation, asthenia, ataxia, lethargy, and confusion. Less common adverse effects include edema, headache, reversible prolongation of bleeding time, and thrombocytopenia. Leukopenia or bone marrow depression and a dose-dependent thrombocytopenia have been reported.

Elevation of liver enzyme values is common but normally transient and dose related. Liver dysfunction, including hepatic failure and fatality, has occasionally been reported, usually in the first few months of treatment and in young children. Baseline testing and routine follow-up of blood counts and liver function are indicated. Life-threatening pancreatitis is a rare but serious adverse event. Valproates are in pregnancy category X, and low concentrations are found in neonates.

Gabapentin

Gabapentin is FDA cleared for the treatment of seizures and postherpetic neuropathy. Off-label uses include the treatment of migraine, diabetic neuropathy, trigeminal neuralgia, short-lasting unilateral neuralgiform headache attacks with conjunctival injection and tearing, and cluster headache. Gabapentin is an amino acid that is structurally related to the inhibitory neurotransmitter GABA. Indeed, gabapentin was designed to be a GABA mimetic with increased lipophilicity to enhance nervous system penetration. Despite the structural similarity, gabapentin and pregabalin do not have an appreciable effect on GABA receptors, although recent findings suggest an effect on presynaptic GABA receptors.[91] Moreover, gabapentin is not converted metabolically into GABA and is not a direct inhibitor of GABA transport.[91]

Efficacy. Gabapentin is an effective agent for the treatment of experimental neuropathies[92,93] and reduces post-injury neuronal activity.[76] Gabapentin prevents pain behavior associated with orofacial pain induced experimentally in rats, which suggests that it may be useful in the treatment of trigeminal neuropathies.[94,95] Gabapentin is a good alternative analgesic in the management of perioperative pain.[96,97] Gabapentin 250 to 500 mg provided significant pain relief to patients undergoing dental or major orthopedic surgery.[98] However, with an NNT of 11, gabapentin is inferior to standard analgesics used in these settings (see chapter 15). Clinical studies have established gabapentin as an effective therapy for chronic neuropathic pain, with an NNT of 5.8, and it provides high-level pain relief in about a third of patients.[99] However, the evidence for the effectiveness of gabapentin is specifically for postherpetic neuropathy, painful diabetic neuropathy, and fibromyalgia.[99]

Based on available data, it appears that the initial target dosage is 900 mg; treatment should be started at 300 mg/day and increased by 300 mg daily over a period of 3 days, or longer if side effects are prohibitive.[100] Initiation of gabapentin at low doses is associated with reduced side effects once the maintenance dose is achieved. Additional titration to 1,800 mg/day is recommended for greater efficacy. Maintenance doses are taken three times daily, and amounts vary between syndromes: 900 to 3,600 mg/day for diabetic neuropathy, up to 2,400 mg/day for migraine prophylaxis, and up to 1,800 mg/day for postherpetic neuropathy. However, the effective dose should be individualized according to patient response and tolerability.

Adverse effects. Many of the side effects occur within 3 days of initiating therapy but usually subside with continued use of gabapentin. The most commonly reported adverse effects are somnolence, dizziness, ataxia, and fatigue. Visual disturbances, tremor, weight gain, dyspepsia, amnesia, weakness, and paresthesia occur less frequently. Mood swings and hostility have also been reported.

More rarely, seizure, altered liver function tests, erythema multiforme, SJS, myalgia, headache, edema, nausea, and vomiting have been reported. Gabapentin is in pregnancy category C, and although it is probably safe, the exact risk to breastfeeding neonates is unknown.

Pregabalin

Pregabalin is an analog of the inhibitory neurotransmitter GABA and is FDA cleared for the treatment of partial seizures, diabetic peripheral neuropathy/neuropathic pain, postherpetic neuropathy, and pain from spinal cord injury. Pregabalin, which is effective for the management of neuropathic pain,[101] ranked as the 27th most sold prescription drug in 2013 at 6.2 million units sold.

Efficacy. Pregabalin is efficacious for the treatment of postherpetic neuropathy and diabetic neuropathy and has relatively few side effects.[102,103] Initial dosage for the treatment of painful diabetic peripheral neuropathy or postherpetic neuropathy is 50 mg three times daily or 75 mg twice daily. Based on efficacy and tolerability, this may be increased to 100 mg three times a day within 1 week. Patients may be maintained on 75 to 150 mg twice daily or 50 to 100 mg three times a day. For patients who do not experience adequate pain relief after 2 to 4 weeks of treatment with 300 mg/day and are tolerating pregabalin, dosage may be increased up to 300 mg two times a day or 200 mg three times a day for a trial period. Pregabalin has shown efficacy in the postoperative acute pain setting, usually at a dose of 300 mg,[104–110] reducing pain scores and use of escape opioid medication, but see Hegarty and Shorten[111] and Moore et al[112] for more detailed information.

Adverse effects. The most common adverse effects include mild to moderate dizziness and somnolence; confusion, headache, amnesia, ataxia, and weakness are less frequent. Other common adverse effects include constipation, dry mouth, and vomiting. Visual disturbances (blurred vision, diplopia), dose-dependent peripheral edema, and weight gain have been reported. A modest and transient elevation of hepatic enzymes and occasionally a drop in platelet count may be observed. Myopathy secondary to muscle damage and accompanied by increases in plasma creatinine kinase is a rare complication. Pregabalin is in pregnancy category C, and although it is probably safe, the exact risk to breastfeeding neonates is unknown.

Clonazepam

Clonazepam is a benzodiazepine with anticonvulsant properties and is FDA cleared for the treatment of panic disorder and seizures.

Efficacy. Clinical effectiveness of clonazepam has been demonstrated in myofascial pain[113,114] and in some neuropathic pain disorders.[115] The authors primarily use clonazepam in patients with myofascial pain who are not responsive to amitriptyline, in patients with posttraumatic pain who present with panic symptoms, and for burning mouth syndrome (see chapter 12). Clonazepam may be useful as monotherapy or add-on therapy for muscular disorders and, more rarely, to supplement therapy in trigeminal neuralgia. No evidence supports its effectiveness in neuropathic pain.[116] The authors initiate therapy at 0.25 mg at night and increase to 0.5 to 1 mg/day in one or two doses, according to side effects and response. Rarely, patients may benefit from higher doses, but side effects are usually severe. Treatment should be discontinued slowly by decreasing the dose every 3 days. For patients with burning mouth syndrome, a possible topical effect suggests that a 1-mg tablet be sucked and not swallowed, thus avoiding side effects associated with systemic therapy.[117] Alternatively, if sedative/hypnotic and antipanic effects are needed, the tablets may be sucked and subsequently swallowed. This has also been shown to be effective in patients with burning mouth syndrome (see chapter 12).

Adverse effects. The most common adverse effect occurring in about half of patients is drowsiness or somnolence, particularly at the start of therapy. Muscle weakness, ataxia, and slurred speech may occur. Excessive salivation, dizziness, and respiratory depression have been reported. Although the relationship between psychiatric depression and benzodiazepine use is unclear, clonazepam should probably be avoided in patients with depression.[118] Clonazepam is in pregnancy category D, and there is insufficient evidence to rule out risk for breastfeeding neonates.

Topiramate

Topiramate is FDA cleared for the management of seizures and Lennox-Gastaut syndrome (a severe form of childhood epilepsy that is usually refractory to medical management) as well as for migraine prophylaxis. The pharmacologic profile of topiramate includes all the modes of action discussed earlier in addition to mild inhibition of carbonic anhydrase and kainate, which leads to enhanced neuronal stability.

Efficacy. In animal models of neuropathic pain, topiramate is an efficient analgesic.[65,119] Specifically, topiramate has dose-dependent and rapid inhibitory effects on trigeminovascular nociceptive neurons.[120] Clinically, topiramate has been successfully applied to the treatment of a variety of pain syndromes (see Chong and Libretto[121]). These include trigeminal neuralgia,[122] diabetic neuropathy,[123,124] and migraine and other headaches,[125] particularly chronic migraine[55] (see chapter 10). Efficacy has recently been proven for medication-overuse headache, which suggests that topiramate does not need to be withdrawn.[55] The recommended total daily dose of topiramate in migraine prophylaxis is 100 mg/day in two divided doses with a slow titration schedule over a period of 4 weeks.

Adverse effects. Dose-related adverse events in adults include dizziness, fatigue, nervousness, concentration difficulties, confusion, depression, language problems, anxiety, or nervousness. Paresthesia, asthenia, ataxia, tremor, and mood problems are also common. Nausea, abdominal pain, and anorexia have also been reported.

Topiramate inhibits some isoenzymes of carbonic anhydrase and may induce renal tubular acidosis. Therefore, in addition to assessment of renal function (particularly in the elderly), serum bicarbonate levels should be assessed at baseline and periodically during treatment. Topiramate is therefore contraindicated in conditions or therapies that predispose a patient to acidosis, such as renal disease, severe respiratory disorders, status epilepticus, diarrhea,

surgery, ketogenic diet, or drugs. Ocular side effects include diplopia and nystagmus. Moreover, a syndrome consisting of acute myopia associated with secondary angle-closure glaucoma has been reported in patients receiving topiramate within 1 month of initiating therapy. The primary treatment to reverse symptoms is discontinuation of topiramate as rapidly as possible. Other serious but rare side effects include pyrexia, pancreatitis, anemia or leukopenia, hepatitis, liver failure, nephrolithiasis, and dyspnea. Topiramate is in pregnancy category D, and there is insufficient evidence to rule out risk for breastfeeding neonates.

Lamotrigine

Lamotrigine is an AED that is structurally unrelated to other drugs in its class. The drug is FDA cleared for the treatment of bipolar disorder, Lennox-Gastaut syndrome, and seizures.

Efficacy. Studies indicate that lamotrigine is analgesic in experimental setups.[51] However, in a recent review, lamotrigine was not found to be significantly analgesic in painful diabetic neuropathy, central post-stroke pain, chemotherapy-induced neuropathic pain, HIV-related neuropathy, mixed neuropathic pain, and spinal cord injury–related pain.[126] This is contrary to a previous review that found good evidence for an analgesic effect of lamotrigine in neuropathic pain,[127] possibly suggesting that in selected patients and conditions lamotrigine may have a role.

In trigeminal neuralgia that is refractory to standard medical therapy, adding 400 mg lamotrigine was superior to placebo.[128] However, experimental data suggest that lamotrigine may be inferior to gabapentin in the management of traumatic trigeminal neuropathies.[94] The target dose for the treatment of neuropathic pain is somewhat higher than that used for seizure control and may reach 400 to 600 mg. To minimize side effects, the initial dose of 25 mg/day should be increased very slowly, reaching the target in 7 weeks or more. Dose increase is dependent on side effects and therapeutic response observed.

Adverse effects. Most side effects of lamotrigine are dose related and commonly include dizziness, nausea or vomiting, sedation, headache, visual disturbances (blurred vision, diplopia), and ataxia. Maculopapular and erythematous rashes have been reported with therapeutic doses of lamotrigine—serious in 1.1% of patients and nonserious in 7% to 10%.[126] This side effect is related to higher starting doses and is also possibly more common in patients younger than 16 years, when the maximum dose is exceeded, or when the dose is increased at a faster rate than recommended. Any sign of skin rash mandates cessation of lamotrigine to avoid increases in severity; TEN and SJS have also been reported. Rarely, cardiovascular (electrocardiogram changes) and bone marrow suppression with leukopenia, anemia, or thrombocytopenia are observed. Other rare but serious events include hepatic necrosis or liver failure, amnesia, seizure, and angioedema. AHS has been associated with lamotrigine therapy. Lamotrigine is in pregnancy category C, and there is insufficient evidence to rule out risk for breastfeeding neonates.

Antihypertensives

Beta-adrenergic receptor blockers: Propranolol

Propranolol is a noncardioselective beta-blocker that is FDA cleared for the treatment of a number of cardiovascular conditions (eg, angina pectoris, cardiac dysrhythmia, hypertension), essential tremor, migraine, and pheochromocytoma (Table 16-4). The beta-adrenergic blockers (beta-blockers) were originally introduced for the treatment of cardiac arrhythmias and angina pectoris. Serendipitous observation led to their application in the treatment of hypertension and migraine. Propranolol does not possess intrinsic sympathomimetic activity.

Mode of action

Sympathetic hyperactivity in regional and generalized muscle disorders, such as fibromyalgia, suggests that beta-blockers may be useful therapeutic agents (see chapter 8). Experimental inhibition of catechol-O-methyltransferase, an enzyme that metabolizes catecholamines,

leads to increased measures of inflammatory pain in rodents.[129] Administration of propranolol reversed this effect, which suggests that beta-blockers may have a role in the management of pain that is modulated by sympathetic hyperactivity. Experimental data demonstrate that propranolol can reduce serotonin-induced masseter muscle pain.[130] Pindolol, also a nonselective beta-blocker, was shown to be effective in the management of fibromyalgia; however, the study was not placebo controlled.[131] Early data suggest that propranolol may be useful in masticatory myofascial pain, but no controlled trials have been published.[132]

The exact role of vasodilation in neurovascular pain is questionable, and propranolol does not constrict cerebral arteries; thus, beta-blockers probably act via additional mechanisms.[133] Beta-blockers seem to exert some of their therapeutic effects in migraine via actions at sites in the central nervous system that are intimately involved with nociception (locus coeruleus, thalamus). Propranolol has a high affinity for 5-HT binding sites in the central nervous system and antagonizes $5-HT_{1A}$ and $5-HT_{2B}$ receptors, thus reducing neuronal hyperexcitability. The production of nitric oxide is inhibited by beta-blockers (beta-2 action). Nitric oxide is intimately associated with the pathophysiology of neurovascular craniofacial pain, such as cluster and migraine headache (see chapters 10 and 11). The membrane-stabilizing properties of propranolol result in neuronal stability. This may be related to inhibition of kainate-induced currents and is synergistic with NMDA blockers.[90]

Some evidence suggests that beta-blockers exert their effect via the central catecholaminergic system. Inhibition of beta-1-mediated noradrenaline release leads to reduced central catecholaminergic hyperexcitability and may be a possible mode of action for propranolol.[134] The reduction is delayed and parallels that often observed clinically in the prophylactic treatment of migraine with propranolol. Migraineurs exhibit an enhanced centrally mediated secretion of epinephrine after exposure to light that returns to normal after treatment with propranolol.[135] This finding therefore supports the conclusion that migraineurs with signs of central catecholaminergic hyperexcitability will respond well to propranolol.

Table 16-4 **Antihypertensives**

Drug	Initial dose (mg)	Target or maximum dose (mg)*	Dose increase (titration)*	Schedule	Pregnancy category	Breastfeeding
Propranalol	40 to 80	240	40 mg/wk	Two or three times per day	C	Risk unclear
Propranalol sustained release	80	160 to 240	80 mg every 1 or 2 wks	Once daily		
Verapamil	120	120 to 480	40 to 80 mg every 1 or 2 wks	Two or three times per day	C	Risk unclear
Verapamil sustained release	120	120 to 480	120 mg every 1 or 2 wks	One or two times per day		

*This is a rough guideline; clinicians should clinically titrate based on therapeutic response versus side effects.

Cortical potentials in response to various stimuli are abnormal in migraineurs relative to control subjects, and after 3 or 4 months of treatment with propranolol, potentials are normalized.[136] Increased thalamocortical activity in response to superior sagittal sinus stimulation is inhibited by beta-blockers through beta-1 adrenoceptor antagonist actions.[137] No effect of propranolol on experimental neurogenic inflammation has been found.[138] In summary, these studies suggest that propranolol may act primarily within the central nervous system.

Efficacy

The positive effect of beta-blockers in migraine and neurovascular orofacial pain has been repeatedly shown (see chapter 10). Propranolol may be prescribed in sustained-release format, although the standard formulation is often used initially as trial therapy. For the prophylaxis of neurovascular pain (eg, neurovascular orofacial pain, migraine), an initial dose of 40 to 80 mg daily is often used in two or three doses. The dose can be increased at weekly intervals up to 240 mg daily if needed. Most often patients are transferred to the slow-release formula, usually 80 to 160 mg daily in a single dose.

Adverse effects

Fatigue, dizziness, coldness of the extremities, dermatitis, and pruritic rashes are common and troublesome side effects experienced with beta-blockers. The most frequent and serious adverse effects are related to their beta-adrenergic blocking activity and include heart failure, hypotension, heart block, and bradycardia. Use of beta-blockers in patients with cardiovascular disease requires a medical consult and monitoring. Bronchospasm with dyspnea or wheezing is a serious side effect, and nonselective beta-blockers, such as propranolol, are therefore contraindicated for patients with asthma. Atenolol, a cardioselective beta-blocker, is a possible alternative in these patients. Paresthesia, peripheral neuropathy, arthralgia, and myopathies, including muscle cramps, have been reported. Adverse GI effects include nausea and vomiting, diarrhea, loss of appetite, constipation, and abdominal cramping. Propranolol also commonly causes sleepiness and depression.

Beta-blockers interfere with carbohydrate and lipid metabolism and can produce hypoglycemia or hyperglycemia as well as changes in blood concentrations of triglycerides and cholesterol. The beta-blockers can reduce the response to insulin and oral hypoglycemics through their effects on pancreatic beta-receptors; their use, therefore, is contraindicated in patients with diabetes. Blockade of peripheral beta-receptors interferes with the effects of sympathomimetics; thus, patients on beta-blockers, especially nonselective beta-blockers, may develop elevated blood pressure if they are given adrenaline. The bronchodilator effects of adrenaline are also inhibited. Propranolol is in pregnancy category C and is considered safe for breastfeeding neonates.

Medical contraindications	Drug interactions	Common side effects
Asthma, cardiovascular problems, diabetes, hepatic/renal problems, hyperlipidemia, peripheral vascular disease	Anticoagulants, antiarrhythmics, calcium-channel blockers, cimetidine, epinephrine, NSAIDs, thyroid hormones, triptans	Arrhythmias, dermatitis, pruritus, rash, loss of appetite, nausea, vomiting, sleepiness, paresthesia, depression, dyspnea, wheezing
Cardiovascular problems, hepatic/renal problems	Antiarrhythmics, antiplatelets, beta-blockers, carbamazepine, cimetidine	Edema, hypotension, constipation, nausea, dizziness, headache

Calcium antagonists: Verapamil and flunarizine

Calcium-channel antagonists, such as verapamil and flunarizine, are FDA cleared for the treatment of angina, hypertension, and supraventricular tachycardia.

Mode of action

The mechanisms underlying the effect of calcium antagonists in neurovascular pain are unclear. Flunarizine inhibits the synthesis and release of nitric oxide (involved in the pathophysiology of headaches) in perivascular neurons.[139] Calcium antagonists may inhibit the release of substance P and calcitonin gene-related peptide (CGRP).[140] Both substance P and CGRP are involved in nociceptive transmission and neurogenic inflammation.[141]

Efficacy

At present there is insufficient evidence to support verapamil as a first-line drug for migraine, but it may be considered when other first-line prophylactics have been ineffective. However, verapamil is a drug of choice in the prophylaxis of cluster headache and is usually effective at doses between 200 and 480 mg, although occasionally higher doses are needed.[142] Flunarizine at a dose of 5 to 10 mg daily has proven highly effective in the prophylaxis of migraine and is usually considered when beta-blockers are contraindicated or ineffective.[143]

Adverse effects

Cardiac effects include bradycardia, atrioventricular block, worsening heart failure, and transient asystole. Rarely, these may induce angina or myocardial infarction. Cardiac effects are particularly severe in patients with hypertrophic cardiomyopathies. The most troublesome noncardiac adverse effect is constipation. Nausea may occur but is less frequent. Other adverse effects include hypotension, dizziness, flushing, headaches, fatigue, dyspnea, peripheral edema, and, rarely, syncope. Reports of skin reactions and some cases of abnormal liver function and hepatotoxicity have been recorded. Gingival hyperplasia is reported as in other calcium-channel blockers. Verapamil is in pregnancy category C and considered safe in breastfeeding neonates. Insufficient data are available for flunarizine.

Muscle Relaxants

Muscle relaxants are a heterogenous group of drugs whose therapeutic use is based on their ability to prevent or alleviate increased muscle tone and activity (Table 16-5). Some of these drugs, however, possess additional modes of action that may be important in the management of pain. Benzodiazepines are sometimes used based on their putative muscle-relaxing properties, although they decrease muscle tone at doses that produce unacceptable side effects. However, there is evidence for short-term

Table 16-5	Muscle relaxants					
Drug	**Initial dose (mg)**	**Target or maximum dose (mg)***	**Dose increase (titration)***	**Schedule**	**Pregnancy category**	**Breastfeeding**
Cyclobenzaprine	5 to 10	30 to 60	< 3 wks total treatment	Three times per day	B	Unknown
Baclofen	5 to 15	30 to 60	5 mg every 3 days	Three times per day	C	Safe

*This is a rough guideline; clinicians should clinically titrate based on therapeutic response versus side effects.

benzodiazepine efficacy for acute muscular conditions, such as low back pain.[144] Cyclobenzaprine is considered of significant therapeutic value for painful muscular conditions[145] and is recommended for similar orofacial pain syndromes. Other muscle relaxants have been proven effective in experiments on masticatory muscle pain.[146] Baclofen has shown efficacy in trigeminal neuralgia.

Cyclobenzaprine

Cyclobenzaprine is a centrally acting skeletal muscle relaxant related to the TCAs. The drug is FDA cleared for the treatment of skeletal spasticity and is often used as an adjunct in the symptomatic treatment of painful muscle spasm associated with musculoskeletal conditions.

Mode of action

Cyclobenzaprine acts mainly at the brainstem to decrease tonic somatic motor activity, thereby influencing both alpha and gamma motor systems, but additional activity at spinal cord sites may be involved. Effects begin within 1 hour of an oral dose, and the effects of a single dose have been reported to last as long as 12 to 24 hours. No specific antinociceptive properties are associated with cyclobenzaprine.

Efficacy

Whether cyclobenzaprine is superior to other drugs for the management of acute myofascial strain is unclear; it usually adds more side effects with little therapeutic gain.[147] For neck pain, however, mixed results are obtained.[148] No extensive studies have examined the use of cyclobenzaprine in the management of chronic painful musculoskeletal conditions, but in general, lidocaine trigger-point injections are superior.[149] A study on patients with orofacial myofascial pain found that cyclobenzaprine is superior to placebo and clonazepam when added to self-care and education for the management of jaw pain upon awakening.[150] Cyclobenzaprine (10 mg/day) failed to significantly improve sleep in the short term, but this may be due to the relatively low dose used. The usual dose is 5 to 10 mg three times daily, and treatment for more than 2 or 3 weeks is not recommended.

A meta-analysis concluded that in the short term, cyclobenzaprine at 10 to 60 mg daily (median, 30 mg daily) improves low back pain.[151] Moderate improvement was observed in the first 4 days of treatment and gradually declined with time. Some evidence of continued improvement was found at 2 weeks. Cyclobenzaprine has modest benefits in fibromyalgia: Patients reported overall improvement and moderate reductions in individual symptoms, particularly sleep disturbance.[152]

Adverse effects

Side effects are common, with at least one occurring in 53% of patients, and are similar to those observed with TCAs. Common side effects include dysgeusia, constipation, dyspepsia, nausea, xerostomia, confusion, dizziness, headache, somnolence, blurred vision, and nervousness. Particular care should be exercised in the elderly, in whom cyclobenzaprine may induce hallucinations. Additionally, some rare but serious side effects include cardiac dysrhythmia, hepatitis, and anaphylaxis. Cyclobenzaprine is in pregnancy category B, but risk to breastfeeding neonates is unknown.

Medical contraindications	Drug interactions	Common side effects
Cardiovascular problems, epilepsy, glaucoma, hepatic problems, hyperthyroidism, urinary retention	Alcohol, antidepressants	Dysgeusia, constipation, dyspepsia, nausea, xerostomia, confusion, dizziness, headache, somnolence, blurred vision, nervousness
Cerebrovascular accident, epilepsy, psychiatric problems, renal problems	Alcohol, antidepressants	Constipation, nausea, vomiting, asthenia, dizziness, headache, somnolence

Baclofen

Baclofen is a derivative of GABA that is FDA cleared for the treatment of spasticity but does not appear to possess conventional analgesic activity.[153]

Mode of action

Baclofen acts specifically at the spinal end of the upper motor neurons to cause muscle relaxation. The drug inhibits monosynaptic and polysynaptic reflexes at the spinal level, probably by effects on the afferent terminal, but it may also affect supraspinal sites. Baclofen increases the stimulus threshold for inducing reflexes, increases the latency between stimulus and reflex, and decreases the amplitude of the muscle response. In the trigeminal nucleus, baclofen depresses excitatory transmission and facilitates segmental inhibition, most probably via GABA-B receptor actions.[154]

Efficacy

Experimentally, baclofen demonstrates antinociceptive properties in neuropathies of sciatic and trigeminal nerves.[77,155] In humans, baclofen is effective intrathecally for intractable pain of the lower back and/or lower extremities.[156] Modest doses of baclofen (15 to 40 mg/day) have also been successfully used in open trials for the treatment of cluster headache and migraine.[157,158] Baclofen relieves pain in facial postherpetic neuropathy and potentiates opioid analgesia.[156,159] At doses ranging between 30 and 80 mg/day, baclofen has proven efficacious in patients with trigeminal neuralgia[160,161] and appears to enhance the effectiveness of carbamazepine and phenytoin.[162] Baclofen is mainly used as add-on therapy when side effects prevent the increase of carbamazepine, but it is also used as single therapy for trigeminal neuralgia. The authors initiate therapy at 5 mg (half a tablet) daily in the evening and increase to 15 mg in three doses within 3 days. Dose escalation is continued by 5 mg per dose every 3 days until there is a positive response or prohibitive side effects.

Adverse effects

Common side effects reported with baclofen include constipation, nausea, vomiting, asthenia, dizziness, headache, and somnolence. Informing patients that abrupt discontinuation of baclofen may produce severe side effects, including seizures, hallucinations, paranoia, delusions, psychosis, anxiety, confusion, and agitation, is extremely important.[163] Dosage should be reduced gradually over at least 10 to 14 days, or longer if symptoms occur. Baclofen is in pregnancy category C and considered safe in breastfeeding neonates.

Triptans

Because of the highly specific actions of triptans in neurovascular headaches, the clinical aspects of triptan use are discussed in chapters 10 and 11. The triptans are agonists of 5-HT$_1$ receptors located at trigeminal and vascular sites. The drugs are in pregnancy category C. Sumatriptan is probably safe for breastfeeding neonates, but the safety of zolmitriptan and rizatriptan is unknown.

Mode of action

The antimigraine effect of the triptans has several sites of action.[164] Peripherally, triptans cause vasoconstriction, a 5HT$_{1B}$ receptor postjunctional effect.[165] Triptans also diminish trigeminal neuropeptide release (5-HT$_{1D}$, 5-HT$_{2B}$, and 5-HT$_7$ effects) and block trigeminal-induced dural plasma-protein extravasation.[166,167] However, antimigraine efficacy is not dependent on this action, as other drugs with a specific effect on extravasation are ineffective in migraine.[164] Centrally, triptans inhibit transmission in the trigeminal nucleus caudalis (effects on 5-HT$_{1B}$, 5-HT$_{1D}$, 5-HT$_{1F}$), reducing afferent stimulation of second-order neurons, possibly by blocking the action of CGRP.[168,169] In clinical trials, abortive therapy with triptans resulted in relief of pain and symptoms as well as a concomitant reduction in the jugular levels of CGRP, which usually increase during migraine episodes. In the periaqueductal gray, triptans induce selective inhibition of trigeminovascular nociceptive afferent input.[170] This occurs for dural but not facial nociceptors and raises an interesting question on whether triptans will be as effective in facial neurovascular pain (eg, neurovascular orofacial pain) as they are in migraine. However, in the only known case series, triptans were effective in facial migraine.[171] In addition to inhibitory effects on the trigeminal nucleus, triptans seem to activate descending pain modulatory pathways, augmenting analgesia.[170,172] However, this effect is dependent on the inherent ability of individual drugs to penetrate the blood-brain barrier, which is low for some triptans. Alternatively, the blood-brain barrier is disrupted during migraine, allowing triptan penetration.[166] In animal models, early administration of triptans blocks the development of central sensitization.[173]

Cannabinoids

Cannabis and its subcompounds, the cannabinoids, have been used in medicine for many years. The best-known cannabinoids are the tetrahydrocannabinoids and their metabolites, which induce the major psychoactive effects.

Mode of action

Two cannabinoid receptors have been cloned: CB1 and CB2. CB1 is located in the brain, spi-

nal cord, and peripheral nervous system. CB2 is found in immune cells and microglia but is expressed in the spinal cord and the peripheral nervous system, particularly after injury. Research indicates that more cannabinoid receptors exist. Cannabis may be administered through the lungs (smoked), via the gut (swallowed), or by topical application on the skin or mucosa. The pharmacokinetics differ significantly among these routes.

The analgesic effects of cannabinoids are mediated largely by activation of the CB1 receptor, which probably leads to the inhibition of neuropeptide and inflammatory agent release, but CB2 activation is also involved. Anandamide (an endogenous cannabinoid) is able to modulate the release of CGRP from sensory fibers.[174] Interestingly, certain nonsteroidal anti-inflammatory agents seem to act by inhibiting the breakdown of anandamide.[175] Topical cannabinoid receptor agonists reverse sensory hypersensitivity,[176] but supraspinal and particularly spinal sites of action are considered important.[177,178] Systemic CB1 agonists reverse behavioral pain parameters and reduce levels of peptides associated with the initiation and maintenance of pain.[179] CB1 receptors in the spinal cord are persistently upregulated after experimental neuropathy, thereby offering a good target for analgesia.[180,181] Combinations of cannabinol with opioids reveal synergistic effects in animal pain models that suggest a useful clinical application.[182,183] In the trigeminal system, cannabinoids act as negative modulators of pain transmission peripherally and centrally, which suggests that they may be useful in orofacial pain syndromes.[184]

Efficacy

Exogenous cannabinoids are analgesic in models of persistent inflammatory,[185] neuropathic,[186] and cancer pain.[187] In humans, cannabinoids have analgesic, muscle relaxant, and appetite-stimulant effects and reduce intraocular pressure. In a recent trial on patients with treatment-resistant neuropathic pain, vaporized cannabis, even at low doses, was an effective option.[188] Synthetic cannabinoids are available for the control of chemotherapy-induced nausea and vomiting, and an oral mucosal formulation seems effective in chemotherapy-induced neuropathic pain.[189] Furthermore, two systematic reviews have found evidence that cannabinoids are modestly effective in patients with neuropathic pain and some evidence for efficacy in fibromyalgia and rheumatoid arthritis.[190–192] Some still raise concerns regarding side effects and safety.[191] Anecdotal reports suggest that cannabinoids are beneficial in a variety of disorders, including glaucoma, multiple sclerosis, and wasting in patients with AIDS and malignant neoplasms.

Cannabinoids have been shown to be efficacious in various pain states, and reports indicate that more than a third of patients with chronic pain have used herbal cannabinoids for symptom relief.[192–194] Acute states tested include experimental[195] and postoperative[196] pain, though results have been inconsistent. In chronic neuropathic pain syndromes (including pain secondary to multiple sclerosis), cannabinoids were effective analgesics.[197-199] Cannabinoids may be useful in headaches according to some indications.[200]

Adverse effects

Not enough information is available on the adverse-effect profile of cannabinoids within a medical setting. Often, the data are derived from nonmedical use. Common serious side effects of cannabinoids reported in clinical trials include relapse of multiple sclerosis, vomiting, and urinary tract infection.[192] Mild side effects included dizziness, somnolence, muscle spasm, pain, dry mouth, bladder disorders, euphoria, delusions, and sedation. As they are psychoactive drugs, cannabinoids potentially have adverse effects related to overdosing, abuse, dependence, addiction, psychomotor effects, cognitive effects, and short-term/long-term psychiatric and medical adverse effects.[192] Although addiction and abuse occur, the evidence points to common risk factors associated with other forms of substance abuse, particularly antisocial behavior and conduct disorders.[192]

As pharmacologic (ie, side effects, addiction), cultural, and legal obstacles are overcome, cannabinoids will no doubt become an integral part of pain medicine. Efforts have begun to delineate guidelines for their use in the management of chronic pain.

NMDA Receptor Antagonists

The role of the NMDA receptor in chronic pain mechanisms makes it an attractive therapeutic target. Clinically available NMDA receptor antagonists include ketamine and dextromethorphan. Ketamine is largely used as an anesthetic, and trials of subanesthetic doses reveal that it provides effective analgesia in patients with orofacial pain, glossopharyngeal neuralgia, and other neuropathic pains.[201–203] However, the severe side effects associated with ketamine limit their clinical use. Dextromethorphan is used extensively as an antitussive (FDA cleared) and acts by elevating the cough threshold in the cough center located in the medulla oblongata. In humans, dextromethorphan is analgesic, but because it is accompanied by limiting side effects,[204] it is rarely used.

Onabotulinumtoxin A

Onabotulinumtoxin A is one of seven antigenically distinct serotypes of botulinum neurotoxins (BoNT-A to -G) making up the clostridial family. BoNT-A is available commercially in the United States (Botox, Allergan). BoNT-A is FDA cleared for the treatment of chronic migraine, cervical dystonia, axillary hyperhidrosis, adult upper limb spasticity, strabismus, and blepharospasm associated with dystonia.

The toxin affects the nervous system predominantly by inhibiting the release of neurotransmitters from nerve terminals. This occurs through a three-stage process that begins with binding to the target nerve terminal membrane and internalization, translocation, and finally, cleavage of a target protein that is involved in neurotransmitter release.[205] The best-studied site of action of the toxin is the neuromuscular junction, where it inhibits the release of acetylcholine from the presynaptic neuron, causing a dose-dependent, reversible muscle relaxation or paralysis. The effect of the toxin is terminated within 2 to 6 months because of the process of axonal sprouting, which is triggered by the toxin's entrance into the cell.

In one double-blind RCT, patients with focal painful neuropathies and mechanical allodynia received a one-time intradermal administration of BoNT-A (20 to 190 units) into the painful area.[206] The results reported suggest a direct analgesic effect independent of its effects on muscle tone. This has also been confirmed in patients with painful diabetic neuropathy.[207]

Clinical and electrophysiologic data support a distinct mechanism of the analgesic effect of BoNT vis-à-vis those involved in muscle relaxation.[208] Often, the toxin's analgesic effect occurs earlier and lasts longer than its effect on muscle tone.[208] In support, there seems to be no correlation between the decrease in migraine frequency and the amplitude of the compound muscle action potentials measured in the corrugator muscles after BoNT-A injection.[209]

BoNT and migraine

The mechanisms by which BoNT-A is effective in migraine prophylaxis are unclear.[208] BoNT-A can affect the release of various neurotransmitters, particularly those involved in pain (eg, substance P, glutamate, and CGRP).[210,211] A recent study provides evidence for the ability of BoNT-A to inhibit mechanical nociception (suprathreshold) in peripheral trigeminovascular C-fiber neurons.[212] Threshold (non-nociceptive) stimuli were not inhibited. These findings suggest that BoNT-A interferes with neuronal surface expression of high-threshold mechanosensitive ion channels linked preferentially to mechanical pain by preventing their fusion into the nerve terminal membrane.[212] This would inhibit nociceptive flow from the periphery to the spinal trigeminal nucleus and suppress pain.

Evidence of retrograde axonal transport of active BoNT-A and transfer of the toxin to afferent synapses suggest that central mechanisms may also be involved.[213] Thus, a possible mechanism of action of BoNT-A in migraine is via the modulation of neural transmission at the sensory afferents of the trigeminocervical complex.[208] These are largely unmyelinated C fibers, and BoNT-A may be able to diffuse into these nerve endings and inhibit the release of neurotransmitters, such as glutamate and CGRP.[208]

Based on current data, the use of BoNT-A in migraine should be restricted to the chronic form.[214,215] The recommended injection paradigm appears on the manufacturer's website (http://www.botoxchronicmigraine.com/HCP/botox-injection-paradigm/) and consists of a total dose of 155 U administered as 5-U injections per site (31 sites) using a sterile 30-gauge, short (0.5-inch) needle.[216] The sites injected are the corrugator, procerus, frontalis, temporalis, occipital, cervical paraspinal group, and trapezius muscles bilaterally (Table 16-6 and Fig 16-2). The aim of injection is not to get into deep tissues or muscle; therefore, the recommended technique is to deliver a more superficial injection that may be taken up by the peripheral innervation. This also minimizes side effects, such as muscle weakness and hematomas.

BoNT in trigeminal neuralgia and other neuropathic pain

A number of studies have examined the effect of BoNT-A in trigeminal neuralgia.[217] Most studies used 20 to 50 U injected into the trigger zones, although lower (5 to 9 U)[218,219] and higher doses (75 U)[220] have been successfully used. Overall, more than 60% of patients reported an improvement of 50% or greater in pain frequency and intensity. The major events reported were transient facial asymmetry, edema, ptosis, dysesthesia, and chewing difficulties, but these were very rare.[217] The effect was achieved less rapidly than by using pharmacotherapy and usually appeared after 1 or 2 weeks. This would suggest that combined approaches may be indicated, including early pharmacotherapeutic intervention for rapid control that is continued until the BoNT-A effect occurs. Although more research is needed, particularly to elucidate the minimum effective dose and the number and sites of injection points, data suggest that BoNT-A is a significant addition to the ways in which trigeminal neuralgia is managed.

Intradermal injection of BoNT-A in patients with chronic neuropathic pain resulted in an analgesic effect that lasted from week 2 to week 14 after injection and that decreased mechanical and thermal allodynia.[206] In patients with diabetic neuropathy, BoNT-A treatment resulted in a significant analgesic effect for 12 weeks.[207]

Table 16-6 Recommended order of injections with BoNT-A*

Order of injection	Muscle	Recommended dose and number of sites
1	Corrugator	10 U divided in two sites
2	Procerus	5 U in one site
3	Frontalis	20 U divided in four sites
4	Temporalis	40 U divided in eight sites
5	Occipitalis	30 U divided in six sites
6	Cervical paraspinal muscles	20 U divided in four sites
7	Trapezius	30 U divided in six sites

*Each injection site = 0.1 mL = 5 U BoNT-A. All muscles should have the dose distributed bilaterally. Total dose is 155 U divided in 31 sites.

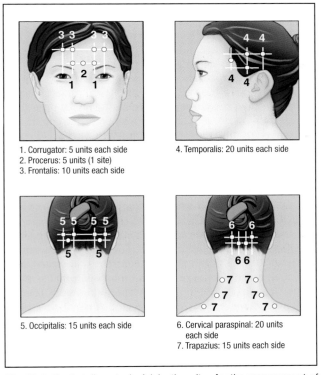

1. Corrugator: 5 units each side
2. Procerus: 5 units (1 site)
3. Frontalis: 10 units each side

4. Temporalis: 20 units each side

5. Occipitalis: 15 units each side

6. Cervical paraspinal: 20 units each side
7. Trapazius: 15 units each side

Fig 16-2 Onabotulinumtoxin A injection sites for the management of chronic migraine: 31 injection sites are divided across seven head and neck muscles (see Table 16-6).

BoNT and muscle pain

BoNT treatment of chronic masticatory muscle pain has yielded good therapeutic outcomes,[221-223] but with an NNT of 11 this is of questionable clinical significance.[224] Moreover, when looking at studies in the management of chronic muscle pain in the neck or other regions, there is insufficient evidence to support the use of BoNT.[225,226] The role of BoNT in the management of chronic muscle pain seems to await further research but may be useful in selected cases.

Topical Therapy for the Management of Pain

Targeted peripheral (or topical) analgesics refer to a number of drugs that have a mechanism of action primarily aimed at peripherally modulating pain mechanisms (inflammatory or neuropathic). The analgesics are therefore most effective in conditions with a primarily peripheral component. These drugs are distinct from transdermal analgesics that require effective systemic concentrations accompanied by an increased risk of adverse effects.[227]

Topical application aims to induce a high local concentration of the active drug at the affected site with minimal or no systemic absorption. Drug interactions are reduced, which is of benefit to patients on multiple drugs or when specific side effects are problematic (eg, NSAIDs and gastric ulcers). Moreover, local application is easy to use and does not require the dose titration that is commonly needed in systemic therapies.[228] Localized reactions, such as rash, may occur but are uncommon[229]; some topicals (eg, capsaicin), may induce local pain on application. Topical agents must be able to cross the epithelium or mucosa to induce an effect. The effectiveness of this barrier is dependent on its integrity as well as its age-related and disease-related changes. Depending on thickness and keratinization, the oral mucosa is up to 10 times more permeable than skin, thereby allowing rapid drug penetration.[230] The effects of saliva will limit the contact time between drug and mucosa and may significantly limit efficacy. Intraorally, the use of topical agents requires either prolonged isolation of the area or the construction of an intraoral appliance (stent) that will allow optimal concentrations for an adequate period.[230] Local application of drugs to facial areas may also be problematic as resultant rashes or dressings may be unsightly. For these reasons, there are fewer studies on the use of topical medications for orofacial conditions, but their use is expanding.

Various topical analgesics are commercially available; most are single drugs, but some combinations are available. Many practitioners use single drugs in combination or have these specifically compounded into gels or creams by specialized pharmacies.[231] The most commonly used agents are NSAIDs and local anesthetics, but a wide variety of topical formulations are in use, including anticonvulsants, antidepressants, opioids, and corticosteroids.[231] In a retrospective study, a compounded mixture of carbamazepine 4%, lidocaine 1%, ketoprofen 4%, ketamine 4%, and gabapentin 4% was applied topically to patients with painful trigeminal neuropathies.[232] The mixture was used on its own or in combination with systemic therapy and was found to significantly relieve pain. The analgesic effects were inferior to those observed with systemic or mixed therapy, but the introduction of the topical drug consistently provided earlier pain relief. The efficacy of topical therapy on trigeminal neuropathies has been confirmed in animal studies.[233]

Topical anesthetics

Topical anesthetics are routinely used in dentistry to attenuate the pain associated with local anesthetic injections. Moreover, topical anesthetics are found in creams used for the treatment of mouth ulcers and erosive conditions of the oral mucosa. The duration of relief is dependent on the carrier's resistance to the effects of mechanical movement and saliva. Topical anesthetic mouthwashes are at times integrated into the management of more generalized ulcerative mucosal conditions, such as mucositis, but they provide doubtful benefit.

The use of 5% lidocaine patches for the treatment of postherpetic neuropathy, painful diabetic neuropathy, and low back pain is effective and safe.[234] Only 10% of patients experienced treatment-related adverse effects; most were local reactions, though some patients suffered headache, raised enzyme levels, and local burning or paresthesia. None of the patients demonstrated changes in gross sensory parameters.[234] Lidocaine patches have been tested intraorally and demonstrated no adverse effects and very low plasma levels.[235] Intraoral lidocaine (10% to 20%) patches provide relatively rapid topical analgesia that may last for up to 45 minutes.[235,236] A benzocaine patch is effective in reducing the intensity of acute toothache when applied to the periapical mucosa.[237] Topical application of a viscous lidocaine gel significantly alleviated pain in patients who underwent tooth socket curettage for alveolar osteitis.[238] These studies suggest that topical anesthetics may be successfully used in the management of painful intraoral syndromes, such as neuropathies.

The actions of topical anesthetics are mediated by their sodium channel–blocking properties, which inhibit signal transduction. Moreover, in injured and inflamed tissue, pain and sensitivity are thought to occur partly because of an upregulation in the numbers of sodium channels and a reduction in their thresholds. Effective concentrations at the injured site must be balanced with the possible systemic toxicity of topical anesthetics, which includes central nervous system and cardiac effects. However, no significant absorption of topical lidocaine mouthwashes was shown even in patients with mucosal breakdown.[239]

More recently, a prescription pain patch (Synera, Galen US [USA]/Rapydan, EUSA Pharma [Europe]) that combines lidocaine, tetracaine, and heat to provide local dermal analgesia has been marketed.[240,241] The primary use is to reduce pain associated with superficial venous access and superficial dermatologic procedures, but it may prove useful for neuropathic pain.

Topical NSAIDs

Systemic NSAIDs are extensively used in medicine and dentistry, both as analgesics and anti-inflammatory agents, but are associated with considerable morbidity and mortality (see chapter 15). Local delivery reduces plasma drug levels to 5% to 15% of that observed after systemic administration while maintaining high concentrations in the dermis and muscle.[242] In clinical situations of cutaneous, neuropathic, and acute and chronic musculoskeletal pain, topical NSAIDs as gel, spray, or patch produce effective analgesia with few side effects.[243–246] Adverse events associated with topical NSAIDs occur in 10% to 15% of patients and are mostly cutaneous—rash and local itching. Systemic effects are rare and tend to occur in patients with a previous history of side effects to systemic NSAIDs.

In patients with painful temporomandibular joints (TMJs), topical diclofenac was as effective as 100 mg oral diclofenac in reducing symptoms.[247] Topical application of 5% ibupro-

fen (three times a day) was as effective as ibuprofen 400 mg (three times a day) taken orally in relieving postexercise jaw pain and maximum voluntary occlusal force of patients with temporomandibular disorders.[248] At the end of the 3-day trial, topical application seemed to offer some advantages over the systemic formulation.[248]

After third molar extraction, topical aspirin or acetaminophen had a significant analgesic effect.[249] Using the same dental extraction model, locally applied ketoprofen (10 mg) was more effective than 10 mg taken orally and was associated with lower plasma levels, which suggests a reduced potential for drug toxicity.[250] A later study with the same experimental model examined flurbiprofen in a slow-release formulation and found that it delayed the onset and lowered the intensity of postoperative pain at lower doses than usually administered orally.[251]

Capsaicin

Topical capsaicin has not been extensively used for oral or perioral application. Low-concentration capsaicin (< 1%) is available and may be applied sparingly three or four times daily. Therapeutic response may not be evident for 1 to 2 weeks for arthritic disorders, or 2 to 4 weeks for neuralgias. More recently, high-concentration (8%) capsaicin has been applied clinically, the aim being to obtain long-term relief (~12 weeks) from a single application and avoid repeated applications. Higher concentrations (10% and 20%) are currently under investigation.[252]

Low-concentration capsaicin

The major adverse event affecting patient compliance is the extreme and immediate burning sensation capsaicin causes (this is also a problem in clinical trials, where blinding becomes very difficult). Burning may last for up to 1 week, but this effect is reduced with repeated applications.

Low-concentration capsaicin seems moderately effective in painful diabetic neuropathy and neuropathic pain, but the evidence for efficacy in postherpetic neuropathy is less convincing.[253,254] A recent systematic review concluded that topical low-concentration capsaicin has unclear efficacy in the treatment of neuropathic pain[255]; however, it may be useful in cases resistant to other modes of therapy or as adjunct therapy.[256]

A positive effect has also been observed in patients with oral neuropathic pain.[257,258] Researchers found that trigeminal neuralgia with an intraoral trigger was less responsive to topical therapy than other neuropathic pain. An open trial of capsaicin in patients with traumatic trigeminal dysesthesia demonstrated a positive clinical effect.[259] Capsaicin in a hard candy–like carrier provided only temporary and incomplete relief for patients with mucositis.[260] Although originally considered potentially useful in the management of temporomandibular disorders,[261] topical application of low-concentration capsaicin cream (0.025%) to painful TMJs produced no statistically significant influence on pain parameters, muscle and joint sensitivity, and maximal mouth opening, compared with placebo.[262] Capsaicin, or its isomer civamide, has been applied to the nasal mucosa for the prevention of cluster headache with modest effects.[263]

Capsaicin 8%

High concentrations provide improved pain relief in patients with postherpetic neuralgia and HIV-related neuropathies but have an NNT of 8.8.[264] The capsaicin 8% patch (Qutenza, Acorda Therapeutics) as a single 30- or 60-minute application significantly reduced pain for up to 3 months in patients with HIV-associated neuropathy or postherpetic neuralgia, and retreatment is effective. Pain reduction occurs rapidly after treatment with capsaicin 8% and is significant from 7 days after treatment.[265] The patch may be used as monotherapy or with systemic medications. Most adverse events are mild to moderate, mostly pain and erythema.[266–268] Safety studies have shown that patients who received repeated treatments with the capsaicin 8% patch over a period of 1 year had no neurologic or sensory impairment.[266,268] Local application of the 8% formulation may be extremely painful and may require topical analgesics such as prilocaine/lidocaine gels.

Application to the facial region is not approved because eye contact is a real concern. However, the capsaicin 8% patch has been successfully used in the treatment of facial neuropathies, under very stringent conditions.[265,269]

Mode of action

Capsaicin, the active component of chili peppers, is an agonist of transient receptor potential vanilloid 1 (TRPV1) channels, which play an important role in pain transmission. TRPV1 is a nonselective cation channel present on C fibers and Aδ fibers. Receptor activation results in an influx of sodium and calcium ions and an action potential. After capsaicin application, substance P is released from peripheral and central terminals. Depending on drug concentration, capsaicin is able to selectively activate, desensitize, or be neurotoxic to small-diameter sensory fibers. Repeated application induces desensitization, inhibits substance P release, and is the basis for its topical therapeutic use.[228] Continuous activation of TRPV1 will induce nociceptor defunctionalization, accompanied by a reversible reduction in epidermal nerve fiber density.[270]

Antidepressants

The peripheral mode of action of antidepressants is multifactorial (see the systemic treatment section) and includes sodium-channel blockade and enhancement of opioid effects.[271]

Topical amitriptyline, alone or combined with ketamine, relieves neuropathic pain.[272–275] Recently, a topical formulation of 10% amitriptyline was successfully used to treat two patients with neuropathic pain in the extremities,[276] which suggests that alternative concentrations need to be examined. Topical application of doxepin significantly relieves chronic neuropathic pain, and when mixed with capsaicin, the effect was observed significantly earlier.[277] In an open, one-dose study, doxepin mouthrinses were shown to be effective in providing analgesia for patients with mucositis.[278] Some patients reported sedation attributed to systemic absorption, but no assays were performed.

Opioids

Topical opioids are being increasingly applied for the relief of pain.[279] The μ-receptor agonists are the most potent topical opioid analgesics;

δ- and κ-receptors are less effective.[228] Opioid receptors are present on the peripheral terminals of thinly myelinated and unmyelinated cutaneous sensory fibers.[280] However, peripheral opioid actions are not prominent in healthy tissue and appear after the induction of inflammation due to enhanced opioid receptor expression.[281] The analgesic opioid effect precedes these changes and is thought to result from the disruption of the perineurial barrier that normally limits access to the nerve.[282] The lowered pH at inflammatory sites may also enhance opioid receptor actions.[228] In the presence of inflammation, morphine (1 mg) added to a local anesthetic for dental surgery results in significant improvement of postoperative analgesia.[283,284] However, application of morphine along the axon (perineurally) or into noninflamed tissue resulted in no reduction in pain scores, which underscores that an inflammatory process is required for peripheral opioid effects.[284] Because oral surgery procedures are accompanied by an inflammatory reaction, supplemental topical morphine may be of benefit for the relief of postoperative pain.[283,284] Low doses of morphine administered into the intraligamentary space of a chronically inflamed hyperalgesic tooth produced a dose-related naloxone-reversible analgesia.[285] The effect was significantly higher than in acute inflammation, which suggests that the effects of topical opioids are related to the time-dependent expression of peripheral receptors. However, these results have not been uniform; morphine applied locally after third-molar surgery was ineffective in providing analgesia.[286]

When administered via intra-articular injection, opioids are effective in controlling joint pain and have few systemic side effects.[287,288] An increased level of opioids in the TMJs of patients with disc displacement without reduction suggests peripheral upregulation and lends support to the use of intra-articular opioids for TMJ pain.[289] In uncontrolled studies, 10 mg of intra-articular morphine injected after arthrocentesis provided excellent pain relief.[290] However, randomized controlled studies in patients with unilateral TMJ arthralgia/osteoarthritis or after arthroscopy have been inconclusive. Morphine may not be superior to placebo[291] or bupivicaine[292]: No dose-effect relation has been shown,[293] no significant short-term analgesic effect occurs,[292,293] and the magnitude of pain relief is often not clinically relevant at long-term follow-up.[293]

In patients with chemoradiotherapy-induced stomatitis, topical morphine (mouthwash) significantly alleviated pain and had a clear dose response.[294] No systemically active detectable levels of morphine were found, which suggests that this may be a useful and safe method to alleviate mucositis pain.

Corticosteroids (steroids)

Steroids are commonly used in the symptomatic management of ulcerative mucosal lesions to reduce both pain and lesion size.[295,296] Intra-articular injection of steroids has been advocated for the management of inflammatory conditions of the TMJ; in this fashion, the systemic side effects may be avoided.[297–301] However, findings of steroid-induced joint damage[302,303] and the high efficacy of standard arthrocentesis have discouraged the use of intra-articular steroids (see chapter 9). The available literature therefore suggests therefore that this modality may be useful in the management of TMJ rheumatoid arthritis, for advanced arthritis that is irresponsive to conservative management, or in patients who are unable to take systemic medication. The potential damage to joint structure must be balanced with the therapeutic effects. In summary, for specific patients and conditions, topically applied drugs are an attractive option in the management of chronic pain.

References

1. Hall GC, Morant SV, Carroll D, Gabriel ZL, McQuay HJ. An observational descriptive study of the epidemiology and treatment of neuropathic pain in a UK general population. BMC Fam Pract 2013;14:28.
2. Green CR, Wheeler JR, LaPorte F, Marchant B, Guerrero E. How well is chronic pain managed? Who does it well? Pain Med 2002;3:56–65.
3. Meghani SH, Kang Y, Chittams J, McMenamin E, Mao JJ, Fudin J. African Americans with cancer pain are more likely to receive an analgesic with toxic metabolite despite clinical risks: A mediation analysis study. J Clin Oncol 2014;32:2773–2779.

4. Bedson J, Belcher J, Martino OI, et al. The effectiveness of national guidance in changing analgesic prescribing in primary care from 2002 to 2009: An observational database study. Eur J Pain 2013;17:434–443.

5. Dworkin RH, Turk DC, Peirce-Sandner S, et al. Considerations for improving assay sensitivity in chronic pain clinical trials: IMMPACT recommendations. Pain 2012;153:1148–1158.

6. Dworkin RH, Turk DC, McDermott MP, et al. Interpreting the clinical importance of group differences in chronic pain clinical trials: IMMPACT recommendations. Pain 2009;146:238–244.

7. Wiener CP, Buhimschi C (eds). Drugs for Pregnant and Lactating Women. New York: Churchill Livingstone, 2004.

8. Saarto T, Wiffen PJ. Antidepressants for neuropathic pain. Cochrane Database Syst Rev 2005;(3).

9. Moore RA, Derry S, Aldington D, Cole P, Wiffen PJ. Amitriptyline for neuropathic pain and fibromyalgia in adults. Cochrane Database Syst Rev 2012;12.

10. Mochizuki D. Serotonin and noradrenaline reuptake inhibitors in animal models of pain. Hum Psychopharmacol 2004;19(suppl 1):S15–S19.

11. Gray AM, Pache DM, Sewell RD. Do alpha2-adrenoceptors play an integral role in the antinociceptive mechanism of action of antidepressant compounds? Eur J Pharmacol 1999;378:161–168.

12. Schreiber S, Backer MM, Pick CG. The antinociceptive effect of venlafaxine in mice is mediated through opioid and adrenergic mechanisms. Neurosci Lett 1999;273:85–88.

13. Hamon M, Gozlan H, Bourgoin S, et al. Opioid receptors and neuropeptides in the CNS in rats treated chronically with amoxapine or amitriptyline. Neuropharmacology 1987;26:531–539.

14. Sacerdote P, Brini A, Mantegazza P, Panerai AE. A role for serotonin and beta-endorphin in the analgesia induced by some tricyclic antidepressant drugs. Pharmacol Biochem Behav 1987;26:153–158.

15. Luccarini P, Perrier L, Dégoulange C, Gaydier AM, Dallel R. Synergistic antinociceptive effect of amitriptyline and morphine in the rat orofacial formalin test. Anesthesiology 2004;100:690–696.

16. Cai Z, McCaslin PP. Amitriptyline, desipramine, cyproheptadine and carbamazepine, in concentrations used therapeutically, reduce kainate- and N-methyl-D-aspartate-induced intracellular Ca2+ levels in neuronal culture. Eur J Pharmacol 1992;219:53–57.

17. Ogata N, Yoshii M, Narahashi T. Psychotropic drugs block voltage-gated ion channels in neuroblastoma cells. Brain Res 1989;476:140–144.

18. Gerner P, Haderer AE, Mujtaba M, et al. Assessment of differential blockade by amitriptyline and its N-methyl derivative in different species by different routes. Anesthesiology 2003;98:1484–1490.

19. Wang GK, Russell C, Wang SY. State-dependent block of voltage-gated Na+ channels by amitriptyline via the local anesthetic receptor and its implication for neuropathic pain. Pain 2004;110:166–174.

20. McCarson KE, Duric V, Reisman SA, Winter M, Enna SJ. GABA(B) receptor function and subunit expression in the rat spinal cord as indicators of stress and the antinociceptive response to antidepressants. Brain Res 2006;1068:109–117.

21. Nakashita M, Sasaki K, Sakai N, Saito N. Effects of tricyclic and tetracyclic antidepressants on the three subtypes of GABA transporter. Neurosci Res 1997;29:87–91.

22. Abdel-Salam OM, Baiuomy AR, Arbid MS. Studies on the anti-inflammatory effect of fluoxetine in the rat. Pharmacol Res 2004;49:119–131.

23. Ferjan I, Erjavec F. Changes in histamine and serotonin secretion from rat peritoneal mast cells caused by antidepressants. Inflamm Res 1996;45:141–144.

24. Irman-Florjanc T, Stanovnik L. Tricyclic antidepressants change plasma histamine kinetics after its secretion induced by compound 48/80 in the rat. Inflamm Res 1998;47(1, suppl):S26–S27.

25. Crews FT, Scott JA, Shorstein NH. Rapid down-regulation of serotonin2 receptor binding during combined administration of tricyclic antidepressant drugs and alpha 2 antagonists. Neuropharmacology 1983;22:1203–1209.

26. Winocur E, Gavish A, Voikovitch M, Emodi-Perlman A, Eli I. Drugs and bruxism: A critical review. J Orofac Pain 2003;17:99–111.

27. Peter C, Watson N, Gilron I, Pollock BG, Lipman AG, Smith MT. Antidepressant analgesics. In: McMahon SB, Koltzenburg M, Tracey I, Turk DC (eds). Wall and Melzack's Textbook of Pain. Philadelphia: Saunders, 2013:465–490.

28. Schenk PW, van Fessem MA, Verploegh-Van Rij S, et al. Association of graded allele-specific changes in CYP2D6 function with imipramine dose requirement in a large group of depressed patients. Mol Psychiatry 2008;13:597–605.

29. Steimer W, Zöpf K, von Amelunxen S, et al. Amitriptyline or not, that is the question: Pharmacogenetic testing of CYP2D6 and CYP2C19 identifies patients with low or high risk for side effects in amitriptyline therapy. Clin Chem 2005;51:376–385.

30. Zhou SF, Liu JP, Chowbay B. Polymorphism of human cytochrome P450 enzymes and its clinical impact. Drug Metab Rev 2009;41:89–295.

31. Bendtsen L, Jensen R. Amitriptyline reduces myofascial tenderness in patients with chronic tension-type headache. Cephalalgia 2000;20:603–610.

32. Max MB, Lynch SA, Muir J, Shoaf SE, Smoller B, Dubner R. Effects of desipramine, amitriptyline, and fluoxetine on pain in diabetic neuropathy. N Engl J Med 1992;326:1250–1256.

33. Sharav Y, Singer E, Schmidt E, Dionne RA, Dubner R. The analgesic effect of amitriptyline on chronic facial pain. Pain 1987;31:199–209.

34. Veldhuijzen DS, Kenemans JL, van Wijck AJ, Olivier B, Kalkman CJ, Volkerts ER. Acute and subchronic effects of amitriptyline on processing capacity in neuropathic pain patients using visual event-related potentials: Preliminary findings. Psychopharmacology (Berl) 2006;183:462–470.

35. Ray WA, Meredith S, Thapa PB, Hall K, Murray KT. Cyclic antidepressants and the risk of sudden cardiac death. Clin Pharmacol Ther 2004;75:234–241.

36. Berilgen MS, Bulut S, Gonen M, Tekatas A, Dag E, Mungen B. Comparison of the effects of amitriptyline and flunarizine on weight gain and serum leptin, C peptide and insulin levels when used as migraine preventive treatment. Cephalalgia 2005;25:1048–1053.

37. Dalton SO, Johansen C, Mellemkjaer L, Norgård B, Sorensen HT, Olsen JH. Use of selective serotonin reuptake inhibitors and risk of upper gastrointestinal tract bleeding: A population-based cohort study. Arch Intern Med 2003;163:59–64.

38. Yang LP, Plosker GL. Desvenlafaxine extended release. CNS Drugs 2008;22:1061–1069.

39. Adelman LC, Adelman JU, Von Seggern R, Mannix LK. Venlafaxine extended release (XR) for the prophylaxis of migraine and tension-type headache: A retrospective study in a clinical setting. Headache 2000;40:572–580.

40. Ozyalcin SN, Talu GK, Kiziltan E, Yucel B, Ertas M, Disci R. The efficacy and safety of venlafaxine in the prophylaxis of migraine. Headache 2005;45:144–152.

41. Kiayias JA, Vlachou ED, Lakka-Papadodima E. Venlafaxine HCl in the treatment of painful peripheral diabetic neuropathy. Diabetes Care 2000;23:699.

42. Sumpton JE, Moulin DE. Treatment of neuropathic pain with venlafaxine. Ann Pharmacother 2001;35:557–559.

43. Rowbotham MC, Goli V, Kunz NR, Lei D. Venlafaxine extended release in the treatment of painful diabetic neuropathy: A double-blind, placebo-controlled study. Pain 2004;110:697–706.

44. Sindrup SH, Bach FW, Madsen C, Gram LF, Jensen TS. Venlafaxine versus imipramine in painful polyneuropathy: A randomized, controlled trial. Neurology 2003;60:1284–1289.

45. Forssell H, Tasmuth T, Tenovuo O, Hampf G, Kalso E. Venlafaxine in the treatment of atypical facial pain: A randomized controlled trial. J Orofac Pain 2004;18:131–137.

46. Bomholt SF, Mikkelsen JD, Blackburn-Munro G. Antinociceptive effects of the antidepressants amitriptyline, duloxetine, mirtazapine and citalopram in animal models of acute, persistent and neuropathic pain. Neuropharmacology 2005;48:252–263.

47. Jones CK, Peters SC, Shannon HE. Efficacy of duloxetine, a potent and balanced serotonergic and noradrenergic reuptake inhibitor, in inflammatory and acute pain models in rodents. J Pharmacol Exp Ther 2005;312:726–732.

48. Lunn MP, Hughes RA, Wiffen PJ. Duloxetine for treating painful neuropathy, chronic pain or fibromyalgia. Cochrane Database Syst Rev 2014;1.

49. Goldstein DJ, Lu Y, Detke MJ, Lee TC, Iyengar S. Duloxetine vs. placebo in patients with painful diabetic neuropathy. Pain 2005;116:109–118.

50. Raskin J, Pritchett YL, Wang F, et al. A double-blind, randomized multicenter trial comparing duloxetine with placebo in the management of diabetic peripheral neuropathic pain. Pain Med 2005;6:346–356.

51. Shannon HE, Eberle EL, Peters SC. Comparison of the effects of anticonvulsant drugs with diverse mechanisms of action in the formalin test in rats. Neuropharmacology 2005;48:1012–1020.

52. Fox A, Gentry C, Patel S, Kesingland A, Bevan S. Comparative activity of the anti-convulsants oxcarbazepine, carbamazepine, lamotrigine and gabapentin in a model of neuropathic pain in the rat and guinea-pig. Pain 2003;105:355–362.

53. Bianchi M, Rossoni G, Sacerdote P, Panerai AE, Berti F. Carbamazepine exerts anti-inflammatory effects in the rat. Eur J Pharmacol 1995;294:71–74.

54. Soderpalm B. Anticonvulsants: Aspects of their mechanisms of action. Eur J Pain 2002;6(suppl A):3–9.

55. Hoffmann J, Akerman S, Goadsby PJ. Efficacy and mechanism of anticonvulsant drugs in migraine. Expert Rev Clin Pharmacol 2014;7:191–201.

56. Moshe SL. Mechanisms of action of anticonvulsant agents. Neurology 2000;55(5, suppl):S32–S40.

57. Foong FW, Satoh M. The periaqueductal gray is the site of the antinociceptive action of carbamazepine as related to bradykinin-induced trigeminal pain. Br J Pharmacol 1984;83:493–497.

58. Leker RR, Neufeld MY. Anti-epileptic drugs as possible neuroprotectants in cerebral ischemia. Brain Res Brain Res Rev 2003;42:187–203.

59. Yang Y, Shuaib A, Li Q, Siddiqui MM. Neuroprotection by delayed administration of topiramate in a rat model of middle cerebral artery embolization. Brain Res 1998;804:169–176.

60. Coderre TJ, Kumar N, Lefebvre CD, Yu JS. Evidence that gabapentin reduces neuropathic pain by inhibiting the spinal release of glutamate. J Neurochem 2005;94:1131–1139.

61. Ambrósio AF, Silva AP, Malva JO, Soares-da-Silva P, Carvalho AP, Carvalho CM. Inhibition of glutamate release by BIA 2-093 and BIA 2-024, two novel derivatives of carbamazepine, due to blockade of sodium but not calcium channels. Biochem Pharmacol 2001;61:1271–1275.

62. Waldmeier PC, Baumann PA, Wicki P, Feldtrauer JJ, Stierlin C, Schmutz M. Similar potency of carbamazepine, oxcarbazepine, and lamotrigine in inhibiting the release of glutamate and other neurotransmitters. Neurology 1995;45:1907–1913.

63. Li X, Ketter TA, Frye MA. Synaptic, intracellular, and neuroprotective mechanisms of anticonvulsants: Are they relevant for the treatment and course of bipolar disorders? J Affect Disord 2002;69:1–14.

64. Cha BH, Silveira DC, Liu X, Hu Y, Holmes GL. Effect of topiramate following recurrent and prolonged seizures during early development. Epilepsy Res 2002;51:217–232.

65. Bischofs S, Zelenka M, Sommer C. Evaluation of topiramate as an anti-hyperalgesic and neuroprotective agent in the peripheral nervous system. J Peripher Nerv Syst 2004;9:70–78.

66. Vinik AI, Pittenger GL, Burcus NI, et al. Topiramate improves in vitro and in vivo measures of nerve fiber loss in patients with diabetic neuropathy. J Peripher Nerv Syst 2003;8:72–73.

67. Knowles SR, Shapiro LE, Shear NH. Anticonvulsant hypersensitivity syndrome: Incidence, prevention and management. Drug Saf 1999;21:489–501.

68. Mockenhaupt M, Messenheimer J, Tennis P, Schlingmann J. Risk of Stevens-Johnson syndrome and toxic epidermal necrolysis in new users of antiepileptics. Neurology 2005;64:1134–1138.

69. Tennis P, Stern RS. Risk of serious cutaneous disorders after initiation of use of phenytoin, carbamazepine, or sodium valproate: A record linkage study. Neurology 1997;49:542–546.

70. Hung SI, Chung WH, Jee SH, et al. Genetic susceptibility to carbamazepine-induced cutaneous adverse drug reactions. Pharmacogenet Genomics 2006;16:297–306.

71. Lonjou C, Thomas L, Borot N, et al. A marker for Stevens-Johnson syndrome: Ethnicity matters. Pharmacogenomics J 2006;6:265–268.

72. Man CB, Kwan P, Baum L, et al. Association between HLA-B*1502 allele and antiepileptic drug-induced cutaneous reactions in Han Chinese. Epilepsia 2007;48:1015–1018.

73. Alfirevic A, Jorgensen AL, Williamson PR, Chadwick DW, Park BK, Pirmohamed M. HLA-B locus in Caucasian patients with carbamazepine hypersensitivity. Pharmacogenomics 2006;7:813–818.

74. Pinelli A, Trivulzio S, Tomasoni L. Effects of carbamazepine treatment on pain threshold values and brain serotonin levels in rats. Pharmacology 1997;54:113–117.

75. Satoh M, Foong FW. A mechanism of carbamazepine-analgesia as shown by bradykinin-induced trigeminal pain. Brain Res Bull 1983;10:407–409.

76. Chapman V, Suzuki R, Chamarette HL, Rygh LJ, Dickenson AH. Effects of systemic carbamazepine and gabapentin on spinal neuronal responses in spinal nerve ligated rats. Pain 1998;75:261–272.

77. Idanpaan-Heikkila JJ, Guilbaud G. Pharmacological studies on a rat model of trigeminal neuropathic pain: Baclofen, but not carbamazepine, morphine or tricyclic antidepressants, attenuates the allodynia-like behaviour. Pain 1999;79:281–290.

78. Tomić MA, Vucković SM, Stepanović-Petrović RM, Ugresić N, Prostran MS, Bosković B. The anti-hyperalgesic effects of carbamazepine and oxcarbazepine are attenuated by treatment with adenosine receptor antagonists. Pain 2004;111:253–260.

79. Kiguchi S, Imamura T, Ichikawa K, Kojima M. Oxcarbazepine antinociception in animals with inflammatory pain or painful diabetic neuropathy. Clin Exp Pharmacol Physiol 2004;31:57–64.

80. Jang Y, Kim ES, Park SS, Lee J, Moon DE. The suppressive effects of oxcarbazepine on mechanical and cold allodynia in a rat model of neuropathic pain. Anesth Analg 2005;101:800–806.

81. Farago F. Trigeminal neuralgia: Its treatment with two new carbamazepine analogues. Eur Neurol 1987;26:73–83.

82. Zakrzewska JM, Patsalos PN. Oxcarbazepine: A new drug in the management of intractable trigeminal neuralgia. J Neurol Neurosurg Psychiatry 1989;52:472–476.

83. Zakrzewska JM, Patsalos PN. Long-term cohort study comparing medical (oxcarbazepine) and surgical management of intractable trigeminal neuralgia. Pain 2002;95:259–266.

84. Löscher W. Valproate: A reappraisal of its pharmacodynamic properties and mechanisms of action. Prog Neurobiol 1999;58:31–59.

85. Cutrer FM, Moskowitz MA. Wolff Award 1996. The actions of valproate and neurosteroids in a model of trigeminal pain. Headache 1996;36:579–585.

86. Kalita J, Bhoi SK, Misra UK. Amitriptyline vs divalproate in migraine prophylaxis: A randomized controlled trial. Acta Neurol Scand 2013;128:65–72.

87. Linde M, Mulleners WM, Chronicle EP, McCrory DC. Valproate (valproic acid or sodium valproate or a combination of the two) for the prophylaxis of episodic migraine in adults. Cochrane Database Syst Rev 2013;6.

88. Freitag FG, Diamond S, Diamond ML, Urban GJ. Divalproex in the long-term treatment of chronic daily headache. Headache 2001;41:271–278.

89. Klapper J. Divalproex sodium in migraine prophylaxis: A dose-controlled study. Cephalalgia 1997;17:103–108.

90. Silberstein SD, Goadsby PJ. Migraine: Preventive treatment. Cephalalgia 2002;22:491–512.

91. Sills GJ. The mechanisms of action of gabapentin and pregabalin. Curr Opin Pharmacol 2006;6:108–113.

92. Yasuda T, Miki S, Yoshinaga N, Senba E. Effects of amitriptyline and gabapentin on bilateral hyperalgesia observed in an animal model of unilateral axotomy. Pain 2005;115:161–170.

93. Blackburn-Munro G, Erichsen HK. Antiepileptics and the treatment of neuropathic pain: Evidence from animal models. Curr Pharm Des 2005;11:2961–2976.

94. Christensen D, Gautron M, Guilbaud G, Kayser V. Effect of gabapentin and lamotrigine on mechanical allodynia-like behaviour in a rat model of trigeminal neuropathic pain. Pain 2001;93:147–153.

95. Grabow TS, Dougherty PM. Gabapentin produces dose-dependent antinociception in the orofacial formalin test in the rat. Reg Anesth Pain Med 2002;27:277–283.

96. Pandey CK, Singhal V, Kumar M, et al. Gabapentin provides effective postoperative analgesia whether administered pre-emptively or post-incision. Can J Anaesth 2005;52:827–831.

97. Turan A, White PF, Karamanlioglu B, et al. Gabapentin: An alternative to the cyclooxygenase-2 inhibitors for perioperative pain management. Anesth Analg 2006;102:175–181.

98. Straube S, Derry S, Moore RA, Wiffen PJ, McQuay HJ. Single dose oral gabapentin for established acute postoperative pain in adults. Cochrane Database Syst Rev 2010;(5).

99. Moore RA, Wiffen PJ, Derry S, Toelle T, Rice AS. Gabapentin for chronic neuropathic pain and fibromyalgia in adults. Cochrane Database Syst Rev 2014;4.

100. Backonja M, Glanzman RL. Gabapentin dosing for neuropathic pain: Evidence from randomized, placebo-controlled clinical trials. Clin Ther 2003;25:81–104.

101. Wiffen PJ, Derry S, Moore RA, et al. Antiepileptic drugs for neuropathic pain and fibromyalgia—An overview of Cochrane reviews. Cochrane Database Syst Rev 2013;11.

102. Freynhagen R, Strojek K, Griesing T, Whalen E, Balkenohl M. Efficacy of pregabalin in neuropathic pain evaluated in a 12-week, randomised, double-blind, multicentre, placebo-controlled trial of flexible- and fixed-dose regimens. Pain 2005;115:254–263.

103. Richter RW, Portenoy R, Sharma U, Lamoreaux L, Bockbrader H, Knapp LE. Relief of painful diabetic peripheral neuropathy with pregabalin: A randomized, placebo-controlled trial. J Pain 2005;6:253–260.

104. Hill CM, Balkenohl M, Thomas DW, Walker R, Mathé H, Murray G. Pregabalin in patients with postoperative dental pain. Eur J Pain 2001;5:119–124.

105. Joshi SS, Jagadeesh AM. Efficacy of perioperative pregabalin in acute and chronic post-operative pain after off-pump coronary artery bypass surgery: A randomized, double-blind placebo controlled trial. Ann Card Anaesth 2013;16:180–185.

106. Zhang J, Ho KY, Wang Y. Efficacy of pregabalin in acute postoperative pain: A meta-analysis. Br J Anaesth 2011;106:454–462.

107. Mathiesen O, Jorgensen DG, Hilsted KL, et al. Pregabalin and dexamethasone improves post-operative pain treatment after tonsillectomy. Acta Anaesthesiol Scand 2011;55:297–305.

108. Ghai A, Gupta M, Hooda S, Singla D, Wadhera R. A randomized controlled trial to compare pregabalin with gabapentin for postoperative pain in abdominal hysterectomy. Saudi J Anaesth 2011;5:252–257.

109. Kim SY, Jeong JJ, Chung WY, Kim HJ, Nam KH, Shim YH. Perioperative administration of pregabalin for pain after robot-assisted endoscopic thyroidectomy: A randomized clinical trial. Surg Endosc 2010;24:2776–2781.

110. Durkin B, Page C, Glass P. Pregabalin for the treatment of postsurgical pain. Expert Opin Pharmacother 2010;11:2751–2758.

111. Hegarty DA, Shorten GD. A randomised, placebo-controlled trial of the effects of preoperative pregabalin on pain intensity and opioid consumption following lumbar discectomy. Korean J Pain 2011;24:22–30.

112. Moore RA, Straube S, Wiffen PJ, Derry S, McQuay HJ. Pregabalin for acute and chronic pain in adults. Cochrane Database Syst Rev 2009;(3).

113. Fishbain DA, Cutler RB, Rosomoff HL, Rosomoff RS. Clonazepam open clinical treatment trial for myofascial syndrome associated chronic pain. Pain Med 2000;1:332–339.

114. Harkins S, Linford J, Cohen J, Kramer T, Cueva L. Administration of clonazepam in the treatment of TMD and associated myofascial pain: A double-blind pilot study. J Craniomandib Disord 1991;5:179–186.

115. Wiffen P, Collins S, McQuay H, Carroll D, Jadad A, Moore A. Anticonvulsant drugs for acute and chronic pain. Cochrane Database Syst Rev 2005;(3).

116. Corrigan R, Derry S, Wiffen PJ, Moore RA. Clonazepam for neuropathic pain and fibromyalgia in adults. Cochrane Database Syst Rev 2012;5.

117. Gremeau-Richard C, Woda A, Navez ML, et al. Topical clonazepam in stomatodynia: A randomised placebo-controlled study. Pain 2004;108:51–57.

118. Patten SB, Love EJ. Drug-induced depression. Incidence, avoidance and management. Drug Saf 1994;10:203–219.

119. Wieczorkiewicz-Plaza A, Plaza P, Maciejewski R, Czuczwar M, Przesmycki K. Effect of topiramate on mechanical allodynia in neuropathic pain model in rats. Pol J Pharmacol 2004;56:275–278.

120. Storer RJ, Goadsby PJ. Topiramate inhibits trigeminovascular neurons in the cat. Cephalalgia 2004;24:1049–1056.

121. Chong MS, Libretto SE. The rationale and use of topiramate for treating neuropathic pain. Clin J Pain 2003;19:59–68.

122. Zvartau-Hind M, Din MU, Gilani A, Lisak RP, Khan OA. Topiramate relieves refractory trigeminal neuralgia in MS patients. Neurology 2000;55:1587–1588.

123. Carroll DG, Kline KM, Malnar KF. Role of topiramate for the treatment of painful diabetic peripheral neuropathy. Pharmacotherapy 2004;24:1186–1193.

124. Raskin P, Donofrio PD, Rosenthal NR, et al. Topiramate vs placebo in painful diabetic neuropathy: Analgesic and metabolic effects. Neurology 2004;63:865–873.

125. Linde M, Mulleners WM, Chronicle EP, McCrory DC. Topiramate for the prophylaxis of episodic migraine in adults. Cochrane Database Syst Rev 2013;6.

126. Wiffen PJ, Derry S, Moore RA. Lamotrigine for chronic neuropathic pain and fibromyalgia in adults. Cochrane Database Syst Rev 2013;12.

127. Eisenberg E, Shifrin A, Krivoy N. Lamotrigine for neuropathic pain. Expert Rev Neurother 2005;5:729–735.

128. Zakrzewska JM, Chaudhry Z, Nurmikko TJ, Patton DW, Mullens EL. Lamotrigine (lamictal) in refractory trigeminal neuralgia: Results from a double-blind placebo controlled crossover trial. Pain 1997;73:223–230.

129. Nackley AG, Tan KS, Fecho K, Flood P, Diatchenko L, Maixner W. Catechol-O-methyltransferase inhibition increases pain sensitivity through activation of both beta2- and beta3-adrenergic receptors. Pain 2007;128:199–208.

130. Ernberg M, Lundeberg T, Kopp S. Effect of propranolol and granisetron on experimentally induced pain and allodynia/hyperalgesia by intramuscular injection of serotonin into the human masseter muscle. Pain 2000;84:339–346.

131. Wood PB, Kablinger AS, Caldito GS. Open trial of pindolol in the treatment of fibromyalgia. Ann Pharmacother 2005;39:1812–1816.

132. Bhalang K, Light K, Maixner W. Effect of propranolol on TMD and fibromyalgia pain: preliminary findings. Presented at the 82nd General Session of the IADR, Honolulu, Hawaii, March 2004.

133. Tvedskov JF, Thomsen LL, Iverson HK, et al. The effect of propranolol on glyceryltrinitrate-induced headache and arterial response. Cephalalgia 2004;24:1076–1087.

134. Ablad B, Dahlof C. Migraine and beta-blockade: Modulation of sympathetic neurotransmission. Cephalalgia 1986;6(suppl 5):7–13.

135. Stoica E, Enulescu O. Propranolol corrects the abnormal catecholamine response to light during migraine. Eur Neurol 1990;30:19–22.

136. Sandor PS, Afra J, Ambrosini A, Schoenen J. Prophylactic treatment of migraine with beta-blockers and riboflavin: Differential effects on the intensity dependence of auditory evoked cortical potentials. Headache 2000;40:30–35.

137. Shields KG, Goadsby PJ. Propranolol modulates trigeminovascular responses in thalamic ventroposteromedial nucleus: A role in migraine? Brain 2005;128(Pt 1):86–97.

138. Akerman S, Williamson DJ, Hill RG, Goadsby PJ. The effect of adrenergic compounds on neurogenic dural vasodilatation. Eur J Pharmacol 2001;424:53–58.

139. Ayajiki K, Okamura T, Toda N. Flunarizine, an anti-migraine agent, impairs nitroxidergic nerve function in cerebral arteries. Eur J Pharmacol 1997;329:49–53.

140. Asakura K, Kanemasa T, Minagawa K, et al. Alpha-eudesmol, a P/Q-type Ca(2+) channel blocker, inhibits neurogenic vasodilation and extravasation following electrical stimulation of trigeminal ganglion. Brain Res 2000;873:94–101.

141. Olesen J, Diener HC, Husstedt IW, et al. Calcitonin gene-related peptide receptor antagonist BIBN 4096 BS for the acute treatment of migraine. N Engl J Med 2004;350:1104–1110.

142. Blau JN, Engel HO. Individualizing treatment with verapamil for cluster headache patients. Headache 2004;44:1013–1018.

143. Andersson KE, Vinge E. Beta-adrenoceptor blockers and calcium antagonists in the prophylaxis and treatment of migraine. Drugs 1990;39:355–373.

144. van Tulder MW, Touray T, Furlan AD, Solway S, Bouter LM. Muscle relaxants for non-specific low back pain. Cochrane Database Syst Rev 2003;(2).

145. Chou R, Peterson K, Helfand M. Comparative efficacy and safety of skeletal muscle relaxants for spasticity and musculoskeletal conditions: A systematic review. J Pain Symptom Manage 2004;28:140–175.

146. Svensson P, Wang K, Arendt-Nielsen L. Effect of muscle relaxants on experimental jaw-muscle pain and jaw-stretch reflexes: A double-blind and placebo-controlled trial. Eur J Pain 2003;7:449–456.

147. Turturro MA, Frater CR, D'Amico FJ. Cyclobenzaprine with ibuprofen versus ibuprofen alone in acute myofascial strain: A randomized, double-blind clinical trial. Ann Emerg Med 2003;41:818–826.

148. Peloso P, Gross A, Haines T, Trinh K, Goldsmith CH, Aker P. Medicinal and injection therapies for mechanical neck disorders. Cochrane Database Syst Rev 2005;(2).

149. Leite FM, Atallah AN, El Dib R, et al. Cyclobenzaprine for the treatment of myofascial pain in adults. Cochrane Database Syst Rev 2009;(3).

150. Herman CR, Schiffman EL, Look JO, Rindal DB. The effectiveness of adding pharmacologic treatment with clonazepam or cyclobenzaprine to patient education and self-care for the treatment of jaw pain upon awakening: A randomized clinical trial. J Orofac Pain 2002;16:64–70.

151. Browning R, Jackson JL, O'Malley PG. Cyclobenzaprine and back pain: A meta-analysis. Arch Intern Med 2001;161:1613–1620.

152. Tofferi JK, Jackson JL, O'Malley PG. Treatment of fibromyalgia with cyclobenzaprine: A meta-analysis. Arthritis Rheum 2004;51:9–13.

153. Terrence CF, Fromm GH, Tenicela R. Baclofen as an analgesic in chronic peripheral nerve disease. Eur Neurol 1985;24:380–385.

154. Fromm GH, Sato K, Nakata M. The action of GABAB antagonists in the trigeminal nucleus of the rat. Neuropharmacology 1992;31:475–480.

155. Santos Tde J, de Castro-Costa CM, Giffoni SD, Santos FJ, Ramos RS, Gifoni MA. The effect of baclofen on spontaneous and evoked behavioural expression of experimental neuropathic chronic pain. Arq Neuropsiquiatr 1999;57:753–760.

156. Zuniga RE, Schlicht CR, Abram SE. Intrathecal baclofen is analgesic in patients with chronic pain. Anesthesiology 2000;92:876–880.

157. Freitag FG. Preventative treatment for migraine and tension-type headaches: Do drugs having effects on muscle spasm and tone have a role? CNS Drugs 2003;17:373–381.

158. Hering-Hanit R, Gadoth N. Baclofen in cluster headache. Headache 2000;40:48–51.

159. Fromm GH. Baclofen as an adjuvant analgesic. J Pain Symptom Manage 1994;9:500–509.

160. Fromm GH, Terrence CF. Comparison of L-baclofen and racemic baclofen in trigeminal neuralgia. Neurology 1987;37:1725–1728.

161. Fromm GH, Terrence CF, Chattha AS, Glass JD. Baclofen in trigeminal neuralgia: Its effect on the spinal trigeminal nucleus: A pilot study. Arch Neurol 1980;37:768–771.

162. Fromm GH, Terrence CF, Chattha AS. Baclofen in the treatment of trigeminal neuralgia: Double-blind study and long-term follow-up. Ann Neurol 1984;15:240–244.

163. Terrence CF, Fromm GH. Complications of baclofen withdrawal. Arch Neurol 1981;38:588–589.

164. Saxen PR, Tfelt-Hansen P. Triptans. 5-HT1B/1D receptor agonists in the acute treatment of migraine. In: Olesen J, Goadsby PJ, Ramadan NM, Tfelt-Hansen P, Welch KMA (eds). The Headaches, ed 3. Philadelphia: Lippincott Williams & Wilkins, 2006:469–503.

165. de Hoon JN, Willigers JM, Troost J, Struijker-Boudier HA, Van Bortel LM. Vascular effects of 5-HT1B/1D-receptor agonists in patients with migraine headaches. Clin Pharmacol Ther 2000;68:418–426.

166. Ahn AH, Basbaum AI. Where do triptans act in the treatment of migraine? Pain 2005;115:1–4.

167. Jennings EA, Ryan RM, Christie MJ. Effects of sumatriptan on rat medullary dorsal horn neurons. Pain 2004;111:30–37.

168. Donaldson C, Boers PM, Hoskin KL, Zagami AS, Lambert GA. The role of 5-HT1B and 5-HT1D receptors in the selective inhibitory effect of naratriptan on trigeminovascular neurons. Neuropharmacology 2002;42:374–385.

169. Storer RJ, Akerman S, Connor HE, Goadsby PJ. 4991W93, a potent blocker of neurogenic plasma protein extravasation, inhibits trigeminal neurons at 5-hydroxytryptamine (5-HT1B/1D) agonist doses. Neuropharmacology 2001;40:911–917.

170. Bartsch T, Knight YE, Goadsby PJ. Activation of 5-HT(1B/1D) receptor in the periaqueductal gray inhibits nociception. Ann Neurol 2004;56:371–381.

171. Obermann M, Mueller D, Yoon MS, Pageler L, Diener H, Katsarava Z. Migraine with isolated facial pain: A diagnostic challenge. Cephalalgia 2007;27:1278–1282.

172. Cumberbatch MJ, Hill RG, Hargreaves RJ. Rizatriptan has central antinociceptive effects against durally evoked responses. Eur J Pharmacol 1997;328:37–40.

173. Burstein R, Jakubowski M. Analgesic triptan action in an animal model of intracranial pain: A race against the development of central sensitization. Ann Neurol 2004;55:27–36.

174. De Petrocellis L, Melck D, Bisogno T, Di Marzo V. Endocannabinoids and fatty acid amides in cancer, inflammation and related disorders. Chem Phys Lipids 2000;108:191–209.

175. Anand P, Whiteside G, Fowler CJ, Hohmann AG. Targeting CB2 receptors and the endocannabinoid system for the treatment of pain. Brain Res Rev 2009;60:255–266.

176. Guindon J, Beaulieu P. Antihyperalgesic effects of local injections of anandamide, ibuprofen, rofecoxib and their combinations in a model of neuropathic pain. Neuropharmacology 2006;50:814–823.

177. Calignano A, La Rana G, Giuffrida A, Piomelli D. Control of pain initiation by endogenous cannabinoids. Nature 1998;394:277–281.

178. Martin WJ, Hohmann AG, Walker JM. Suppression of noxious stimulus-evoked activity in the ventral posterolateral nucleus of the thalamus by a cannabinoid agonist: Correlation between electrophysiological and antinociceptive effects. J Neurosci 1996;16:6601–6611.

179. Costa B, Colleoni M, Conti S, et al. Repeated treatment with the synthetic cannabinoid WIN 55,212-2 reduces both hyperalgesia and production of pronociceptive mediators in a rat model of neuropathic pain. Br J Pharmacol 2004;141:4–8.

180. Farquhar-Smith WP, Egertová M, Bradbury EJ, McMahon SB, Rice AS, Elphick MR. Cannabinoid CB(1) receptor expression in rat spinal cord. Mol Cell Neurosci 2000;15:510–521.

181. Lim G, Sung B, Ji RR, Mao J. Upregulation of spinal cannabinoid-1-receptors following nerve injury enhances the effects of WIN 55,212-2 on neuropathic pain behaviors in rats. Pain 2003;105:275–283.

182. Cichewicz DL. Synergistic interactions between cannabinoid and opioid analgesics. Life Sci 2004;74:1317–1324.

183. Yesilyurt O, Dogrul A, Gul H, et al. Topical cannabinoid enhances topical morphine antinociception. Pain 2003;105:303–308.

184. Liang YC, Huang CC, Hsu KS. Therapeutic potential of cannabinoids in trigeminal neuralgia. Curr Drug Targets CNS Neurol Disord 2004;3:507–514.

185. Jaggar SI, Hasnie FS, Sellaturay S, Rice AS. The anti-hyperalgesic actions of the cannabinoid anandamide and the putative CB2 receptor agonist palmitoylethanolamide in visceral and somatic inflammatory pain. Pain 1998;76:189–199.

186. Herzberg U, Eliav E, Bennett GJ, Kopin IJ. The analgesic effects of R(+)-WIN 55,212-2 mesylate, a high affinity cannabinoid agonist, in a rat model of neuropathic pain. Neurosci Lett 1997;221:157–160.

187. Kehl LJ, Hamamoto DT, Wacnik PW, et al. A cannabinoid agonist differentially attenuates deep tissue hyperalgesia in animal models of cancer and inflammatory muscle pain. Pain 2003;103:175–186.

188. Wilsey B, Marcotte T, Deutsch R, Gouaux B, Sakai S, Donaghe H. Low-dose vaporized cannabis significantly improves neuropathic pain. J Pain 2013;14:136–148.

189. Lynch ME, Cesar-Rittenberg P, Hohmann AG. A double-blind, placebo-controlled, crossover pilot trial with extension using an oral mucosal cannabinoid extract for treatment of chemotherapy-induced neuropathic pain. J Pain Symptom Manage 2014;47:166–173.

190. Lynch ME, Campbell F. Cannabinoids for treatment of chronic non-cancer pain; A systematic review of randomized trials. Br J Clin Pharmacol 2011;72:735–744.

191. Martín-Sánchez E, Furukawa TA, Taylor J, Martin JL. Systematic review and meta-analysis of cannabis treatment for chronic pain. Pain Med 2009;10:1353–1368.

192. Aggarwal SK. Cannabinergic pain medicine: A concise clinical primer and survey of randomized-controlled trial results. Clin J Pain 2013;29:162–171.

193. Clark AJ, Lynch ME, Ware M, Beaulieu P, McGilveray IJ, Gourlay D. Guidelines for the use of cannabinoid compounds in chronic pain. Pain Res Manag 2005;10(suppl A):44A–46A.

194. Ware M, Beaulieu P. Cannabinoids for the treatment of pain: An update on recent clinical trials. Pain Res Manag 2005;10(suppl A):27A–30A.

195. Naef M, Curatolo M, Petersen-Felix S, Arendt-Nielsen L, Zbinden A, Brenneisen R. The analgesic effect of oral delta-9-tetrahydrocannabinol (THC), morphine, and a THC-morphine combination in healthy subjects under experimental pain conditions. Pain 2003;105:79–88.

196. Buggy DJ, Toogood L, Maric S, Sharpe P, Lambert DG, Rowbotham DJ. Lack of analgesic efficacy of oral delta-9-tetrahydrocannabinol in postoperative pain. Pain 2003;106:169–172.

197. Berman JS, Symonds C, Birch R. Efficacy of two cannabis based medicinal extracts for relief of central neuropathic pain from brachial plexus avulsion: Results of a randomised controlled trial. Pain 2004;112:299–306.

198. Karst M, Salim K, Burstein S, Conrad I, Hoy L, Schneider U. Analgesic effect of the synthetic cannabinoid CT-3 on chronic neuropathic pain: a randomized controlled trial. JAMA 2003;290:1757–1762.

199. Rog DJ, Nurmikko TJ, Friede T, Young CA. Randomized, controlled trial of cannabis-based medicine in central pain in multiple sclerosis. Neurology 2005;65:812–819.

200. Evans RW, Ramadan NM. Are cannabis-based chemicals helpful in headache? Headache 2004;44:726–727.

201. Eide PK, Stubhaug A. Relief of glossopharyngeal neuralgia by ketamine-induced N-methyl-aspartate receptor blockade. Neurosurgery 1997;41:505–508.

202. Felsby S, Nielsen J, Arendt-Nielsen L, Jensen TS. NMDA receptor blockade in chronic neuropathic pain: A comparison of ketamine and magnesium chloride. Pain 1996;64:283–291.

203. Mathisen LC, Skjelbred P, Skoglund LA, Oye I. Effect of ketamine, an NMDA receptor inhibitor, in acute and chronic orofacial pain. Pain 1995;61:215–220.

204. Carlsson KC, Hoem NO, Moberg ER, Mathisen LC. Analgesic effect of dextromethorphan in neuropathic pain. Acta Anaesthesiol Scand 2004;48:328–336.

205. Turton K, Chaddock JA, Acharya KR. Botulinum and tetanus neurotoxins: Structure, function and therapeutic utility. Trends Biochem Sci 2002;27:552–558.

206. Ranoux D, Attal N, Morain F, Bouhassira D. Botulinum toxin type A induces direct analgesic effects in chronic neuropathic pain. Ann Neurol 2008;64:274–283.

207. Yuan RY, Sheu JJ, Yu JM, et al. Botulinum toxin for diabetic neuropathic pain: A randomized double-blind crossover trial. Neurology 2009;72:1473–1478.

208. Ashkenazi A, Blumenfeld A. OnabotulinumtoxinA for the treatment of headache. Headache 2013;53(2, suppl):54–61.

209. Smuts JA, Schultz D, Barnard A. Mechanism of action of botulinum toxin type A in migraine prevention: A pilot study. Headache 2004;44:801–805.

210. Durham PL, Cady R. Insights into the mechanism of onabotulinumtoxinA in chronic migraine. Headache 2011;51:1573–1577.

211. Durham PL, Masterson CG. Two mechanisms involved in trigeminal CGRP release: Implications for migraine treatment. Headache 2013;53:67–80.

212. Burstein R, Zhang X, Levy D, Aoki KR, Brin MF. Selective inhibition of meningeal nociceptors by botulinum neurotoxin type A: Therapeutic implications for migraine and other pains. Cephalalgia 2014;34:853–869.

213. Antonucci F, Rossi C, Gianfranceschi L, Rossetto O, Caleo M. Long-distance retrograde effects of botulinum neurotoxin A. J Neurosci 2008;28:3689–3696.

214. Aurora SK, Dodick DW, Diener HC, et al. OnabotulinumtoxinA for chronic migraine: Efficacy, safety, and tolerability in patients who received all five treatment cycles in the PREEMPT clinical program. Acta Neurol Scand 2014;129:61–70.

215. Jackson JL, Kuriyama A, Hayashino Y. Botulinum toxin A for prophylactic treatment of migraine and tension headaches in adults: A meta-analysis. JAMA 2012;307:1736–1745.

216. Blumenfeld A, Silberstein SD, Dodick DW, Aurora SK, Turkel CC, Binder WJ. Method of injection of onabotulinumtoxinA for chronic migraine: A safe, well-tolerated, and effective treatment paradigm based on the PREEMPT clinical program. Headache 2010;50:1406–1418.

217. Hu Y, Guan X, Fan L, et al. Therapeutic efficacy and safety of botulinum toxin type A in trigeminal neuralgia: A systematic review. J Headache Pain 2013;14:72.

218. Shehata HS, El-Tamawy MS, Shalaby NM, Ramzy G. Botulinum toxin-type A: Could it be an effective treatment option in intractable trigeminal neuralgia? J Headache Pain 2013;14:92.

219. Piovesan EJ, Teive HG, Kowacs PA, Della Coletta MV, Werneck LC, Silberstein SD. An open study of botulinum-A toxin treatment of trigeminal neuralgia. Neurology 2005;65:1306–1308.

220. Wu CJ, Lian YJ, Zheng YK, et al. Botulinum toxin type A for the treatment of trigeminal neuralgia: Results from a randomized, double-blind, placebo-controlled trial. Cephalalgia 2012;32:443–450.

221. Guarda-Nardini L, Manfredini D, Salamone M, Salmaso L, Tonello S, Ferronato G. Efficacy of botulinum toxin in treating myofascial pain in bruxers: A controlled placebo pilot study. Cranio 2008;26:126–135.

222. Kurtoglu C, Gur OH, Kurkcu M, Sertdemir Y, Guler-Uysal F, Uysal H. Effect of botulinum toxin-A in myofascial pain patients with or without functional disc displacement. J Oral Maxillofac Surg 2008;66:1644–1651.

223. Sidebottom AJ, Patel AA, Amin J. Botulinum injection for the management of myofascial pain in the masticatory muscles. A prospective outcome study. Br J Oral Maxillofac Surg 2013;51:199–205.

224. Ernberg M, Hedenberg-Magnusson B, List T, Svensson P. Efficacy of botulinum toxin type A for treatment of persistent myofascial TMD pain: A randomized, controlled, double-blind multicenter study. Pain 2011;152:1988–1996.

225. Soares A, Andriolo RB, Atallah AN, da Silva EM. Botulinum toxin for myofascial pain syndromes in adults. Cochrane Database Syst Rev 2012;4.

226. Langevin P, Lowcock J, Weber J, et al. Botulinum toxin intramuscular injections for neck pain: A systematic review and metaanalysis. J Rheumatol 2011;38:203–214.

227. Argoff CE. Targeted peripheral analgesics therapy for neuropathic pain. Curr Pain Headache Rep 2004;8:199–204.

228. Sawynok J. Topical and peripherally acting analgesics. Pharmacol Rev 2003;55:1–20.

229. Galer BS. Topical medications. In: Loeser JD (ed). Bonica's Management of Pain. Philadelphia: Lippincott Williams & Wilkins, 2001:1736–1741.

230. Padilla M, Clark GT, Merrill RL. Topical medications for orofacial neuropathic pain: A review. J Am Dent Assoc 2000;131:184–195.

231. Ness TJ, Jones L, Smith H. Use of compounded topical analgesics—Results of an Internet survey. Reg Anesth Pain Med 2002;27:309–312.

232. Heir G, Karolchek S, Kalladka M, et al. Use of topical medication in orofacial neuropathic pain: A retrospective study. Oral Surg Oral Med Oral Pathol Oral Radiol Endod 2008;105:466–469.

233. Plaza-Villegas F, Heir G, Markman S, et al. Topical pregabalin and diclofenac for the treatment of neuropathic orofacial pain in rats. Oral Surg Oral Med Oral Pathol Oral Radiol 2012;114:449–456.

234. Argoff CE, Galer BS, Jensen MP, Oleka N, Gammaitoni AR. Effectiveness of the lidocaine patch 5% on pain qualities in three chronic pain states: Assessment with the Neuropathic Pain Scale. Curr Med Res Opin 2004;20(2, suppl):S21S28.

235. Hersh EV, Houpt MI, Cooper SA, Feldman RS, Wolff MS, Levin LM. Analgesic efficacy and safety of an intraoral lidocaine patch. J Am Dent Assoc 1996;127:1626–1634.

236. Houpt MI, Heins P, Lamster I, Stone C, Wolff MS. An evaluation of intraoral lidocaine patches in reducing needle-insertion pain. Compend Contin Educ Dent 1997;18:309–310;312–314;316.

237. Hersh EV, DeRossi SS, Ciarrocca KN, Secreto SA, Ghassemi A. Efficacy and tolerability of an intraoral benzocaine patch in the relief of spontaneous toothache pain. J Clin Dent 2003;14:1–6.

238. Betts NJ, Makowski G, Shen YH, Hersh EV. Evaluation of topical viscous 2% lidocaine jelly as an adjunct during the management of alveolar osteitis. J Oral Maxillofac Surg 1995;53:1140–1144.

239. Elad S, Cohen G, Zylber-Katz E, et al. Systemic absorption of lidocaine after topical application for the treatment of oral mucositis in bone marrow transplantation patients. J Oral Pathol Med 1999;28:170–172.

240. Masud S, Wasnich RD, Ruckle JL, et al. Contribution of a heating element to topical anesthesia patch efficacy prior to vascular access: Results from two randomized, double-blind studies. J Pain Symptom Manage 2010;40:510–519.

241. Sawyer J, Febbraro S, Masud S, Ashburn MA, Campbell JC. Heated lidocaine/tetracaine patch (Synera, Rapydan) compared with lidocaine/prilocaine cream (EMLA) for topical anaesthesia before vascular access. Br J Anaesth 2009;102:210–215.

242. Barkin RL. The pharmacology of topical analgesics. Postgrad Med 2013;125(4, suppl):7–18.

243. Derry S, Moore RA, Rabbie R. Topical NSAIDs for chronic musculoskeletal pain in adults. Cochrane Database Syst Rev 2012;9.

244. Massey T, Derry S, Moore RA, McQuay HJ. Topical NSAIDs for acute pain in adults. Cochrane Database Syst Rev 2010;(6).

245. Stanos SP, Galluzzi KE. Topical therapies in the management of chronic pain. Postgrad Med 2013;125(4, suppl):25–33.

246. McCarberg B, D'Arcy Y. Options in topical therapies in the management of patients with acute pain. Postgrad Med 2013;125(4, suppl):19–24.

247. Di Rienzo Businco L, Di Rienzo Businco A, D'Emilia M, Lauriello M, Coen Tirelli G. Topical versus systemic diclofenac in the treatment of temporo-mandibular joint dysfunction symptoms. Acta Otorhinolaryngol Ital 2004;24:279–283.

248. Svensson P, Houe L, Arendt-Nielsen L. Effect of systemic versus topical nonsteroidal anti-inflammatory drugs on postexercise jaw-muscle soreness: A placebo-controlled study. J Orofac Pain 1997;11:353–362.

249. Moore UJ, Seymour RA, Rawlins MD. The efficacy of locally applied aspirin and acetaminophen in postoperative pain after third molar surgery. Clin Pharmacol Ther 1992;52:292–296.

250. Dionne RA, Gordon SM, Tahara M, Rowan J, Troullos E. Analgesic efficacy and pharmacokinetics of ketoprofen administered into a surgical site. J Clin Pharmacol 1999;39:131–138.

251. Dionne RA, Haynes D, Brahim JS, Rowan JS, Guivarc'h PH. Analgesic effect of sustained-release flurbiprofen administered at the site of tissue injury in the oral surgery model. J Clin Pharmacol 2004;44:1418–1424.

252. Peppin JF, Pappagallo M. Capsaicinoids in the treatment of neuropathic pain: A review. Ther Adv Neurol Disord 2014;7:22–32.

253. Kingery WS. A critical review of controlled clinical trials for peripheral neuropathic pain and complex regional pain syndromes. Pain 1997;73:123–139.

254. Zhang WY, Li Wan Po A. The effectiveness of topically applied capsaicin. A meta-analysis. Eur J Clin Pharmacol 1994;46:517–522.

255. Derry S, Moore RA. Topical capsaicin (low concentration) for chronic neuropathic pain in adults. Cochrane Database Syst Rev 2012;9.

256. Mason L, Moore RA, Derry S, Edwards JE, McQuay HJ. Systematic review of topical capsaicin for the treatment of chronic pain. BMJ 2004;328:991.

257. Epstein JB, Marcoe JH. Topical application of capsaicin for treatment of oral neuropathic pain and trigeminal neuralgia. Oral Surg Oral Med Oral Pathol 1994;77:135–140.

258. Pastre T, Faot F, Westphalen FH, da Rosa RS. Treatment of painful post-traumatic peripheral neuropathy with capsaicin in an edentulous patient with extreme resorption in the mental region: A case report. J Contemp Dent Pract 2008;9:106–113.

259. Canavan D, Graff-Radford SB, Gratt BM. Traumatic dysesthesia of the trigeminal nerve. J Orofac Pain 1994;8:391–396.

260. Berger A, Henderson M, Nadoolman W, et al. Oral capsaicin provides temporary relief for oral mucositis pain secondary to chemotherapy/radiation therapy. J Pain Symptom Manage 1995;10:243–248.

261. Hersh EV, Pertes RA, Ochs HA. Topical capsaicin-pharmacology and potential role in the treatment of temporomandibular pain. J Clin Dent 1994;5:54–59.

262. Winocur E, Gavish A, Halachmi M, Eli I, Gazit E. Topical application of capsaicin for the treatment of localized pain in the temporomandibular joint area. J Orofac Pain 2000;14:31–36.

263. Saper JR, Klapper J, Mathew NT, Rapoport A, Phillips SB, Bernstein JE. Intranasal civamide for the treatment of episodic cluster headaches. Arch Neurol 2002;59:990–994.

264. Derry S, Sven-Rice A, Cole P, Tan T, Moore RA. Topical capsaicin (high concentration) for chronic neuropathic pain in adults. Cochrane Database Syst Rev 2013;2.

265. Wagner T, Poole C, Roth-Daniek A. The capsaicin 8% patch for neuropathic pain in clinical practice: A retrospective analysis. Pain Med 2013;14:1202–1211.

266. Backonja MM, Malan TP, Vanhove GF, Tobias JK. NGX-4010, a high-concentration capsaicin patch, for the treatment of postherpetic neuralgia: A randomized, double-blind, controlled study with an open-label extension. Pain Med 2010;11:600–608.

267. Clifford DB, Simpson DM, Brown S, et al. A randomized, double-blind, controlled study of NGX-4010, a capsaicin 8% dermal patch, for the treatment of painful HIV-associated distal sensory polyneuropathy. J Acquir Immune Defic Syndr 2012;59:126–133.

268. Simpson DM, Gazda S, Brown S, et al. Long-term safety of NGX-4010, a high-concentration capsaicin patch, in patients with peripheral neuropathic pain. J Pain Symptom Manage 2010;39:1053–1064.

269. Sayanlar J, Guleyupoglu N, Portenoy R, Ashina S. Trigeminal postherpetic neuralgia responsive to treatment with capsaicin 8% topical patch: A case report. J Headache Pain 2012;13:587–589.

270. Kennedy WR, Vanhove GF, Lu SP, et al. A randomized, controlled, open-label study of the long-term effects of NGX-4010, a high-concentration capsaicin patch, on epidermal nerve fiber density and sensory function in healthy volunteers. J Pain 2010;11:579–587.

271. Sawynok J, Esser MJ, Reid AR. Antidepressants as analgesics: An overview of central and peripheral mechanisms of action. J Psychiatry Neurosci 2001;26:21–29.

272. Lynch ME, Clark AJ, Sawynok J. A pilot study examining topical amitriptyline, ketamine, and a combination of both in the treatment of neuropathic pain. Clin J Pain 2003;19:323–328.

273. Lynch ME, Clark AJ, Sawynok J, Sullivan MJ. Topical amitriptyline and ketamine in neuropathic pain syndromes: An open-label study. J Pain 2005;6:644–649.

274. Kopsky DJ, Liebregts R, Keppel Hesselink JM. Central neuropathic pain in a patient with multiple sclerosis treated successfully with topical amitriptyline. Case Rep Med 2012;2012.

275. Liebregts R, Kopsky DJ, Hesselink JM. Topical amitriptyline in post-traumatic neuropathic pain. J Pain Symptom Manage 2011;41:e6–e7.

276. Kopsky DJ, Hesselink JM. High doses of topical amitriptyline in neuropathic pain: Two cases and literature review. Pain Pract 2012;12:148–153.

277. McCleane G. Topical application of doxepin hydrochloride, capsaicin and a combination of both produces analgesia in chronic human neuropathic pain: A randomized, double-blind, placebo-controlled study. Br J Clin Pharmacol 2000;49:574–579.

278. Epstein JB, Truelove EL, Oien H, Allison C, Le ND, Epstein MS. Oral topical doxepin rinse: Analgesic effect in patients with oral mucosal pain due to cancer or cancer therapy. Oral Oncol 2001;37:632–637.

279. Oeltjenbruns J, Schäfer M. Peripheral opioid analgesia: Clinical applications. Curr Pain Headache Rep 2005;9:36–44.

280. Coggeshall RE, Zhou S, Carlton SM. Opioid receptors on peripheral sensory axons. Brain Res 1997;764:126–132.

281. Zhou L, Zhang Q, Stein C, Schäfer M. Contribution of opioid receptors on primary afferent versus sympathetic neurons to peripheral opioid analgesia. J Pharmacol Exp Ther 1998;286:1000–1006.

282. Antonijevic I, Mousa SA, Schäfer M, Stein C. Perineurial defect and peripheral opioid analgesia in inflammation. J Neurosci 1995;15(Pt 1):165–172.

283. Likar R, Sittl R, Gragger K, et al. Peripheral morphine analgesia in dental surgery. Pain 1998;76:145–150.

284. Likar R, Koppert W, Blatnig H, et al. Efficacy of peripheral morphine analgesia in inflamed, non-inflamed and perineural tissue of dental surgery patients. J Pain Symptom Manage 2001;21:330–337.

285. Dionne RA, Lepinski AM, Gordon SM, Jaber L, Brahim JS, Hargreaves KM. Analgesic effects of peripherally administered opioids in clinical models of acute and chronic inflammation. Clin Pharmacol Ther 2001;70:66–73.

286. Moore UJ, Seymour RA, Gilroy J, Rawlins MD. The efficacy of locally applied morphine in post-operative pain after bilateral third molar surgery. Br J Clin Pharmacol 1994;37:227–230.

287. Likar R, Kapral S, Steinkellner H, Stein C, Schafer M. Dose-dependency of intra-articular morphine analgesia. Br J Anaesth 1999;83:241–244.

288. Likar R, Schäfer M, Paulak F, et al. Intraarticular morphine analgesia in chronic pain patients with osteoarthritis. Anesth Analg 1997;84:1313–1317.

289. Kajii TS, Okamoto T, Yura S, Mabuchi A, Iida J. Elevated levels of beta-endorphin in temporomandibular joint synovial lavage fluid of patients with closed lock. J Orofac Pain 2005;19:41–46.

290. Kunjur J, Anand R, Brennan PA, Ilankovan V. An audit of 405 temporomandibular joint arthrocentesis with intra-articular morphine infusion. Br J Oral Maxillofac Surg 2003;41:29–31.

291. Bryant CJ, Harrison SD, Hopper C, Harris M. Use of intra-articular morphine for postoperative analgesia following TMJ arthroscopy. Br J Oral Maxillofac Surg 1999;37:391–396.

292. Furst IM, Kryshtalskyj B, Weinberg S. The use of intra-articular opioids and bupivacaine for analgesia following temporomandibular joint arthroscopy: A prospective, randomized trial. J Oral Maxillofac Surg 2001;59:979–983.

293. List T, Tegelberg A, Haraldson T, Isacsson G. Intra-articular morphine as analgesic in temporomandibular joint arthralgia/osteoarthritis. Pain 2001;94:275–282.

294. Cerchietti LC, Navigante AH, Körte MW, et al. Potential utility of the peripheral analgesic properties of morphine in stomatitis-related pain: A pilot study. Pain 2003;105:265–273.

295. Hegarty AM, Hodgson TA, Lewsey JD, Porter SR. Fluticasone propionate spray and betamethasone sodium phosphate mouthrinse: A randomized crossover study for the treatment of symptomatic oral lichen planus. J Am Acad Dermatol 2002;47:271–279.

296. Lo Muzio L, della Valle A, Mignogna MD, et al. The treatment of oral aphthous ulceration or erosive lichen planus with topical clobetasol propionate in three preparations: A clinical and pilot study on 54 patients. J Oral Pathol Med 2001;30:611–617.

297. Arabshahi B, Dewitt EM, Cahill AM, et al. Utility of corticosteroid injection for temporomandibular arthritis in children with juvenile idiopathic arthritis. Arthritis Rheum 2005;52:3563–3569.

298. Kopp S, Carlsson GE, Haraldson T, Wenneberg B. Long-term effect of intra-articular injections of sodium hyaluronate and corticosteroid on temporomandibular joint arthritis. J Oral Maxillofac Surg 1987;45:929–935.

299. Toller PA. Use and misuse of intra-articular corticosteroids in treatment of temporomandibular joint pain. Proc R Soc Med 1977;70:461–463.

300. Vallon D, Akerman S, Nilner M, Petersson A. Long-term follow-up of intra-articular injections into the temporomandibular joint in patients with rheumatoid arthritis. Swed Dent J 2002;26(4):149–158.

301. Wenneberg B, Kopp S, Gröndahl HG. Long-term effect of intra-articular injections of a glucocorticosteroid into the TMJ: A clinical and radiographic 8-year follow-up. J Craniomandib Disord 1991;5:11–18.

302. Schindler C, Paessler L, Eckelt U, Kirch W. Severe temporomandibular dysfunction and joint destruction after intra-articular injection of triamcinolone. J Oral Pathol Med 2005;34:184–186.

303. El-Hakim IE, Abdel-Hamid IS, Bader A. Tempromandibular joint (TMJ) response to intra-articular dexamethasone injection following mechanical arthropathy: A histological study in rats. Int J Oral Maxillofac Surg 2005;34:305–310.

Complementary and Alternative Medicine

Yair Sharav, DMD, MS
Rafael Benoliel, BDS

17

Complementary and alternative medicine (CAM) has become increasingly popular. In 1990, Americans made an estimated 425 million visits to providers of unconventional therapy, a number that exceeds the number of visits to all US primary care physicians (388 million) in the same year.[1] A national survey of CAM use showed an increase in use of alternative therapies from 33.8% in 1990 to 42.1% of the US population in 1997.[2] However, in the United States there was no evidence to suggest a change in 12-month prevalence of CAM use (excluding prayer) from 2002 to 2007.[3] In 1997, expenditures for professional CAM services in the United States were conservatively estimated at $21.2 billion, and at least $12.2 billion was paid out of pocket.[2] This figure is apparently growing fast: for the period 1999 to 2004, out-of-pocket expenditures were estimated at more than $34 billion per year in the United States.[4] In 2007, more than 30 million adults reported out-of-pocket expenditures on CAM services, and of these, 7.2 million were heavy CAM spenders with a mean annual expenditure of $1,385.[5]

Alternative medicine is most frequently used for chronic conditions, including pain and, in particular, back problems and headache. Surveys of general population samples indicate that chronic pain symptoms are significant predictors of CAM use.[6] In a national survey of 2,055 adults, of those reporting back or neck pain in the previous 12 months, 37% had seen a conventional provider and 54% had used complementary therapies to treat the condition.[7] More than three-quarters (76.1%) of studied patients in a dental school clinic reported using at least one CAM treatment in the previous 12 months, and there were high rates of chiropractic use.[8] Chiropractic, massage, and relaxation techniques were the most commonly used complementary treatments for back or neck pain. Higher education, pain severity, and pain duration are persistent correlates of CAM usage, regardless of the therapy considered.[9] In terms of cost for treatment of painful conditions, acupuncture for migraine and manual therapy for neck pain were cost-effective CAM therapies.[4] Clearly, CAM is increasingly in demand, and the more severe and long lasting the pain, the more demand increases.

CAM

CAM is often used in situations in which conventional medicine fails to provide adequate relief.[10] Common examples include back and neck pain, arthritis, and fibromyalgia. People who use CAM are better educated but often less healthy than those who do not.[6] Most alternative medicine users appear to be doing so largely because they find these health care alternatives to be more (congruent) with their own values, beliefs, and philosophic orientation toward health and life. This is contrary to the common belief that people who use CAM are dissatisfied with conventional medicine.

In addition to increasing patient awareness, interest in CAM among medical schools and physicians has grown worldwide.[11-14] Twenty-five years ago, not a single CAM course was taught in any US medical school; by 1996, 64% offered courses in CAM.[15] The percentage of British medical schools offering CAM courses increased from 10% in 1995 to 40% in 1997.[16] Furthermore, the International Association for the Study of Pain's core curriculum for professional education in pain now includes a chapter on complementary therapies.[17]

What Is CAM?

The definition of CAM is more complex than one would expect. One broad and loose definition refers to it as "medical practices that are not in conformity with the standards of the medical community."[1] The definition "medical interventions not taught widely at US medical schools or generally available at US hospitals"[2] is not much of an improvement. According to these definitions, the list of what is considered to be CAM changes continually; new approaches to health care emerge, and CAM therapies that are proven to be safe and effective are adopted into conventional health care.

Clearly, CAM therapies are difficult to define and include a changing, broad spectrum of practices and beliefs ranging from spiritual healing to relaxation techniques, homeopathy, hypnosis, acupuncture, and chiropractic manipulation.[17] More recently, CAM has been classified as including five major approaches: *(1)* alternative medical systems (eg, traditional Chinese medicine, including acupuncture, naturopathic medicine, homeopathy);

(2) biologic-based therapies (eg, herbal, special dietary); *(3)* energy therapies (eg, Reiki, therapeutic touch, magnet therapy); *(4)* manipulative and body-based systems (eg, chiropractic, osteopathy, and massage); and *(5)* mind-body interventions (eg, meditation, biofeedback, hypnotherapy, relaxation).[18]

As CAM has developed extensively, uncertainty about the appropriateness of the term *CAM* and other CAM-related terms has grown in both the research and practice communities. Various terms and definitions have been proposed over the past three decades, which highlights how little agreement exists in the field. Moreover, all terms that have been introduced so far are to some extent problematic, though *CAM* and *integrative healthcare* remain the most popular and accepted terms.[19] A new term was recently introduced: *complementary and integrative medicine*[20]; replacing the term *alternative* with *integrative* may reflect a change in attitudes toward CAM.

The widespread use of CAM has intensified the need to evaluate its safety and efficacy. Although scientific evidence exists for some CAM therapies, most key questions remain unanswered by well-designed scientific studies, including whether these therapies are safe and whether they work for the diseases or medical conditions for which they are used. In the absence of such evidence for effectiveness, a heated debate results each time CAM departments are introduced in public hospitals or health organizations suggest offering such services. Contributing to the controversy is that in most of these institutions the standard demanded for introducing a new technology or conventional drug is far higher than that demanded for CAM modalities.[21] Complicating the problem is that patients have access to many websites advertising different therapies, but practitioners know that this information must be approached with caution because the evidence often fails to stand up to currently accepted levels of medical scrutiny.[22]

Although the gold standard for biomedical research is considered to be the double-blind, randomized controlled trial (RCT), such an approach is not always easy or feasible for CAM.[23] In conventional biomedical research, the placebo is often considered to be an ideal control, but because many CAM care systems are mul-

* RCT

timodal (eg, combinations of change in diet, exercise, spiritual practice, and interventions such as herbal therapy and acupuncture), it may be impractical, if not impossible, to control for every aspect of treatment. Other aspects, such as inclusion and exclusion criteria, may impose additional difficulties; CAM systems have considerably different diagnostic definitions from those that apply to classic biomedical research. The definition of outcome may also differ; in CAM, subjective evaluations, such as improvement in quality of life or the activities of daily living, are often considered more important than objective outcomes.[23] At the heart of many critiques of CAM are two fundamental beliefs: (1) in most instances, any positive effects of CAM are the result of the placebo effect rather than the clinical effects of the intervention, and (2) such treatment is either potentially harmful because it diverts patients away from real medicine or unethical and dishonest because it knowingly advocates and administers sham medicine.[24] However, some patients with such conditions as chronic pain, chronic fatigue, irritable bowel syndrome, stress, and anxiety have found CAM to be successful in treating or ameliorating these conditions. The argument that such treatment is no better than placebo was not necessarily seen as being negative.[24] Moreover, many elements of the health care encounter that are categorized as incidental (placebo) in the context of drug trials are characteristic (intrinsic) of the complex nonpharmacologic interventions of CAM.[25] Thus, the use of placebo- or sham-controlled trial designs for complex CAM interventions will not detect the whole characteristic effect of the intervention and may generate false-negative results.[25] The implications derived from these methodologic considerations of CAM treatments emphasize the importance of the placebo effect as an integral part of the treatment. The placebo effect phenomenon is discussed in the next section.

The Placebo Effect and CAM

Attitudes toward placebo have changed dramatically since the introduction of the double-blind RCT around 1955.[26] In the pre-RCT period, the placebo was looked upon as a benevolent deception to comfort and please the patient (hence the name *placebo*, which is Latin for "I shall please") and sometimes as a diagnostic tool to separate imaginary problems from real ones. Interestingly, even today many US family physicians use placebos, believe the placebo effect is therapeutic, and often use real drugs as placebos, attributing psychologic and physical benefits to the placebo effect.[27] In 1955, Beecher[28] explicitly assumed an additive model of placebo effects, whereby the total drug effect is equal to its active effect plus its placebo effect. Therefore, to find the true effect of a treatment, results should be subtracted from the placebo effect as derived from an RCT. In the current RCT era, a legitimate therapy must therefore demonstrate an effect greater than that of a decoy disguised as a real intervention. Thus, the placebo has value only as a comparison marker, and the magnitude of its absolute power has an incidental significance.[26] Very elegantly, the placebo effect can be demonstrated without using a placebo group, which may be denied the active drug.[29] This was discovered in studies that assessed postsurgical treatment efficacy by comparing pump-delivered intravenous analgesic (ie, hidden administration) with the same intervention administered by a physician (ie, open administration). Open administration was found to be more effective than hidden administration, and the difference between the two results is attributed to a placebo effect.[29] In postoperative pain after extraction of the third molars, researchers found that a hidden injection of a 6- to 8-mg intravenous dose of morphine corresponded to an open injection of saline solution in full view of the patient (placebo). Thus, the placebo effect in this trial was as powerful as 6 to 8 mg of morphine.[30] Yet the placebo effect is not constant, and its power, especially as an analgesic treatment, is context dependent and can vary under different circumstances.[31,32] Additionally, people may respond to unique placebo-related healing rituals in different ways, further suggesting that the placebo response may be a complex behavioral phenomenon with properties that constitute a state, rather than a trait, characteristic.[33] Studies have shown that expectation and conditioning mediate placebo effects.[34–37] For instance, it was reported that after chest surgery patients received a basal saline infusion under three conditions: *(1)* they were told they would receive a potent painkiller, *(2)* they were told they might receive a placebo or a painkiller, or *(3)* they were told nothing.[36] All three groups also received, on demand, the same opioid analgesic medication (buprenorphine), and the researchers found that the dose demand differed; those who believed they were already receiving a potent painkiller requested the least, and those who were told nothing about their medication requested the most. These results clearly indicate that higher expectation for analgesia resulted in a smaller demand for the opioid analgesic.[36]

Pain is the field in which most of the placebo research has been performed, and its neurobiologic mechanisms were made significant when Levine et al[38] showed that placebo analgesia was reversed by the opioid antagonist naloxone, suggesting a role for endogenous opioids. The role of endogenous opioids was further supported by brain-imaging studies using positron emission tomography, which showed similar activation in descending opioid-mediated pain-modulating pathways by placebo or opioid injections.[39] Functional magnetic resonance imaging studies also found brain activation patterns in the prefrontal cortex in anticipation to analgesia after placebo administration.[40] Currently, analgesia is known to be mediated by both opioid and nonopioid mechanisms. Benedetti. et al[41] showed that a specific cannabinoid 1 (CB1) receptor antagonist (rimonabant or SR141716) blocks nonopioid placebo analgesic responses but has no effect on opioid placebo responses. They concluded that the endocannabinoid system has a pivotal role in placebo analgesia in some circumstances, when the opioid system is not involved and is mediated by CB1 receptors.[41]

In alternative medicine, the main question regarding placebo has been whether a given therapy has more than a placebo effect. For example, an analysis that reviewed the effect of homeopathy concluded that it has no more than a placebo effect.[42] However, just as mainstream medicine ignores the clinical significance of its own placebo effect,[43-45] the placebo effect of unconventional medicine is also ignored and disregarded, except for polemics.[46] In other words, those aspects of healing regarded as fake or sham by the medical profession are fascinating, powerful, and efficacious and are embraced by CAM. The term *placebo effect* is taken to mean not only an imitation intervention but also the broad mixture of nonspecific effects present in the clinical setup. For instance, in a study comparing acupuncture to massage for back pain, subjects were randomly assigned to one of the two treatments regardless of expectations of efficacy of the type of treatment. Overall, there was no difference in outcomes between the acupuncture and massage groups, but there was a significant and clinically important difference between the high- and low-expectancy groups; subjects administered the treatment they believed was best for their back pain, whether massage or acupuncture, had outcomes superior to subjects given the opposite treatment.[47] In this sense, the concept of placebo has shifted from the inert content of the placebo agent to the concept of simulation of an active therapy within a psychosocial context. Attending to the patient's belief or, alternatively, convincing the patient that the treatment allocated is the most appropriate, may improve the outcome of the treatment. Physicians will generally be most justified in recommending a treatment primarily for its placebo properties when evidence shows that the modality is associated with a pronounced placebo response and when the risk of adverse reactions is low.[48] An ethical tension is built in between the need to share decision-making information with the patient and any health outcomes produced by therapy that can directly alter therapeutic outcomes produced via placebo responses.[48] However, disclosure of the physician's goal of enhancing the placebo response may be perceived by the patient as a positive pep talk and may actually augment the placebo reaction by reinforcing positive expectations. Researchers concluded that placebos administered without deception may be an effective treatment and significantly better than no treatment.[49] Yet, the informed consent presented to participants in most recent high-quality clinical trials emphasized the benefits and adverse effects of the target treatment while largely ignoring the possible effects of the placebo. Moreover, 18% of these trials explicitly stated that the placebo treatment was undesirable or ineffective, thereby providing incomplete and at times inaccurate information about placebos.[50] Furthermore, in placebo-controlled clinical trials, patients receiving placebo often reported side effects similar to those experienced by patients receiving the study treatment. This could be attributable to the mere communication of potential adverse effects in the informed consent process, which develops because of a nocebo effect.[51]

The *nocebo effect*, that is, undesired outcomes resulting from the patient's negative expectations, also has important implications for treatment outcome. For example, informing a patient that a prescribed drug may cause a side effect may itself produce the same side effect independent of the pharmacologic properties of the drug.[52] The nocebo response is influenced by the information given to patients and the way that information is presented. Specifically, research on the nocebo effect indicates that information disclosure about potential side effects can itself contribute to producing adverse effects.[53] The nocebo effect adversely influences quality of life and therapy adherence, emphasizing the need for minimizing these responses to the extent possible.[54] Giving information in an appropriate way may help prevent nocebo effects. For example, in a study of influenza immunization, those told that 5% of patients suffered reactions ended up reporting more side effects than those told that 95% would suffer no such reactions.[55]

Conclusions

Many elements are at work during a placebo response, such as the relationship between the physician and patient, the patient's expectations and needs, the patient's personality and psychologic state, the severity and discomfort of the symptoms, the type of verbal instructions, the preparation characteristics, and the environmental milieu.[56] A question of interest is whether the setup of CAM creates more of these nonspecific effects and therefore an enhanced placebo effect. This question, reviewed by Kaptchuk,[46] examines such aspects as patient and practitioner characteristics and the interaction between the two and concludes that there is scant empiric evidence that any particular type of CAM has an augmented placebo effect. Undoubtedly, interventions of mainstream medicine possess no less of a placebo effect.

A summary of the role of the physician-patient relationship as it relates to the physiology of the placebo effect can be found in a recent review.[56]

Physicians today can treat and prevent a number of diseases through pharmacology, genetics, and physical interventions. In addition, the patient's mind, cognition, and emotions play a central part in any therapeutic outcome. Patients must be both cured and cared for. Only curing the disease is not sufficient; care of the patient is of no less importance. Moreover, a warm relationship between practitioner and patient can add to the placebo response.[57] Also, it is important to consider the patient's preferred treatment because treatment choice contributes to its efficacy, especially if the patient believes in its potency.[47] Notably, patients usually do not care if they get better because of a placebo effect as long as it works,[48] even if the placebo is delivered without deception. For example, patients with irritable bowel syndrome randomized to receive open-label placebo pills who were told that such pills often relieve symptoms through a "mind-body self-healing process" experienced more relief than control subjects who received no treatment.[49]

Moreover, one of the most fascinating concepts emerging from recent physiologic understanding of placebos and expectations is related to the reduced efficacy of drugs when administered covertly; drugs without therapeutic rituals are less effective. In effect, if the placebo/expectation component of a treatment is eliminated by means of a hidden administration (uninformed by the patient) drug efficacy is very much reduced.[32] Therefore, the way the information is presented to the patient is of utmost importance,[36] as well as the mode of drug delivery.[32]

CAM and Chronic Facial Pain

Relatively little is known about the prevalence of use of CAM to treat chronic facial pain. In a survey of 192 patients with documented temporomandibular disorders (TMDs), it was found that about 36% reported using CAM therapies, although most (96%) used conventional care simultaneously.[58] In another study, 14 of 63

(22%) women with TMDs who were recruited to a study on oral splints reported on the previous use of CAM therapy. Users of CAM were significantly more likely to report work or social disability associated with their facial pain and were more likely to report onset associated with an accident.[59] Recently, it was found that more than three-quarters (76.1%) of patients surveyed at a dental school clinic had used at least one CAM treatment in the previous 12 months, and there were high rates of chiropractic use.[8]

Myers et al[60] reviewed randomized clinical trials of patients with chronic facial pain who were subjected to a CAM intervention or to a control comparison group. Across studies, results suggested that acupuncture, biofeedback, and relaxation were comparable to conservative treatment (eg, an intraoral appliance) and warranted further study. They were unable to comment on other modes of CAM therapy because they could not locate any RCT that tested the effects of treatments such as homeopathy, massage, chiropractic, or herbal remedies on chronic facial pain.[60] In a later review, it was concluded that selected complementary therapies, such as biofeedback, relaxation, and acupuncture, seemed promising[61]; however, there were more unanswered than answered questions about cost-effectiveness, efficacy, and mechanisms of action related to CAM for persistent facial pain. In general, the hands-on CAM therapies (massage, acupuncture, and chiropractic care) were the most satisfactory of the CAM therapies used.[58]

Facial pain and acupuncture

In a systematic review of the use of acupuncture as a treatment for TMDs, three trials met the criteria for inclusion as RCTs, and it was concluded that acupuncture might be an effective therapy for TMDs, although none of the studies controlled for a placebo effect.[62] Raustia et al[63] compared acupuncture with various treatments for 50 subjects with temporomandibular joint dysfunction, including counseling, occlusal adjustment, muscle exercises, and occlusal splints in two parallel groups. The two treatment modalities had similar positive effects on the dysfunction index. Acupuncture was found to be superior to standard therapy on mouth opening with initial significant limitation

of opening, but standard therapy was superior when the initial limitation was less marked.

In another study, acupuncture was compared with a maxillary occlusal splint or no treatment in 45 patients with myogenous facial pain.[64] Ninety percent of the acupuncture group and 86% of those who received occlusal splints improved, and scored significantly better than the no-treatment group, on both the subjective symptoms and objective clinical examination scores, and there was no significant difference between the two active groups.[64] In a similar study, 110 patients with a median 4-year duration of craniomandibular disorders were allocated to one of three groups: acupuncture treatment, maxillary occlusal splint therapy, and a no-treatment control group.[65] Scores of the acupuncture and splint therapy groups were superior to those of the control group on the pain visual analog scale (VAS) and clinical dysfunction index, but there was significant reduction in pain frequency only in the acupuncture group. Six-month and 1-year follow-up studies were carried out only for the patients in the two treatment groups who improved.[66] Long-term improvement was noted in both groups, and there was no significant difference between the groups for any end point. A third study by the same group on 55 of the original 110 subjects (criteria for selecting these 55 subjects were not clear) found increased thresholds to a pressure algometer applied to the belly of the masseter muscle that were significantly higher in the treatment groups than the no-treatment group.[67] This change was maintained in a repeated measure 6 months later.

Based on traditional Chinese medicine, seven local acupuncture points and one distant point have been recommended for the use of acupuncture in the treatment of TMDs.[68] However, both acupuncture and sham acupuncture (dry needling in skin areas not recognized as acupuncture points) equally reduced pain evoked by mechanical stimulation of the masseter muscles in patients with myofascial pain, and this effect may not be specific to the location of the stimulus as predicted by the classic acupuncture literature.[69] On the other hand, a study was conducted on nine patients with chronic myofascial pain who received real acupuncture and six subjects who received sham acupuncture conducted by lightly pricking the skin with a shortened, blunted acupuncture needle through a foam pad without penetrating the skin.[70] They reported a statistically significant difference in pain tolerance only with real acupuncture ($P = .027$) as well as a significant reduction in facial pain ($P = .003$), neck pain ($P = .011$), and headache ($P = .015$).[70] Different types of sham acupuncture therefore may result in different outcomes. Recently, pain reduction measured by VAS was found to be significantly more pronounced after acupuncture than after placebo (sham laser treatment; $P = .031$), and the sum of pain scores across 14 muscles was considerably more reduced after acupuncture than after sham laser treatment.[71]

Facial pain, relaxation, and hypnosis

The effects of behavioral treatments and occlusal splint therapy were compared in 122 adolescent patients with TMDs who were divided into three groups of treatment: brief information, brief information plus relaxation training, and brief information plus an occlusal appliance. The groups that used relaxation or an occlusal appliance showed significant improvement, but the group that used brief information alone did not.[72] Seventy-two patients with TMDs took part in a study that evaluated the efficacy of cognitive-behavioral therapy (CBT), including hypnosis. All patients received conservative standard treatment for TMDs; in addition, the experimental group received six sessions of CBT. The groups showed significant differences: 90% of the patients under CBT reported a significant reduction in frequency of pain and 70% in emotional distress. CBT, including hypnosis, significantly improved conservative standard treatment outcome in patients with TMDs. The improvement was stable over time, and there were no significant differences between posttreatment and 9-month follow-ups.[73]

Twenty-eight patients who were recalcitrant to conservative treatment for TMDs participated in a medical hypnosis treatment program and completed measures of their pain symptoms on four separate occasions: during wait list, before treatment, after treatment, and at a 6-month follow-up. Hypnosis for treatment of TMDs was effective in decreasing pain frequency, intensity, and duration ($P < .001$) as well as improving daily functioning. Analysis suggested that treatment gains were maintained for 6 months after hypnosis treatment and that patients also exhibited a significant reduction in medical use.[74] Forty-one patients with persistent idiopathic orofacial pain were randomized to active hypnotic intervention or simple relaxation as a control measure for five individual 1-hour sessions. The change in VAS pain scores from baseline to the last treatment was ($33.1\% \pm 7.4\%$) in the hypnosis group and ($3.2\% \pm 5.4\%$) in the control group ($P < .03$). Moreover, the pain reduction was dependent on hypnotic susceptibility; in the hypnosis group, highly hypnotic susceptible patients had greater decreases in VAS pain scores ($55.0\% \pm 12.3\%$) compared with less susceptible patients ($17.9\% \pm 6.7\%$) ($P < .02$).[75] In a later study, the same authors studied the effect of hypnosis on oral function and psychologic factors in patients with TMDs.[76] In the hypnosis group, daily scores on the numeric rating scale significantly decreased from 4.5 ± 2.1 at baseline to 2.9 ± 2.4 after treatment ($P < .001$) compared with the control group, where no significant changes were found (4.2 ± 1.4 at baseline and 3.9 ± 1.5 after treatment) ($P = .733$). The number needed to treat for a 50% pain reduction was 4.0.[76]

Conclusions

About a third of patients seen for chronic facial pain (mostly patients with TMDs) were concomitantly using CAM therapy. Acupuncture was the most frequently used mode of therapy, and its effect seemed to be comparable with that of conventionally used therapy, such as intraoral splints. However, this reduction in pain was not dependent on whether the acupuncture needling was performed at standard acupuncture points or in other areas of the skin. Hypnosis was more effective than simple relaxation and was more effective in subjects who were highly susceptible to hypnosis. The effect of hypnotic treatment is long lasting, at least 6 months after termination of treatment. CBT for orofacial pain is discussed in detail in chapter 4.

CAM and Headaches

A survey of CAM utilization by migraine patients in Italy found that about 31% of 481 patients attending a headache clinic reported using CAM in the past.[77] Around 40% of patients who used CAM considered it beneficial, but it was less effective for transformed than for episodic migraine.[77] In another survey of 73 headache patients, it was found that 85% used CAM therapy for their headache, and 60% found it to be beneficial.[78] Although it is apparent that there are cultural differences in the rate of CAM utilization for headache, there is no doubt that many patients with headache around the world seek alternatives to conventional medical therapy. Therapists should be aware of this fact, especially because more than 60% of patients did not report their CAM treatments to their physician.[77] A recent survey on the use of CAM therapy for chronic headache reported that 62% had used CAM for primary and 73% for secondary chronic headache, but self-reported efficacy ranged from 0% to 43%.[79] An estimated 30% of patients do not respond to pharmacologic interventions for headache, and among the alternative therapies used are behavioral treatments, acupuncture, and nutritional therapies.[80] A systematic review of 24 RCTs examined the effects of CAM therapies (acupuncture, spinal manipulation, and physiotherapy) for nonmigraineur's headaches (tension-type headache, cervicogenic headache, and posttraumatic headache). Evidence from a subset of high-quality studies indicates that some CAM therapies may be useful in the treatment of these conditions.[81] Stress management, relaxation, and cognitive coping were applied for headaches, but most studies involved acupuncture therapy.

Headaches and acupuncture

In an early systematic review on acupuncture and headache, it was concluded that the existing evidence supports the value of acupuncture for the treatment of idiopathic headache but that the quality and amount of evidence are not fully convincing.[82] In later studies, the effect of acupuncture for abortive treatment of migraine was compared with that of sumatriptan.[83] A total of 179 inpatient migraineurs were allocated into three groups: traditional Chinese acupuncture, sumatriptan (6 mg subcutaneously), or placebo injection. A full migraine attack was prevented in 21 of 60 (35%) patients

by acupuncture, in 21 of 58 (36%) patients by sumatriptan, and in 11 of 61 (18%) patients by placebo. Response to a second intervention in patients who developed a full attack was significantly better with sumatriptan than with acupuncture. In a more recent study of 302 patients by the same group, the prophylactic effects of acupuncture and sham acupuncture (superficial needling at non-acupuncture points) were compared with a control group.[84] Acupuncture and sham acupuncture consisted of 12 sessions over 8 weeks, and differences in number of days with headache were compared on diaries from 4 weeks before to 9 to 12 weeks after randomization. Days of headache decreased significantly over the 8-week period by 2.2 in the acupuncture and sham acupuncture groups compared with 0.8 in the control group. A study with a similar design by the same group also tested the effect of acupuncture and sham acupuncture on tension-type headache.[84] Acupuncture reduced the number of days with headache by 7.2 and sham acupuncture by 6.6; in the control group, the number of days was reduced by 1.5. In both studies, it was concluded that acupuncture intervention or sham acupuncture was more effective than no treatment.[84,85] In a recent Cochrane review, Linde et al[86] examined the effect of acupuncture on migraine prophylaxis in 22 trials with 4,419 participants and concluded that there is no evidence for an effect of acupuncture over sham interventions as both interventions were equally effective, though this is difficult to interpret because exact points of accupuncture location could be of limited importance. Available studies suggest that acupuncture is at least as effective as, or possibly more effective than, prophylactic drug treatment and has fewer adverse effects. Linde et al[87] also reviewed the effect of acupuncture on tension-type headache and concluded that acupuncture could be a valuable nonpharmacologic tool in patients with frequent episodic or chronic tension-type headaches. A sham-controlled trial of acupuncture as an adjunct, add-on therapy in migraine prophylaxis was conducted in 100 patients in whom prophylactic drugs had not produced a decrease of at least 50% in the number of attacks.[88] The frequency of attacks decreased significantly with this add-on therapy, but there was no significant difference between sham and true acupuncture.[88] On the other hand, the efficacy of acupuncture compared with sham acupuncture for acute migraine attacks suggested that the true acupuncture group was superior to the sham acupuncture group for relieving pain and reducing the usage of acute medication.[89] However, the study was a multicenter, single-blinded study and most probably culturally biased. The effect of acupuncture was also tested in chronic daily headache.[90] An RCT on 74 patients compared medical management provided by neurologists to medical management plus 10 acupuncture treatments. Patients with chronic daily headache who received medical treatment only did not have improved daily pain severity and headache-related quality of life. On the other hand, patients who also received acupuncture were 3.7 times more likely to report less suffering from headaches at 6 weeks. Thus, supplementing medical management with acupuncture resulted in improvement in both quality of life and the patients' perception that they suffered less from headaches.[90]

The cost-effectiveness of acupuncture for chronic headache was reported in two British studies in which 401 patients with chronic headache, predominantly migraine, were randomly allocated to receive up to 12 acupuncture treatments or a control intervention offering usual care by the National Health Service.[91,92] Headache score at 12 months, the primary end point, was significantly lower in the acupuncture group than in the control group (34% and 16% reduction from baseline, respectively). Patients in the acupuncture group experienced 22 fewer days of headache per year than control subjects and used 15% less medication ($P = .02$).[91] Total costs during the 1-year study period were, on average, higher for the acupuncture group than for the control group (£403 and £217, respectively) because of the acupuncture practitioners' fees. However, the mean health gain, as measured in terms of incremental cost per quality of adjusted life year (QALY) during the first year of the trial was 0.021 QALYs, leading to a base case estimate of approximately £9,180 per QALY gained.[92] The authors concluded that acupuncture is beneficial for primary-care patients with chronic headache and improves health-related quality of life at a small additional cost.

Headaches and behavioral management

In a meta-analysis of 50 clinical trials (2,445 patients collectively), it was found that both propranolol and relaxation/biofeedback yielded a 43% reduction in migraine headache activity compared with 14% with placebo medication.[93] Holroyd et al[94] compared the effects of tricyclic antidepressants with stress management on chronic tension-type headache (a mean of 26 headache days per month). Four groups were allocated: antidepressants (amitriptyline up to 100 mg/day or nortriptyline up to 75 mg/day), placebo, stress management (eg, relaxation, cognitive coping) plus placebo, and stress management plus antidepressants. All three active treatments, but not the placebo, yielded improvement in headache activity by the 6-month evaluation, but improvement occurred more rapidly with antidepressants than with stress management. Combined therapy was more likely to produce clinically significant (> 50%) reduction in headache index scores (64% of participants) than antidepressants (38% of participants), stress management (35% of participants), or placebo (29% of participants).[94]

Conclusions

Acupuncture is effective for abortive and prophylactic treatment of migraine and comparable with pharmacotherapy. Available studies suggest that acupuncture is at least as effective as, or possibly more effective than, prophylactic drug treatment and has fewer adverse effects. Overall, it seems that there is no significant difference between sham and true acupuncture, but cultural variations may exist. Nonetheless, combined therapy is more likely to produce clinically significant (> 50%) reduction in headache index scores. This combined therapy has a special beneficial effect in chronic daily headache, a usually most resistant condition.

Mechanisms of Acupuncture

The use of acupuncture for the treatment of pain has become widespread in the past few decades. The introduction of the gate control

Q#9, "B"

Q#9, "C"

theory lent theoretic support for possible pain control by means of an external stimulus applied to the body, such as acupuncture.[95] Later investigations have demonstrated that the nervous system, neurotransmitters, and endogenous substances respond to needling stimulation.[96] Cheng and Pomeranz[97] established that acupuncture analgesia is mediated by opioid peptides produced in the periaqueductal gray and can be reversed by naloxone, an opioid antagonist. The periaqueductal gray and other supraspinal sites of the descending pain modulatory system exert powerful inhibitory effects on the response at the spinal level.[98,99] Evidence suggests that acupuncture also increases neuronal nitric acid expression in the gracile nucleus.[100] This nitric acid expression plays an important role in mediating the cardiovascular response to acupuncture, may participate in central autonomic regulation of somatosympathetic reflex activities, and could contribute to the therapeutic effects of acupuncture.[99] Some recent studies also point to the possible role of CB1 and CB2 receptor activation in contributing to the antinociceptive and anti-inflammatory effects of electroacupuncture.[101–103]

Acupuncture research has also been the subject of a recent systematic review focusing on three-armed RCTs (comparing acupuncture, placebo acupuncture, and no treatment) testing acupuncture treatment for pain.[104] The resulting assessments of the clinical benefits of acupuncture were either negative or equivocal. The authors concluded that the analgesic effects of acupuncture are small and "below a clinically relevant pain improvement," and they end their review by suggesting that future research should try to disentangle the physiologic effects of acupuncture from the psychologic and ritual elements of treatment.

Omega-3 Fatty Acids

The anti-inflammatory effect of omega-3 fatty acids has recently been demonstrated, and the possibility emerges for their long-term use as an alternative to nonsteroidal anti-inflammatory drugs (NSAIDs).[105,106] A search for an alternative and safer anti-inflammatory agent became even more important as the concept of safe NSAIDs collapsed. Multiple observations have

clearly established an increased risk for cardiovascular events associated with use of the new cyclooxygenase (COX) 2 selective NSAIDs and for other nonselective NSAIDs. This is in addition to the renal, gastrointestinal, and other side effects associated with NSAID use (see chapter 15).

Fish oils contain long-chain omega-3 eicosapentaenoic acid (EPA) and docosahexaenoic acid, which produce competitive inhibition of arachidonic acid metabolism by COX.[107] EPA is a natural homolog of arachidonic acid, which has a structural difference of only one additional double bond (the omega-3 bond). Not surprisingly, it is an alternative substrate and inhibitor of arachidonic acid metabolism by COX.[108] Whereas prostaglandin (PG) H_2 is the COX metabolite of arachidonic acid, PGH_3 is the COX metabolite of EPA. Studies of prostanoid metabolism in the presence of dietary EPA or exogenous EPA added in vitro suggest that PGH_3 is a poor substrate and an inhibitor of PGE synthase[109] and thromboxane (TX) A synthase[110] as well as a potential substrate without inhibitory effect on PGI synthase. Indeed, the increased PGI_2 synthesis seen with anti-inflammatory doses of fish oils raises the possibility of shunting of PGH_2 from blocked PGE synthase and TX synthase to uninhibited PGI synthase.[111] Thus, the overall effect of EPA is suppression of PGE_2 synthesis and shifting of the TXA2/PGI_2 balance in favor of PGI_2. In contrast, selective COX-2 inhibitors shift the TXA2/PGI_2 balance in favor of TXA2 and may cause a prothrombotic effect (see chapter 15). EPA and docosahexaenoic acid inhibit the activity of COX-1 and COX-2 with a dissociation constant of approximately 2 µm, which is similar to that for ibuprofen.[112]

Although not suitable for on-demand use, fish oils have a number of advantages over NSAIDs. First, they have not been associated with serious upper gastrointestinal complications.[113] Second, they have been shown to reduce risk for cardiovascular events, including cardiac death, through multiple actions,[114] in contrast with the increased risk seen with most NSAIDs.[115,116] Third, fish oils have been shown to reduce synthesis of the pro-inflammatory cytokines tumor necrosis factor and interleukin (IL)-1 by mononuclear cells[117,118]; in contrast, NSAIDs can increase synthesis of these cytokines.[119] Thus, long-term fish oil treatment may reduce NSAID use and reduce gastrointestinal and cardiovascular events in potential NSAID users.

To date, more than 10 randomized controlled studies have been performed in patients with rheumatoid arthritis, most in patients with disease duration of more than 10 years.[108] The most consistent benefits were reduced morning stiffness and decreased tender joint count, and NSAIDs given on an as-required basis could be reduced.[108]

Thus, for example, in a double-blind, placebo-controlled, prospective study of fish oil supplementation,[120] patients with active rheumatoid arthritis took either 130 mg/kg per day of omega-3 fatty acids or nine capsules of corn oil per day while on diclofenac (75 mg twice a day). Placebo diclofenac was substituted at week 18 or 22, and fish oil supplements were continued for another 8 weeks. Patients who took dietary supplements of fish oil but not corn oil exhibited improvements in clinical parameters of disease activity from baseline, including the number of tender joints. These improvements were also associated with significant decreases in levels of IL-1β. The researchers concluded that patients who took fish oil were able to discontinue NSAIDs without experiencing a disease flare. Similarly, about 60% of patients with nonsurgical neck or back discogenic pain who took a daily total of 1,200 mg of omega-3 EFAs (eicosapentaenoic acid and docosahexaenoic acid) for 1 month could stop taking their NSAIDs.[106] In a long-term, 12-month study, 90 patients with active diclofenac were enrolled in a double-blind, randomized study comparing daily supplementation with 2.6 g of omega-3, 1.3 g of omega-3 plus 3 g of olive oil, or 6 g of olive oil. Significant improvement in the patient's global evaluation and in the physician's assessment of pain was observed only in those taking 2.6 g of omega-3 per day.[121] Another study conducted on 43 patients with rheumatoid arthritis showed that 3 g of fish oil omega-3 per day relieved many clinical signs significantly more than soy-oil controls. However, the combination of 3 g of fish oil and 9.6 mL of olive oil per day was superior to fish oil alone.[122] The conflicting findings of these two studies may result from the difference in the

amount of omega-3 (1.3 g and 3 g, respectively) used in combination with the olive oil. The amount of 1.3 g per day was apparently lower than the recommended omega-3 fatty acid dose of about 2.5 g per day for the treatment of adult rheumatoid arthritis.[108] A recent meta-analysis[123] also suggests that the use of omega-3 polyunsaturated fatty acids at dosages greater than 2.7 g per day for more than 3 months reduces NSAID consumption by patients with rheumatoid arthritis, and clinical signs showed a trend to improve more in patients treated with omega-3 polyunsaturated fatty acids than in placebo-treated control subjects.

Significant improvement was noticed under the effects of fish oil and olive oil on the frequency and severity of recurrent migraine in adolescents, although no difference was found between the two treatments.[124] Because no additional control (eg, corn or soy oil) was used, these findings are difficult to interpret. In a recent study,[125] 56 ambulatory patients with chronic daily headache undergoing usual care were randomized to one of two intensive, food-based, 12-week dietary interventions: a high omega-3 plus low omega-6 intervention or a low omega-6 intervention. In an intention-to-treat analysis, the high omega-3 plus low omega-6 intervention produced significantly greater improvement in clinical outcomes than the low omega-6 group. The authors concluded that a dietary intervention increasing omega-3 and reducing omega-6 fatty acids reduced headache pain, altered antinociceptive lipid mediators, and improved quality of life in this population.[125]

Treatment of recurrent aphthous stomatitis with 3 g of omega-3 per day achieved a significant reduction in the number of ulcers, the duration of ulcers, and the level of pain at 3 months that persisted for 6 months.[126]

Conclusions

Other than for rheumatoid arthritis, not enough data are available to recommend the proper clinical utilization (eg, amount, frequency, duration) of omega-3 fatty acids for chronic orofacial pain. Some preliminary evidence also suggests that omega-3 may be used for chronic headache and prophylaxis of aphthous lesions.

Because of its anti-inflammatory effect, coupled with a high safety profile, omega-3 should be considered for long-term use in painful arthritis of the temporomandibular joint. Furthermore, its antiplatelet and anticoagulant effects should be taken into account when performing oral surgery.

References

1. Eisenberg DM, Kessler RC, Foster C, Norlock FE, Calkins DR, Delbanco TL. Unconventional medicine in the United States. Prevalence, costs, and patterns of use. N Engl J Med 1993;328:246–252.
2. Eisenberg DM, Davis RB, Ettner SL, et al. Trends in alternative medicine use in the United States, 1990–1997: Results of a follow-up national survey. JAMA 1998;280:1569–1575.
3. Harris PE, Cooper KL, Relton C, Thomas KJ. Prevalence of complementary and alternative medicine (CAM) use by the general population: A systematic review and update. Int J Clin Pract 2012;66:924–939.
4. Herman PM, Craig BM, Caspi O. Is complementary and alternative medicine (CAM) cost-effective? A systematic review. BMC Complement Altern Med 2005;5:11.
5. Davis MA, Weeks WB. The concentration of out-of-pocket expenditures on complementary and alternative medicine in the United States. Altern Ther Health Med 2012;18(5):36–42.
6. Astin JA. Why patients use alternative medicine: Results of a national study. JAMA 1998;279:1548–1553.
7. Wolsko PM, Eisenberg DM, Davis RB, Kessler R, Phillips RS. Patterns and perceptions of care for treatment of back and neck pain: Results of a national survey. Spine 2003;28:292–297.
8. Spector ML, Fischer M, Dawson DV, et al. Complementary and alternative medicine usage by patients of a dental school clinic. Spec Care Dentist 2012;32:177–183.
9. Ndao-Brumblay SK, Green CR. Predictors of complementary and alternative medicine use in chronic pain patients. Pain Med 2010;11:16–24.
10. Weintraub MI. Complementary and alternative methods of treatment of neck pain. Phys Med Rehabil Clin N Am 2003;14:659–674.
11. Gracely EJ, O'Connor B. Students' attitudes toward alternative health care. Acad Med 1996;71:109–110.
12. Oberbaum M, Notzer N, Abramowitz R, Branski D. Attitude of medical students to the introduction of complementary medicine into the medical curriculum in Israel. Isr Med Assoc J 2003;5:139–142.
13. Goldszmidt M, Levitt C, Duarte-Franco E, Kaczorowski J. Complementary health care services: A survey of general practitioners' views. CMAJ 1995;153:29–35.
14. Visser GJ, Peters L. Alternative medicine and general practitioners in the Netherlands: Towards acceptance and integration. Fam Pract 1990;7:227–232.
15. Wetzel MS, Eisenberg DM, Kaptchuk TJ. Courses involving complementary and alternative medicine at US medical schools. JAMA 1998;280:784–787.
16. Zollman C, Vickers A. ABC of complementary medicine. Users and practitioners of complementary medicine. BMJ 1999;319:836–838.
17. Charlton JE. Complementary therapies. In: Charlton, JE (ed). Core Curriculum for Professional Education in Pain, ed 3. Seattle: IASP, 2005.
18. Staud R. Effectiveness of CAM therapy: Understanding the evidence. Rheum Dis Clin North Am 2011;37:9–17.
19. Gaboury I, April KT, Verhoef M. A qualitative study on the term CAM: Is there a need to reinvent the wheel? BMC Complement Altern Med 2012;12:131.
20. Herman PM, Poindexter BL, Witt CM, Eisenberg DM. Are complementary therapies and integrative care cost-effective? A systematic review of economic evaluations. BMJ Open 2012;2.
21. Glick S. CAM—Image vs. reality: A personal perspective. Isr Med Assoc J 2005;7:604–606.
22. Morris CA, Avorn J. Internet marketing of herbal products. JAMA 2003;290:1505–1509.
23. Eskinazi D. Methodologic considerations for research in traditional (alternative) medicine. Oral Surg Oral Med Oral Pathol Oral Radiol Endod 1998;86:678–681.
24. Segar J. Complementary and alternative medicine: Exploring the gap between evidence and usage. Health (London) 2012;16:366–381.
25. Paterson C, Dieppe P. Characteristic and incidental (placebo) effects in complex interventions such as acupuncture. BMJ 2005;330:1202–1205.
26. Kaptchuk TJ. Powerful placebo: The dark side of the randomised controlled trial. Lancet 1998;351(9117):1722–1725.
27. Kermen R, Hickner J, Brody H, Hasham I. Family physicians believe the placebo effect is therapeutic but often use real drugs as placebos. Fam Med 2010;42:636–642.
28. Beecher HK. The powerful placebo. J Am Med Assoc 1955;159:1602–1606.
29. Colloca L, Lopiano L, Lanotte M, Benedetti F. Overt versus covert treatment for pain, anxiety, and Parkinson's disease. Lancet Neurol 2004;3:679–684.
30. Levine JD, Gordon NC, Smith R, Fields HL. Analgesic responses to morphine and placebo in individuals with postoperative pain. Pain 1981;10:379–389.
31. Price DD. Psychological Mechanisms of Pain and Analgesia, vol 15. Seattle: IASP, 1999.
32. Pollo A, Benedetti F. Neural mechanisms of placebo-nduced analgesia. In: Price DD, Bushnell MC (eds). Psychological Methods of Pain Control. Seattle: IASP, 2004:171–186.
33. Kong J, Spaeth R, Cook A, et al. Are all placebo effects equal? Placebo pills, sham acupuncture, cue conditioning and their association. PLoS One 2013;8:e67485.
34. Montgomery GH, Kirsch I. Classical conditioning and the placebo effect. Pain 1997;72:107–113.
35. Price DD, Milling LS, Kirsch I, Duff A, Montgomery GH, Nicholls SS. An analysis of factors that contribute to the magnitude of placebo analgesia in an experimental paradigm. Pain 1999;83:147–156.
36. Pollo A, Amanzio M, Arslanian A, Casadio C, Maggi G, Benedetti F. Response expectancies in placebo analgesia and their clinical relevance. Pain 2001;93:77–84.

37. De Pascalis V, Chiaradia C, Carotenuto E. The contribution of suggestibility and expectation to placebo analgesia phenomenon in an experimental setting. Pain 2002;96:393–402.

38. Levine JD, Gordon NC, Fields HL. The mechanism of placebo analgesia. Lancet 1978;2(8091):654–657.

39. Petrovic P, Kalso E, Petersson KM, Ingvar M. Placebo and opioid analgesia—Imaging a shared neuronal network. Science 2002;295(5560):1737–1740.

40. Wager TD, Rilling JK, Smith EE, et al. Placebo-induced changes in FMRI in the anticipation and experience of pain. Science 2004;303(5661):1162–1167.

41. Benedetti F, Amanzio M, Rosato R, Blanchard C. Non-opioid placebo analgesia is mediated by CB1 cannabinoid receptors. Nat Med 2011;17:1228–1230.

42. Shang A, Huwiler-Müntener K, Nartey L, et al. Are the clinical effects of homoeopathy placebo effects? Comparative study of placebo-controlled trials of homoeopathy and allopathy. Lancet 2005;366(9487):726–732.

43. Hróbjartsson A, Gøtzsche PC. Is the placebo powerless? An analysis of clinical trials comparing placebo with no treatment. N Engl J Med 2001;344:1594–1602.

44. Hróbjartsson A, Gøtzsche PC. Is the placebo powerless? Update of a systematic review with 52 new randomized trials comparing placebo with no treatment. J Intern Med 2004;256:91–100.

45. Vase L, Riley JL 3rd, Price DD. A comparison of placebo effects in clinical analgesic trials versus studies of placebo analgesia. Pain 2002;99:443–452.

46. Kaptchuk TJ. The placebo effect in alternative medicine: Can the performance of a healing ritual have clinical significance? Ann Intern Med 2002;136:817–825.

47. Kalauokalani D, Cherkin DC, Sherman KJ, Koepsell TD, Deyo RA. Lessons from a trial of acupuncture and massage for low back pain: Patient expectations and treatment effects. Spine 2001;26:1418–1424.

48. Brody H, Colloca L, Miller FG. The placebo phenomenon: Implications for the ethics of shared decision-making. J Gen Intern Med 2012;27:739–742.

49. Kaptchuk TJ, Friedlander E, Kelley JM, et al. Placebos without deception: A randomized controlled trial in irritable bowel syndrome. PLoS One 2010;5:e15591.

50. Bishop FL, Adams AE, Kaptchuk TJ, Lewith GT. Informed consent and placebo effects: A content analysis of information leaflets to identify what clinical trial participants are told about placebos. PLoS One 2012;7:e39661.

51. Barsky AJ, Saintfort R, Rogers MP, Borus JF. Nonspecific medication side effects and the nocebo phenomenon. JAMA 2002;287:622–627.

52. Flaten MA, Simonsen T, Olsen H. Drug-related information generates placebo and nocebo responses that modify the drug response. Psychosom Med 1999;61:250–255.

53. Rief W, Nestoriuc Y, von Lilienfeld-Toal A, et al. Differences in adverse effect reporting in placebo groups in SSRI and tricyclic antidepressant trials: A systematic review and meta-analysis. Drug Saf 2009;32:1041–1056.

54. Colloca L, Miller FG. The nocebo effect and its relevance for clinical practice. Psychosom Med 2011;73:598–603.

55. O'Connor AM, Pennie RA, Dales RE. Framing effects on expectations, decisions, and side effects experienced: The case of influenza immunization. J Clin Epidemiol 1996;49:1271–1276.

56. Benedetti F. Placebo and the new physiology of the doctor-patient relationship. Physiol Rev 2013;93:1207–1246.

57. Kaptchuk TJ, Kelley JM, Conboy LA, et al. Components of placebo effect: Randomised controlled trial in patients with irritable bowel syndrome. BMJ 2008;336:999–1003.

58. DeBar LL, Vuckovic N, Schneider J, Ritenbaugh C. Use of complementary and alternative medicine for temporomandibular disorders. J Orofac Pain 2003;17:224–236.

59. Raphael KG, Klausner JJ, Nayak S, Marbach JJ. Complementary and alternative therapy use by patients with myofascial temporomandibular disorders. J Orofac Pain 2003;17:36–41.

60. Myers CD, White BA, Heft MW. A review of complementary and alternative medicine use for treating chronic facial pain. J Am Dent Assoc 2002;133:1189–1196.

61. Myers CD. Complementary and alternative medicine for persistent facial pain. Dent Clin North Am 2007;51:263–274.

62. Ernst E, White AR. Acupuncture as a treatment for temporomandibular joint dysfunction: A systematic review of randomized trials. Arch Otolaryngol Head Neck Surg 1999;125:269–272.

63. Raustia AM, Pohjola RT, Virtanen KK. Acupuncture compared with stomatognathic treatment for TMJ dysfunction. Part I: A study. J Prosthet Dent 1985;54:581–585.

64. Johansson A, Wenneberg B, Wagersten C, Haraldson T. Acupuncture in treatment of facial muscular pain. Acta Odontol Scand 1991;49:153–158.

65. List T, Helkimo M, Andersson S, Carlsson GE. Acupuncture and occlusal splint therapy in the treatment of craniomandibular disorders. Part I. A comparative study. Swed Dent J 1992;16(4):125–141.

66. List T, Helkimo M. Acupuncture and occlusal splint therapy in the treatment of craniomandibular disorders. II. A 1-year follow-up study. Acta Odontol Scand 1992;50:375–385.

67. List T, Helkimo M, Karlsson R. Pressure pain thresholds in patients with craniomandibular disorders before and after treatment with acupuncture and occlusal splint therapy: A controlled clinical study. J Orofac Pain 1993;7:275–282.

68. Rosted P. Practical recommendations for the use of acupuncture in the treatment of temporomandibular disorders based on the outcome of published controlled studies. Oral Dis 2001;7:109–115.

69. Goddard G, Karibe H, McNeill C, Villafuerte E. Acupuncture and sham acupuncture reduce muscle pain in myofascial pain patients. J Orofac Pain 2002;16:71–76.

70. Shen YF, Goddard G. The short-term effects of acupuncture on myofascial pain patients after clenching. Pain Pract 2007;7:256–264.

71. Simma I, Gleditsch JM, Simma L, Piehslinger E. Immediate effects of microsystem acupuncture in patients with oromyofacial pain and craniomandibular disorders (CMD): A double-blind, placebo-controlled trial. Br Dent J 2009;207:e26.

72. Wahlund K, List T, Larsson B. Treatment of temporomandibular disorders among adolescents: A comparison between occlusal appliance, relaxation training, and brief information. Acta Odontol Scand 2003;61:203–211.

73. Ferrando M, Galdón MJ, Durá E, Andreu Y, Jiménez Y, Poveda R. Enhancing the efficacy of treatment for temporomandibular patients with muscular diagnosis through cognitive-behavioral intervention, including hypnosis: A randomized study. Oral Surg Oral Med Oral Pathol Oral Radiol 2012;113:81–89.

74. Simon EP, Lewis DM. Medical hypnosis for temporomandibular disorders: Treatment efficacy and medical utilization outcome. Oral Surg Oral Med Oral Pathol Oral Radiol Endod 2000;90:54–63.

75. Abrahamsen R, Baad-Hansen L, Svensson P. Hypnosis in the management of persistent idiopathic orofacial pain—Clinical and psychosocial findings. Pain 2008;136:44–52.

76. Abrahamsen R, Zachariae R, Svensson P. Effect of hypnosis on oral function and psychological factors in temporomandibular disorders patients. J Oral Rehabil 2009;36:556–570.

77. Rossi P, Di Lorenzo G, Malpezzi MG, et al. Prevalence, pattern and predictors of use of complementary and alternative medicine (CAM) in migraine patients attending a headache clinic in Italy. Cephalalgia 2005;25:493–506.

78. von Peter S, Ting W, Scrivani S, et al. Survey on the use of complementary and alternative medicine among patients with headache syndromes. Cephalalgia 2002;22:395–400.

79. Kristoffersen ES, Aaseth K, Grande RB, Lundqvist C, Russell MB. Self-reported efficacy of complementary and alternative medicine: The Akershus study of chronic headache. J Headache Pain 2013;14:36.

80. Holroyd KA, Mauskop A. Complementary and alternative treatments. Neurology 2003;60(6, suppl):S58–S62.

81. Vernon H, McDermaid CS, Hagino C. Systematic review of randomized clinical trials of complementary/alternative therapies in the treatment of tension-type and cervicogenic headache. Complement Ther Med 1999;7:142–155.

82. Melchart D, Linde K, Fischer P, et al. Acupuncture for idiopathic headache. Cochrane Database Syst Rev 2001;(1).

83. Melchart D, Thormaehlen J, Hager S, Liao J, Linde K, Weidenhammer W. Acupuncture versus placebo versus sumatriptan for early treatment of migraine attacks: A randomized controlled trial. J Intern Med 2003;253:181–188.

84. Linde K, Streng A, Jurgens S, et al. Acupuncture for patients with migraine: A randomized controlled trial. JAMA 2005;293:2118–2125.

85. Melchart D, Streng A, Hoppe A, et al. Acupuncture in patients with tension-type headache: Randomised controlled trial. BMJ 2005;331:376–382.

86. Linde K, Allais G, Brinkhaus B, Manheimer E, Vickers A, White AR. Acupuncture for migraine prophylaxis. Cochrane Database Syst Rev 2009;(1).

87. Linde K, Allais G, Brinkhaus B, Manheimer E, Vickers A, White AR. Acupuncture for tension-type headache. Cochrane Database Syst Rev 2009;(1).

88. Foroughipour M, Golchian AR, Kalhor M, Akhlaghi S, Farzadfard MT, Azizi H. A sham-controlled trial of acupuncture as an adjunct in migraine prophylaxis. Acupunct Med 2014;32:12–16.

89. Wang LP, Zhang XZ, Guo J, et al. Efficacy of acupuncture for acute migraine attack: A multicenter single blinded, randomized controlled trial. Pain Med 2012;13:623–630.

90. Coeytaux RR, Kaufman JS, Kaptchuk TJ, et al. A randomized, controlled trial of acupuncture for chronic daily headache. Headache 2005;45:1113–1123.

91. Vickers AJ, Rees RW, Zollman CE, et al. Acupuncture for chronic headache in primary care: Large, pragmatic, randomised trial. BMJ 2004;328:744.

92. Wonderling D, Vickers AJ, Grieve R, McCarney R. Cost effectiveness analysis of a randomised trial of acupuncture for chronic headache in primary care. BMJ 2004;328:747.

93. Holroyd KA, Penzien DB. Pharmacological versus non-pharmacological prophylaxis of recurrent migraine headache: A meta-analytic review of clinical trials. Pain 1990;42:1–13.

94. Holroyd KA, O'Donnell FJ, Stensland M, Lipchik GL, Cordingley GE, Carlson BW. Management of chronic tension-type headache with tricyclic antidepressant medication, stress management therapy, and their combination: A randomized controlled trial. JAMA 2001;285:2208–2215.

95. Melzack R, Wall PD. Pain mechanisms: A new theory. Science 1965;150(3699):971–979. *Gate Control*

96. Foster JM, Sweeney BP. The mechanisms of acupuncture analgesia. Br J Hosp Med 1987;38:308–312.

97. Cheng RS, Pomeranz BH. Electroacupuncture analgesia is mediated by stereospecific opiate receptors and is reversed by antagonists of type I receptors. Life Sci 1980;26:631–638.

98. Fields HL, Basbaum AI. Brainstem control of spinal pain-transmission neurons. Annu Rev Physiol 1978;40:217–248.

99. Nicholson K, Martelli MF. The problem of pain. J Head Trauma Rehabil 2004;19:2–9.

100. Abou-Donia MB, Dechkovskaia AM, Goldstein LB, Bullman SL, Khan WA. Sensorimotor deficit and cholinergic changes following coexposure with pyridostigmine bromide and sarin in rats. Toxicol Sci 2002;66:148–158.

101. Zhang J, Chen L, Su T, et al. Electroacupuncture increases CB2 receptor expression on keratinocytes and infiltrating inflammatory cells in inflamed skin tissues of rats. J Pain 2010;11:1250–1258.

102. Su TF, Zhao YQ, Zhang LH, et al. Electroacupuncture reduces the expression of proinflammatory cytokines in inflamed skin tissues through activation of cannabinoid CB2 receptors. Eur J Pain 2012;16:624–635.

103. Gondim DV, Araújo JC, Cavalcante AL, et al. CB1 and CB2 contribute to antinociceptive and anti-inflammatory effects of electroacupuncture on experimental arthritis of the rat temporomandibular joint. Can J Physiol Pharmacol 2012;90:1479–1489.

104. Madsen MV, Gøtzsche PC, Hróbjartsson A. Acupuncture treatment for pain: Systematic review of randomised clinical trials with acupuncture, placebo acupuncture, and no acupuncture groups. BMJ 2009;338:a3115.

105. Cleland LG, James MJ. Marine oils for antiinflammatory effect—Time to take stock. J Rheumatol 2006;33:207–209.

106. Maroon JC, Bost JW. Omega-3 fatty acids (fish oil) as an anti-inflammatory: An alternative to nonsteroidal anti-inflammatory drugs for discogenic pain. Surg Neurol 2006;65:326-331.

107. Cleland LG, James MJ, Proudman SM. Fish oil: What the prescriber needs to know. Arthritis Res Ther 2005;8:202.

108. Cleland LG, James MJ, Proudman SM. The role of fish oils in the treatment of rheumatoid arthritis. Drugs 2003;63:845–853.

109. Hawkes JS, James MJ, Cleland LG. Separation and quantification of PGE3 following derivatization with panacyl bromide by high pressure liquid chromatography with fluorometric detection. Prostaglandins 1991;42:355–368.

110. von Schacky C, Fischer S, Weber PC. Long-term effects of dietary marine omega-3 fatty acids upon plasma and cellular lipids, platelet function, and eicosanoid formation in humans. J Clin Invest 1985;76:1626–1631.

111. DeCaterina R, Giannessi D, Mazzone A, et al. Vascular prostacyclin is increased in patients ingesting omega-3 polyunsaturated fatty acids before coronary artery bypass graft surgery. Circulation 1990;82:428–438.

112. Lands WE. Biosynthesis of prostaglandins. Annu Rev Nutr 1991;11:41–60.

113. Kremer JM, Malamood H, Maliakkal B, Rodgers JB, Ross JS, Cooper JA. Fish oil dietary supplementation for prevention of indomethacin induced gastric and small bowel toxicity in healthy volunteers. J Rheumatol 1996;23:1770–1773.

114. Kris-Etherton PM, Harris WS, Appel LJ. Fish consumption, fish oil, omega-3 fatty acids, and cardiovascular disease. Circulation 2002;106:2747–2757.

115. Solomon DH. Selective cyclooxygenase 2 inhibitors and cardiovascular events. Arthritis Rheum 2005;52:1968–1978.

116. Hippisley-Cox J, Coupland C. Risk of myocardial infarction in patients taking cyclo-oxygenase-2 inhibitors or conventional non-steroidal anti-inflammatory drugs: Population based nested case-control analysis. BMJ 2005;330:1366.

117. James MJ, Gibson RA, Cleland LG. Dietary polyunsaturated fatty acids and inflammatory mediator production. Am J Clin Nutr 2000;71(suppl 1):343S–348S.

118. Simopoulos AP. Omega-3 fatty acids in inflammation and autoimmune diseases. J Am Coll Nutr 2002;21:495–505.

119. Demasi M, Cleland LG, Cook-Johnson RJ, Caughey GE, James MJ. Effects of hypoxia on monocyte inflammatory mediator production: Dissociation between changes in cyclooxygenase-2 expression and eicosanoid synthesis. J Biol Chem 2003;278:38607–38616.

120. Kremer JM, Lawrence DA, Petrillo GF, et al. Effects of high-dose fish oil on rheumatoid arthritis after stopping nonsteroidal antiinflammatory drugs. Clinical and immune correlates. Arthritis Rheum 1995;38:1107–1114.

121. Geusens P, Wouters C, Nijs J, Jiang Y, Dequeker J. Long-term effect of omega-3 fatty acid supplementation in active rheumatoid arthritis. A 12-month, double-blind, controlled study. Arthritis Rheum 1994;37:824–829.

122. Berbert AA, Kondo CR, Almendra CL, Matsuo T, Dichi I. Supplementation of fish oil and olive oil in patients with rheumatoid arthritis. Nutrition 2005;21:131–136.

123. Lee YH, Bae SC, Song GG. Omega-3 polyunsaturated fatty acids and the treatment of rheumatoid arthritis: A meta-analysis. Arch Med Res 2012;43:356–362.

124. Harel Z, Gascon G, Riggs S, Vaz R, Brown W, Exil G. Supplementation with omega-3 polyunsaturated fatty acids in the management of recurrent migraines in adolescents. J Adolesc Health 2002;31:154–161.

125. Ramsden CE, Faurot KR, Zamora D, et al. Targeted alteration of dietary n-3 and n-6 fatty acids for the treatment of chronic headaches: A randomized trial. Pain 2013;154:2441–2451.

126. El Khouli AM, El Gendy EA. Efficacy of omega-3 in treatment of recurrent aphthous stomatitis and improvement of quality of life: A randomized, double-blind, placebo-controlled study. Oral Surg Oral Med Oral Pathol Oral Radiol 2014;117:191–196.

Index

Handwritten annotations: AVASCULAR – p.267; ANAMNESTIC – p.262; ATTENUATED – p.267

Handwritten bottom margin: Acid-Reflux p.169   Augmentin – p.155

Azithromycin - p.169

Astrocytes - p.66

Bupivacaine p.211

Anosmia – p.173

Avascular – p.265

Bonain's liquid p.184

Beta-Lactamase – p.155

Tongue Cancer - p.164

Class III Lever - p.266

CAM - p.623

Cystic Fibrosis - p.
Crocodile tears - p.168

CMV - p.234

CBT - p. 237
210

Conversion - p.98

Chronic
Daily Headache - 225, 226

GINGLYMOARTHRODIAL p.265

HARd end-feel p.260
HodgKin disease p.425
HZ - Herpes Zoster - p.425
Hinge - p.265
IMPACT LOADING p.268

INFERIOR SALIVARY Nucleus - p.46

IMMOBILIZATION - p.288

Leishmaniasis p.67

Leptin - p 288

JAPAN - p.500

LTM's - p. 39, 41, 67
(LOW-Threshold Mechanoreceptors)

LUPUS - p.237

MACROGLOSSIA p.517

MAST cells - p.150

Lever - Class III p.266

Load Test - p.274

2,83

LTB4 p.149

LATERAL Pterygoid p.266, 276

(LINGUAL NERVE) - p.38

MesV - p. 35, 44

MelZACK + WALL p.53

NMDA - p.47

OCCULOMOTOR NERVE
CC.N. III p. 45

I N Index

Nucleus Caudalis - p. 34
(SPC 5) p. 36

OTIC GANGLION - p. 38.4 -286

"opening" muscles - p.202

ORDINAL - p.260
scale

PANORAMIC - p.261
X-RAY
(Limited use)

Periodontal disease -
Abscence
of pain   Index P
P.67

- Prednisolone, 373t
- Prednisone
  - cluster headaches treated with, 373
  - giant cell arteritis treated with, 499
- Preeclampsia, 502
- Pregabalin, 418, 418t, 437–438, 592t–593t, 599
- Preganglionic parasympathetic fibers, 45
- Pregnancy
  - acetaminophen use during, 547, 573
  - analgesic use during, 572–573
  - diclofenac contraindications during, 553
  - FDA pregnancy category for drugs in, 586t
  - migraine treatment during, 339
  - nonsteroidal anti-inflammatory drugs during, 339, 572–573
- Pre-pain, 42
- Pressure algometers, 87
- Pretrigeminal neuralgia, 395, 413–415
- Preventive analgesia, 437
- Primary otalgia. *See* Otalgia, primary.
- Progressive systemic sclerosis, 494
- Proinflammatory cytokines, 65
- Propranolol, 336t, 340, 601–603, 602t–603t
- Proprioception, 87
- Prostacyclin, 565, 569
- Prostaglandin-endoperoxide synthase 1, 223
- Prostaglandins
  - description of, 564–565, 632
  - E2, 149, 153, 270, 548
- Prosthetic temporomandibular joint, 303
- Protease-activated receptor-2, 150
- Proton pump inhibitors, 567
- Pseudomonas aeruginosa, 168
- Psoriatic arthritis, 291t, 490
- Psychiatric disorders
  - chronic orofacial pain and, 98
  - depression. *See* Depression.
  - mental health provider referral for, 114–115
  - orofacial pain and, shared pathogenesis of, 105
  - screening for, 113–115, 114b
- Psychogenic facial pain, 105
- Psychogenic model, 98–100
- Psychogenic pain, 98–99
- Psychologic management, of chronic orofacial pain, 106–115
- Psychophysical testing, 89–91
- Psychosocial assessment, 17
- Psychosocial characteristics
  - orofacial pain disorder outcome and, 105
  - pain onset and, 102–103
  - temporomandibular disorder outcome and, 103–104
- Psychosocial stress, 100–102
- Pterygopalatine fossa segment neurectomy, 420
- Pterygopalatine ganglion, 37, 58
- Pulmonary diseases, 506
- Pulp, stimulus transduction in, 42
- Pulpal pain
  - characteristics of, 145
  - irreversible pulpitis, 146, 146t
  - mechanisms of, 149
  - physical signs of, 146
  - radiographic signs of, 146
  - reversible pulpitis, 146, 146t
  - symptoms of, 145–146
  - treatment of, 146, 146t
- Pulpitis, 146t, 146–147, 149
- Pyrazolone, 558–559
- Pyriform sinus carcinoma, 164

Q

- Quality of life, 15
- Quantitative sensory testing (QST)
  - bilateral mental neuropathy evaluation using, 85
  - clinical relevance of, 91–92
  - definition of, 84
  - methods of, 84–86
    - levels-based, 85
    - limits-based, 84–85
    - stimulus-dependent methods, 84
    - two-point discrimination test, 85
  - neuropathic pain evaluations, 408–409
  - pain perception measured by, 125
  - sensation levels, 86–87
  - standardization of, 91–92
  - stimulus modalities for
    - chemical, 89
    - dynamic psychophysical testing, 89–91
    - electrical, 89
    - mechanical, 87–88
    - thermal, 88–89
  - temporomandibular disorder evaluations, 215
  - variables that affect, 84

R

- Radiofrequency rhizolysis, 477–478, 480–481
- Radiosurgery
  - headache caused by, 523
  - stereotactic, 421–422, 480
- Radiotherapy-related pain, 508–509
- Ramsay Hunt syndrome, 168, 450
- Randomized controlled trials, 584–585
- Reactive oxygen species, 269
- Recombinant human keratinocyte growth factor-1, 512t
- Recurrent acute rhinosinusitis, 177–178
- Recurrent aphthous stomatitis, 156
- Referrals
  - mental health provider, 114–115
  - for pain, 17, 26
- Referred pain
  - definition of, 11
  - odontalgia caused by, 149
- Reiter syndrome, 291t, 492
- Relapsing polychondritis, 167
- Relaxation, 111–113, 629, 631
- Relocated migraine, 343
- REM sleep, 123–124
- Renal disorders, 505
- Repetitive transcranial magnetic stimulation, 58
- Research Diagnostic Criteria for Temporomandibular Disorders, 5–6, 82–83
- Restless legs syndrome, 130
- Reticulothalamocortical network, 52
- Retropharyngeal space infection, 188–189
- Reversible pulpitis, 146, 146t
- Rheumatoid arthritis, 291t, 489–490, 633
- Rhinosinusitis
  - acute
    - analgesics for, 177
    - bacterial, 173–174
    - clinical criteria for, 174b, 175
    - diagnosis of, 174b, 174–175
    - frontal, 176–177, 177f
    - headache caused by, 175, 175b
    - health care costs for, 172–173
    - maxillary, 176, 176f
    - pain assessment of, 177
    - radiographic findings, 176f
    - recurrent, 177–178
    - symptoms of, 173
    - treatment of, 176
    - viral, 173–175
  - chronic, 178b, 178–179
    - classification of, 173
    - definition of, 172
    - dental implants as cause of, 180, 181f
    - development of, 173
    - diagnosis of, 173–174
    - epidemiology of, 172
    - frontal acute, 176–177, 177f, 179
    - maxillary acute, 176, 176f, chronic, 179, 181f
    - migraine versus, 184
    - odontogenic, 179–180, 181f
    - sinonasal toothache as cause of, 176
    - sinus elevation complications as cause of, 180, 181f
  - subacute, 177
- Rhinovirus, 185
- Rhizolysis, 477–478, 480–482
- Rhythmic masticatory muscle activity, 221
- Rizatriptan, 331, 332t, 333
- Rofecoxib, 554–555
- Root canal therapy, 433
- Root fracture, vertical, 154
- Rostral ventromedial medulla, 54–56
- Ruffini corpuscles, 42

Handwritten annotations (top): Shift-to-the-left - p. 186, 189 / Superoxide - p.269 / Subacute 173 / RINE PROTEASES - p.270 / SURFACTANT p.269 / SSN p.58, 184, 352, 351, 396

Handwritten annotations (right margin): SRD / P. 41, 44, 60 / Sumatriptan - p.183 / 225 TTH / Superior salivary nucleus, 58, p.184 / Sympathetic Nervous System - p.210

Handwritten annotations (bottom): Sjögren-syndrome - p.237 / soft end-feel p.204 / SURFACTANT p.269

Sudomotor - p. 45
(sweat)

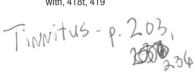

Handwritten notes (top):
- TNFα - p. 149
- TNFα p. 154
- good description → p. 270
- Verapamil - p. 130
- Valsalva maneuver - p. 234
- Viral illness - p 233 234

Handwritten: Turkey - p. 500

Handwritten: Vertigo - p 233

Handwritten: - p. 170

Handwritten notes (bottom):
- URI - upper respiratory infection - p. 168 169
- p. 168
- Tryptase p. 150

→ Vestibulocochlear Nerve
~~XII~~ VIII

, Table 7-4
Whiplash p.277